PATRICK C. WALSH, M.D.
Urologist-in-Chief, James Buchanan Brady
   Urological Institute
The Johns Hopkins Hospital
Professor and Director
   Department of Urology
The Johns Hopkins University
   School of Medicine
Baltimore, Maryland

RUBEN F. GITTES, M.D.
Urologist-in-Chief
Brighman and Women's Hospital
Professor of Urological Surgery
Harvard Medical School
Boston, Massachusetts

ALAN D. PERLMUTTER, M.D.
Chief, Department of Pediatric Urology
Children's Hospital of Michigan
Professor of Urology
Wayne State University School of Medicine
Detroit, Michigan

THOMAS A. STAMEY, M.D.
Professor of Surgery and
Chairman, Division of Urology
Stanford University School of Medicine
Stanford, California

Volume 3

Campbell's

UROLOGY

FIFTH EDITION

1986
W.B. SAUNDERS COMPANY

Philadelphia • London • Toronto • Mexico City • Rio de Janeiro • Sydney • Tokyo • Hong Kong

W. B. Saunders Company: West Washington Square
Philadelphia, PA   19105

Library of Congress Cataloging in Publication Data

Urology.

Campbell's Urology.

1. Urology.   I. Campbell, Meredith Fairfax, 1894-
1968.   II. Walsh, Patrick C.   III. Title. [DNLM:
1. Urologic diseases. WJ 100 C192]

RC871.U758 1986   616.6   83–20427

ISBN 0–7216–9088–2 (set)

Listed here is the latest translated edition of this book together with the language of the translation and the publisher.

Italian (3rd Edition)—   Casa Editrice Universo,
Rome, Italy

Portuguese (1st Edition)—Editora Guanabara Koogan,
Rio de Janeiro, Brazil

Editor: Carroll Cann
Cover Designer: Terri Siegel
Production Manager: Bob Butler
Manuscript Editor: Connie Burton
Illustration Coordinator: Walt Verbitski

Volume 1 ISBN   0–7216–9085–8
Volume 2 ISBN   0–7216–9086–6
Volume 3 ISBN   0–7216–9087–4
Set ISBN   0–7216–9088–2

Campbell's Urology

Last digit is the print number: 9   8   7   6   5   4   3   2   1

CONTRIBUTORS

HERBERT L. ABRAMS, M.D.

Philip H. Cook Professor of Radiology, Harvard
Medical School; Senior Radiologist, Brigham and
Women's Hospital, Boston, Massachusetts.

*Computed Tomography of the Kidney; Renal
and Adrenal Angiography; Renal Venography*

DOUGLASS E. ADAMS, M.D.

Professor of Radiology, Harvard Medical School;
Director, NMR Division, Department of Radiol-
ogy, Brigham and Women's Hospital, Boston,
Massachusetts.

Renal and Adrenal Angiography

**S. JAMES ADELSTEIN, M.D.,
Ph.D.**

Professor of Radiology, Harvard Medical School;
Director, Joint Program in Nuclear Medicine,
Brigham and Women's Hospital, Beth Israel Hospital, The Children's Hospital, Dana Farber Cancer Institute, Boston, Massachusetts.

Radionuclides in Genitourinary Disorders

ERNEST H. AGATSTEIN, M.D.

Senior Resident, Division of Urology, University
of California, Los Angeles, School of Medicine;
Staff, UCLA Medical Center, Los Angeles, California.

*Imperforate Anus, Persistent Cloaca, and
Urogenital Sinus Outlet Obstruction*

RODNEY U. ANDERSON, M.D.

Associate Professor of Surgery (Urology), Stan-
ford University School of Medicine; Chief of
Urology, Santa Clara Valley Medical Center, San
Jose, California.

*Urinary Tract Infections in Spinal Cord Injury
Patients*

STUART B. BAUER, M.D.

Assistant Professor of Urology (Surgery), Harvard Medical School; Associate in Surgery (Urology), The Children's Hospital Medical Center,
Boston, Massachusetts.

Anomalies of the Upper Urinary Tract

RICHARD E. BERGER, M.D.

Associate Professor, Department of Urology,
University of Washington School of Medicine;
Chief, Department of Urology, Harborview Med-
ical Center, Seattle, Washington.

Sexually Transmitted Diseases

JAY BERNSTEIN, M.D.

Clinical Professor of Pathology, Wayne State University School of Medicine; Director, Department
of Anatomic Pathology, William Beaumont Hospital, Royal Oak, Michigan.

Renal Cystic Disease and Renal Dysplasia

WILLIAM E. BRADLEY, M.D.

Professor, Department of Neurology, University
of California, Irvine, School of Medicine; Neurology Service, Veterans Administration Medical
Center, Long Beach, California.

Physiology of the Urinary Bladder

CHARLES B. BRENDLER, M.D.

Assistant Professor of Urology, The Johns Hopkins University School of Medicine, Baltimore,
Maryland.

Perioperative Care

v

C. EUGENE CARLTON, Jr., M.D.

Russell and Mary Hugh Scott Professor and Chairman, Department of Urology, Baylor College of Medicine; Chief, Urology Service, Methodist Hospital; Active Staff, Ben Taub General Hospital, St. Luke's Episcopal Hospital, Texas Children's Hospital; Consulting Staff, Veterans Administration Hospital, Houston, Texas.

Initial Evaluation, Including History, Physical Examination, and Urinalysis.

WILLIAM J. CATALONA, M.D.

Professor and Chief, Division of Urologic Surgery, Washington University Medical Center; Attending Urologist, Barnes Hospital, Jewish Hospital, St. Louis Children's Hospital, St. Louis County Hospital, Veterans Administration Hospital, St. Louis, Missouri.

Carcinoma of the Prostate

THOMAS S. K. CHANG, Ph.D.

Assistant Professor, James Buchanan Brady Urological Institute, The Johns Hopkins University School of Medicine, Baltimore, Maryland.

The Testis, Epididymis, and Ductus Deferens

DONALD S. COFFEY, Ph.D.

Professor of Urology, Professor of Oncology, and Professor of Pharmacology and Experimental Therapeutics, The Johns Hopkins University School of Medicine; Director of the Research Laboratories of the Department of Urology, The Johns Hopkins Hospital, Baltimore, Maryland.

Biochemistry and Physiology of the Prostate and Seminal Vesicles.

GIULIO J. D'ANGIO, M.D.

Professor of Radiology, Radiation Therapy, and Pediatric Oncology, University of Pennsylvania School of Medicine; Director, Children's Cancer Research Center, Children's Hospital of Philadelphia, Philadelphia, Pennsylvania.

Pediatric Oncology

JEAN B. DE KERNION, M.D.

Professor of Surgery/Urology, and Head of Urologic Oncology, University of California, Los Angeles, School of Medicine; Director for Clinical Programs, Jonsson Cancer Center; Attending Physician, UCLA Hospital, Wadsworth Veterans Administration Hospital, Los Angeles, California.

Renal Tumors

FRANCESCO DEL GRECO, M.D.

Chief, Section of Nephrology-Hypertension, and Professor of Medicine, Northwestern University Medical School, Chicago, Illinois.

Other Renal Diseases of Urologic Significance

CHARLES J. DEVINE, Jr., M.D., F.A.C.S., F.A.A.P.

Professor and Chairman, Department of Urology, Eastern Virginia Medical School; Staff, Medical Center Hospitals, Norfolk General Hospital, De Paul Hospital, Leigh Memorial Hospital; Consultant in Urology, U.S. Naval Regional Medical Center, Portsmouth; Chief of Urology, Children's Hospital of the King's Daughters, Norfolk, Virginia.

Surgery of the Urethra

ROBERT G. DLUHY, M.D.

Associate Professor of Medicine, Harvard Medical School; Physician, Brigham and Women's Hospital, Boston, Massachusetts.

The Adrenals.

GEORGE W. DRACH, M.D.

Professor of Surgery and Chief of Urology, University of Arizona College of Medicine, Tucson, Arizona.

Urinary Lithiasis.

MICHAEL J. DROLLER, M.D.

Professor and Chairman, Department of Urology, Mount Sinai Medical School; Consultant, Bronx Veterans Administration Medical Center, Elmhurst General Hospital; Director of Urology, Mount Sinai Medical Center, New York, New York.

Transitional Cell Cancer: Upper Tracts and Bladder

JOHN W. DUCKETT, M.D.

Professor of Urology, University of Pennsylvania School of Medicine; Director, Division of Urology, Children's Hospital of Philadelphia, Philadelphia, Pennsylvania.

Hypospadias; Disorders of the Urethra and Penis

RICHARD M. EHRLICH, M.D., F.A.C.S., F.A.A.P.

Professor of Surgery/Urology, University of California, Los Angeles, School of Medicine; Staff, UCLA Medical Center, Los Angeles, California.

Imperforate Anus, Persistent Cloaca, and Urogenital Sinus Outlet Obstruction

AUDREY E. EVANS, M.D.

Professor of Pediatrics, University of Pennsylvania School of Medicine; Director, Division of Oncology, Children's Hospital of Philadelphia, Philadelphia, Pennsylvania.

Pediatric Oncology

LARRY L. EWING, Ph.D.

Professor, The Johns Hopkins University School of Hygiene and Public Health, Baltimore, Maryland.

The Testis, Epididymis, and Ductus Deferens

STEWART FELDMAN, M.D.

Formerly, Resident in Urology, Case Western Reserve University School of Medicine, Cleveland, Ohio.

Extrinsic Obstruction of the Ureter

JOHN F. GAETA, M.D.

Professor of Pathology and Associate Professor of Urology, State University of New York at Buffalo School of Medicine; Director, Tissue Pathology, Buffalo General Hospital, Buffalo, New York.

Tumors of Testicular Adnexal Structures and Seminal Vesicles

KENNETH D. GARDNER, Jr., M.D.

Professor of Medicine, University of New Mexico School of Medicine; Chief of Renal Diseases, Department of Medicine, University of New Mexico Hospital, Albuquerque, New Mexico.

Renal Cystic Disease and Renal Dysplasia

FREDRICK W. GEORGE, Ph.D.

Assistant Professor of Cell Biology, University of Texas Health Science Center at Dallas, Southwestern Medical School, Dallas, Texas.

Embryology of the Genital Tract

JAY Y. GILLENWATER, M.D.

Professor and Chairman, Department of Urology, University of Virginia School of Medicine; Chief of Urology, University of Virginia Hospital, Charlottesville, Virginia.

The Pathophysiology of Urinary Obstruction

RUBEN F. GITTES, M.D.

Elliot C. Cutler Professor of Urological Surgery, Harvard Medical School; Chief of Urology, Brigham and Women's Hospital, Boston, Massachusetts.

Partial Nephrectomy: In Situ or Extracorporeal; The Adrenals

JAMES G. GOW, M.D., Ch.M., F.R.C.S.

Formerly, Clinical Lecturer, University of Liverpool; Lourdes Private Hospital, Liverpool, England.

Genitourinary Tuberculosis

HARRY GRABSTALD, M.D., F.A.C.S.

Professor of Urology, Mount Sinai School of Medicine; Acting Director, Department of Urology, Beth Israel Medical Center, New York, New York.

Benign and Malignant Tumors of the Male and Female Urethra; Surgery of Penile and Urethral Carcinoma

JOHN T. GRAYHACK, M.D.

Professor and Chairman, Department of Urology, Northwestern University Medical School; Chief, Northwestern Memorial Hospital; Consultant, Veterans Administration Lakeside Hospital, Chicago, Illinois.

Surgical Management of Ureteropelvic Junction Obstruction.

LAWRENCE F. GREENE, M.D., Ph.D.*

Formerly, Clinical Professor of Surgery/Urology, University of California, San Diego, School of Medicine; Chief of Urology, Veterans Administration Hospital, San Diego, California.

Transurethral Surgery

JAMES E. GRIFFIN, M.D.

Associate Professor of Internal Medicine, University of Texas Health Science Center at Dallas, Southwestern Medical School; Attending Physician, Parkland Memorial Hospital, Dallas, Texas.

Disorders of Sexual Differentiation

H. ROGER HADLEY, M.D.

Assistant Professor, Loma Linda University School of Medicine; Consultant, Riverside General Hospital; Staff, Jerry Pettis Veterans Hospital, San Bernardino County Hospital, Loma Linda University Medical Center, Loma Linda, California.

The Treatment of Male Urinary Incontinence

W. HARDY HENDREN, M.D.

Professor of Surgery, Harvard Medical School; Chief of Surgery, The Children's Hospital; Visiting Surgeon, Massachusetts General Hospital, Boston, Massachusetts.

Urinary Undiversion: Refunctionalization of the Previously Diverted Urinary Tract

STANLEY C. HOPKINS, M.D., C.M., F.R.C.S.(C)

Assistant Professor of Surgery, Division of Urology, University of South Florida College of Medicine; Acting Chief, Urology Section, James A. Haley Veterans Administration Hospital, Tampa, Florida.

Benign and Malignant Tumors of the Male and Female Urethra

*Deceased.

STUART S. HOWARDS, M.D.

Professor of Urology and Physiology, University of Virginia School of Medicine; Urologist, University of Virginia Medical Center, Charlottesville, Virginia.

Male Infertility; Surgery of the Scrotum and Its Contents

DOMINIK J. HUBER, M.D.

Radiologist, Long Island Jewish Medical Center, New Hyde Park, New York.

Computed Tomography of the Kidney

PERRY B. HUDSON, M.D.

Professor of Surgery, University of South Florida College of Medicine; Chief, Urology Section, Veterans Administration Medical Center, Bay Pines, Florida

Perineal Prostatectomy

SARWAT HUSSAIN, M.B.B.S.

Department of Radiology, Aga Khan University Medical College, Islamabad, Pakistan.

Computed Tomography of the Adrenal Gland

ROBERT D. JEFFS, M.D., F.R.C.S.(C)

Professor of Pediatric Urology, The Johns Hopkins University School of Medicine; Director of Pediatric Urology, The Johns Hopkins Hospital; Consultant in Pediatric Urology, Francis Scott Key Medical Center, University of Maryland Hospital, John F. Kennedy Institute, Baltimore, Maryland.

Management of the Exstrophy-Epispadias Complex and Urachal Anomalies

JOSEPH J. KAUFMAN, M.D.

Professor of Surgery/Urology, and Chief, Division of Urology, University of California, Los Angeles, School of Medicine; Chief, UCLA Urology Hospital; Director, Clark UCLA Urological Center; Consultant, Wadsworth Veterans Administration Hospital, Sepulveda Veterans Administration Hospital, Cedars/Sinai Hospital, Los Angeles, California.

Surgical Treatment of Renovascular Hypertension

ROBERT W. KINDRACHUK, M.D.

Chief Resident in Urology, Stanford University Medical School; Staff, Stanford University Medical Center, Stanford, California.

Urinalysis

LOWELL R. KING, M.D.

Professor of Urology and Associate Professor of Pediatrics; Head, Section on Pediatric Urology, Duke University School of Medicine; Division of Urology, Duke University Medical Center, Durham, North Carolina.

Vesicoureteral Reflux, Megaureter, and Ureteral Reimplantation

FREDERICK A. KLEIN, M.D.

Assistant Professor of Urology, Virginia Commonwealth University Medical College of Virginia School of Medicine; Staff, Medical College of Virginia Hospitals, Richmond, Virginia.

Surgery of the Ureter

STEPHEN A. KOFF, M.D.

Associate Professor of Surgery; Head, Section of Pediatric Urology, Ohio State University Medical College, Columbus, Ohio.

Enuresis

WARREN W. KOONTZ, Jr., M.D.

Professor and Chairman, Division of Urology, Associate Dean for Clinical Affairs, Virginia Commonwealth University Medical College of Virginia School of Medicine; Staff, Medical College of Virginia Hospitals, Richmond, Virginia.

Surgery of the Ureter

ROBERT J. KRANE, M.D.

Professor and Chairman, Department of Urology, Boston University School of Medicine; Urologist-in-Chief, University Hospital, Boston, Massachusetts.

Sexual Function and Dysfunction.

R. LAWRENCE KROOVAND, M.D.

Associate Professor of Surgery (Pediatric Urology) and Pediatrics, and Director of Pediatric and Reconstructive Urology, Bowman Gray School of Medicine of Wake Forest University; Director of Pediatric and Reconstructive Urology, North Carolina Baptist Hospital, Winston-Salem, North Carolina.

Myelomeningocele

ELROY D. KURSH, M.D.

Associate Professor of Urology, Case Western Reserve University School of Medicine; Staff, University Hospitals of Cleveland, Cleveland, Ohio.

Extrinsic Obstruction of the Ureter

PAUL H. LANGE, M.D.

Professor of Urologic Surgery, University of Minnesota Medical School; Chief, Urology Section, Veterans Administration Medical Center, Minneapolis, Minnesota.

Diagnostic and Therapeutic Urologic Instrumentation

JAY STAUFFER LEHMAN, M.D.*

Formerly, Assistant Director, The Edna McConnell Clark Foundation, New York, New York.

Parasitic Diseases of the Genitourinary System

_____

*Deceased.

HERBERT LEPOR, M.D.

Postdoctoral Fellow, Department of Urology, The Johns Hopkins University School of Medicine; Chief Resident, Department of Urology, The Johns Hopkins Hospital, Baltimore, Maryland.

Management of the Exstrophy-Epispadias Complex and Urachal Anomalies

BRUCE R. LESLIE, M.D.

Staff Physician, Division of Hypertensive Diseases, Ochsner Medical Institutions, New Orleans, Lousiana.

Normal Renal Physiology

SELWYN B. LEVITT, M.D.

Adjunct Clinical Professor of Urology, New York Medical College; Attending Pediatric Urologist, Albert Einstein College Hospital; Co-Director, Section of Pediatric Urology, Westchester County Medical Center; Attending Pediatric Urologist, Montefiore Hospital and Medical Center and Bronx Municipal Hospital Center, New York, New York.

Vesicoureteral Reflux, Megaureter, and Ureteral Reimplantation

MICHAEL M. LIEBER, M.D.

Associate Professor of Urology, Mayo Medical School, Consultant in Urology, Mayo Clinic; Staff, Methodist Hospital, St. Mary's Hospital, Rochester, Minnesota.

Open Bladder Surgery

GARY LIESKOVSKY, M.D.

Assistant Professor of Surgery/Urology, University of Southern California School of Medicine, Los Angeles, California.

Use of Intestinal Segments in the Urinary Tract

BERNARD LYTTON, M.B., F.R.C.S.

Professor of Surgery/Urology, Yale University School of Medicine; Chief of Urology, Yale–New Haven Medical Center, New Haven, Connecticut.

Surgery of the Kidney

MAX MAIZELS, M.D.

Assistant Professor of Urology, Northwestern University Medical School; Staff, Children's Memorial Hospital, Northwestern Memorial Hospital, Chicago, Illinois.

Normal Development of the Urinary Tract

TERRENCE R. MALLOY, M.D.

Professor of Urology, University of Pennsylvania School of Medicine; Chief, Section of Urology, Pennsylvania Hospital, Philadelphia, Pennsylvania.

Surgery of the Penis

FRAY F. MARSHALL, M.D.

Associate Professor of Urology, The Johns Hopkins University School of Medicine; Active Staff, The Johns Hopkins Hospital, Baltimore, Maryland.

Anatomy of the Retroperitoneum and Adrenal

VICTOR F. MARSHALL, M.D., D.Sc.

Emeritus Professor of Surgery (Urology), Cornell University Medical College; Professor of Urology, University of Virginia; Emeritus Attending Surgeon, Memorial Hospital for Cancer and Allied Diseases; Consultant in Urology, University of Virginia Hospital, Charlottesville, Virginia.

Suprapubic Vesicourethral Suspension (Marshall-Marchetti-Krantz) for Stress Incontinence.

EDWARD J. McGUIRE, M.D.

Professor of Surgery and Head, Section of Urology, University of Michigan Medical School, Ann Arbor, Michigan.

Neuromuscular Dysfunction of the Lower Urinary Tract

EDWIN M. MEARES, Jr., M.D.

Charles M. Whitney Professor of Urology, and Chairman, Division of Urology, Tufts University School of Medicine; Chairman, Department of Urology, and Urologist-in-Chief, New England Medical Center Hospitals, Boston, Massachusetts.

Prostatitis and Related Disorders

HARRY Z. MELLINS, M.D.

Professor of Radiology, Harvard Medical School; Director, Diagnostic Radiology, Brigham and Women's Hospital, Boston, Massachusetts.

Urography and Cystourethrography

EDWARD M. MESSING, M.D.

Assistant Professor of Surgery and Human Oncology, Division of Urology, University of Wisconsin School of Medicine; Attending Surgeon, University of Wisconsin Hospital and Clinics; Consulting Surgeon, Middleton Veterans Administration Hospital, Madison, Wisconsin.

Interstitial Cystitis and Related Syndromes

BRUCE A. MOLITORIS, M.D.

Assistant Professor of Medicine, Division of Renal Diseases, University of Colorado School of Medicine; Staff, University Hospital, Denver Veterans Administration Medical Center, Denver, Colorado.

Etiology, Pathogenesis, and Management of Renal Failure

MICHAEL J. MORSE, M.D.

Assistant Professor of Surgery (Urology), Cornell University Medical College; Clinical Assistant Attending, Urologic Service, Memorial Sloan-Kettering Cancer Center, New York, New York.

Neoplasms of the Testis; Surgery of Testicular Neoplasms

EDWARD C. MUECKE, M.D.

Clinical Professor of Surgery (Urology), Cornell University Medical College; Attending Surgeon (Urology), The New York Hospital; Associate Attending Surgeon (Urology), Lenox Hill Hospital, New York, New York.

Exstrophy, Epispadias, and Other Anomalies of the Bladder

GERALD P. MURPHY, M.D.

Professor of Surgery, State University of New York at Buffalo School of Medicine; Director, Roswell Park Memorial Institute, Buffalo, New York.

Tumors of Testicular Adnexal Structures and Seminal Vesicles

JOHN B. NANNINGA, M.D.

Associate Professor of Urology, Northwestern University Medical School; Attending Urologist, Northwestern Memorial Hospital; Consultant in Urology, Veterans Administration Lakeside Hospital; Chief, Division of Surgery, Rehabilitation Institute of Chicago, Chicago, Illinois.

Suprapubic and Retropubic Prostatectomy

WALTER R. NICKEL, M.D.

Clinical Professor of Dermatology and Pathology, University of California, San Diego, School of Medicine; Civilian Consultant, U.S. Naval Regional Medical Center, San Diego, California.

Visible Lesions of the Male Genitalia; Cutaneous Diseases of External Genitalia

VINCENT J. O'CONOR, Jr., M.D.

Professor of Urology, Northwestern University Medical School; Chief of Urology, Northwestern Memorial Hospital; Attending Urologist, Veterans Administration Lakeside Hospital, Chicago, Illinois.

Suprapubic and Retropubic Prostatectomy

CARL A. OLSSON, M.D.

Lattimer Professor and Chairman, Department of Urology, College of Physicians and Surgeons, Columbia University; Chief of Urology and Director, Squier Urologic Clinic, Presbyterian Hospital, New York, New York.

Anatomy of the Upper Urinary Tract

JOHN M. PALMER, M.D.

Professor of Urology, University of California, Davis, School of Medicine; Consultant, Veterans Administration Medical Center, Kaiser Permanente Medical Center, Sutter Community Hospitals Cancer Center, Sacramento, California.

Surgery of The Seminal Vesicles

JEROME P. PARNELL, II, M.D.

Clinical Assistant Professor of Surgery-Urology, University of North Carolina at Chapel Hill School of Medicine, Chapel Hill, North Carolina.

Suprapubic Vesicourethral Suspension (Marshall-Marchetti-Krantz) for Stress Incontinence

DAVID F. PAULSON, M.D.

Professor and Chief, Division of Urology, Department of Surgery, Duke University Medical Center, Durham, North Carolina.

Principles of Oncology

ALAN D. PERLMUTTER, M.D.

Professor of Urology, Wayne State University School of Medicine; Chief, Department of Pediatric Urology, Children's Hospital of Michigan, Detroit, Michigan.

Anomalies of the Upper Urinary Tract; Management of Intersexuality; Temporary Urinary Diversion in Infants and Young Children

LESTER PERSKY, M.D.

Clinical Professor of Urology, Case Western Reserve University School of Medicine; Staff, University Hospitals of Cleveland, St. Luke's Hospital, Cleveland, Ohio.

Extrinsic Obstruction of the Ureter

PAUL C. PETERS, M.D.

Professor and Chairman, Division of Urology, The University of Texas Health Science Center at Dallas, Southwestern Medical School; Chief of Urology, Parkland Memorial Hospital, Children's Medical Center; Attending Staff, Baylor University Medical Center, Presbyterian Hospital, Medical Arts Hospital, John Peter Smith Hospital (Ft. Worth), Dallas Veterans Administration Hospital, Dallas, Texas.

Genitourinary Trauma

ROBERT T. PLUMB, M.D.

Clinical Professor of Surgery (Urology), University of California, San Diego, School of Medicine; Senior Staff, Mercy Hospital, Donald N. Sharp Memorial Community Hospital, Coronado Hospital, San Diego, California.

Visible Lesions of the Male Genitalia; Cutaneous Diseases of External Genitalia

JACOB RAJFER, M.D.

Associate Professor of Surgery/Urology, University of California, Los Angeles; School of Medicine; Chief, Division of Urology, Harbor/UCLA Medical Center, Los Angeles, California.

Congenital Anomalies of the Testis

R. BEVERLY RANEY, Jr., M.D.

Associate Professor of Pediatrics, The University of Pennsylvania School of Medicine; Associate Director for Education and Training, and Senior Physician, Division of Oncology, Department of Pediatrics, Children's Hospital of Philadelphia, Philadelphia, Pennsylvania.

Pediatric Oncology

VASSILIOS RAPTOPOULOS, M.D.

University of Massachusetts Medical School; University of Massachusetts Medical Center, Worcester, Massachusetts.

Ultrasound

SHLOMO RAZ, M.D.

Associate Professor of Surgery/Urology, University of California, Los Angeles, School of Medicine; UCLA Center for the Health Sciences, Los Angeles, California.

The Treatment of Male Urinary Incontinence

MARTIN I. RESNICK, M.D.

Professor and Chairman, Division of Urology, Case Western Reserve University School of Medicine; Staff, University Hospitals of Cleveland, Cleveland, Ohio.

Extrinsic Obstruction of the Ureter

ALAN B. RETIK, M.D.

Professor of Surgery (Urology), Harvard Medical School; Chief, Division of Urology, The Children's Hospital, Boston, Massachusetts.

Anomalies of the Upper Urinary Tract; Ectopic Ureter and Ureterocele; Temporary Urinary Diversion in Infants and Young Children

JEROME P. RICHIE, M.D.

Associate Professor of Urological Surgery, Harvard Medical School; Chief, Urologic Oncology, Brigham and Women's Hospital, Boston, Massachusetts.

Ureterointestinal Diversion

ARTHUR I. SAGALOWSKY, M.D.

Associate Professor, Division of Urology, and Surgical Director, Renal Transplant, The University of Texas Health Science Center at Dallas, Southwestern Medical School; Attending Staff, Dallas Veterans Administration Hospital, Children's Medical Center, St. Paul Hospital, Baylor University Medical Center Hospital, Parkland Memorial Hospital, Dallas, Texas.

Genitourinary Trauma

OSCAR SALVATIERRA, Jr., M.D.

Professor of Surgery and Urology, and Chief, Transplant Service, University of California, San Francisco, School of Medicine, San Francisco, California.

Renal Transplantation

PETER T. SCARDINO, M.D.

Associate Professor of Urology, Baylor College of Medicine; Active Staff, The Methodist Hospital, Ben Taub General Hospital; Assistant Staff, St. Luke's Episcopal Hospital; Courtesy Staff, Veterans Administration Hospital, Texas Children's Hospital, Houston, Texas.

Initial Evaluation, Including History, Physical Examination, and Urinalysis

ANTHONY J. SCHAEFFER, M.D.

Associate Professor, Northwestern University Medical School; Attending, Northwestern Memorial Hospital; Associate Attending, Children's Memorial Hospital; Consultant in Urology, Veterans Administration Lakeside Hospital, Chicago, Illinois.

Other Renal Diseases of Urologic Significance; Surgical Management of Ureteropelvic Junction Obstruction

PAUL F. SCHELLHAMMER, M.D.

Professor of Urology, Eastern Virginia Medical School; Director, Urology Training Program, Eastern Virginia Graduate School of Medicine; Active Staff, General Hospital of Virginia Beach, Norfolk General Hospital, Leigh Memorial Hospital, Children's Hospital of the King's Daughters, DePaul Hospital, Norfolk, Virginia.

Tumors of the Penis

JAN SCHÖNEBECK, M.D.

Associate Professor of Urology, University of Linköping, Sweden; Head of Urology, Department of Surgery, Central Hospital, Norrköping, Sweden.

Fungal Infections of the Urinary Tract

ROBERT W. SCHRIER, M.D.

Professor and Chairman, Department of Medicine, University of Colorado School of Medicine; Head, Division of Renal Diseases; Staff, University Hospital, Denver Veterans Administration Medical Center, Denver General Hospital, Rose Medical Center, Denver, Colorado

Etiology, Pathogenesis, and Management of Renal Failure

WILLIAM W. SCOTT, Ph.D., M.D., D.Sc.

Professor of Urology, Emeritus, The Johns Hopkins University School of Medicine; The Johns Hopkins Hospital, Baltimore, Maryland.

Carcinoma of the Prostate

STEVEN E. SELTZER, M.D.

Associate Professor of Radiology, Harvard Medical School; Radiologist and Director, Computed Tomography, Brigham and Women's Hospital, Boston, Massachusetts.

Computed Tomography of the Kidney

RICHARD J. SHERINS, M.D.

Chief, Section on Reproductive Endocrinology, Developmental Endocrinology Branch, National Institute of Child Health and Human Development, Bethesda, Maryland.

Male Infertility

LINDA M. DAIRIKI SHORTLIFFE, M.D.

Assistant Professor of Surgery (Urology), Stanford University School of Medicine; Chief, Urology Section, Veterans Administration Medical Center, Palo Alto, California.

Infections of the Urinary Tract: Introduction and General Principles; Urinary Infections in Adult Women; Urinary Incontinence in the Female: Stress Urinary Incontinence

DONALD G. SKINNER, M.D.

Professor and Chairman, Division of Urology (Surgery), University of Southern California School of Medicine; Chief of Staff, Kenneth Norris, Jr., Cancer Hospital and Research Institute, Los Angeles, California.

Ureterointestinal Diversion; Use of Intestinal Segments in the Urinary Tract

EDWARD H. SMITH, M.D.

Professor and Chairman, Department of Radiology, University of Massachusetts Medical School, Worcester, Massachusetts.

Ultrasound

BRENT W. SNOW, M.D.

Assistant Professor, University of Utah School of Medicine, Salt Lake City, Utah.

Disorders of the Urethra and Penis

HOWARD McC. SNYDER, III, M.D.

Assistant Professor of Urology in Surgery, University of Pennsylvania School of Medicine; Assistant Surgeon, Division of Urology, Children's Hospital of Philadelphia, Philadelphia, Pennsylvania.

Pediatric Oncology

JOSEPH T. SPAULDING, M.D.

Assistant Clinical Professor of Urology, University of California, San Francisco, School of Medicine; Active Staff, St. Francis Memorial Hospital, St. Mary's Medical Center, Pacific Presbyterian Medical Center, San Francisco, California.

Surgery of Penile and Urethral Carcinoma

THOMAS A. STAMEY, M.D.

Professor of Surgery and Chairman, Division of Urology, Stanford University School of Medicine, Stanford, California.

Urinalysis; Infections of the Urinary Tract: Introduction and General Principles; Urinary Infections in Adult Women; Urinary Incontinence in the Female: Stress Urinary Incontinence

RALPH A. STRAFFON, M.D.

Chairman, Division of Surgery; Member, Department of Urology, Cleveland Clinic Foundation, Cleveland, Ohio.

Surgery for Calculus Disease of the Urinary Tract

RONALD S. SWERDLOFF, M.D.

Professor of Medicine, University of California, Los Angeles, School of Medicine; Chief, Division of Endocrinology, Harbor-UCLA Medical Center, Los Angeles, California.

Physiology of Male Reproduction: Hypothalamic-Pituitary Function

EMIL A. TANAGHO, M.D.

Professor and Chairman, Department of Urology, University of California, San Francisco, School of Medicine, San Francisco, California.

Anatomy of the Lower Urinary Tract

SALVATOR TREVES, M.D.

Associate Professor of Radiology, Harvard Medical School; Chief, Division of Nuclear Medicine, The Children's Hospital Medical Center, Boston, Massachusetts.

Radionuclides in Genitourinary Disorders

TIMOTHY S. TRULOCK, M.D.

Fellow in Pediatric Urology, Emory University School of Medicine, Atlanta, Georgia.

Prune-Belly Syndrome

SABAH S. TUMEH, M.D.

Assistant Professor of Radiology, Harvard Medical School; Radiologist, Brigham and Women's Hospital; Consultant in Oncodiagnostic Radiology and Nuclear Medicine; Dana Farber Cancer Institute, Boston, Massachusetts.

Radionuclides in Genitourinary Disorders

RICHARD TURNER-WARWICK, B.Sc., D.M. (Oxon.), M.Ch., F.R.C.S., F.R.C.P., F.A.C.S.

Consultant Urological Surgeon, The London University Institute of Urology, Middlesex Hospital, St. Peter's Group Hospitals, Royal National Orthopaedic Hospital, London, England.

Urinary Fistulae in the Female

DAVID C. UTZ, M.D.

Anson L. Clark Professor of Urology, Mayo Clinic and Mayo Medical School; Staff, Methodist Hospital, Saint Mary's Hospital, Rochester, Minnesota.

Open Bladder Surgery

E. DARRACOTT VAUGHAN, Jr., M.D.

James J. Colt Professor of Urology in Surgery, Cornell University Medical College; Attending Surgeon, The New York Hospital, Memorial Sloan-Kettering Cancer Center; Visiting Physician, The Rockefeller University Hospital, New York, New York

Normal Renal Physiology; Renovascular Hypertension; Suprapubic Vesicourethral Suspension (Marshall-Marchetti-Krantz) for Stress Incontinence

M. J. VERNON SMITH, M.D., Ph.D.

Professor of Urology, Virginia Commonwealth University Medical College of Virginia School of Medicine; Staff, Medical College of Virginia Hospitals, Richmond, Virginia.

Surgery of the Ureter

FRANZ VON LICHTENBERG, M.D.

Professor of Pathology, Harvard Medical School; Pathologist, Brigham and Women's Hospital, Boston, Massachusetts.

Parasitic Diseases of the Genitourinary System

PATRICK C. WALSH, M.D.

David Hall McConnell Professor and Director, Department of Urology, The Johns Hopkins University School of Medicine; Urologist-In-Chief, The James Buchanan Brady Urological Institute, the Johns Hopkins Hospital, Baltimore, Maryland.

Benign Prostatic Hyperplasia; Radical Retropubic Prostatectomy

ALAN J. WEIN, M.D.

Professor of Urology and Chairman, Section of Urology, University of Pennsylvania School of Medicine, Philadelphia, Pennsylvania.

Surgery of the Penis

LESTER WEISS, M.D.

Clinical Professor of Pediatrics, University of Michigan, Medical School; Director, Medical Genetics and Birth Defects Center, Henry Ford Hospital, Detroit, Michigan.

Genetic Determinants of Urologic Disease

ROBERT M. WEISS, M.D.

Professor, Department of Surgery/Urology, Yale University School of Medicine; Adjunct Professor, Department of Pharmacology, Columbia University, College of Physicians and Surgeons, New York, New York; Medical Staff, Gaylord Hospital, Wallingford; Attending, Yale–New Haven Hospital; Consulting, West Haven Veterans Administration Hospital, Waterbury Hospital, Sharon Hospital, William Backus Hospital, Norwalk Hospital, St. Raphael's Hospital, New Haven, Connecticut.

Physiology and Pharmacology of the Renal Pelvis and Ureter

WILLET F. WHITMORE, Jr., M.D.

Professor of Surgery (Urology), Cornell University Medical College; Attending Surgeon, Urologic Service, Memorial Sloan-Kettering Cancer Center, New York, New York.

Neoplasms of the Testis; Surgery of Testicular Neoplasms

JEAN D. WILSON, M.D.

Professor of Internal Medicine, University of Texas Health Science Center at Dallas, Southwestern Medical School; Attending Physician, Parkland Memorial Hospital, Dallas, Texas.

Embryology of the Genital Tract; Disorders of Sexual Differentiation

JAN WINBERG, M.D.

Professor of Pediatrics, Karolinska Institute; Chairman, Department of Pediatrics, Karolinska Hospital, Stockholm, Sweden.

Urinary Tract Infections in Infants and Children

JOHN R. WOODARD, M.D.

Professor of Surgery (Urology) and Director of Pediatric Urology, Emory University School of Medicine; Chief, Urology Service, Henrietta Egleston Hospital for Children, Atlanta, Georgia.

Prune-Belly Syndrome; Neonatal and Perinatal Emergencies

PHILIPPE E. ZIMMERN, M.D.

Resident in Urology, University of California, Los Angeles, School of Medicine, Los Angeles, California.

The Treatment of Male Urinary Incontinence

PREFACE

Urology has undergone remarkable growth and change since the Fourth Edition of this textbook was published. In creating this edition we recognized the need for an authoritative textbook incorporating the new advances in basic science, clinical medicine, instrumentation, and surgical technique. At the outset we knew we had the opportunity to create the best textbook of urology ever written and, in doing so, to improve the quality of care provided by all urologists for their patients.

We began by re-evaluating every chapter in the Fourth Edition with the help of our residents. No one is more critical or frank than the resident in training, and these evaluations were helpful in focusing new goals. We recognized that it was possible to consolidate the pathophysiologic material contained in the early chapters into a smaller space while providing more information. This enabled us to expand the clinical and surgical sections.

In keeping with past tradition there has been a significant turnover of participants in the book in order to ensure fresh approaches to specific topics. In this edition, for example, there are 26 new authors and 9 new chapters. The anatomy chapter has been subdivided into three sections: the retroperitoneum and adrenal, the upper urinary tract, and the lower urinary tract and genitalia. All three sections are now under new authorship and have new illustrations, new depth, and new emphasis on surgical considerations. The sections on normal renal function; renovascular hypertension; the etiology, pathogenesis, and management of renal failure; and renal diseases of urologic significance have new authorship. They have been completely updated and modernized and contain succinct, factual, specific applications for the urologist. A new chapter on diagnostic and therapeutic urologic instrumentation has been provided. This excellent chapter on endourology incorporates all the new information in this rapidly developing field. The section on sexual function and dysfunction, which also has new authorship, contains the newer concepts of physiology of penile erection along with extensive recommendations regarding the evaluation and management of patients with sexual dysfunction. In the recognition that a major portion of the urologist's practice involves the management of patients with cancer, a new chapter, "Principles of Oncology," has been included. Urologists have been called upon to provide an ever increasing level of sophisticated care for cancer patients. This chapter will enable the urologist to have a more informed understanding of the principles of oncology and their applications to clinical care. A new chapter on pre- and postoperative care of the urologic patient is also included. This chapter amounts to a "mini-textbook" of medicine and is an excellent synopsis of the modern concepts of pre- and postoperative care that the urologic surgeon should know.

Over 50 per cent of the chapters on urologic surgery have new authors and new illustrations. Examples from this section of the book include new chapters on urinary undiversion and the surgery of calculus disease. In addition, new approaches are presented to the management of extracorporeal renal surgery and partial nephrectomy, the surgical management of ureteropelvic junction obstruction, the surgical management of the ureter, open bladder surgery, transurethral prostatectomy, surgery of the penis, and surgery of the scrotum and its contents. The chapter on the use of intestinal segments provides an excellent description of the Kock pouch, a technique that has received widespread attention from urologists because it provides a form of urinary diversion that does not require an external appliance. In addition, the chapter on radical retropubic prostatectomy emphasizes the new "nerve-sparing" modifications that preserve postoperative potency following radical prostatectomy and cystoprostatectomy.

We wish to thank the authors of prior editions, since this new edition has been built upon the solid foundation they laid. Our gratitude is greatest for the contingent of contributing authors who collectively represent the finest scientists and clinicians associated with the field of urology. We wish to pay tribute to the late J. Hartwell Harrison, who coedited the Third Edition with the late Meredith Campbell and who led all of us through the major transition incorporated in the Fourth Edition. His untimely death prevents his witnessing our present efforts.

A work of this scope and magnitude cannot be accomplished without the assistance of a great number of persons whose efforts may not be specifically attributed within this book. Finally, we wish to express our thanks to Carroll C. Cann, Robert Butler, Constance Burton, Carolyn Naylor, and the staff of the W. B. Saunders Company for their patience and help in bringing this ambitious undertaking to publication.

PATRICK C. WALSH, M.D.
For the Editors

CONTENTS

VOLUME 1

SECTION I. ANATOMY AND PHYSIOLOGY

SECTION II. THE UROLOGIC EXAMINATION AND DIAGNOSTIC TECHNIQUES

SECTION III. THE PATHOPHYSIOLOGY OF URINARY OBSTRUCTION

9

10

SECTION IV. NEUROGENIC BLADDER

SECTION V. INFERTILITY

SECTION VI. SEXUAL FUNCTION

SECTION VII. INFECTIONS AND INFLAMMATIONS OF THE GENITOURINARY TRACT

SECTION VIII. URINARY LITHIASIS

SECTION IX. GENITOURINARY TRAUMA

VOLUME 2

SECTION X. BENIGN PROSTATIC HYPERPLASIA

SECTION XI. TUMORS OF THE GENITOURINARY
TRACT IN THE ADULT

SECTION XII. EMBRYOLOGY AND ANOMALIES OF THE GENITOURINARY TRACT

VOLUME III

SECTION XIV. RENAL DISEASES OF UROLOGIC SIGNIFICANCE

SECTION XV. UROLOGIC SURGERY

RENAL DISEASES OF UROLOGIC SIGNIFICANCE

CHAPTER 58

Renovascular Hypertension

E. DARRACOTT VAUGHAN, JR., M.D.

INTRODUCTION

Renovascular disease is one of the most common causes of secondary hypertension, with a rising rate of detection as more definitive diagnostic tests are developed. The need for identification of the entity is apparent, since this type of hypertension is difficult to manage with medical therapy (Hunt and Strong, 1973) and many renal lesions are progressive (Schreiber et al., 1984), leading to renal damage.

Fortunately, newer diagnostic tests, which often do not require hospitalization to identify these patients (Vaughan et al., 1984), have reduced the previous high cost of evaluation (McNeil and Adelstein, 1975; McNeil et al., 1975), resulting in a more aggressive diagnostic approach. In this chapter I will review the current strategies that are useful in identifying patients with renovascular hypertension, with emphasis upon renin determinations and the use of angiotensin-converting enzyme inhibitors for diagnostic purposes.

HISTORICAL BACKGROUND

Richard Bright, Physician Extraordinary to the Queen of England, was the first to associate proteinuria, fullness and hardness of the pulse, and dropsy with "hardening of the kidneys" (Bright, 1827). In 1856, Traube, from an analysis of pulse tracings, suggested that the abnormality might be high blood pressure (Traub, 1856), and Mohomed demonstrated "high tension in the arterial system" in association with renal disease (Mohomed, 1874).

The critical experimental work was the dis-covery of renin by Tigerstedt and Bergmann (1898), who noted an increase in arterial blood pressure in rabbits when they were injected with a saline renal extract. They reasoned that the renal extract contained a pressor substance and coined the term "renin." However, the significance of their work was not recognized until the critical experiments by Goldblatt et al. (1934). They produced diastolic hypertension in the dog by clamping the main renal arteries and corrected the hypertensive state by clamp removal.

Soon thereafter, Butler (1937) reported the first reversal of hypertension following nephrectomy in a patient with a small "pyelonephritic kidney"; one year later Leadbetter reported another cure of hypertension in a child with pathology demonstrating a renal arterial lesion (Leadbetter and Burkland, 1938).

These clinical observations were paralleled by laboratory investigation, and in 1940 Page and Braun-Menendez independently reported that renin itself was not a pressor substance but acted as an enzyme to release a pressor peptide, now called angiotensin, from a circulating plasma globulin (Page and Helmer, 1940; Braun-Menendez et al., 1940). Goormaghtigh, who had previously described the juxtaglomerular cells, then described increased granularity of these cells in both animals and man with renal hyertension and postulated that these cells were secreting excessive amounts of renin (Goormaghtigh and Grimson, 1939).

There followed an aggressive yet disappointing clinical experience with nephrectomy for cure of hypertension in patients with unilateral renal disease. This experience led to the search for a way of proving that a renal lesion was actually causing the hypertension. Homer

Smith, reviewing the literature, reported relief of hypertension in only 19 per cent of 200 patients whose elevated blood pressure was thought to result from unilateral renal disease (Smith, 1948). Thus it became apparent that even if pressor mechanisms did underlie some forms of renal hypertension, there were no ways to measure them.

This challenge led to studies of the effect of renal artery constriction on renal function. In dogs, renal artery constriction resulted in a marked decrease in sodium and water excretion from the affected kidney (Blake et al., 1950; Pitts and Duggan, 1950). In 1954, Howard utilized these observations to develop a differential renal function test based on bilateral ureteral catheterization to identify the "ischemic kidney" (Howard and Conner, 1954). Another major advance was the development of translumbar aortography and demonstration of its value in visualizing renal arterial lesions (Smith et al., 1952). By 1957, the first large series of patients with renal arterial lesions was reported (Poutasse and Dustan, 1957).

In addition, interest in what would become the renin-angiotensin-aldosterone system was also emerging as new discoveries were made. Accordingly, it was determined that there were two forms of angiotensin (Skeggs et al., 1954), and that angiotensin was sequenced (Skeggs et al., 1956) and synthesized (Bumpus et al., 1957). These critical advancements have led to accurate radioimmunoassay for angiotensin, the development of angiotensin analogs, and, more recently, angiotensin-converting enzyme inhibitors, all major tools now utilized to identify the patient with renovascular hypertension.

DEFINITIONS

Hypertension

As strange as it may seem, it has been difficult to establish a precise definition of hypertension. The problem was best stated by Sir George Pickering, who wrote that "there is no dividing line. The relationship between arterial blood pressure and mortality is quantitative; the higher the pressure, the worse the prognosis" (Pickering, 1973). Indeed, cumulative data obtained from insurance companies have validated this point! Untreated blood pressure in excess of 140/90 is associated with excess mortality, and diastolic pressures below 70 mm Hg are optimal (Lew, 1973). For operational purposes, the World Health Organization has defined hypertension in adults as a systolic pressure greater than 160 mm Hg and/or diastolic pressure greater than 95 mm Hg. However, the benefit of treating mild hypertension remains controversial (Pickering et al., 1983). In addition, consistent elevation of blood pressure should be established with repeated readings before evaluation is instituted. In our hypertension detection survey in Charlottesville, Virginia, we found that one half the patients identified as hypertensive in a house-to-house survey were normotensive on a repeat blood pressure measurement (Carey et al., 1976).

In children there is a rise in blood pressure with age, with an upper limit of normal reaching 130/80 by age 12 to 15 years. The most accurate evaluation, utilizing an appropriately small cuff, requires comparison of the measured blood pressure with a standard nomogram showing blood pressure related to age (Fig. 58–1).

Renal Arterial Disease Versus Renovascular Hypertension

The development of arteriography gave us an accurate means of identifying renal arterial disease and heralded the advent of renal arterial vascular repair (Freeman et al., 1954), which led to renewed enthusiasm for surgical management of the disease. However, it soon became apparent that normotensive patients undergoing arteriography for other reasons often had renal arterial disease (Eyler et al., 1962), and autopsy figures subsequently confirmed the radiologic findings (Holley et al, 1964). Accordingly, the finding of renal arterial disease alone is not sufficient justification to warrant correction in a hypertensive patient. The lesion must be functionally significant, i.e., it must reduce blood flow by an amount sufficient to activate renin release, initiating renovascular hypertension. Hence, a practical definition of renovascular hypertension is hypertension resulting from a renal arterial lesion that is relieved by correction of the offending lesion or removal of the kidney.

It is not surprising that all renal arterial lesions do not cause renovascular hypertension. Mann and coworkers (1958) showed that the internal diameter of the carotid artery could be reduced 70 per cent before a significant fall in blood flow occurred (Fig. 58–2). Similarly, Goldblatt et al. (1934) realized that a critical degree of renal arterial stenosis had to be reached before there was sufficient pressure gradient and flow reduction to initiate hypertension. This observation was carried further by

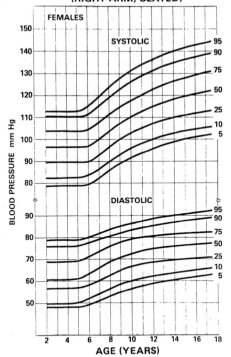

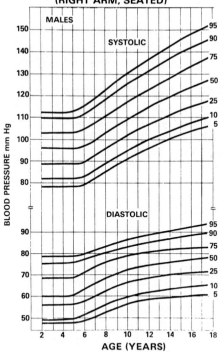

PERCENTILES OF BLOOD PRESSURE MEASUREMENT (RIGHT ARM, SEATED)

PERCENTILES OF BLOOD PRESSURE MEASUREMENT (RIGHT ARM, SEATED)

Figure 58–1. Distribution curves for seated blood pressure readings in male and female children from ages 2 to 18 years. (From Loggie, J. H.: *In* Brunner, H. F., et al. (Eds.): Hypertension in the Child and Adolescent. New York, Marcel Dekker, 1982.)

Selkurt (1951), who showed that a 40 mm Hg gradient across a renal artery stenosis was required before there was a change in renal plasma flow, glomerular filtration, sodium excretion, and urinary flow rate. Taken altogether, the renal vascular anatomy is important as a guide for choice of transluminal angioplasty or surgical repair, but the demonstration of a renal vascular lesion alone is inadequate to predict the blood pressure response following correction of the obstructing lesion.

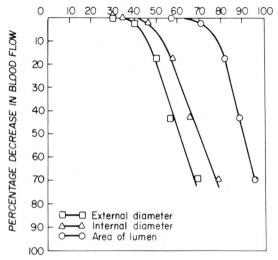

Figure 58–2. The effect of progressive arterial constriction on blood flow distal to the stenotic area. (From Mann, F. C., et al.: Surgery, *4*:249, 1938).

Cure Following Correction of Renal Artery Stenosis

Inherent in the care of patients with renovascular hypertension is close and continuing postoperative blood pressure recording. In fact, sustained blood pressure response at least 1 year after surgical correction is mandatory before the diagnosis of renovascular hypertension is validated. In the past, the definition of "successful" revascularization was often arbitrary, especially in terms of the category "improvement," defined as a 15 per cent decrease in diastolic pressure or "blood pressure easier to control with antihypertensive medications" (Foster et al., 1975).

The definition of a surgical response now should be predicted on reversal of the pathophysiologic abnormalities underlying renovascular hypertension. Hence, patients with inadequate blood pressure responses to surgical intervention require repeat plasma renin activity (PRA) determinations and/or anti-angiotensin testing with saralasin or captopril. We have found that persistence of the criteria characteristic of renovascular hypertension (postoperatively) signifies technical failure of renal revascularization (Vaughan et al., 1979). In contrast, following successful renal angioplasty and normalization of blood pressure, the peripheral plasma renin activity indexed to sodium excretion usually returns to normal and bilateral symmetric renal renin secretion returns (Pickering et al., 1984).

PATHOLOGY

The two major pathologic entities that cause renal arterial disease are atherosclerosis and fibromuscular disease. The Cleveland Clinic group has emphasized the importance of the various distinct histologic patterns, identifiable by angiographic techniques, that have predictable natural histories (Stewart et al., 1970; Harrison and McCormack, 1971; Schreiber et al., 1984). Their classification is shown in Table 58–1.

ATHEROSCLEROSIS

Atheromatous lesions of the renal artery are common and account for about 60 per cent of the lesions that cause renovascular hypertension. They usually occur in the proximal 2 cm of the renal artery but can involve the distal artery or branches. The natural history of this disease has been described, and the stage of the disease may prove to be a major factor in the response to transluminal renal angioplasty (Ratliff, 1984). Atherosclerosis begins as a proliferation of smooth muscle or myointimal cells in the intima. As they proliferate they form a rounded eccentric mound that protrudes into the lumen (Fig. 58–3). The fully formed initial lesion consists of a mass of smooth muscle cells with a varying amount of connective tissue. Subsequently lipid deposition occurs, with necrosis, inflammation, and the formation of an atherosclerotic plaque. Local complications of hemorrhage, calcification, or surface erosion with secondary thrombus formation may ensue (Fig. 58–4). Accordingly, the early lesion may be amenable to percutaneous angioplasty, whereas the mature lesion is more difficult to traverse, more rigid, and more likely to shed atheromatous emboli (Ratliff, 1984). Total reversal of hypertension following correction of atherosclerotic lesions is less common than in patients with fibromuscular disease. These patients often have diffuse atherosclerotic disease and underlying essential hypertension. In the cooperative study of renovascular hypertension, patients with bilateral atherosclerotic disease had the lowest cure rate and the highest morbidity of the various groups operated upon (Foster et al., 1975). However, attention to concurrent carotid and coronary disease prior to renal revascularization and avoidance of a severely diseased aorta have markedly reduced the morbidity of reconstructive surgery in this group (Novick et al., 1981).

INTIMAL FIBROPLASIA

This lesion is characterized by circumferential accumulation of collagen compromising

TABLE 58–1. CLASSIFICATION AND NATURAL HISTORY OF RENOVASCULAR DISEASE

Atherosclerosis: Proximal intimal plaques. Seen predominantly in males and usually in older age groups. Progressive in about 40 per cent of patients; may dissect or thrombose. May involve renal arteries only or may involve carotid and coronary arteries, aorta, and other vessels.

Intimal Fibroplasia: Collagenous disease involving intima; seen in children and young male adults. Progressive; may dissect. May involve other vessels.

True Fibromuscular Hyperplasia: Diffusely involves media. Seen in children and young adults. Progressive. Radiographically indistinguishable from intimal fibroplasia. Very rare.

Medial Fibroplasia: Series of collagenous rings involving media of main renal artery, often extending into branches. Usually seen in women in the thirties and forties. Produces typical "string of beads" pattern on angiography. Does not dissect, thrombose, or rupture and seldom progresses after age 40. May involve other vessels.

Perimedial (Subadventitial) Fibroplasia: Dense collagenous collar involving outer media, just beneath adventitia of vessel. Tightly stenotic, with extensive collateral circulation on angiography. Seen mostly in young women ("girlie disease"). Progressive. Involves renal arteries only.

Miscellaneous: Renal artery aneurysms, middle aortic syndrome, periarterial fibrosis, and post-traumatic intimal or medial disease. Variable in location and obstruction; occurs in diverse clinical settings.

From Stewart, B. H., Dustan, H. P., Kiser, W. S., et al. J. Urol., *104*:231, 1970.

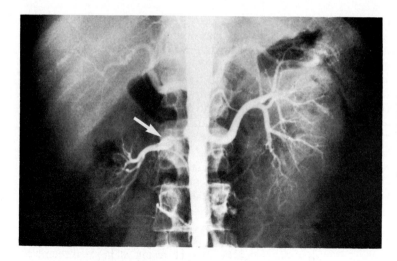

Figure 58–3. Severe atherosclerotic stenosis of the proximal right renal artery in an elderly man. Note the poststenotic arterial dilatation (arrow). (From Walter, J. F., and Bookstein, J. J.: *In* Stanley, J. C. et al. (Eds.): Renovascular Hypertension. Philadelphia, W. B. Saunders Co., 1984.)

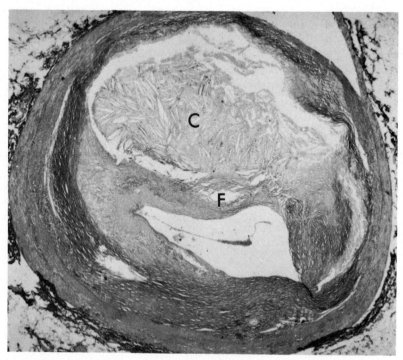

Figure 58–4. Atheromatous plaque. F, fibrous cap; C, central lipid core with typical cholesterol clefts. (Courtesy of Dr. C. Haudenschild, Boston University Medical Center. From Robbins, S. L. et al. (Eds.): Pathologic Basis of Disease. Philadelphia, W. B. Saunders Co., 1984.)

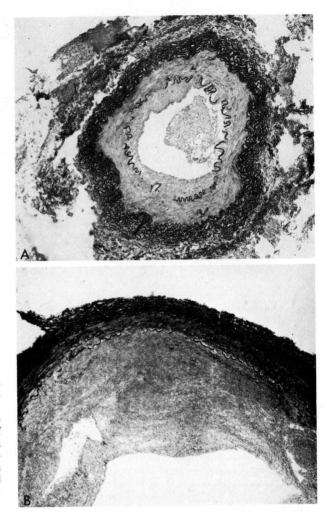

Figure 58–5. *A*, Photomicrograph cross section demonstrating intimal fibroplasia with focal fragmentation and partial absence of the elastica interna. *B*, Photomicrograph cross section demonstrating severe renal arterial intimal fibroplasia with a dense cuff of intimal collagen apposed to the luminal surface of a partially disrupted elastica interna. A small recannulized channel is noted in the lower left. (From Novick, A. C.: *In* Kelalis, P. P., King, L. R., and Belman, A. B. (Eds.): Clinical Pediatric Urology. Philadelphia, W. B. Saunders Co., 1984.)

the lumen inside the internal elastic membrane (Fig. 58–5). It occurs in children and young adults, is almost always progressive, may be complicated by dissection, and accounts for 10 per cent of the total number of fibrous lesions. Angiography reveals a smooth, fairly focal stenosis usually involving the midportion of the vessel or its branches (Fig. 58–6). Because of progression and dissection the lesion should be corrected when identified.

FIBROMUSCULAR HYPERPLASIA

This rare lesion, composing only 2 to 3 per cent of the total, is the only one in which true hyperplasia of the smooth muscle and fibrous tissue is present. The angiographic picture may be indistinguishable from intimal fibroplasia. It also occurs in children and young adults, and, since it is progressive, intervention is warranted.

MEDIAL FIBROPLASIA

This lesion is usually referred to as fibromuscular hyperplasia, a misnomer because it does not consist of true muscle hyperplasia. It gives the typical "string of beads" pattern (Fig. 58–7) on angiography, which is caused by the presence of a series of fibrous rings interspersed with aneurysmal dilatations. The aneurysms themselves are greater in diameter than the normal renal artery, and the actual degree of stenosis is difficult to assess. It is the most common fibrous lesion, constituting 75 to 80 per cent of the total, and characteristically occurs in women between the ages of 20 and 50 years. The lesion does not hemorrhage or dissect but may progress (Schreiber et al., 1984). Intervention is indicated in the younger patient, but the older patient probably can be treated with antihypertensive agents if renal function and renal size are carefully monitored.

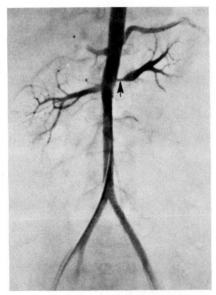

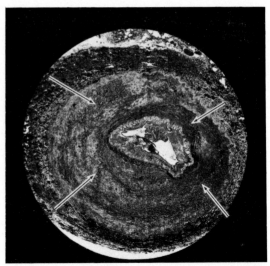

Figure 58–6. Aortogram of a 6-year-old boy demonstrates proximal left renal artery stenosis (arrow) from intimal fibroplasia. (From Novick, A. C.: *In* Kelalis, P. P., King, L. R., and Belman, A. B. (Eds.): Clinical Pediatric Urology. Philadelphia, W. B. Saunders Co., 1984.)

Figure 58–8. Cross section of the main renal artery in a girl with perimedial fibroplasia, demonstrating a dense collagenous collar involving the outer media of the vessel, which causes a severe progressive stenosis. (From Novick, A. C.: *In* Kelalis, P. P., King, L. R., and Belman, A. B. (Eds.): Clinical Pediatric Urology. Philadelphia, W. B. Saunders Co., 1984.)

PERIMEDIAL (SUBADVENTITIAL) FIBROPLASIA

This is a tightly stenotic lesion with dense collagen within intact adventitia (Fig. 58–8). In this case, the arterial beading is due to constric-

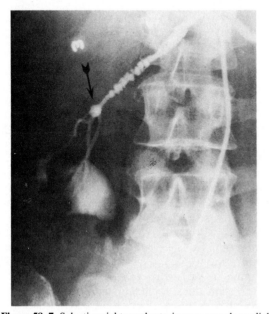

Figure 58–7. Selective right renal arteriogram reveals medial fibroplasia involving the main renal artery with typical "string of beads" appearance. (From Novick, A. C.: *In* Kelalis, P. P., and King, L. R. (Eds.): Clinical Pediatric Urology. Philadelphia, W. B. Saunders Co., 1984.)

tion and the beads are smaller than the diameter of the normal artery (Fig. 58–9). The lesion, accounting for 10 to 15 per cent of the fibrous disorders, is progressive and is seen primarily in young females. It occurs only in the renal artery and predominantly involves the right side. Repair of the lesion is indicated because of progression and the severe hypertension that usually accompanies the disease.

MISCELLANEOUS LESIONS

Saccular renal artery aneurysms not associated with coexisting renal arterial vascular disease rarely cause hypertension and usually have a benign natural history (Tham et al., 1983). Although these lesions can be repaired with a high degree of success (Ortenberg et al., 1983), the current trend favors a conservative approach. If hypertension is present the etiologic role of the aneurysm should be proved before resection is advised.

Takayasu's aortitis is a chronic sclerosing aortitis of unknown etiology that may involve the renal arteries (Rose and Sinclair-Smith, 1980). The disease is progressive and difficult to manage.

Renal vascular lesions can also occur following irradiation (McGill et al., 1979), in association with neurofibromatosis (Halpern and Currarino, 1965), or in association with a variety of other diseases (Gephardt and McCormack, 1982) (Table 58–2). Moreover, hypertension can

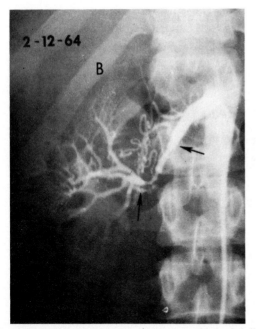

Figure 58–9. Renal arteriogram in patient with perimedial fibroplasia, showing slightly irregular yet severe stenosis of the midrenal artery, associated with extensive collateral circulation to the kidney. The small size of the arterial irregularities and the presence of collateral circulation distinguishes this lesion radiographically from medial fibroplasia. (From Novick, A. C.: *In* Kelalis, P. P., King, L. R., and Belman, A. B. (Eds.): Clinical Pediatric Urology. Philadelphia, W. B. Saunders Co., 1984.)

be caused by a number of unilateral renal parenchymal diseases (Sosa and Vaughan, 1984) (Table 58–2).

NATURAL HISTORY

There have been relatively few reports about the natural history of renal artery lesions. The limited data available have suggested that many patients with both atherosclerotic disease (Wollenweber et al., 1968) and fibromuscular disease (Meaney et al., 1968) will have progressive disease. However, it has been impossible from the initial renal arteriograms to predict which lesions would undergo progression (Stewart et al., 1970). The important question of progression has been addressed by Schreiber and coworkers (1984), and more precise information is now available.

Serial angiographic studies over a mean interval of 52 months in 85 patients with atherosclerotic disease revealed progressive vascular obstruction in 37 patients (44 per cent). Total arterial occlusion occurred in 14 patients, most commonly in those with a greater than 75 per cent stenosis on the initial arteriogram. As would be expected, decline in renal function was more common in patients with progressive disease. Accordingly, the authors suggested that renal revascularization might be indicated for preservation of renal function in individuals whose advanced atherosclerotic disease was a major threat to overall renal function. These patients are characterized by azotemia and high-grade renal artery stenosis (greater than 75 per cent), bilateral high-grade stenosis, and stenosis involving a solitary kidney (Schreiber et al., 1984).

Sixty patients with medial fibroplasia were also followed for a mean interval of 45 months. Progressive renal arterial obstruction was observed in 22 of 66 patients (33 per cent); however, there were no cases of progression to total occlusion. Of particular interest was the similar development of progressive disease in patients greater than 40 years of age (15 of 46). Previously it was felt that the disease was stable in this age group (Meaney et al., 1968). Despite the angiographic progression demonstrated, increases in serum creatinine value or reduction in renal size seldom occurred. Accordingly, the authors did not suggest renal revascularization for preservation of renal function in this group.

NORMAL PHYSIOLOGY OF THE RENIN-ANGIOTENSIN-ALDOSTERONE SYSTEM

The renin-angiotensin system (RAAS) Fig. 58–10) is one of the major renal hormonal systems involved in the regulation of systemic blood pressure, sodium and potassium balance, and regional blood flow. Its main components are renin, angiotensin II (AII), an octapeptide that is a pressor agent, and aldosterone, a mineralocorticoid released from the adrenal cortex. The system is thus involved in both the vasoconstriction and the volume/sodium components of blood pressure control (Laragh and Sealy, 1973; Peach, 1977).

Renin is a proteolytic enzyme formed in the juxtaglomerular (JG) apparatus. The JG apparatus (Fig. 58–11) is a group of cells located on or in very close proximity to the afferent arteriole of the renal glomerulus. Renin has a molecular weight of 48,000 and is released from the juxtaglomerular cells into the renal lymphatics, tubular fluid, urine, and systemic circulation (plasma renin). There are also reports of larger molecular weight renin species (MW 58,000), which exist in the plasma at concentra-

TABLE 58–2. OTHER VASCULAR LESIONS OR DISEASES ASSOCIATED WITH HYPERTENSION

I. INTRINSIC LESIONS
  A. Vascular
    1. Aneurysm (Perry: Arch. Surg., *102*:216, 1971)
    2. Emboli (Arakawa: Arch. Intern. Med., *129*:958, 1972)
    3. Arteritis
      a. Polyarteritis nodosa (Dornfield: JAMA, *215*:1950, 1971)
      b. Takayasu's (Kirshbaum: Am. Heart J., *80*:811, 1970)
    4. Arteriovenous fistula (Bennet: Am. J. Roentgenol. Radium Ther. Nucl. Med., *95*:372, 1965)
    5. Angioma (Farreras-Valenti: Am. J. Med., *34*:735, 1973)
    6. Neurofibromatosis (Halpern: N. Engl. J. Med., *273*:248, 1965)
    7. Tumor thrombus (Jennings: Br. Med. J., *2*:1053, 1964)
    8. Renal transplant rejection (Gunnels: N. Engl. J. Med., *274*:543, 1966)
  B. Renal Parenchymal
    1. Vesicoureteral reflux and renal scarring (Savage: Lancet, *1*:441, 1978)
    2. Renal tuberculosis (Stockigt: Aust. N.Z.J. Med., *6*:229, 1976)
    3. Ask-Upmark kidney (Amat: Virchows Arch., *390*:193, 1981)
    4. "Page kidney" (Sufrin: J. Urol., *113*:450, 1975)
    5. Solitary cyst (Kala: J. Urol., *116*:710, 1976)
    6. Polycystic kidney disease (Nash: Arch. Intern. Med., *137*:1571, 1977)
    7. Radiation nephritis (Shapiro: Arch. Intern. Med., *137*:848, 1977)
    8. Renal cell carcinoma (Hollifield: Arch. Intern. Med., *135*:859, 1975)
    9. Wilms' tumor (Mitchell: Arch. Dis. Child., *45*:376, 1970)
    10. Reninoma (Robertson: Am. J. Med., *43*:963, 1967)
    11. Unilateral hydronephrosis (Riehle: J. Urol., *126*:243, 1981)
    12. Bilateral hydronephrosis (Vaughan: J. Urol., *109*:286, 1973)

II. EXTRINSIC LESIONS
  A. Vascular
    1. Stenosis of celiac axis with "steal of renal blood flow" (Alfidi: Radiology, *102*:545, 1972)
    2. Congenital fibrous band (Lampe: Angiology, *16*:677, 1965)
    3. Hypoplastic aorta (Kaufman: J. Urol., *109*:711, 1973)
    4. Post radiation arteritis (McGill: J. Pediatr. Surg., *14*:831, 1979)
    5. Traumatic occlusion (Cornell: JAMA, *219*:1754, 1972)
    6. Coarctation (Shumaker: N. Engl. J. Med., *295*:148, 1976)
  B. Other Lesions
    1. Pheochromocytoma (Rosenheim: Am. J. Med., *34*:735, 1963)
    2. Metastatic tumors (Weidemann: Am. J. Med., *47*:528, 1969)
    3. Ptosis (Derrick: Am. J. Surg., *106*:673, 1963)

tions at least ten times that of renin and which can also be found in the kidney. The function of other renin species is not known (Sealey et al., 1980). The half-life of plasma renin is usually reported as between 10 and 20 minutes, and its major site of metabolism is in the liver. Release of renin from the juxtaglomerular cells is regulated by several factors to be discussed.

Once in the plasma, renin acts on its substrate angiotensinogen. Angiotensinogen is an α-2 globulin of MW 66,000 to 110,000, which is produced by the liver. Renin splits a leucyl-leucyl peptide bond and causes release of the decapeptide angiotensin I (AI). It is generally agreed that AI itself is basically an inactive species and that its biologic activity results from its conversion to the active species AII. Angiotensin-converting enzyme, also known as kininase II, is a carboxydipeptidase that splits histidyl-leucine from AI, yielding the octapeptide AII, which is the active peptide in the system.

Angiotensin-converting enzyme is found in lung (Ng and Vane, 1967), plasma, or endothelium of vascular beds, including the kidney. It is the discovery of converting enzyme inhibitors that has contributed much to the understanding of the renin-angiotensin system. In summary, angiotensinogen is metabolized to AI by the action of renin. Converting enzyme converts AI to AII. Since all the components of the system are present in the kidney, AII may function as an intrarenal as well as an extrarenal hormone (Levens et al., 1981).

AII is a compound with a wide range of biologic activity. Most of its actions are directed toward maintenance or increase of blood pressure. This control is accomplished through both its direct effect as a vasoconstrictor and its effect on sodium and volume. The data suggest that the renin-angiotensin-aldosterone system is activated by sodium depletion to maintain sodium balance and blood pressure by direct vasocon-

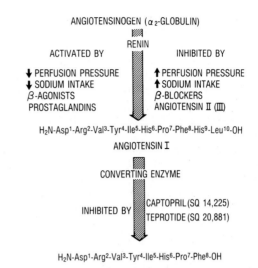

ANGIOTENSINOGEN (α_2-GLOBULIN)

RENIN

ACTIVATED BY		INHIBITED BY
↓ PERFUSION PRESSURE		↑ PERFUSION PRESSURE
↓ SODIUM INTAKE		↑ SODIUM INTAKE
β-AGONISTS		β-BLOCKERS
PROSTAGLANDINS		ANGIOTENSIN II (III)

H_2N-Asp^1-Arg^2-Val^3-Tyr^4-Ile^5-His^6-Pro^7-Phe^8-His^9-Leu^{10}-OH

ANGIOTENSIN I

CONVERTING ENZYME

INHIBITED BY   CAPTOPRIL (SQ 14,225)
                 TEPROTIDE (SQ 20,881)

H_2N-Asp^1-Arg^2-Val^3-Tyr^4-Ile^5-His^6-Pro^7-Phe^8-OH

ANGIOTENSIN II (AII)

A II RECEPTOR

ACTIVATION OF RECEPTOR RESULTS IN:	A II RECEPTOR BLOCKED BY A II ANALOGUES: PROTOTYPE
1. VASOCONSTRICTION	(Sarcosine^1, Valine^5,
2. SODIUM RETENTION	Alanine^8)A II (Saralasin)
3. RELEASE OF ALDOSTERONE	
4. RELEASE OF CATECHOLAMINES	

Figure 58–10. The renin-angiotensin-aldosterone system.

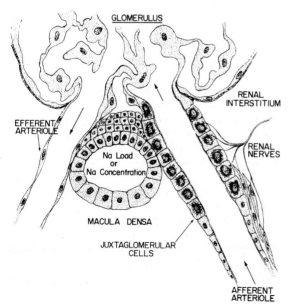

Figure 58–11. Diagram of the juxtaglomerular apparatus. The two intrarenal receptors, the vascular receptor and the macula densa, are depicted in their close physical relationship. According to current theory, the vascular receptor includes the juxtaglomerular cells and adjacent renal afferent arteriole, and this receptor responds to changes in wall tension. A change in renal tubular sodium appears to give the signal for stimulation of the macula densa, with a resulting influence on renin release. The juxtaglomerular cells secrete renin into the lumen of the renal afferent arteriole and into the renal lymph. The renal nerves are shown ending in both the juxtaglomerular cells and the smooth muscle cells of the renal afferent arteriole. Attention is also called to the intimate relationship of the efferent arteriole and the macula densa; granular cells have been observed, but rarely, in the efferent arteriole. (From Davis, J. O.: *In* Laragh, J. H. (Ed.): Hypertension Manual. New York, Yorke Medical Books, 1973.)

striction, aldosterone biosynthesis, and renal conservation of salt and water (see Chapter 2). In 1960, Laragh et al. demonstrated that AII infusion caused a rise in plasma aldosterone. This is a direct effect of AII on the adrenals, since AII increases aldosterone release from isolated adrenal slices and adrenal zona glomerulosa cell suspensions. AII acts by stimulating the conversion of cholesterol to pregnenolone, an early step in aldosterone biosynthesis. Aldosterone, an 18-aldehyde steroid, is secreted in nanogram amounts but is a potent regulator of sodium and potassium balance. Aldosterone acts primarily on the renal tubule to promote the reabsorption of sodium and the excretion of potassium. Fortunately, both plasma and urinary levels of aldosterone can be measured by precise radioimmunoassay (see Chapter 85).

AII also has been shown to have a direct sodium-retaining effect, acting at the ascending limb of the loop of Henle (Munday et al., 1971). Mechanisms that serve to dampen the system are feedback-inhibiting loops. The "long" loop involves inhibition of renin release mediated by aldosterone-induced sodium retention and volume expansion and increased blood pressure. There is also a "short"intrarenal loop, in which AII directly inhibits renin release (Ayers et al., 1977).

Renin release from the juxtaglomerular cells is controlled indirectly by a least three separate mechanisms—baroreceptor, macula densa, or beta-adrenergic—and directly by agents acting at the level of the juxtaglomerular cells. The physiologic control of renin release and its pharmacologic alteration have been reviewed recently, and only the most salient points will be mentioned here (Keeton and Campbell, 1980). The baroreceptor mechanism involves changes in renin release in response to changes in pressure at the afferent arteriole (Tobian et al., 1959). Increased pressure decreases renin release, and decreased pressure increases renin release.

The macula densa mechanism involves changes in electrolyte composition detected at the macula densa, a segment of the distal tubule that is in very close proximity to the vascular pole of the glomerulus (Barajas and Latta, 1964). For many years it was believed that sodium was the ion controlling reactivity of the macula densa. It was known that with decreased salt intake, the filtered fraction of sodium reabsorbed in the proximal tubule increased and less sodium reached the distal tubule. Decreased salt intake is associated with increased plasma renin activity (PRA). The opposite is true of increased sodium intake. This observation led to the conclusion that renin secretion is inversely related to sodium load. Data have been obtained concerning the role of chloride in regulating the macula densa response. Kotchen and coworkers (1978) maintained animals on diets containing identical sodium concentrations but differing chloride compositions; chloride delivery was measured by micropuncture. Increased chloride consumption decreased PRA (Kotchen et al., 1978). Although this suggestion is intriguing, there are some conflicting data and the question remains open.

The juxtaglomerular cells of rats, dogs, and humans are innervated by sympathetic fibers. Vander (1965) demonstrated that electrical stimulation of the renal artery and its associated sympathetics causes renin release. As these studies did not control for other changes in renal function, it was not established that a specific adrenergic receptor was involved. However, later studies established that in dogs with a single nonfiltering kidney, renal nerve stimulation increased renin secretion (Johnson et al., 1971).

Several groups have studied this phenomenon in order to characterize this response pharmacologically. In general, this receptor appears to have the properties of a β-adrenergic receptor. For example, changes in renin release caused by nerve stimulation are blocked by l-propranolol, a β-blocker, but not by its inactive stereoisomer, d-propranolol. In addition, use of β-adrenergic antagonists suppresses basal renin release and these drugs appear to act on the β-receptors of the juxtaglomerular cells (Buhler et al., 1972).

Mechanisms of Experimental Goldblatt Hypertension

The initial work of Goldblatt stimulated a search for a clearer understanding of the relationship between the renin system and renovascular hypertension. The first adancement was the realization that two models of experimental Goldblatt hypertension can be produced. In one model, a renal artery is clamped and the opposite kidney is left in place; in the other, a renal artery is clamped but the other kidney is removed. Although animals are equally hypertensive in both models, in the two-kidney, one-clip model, plasma renin activity and renin content are increased in the kidney with the stenosed artery and decreased in the opposite kidney (Gross, 1971; Mohring et al., 1975). In the one-kidney, one-clip model, Goldblatt hypertension is characterized by volume expansion and normal or suppressed plasma renin activity (Liard et al., 1974).

A second advance in exposing the role of AII in these experimental models was the administration of compounds that either block the conversion of angiotensin I to angiotensin II or are specific AII receptor antagonists (Miller et al., 1972; Brunner et al., 1971). These drugs have been important both in their insights into the role of the renin-angiotensin-aldosterone system in the normal and abnormal state and, in the case of converting enzyme inhibitors, in their clinical use in renovascular hypertension.

Knowledge of the structure of AII and improved methods of peptide synthesis have led to the synthesis of many AII analogs of modified amino acid sequence. In the process, analogs were discovered with differing biologic potencies, which led to an understanding of the contribution of each of the amino acid residues to the action of AII (Peach, 1979). Among those synthesized were two that had considerably reduced biologic activity of their own but that also blocked the action of AII on isolated smooth muscle and in the intact animal. These derivatives were [Phe^4, Tyr^8] AII (Marshall et al., 1970) and [Ala^8] AII (Khairallah et al., 1970). Further modifications led to the synthesis of the [sarcosine^1, Val^5, Ala^8] AII derivative, saralasin (Pals et al., 1971). The substitution of alanine at position 8 resulted in severe reduction of biologic activity without a loss of affinity for the receptor; the presence of sarcosine at the amino terminus allowed for resistance to hydrolysis by peptidases. These characteristics made saralasin a prototype of an AII receptor antagonist with a significant duration of action. Since saralasin is not completely devoid of biologic activity (thus it is a partial agonist), studies in which it is used require careful evaluation (Case and Laragh, 1979).

Captopril (SQ 14,225; D-3-mercapto-2-methylpropanoyl-L-proline) is a clinically used antihypertensive drug that is an angiotensin-converting enzyme inhibitor (CEI) (Rubin et al., 1978). Its synthesis followed by approximately 10 years the discovery of several naturally occurring CEI's found in snake venom (Bakhle, 1968). The active components of snake venom that were CEI's turned out to be small peptides. Synthesis of large numbers of peptide analogs resulted in synthesis of a nonapeptide CEI (SQ 20881, teprotide), the first CEI used in humans (Cheung and Cushman, 1973). Although useful, SQ 20881 was limited in its effectiveness owing to a lack of oral activity. Further modifications led to the synthesis of captopril.

Typically, a CEI blocks the pressor response that occurs following injection of AI (which is due to conversion of AI to AII); blockade of the pressor response to AI occurs without simultaneous blockade of the pressor response to AII or other pressor agents. In addition, since angiotensin-converting enzyme also participates in the metabolism of bradykinin, the depressor effect of bradykinin is potentiated in the presence of a CEI (Rubin et al., 1978).

The animal model with hypertension that is most analogous to human renovascular hypertension is the one-clip, two-kidney Goldblatt preparation. The hypertension in this model is initially dependent on increased renin secretion from the kidney with the clipped vessel, leading to AII formation and arteriolar vasoconstriction. The administration of an AII analog (saralasin) (Brunner et al., 1971) or an AI-converting enzyme inhibitor (captopril) (Weed et al., 1979) can prevent or reverse the hypertension. This early state of one-clip, two-kidney Goldblatt hypertension exhibits four characteristics (Fig. 58–12): increased renin secretion from the damaged kidney; absence of renin secretion from the opposite kidney; decreased renal blood flow to the damaged kidney; and elevated blood pressure secondary to AII-induced vasoconstriction. The identification of these characteristics has permitted the development of a rational approach to the use of plasma renin determinations (PRA) and angiotensin blockade in the diagnosis of renovascular hypertension (Vaughan et al., 1973, 1984).

In contrast, the one-kidney, one-clip Goldblatt model rapidly establishes hypertension unresponsive to AII antagonists (Brunner et al., 1971) or converting enzyme inhibition unless the animal is sodium-depleted (Gavras et al., 1973). In addition, it is apparent that the early phase of experimental one-clip, two-kidney Goldblatt hypertension is transitory (Gavras et al., 1975b; Weed et al., 1979). The blood pressure in these animals subsequently becomes resistant to acute AII blockade unless the animals are subjected to a restriction in dietary sodium. The animals now resemble the one-kidney, one-clip model. However, failure of a blood pressure response to acute AII blockade does not eliminate totally an action of AII in blood pressure maintenance. In fact, chronic administration of captopril (Bengis et al., 1978)

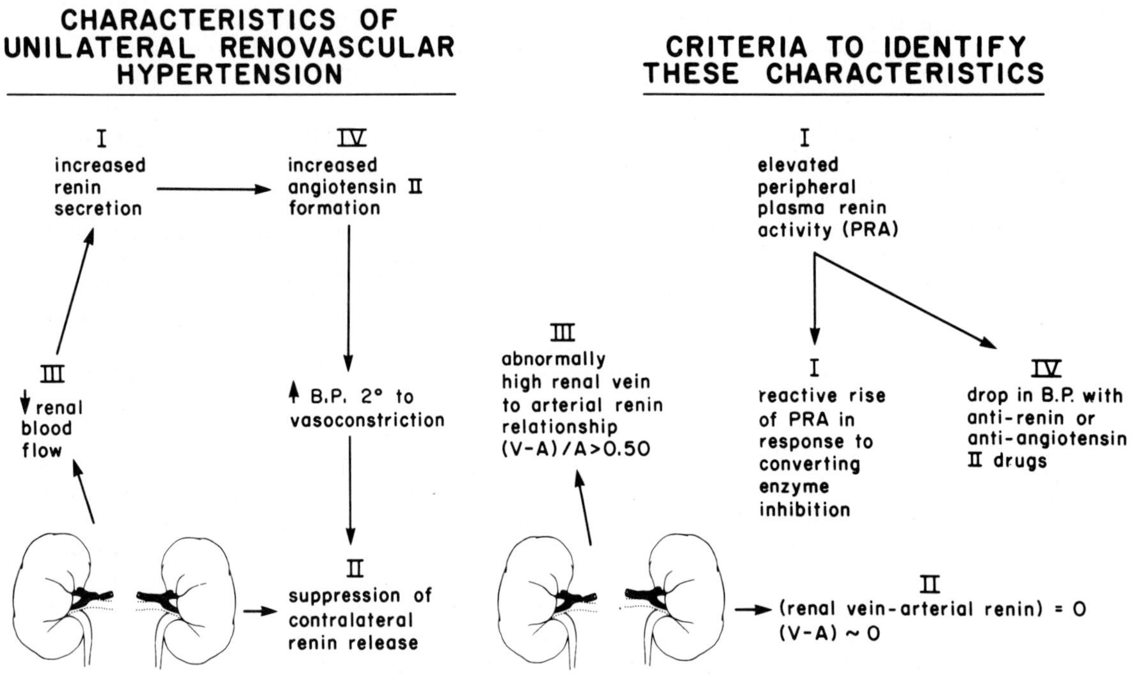

CHARACTERISTICS OF UNILATERAL RENOVASCULAR HYPERTENSION

CRITERIA TO IDENTIFY THESE CHARACTERISTICS

I
increased renin secretion

IV
increased angiotensin II formation

III
↓ renal blood flow

↑ B.P. 2° to vasoconstriction

III
abnormally high renal vein to arterial renin relationship (V-A)/A>0.50

II
suppression of contralateral renin release

I
elevated peripheral plasma renin activity (PRA)

I
reactive rise of PRA in response to converting enzyme inhibition

IV
drop in B.P. with anti-renin or anti-angiotensin II drugs

II
(renal vein-arterial renin) = 0
(V-A) ~ 0

Figure 58–12. Characteristics of the early phase of two-kidney one-clip Goldblatt hypertension in the rat *(left)* and the criteria derived from the animal model that identify the patient with correctable renal hypertension. (From Vaughan, E. D., Jr. et al.: Urol. Clin. North Am. *11*:393, 1984.)

leads to a decrease in blood pressure accompanied by natriuresis and diuresis in "saralasin-resistant" one-kidney, one-clip Goldblatt hypertensive rats.

From use of the animal data as a basis, the patient most likely to be cured following successful correction of a renal arterial lesion will exhibit the characteristics of the early-phase one-clip, two-kidney Goldblatt model. The information gained from the one-kidney model suggests that in any clinical series there will be patients who do not meet defined preoperative criteria used to predict curability who will have reversal of the hypertension following successful revascularization. It is not known whether these patients are analogous to the chronic one-clip, two-kidney model. Blood pressure control could be due either to restoration of renal blood flow, glomerular filtration rate, and sodium excretion or to reversal of an ill-defined role of AII in the presence of normal PRA. It is estimated that 20 per cent of patients with renal artery stenosis whose hypertension is cured by renal angioplasty will have normal peripheral PRA (Pickering et al., 1984).

IDENTIFYING THE PATIENT WITH RENOVASCULAR HYPERTENSION

Clinical means by which patients with functionally significant renal artery stenosis can be identified have proved to be more elusive than might have been predicted. Certainly, there are no pathognomonic clinical characteristics that lead to a reliable diagnosis (Simon et al., 1972). There are, however, a number of clinical features that should arouse suspicion that renovascular hypertension may be present. These are summarized in Table 58–3.

The only laboratory finding of importance is hypokalemia. The low potassium is due to secondary hyperaldosteronism. However, a low serum K^+ is found in less than 20 per cent of patients with renovascular hypertension.

In many patients, none of the usual clinical clues is present to prompt a definitive evaluation. Thus, the unreliability of clinical information led to the development of a variety of approaches to screen for the patient with renovascular hypertension.

TABLE 58–3. CLINICAL CLUES SUGGESTIVE OF RENOVASCULAR HYPERTENSION

History	Comment
Hypertension in the absence of any family history of hypertensive disease	Suspect if family history is negative; however, about one third of patients with renovascular hypertension will have a positive family history
Age of onset of hypertension: less than 25 years or greater than 45 years	The average age of onset for essential hypertension is 31 ± 10 (SD) years. Children and young adults usually will have fibromuscular disease, whereas adults over 45 years are more likely to have atherosclerotic narrowing of arteries.
Abrupt onset of moderate to severe hypertension	While essential hypertension usually begins with a "labile" phase before mild hypertension becomes established, renovascular hypertension usually has a more telescoped natural history, often first appearing as moderate hypertension of recent onset.
Development of severe or malignant hypertension	Renovascular hypertension often becomes moderately severe and is prone to produce acceleration or malignant phase hypertension; both forms of hypertension involve markedly increased renin release.
Headaches	Essential hypertension is usually asymptomatic. There seem to be more headaches with renovascular hypertension, possibly related to its severity or high levels of angiotensin II, a potent cerebrovascular vasoconstrictor.
Cigarette smoking	In a recent survey, 74 per cent of patients with fibromuscular renal artery stenosis were smokers; 88 per cent of those with atherosclerotic disease smoke (Nicholson et al., 1983).
White race	Renovascular hypertension is uncommon in the black population
Resistance to or escape from blood pressure control with standard diuretic therapy or antiadrenergic	Probably the most typical feature of renovascular hypertension is that it responds poorly to diuretics and often only transiently to antiadrenergic drugs.
Excellent antihypertensive response to converting enzyme inhibitors, e.g., captopril	Converting enzyme inhibitors block the renin-angiotensin system most effectively and are, therefore, highly specified agents.
Physical Examination and Routine Laboratory Tests	**Comment**
Retinopathy	Hemorrhages, exudates, or papilledema indicate acceleration or malignant phase.
Abdominal or flank bruit	A helpful clue, but bruits are commonly present in elderly individuals and occasionally present in younger patients who have no apparent vascular stenosis.
Carotid bruits or other evidence of large vessel disease	Commonly, the vascular pathology is not limited to the renal bed.
Hypokalemia—in the untreated state or in response to a thiazide diuretic	Increased aldosterone stimulation by the renin-angiotensin system tends to reduce the serum potassium level. In untreated essential hypertension this does not occur. Thiazide diuretics accentuate this phenomenon in renovascular hypertension.

From Vaughan, E. D., Jr., Case, D. B., Pickering, T. G., Urol. Clin. North Am., *11*:393, 1984.

DIFFERENTIAL RENAL FUNCTION STUDIES

As previously discussed, the observation in animals that partial occlusion of the renal artery resulted in increased fractional reabsorption of sodium and water (Blake et al., 1950) and increased urinary concentration of non-reabsorbable solute led to the development of differential renal function studies (Howard et al., 1954). The initial criterion for a positive test was a 50 per cent decrease in urine flow and a 15 per cent or greater decrease in sodium concentration from the affected kidney. The test underwent numerous modifications (Stamey, 1963); the most popular included the infusion of inulin, PAH, and antidiuretic hormone during a urea-saline diuresis to accentuate the disparity in salt and water reabsorption between the two kidneys (Stamey et al., 1961).

However, the complexity involved in performing differential split renal function studies coupled with the development of more accurate methods to measure activity of the RAAS has almost eliminated the use of this technique. Generally, at this time, differential renal function studies are performed only if renin studies are equivocal or if the patient has unilateral parenchymal disease. In contrast, the Vanderbilt group still feels that in many cases renin studies and split renal function studies are complementary and that the omission of either will increase the false negative rate (Dean, 1984). In the setting of unilateral parenchymal disease, differential function studies are most useful. The treatment choices are nephrectomy or antihypertensive medical management; the latter is preferable if the affected kidney is contributing substantially to the total renal function. Hence, the technique is utilized to measure the glomerular filtration rate of the involved kidney. If the kidney has sufficient function to sustain life, medical treatment should be the first management strategy.

INTRAVENOUS UROGRAM AND RADIONUCLIDE RENOGRAPHY

The rapid-sequence intravenous urogram is actually a radiographic differential renal function study utilizing the contrast material as the indicator. Reduced renal blood flow is indicated by decreased renal mass or size; decreased glomerular filtration rate by delayed calyceal appearance time of contrast agent; and hyper-reabsorption of water by delayed hyperconcentration of non-reabsorbable solute, the iodinated contrast material. The most reliable abnormality seen in patients with proven unilateral renovascular hypertension is delayed calyceal appearance time on the side of the offending lesion (Bookstein et al., 1972). Accordingly, the rapid-sequence series of 1- to 4-minute films after injection is critical if this test is to be utilized.

The accuracy of urography depends upon the population under study. Hence, if the urograms of patients with proven renovascular hypertension are reviewed, 80 to 90 per cent will show positive findings, based on the aforementioned criteria (Maxwell and Lupu, 1968). However, when populations of hypertensive patients have been screened, a false positive rate (a positive study in a patient with essential hypertension) of about 10 per cent has been found. Since greater than 90 per cent of the overall hypertensive population is composed of patients with essential hypertension, this false positive rate is translated into an unacceptably high number of patients falsely identified as having potential renovascular disease (Maxwell and Lupu, 1968).

Moreover, the presence of a positive urogram in a patient with renal arterial disease does not predict the blood pressure response to surgery. In the Cooperative Study of Renovascular Hypertension, abnormal urograms were found in 80 per cent of both the cured patients and the patients whose blood pressure failed to respond to surgical repair (Bookstein et al., 1972). Similarly, the radionuclide renogram, despite numerous modifications, has been plagued with variability that has led to even less specificity. In fact, review of a variety of techniques disclosed a false positive rate of 25 per cent (Maxwell et al., 1968), while a later study utilizing a refined technique reduced the false positive rate to 10 per cent—still no better than the urogram (Franklin and Maxwell, 1975). In summary, both the intravenous urogram and the nuclide studies have failed to achieve suitable sensitivity and specificity to be reliable screening tests for renovascular hypertension.

INCREASED RENIN SECRETION—THE PERIPHERAL PLASMA RENIN

After the initial work of Dr. Harry Goldblatt, it was assumed that excess renin secretion, leading to excess angiotensin II (AII) formation, was the underlying derangement in renovascular hypertension. Unfortunately, this possibility was soon challenged when circulating PRA was found to be normal in both animal models (Ayers et al., 1969) and a fraction of patients with renovascular hypertension (Marks and Maxwell, 1975). This latter review of the literature found the peripheral PRA to be elevated in only 109 of 196 patients (56 per cent) with verified cases of correctable renovascular hypertension. However, upon careful review of the primary papers it is apparent that these samples were often obtained under conditions that are now recognized to invalidate or limit accurate interpretation of the values obtained. For example, it is now recognized that PRA is inversely related to sodium intake and must be indexed in some fashion to the state of sodium balance (Fig. 58–13). Moreover, all antihypertensive drugs influence PRA and must be stopped 2 weeks before blood sampling for PRA. Aids to increase the accuracy of determinations of peripheral PRA are shown in Table 58–4.

The peripheral PRA is emphasized because it represents an index of renin secretion (Sealey et al., 1973). There is a common misconception

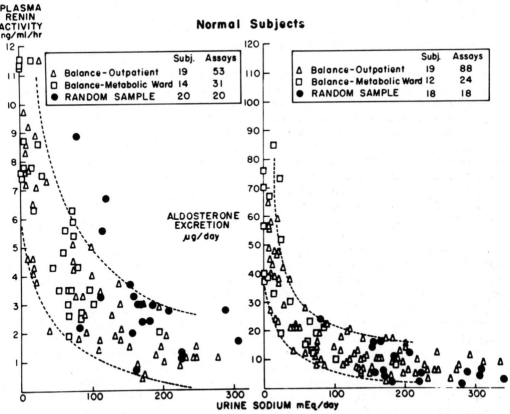

Figure 58–13. Relationship of renin activity in plasma samples obtained at noon and the corresponding 24-hour urinary excretion of aldosterone to the concurrent daily rate of sodium excretion. For these normal subjects, the data describe a similar dynamic hyperbolic relationship between each hormone and sodium excretion. Of note is the fact that subjects studied on random diets outside the hospital exhibited similar relationships, a finding that validates the use of this nomogram in studying outpatients or subjects not receiving constant diets. (From Laragh, J. H. et al.: *In* Laragh, J. H. (Ed.): Hypertension Manual. New York, Yorke Medical Books, 1973.)

TABLE 58–4.   AIDS TO INCREASE THE ACCURACY OF DETERMINATIONS OF PERIPHERAL PLASMA
RENIN ACTIVITY (PRA)

Problems	Solution
The "normal" value for PRA varies from laboratory to laboratory.	Clearly understand the factors that affect "normal" values in your laboratory: time of sampling, state of ambulation (upright posture influences PRA), state of sodium intake.
The method of collection of blood samples from patients may vary from that used to collect samples designed to establish normal range.	Utilize identical conditions for sampling.
All antihypertensive and diuretic drugs alter PRA.	Stop all treatment 2 weeks prior to blood sampling for PRA.
PRA is inversely related to sodium intake/excretion.	Collect a 24-hr urine for sodium determinations at the time that you collect blood for PRA; use the sodium intake level that your laboratory uses to define their normal range.*
Inferior vena cava renin used as "peripheral."	Obtain peripheral blood for PRA as described on a day separate from renal vein sampling.

*If a new methodology is being established, suggest the development of a renal/sodium index.
Adapted from Vaughan, E. D., Jr.: Urol. Clin. North Am., 6:485, 1979.

that increased renin secretion is determined from differential renal vein renin measurements. Actual renin secretion (renal vein renin concentration minus arterial renin concentration multiplied by renal blood flow) is rarely determined. Accordingly, a high renal venous renin concentration may reflect increased secretion with normal renal blood flow or, alternatively, a normal amount of renin secreted into reduced renal blood flow (i.e., secretion = concentration × flow).

Increased secretion of renin is characteristic of renovascular hypertension and should therefore be reflected by elevated peripheral PRA as compared with PRA values obtained from normotensive controls that are collected and analyzed under exactly the same conditions. Peripheral PRA (determined in blood collected at noon after 4 hours of patient ambulation), when indexed against the rate of urinary sodium excretion, is an excellent tool for identifying abnormally high renin secretion. In a recent study of patients who subsequently had successful transluminal angioplasty, the peripheral PRA was elevated in 80 per cent (Fig. 58–14). Moreover, the PRA always decreased and often returned to normal following successful renal angioplasty, thereby confirming the hypothesis that the peripheral PRA is an indicator of increased renin secretion, which is corrected following relief of the offending stenotic lesion (Pickering et al., 1984).

Measurement of PRA in this manner as a *screening* test for renovascular hypertension has important limitations. In addition to a 20 per cent false negative rate (i.e., a normal PRA indexed against sodium excretion) in patients with proven renovascular hypertension, there is a technical problem. Many patients with reno-

vascular hypertension have severe life-threatening hypertension or coexistent heart disease that precludes cessation of antihypertensive medication prior to collecting blood for peripheral PRA determinations. Thus, sampling blood while patients are on drugs invalidates the accuracy of peripheral PRA as a practical screening tool. In addition, 16 per cent of the large population of patients with essential hypertension have high PRA (Brunner et al., 1972). Taken altogether, these problems have led to the search for an additional test to screen for renovascular hypertension.

ENHANCED ACCURACY OF PERIPHERAL PLASMA RENIN ACTIVITY BY STIMULATION WITH ANGIOTENSIN-BLOCKING DRUGS

The first angiotensin-blocking agent used for testing in human hypertension was saralasin. The initial results demonstrated that the compound did, as predicted, lower blood pressure in high-renin forms of hypertension, including renovascular hypertension (Brunner et al., 1973). In a second generation of human studies with saralasin, the partial agonist activity of the drug was exposed (Case et al., 1976a; Carey et al., 1978). Thus, in clinical settings in which PRA was low, the drug actually increased blood pressure. Moreover, the blood pressure–lowering effect of the drug was found to be inversely proportional to the sodium intake. Accordingly, although reasonably accurate in identifying patients with renovascular hypertension (Horn et al., 1979), the test is limited because of the need for intravenous infusion, the agonist effect of the drug, and the influence of sodium balance on the blood pressure response to the agent.

A second approach to the use of angiotensin blockade to expose renovascular hyperten-

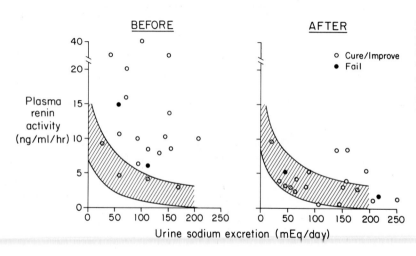

Figure 58–14. Effect of angioplasty on peripheral plasma renin activity indexed against 24-hour sodium excretion. *Left,* Before angioplasty; *right,* 6 months after angioplasty. Hatched area shows normal range. (From Pickering, T. G. et al.: Am. J. Med. 76:398, 1984.)

sion came from experience following the development of converting enzyme inhibitors that block angiotensin II formation. A nonapeptide obtained from the venom of the *Bothrops jararaca* viper, teprotide or SQ-20881, was shown to block the vasopressor effect of angiotensin I; it was possible to demonstrate a close direct correlation between the pretreatment level of PRA and the magnitude of the depressor response (Case et al., 1976*b*). Moreover, in untreated hypertensive patients on the same normal sodium intake, intravenous teprotide lowered blood pressure to the greatest extent in the group profiled as high-renin by the renin-sodium index but did not lower blood pressure significantly in the low-renin subgroup. From these studies, it was possible to predict that inhibition of converting enzyme might be a useful diagnostic approach for detecting angiotensin-dependent forms of hypertension.

The success of the intravenous converting enzyme inhibitor was a potent stimulus to the development of an orally active form, the first of which to be used in man was captopril (SQ-14225). Captopril has the potential for use as a diagnostic probe, like teprotide, since it has a rapid onset of action (within 10 to 15 minutes), reaching a peak effect by 90 minutes (Case et al., 1978). Initial studies showed a close relationship between the pretreatment plasma-renin activity and the magnitude of the depressor

response induced after the first dose of captopril (Case et al., 1978).

During the early studies of the effect of these agents on blood pressure in hypertensive patients it was noted that angiotensin blockade resulted in a marked rise in PRA in selected patients. Accordingly, the induction of marked rises in plasma renin activity in 31 of 32 renovascular patients, but only 2 of 64 with essential hypertension, appeared to be an even more specific test for renovascular hypertension than the induction of depressor responses. These studies also revealed that prior sodium depletion either with diuretics or by low-sodium diet *abolished* the specificity of this test (Case and Laragh, 1979).

With the availablity of the oral converting enzyme inhibitor captopril, we began using single oral test doses instead of intravenous infusions. Results very similar to those obtained using the intravenous competitive antagonist saralasin or the converting enzyme inhibitor teprotide were found (Case et al., 1979). An additional advantage was the observation that renovascular hypertensive patients being treated with a beta-adrenergic blocker still responded to oral administration of captopril with a fall in blood pressure and a rise in PRA (Fig. 58–15) (Case et al., 1982).

The protocol for using single oral doses of captopril to screen for renovascular hyperten-

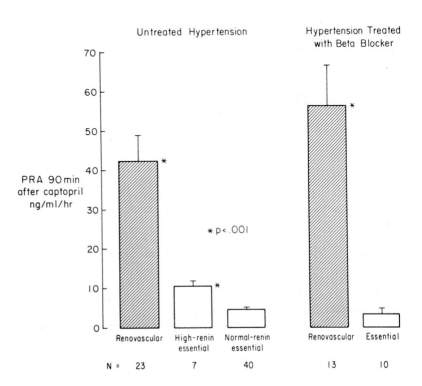

Figure 58–15. Levels of plasma-renin activity in renovascular and essential hypertension 90 minutes after a single dose of captopril. A marked reactive hyperreninemia was found in the group with renovascular hypertension whether they were already receiving β-blocker therapy or not. (From Case, D. B. et al.: *In* Laragh, J. H., et al. (Eds.): Frontiers in Hypertension Research. New York, Springer-Verlag, 1982.)

TABLE 58–5. SINGLE-DOSE CAPTOPRIL TEST

Drugs

The patient should be taken off all medicines for at least 2 weeks, if possible. Otherwise, leave on a beta-blocker but omit all diuretics, converting enzyme inhibitors, or nonsteroidal anti-inflammatory drugs for at least 1 week, ideally 2 weeks.

Diet

A diet with normal or a high salt or sodium content is needed. Too low a sodium intake will produce falsely positive results. If there is a question about diet, a 24-hour urine collection for sodium will closely reflect the intake.

Procedure

The patient may be supine, semi-recumbent, or seated for the test, but measurements must be made with the patient in the same position.

After measurements of blood pressure are stable (this usually takes about 10 to 20 minutes), a blood sample for plasma renin activity is drawn (in lavender-topped Vacutainer kept at room temperature.

Crush a 25-mg tablet of captopril (to ensure that it dissolves) and pour in water to produce a suspension of about 30 ml. Instruct the patient to drink the suspension, wash the contents out twice, and drink those also.

Remeasure blood pressure and PRA after 1 hour.

From Vaughan, E. D., Jr., Case, D. B., Pickering, T. G., et al.: Urol. Clin. North Am., *11*:393, 1984.

---

sion is shown in Table 58–5. Our current criteria for a positive test to identify a patient with renovascular hypertension are: a post-captopril PRA ≥ 12 ng/ml/hr and an increase in renin of ≥10 ng/ml/hr, plus a Δ per cent increase in renin of over 400 per cent if the baseline PRA was <3 and over 150 per cent if the baseline renin was >3 ng/ml/hr. In summary, single-dose captopril appears to accurately separate patients with renovascular or renal hypertension from those with essential hypertension. Moreover, a 24-hour urine collection is not necessary and the patient can remain on beta blockade if the baseline PRA is >1ng/ml/min. The test is not valid if the PRA is lower than one. Hence, the test is complementary to the renin-sodium index to identify renin hypersecretion.

CONTRALATERAL SUPPRESSION OF RENIN SECRETION AND AN ELEVATED RENAL VEIN TO ARTERIAL RENIN RELATIONSHIP—USE OF DIFFERENTIAL RENAL VEIN RENIN DETERMINATIONS

Since the development of the technique (Judson and Helmer, 1965), differential renal vein renin determinations have emerged as the most useful tool in identifying correctable renovascular hypertension. The most common approach has been to calculate the renal vein–renin ratio, that is, stenotic divided by normal side PRA values with some arbitrary "positive" ratio (usually 1.5:1). The major difficulty with this method is in selecting a ratio that has the accuracy to divide precisely patients with renovascular hypertension from those with essential hypertension (Marks and Maxwell, 1975). Generally, a positive renal vein ratio predicts a fall in blood pressure following correction of the vascular lesion in over 90 per cent

of cases. However, a negative ratio does not preclude a successful response to revascularization. In the review of Marks and Maxwell (1975), 49 per cent of patients with negative ratio were cured by appropriate surgical intervention. However, these patients were a minority of the total patients studied, and the actual false negative rate was 15 per cent (62 of 412 patients).

In addition, the collection of renal vein blood alone for PRA is subject to the risk of a sampling error caused either by incorrect catheter placement or by sampling from a renal vein that does not subtend the renal area supplied by the stenotic artery. Sampling from the inferior vena cava below the renal veins is a safeguard against this source of error, and the absence of a 50 per cent renin increment from both kidneys together identifies an inadequate differential renal vein renin study (Vaughan et al., 1973).

Finally, a positive renal vein ratio does not exclude bilateral, albeit asymmetric, renin secretion, which would indicate bilateral renal disease. In this setting, correction of a unilateral lesion may not totally correct the underlying pathology, with subsequent failure of total blood pressure control.

In view of these limitations of the traditional renal vein ratio analysis, another method for analysis of renin values has been devised. It is based on the characteristics of the experimental one-clip, two-kidney Goldblatt hypertension, as detailed in Table 58–6 and Figure 58–12.

Hypersecretion of renin, as determined by the renin-sodium index or captopril stimulation, serves as the primary criterion for the diagnosis of renovascular hypertension. A second criterion is the demonstration of the absence of renin

TABLE 58–6. RENIN VALUES FOR PREDICTING CURABILITY OF RENOVASCULAR HYPERTENSION

Collection of Samples
(moderate sodium intake ± 100 mEq/day)

1. Ambulatory peripheral renin and 24-hour urine sodium excretion under steady-state conditions (i.e., not on day of arteriography)
2. Collection of blood for PRA before and after converting enzyme blockade
3. Collection of Supine
   a. Renal vein renin from suspect kidney (V1) and inferior vena cava renin (A1)
   b. Renal vein from contralateral kidney (V2) and inferior vena cava renin (A2)
4. Enhancement of renin secretion by converting enzyme blockade if initial renin sampling is inconclusive

Criteria for Predicting Cure

High PRA in relation to UNaV	Measurement of hypersecretion of renin
Contralateral kidney: $(V2 - A2) = 0$	An indicator of absent renin secretion from the contralateral kidney
Suspect kidney: $(V1 - A1)/A1 = 0.50$	An indicator of unilateral renin secretion
$(V1 - A1)/A1 = 0.50$	Measurement of reduced renal blood flow
$\dfrac{(V - A)}{A} + \dfrac{(V - A)}{A} < 0.50$	
In patients with high PRA	
Means: a. Incorrect sampling b. Segmental disease	Repeat with segmental sampling

From Vaughan, E. D., Jr., *In* Brenner, B. M., and Stein, J. M. (Eds.): Hypertension. New York, Churchill Livingstone, 1981.

secretion from the contralateral (or noninvolved) kidney. Suppression of renin secretion from this kidney can be determined by subtracting the arterial plasma renin activity (A) from the renal venous renin activity (V). Since the inferior vena caval (IVC) renin and aortic renin are the same, the IVC renin value can be substituted for (A) in this equation (Fig. 58–16)

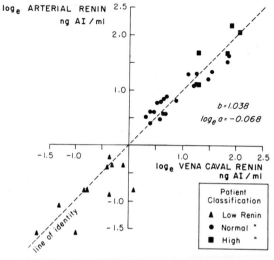

Figure 58–16. Relationship of renin activity in blood collected from the aorta to that found in vena caval blood. The two values do not differ in patients with essential hypertension. (From Sealey, J. E. et al.: Am. J. Med., 55:391, 1973.)

(Sealey et al., 1973). Hence, patients with curable renovascular hypertension exhibit an absence of renin secretion from the opposite kidney, i.e., $(V - A) = 0$, also termed contralateral suppression of renin (Stockigt et al., 1972; Vaughan et al., 1973). Contralateral suppression of renin indicates that the noninvolved kidney is responding in an appropriate "normal" fashion to the elevated blood pressure, increased circulating AII levels, and/or increased sodium chloride at the macula densa by shutting off renin secretion. This phenomenon is at times present not only in patients with unilateral renal arterial lesions but also in patients with bilateral disease demonstrated by arteriograms who have a dominant lesion on one side (Gittes and McLaughlin, 1974; Pickering et al., 1983).

A third criterion is based on studies of renal vein and arterial renin relationships in patients with essential hypertension. The mean renal venous renin level has been determined to be about 25 per cent higher than arterial PRA (Fig. 58–17) (Sealey et al., 1973). Hence, a total renin increment (both kidneys) of approximately 50 per cent is necessary to maintain a given peripheral renin level $(V - A)/A = 50$ per cent. However, a reduction in renal blood flow also influences the renal venous renin level. In this setting, the renal venous renin concentration will be misleadingly high, shifting the renal vein:arterial renin relationships upward.

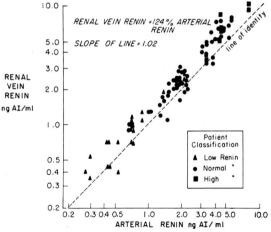

Figure 58–17. Relationship of renal vein renin to arterial (or venous) renin in patients with essential hypertension. The slope of the line does not differ from the line of identity, indicating that the relationship of renal vein renin to arterial renin is constant at all levels of plasma renin activity found in essential hypertension. The intercept of 1.24 indicates that the renal vein renin is 124 per cent of arterial renin. (From Sealey, J. E. et al.: Am. J. Med., 55:391, 1973.)

found in a group of patients managed by renal revascularization is shown in Figure 58–19 (Vaughan et al., 1979).

In a group of 46 hypertensive patients with arteriographically proved unilateral renal artery stenosis who underwent successful angioplasty, 34 had technically successful sampling (Pickering et al., 1984). Twelve patients had studies that were judged to be unsuccessful; 9 sets of values were rejected because the combined increment from the two sides was less than 50 per cent. It is of interest that six of nine patients were taking captopril chronically and exhibited high systemic levels of PRA (between 14 and 99 ng/ml/hr) at the time of sampling. These data suggest that chronic converting enzyme blockade with captopril may invalidate renal vein renin analysis by a mechanism that is unclear at present. In contrast, three patients, two of whom were taking beta blockers, had extremely low peripheral PRA (less than 1 ng/ml/hr) at the time of sampling. This latter situation is potentially clarified by captopril stimulation (see further on).

Of the 34 patients with technically acceptable values, there were 23 true positive, no false positive, 3 true negative, and 8 false negative results. Of the eight false negative findings, four had a $(V - A)/A$ between 40 and 48 per cent, and six showed contralateral suppression. Only

Hence, the elevation of the increment above approximately 50 per cent becomes an index of the severity of the reduction in blood flow consequent to the obstructing vascular lesion (Fig. 58–18). The combination of these criteria

ESSENTIAL HYPERTENSION

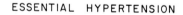

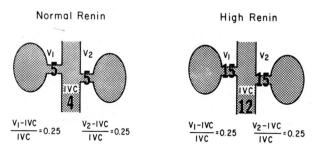

Figure 58–18. Renal vein renin diagnostic patterns. In essential hypertension *(top)* at all levels of renin secretion, the renin level in each renal vein is about 25 per cent greater than either the peripheral arterial or the venous level. In the setting of unilateral renin secretion (curable renovascular hypertension), the active kidney is solely responsible for maintaining the peripheral renin levels. Hence, the increment is 50 per cent (0.5) and becomes progressively greater as renal blood flow is reduced. Unequal bilateral renin secretion *(bottom right)* indicates bilateral disease and decreases the chance of cure following corrective unilateral surgery. (From Laragh, J. H., and Sealey, J. E.: Cardiovas. Med., 2:1053, 1977.)

RENOVASCULAR HYPERTENSION

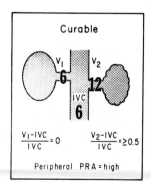

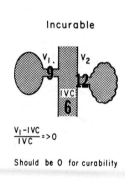

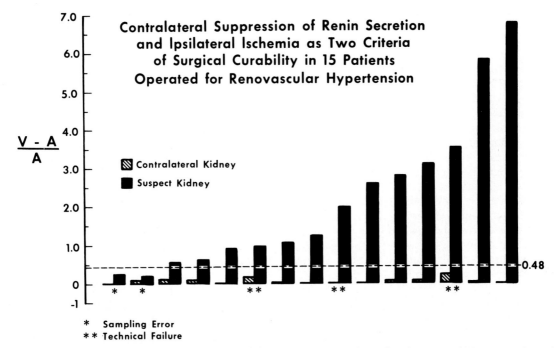

$$\frac{V - A}{A}$$

Contralateral Suppression of Renin Secretion and Ipsilateral Ischemia as Two Criteria of Surgical Curability in 15 Patients Operated for Renovascular Hypertension

▨ Contralateral Kidney

■ Suspect Kidney

0.48

* Sampling Error
** Technical Failure

Figure 58–19. Of 15 patients with renovascular hypertension, 13 exhibited $(V - A)$ A in excess of 48 per cent from the suspect kidney and a suppressed value from the contralateral kidney. V is renal venous PRA; A is arterial or infrarenal inferior vena cava PRA. Asterisks denote the three patients who had values suggesting surgical curability, yet had residual or recurrent hypertension due to technical failure. (From Vaughan, E. D., Jr., et al.: Kid. Int., *15*:S83, 1979.)

two patients had symmetric renal vein renins (Pickering et al., 1984). Hence, the present approach gave a sensitivity of 74 per cent and a specificity of 100 per cent, better indices than found by renin ratio analysis.

An additional aid to renal vein sampling is the utilization of segmental renal venous sampling (Schambelan et al., 1974), especially when sampling of blood from the major renal veins fails to demonstrate a combined renin increment of 50 per cent from both kidneys, suggesting either a technical error or segmental disease. This approach may be particularly helpful in children with segmental parenchymal disease (Parrott et al., 1984).

CONVERTING ENZYME INHIBITION TO ENHANCE THE ACCURACY OF RENAL VEIN RENIN ANALYSIS

Following the initial report of renin stimulation by angiotensin blockade (Re et al., 1978), several groups of investigators have reported increased renin release from the ischemic kidney with converting enzyme inhibition (Lyons et al., 1983; Thibonnier et al., 1984). The magnitude of these induced changes is shown in Figure 58–20. These data were determined from 26 patients with unilateral renovascular hypertension. Not shown in this illustration is the observation that the inferior vena cava levels (sys-

temic or peripheral levels) were comparable to those values measured from the normal side, revealing the continued suppression of renin secretion from that kidney even after stimulation. Although more information is required to distinguish the subtleties (i.e., bilateral renovascular disease, branch lesions, total occlusions,

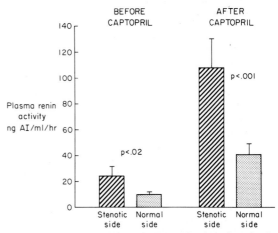

Figure 58–20. Renal vein renin determinations (renal vein levels only) in patients with documented renovascular hypertension before and after captopril stimulation. Captopril accentuates renin secretion from the ischemic kidney. Not shown are the inferior vena cava levels, which are the same as the levels measured from the normal side both before and after captopril stimulation. (From Vaughan, E. D., Jr., et al.: Urol. Clin. North Am. In press.)

coexistent renal parenchymal disease, and so forth), it is clear that stimulation adds to the analysis in certain specific situations: (1) when patients are already on drug therapy, e.g., beta blockers, and the renin levels are generally reduced; (2) when there is a question about the reliability of the PRA measurements, particularly of low levels; (3) when experience in performing renal vein renins is limited and subject to sampling errors; and (4) when equivocal values already exist.

In summary, renal vein renin sampling after captopril stimulation accentuates renin release from ischemic renal tissue, which is particularly useful when values are equivocal, when branch stenoses are present, or when renovascular disease is superimposed on coexisting hypertension or renal disease. We anticipate that the addition of converting enzyme inhibition during renal venous sampling for renin will virtually eliminate the false negative analyses that have previously limited the accuracy of the studies.

Anatomic Confirmation of the Four Criteria. It should be noted that virtually the entire evaluation of the hypertensive patient can now be accomplished without hospitalization, thus avoiding much of the expense previously thought to be too great to warrant evaluation (McNeil et al., 1975). We have performed over 300 renal vein renin samplings on an outpatient basis, 100 of these being accompanied by digital angiography (DIVA), which is about 90 per cent accurate in identifying renal arterial lesions (Osborne et al., 1981). We utilize a central injection for the DIVA, which gives better definition of the renal vasculature. The major error arises with branch or segmental disease involving the smaller renal vessels.

The concept of intravenous angiography is not new. It was first performed in the 1930's (Robb and Steinberg, 1939). In fact, the use of the early technique in urology was reviewed by Steinberg and Marshall in 1961. However, the technique was soon replaced by refinements in catheter angiography. Recently, the combination of equipment designed for image enhancement and computer analysis has revolutionized the field and led to DIVA as a major tool in the management of patients with renovascular hypertension (Hillman et al., 1983).

Accordingly, DIVA can be utilized both to accompany renal vein sampling for renin to give anatomic definition of the renal vasculature and to follow patients following correction of a renovascular lesion (Sos et al., 1983). The only caveat is that because DIVA only detects anatomic vascular disease, the functional significance of the lesion must still be demonstrated.

Screening criteria have been identified to assure both that the patient with renovascular disease will be physiologically and anatomically characterized and that the success of a corrective procedure can be predicted. When these criteria have been met, the patient is admitted to the hospital for definitive management of the offending lesion.

Validation of the Criteria. In addition to a favorable clinical response to renal angioplasty, we have had the unique opportunity to study the effect of restoration of blood flow on renal vein renin concentration and renin secretion (Vaughan et al., 1981; Pickering et al., 1984). To accomplish this goal, we have monitored the immediate effect of successful angioplasty on renal renin secretion. Thirty minutes following angioplasty, there was a marked reduction in the renal vein renin from the previously stenotic side (Fig. 58–21). The residual ipsilateral increment of renal vein renin was about 50 per cent above the peripheral level, while contralateral renin suppression persisted. This 50 per cent increment had been predicted previously to occur in the setting of unilateral renin secretion and normal renal blood flow (Sealey et al., 1973).

Several months after angioplasty, there was a marked fall in peripheral PRA with a return to normal in most patients, indicating a reduction of renin secretion (see Fig. 58–14). Of equal interest is the restoration of bilateral renin increment of about 25 per cent above the inferior vena cava renin level (Fig. 58–21). Hence, con-

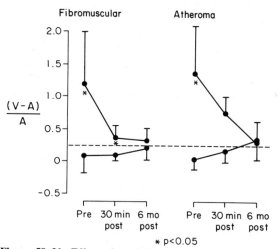

Figure 58–21. Effect of angioplasty on renal vein renin. Samples were taken immediately before angioplasty, 30 minutes after, and 6 months after. The higher values are for the ischemic kidney; the lower values are for the contralateral kidney. Asterisk indicates significant difference between the two kidneys, and the dotted line is the normal level of $(V - A)/A$ (0.24). (From Pickering, T. G. et al.: Am. J. Med. In press. 1984).

tralateral renin suppression was reversed following successful angioplasty. This 25 per cent increment from both kidneys is characteristic of the renin secretory pattern found in patients with essential hypertension (Pickering et al., 1984).

The finding that the renal renin secretory characteristics of renovascular hypertension are reversed following successful angioplasty with correction of the hypertension is strong evidence that they truly reflect the abnormal secretory behavior of renin in curable renovascular hypertension.

Identifying the Potentially Curable Patient: A Cost-Effective Approach

Our current approach is outlined in Figure 58–22. All patients with fixed hypertension are potential candidates for this protocol, since we believe that nearly all patients with renovascular hypertension, when identified, can be best managed by angioplasty or revascularization. With respect to this empirical protocol, it could be argued that highly suspect patients could be

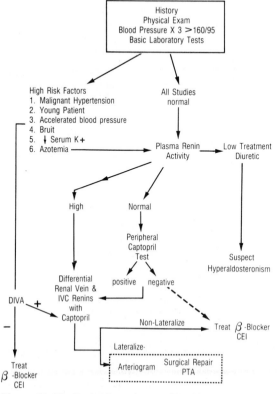

Figure 58–22. Evaluation plan to identify patients with renovascular hypertension. (From Sosa, R. E., and Vaughan, E. D., Jr.: AVA Update Series 2: Lesson 31, 1983.)

screened initially with a digital angiogram. However, the functional significance of an anatomic lesion with respect to ischemia-induced renin release still must be established, so we routinely begin with a peripheral PRA.

In our experience, a low PRA is rarely found in untreated patients with nonazotemic renal arterial disease, and we therefore do not usually continue this evaluation in these patients unless they demonstrate refractoriness to treatment. Patients with high or normal PRA undergo a peripheral captopril test. The test cannot be performed if the patient is taking captopril chronically. If the test is positive, the differential renal vein sampling and digital angiography are performed together. The sampling procedure ideally is done first, and then the catheter is advanced into the superior vena cava for injection of contrast material. This combined study is performed in the radiology suite, following which the patient lies quietly in the hypertension unit for 2 to 4 hours before returning home. After the diagnostic criteria have been established, the patient is briefly hospitalized for selective arteriography and percutaneous transluminal angioplasty.

We continue to believe that the functional significance of a renal artery lesion must be identified before the therapeutic decision is directed toward intervention.

Tailored Therapy for Renovascular Hypertension

The rationale for identifying patients with renovascular hypertension is that their management will differ from the treatment offered patients with essential hypertension. Indeed, hypertension of renal origin is difficult to manage with conventional antihypertensive drugs. In a randomized study (Hunt and Strong, 1973), the morbidity and mortality were greater in patients with renal hypertension treated in the medical group as contrasted to the surgical group. In addition, as previously discussed, most renovascular lesions are progressive with time, and there is little evidence to suggest that successful control of hypertension influences the natural history of the various pathologic entities (Meaney et al., 1968; Schreiber et al., 1984; Goncharenko et al., 1981). Accordingly, for properly selected cases, surgical management has been the preferable choice.

However, with the development of better and more specific antihypertensive drugs, such as converting enzyme inhibitors and beta-blockers, it is now possible to treat cases of renovascular hypertension more effectively. Certainly, in our early experience, captopril appears to be effective in controlling blood pressure in patients who are poor surgical candidates. Although more specific medical management is attractive, it is becoming increasingly apparent that dramatic reduction of blood pressure can lead to rapid progression of renal insufficiency and total renal arterial occlusion (Ying et al., 1984). Indeed, reversible renal failure has been observed in patients with renovascular disease treated with captopril (Mason and Hilton, 1983; Chrysant et al., 1983). Moreover, less dramatic reductions in renal function have been observed in patients with renovascular hypertension randomly selected for nonoperative management, and even in patients with acceptable blood pressure control during the period of observation (Dean et al., 1981).

These observations make a strong argument against noninterventive management in a patient with known renovascular disease, especially in view of the increasing success of either percutaneous transluminal renal angioplasty (PTA) (Sos et al., 1983) or operative renal revascularization (Stanley and Graham, 1984). Moreover, further consideration and study must be addressed toward the concept of PTA or revascularization of renal arterial lesions for the preservation of renal function even in the absence of the criteria for patient selection described herein or perhaps even in the absence of hypertension (Schreiber et al., 1984).

References

Ayers, C. R., Harris, R. H., and Lefer, L. G.: Control of renin release in experimental hypertension. Circ. Res. (Suppl. 1), 24/25:103, 1969.

Ayers, C. R., Katholi, R. E., Vaughan, E. D., Jr., Carey, R. M., Kimbrough, H. M., Jr., Yancey, M. S., and Morton, C. L.: Intrarenal renin-angiotensin-sodium interdependent mechanism controlling post clamp renal artery pressure and renin release in the conscious dog with chronic one-kidney Goldblatt hypertension. Circ. Res., 40:238, 1977.

Bakhle, Y. S.: Conversion of angiotensin I to angiotensin II by cell-free extracts of dog lung. Nature, 220:919, 1968.

Barajas, L., and Latta, H.: The innervation of the juxtaglomerular apparatus: An electron microscopic study of the innervation of the glomerular arterioles. Lab. Invest., 13:916, 1964.

Bengis, R. G., Coleman, T. G., Young, D. B., and McCaa, R. E.: Long term blockade of angiotensin formation in various normotensive and hypertensive rat models using converting enzyme inhibitor (SE 14225). Circ. Res. (Suppl. 1), 43:145, 1978.

Blake, W. D., Wegria, R., Ward, H. P., and Frank, C. W.: Effect of renal arterial constriction on excretion of sodium and water. Am. J. Physiol., 163:422, 1950.

Bookstein, J. J., Abrams, H. L., Buenger, R. E., Lecky, J., Franklin, S. S., Reiss, N. D., Bleifer, K. H., Klatte, E. C., Varady, P. D., and Maxwell, M. H.: Radiologic aspects of renovascular hypertension. Part II. The role of urography in unilateral renovascular disease. J.A.M.A., 220:1225, 1972.

Braun-Menendez, E., Fasciolo, J. C., Leloir, L. R., and Munoz, J. M.: The substance causing renal hypertension. J. Physiol., 98:283, 1940.

Bright, R: Reports of medical cases, selected with a view of illustrating symptoms and cure of disease by reference to morbid anatomy. London, Longman Group, Ltd., 1827.

Brunner, H. R., Gavras, H., Laragh, J. H., and Keenan, R.: Angiotensin II blockade in man by SAR^1-Ala^8-angiotensin II for understanding and treatment of high blood pressure. Lancet, 2:1045, 1973.

Brunner, H. R., Kirshmann, J. D., Sealey, J. E., and Laragh, J. H.: Hypertension of renal origin: Evidence for two different mechanisms. Science, 174:1344, 1971.

Brunner, H. R., Laragh, J. H., Baer, L., Newton, M. A., Goodwin, F. T., Krakoff, L. R., Bard, R. M., and Buhler, F. R.: Essential hypertension: Renin and aldosterone, heart attack, and stroke. N. Engl. J. Med., 286:441, 1972.

Buhler, F. R., Laragh, J. H., Baer, L., Vaughan, E. D., Jr., and Brunner, H. R.: Propranolol inhibition of renin secretion. N. Engl. J. Med., 287:1209, 1972.

Bumpus, F. M., Schwarz, H., and Page, I. H.: Synthesis and pharmacology of the octapeptide angiotensin. Science, 125:886, 1957.

Butler, A. M.: Chronic pyelonephritis and arterial hypertension. J. Clin. Invest., 16:889, 1937.

Carey, R. M., Reid, R. A., Ayers, C. R., Lynch, S. S., McLain, W. L. III, and Vaughan, E. D., Jr.: The Charlottesville blood pressure survey: Value of repeat blood pressure measurement to define the prevalence of labile and sustained hypertension. JAMA, 236:847, 1976.

Carey, R. M., Vaughan, E. D., Jr., Ackerly, J. A., Peach, M. J., and Ayers, C. R.: The immediate pressor effect of saralasin in man. J. Clin. Endocrinol. Metab., 46:36, 1978.

Case, D. B., and Laragh, J. H.: Reactive hyperreninemia following angiotensin blockade with either saralasin or converting enzyme inhibitor: A new approach to screen for renovascular hypertension. Ann. Intern. Med., 91:153, 1979.

Case, D. B., Atlas, S. A., and Laragh, J. H.: Reactive hyperreninemia to angiotensin blockade identified renovascular hypertension. Clin. Sci., 57:313s, 1979.

Case, D. B., Atlas, S. A., and Laragh, J. H.: Physiologic effects and blockade. In Laragh, J. H., Buhler, F. R., and Seldin, D. W. (Eds.): Frontiers in Hypertension Research. New York, Springer-Verlag, 1982, pp. 541–550.

Case, D. B., Atlas, S. A., Laragh, J. H., Sealey, J.E., Sullivan, P. A., and McKinstry, D. N.: Clinical experience with blockade of the renin-angiotensin-aldosterone system by an oral converting enzyme inhibitor (SQ 14225, captopril) in hypertensive patients. Prog. Cardiovasc. Dis., 21:195, 1978.

Case, D. B., Wallace, J. M., Keim, H. J., Sealey, J. E., and Laragh, J. H.: Usefulness and limitations of saralasin, a weak competitive agonist for angiotensin II, for evaluating the renin and sodium factor in hypertensive patients. Am. J. Med., 60:825, 1976a.

Case, D. B., Wallace, J. M., Keim, H. J., Weber, M. A., Drayer, J. I. M., White, R. P., Sealey, J. E., and Laragh, J. H.: Estimating renin participation in hypertension: Superiority of converting enzyme inhibitor over saralasin. Am. J. Med., *61*:790, 1976*b*.

Case, D. B., Wallace, J. M., Keim, H. J., Weber, M. A., Sealey, J. E., and Laragh, J. H.: Possible role of renin in hypertension as suggested by renin-sodium profiling and inhibition of converting enzyme. N. Engl. J. Med., *296*:641, 1977.

Cheung, H. S., and Cushman, D. W.: Inhibition of homogenous angiotensin-converting enzyme of rabbit lung by synthetic venom peptides of Bothrops jararaca. Biochim. Biophys. Acta, *293*:451, 1973.

Chrysant, S. G., Dunn, M., and Marples, D.: Severe reversible azotemia from captopril therapy. Arch. Intern. Med., *143*:437, 1983.

Dean, R. H.: Renovascular hypertension: An overview. *In* Rutherford, R. B. (Ed.): Vascular Surgery. Philadelphia, W. B. Saunders Co., 1984.

Dean, R. H., Kieffer, R. W., Smith, B. M., Oates, J. A., Nadeau, J. H. J., Hollifield, J. U., and DuPont, W. D.: Renovascular hypertension: Anatomic and functional changes during drug therapy. Arch. Surg., *116*:1408, 1981.

Eyler, W. R., Clark, M. D., Garman, J. E., Rian, R. L., and Meininger, D. E.: Angiography of the renal areas including a comparative study of renal arterial stenosis in patients with and without hypertension. Radiology, *78*:879, 1962.

Foster, J. H., Maxwell, M .H., Franklin, S. S., Bleifer, K. H., Trippel, O. H., Julian, O. C., DeCamp, P. T., and Varady, P. Y.: Renovascular occlusive disease: Results of operative treatment. JAMA, *231*:1043, 1975.

Franklin, S. S., and Maxwell, M. H.: Clinical workup for renovascular hypertension. Urol. Clin. North Am., *2*:301, 1975.

Freeman, N. E., Leeds, F. M., and Elliot, W.: Thromboendarterectomy for hypertension due to renal artery occlusion. JAMA, *156*:1077, 1954.

Gavras, H., Brunner, H. R., Laragh, J. H., Gavras, I., and Vukovich, R. A.: The use of angiotensin-converting enzyme inhibitor in the diagnosis and treatment of hypertension. Clin. Sci. Mol. Med., *48*:57S, 1975*a*.

Gavras, H., Brunner, H. R., Thurston, H., and Laragh, J. H.: Reciprocation of renin dependency with sodium volume dependency in renal hypertension. Science, *188*:1316, 1975*b*.

Gavras, H., Brunner, H. R., Vaughan, E. D., Jr., and Laragh, J. H.: Angiotensin-sodium interaction in blood pressure maintenance of renal hypertensive and normotensive rats. Science, *180*:1369, 1973.

Gephardt, G. N., and McCormack, L. J.: Pathology of the renal artery in hypertension. *In* Breslin, D. J., Swinton, N. W., Jr., Libertino, J. A., and Zinman, L. (Eds.): Renovascular Hypertension. Baltimore, Williams & Wilkins Co., 1982, pp. 63–72.

Gittes, R. F., and McLaughlin, A. P.: Unilateral operation for bilateral renovascular disease. J. Urol., *111*:292, 1974.

Goldblatt, H., Lynch, J., Hanzal, R. F., and Summerville, W. W.: Studies on experimental hypertension. I. The production of persistent elevation of systolic blood pressure by means of renal ischemia. J. Exp. Med., *59*:347, 1934.

Goncharenko, V., Gerlock, A. J., Shaff, M. I., and Hollifield, S. W.: Progression of renal artery fibromuscular dysplasia in 42 patients as seen on angiography. Radiology, *139*:45, 1981.

Goormaghtigh, N., and Grimson, K. S.: Vascular changes in renal ischemia, cell mitosis in the media of arteries. Proc. Soc. Exp. Biol. Med., *42*:227, 1939.

Gross, F.: The renin-angiotensin system in hypertension. Ann. Intern. Med., *75*:777, 1971.

Halpern, M , and Currarino, M.: Vascular lesions causing hypertension in neurofibromatosis. N. Engl. J. Med., *73*:248, 1965.

Harrison, E. G., Jr., and McCormack, L. J.: Pathologic classification of renal arterial disease in renovascular hypertension. Mayo Clin. Proc., *46*:161, 1971.

Hillman, B. J., Smith, J. R. L., Pond, G. D., Ovitt, T. W., and Capp, M. P.: Photoelectric radiology. *In* Hanafec, W. N., and Wilson, G. H. (Eds.): Radiology. New York, John Wiley & Sons, 1983.

Holley, K. E., Hunt, J. C., Brown, A. L., Kincaid, O. W., and Sheps, S. G.: Renal artery stenosis: A clinical-pathologic study in normotensive patients. Am. J. Med., *37*:14, 1964.

Horn, M. L., Conklin, V. M., Keenan, R. E., Varady, P. D., and Dinardo, J.: Angiotensin II profiling with saralasin: Summary of the Eaton Collaborative Study. Kidney Int. (Suppl.), *9*:S115, 1979.

Howard, J. E., and Conner, T. B.: Use of differential renal function studies in the diagnosis of renovascular hypertension. Am. J. Surg., *107*:58, 1954.

Howard, J. E., Berthrong, N., Gould, D., and Yendt, E. R.: Hypertension resulting from unilateral renovascular disease and its relief by nephrectomy. Bull. Johns Hopkins Hosp., *94*:51, 1954.

Hunt, J. C., and Strong, C. S.: Renovascular hypertension: Mechanisms, natural history and treatment. Am. J. Cardiol., *32*:562, 1973.

Johnson, J. A., Davis, J. O., and Witty, R. T.: Effects of catecholamines and renal nerve stimulation on renin release in the non-filtering kidney. Circ. Res., *29*:646, 1971.

Judson, W. E., and Helmer, O. M.: Diagnostic and prognostic values of renin activity in renal venous plasma in renovascular hypertension. Hypertension, *13*:79, 1965.

Keetor, T. K., and Campbell, W. B.: The pharmacologic alteration of renin release. Pharmacol. Rev., *32*:81, 1980.

Khairallah, P. A., Toth, A., and Bumpus, F. M.: Analogs of angiotensin II: II. Mechanism of receptor interaction. J. Med. Chem., *13*:181, 1970.

Kotchen, T. A., Galla, J. H., and Luke, R. G.: Contribution of chloride to the inhibition of plasma renin by sodium chloride in the rat. Kidney Int., *13*:201, 1978.

Laragh, J. H., and Sealey, J. E.: The renin-angiotensin-aldosterone hormonal system and regulation of sodium, potassium, and blood pressure homeostasis. *In* Handbook of Physiology. Washington, D.C., American Physiological Society, 1973.

Laragh, J. H., Angers, M., Kelly, W. G., et al.: The effect of epinephrine, norepinephrine, angiotensin II, and others on the secretory rate of aldosterone in man. JAMA, *174*:234, 1960.

Laragh, J. H., Sealey, J. E., Buhler, F. R., Vaughan, E. D., Jr., Brunner, H. R., Gavras, H., and Baer, L.: The renin axis and vasoconstriction volume analysis for understanding and treatment of renovascular and renal hypertension. Am. J. Med., *58*:4, 1975.

Leadbetter, W. F., and Burkland, C. F.: Hypertension in unilateral renal disease. J. Urol., *39*:611, 1938.

Levens, N. R., Peach, M. J., and Carey, R. M.: Role of the intrarenal renin-angiotensin system in the control of renal function. Circ. Res., *48*:157, 1981.

Lew, E. A.: High blood pressure, other risk factors and longevity. *In* Laragh, J. H. (Ed.): The Insurance Viewpoint in Hypertension Manual. New York, Yorke Medical Books, 1973.

Liard, J. F., Cowley, A. W., McCaa, R. E., McCae, C. S., and Guyton, A. C.: Renin, aldosterone, body fluid volumes, and the baroreceptor reflex in the development and reversal of Goldblatt hypertension in conscious dogs. Circ. Res., *34*:549, 1974.

Lyons, D. F., Streck, W. F., Kem, D. C., et al.: Captopril stimulation of differential renins in renovascular hypertension. Hypertension, *5*:65, 1983,

McCormack, L. J., Poutasse, E. F., Meaney, T. F., Noto, T. J., and Dustan, H. P.: A pathologic arteriographic correlation of renal arterial disease. Am. Heart J., *72*:188, 1966.

McGill, C. W., Holder, T. M., and Smith, T. H.: Postradiation renovascular hypertension. J. Pediatr. Surg., *14*:831, 1979.

McNeil, B. J., and Adelstein, S. J.: Measures of clinical efficacy: The value of case finding in hypertensive renovascular disease. N. Engl. J. Med., *293*:221, 1975.

McNeil, B. J., Varady, P. D., and Burrows, B. A.: Measures of clinical efficacy: Cost-effectiveness calculations in the diagnosis and treatment of hypertensive renovascular disease. N. Engl. J. Med., *293*:216, 1975.

Mann, F. C., Herrick, J. F., Essex, H. E., and Baldes, E. J.: The effect on the blood flow of decreasing lumen of a blood vessel. Surgery, *4*:249, 1938.

Marks, L. S., and Maxwell, M. H.: Renal vein renin value and limitations in the prediction of operative results. Urol. Clin. North. Am., *2*:311, 1975.

Marshall, G. R., Vine, W., and Needleman, P.: A specific competitive inhibitor of angiotensin II. Proc. Natl. Acad. Sci. (USA), *67*:1624, 1970.

Mason, J. C., and Hilton, P. J.: Reversible renal failure due to captopril in a patient with transplant artery stenosis. Hypertension, *5*:623, 1983.

Maxwell, M. H., and Lupu, A. N.: Excretory urogram in renal arterial hypertension. J. Urol., *100*:395, 1968.

Maxwell, M. H., Lupu, A. N., and Taplin, G. V.: Radioisotope renogram in renal arterial hypertension. J. Urol., *100*:376, 1968.

Meaney, T. F., Dustan, H. P., and Gilmore, J. P.: Angiotensin I conversion in the kidney and its modulation by sodium balance. Am. J. Physiol., *224*:1104, 1973.

Miller, E. D., Jr., Samuels, A. I., and Haber, E.: Inhibition of angiotensin conversion in experimental renovascular hypertension. Science, *177*:1108, 1972.

Mohomed, F. A.: The etiology of Bright's disease and the prealbuminuric stage. Med. Chir. Trans., *57*:197, 1874.

Mohring, J., Mohring, B., Naumann, J. H., Dauda, G., Kazda, S., Gross, F., Philippi, A., Homsy, E., and Orth, H.: Salt and water balance and renin activity in renal hypertension of rats. Am. J. Physiol., *228*:1847, 1975.

Munday, K. A., Parsons, B. J., and Poàt, J. A.: The effect of angiotensin on cation transport in rat kidney cortex slices. J. Physiol. (Lond.), *215*:269, 1971.

Ng, K. K. F., and Vane, J. R.: Conversion of angiotensin I to angiotensin II. Nature, *215*:762, 1967.

Nicholson, J. P., Alderman, M. H., Pickering, T. G., Teishman, S. L., Sos, T. A., and Laragh, J. H.: Cigarette smoking in renovascular hypertension. Lancet, *2*:765, 1983.

Novick, A. C., Straffon, R. A., Stewart, B. H., Gifford, R. W., and Vidt, D.: Diminished operative morbidity and mortality in renal revascularization. JAMA, *246*:749, 1981.

Ortenberg, J., Novick, A. C., Straffon, R.A., and Stewart, B. H.: Surgical treatment of renal artery aneurysm. Br. J. Urol., *55*:341, 1983.

Osborne, R. W., Jr., Goldstone, J., Hillman, B.J., et al.: Digital video subtraction angiography: Screening technique for renovascular hypertension. Surgery, *90*:932, 1981.

Page, I. H., and Helmer, O. M.: A crystalline pressor substance (angiotonin) resulting from the reaction between renin and renin activator. J. Exp. Med., *71*:29, 1940.

Pals, D. T., Masucci, F. D., Denning, G. S., Jr., et al.: Role of the pressor action of angiotensin II in experimental hypertension. Circ. Res., *29*:673, 1971.

Parrott, T. S., Woodard, J. R., Trulock, T. S., and Glenn, J. F.: Segmental renal vein renins and partial nephrectomy for hypertension. J. Urol., *131*:736, 1984.

Peach, M. J.: Renin-angiotensin system: Biochemistry and mechanisms of action. Physiol. Rev., *57*:313, 1977.

Peach, M. J.: Structural features of angiotensin II which are important for biologic activity. Kidney Int., *15*:S3, 1979.

Pickering, G.: Hypertension definitions, natural histories and consequences. *In* Laragh, J. H. (Ed.): Hypertension Manual. New York, Yorke Medical Books, 1973.

Pickering, T. G.: Treatment of mild hypertension and the reduction of cardiovascular mortality: The "of or by" dilemma. JAMA, *249*:399, 1983.

Pickering, T. G., Case, D. B., Sos, T. A., Vaughan, E. D., Jr., Sealey, J. E., and Laragh, J. H.: Unilateral suppression of renin secretion in patients with bilateral renal artery stenosis. Clin. Res., 1983.

Pickering, T. G., Sos, T. A., Vaughan, E. D., Jr., et al.: Predictive value and changes of renin secretion in hypertensive patients with unilateral renovascular disease undergoing successful renal angioplasty. Am. J. Med., *76*:398, 1984.

Pitts, R. F., and Duggan, J. J.: Studies on diuretics. II. The relationship between glomerular filtration rate, proximal tubular absorption of sodium, and diuretic efficacy of mercurials. J. Clin. Invest., *29*:372, 1950.

Poutasse, E. F., and Dustan, H. P.: Arteriosclerosis and renal hypertension: Indications for aortography in hypertensive patients and results of surgical treatment of obstructive lesions of renal artery. JAMA, *165*:1521, 1957.

Ratliff, N. B.: Renal vascular disease: Pathology of large blood vessel disease. Am. J. Kidney Dis. In press.

Re, R., Noveline, R., Escourrou, M-T., Athanasoulis, C., Burton, J., and Haber, E.: Inhibition of angiotensin-converting enzyme for diagnosis of renal-artery stenosis. N. Engl. J. Med. *298*:582, 1978.

Robb, G. P., and Steinberg, I.: Visualization of the chambers of the heart, the pulmonary circulation and the great vessels in man. Am. J. Roentgenol., *41*:1, 1939.

Rose, A. G., and Sinclair-Smith, C. C.: Takayasu's arteritis. A study of sixteen autopsy patients. Arch. Pathol. Lab. Med., *104*:231, 1980.

Rubin, B., Laffan, R. J., Kotler, D. G., et al.: SQ 14225 (D-3-mercapto-2-methylpropanoyl-L-proline), a novel orally active inhibitor of angiotensin I–converting enzyme. J. Pharm. Exp. Ther., *204*:271, 1978.

Schambelan, M., Glickman, M., Stockigt, J. R., and Biglieri, E. G.: The selective renal vein renin sampling in hypertensive patients with segmental renal lesions. N. Engl. J. Med., *290*:1153, 1974.

Schreiber, M. J., Pohl, M. A., and Novick, A. C.: The natural history of atherosclerotic and fibrous renal artery disease. Urol. Clin. North Am., *11*:383, 1984.

Sealey, J. E., Atlas, S. A., and Laragh, J. H.: Prorenin and other large molecular weight forms of renin. Endocrine Rev., *1*:365, 1980.

Sealey, J. E., Buhler, F. R., Laragh, J. H., and Vaughan, E. D., Jr.: The physiology of renin secretion in essential hypertension: Estimation of renin secretion rate and renal plasma flow from peripheral and renal vein renin levels. Am. J. Med., *55*:391, 1973.

Selkurt, E. E.: The effect of pulse pressure and mean arterial pressure modification of renal hemodynamics and electrolyte and water excretion. Circulation, *4*:541, 1951.

Simon, N., Franklin, S. S., Bleifer, K. H., and Maxwell, M. H.: Clinical characteristics of renovascular hypertension. JAMA, *220*:1209, 1972.

Skeggs, L. T., Jr., Lentz, K. E., Kahn, J. R., Shumway, N. P., and Woods, K. R.: Amino acid sequence of hypertension II. J. Exp. Med., *104*:193, 1956.

Skeggs, L. T., Marsh, W. H., Kahn, J. R., and Shumway, N. P.: The existence of two forms of hypertension. J. Exp. Med., *99*:275, 1954.

Smith, H. W.: Hypertension and urologic disease. Am. J. Med., *4*:724, 1948.

Smith, P., Rush, T. W., and Evans, A. T.: The technique of translumbar arteriography. JAMA, *148*:255, 1952.

Sos, T. A., Sniderman, K. W., Pickering, T. G., et al.: Percutaneous transluminal renal angioplasty in renovascular hypertension due to atheroma or fibromuscular dysplasia. N. Engl. J. Med., *309*:274, 1983.

Sosa, R. E., and Vaughan, E. D., Jr.: Evaluation for surgically curable hypertension. AUA Update Series, *2*:Lesson 31, 1983.

Stamey, T. A.: Renovascular Hypertension. Baltimore, The Williams & Wilkins Co., 1963.

Stamey, T. A., Nudelman, I. J., Good, T. H., Schwentker, E. N., and Hendricks, F.: Functional characteristics of renovascuar hypertension. Medicine, *40*:347, 1961.

Stanley, J. C., and Graham, L. M.: Renal artery fibrodysplasia and renovascular hypertension. *In* Rutherford, R. B. (Ed.): Vascular Surgery. Philadelphia, W. B. Saunders Co., 1984.

Steinberg, I., and Marshall, V. F.: Intravenous abdominal aortography in urologic diagnosis. J. Urol., *86*:456, 1961.

Stewart, B. H., and Dustan, H. P., Kiser, W. S., Meaney, T. F., Straffon, R. A., and McCormack, L. J.: Correlation of angiography and natural history in evaluation of patients with renovascular hypertension. J. Urol., *104*:231, 1970.

Stockigt, J. R., Noakes, C. A., Collins, R. D., Schambelan, M., and Biglieri, E. G.: Renal-vein renin in various forms of renal hypertension. Lancet, *1*:1194, 1972.

Tham, G., Ekelund, L., Herrlin, K., Lindstedt, E. L., Olin, T., and Bergentz, S-E.: Renal artery aneurysms: Natural history and prognosis. Ann. Surg., *197*:348, 1983.

Thibonnier, M., Joseph, A., Sassano, P., Guyenne, T. T., Corvol, P., Raynaud, A., Seurot, M., and Gaux, J. C.: Improved diagnosis of unilateral renal artery lesions after captopril administration. JAMA, *251*:56, 1984.

Tigerstedt, R., and Bergmann, T. G.: Niere und kreislauf. Skand. Arch. Physiol., *8*:233, 1898.

Tobian, L., Tomboulian, A., and Janecek, J.: Effect of high perfusion pressure on the granulation of juxtaglomerular cells in an isolated kidney. J. Clin. Invest., *38*:605, 1959.

Traube, L.: Uber den Zusammenhang von Herz- und Nieren-Krankheiten. *In* Gesammelte Beitraege zur Pathologie und Physiologie, Vol. II, Part I, Clinical Investigations. Berlin, A. Hirschwalt, 1856.

Vander, A. J.: Effect of catecholamines and the renal nerves on renin secretion in anesthetized dogs. Am. J. Physiol., *209*:659, 1965.

Vaughan, E. D., Jr.: Renal artery stenosis. *In* Brenner, B. M., and Stein, J. H. (Eds.): Hypertension. New York, Churchill Livingstone, 1981.

Vaughan, E. D., Jr., Buhler, F. R., Laragh, J. H., Sealey, J. E., Baer, L., and Bard, R. H.: Renovascular hypertension; renin measurements to indicate hypersecretion and contralateral suppression, estimate renal plasma flow and score for surgical curability. Am. J. Med., *55*:402, 1973.

Vaughan, E. D., Jr., Carey, R. M., Ayers, C. R., Peach, M. J., Tegtmeyer, C. J., and Wellons, M. A., Jr.: A physiologic definition of blood pressure response to renal revascularization in patients with renovascular hypertension. Kidney Int., *15*:S83, 1979.

Vaughan, E. D., Jr., Case, D. B., Pickering, T. G., Sosa, R. E., Sos, T. A., and Laragh, J. H.: Clinical evaluation for renovascular hypertension and therapeutic decisions. Urol. Clin. North Am., *11*:393, 1984.

Vaughan, E. D., Jr., Sos, T. A., Sniderman, K. W., Pickering, T. G., Case, D. B., Sealey, J. E., and Laragh, J. H.: Renal venous renin secretory patterns before and after percutaneous transluminal angioplasty: Verification of analytic criteria. *In* Laragh, J. H. (Ed.): Frontiers in Hypertension Research. New York, Springer-Verlag, 1981.

Weed, W. C., Vaughan, E. D., Jr., and Peach, M. J.: Prolongation of the saralasin responsive state of two-kidney, one-clip hypertension in the rat by the orally administered converting enzyme inhibitor captopril (SQ 14225). Hypertension, *1*:8, 1979.

Wollenweber, J., Sheps, S. G., and David, D. G.: Clinical course of atherosclerotic renovascular disease. Am. J. Cardiol., *21*:60, 1968.

Ying, C. Y., Tifft, C. P., Gavras, H., et al.: Renal revascularization in the azotemic hypertensive patient resistant to therapy. N. Engl. J. Med., *311*:1070, 1984.

CHAPTER 59

Etiology, Pathogenesis, and Management of Renal Failure

BRUCE A. MOLITORIS, M.D.
ROBERT W. SCHRIER, M.D.

INTRODUCTION

Renal failure is defined as the deterioration of renal function associated with the accumulation of nitrogenous wastes in the body (azotemia) that is not due to extrarenal factors. Acute renal failure is characterized by rapid deterioration over a period of days. It is usually reversible, although temporary dialysis may be required.

Acute renal failure* is therefore differentiated from prerenal and postrenal azotemia. Prerenal azotemia refers to diminished glomerular filtration resulting from inadequate perfusion of the kidneys and is reversible within 24 hours, with correction of the hypoperfusion. Postrenal azotemia results from mechanical or functional obstruction of the urinary tract, and renal function can be restored or improved if the obstruction is removed. However, both prerenal and postrenal azotemia can result in acute renal failure if the duration and degree of the insult are severe enough.

Classification of acute renal failure into oliguric (< 400 ml/24 hours) or nonoliguric (> 400 ml/24 hours) has recently proved clinically important since nonoliguric acute renal failure has a more benign course. Also, the setting in which acute renal failure develops has

*The authors prefer the term "acute renal failure" to "acute tubular necrosis" to describe the rapid deterioration in renal function due to tubular dysfunction. Acute tubular necrosis describes a histologic condition that is not present in some cases of acute renal failure.

some influence on outcome, as surgically related acute renal failure has a higher rate of mortality than acute renal failure arising in a medical setting.

Chronic renal failure, on the other hand, occurs over months to years. It is caused by irreversible loss of renal function, and the majority of sufferers have chronic progressive renal disease. Dietary maneuvers to decrease the rate of renal deterioration are now being actively investigated. Also, the improved graft survival and increased availability of renal transplantation are changing the therapy of chronic renal failure.

ACUTE RENAL FAILURE

Causes

The causes of acute renal failure are quite diverse and are listed in Table 59–1. The specific disorders can be grouped into four major classes, which include ischemia, nephrotoxins, and diseases of large and small renal vessels. Acute renal failure can also be classified according to the nephron segment involved. Involvement of the glomerulus (acute glomerular nephritis), tubule (acute tubular necrosis), or the surrounding interstitium (acute interstitial nephritis) can occur alone or in combination. Discussion of all the causes of acute renal failure is beyond the scope of this chapter. Therefore, unique characteristics of specific causes of acute

TABLE 59–1. SPECIFIC DISORDERS THAT CAUSE
ACUTE RENAL FAILURE

Ischemic Disorders
  Major trauma
  Massive hemorrhage
  Crush syndrome
  Septic shock
  Transfusion reactions
  Myoglobinuria
  Pregnancy: postpartum hemorrhage
  Postoperative: particularly cardiac, aortic, and biliary
    surgery
  Medical: pancreatitis, gastroenteritis

Nephrotoxins, Including Hypersensitivity Reactions
  Heavy metals: mercury, arsenic, lead, bismuth,
    uranium, cadmium
  Carbon tetrachloride
  Ethylene glycol
  Other organic solvents
  X-ray contrast media (particularly in patients with
    diabetes mellitus)
  Pesticides
  Fungicides
  Antibiotics: aminoglycosides, penicillins, tetracyclines,
    amphotericin
  Other drugs and chemical agents: phenytoin,
    phenylbutazone, uric acid, calcium

Diseases of Glomeruli and Small Blood Vessels
  Acute poststreptococcal glomerulonephritis
  Systemic lupus erythematosus
  Polyarteritis nodosa
  Henoch-Schönlein purpura
  Subacute bacterial endocarditis
  Serum sickness
  Goodpasture syndrome
  Malignant hypertension
  Hemolytic-uremic syndrome
  Drug-related vasculitis
  Pregnancy: abruptio placentae; abortion with and
    without gram-negative sepsis; post-partum renal
    failure
  Rapidly progressive glomerulonephritis, unknown
    etiology

Major Blood Vessel Disease
  Renal artery thrombosis, embolism, or stenosis
  Bilateral renal vein thrombosis

From Schrier, R. W., and Conger, J. D.: *In* Schrier, R. W. (Ed.): Renal and Electrolyte Disorders. Boston, Little, Brown & Co., 1980, p. 376. Used by permission.

renal failure that are of particular importance to urologists will be considered in some detail.

Aminoglycosides. Aminoglycosides are a commonly used class of antibiotics known to induce both nephrotoxicity and ototoxicity. Although the clinical characteristics of aminoglycoside-induced acute renal failure have been known for some time, the cellular mechanisms are only now beginning to be understood. Aminoglycosides are principally excreted by the kidneys, and therefore the serum half-life is inversely related to renal function. Since amino-glycosides have a low toxic-to-therapeutic index and other factors in addition to renal function influence serum levels, careful monitoring of serum creatinine levels is important, especially when renal function is changing. Clinically apparent renal functional deterioration is usually encountered only after 8 to 10 days of administration of the drug and is usually associated with nonoliguric acute renal failure. Therefore, urinary volume is a poor indicator of renal function in this setting. If nephrotoxicity secondary to aminoglycosides does develop, the drug should be discontinued if at all possible. However, even with discontinuation of the offending drug, renal function will probably continue to deteriorate for several days, as the drug tissue half-life is greater than 100-fold the serum half-life.

Several predisposing factors for developing nephrotoxicity have been determined and include duration, dose and type of aminoglycoside, advancing age of the patient, volume depletion, preexisting renal dysfunction, potassium depletion, prior administration of other nephrotoxins, and the concomitant administration of cephalothin. The relative nephrotoxic potential (in order from greatest to least) for the four commonly used aminoglycosides is gentamicin, tobramycin, amikacin, and netilmicin. Subclinical (early) aminoglycoside nephrotoxicity includes brush-border and lysosomal enzymuria and proximal tubular transport defects for amino acids, glucose, and the tubular protein β_2-microglobulin. Additionally, hypokalemia and hypomagnesemia may result from renal magnesium and potassium wasting. Finally, nephrogenic diabetes insipidus (inability to respond to antidiuretic hormone) may ensue, resulting in normal or increased urine production during the acute renal failure phase.

The management of aminoglycoside nephrotoxicity should be directed toward prevention. These drugs should only be used if less toxic alternatives are not available. Prior to the initiation of therapy, the patient should be well hydrated and hypokalemia should be corrected, if present. Other drugs known to increase the nephrotoxic potential of aminoglycosides should be discontinued if possible. Although the loading dose is independent of renal function, the maintenance dose should be determined by each patient's creatinine clearance. Blood levels should be monitored to ensure adequate antimicrobial action. The drug should be discontinued if cultures reveal an organism with sensitivities to less-toxic drugs. Once established, the management of aminoglycoside-induced acute renal failure is similar to other forms of acute renal failure.

Radiocontrast-Induced Nephropathy. This is an area that has received considerable attention recently. The clinical course is one of onset within 24 hours, maximal renal dysfunction in 4 to 5 days, and recovery in 10 to 14 days. Seventy to 90 per cent of individuals who develop acute renal failure secondary to contrast dye remain nonoliguric. Therefore, urine volume is again not an adequate method to clinically evaluate these patients. The extent of recovery depends on the preexisting disease states. Patients with diabetes mellitus, multiple myeloma, or prior renal insufficiency have a less likely chance for complete recovery of renal function. The incidence in all patients undergoing contrast studies is probably < 1 per cent. However, numerous risk factors have been identified, and their presence may increase the risk of transient dysfunction to as high as 90 per cent. These factors include diabetes mellitus, multiple myeloma, prior renal insufficiency, advanced age, volume depletion, hyperuricemia, proteinuria (> 1 gm in 24 hours) and additional contrast exposure within 24 hours.

Numerous theories have been advanced to explain the pathophysiology of contrast-induced nephropathy. However, to date no single theory adequately explains all of the observed phenomena associated with this reaction. As the commonly used contrast agents are organic salts of triiodobenzoic acid and have molecular weights of < 1000 and high osmolality (1500 mOsm/kg H_2O), direct renal toxicity seems likely. Indeed, renal enzymuria and proximal tubule vacuolization with necrosis have been noted. Also, a sustained reduction in renal blood flow has been reported. However, no clear relationship exists between dose or site of administration and the induction of acute renal failure. Additional theories center around intratubular obstruction with uric acid crystals, oxalate, and urine proteins.

Management again centers around prevention, with hydration recommended prior to any radiocontrast dye study, particularly in the presence of renal impairment. However, hydration alone is not adequate unless extremely large volumes of fluid are administered (1000 ml/hour prior to and following the procedure). Mannitol given either just prior to or within 60 minutes of the study has been shown to reduce the incidence of acute renal failure. In patients with pre-existing hypervolemia, the use of furosemide to induce diuresis may be of benefit, although no published data exist to verify this

theory. The mechanism of mannitol-induced protection is unknown. Mannitol could work by causing an osmotic diuresis, thereby reducing exposure of the proximal tubular cells to the dye. Mannitol is also known to reduce tubular obstruction, and this could also be responsible for its beneficial effects. Finally, most radiologists prefer to use the minimal amount of contrast medium necessary for an adequate study. The utility of this latter point is debatable.

Cis-diamminedichloroplatinum (cisplatin) is a chemotherapeutic agent that is known to be nephrotoxic. Elevation in serum creatinine is noted approximately 7 days after administration of *cis*-diamminedichloroplatinum. Proteinuria and enzymuria precede overt renal failure by 1 to 2 days. The incidence of acute renal failure is dose dependent, and renal toxicity is one of the major dose-limiting toxicities of *cis*-diamminedichloroplatinum. A patient's volume status prior to and during drug administration is a major factor influencing nephrotoxicity. Hydration reduces nephrotoxicity from 39 to 12 to 3 per cent prior to as well as during drug administration, respectively. *Cis*-diamminedichloroplatinum is believed to be a direct nephrotoxin. Renal pathology shows proximal tubular epithelia brush-border loss with cellular vacuolization. Also, distal convoluted tubule and collecting duct changes are noted. Additional complications include severe magnesium wasting and polyuria, with the latter at least initially due to decreased vasopressin release.

Management has centered around prevention with prehydration and the use of mannitol. Although mannitol does not reduce the cytotoxicity of *cis*-diamminedichloroplatinum, it has been shown in humans to significantly reduce the incidence and severity of acute renal failure. In animals, mannitol increases the dose of *cis*-diamminedichloroplatinum needed to cause acute renal failure. Mannitol does not decrease the serum concentration, serum half-life, or renal excretion of *cis*-diamminedichloroplatinum but does decrease the urine concentration of the drug. Furosemide has also been used successfully alone or in conjunction with mannitol. Therefore, prior and continued (24 hour) hydration with saline plus mannitol before *cis*-diamminedichloroplatinum infusion is necessary for the maximal protective effect. Urine output should be > 3 L during the first 24 hours.

Acute Urate Nephropathy. This is potentially a rapidly reversible and even preventable cause of acute renal failure, especially in chemotherapy-induced hyperuricemia. Onset of acute renal failure is sudden and almost universally oliguric. Tubular obstruction from precipitation of urate crystals is the underlying mechanism. Casts occur characteristically in the medullopapillary collecting ducts, where both the urine pH and maximal urinary concentration favor precipitation. Risk factors include tumor load and volume depletion. Management is aimed at limiting the production of uric acid by administering allopurinol, maintaining adequate hydration, and the use of mannitol or furosemide or both to ensure adequate urine volumes to reduce distal uric acid crystal concentrations.

Rhabdomyolysis and Myoglobinuria. Rhabdomyolysis is an acute syndrome resulting from skeletal muscle injury, lysis and subsequent release of cell contents into the plasma. This sequence leads to hyperphosphatemia, hypocalcemia (due to precipitation of calcium phosphate), hyperkalemia, hyperuricemia, and a rapid rise in serum creatinine that is out of proportion to the duration and severity of the renal failure. The causes of rhabdomyolysis are classified as traumatic and nontraumatic. Traumatic causes are further classified as attributable to excessive muscle activity, direct muscle injury, and ischemic muscle disorders. Nontraumatic causes include immunologic disorders, metabolic disorders (hypokalemia, hypophosphatemia), drugs (i.e., succinylcholine), toxins (i.e., ethylene glycol, ethanol), infections (viral, bacterial), and genetic disorders. Myoglobin, also released from skeletal cells, is a direct nephrotoxin, with its toxicity related to both concentration and urine pH. As urine pH decreases below 6.0, cell uptake occurs and therefore nephrotoxicity increases. Tubular obstruction also occurs in rhabdomyolysis and may be potentiated by the high urine excretion of uric acid. Management of rhabdomyolysis centers around maintaining a high urine flow rate. This minimizes myoglobin concentrations in the urine and helps keep urine pH above 6.0. Use of normal saline to expand the extracellular fluid volume followed by either furosemide or mannitol to induce diuresis is the preferred therapy. The use of bicarbonate to alkalize the urine can be hazardous if systemic alkalemia results.

Pathogenesis of Renal Failure

The actual mechanisms by which different renal insults induce acute renal failure remain controversial. Any proposed pathogenic mechanism must account for a variety of observed clinical phenomena, including a severe reduction in glomerular filtration rate (GFR) and

renal blood flow, the variability in renal histologic changes, and finally the potential for complete recovery. Acute renal failure has been divided into an initiation phase and maintenance phase. During the initiation phase of ischemia or toxin-induced acute renal failure, experimental and clinical evidence is accumulating to indicate direct tubular cell injury. Loss of apical (luminal) membrane, cell swelling, altered intracellular electrolytes, and reduced mitochondrial function have been documented. It is possible to visualize how this results in reduced GFR and renal tubular cell functioning during the acute insult. However, the maintenance phase of acute renal failure has been more difficult to explain. The four proposed mechanisms that have been suggested include tubular obstruction from cell debris, an alteration in renal vascular hemodynamics, glomerular permeability barrier alterations, and the backleak of reabsorbed tubular fluid through defective epithelium.

Tubular obstruction would lead to a reduction in GFR by increasing intratubular pressure, thereby reducing the Starling forces favoring filtration. Mannitol and furosemide may afford protection against ischemic-induced acute renal failure by limiting tubular obstruction. However, collapsed proximal tubules have been noted in both clinical and experimental nephrons of kidneys with acute renal failure, which is evidence against obstruction as a critical factor in all forms of acute renal failure.

Alterations in renal blood flow are known to occur during acute renal failure. Renal blood flow is reduced to between 25 and 50 per cent of normal values in humans with acute renal failure. In addition, micropuncture studies on rats have shown markedly reduced glomerular filtration due to reduced blood flow. Two mechanisms have been proposed to explain this finding. Either afferent arteriolar constriction or efferent arteriolar dilatation can lead to a reduction in GFR by reducing the hydrostatic pressure favoring filtration. In addition, a redistribution of renal blood flow away from the cortex has been observed. However, experiments using vasodilator drugs to return renal blood flow to control values have not caused parallel changes in the GFR during acute renal failure. These experiments then dissociated altered renal blood flow from glomerular filtration and made the term "vasomotor nephropathy" not totally acceptable.

Glomerular filtration could also be reduced if glomerular permeability were decreased. Early morphologic data using scanning electron

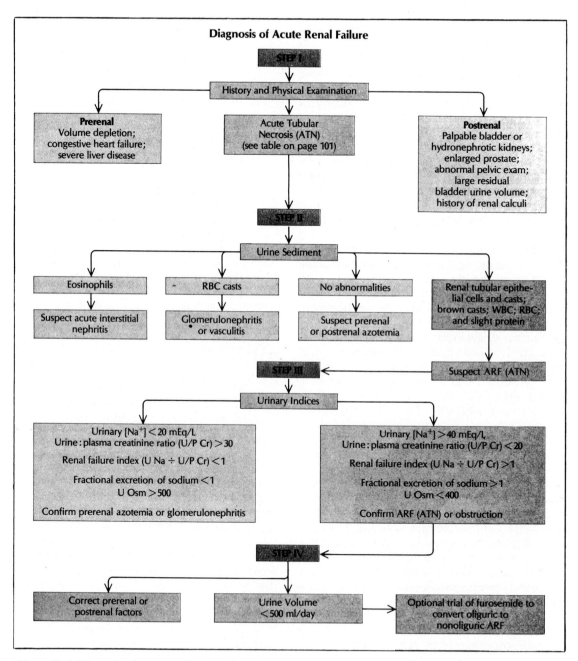

Figure 59–1. Diagnosis of acute renal failure. (From Schrier, R. W.: Hosp. Pract. *20*:103, 1981. Used by permission.)

microscopy revealed collapsed tubules and capillary epithelial cell alterations in an ischemic model of acute renal failure. However, these data were not confirmed by subsequent investigations. Also, glomerular functional alterations could not be documented in acute renal failure. These data therefore make glomerular permeability alterations an unlikely explanation for the decreased GFR in acute renal failure.

The final theory invokes back-leak of reabsorbed glomerular filtrate through or around damaged tubular epithelial cells. The back-leak could occur because the functional integrity of the transporting epithelia would have been destroyed by the initiating event. Morphologic studies revealing normal glomeruli and disrupted tubular cells, together with early micropuncture studies, lend support to this theory. However, more recent studies using inulin, a nonreabsorbed marker of glomerular filtration, could not demonstrate a lack of epithelial functional integrity.

In summary there is no one mechanism that totally explains the pathophysiology of acute renal failure. Multiple mechanisms may be involved in the same model, and different mechanisms may play variable roles in different models of acute renal failure. For example, obstruction probably plays a major part in the acute renal failure induced by ischemia and rhabdomyolysis, whereas tubular disruption and back-leak may contribute in various nephrotoxic models.

Diagnosis of Acute Renal Failure

The diagnosis of acute renal failure involves several processes, using information gained from the history and physical examination, careful analysis of the urine, and laboratory data. A summary of this process is shown in Figure 59–1. A careful history and physical examination are necessary to help rule out both prerenal and postrenal states. Prerenal azotemia results from renal underperfusion due to decreased renal perfusion pressure or increased renal vasculature resistance. Conditions causing prerenal azotemia are listed in Table 59–2 and include hypovolemia, decreased cardiac output, vasodilatation, and incomplete bilateral vascular obstruction. The renal functional impairment is rapidly reversed with correction of the underlying process. Clues to search for during the history-taking and physical examination include rapid weight loss, postural blood pressure changes, decreased urine output, and decreased

TABLE 59–2. CONDITIONS CAUSING PRERENAL AZOTEMIA

Hypovolemia
  Hemorrhage
  Gastrointestinal losses
  Third space
    Burns
    Peritonitis
    Traumatized tissue
  Diuretic abuse

Impaired Cardiac Function
  Congestive heart failure
  Myocardial infarction
  Pericardial tamponade
  Acute pulmonary embolism

Peripheral Vasodilatation
  Bacteremia
  Antihypertensive medications

Increased Renal Vascular Resistance
  Anesthesia
  Surgical operation
  Hepatorenal syndrome

Renal Vascular Obstruction, Bilateral
  Embolism
  Thrombosis

From Schrier, R. W., and Conger, J. D.: *In* Schrier, R. W. (Ed.): Renl and Electrolyte Disorders. Boston, Little, Brown & Co., 1980, p. 392. Used by permission.

skin turgor. A blood urea nitrogen to creatinine ratio of > 10:1 is also indicative of the prerenal or postrenal state. However, a volume challenge or hemodynamic monitoring is a more specific way to rule out the prerenal state.

The second step involves determining that the patient does not have bladder outlet obstruction causing postrenal azotemia. The causes of postrenal azotemia are listed in Table 59–3. It

TABLE 59–3. CONDITIONS CAUSING POSTRENAL AZOTEMIA

Urethral Obstruction
Bladder Neck Obstruction
  Prostatic hypertrophy
  Bladder carcinoma
  Bladder infection
  Functional: neuropathy or ganglionic blocking agents

Obstruction of Ureters, Bilateral
  Intraureteral
    Sulfonamide and uric acid crystals
    Blood clots
    Pyogenic debris
    Stones
    Edema
    Necrotizing papillitis
  Extraureteral
    Tumor-cervix, prostate, endometriosis
    Periureteral fibrosis
    Accidental ureteral ligation during pelvic operation

From Schrier, R. W., and Conger, J. D.: *In* Schrier, R. W. (Ed.): Renal and Electrolyte Disorders. Boston, Little, Brown & Co., 1980, p. 393. Used by permission.

is important to remember that 10 per cent of all cases of acute renal failure are due to outlet obstruction, and this is usually a reversible cause of acute renal failure. Indications of urinary tract obstruction include a palpable bladder, hydronephrotic kidneys, enlarged prostate, history of anuria, variable or unusually copious urine output, calculi, or abnormal findings on pelvic examination. The evaluation to rule out obstruction is dealt with in Chapter 7 and will therefore not be discussed here.

Once the prerenal and postrenal states have been ruled out, the physician is ready to determine the cause of the acute renal failure. Although a complete history and physical examination are often quite revealing, an accurate urinalysis is absolutely essential. The urinalysis often allows classification of the cause of acute renal failure as due to either nephrotoxic damage, interstitial nephritis, or glomerulonephritis. Ischemic disorders and nephrotoxins leading to tubular damage usually cause characteristic changes in the urine cell components. Renal tubular epithelial cells, pigmented brown tubular casts, and mild proteinuria are commonly seen. A heme-positive dipstick without red blood cells in a fresh urine sample is strong evidence supporting the diagnosis of rhabdomyolysis. Glomerular and vascular diseases, on the other hand, frequently produce large amounts of urine protein (> 3 gm/24 hours) associated with numerous red blood cells, white blood cells, and cell casts. A red blood cell cast, although not pathognomonic, is extremely strong evidence for either a glomerular or vascular disease process. Interstitial disease processes also cause specific urine abnormalities. Urine eosinophils (seen with a Wright stain of the spun, alkalinized urine) are strongly suggestive of acute interstitial nephritis. Also, red blood cells, white blood cells, and white blood cell casts can be noted along with mild proteinuria in acute interstitial disease processes.

Urine composition is also extremely important in determining first if acute renal failure

exists and, second, the cause of the acute renal failure. Urine composition is determined by intake and tubular function. Since tubular function differs markedly between prerenal azotemia and acute renal failure, urinary indices have become quite helpful in the diagnosis of acute renal failure. In prerenal azotemia the tubule is functioning maximally to reabsorb sodium and water in an effort to restore extracellular fluid volume. Therefore, the urine concentration of sodium is quite low and urinary osmolality is high. The ratios of urine to plasma creatinine and urea nitrogen are also measures of tubular concentrating ability and are elevated in prerenal azotemia. Finally, the renal failure index (i.e., urine sodium divided by the ratio of urine to serum creatinine) combines two determinations varying in opposite directions to provide a more sensitive value. In prerenal azotemia the renal failure index is < 1. In acute renal failure, due to direct tubular damage the ability of the tubule to conserve sodium and water is severely impaired. Thus the urine will not be maximally concentrated, and its composition more closely reflects that of plasma. Therefore, the urine osmolality and the ratio of urine to plasma creatinine are low and urine sodium and the renal failure index are elevated. These data are summarized in Table 59–4. These values may not be valid in a patient who has received diuretics, mannitol, or large amounts of glucose and water within a few hours of the urine collection. Also, in metabolic alkalosis with an elevated urine pH, the obligate loss of sodium with bicarbonate makes the urine sodium concentration less valid. In this case the urine chloride concentration can be used to differentiate prerenal azotemia from acute renal failure, as it will more adequately reflect tubular functional ability. In obstructive uropathy the urine composition depends on the severity and duration of the obstruction and cannot be used to make the diagnosis of postrenal azotemia. In early acute glomerulonephritis or vasculitis, the urine indices resemble those of prerenal azo-

TABLE 59–4. SUMMARY OF URINE INDICES IN OLIGURIC RENAL FAILURE

	Prerenal Azotemia	Acute Oliguric Renal Failure
Urine osmolality, mOsm/kg H_2O	>500	<350
Urine sodium, mEq/L	<20	>40
Urine/plasma creatinine	>40	<20
Urine/plasma urea nitrogen	>8	<3
Renal failure index	<1	>1
Fractional excretion of filtered sodium	<1	>1

From Miller, T. R., et al.: Ann. Intern. Med., *89:*49, 1978. Used by permission.

temia as tubular function is intact. However, as the glomerulonephritis or vasculitis worsens tubular function may be impaired. This then leads to urine composition changes similar to those noted to occur during acute renal failure.

Clinical Course

The natural history of acute renal failure is determined by multiple factors including cause, severity, daily urine volume, and the previous health of the patient. Acute renal failure secondary to renal ischemia usually carries a higher morbidity and mortality rate than does nephrotoxin-induced acute renal failure. This probably relates to a higher incidence of multiple organ failure in ischemia-induced renal failure. In addition, nephrotoxin-induced acute renal failure is more likely to occur in hospitalized patients who are being screened for alterations in renal function (i.e., aminoglycoside-induced acute renal failure). Recent studies have shown that nonoliguric acute renal failure also portends a better prognosis. Patients with nonoliguric acute renal failure have shorter hospital stays, less need for dialysis, reduced mortality rate, and a decreased incidence of gastrointestinal bleeding and sepsis. The age and previous health of the patient are also important determinants. Older patients and patients with multiple organ dysfunction have increased morbidity and mortality.

Stages of acute tubular injury can be described as consisting of the renal failure, diuretic, and recovery phases. The renal failure phase consists of initiation and maintenance phases. However, distinguishing between those two events clinically is often impossible, as the initiation phase lacks characteristic signs. The detection of tubular injury early in its course is becoming increasingly important, as specific maneuvers instituted early may be capable of decreasing the severity or alleviating the tubular injury altogether. The initiation phase merges into the maintenance phase when the tubular injury is no longer immediately reversible. Once established, tubular injury can persist for a variable period of time lasting as long as 6 weeks. However, the mean duration of nonoliguric acute renal failure is approximately 7 days, whereas the duration of oliguric renal failure averages approximately 2 weeks. During the renal failure phase, renal function is below that required to maintain metabolic balance of nitrogenous wastes and certain electrolytes. The extent of the ensuing biochemical abnormalities depends on the severity of the tubular injury, the catabolic state of the patient, and whether the patient has oliguric or nonoliguric acute renal failure. In hypercatabolic states such as those associated with trauma, starvation, fever, sepsis, burns, surgery, and glucocorticoid administration, biochemical abnormalities develop and proceed at a much faster rate than in noncatabolic states. The differences are shown in Table 59–5. These catabolic variables reduce the time interval between the onset of acute renal failure and the necessity for dialysis and thus should be alleviated when possible (e.g., by treating fever).

The second stage of acute renal failure secondary to tubular injury is the diuretic phase. During this phase the GFR increases, but tubular function remains depressed. As a result, urine volume increases and inappropriate loss of sodium and water can occur. In the absence of adequate intake, hypovolemia may result. The hypovolemia can then potentiate the underlying tubular dysfunction, worsen the renal failure, and prevent complete recovery. It is therefore particularly important to maintain a state of euvolemia during this phase of acute renal failure.

At the end of the recovery phase, tubular function returns toward normal and once again urine output is dictated by input. In those patients who recover from acute renal failure, renal function returns to, or close to, the preinsult level. However, the mortality during acute

TABLE 59–5. BIOCHEMICAL ABNORMALITIES IN ACUTE RENAL FAILURE

	Noncatabolic	Catabolic
Daily rise in blood urea nitrogen (mg/dl)	<20	>30
Daily rise in creatinine (mg/dl)	<1.5	>2
Daily rise in serum potassium (mEq/L)	<0.5	>0.5
Daily decrease in serum HCO_3^- (mEq/L)	<1	>2
Daily rise in uric acid (mg/dl)	<1	>1

From Conger, J. D., Anderson, R. J.: *In* Massry, S. G., and Glassock, R. J. (eds.): Textbook of Nephrology. Baltimore, The Williams & Wilkins Co., 1983, p. 6.224. Used by permission.

renal failure is approximately 50 per cent. This value has remained stable since the introduction of dialysis. Gastrointestinal bleeding and sepsis are the two main complications leading to death during acute renal failure. Therefore, it is clinically important to prevent or limit the severity and duration of acute renal failure, and sources of infection (i.e., urinary and intravenous catheters) should be carefully monitored.

A complete discussion of acute renal failure due to renal parenchymal disease is beyond the scope of this chapter. However, a few clinical associations will be discussed. Acute renal failure due to interstitial nephritis is now recognized with increasing frequency. Many drugs, such as methicillin, other penicillins, and nonsteroidal anti-inflammatory drugs, can cause acute interstitial nephritis. This entity may be associated with a maculopapular rash, fever, pyuria and eosinophiluria, although this constellation of signs and symptoms may be absent. Withdrawal of the offending agent usually leads to complete recovery of renal function, although dialysis may be necessary for a short period of time. The use of high-dose glucocorticoids has been shown to reduce the duration of the altered renal function and has been suggested, but not proved, to influence the eventual outcome.

The outcome of acute renal failure due to glomerulonephritis is dependent on the cause, duration prior to diagnosis, and use of adequate therapy. The use of immunosuppressive therapy is becoming increasingly important, depending on the cause of the glomerulonephritis. Vasculitides, such as Wegener granulomatosis, have been shown to be quite responsive to cyclophosphamide, and idiopathic rapidly progressive glomerulonephritis has been shown to respond to aggressive pulse therapy with glucocorticoids. In addition, the use of plasmapheresis in glomerulonephritis secondary to circulating immune complex deposition (i.e., mixed cyroglobulinemia) is also showing promising results. However, multiple controlled studies need to be carried out prior to the widespread clinical use of plasmapheresis.

Complications secondary to acute renal failure can be classified as metabolic, hematologic, neurologic, and infectious. Metabolic complications are universal. Their magnitude and onset are determined by the catabolic state and type of acute renal failure (oliguric versus nonoliguric) observed. Hyperkalemia is particularly important and may be a life-threatening complication, occurring in more than half of the patients with acute renal failure. The continuous elevation in serum potassium is due to the limited ability to excrete potassium via the urine. Factors that cause a particularly rapid increase in serum potassium include excessive intake (medications, diet, intravenous fluids), blood transfusions, hypercatabolism, hemolysis, and acidosis (which causes a shift of potassium out of cells). When the serum potassium level exceeds 6.0 mg/I, electrocardiographic abnormalities can develop. These may include peaked T waves, prolonged or absent P waves, widened QRS complexes, and lengthening of the QT interval; if untreated, cardiac arrest can ensue.

Hyponatremia, which can lead to central nervous system dysfunction, is another frequently encountered metabolic abnormality. The cause is usually the inability to excrete the excess amount of free water administered to patients with acute renal failure. Hyperphosphatemia due to decreased urinary excretion of phosphate and occasionally increased release from traumatized or ischemic muscles is often noted. The hyperphosphatemia can lead to hypocalcemia because of soft tissue deposition of calcium and phosphate. The skeletal resistance to parathyroid hormone and decreased production of 1,25-dihydroxyvitamin D_3 also plays a role in the hypocalcemia of acute renal failure. An anion gap metabolic acidosis occurs commonly during acute renal failure as a result of a reduced capacity to excrete nonvolatile acids, which are produced daily by the body.

Cardiovascular complications are due primarily to volume overload resulting in pulmonary congestion and hypertension. The volume overloaded state is due to excessive accumulation of sodium and water during diminished excretion. Patients with oliguric renal failure are especially prone to these complications. In addition, arrhythmias (especially supraventricular) may occur. Pericarditis is noted only rarely in acute renal failure when dialysis is available.

Hematologic abnormalities include a normochromic normocytic anemia, thrombocytopenia, diminished platelet function, and a poorly characterized coagulopathy. Marrow suppression and hemodilution play a role in the anemia and thrombocytopenia, but gastrointestinal bleeding must always be considered as a potential cause of the anemia. Neurologic disorders include lethargy, somnolence, confusion, asterixis, myoclonic muscle twitching, and seizures. Although the pathogenesis of these disorders is not known, they usually respond rapidly to dialysis therapy. However, causes such as hypoglycemia, hyponatremia, acidosis, and delayed elimination of drugs known to depress central nervous system function must be ruled out in patients with neurologic disorders.

Gastrointestinal bleeding is a major complication during acute renal failure and portends a poorer prognosis. Multiple factors including stress, platelet dysfunction, and the coagulopathy of acute renal failure are involved in the 20 to 30 per cent incidence of gastrointestinal bleeding that occurs. Finally, infectious complications are the leading cause of mortality in acute renal failure. Clinically significant infections occur in as many as 70 per cent of patients with acute renal failure. This high incidence is due to several factors, including altered cellular and humoral immune function during acute renal failure.

Therapy

Prevention of acute renal failure should be the goal and is now possible in many clinical situations. Mannitol has been used successfully in treating patients receiving radiocontrast agents to prevent or limit the degree of renal failure induced. In experimental models of ischemic-induced acute renal failure, mannitol, furosemide, verapamil, and adenosine triphosphate magnesium chloride have all been shown to limit the degree of acute renal failure. The pathophysiologic mechanisms underlying this prevention are presently under intense investigation. In addition the conversion of oliguric to nonoliguric acute renal failure, using either mannitol or furosemide, may be beneficial, as recent prospective studies indicate nonoliguric acute renal failure has an improved prognosis. This, however, remains to be proved. Finally, in all cases the diagnosis of acute renal failure must be confirmed by ruling out prerenal and postrenal azotemia.

Once acute renal failure due to tubular injury is established, little can be done to ameliorate its natural course. Therapy is aimed at minimizing the complications known to occur during acute renal failure. Patients should be maintained in a state of adequate hydration, with alterations in metabolic abnormalities limited by reducing the catabolic rate. Daily management includes monitoring electrolytes, input-output, and restricting input based on urine output and insensible losses. In addition, intravenous fluids that approximate urine and sweat electrolyte losses should be administered. Serum sodium in the absence of hyperglycemia or hyperlipidemia can be used to monitor free-water administration. Hyponatremia denotes an excess of free water, whereas hypernatremia indicates a relative lack of body water. Fluid therapy is therefore directed partially by the serum sodium concentration on a day-to-day

basis. Elevations in serum potassium are best controlled by limiting the oral and intravenous intake of potassium. Potassium exchange resins can be used when excessive volume will not be a problem for the patient to handle (nonoliguric acute renal failure), as the resin exchanges sodium for potassium. Serum potassium values of < 6.0 mEq/L may only require careful monitoring. If the serum potassium levels exceed 6.5 mEq/L, severe complications can ensue, especially if any electrocardiographic changes occur. Therapy for hyperkalemia is described in Table 59–6.

The hypocalcemia observed during acute renal failure is usually mild and rarely requires specific therapy. Correction of the hyperphosphatemia using gastrointestinal phosphate binders (aluminum-containing antacids) with meals and at bedtime will reduce soft tissue calcification and also limit the decrement in serum calcium. Magnesium-containing antacids should be avoided, as magnesium intoxication can occur as a result of decreased renal magnesium excretion.

Nutrition is another important aspect in the management of patients with acute renal failure. The minimal amount of high-biologic-value protein to maintain nitrogen balance should be given. Additional calories are necessary to minimize the protein requirement and are best supplied as carbohydrates. This will reduce endogenous catabolism and thereby minimize increases in serum nitrogenous wastes. Hyperalimentation has been shown to be useful in catabolic patients, but possible infectious and metabolic complications must be weighed prior to its use.

As already mentioned, the incidence of infection can be minimized by giving meticulous care to all indwelling catheters, which should be used only when necessary. The indiscriminate use of antibiotics must be avoided. Suspected infections must be thoroughly evaluated by obtaining Gram stains and cultures. Antibiotic therapy must be directed as specifically as possible. The doses of all drugs eliminated by the kidneys must be reduced and administered according to the reduction in renal function. It is important to remember that renal function during the initiation and maintenance phases of acute renal failure is minimal even if the serum creatinine is not yet severely elevated. Numerous charts are available to direct alterations in drug dosage during both acute and chronic renal failure. Close monitoring for gastrointestinal bleeding and neurologic alterations is essential, as either one of these complications may be an indication for dialysis. Monitoring for blood in

TABLE 59–6. THERAPY OF HYPERKALEMIA IN PATIENTS WITH ACUTE RENAL FAILURE

Therapy	Mechanism	Onset	Duration	Limiting Factors
Calcium gluconate intravenously (10% solution, 1 to 3 ampules, 10 to 30 ml)	Direct antagonism	Immediate	Brief	Calcium load
NaHCO₃ intravenously (1 to 3 ampules, 45 to 135 mEq)	Redistribution	Minutes	Hours	Sodium load, alkali load
Glucose 10%, 500 ml, plus regular insulin, 10 units	Redistribution	Minutes	Hours	Volume expansion, low blood glucose
Potassium-exchange resin 20 to 50 gm plus sorbitol 70% (20 ml oral, 50 ml rectal)	Elimination	Hours	Hours	Sodium load, gastrointestinal symptoms
Hemodialysis	Elimination	Hours	Hours	Facilities

From Conger, J. D., Anderson, R. J.: In Massry, S. G., and Glassock, R. J. (Eds.): Textbook of Nephrology. Baltimore, The Williams & Wilkins Co., 1982, p. 6.227. Used by permission.

the stool and rapid changes in the hematocrit will screen for occult bleeding. The use of non–magnesium-containing antacids and cimetidine (one-half normal dose during acute renal failure) to reduce stress gastritis has been used in treating seriously ill patients with acute renal failure. Serial physical examinations are necessary for early detection of hypertension, pulmonary edema, pericarditis, and early neurologic abnormalities.

Greater than half of all patients who develop acute renal failure will require dialytic therapy. Absolute indications for dialysis are listed in Table 59–7. Neurologic disorders, hemorrhagic disorders, and pericarditis are all considered to be secondary to the uremic state. These complications respond rapidly to dialysis if indeed they are secondary to uremia. However, the incidence of potential complications during dialysis increases as uremia advances. For example, hemodialysis, which requires heparinizing the patient, may temporarily worsen hemorrhagic disorders. Therefore, emphasis has recently been placed on preventing, not treating, these disorders through "prophylactic" dialysis. Although the value of this therapy has never been shown in a sizable prospective controlled study, the overwhelming clinical impres-

sion, based on published literature and consensus of clinical experience, supports this approach. Dialysis is employed as often as is required to maintain serum creatinine and blood urea nitrogen below 8 and 100 mg/dl, respectively. This approach also allows more liberal intake and supplementation to oliguric patients, as their volume status can be controlled more easily.

The choice of either peritoneal dialysis or hemodialysis depends on the clinical situation and the availability of equipment and trained personnel for hemodialysis. For catabolic patients, hemodialysis is the therapy of choice since it is much more efficient than peritoneal dialysis. Also, hemodialysis is preferred for patients with recent abdominal surgery or undiagnosed intraabdominal disease. Disadvantages of hemodialysis include greater hemodynamic stress, the requirement for anticoagulation, a need for vascular access, and a higher incidence of the dysequilibrium syndrome. Peritoneal dialysis is a simpler, more economic form of dialysis and is quite useful for the noncatabolic patient. Factors that favor peritoneal dialysis include hemodynamic instability and an absolute contraindication to heparin.

Again, it should be emphasized that prevention of acute renal failure should be the goal of all clinicians. The incidence and severity of acute renal failure can be minimized by first identifying those patients at high risk of developing acute renal failure. These include patients receiving potential nephrotoxins, patients undergoing operative procedures requiring interruption of renal blood flow, and patients with multiple trauma, burns, intravascular hemolysis,

TABLE 59–7. ABSOLUTE INDICATIONS FOR DIALYSIS

Central nervous system disorders
Gastrointestinal hemorrhage
Pericarditis
Refractory hyperkalemia
Volume overload refractory to medical therapy

renal insufficiency, diabetes mellitus, and rhabdomyolysis. These patients require optimal intravascular volume maintenance, carefully considered use of nephrotoxic agents, careful monitoring of renal function, and possibly the use of agents known to limit potential renal damage (e.g., mannitol).

CHRONIC RENAL FAILURE

Many types of renal parenchymal disease unfortunately are progressive and eventually lead to chronic renal failure. Specific therapy for the underlying disease is often not available, and therefore chronic renal failure is unavoidable. The major causes of chronic renal failure are listed in Table 59–8. Glomerulonephritis can be subdivided into primary glomerulonephritis or glomerulonephritis associated with a number of systemic illnesses. Primary glomerulopathies potentially leading to chronic renal failure can be subdivided into those presenting with a nephrotic sediment (heavy proteinuria with minimal cell components in the urine sediment) and disorders with nephritic sediment (variable proteinuria but numerous cells and cell casts in the urine sediment). Those having nephrotic sediment include membranous nephropathy, focal glomerulosclerosis, and minimal change disease. Primary glomerular disorders having nephritic sediment include chronic glomerulonephritis, IgA nephropathy, membranoproliferative glomerulonephritis, idiopathic rapidly progressive glomerulonephritis, and postinfectious glomerulonephritis. In general no universally effective therapy is available for any of these disorders, with the exception of minimal change disease, which usually responds to glucocorticoids and rarely leads to chronic renal failure.

Systemic disorders associated with glomer-

TABLE 59–8. Major Causes of Chronic Renal Failure

Glomerulopathies
Primary
Associated with systemic illness
Diabetes
Amyloidosis
Hereditary renal disease
Hypertension
Obstructive uropathy
Infection
Interstitial nephritis

From Alfrey, A. C.: *In* Schrier, R. W. (Ed.): Renal and Electrolyte Disorders. Boston, Little, Brown & Co., 1980, p. 410. Used by permission.

ular disease and chronic renal failure can also be classified on the basis of urine sediment. Disorders causing primarily a nephrotic sediment include diabetes mellitus, amyloidosis, and preeclampsia. Those presenting with nephritic sediment include vasculitides (e.g., Wegener granulomatosis, polyarteritis nodosa), hemolytic-uremic syndrome, thrombolic thrombocytopenic purpura, mixed cryoglobulinemia, Henoch-Schönlein purpura, hereditary nephritis (e.g., Alport syndrome), bacterial endocarditis, and systemic lupus erythematosus. Systemic lupus erythematosus is unusual in that it has been associated with five different morphologic glomerular patterns: mesangial, membranous, membranoproliferative, focal proliferative, and diffuse proliferative. The responsiveness to therapy and the prognosis are somewhat dependent on the morphologic type.

Patients with glomerulonephritis characteristically present with edema, hypertension, and normal to decreased urine output. Acute glomerulonephritis is often associated with fever, leukocytosis, an elevated erythrocyte sedimentation rate, and oliguria.

Interstitial nephritis is a term derived from the microscopic appearance of fibrosis and inflammation in the renal interstitium. Glomerular involvement occurs only secondarily as a result of the fibrosis and vascular alterations. A number of compounds can cause interstitial nephritis, and these are listed in Table 59–9. The associated renal failure may either be acute or chronic in onset. The importance of this diagnosis lies in the potential reversibility of the renal function once the initiating agent is removed. Features differentiating interstitial nephritis and glomerulonephritis are listed in Table 59–10. Clinically, patients with chronic interstitial nephritis have a history of polyuria and nocturia, as the kidney's ability to concentrate urine is diminished. Fatigue is another common symptom, since these patients suffer anemia that is disproportionately severe for the degree of renal failure. Hypertension and peripheral edema are much less common than in patients with glomerulonephritis. Inspection of the urine reveals much less proteinuria, with the proteins predominantly of the $\alpha2$ or β-globulin types, and not albumin, as is seen in glomerulonephritis. In interstitial nephritis the cellularity of the urine is often reduced. However, eosinophils in the urine and eosinophilia are common. Finally, patients with interstitial nephritis tend to have markedly elevated uric acid and hyperchloremic metabolic acidosis.

Hereditary renal disease is another class of

TABLE 59–9. VARIOUS CAUSES OF INTERSTITIAL NEPHRITIS

Analgesics
Other Drugs
Sulfonamide
Penicillin and homologs
Furosemide, thiazides
Phenindione
Phenytoin
Calcium Disorders
Hyperparathyroidism
Milk-alkali syndrome
Sarcoid
Neoplasms
Multiple myeloma
Uric Acid
Gouty nephropathy
Hematologic disorders
Oxalate Deposition
Associated with small bowel disease
Hereditary
Anesthetic agents: methoxyflurane
Ethylene glycol
Heavy Metals
Lead
Cadmium
Uranium
Copper
Reflux Nephropathy

From Alfrey, A. C.: *In* Schrier, R. W. (Ed.): Renal and Electrolyte Disorders. Boston, Little, Brown & Co., 1980, p. 412. Used by permission.

disorders leading to end-stage renal disease. This group of disorders includes Alport syndrome, Fabry disease, polycystic kidney disease, and medullary cystic disease, which together probably account for between 10 and 15 per cent of all chronic renal failure cases. No specific therapy is available.

The progressive deterioration in renal function associated with hypertension-induced renal disease (arteriolar nephrosclerosis) can be pre-

vented with early and adequate control of blood pressure.

In the initial evaluation of patients with chronic renal failure, it is essential to document the cause of the renal failure and eliminate any potentially reversible factor contributing to renal functional deterioration. These factors are listed in Table 59–11. A urine culture should be obtained on all patients with chronic renal failure, as urinary tract infections can be asymptomatic. Obstruction should be evaluated with postvoid residual urine to exclude bladder outlet obstruction (> 50 ml of residual urine). Ultrasound studies of the upper urinary tract have made retrograde pyelography less necessary to rule out obstruction. Intravenous pyelography should be avoided, as patients with chronic renal failure are more prone to the nephrotoxic complications of contrast media. Radiopaque calculi should be ruled out with nephrotomograms; uric acid stones are, however, radiolucent. This procedure will also yield useful information regarding renal size and contour. It is particularly important to exclude extracellular volume depletion in a patient with preexisting renal insufficiency. A patient may be asymptomatic but yet have enough volume depletion to cause an additional decrement in renal function. Often a trial of intravenous normal saline is necessary to completely rule out volume depletion. All potential nephrotoxic agents should be discontinued if at all possible. The doses of all drugs should be altered as determined by the level of renal function.

Diminished cardiac output secondary to any number of causes (e.g., myocardial infarction, pericardial tamponade, constrictive pericarditis) can also result in accelerated renal deterioration. Correction of these underlying causes often results in improved renal function. Hypertension, if not treated, can result in arteriolar

TABLE 59–10. FEATURES DIFFERENTIATING GLOMERULONEPHRITIS AND INTERSTITIAL NEPHRITIS

Feature	Glomerulonephritis	Interstitial Nephritis
Proteinuria	>3 gm	<1.5 gm
Sediment	Numerous cells and red blood cell casts	Few cells and casts
Sodium-handling	Normal until late	Sodium-wasting
Anemia	Moderate severity until late	Disproportionately severe for degree of renal failure
Hypertension	Common	Less common
Acidosis	Normochloremic	Hyperchloremic
Uric acid	Slightly elevated	Markedly elevated
Urine volume	Normal	Increased

From Alfrey, A. C.: *In* Schrier, R. W. (Ed.): Renal and Electrolyte Disorders. Boston, Little, Brown & Co., 1980, p. 412. Used by permission.

TABLE 59–11. REVERSIBLE FACTORS RESPONSIBLE FOR RENAL FUNCTION DETERIORATION

Infection
Obstruction
Extracellular fluid volume depletion
Nephrotoxic agents
Congestive heart failure
Hypertension
Pericardial tamponade
Hypercalcemia
Hyperuricemia (>15 to 20 mg/dl)
Hypokalemia

From Alfrey, A. C.: *In* Schrier, R. W. (Ed.): Renal and Electrolyte Disorders. Boston, Little, Brown & Co., 1980, p. 412. Used by permission.

nephrosclerosis and can accelerate the loss of renal function. Finally, correction of hypercalcemia, hypocalcemia, and hyperuricemia is also important in minimizing renal functional deterioration. Careful and frequent measurements of renal function are necessary to allow the physician to detect an unusual change in a patient's course. For clinical purposes, renal function is estimated by using the creatinine clearance as a measure of the GFR. The daily metabolism of muscle produces creatinine, which is then eliminated via the urine. As the ratio of muscle metabolized to creatinine produced (20 gm/1 mg) is relatively constant, the amount of creatinine excreted depends on body muscle mass. Therefore, the amount of creatinine excreted daily is relatively constant for a given individual and can be used to determine the adequacy of a 24-hour urine collection. Also, males have a higher daily creatinine production rate (20 to 25 mg/kg body weight) than females (15 to 20 mg/kg body weight), which has to be considered when calculating the adequacy of a 24-hour urine collection. If lean body mass remains constant, daily production and excretion of creatinine remain constant, and serum creatinine can be used as an estimate of renal function. It is important to realize that the serum creatinine doubles if the GFR is reduced by 50 per cent. Since the rate of renal functional deterioration is constant for many diseases causing chronic renal failure, a convenient way to monitor a patient's renal function is to plot the reciprocal of serum creatinine against time. This will form a straight line if renal deterioration proceeds at a constant rate. Reciprocal values of serum creatinine falling below the observed line will then alert the physician to evaluate for potentially reversible causes of renal deterioration.

Symptoms of chronic uremia rarely occur until the GFR is < 25 ml/minute (25 per cent of normal). Earlier findings usually only include hypertension and the nephrotic syndrome. Numerous gastrointestinal, neuromuscular, and skeletal symptoms do occur with further deterioration in renal function. Gastrointestinal symptoms include nausea, vomiting, anorexia, a metallic taste, and uremic stomatitis. Neuromuscular symptoms consist of emotional lability, insomnia, decreased ability to think abstractly, distal paresthesias, and hypalgesia (especially of the lower extremities). Affected persons have increased deep-tendon reflexes, clonus, and in severe cases can progress on to asterixis, stupor, coma, seizures, and finally death. Skeletal abnormalities include severe rickets and growth retardation in children, osteomalacia, osteoporosis, and metastatic calcification (vascular, periarticular, and visceral).

Metabolic abnormalities also begin to occur when the GFR declines below 25 ml per minute. Phosphate and magnesium retention occur, with the former leading to reduced serum calcium concentrations by causing calcium to precipitate out of solution (metastatic calcifications). Calcium concentrations also fall as the ability of the kidney to hydroxylate 25-dihydroxyvitamin D_3 to 1,25-dihydroxyvitamin D_3 is reduced. This results in reduced gastrointestinal absorption of calcium.

A normocytic normochronic anemia develops when the blood urea nitrogen exceeds 60 to 80 mg/100 ml. The cause of the anemia is multifactorial, including reduced erythropoietin activity, shortened erythrocyte life span, and inhibition of bone marrow response to erythropoietin secondary to unidentified circulating factors. The hematocrit rarely goes below 18 to 20 per cent, rarely requires transfusions, and tends to rise with institution of dialysis. Uremia also induces thrombocytopenia and platelet dysfunction, which usually respond to dialysis.

Sodium and water balance are also affected when the GFR falls below 25 ml/minute. The renal capacity to respond to wide variations in sodium and water intake is altered and results in very slow renal adaptation to alterations in water and sodium intake. This slow adaptation can result in severe volume depletion or volume overload if the sodium intake is decreased or increased rapidly. The renal ability to dilute or concentrate urine is also impaired. A normal individual can rapidly vary the final urine osmolality between 50 and 1200 mOsm, allowing for wide variation in water intake. Patients with severe chronic renal failure have a markedly reduced ability to dilute or concentrate their urine. Therefore, wide fluctuations in water intake can lead to life-threatening hyponatremia or hypernatremia.

Acidosis is another common disorder in chronic renal failure. The ability of a normal kidney to excrete 60 to 70 mEq of hydrogen ions per day is reduced to 30 to 40 mEq in advanced renal failure. This reduction is due to a decreased ability of the kidneys to produce ammonia. The excess hydrogen ions are buffered by bone salts, and an anion gap metabolic acidosis ensues. The degree of the acidosis is usually mild until very severe renal failure ensues.

Potassium balance is maintained until the GFR is reduced to below 5 ml/minute. This adaptation is due, at least in part, to increased aldosterone-induced renal tubular secretion of potassium and increased fecal potassium loss. However, rapid wide variations in the daily potassium intake or acute alterations in pH can cause acute life-threatening hypokalemia or hyperkalemia. Glucose intolerance and hypertriglyceridemia are also disorders that may accompany chronic renal failure. The glucose intolerance is secondary to peripheral insulin resistance, as fasting glucose levels and the secretion of insulin are normal in uremic patients.

The therapy for patients with chronic renal failure initially centers around minimizing the rate of functional renal deterioration. After excluding any controllable or reversible component that may accelerate renal deterioration, dietary maneuvers to retard the rate of functional impairment have been proposed. To date, controlling protein and phosphate intake have been the principle promising dietary measures. Several experimental animal models have conclusively shown that a high dietary intake of phosphate is associated with more rapid renal deterioration. Excretion of phosphate is severely reduced as the number of functioning nephrons decreases. This leads to elevations in serum phosphate, metastatic calcification, and reduced serum calcium, which in turn increases the secretion of parathyroid hormone. Elevations of parathyroid hormone have been correlated with many of the biochemical alterations that accompany uremia. Therefore, control of serum phosphate by reducing dietary phosphate intake and decreasing gastrointestinal phosphate absorption using aluminum hydroxide binders (30 to 60 ml with meals and at bedtime) is essential in patients with chronic renal failure. There is also data from human studies indicating severe phosphate restriction may reduce the rate of renal functional deterioration. Finally, recent evidence indicates a compound that inhibits calcium phosphate deposition within tissues (3-phosphocitric acid) is also effective in reducing phosphate-induced deterioration of renal function.

Protein restriction has been used for many years to curtail the rate of renal functional deterioration. Using high-biologic-value protein (eggs, milk, or essential amino acid substitutes), the minimal daily protein requirement necessary to maintain nitrogen balance can be significantly reduced. Blood urea nitrogen may also be utilized for the synthesis of nonessential amino acids and thereby spare additional protein intake if the caloric intake is adequate. The mechanism by which dietary protein restriction limits renal deterioration is subject to debate. Restricting dietary protein intake also limits phosphate intake, as protein is high in phosphate. Recently, however, protein restriction has been shown to reverse the altered glomerular hemodynamics associated with chronic renal failure. As altered glomerular hemodynamics has been correlated with glomerular functional changes, protein restriction may invoke a protective mechanism independent of the attendant phosphate restriction.

If a patient reaches end-stage renal disease, a decision regarding dialytic therapy or transplantation must be made. In general, young, otherwise healthy individuals should be encouraged to undergo transplantation. Significant strides have recently been accomplished in this field, allowing increased graft survival from cadaver kidneys. Also, continued advances in immunosuppressive therapy have reduced side effects.

Chronic dialysis remains a viable long-term alternative and can also be used to stabilize a patient prior to transplantation. Both hemodialysis and peritoneal dialysis can be used, and the type of dialysis depends on the patient's decision and availability of certain resources.

References

Alfrey, A. C.: Chronic renal failure: Manifestations and pathogenesis. *In* Schrier, R. W. (Ed.): Renal and

Electrolyte Disorders. Boston, Little, Brown & Co., 1980 (in press.

Anderson, R. J., Linas, S. L., Berns, A. S., Henrich, W. L., Miller, T. R., Gabow, P. A., and Schrier, R. W.: Nonoliguric acute renal failure. N. Engl. J. Med., 296:1134–1138, 1977.

Conger, J. D.: A controlled evaluation of prophylactic dialysis in posttraumatic acute renal failure. J. Trauma, 15:1056–1060, 1975.

Conger, J. D., and Anderson, R. J.: Acute renal failure including cortical necrosis. *In* Massry, S. G., and Glassock, R. J. (Eds.): Textbook of Nephrology. Baltimore, The Williams & Wilkins Co., 1983.

Miller, T. R., Anderson, R. J., Linas, S. L., Henrich, W. L., Berns, A. S., Gabow, P. A., and Schrier, R. W.: Urinary diagnostic indices in acute renal failure. A prospective study. Ann. Intern. Med., 89:47–50, 1978.

Rose, B. D.: Acute renal failure. *In* Rose, B. D. (Ed.): Pathophysiology of Renal Disease. McGraw-Hill Book Co., 1981.

Schrier, R. W.: Acute renal failure: Pathogenesis, diagnosis, and management. Hosp. Pract., 20:93–112, 1981.

Schrier, R. W., and Conger, J. D.: Acute renal failure: Pathogenesis, diagnosis, and management. *In* Schrier, R. W. (Ed.): Renal and Electrolyte Disorders. Boston, Little, Brown & Co., 1985 (in press).

CHAPTER 60

Other Renal Diseases Of Urologic Significance

ANTHONY J. SCHAEFFER, M.D.
FRANCESCO DEL GRECO, M.D.

INTRODUCTION

Urologists are frequently asked to see patients whose presenting symptoms or signs may be expressions of renal rather than urologic disorders. It is therefore imperative that urologists be familiar with those primary renal diseases that they will frequently encounter in daily practice. Although the clinical presentation of primary renal disease may include hematuria, flank pain, or polyuria, the majority of patients have no obvious symptoms and signs, and the underlying pathology will be revealed by routine screening of urine, blood pressure, and blood chemistries. Important clues to underlying primary renal diseases include microscopic hematuria, cylinduria, proteinuria, glycosuria, elevated serum creatinine, decreased serum bicarbonate, and hypertension. Other renal diseases should be suspected because of their association with systemic conditions that directly or indirectly affect renal function and thus produce clinical features of primary renal disease.

This chapter will focus on the major manifestations of primary renal disease—that is, hematuria, proteinuria, and rising or elevated serum creatinine—those that urologists might encounter most frequently. Urologic conditions such as tumors, stones, or infection, which might also precipitate these signs and symptoms, are discussed in Sections VII, VIII, and XI.

HEMATURIA

Hematuria is defined as the excretion of abnormal quantities of erythrocytes in the urine. Red cells can readily be identified by their color (yellow to red) and their shape (biconcave in isotonic urine and swollen spheres in hypotonic urine). *Candida* spores in the urine mimic red blood cells, but they are usually larger and can be readily distinguished if mycelial forms or buds are appreciated.

Detection and quantitation of red blood cells is best accomplished by microscopic examination of a freshly voided, concentrated urine specimen. A first-voided overnight urine specimen is ideal. Moderate exercise prior to urine collection frequently will accentuate hematuria associated with glomerular disease. Examination of unspun urine may be helpful when gross bleeding is present, in order to identify other formed elements such as casts, white blood cells, or bacteria. In all other instances, examination of unspun urine is not advantageous because of reduced sensitivity. The urine specimen should be centrifuged for 3 to 5 minutes at 2000 to 3000 RPM and the sediment examined by low-power ($\times$ 10) and high-power ($\times$ 40) light microscopy. Approximately 3 per cent of normal individuals will excrete more than 3 erythrocytes per high-power field. Although this value is commonly accepted as the upper limit of normal, in our opinion identification of any number of erythrocytes on several repeated urine specimens from the same individual should be considered abnormal.

Localization of Hematuria

Hematuria may herald either significant nephrologic or urologic disease. Nephrologic disease is frequently indicated by the presence of concomitant casts and is nearly always indicated by the presence of heavy proteinuria. Even heavy bleeding into the urinary tract will generally not elevate the protein concentration into the range of 100 to 300 mg/dl or 2+ to 3+ proteinuria by the dipstick method; this finding is commonly observed in patients with glomerular diseases. Thus, hematuria associated with 2+ to 3+ proteinuria should always be assumed to be of glomerular or interstitial origin.

Morphologic evaluation of the red blood cells provides further localization of their origin. Erythrocytes originating from glomerular diseases are commonly disfigured (dysmorphic) and show a wide range of morphologic alterations. In contrast, hematuria originating from a nonglomerular lesion will usually be associated with two morphologic types, most being undamaged circular cells with normal hemoglobin content and the remainder being red cell "ghosts," which have lost their hemoglobin. Red cells present in the urine of apparently healthy persons invariably exhibit the morphologic changes characteristic of glomerular bleeding, but they are present in very small numbers. Dysmorphic cells are best recognized with phase contrast microscopy, but after some experience they also can be distinguished by light microscopy (Fassett et al., 1982).

Glomerular Hematuria

The most common glomerular disorders in 151 patients with glomerular hematuria are listed in Table 60–1. Of these patients with glomerulonephritis of various types proven by renal biopsy, 24 (21 per cent) had glomerular hematuria not accompanied by red cell casts or proteinuria (Fassett et al., 1982). Assessment of possible glomerular hematuria should begin with a thorough history to elicit symptoms and signs associated with hematuria of glomerular or tubulointerstitial disease (Table 60–2). Poststreptococcal glomerulonephritis should be suspected in a child with recent streptococcal upper respiratory or skin infection. Associated symptoms of rash and arthritis might suggest systemic lupus erythematosus nephritis. Hemoptysis and bleeding tendencies accompanied by microcytic anemia are characteristic of the Goodpasture syndrome. A family history of renal disease, hematuria, or deafness may suggest familial hematuria or familial (Alport) nephropathy. Screening laboratory tests should initially include serum creatinine and creatinine clearance. When proteinuria of 2+ or greater accompanies hematuria, 24-hour urine protein should be

TABLE 60–1. GLOMERULAR DISORDERS IN 115 PATIENTS WITH GLOMERULAR HEMATURIA*

Disorder	Percentage of Patients	Percentage of Patients with Hematuria Alone†
IgA nephropathy (Berger disease)	30	23
Mesangioproliferative GN‡	14	31
Focal segmental proliferative GN	13	27
Familial nephritis (e.g., Alport syndrome)	11	23
Membranous GN	7	0
Mesangiocapillary GN	6	0
Focal segmental sclerosis	4	0
Unclassifiable	4	0
Systemic lupus erythematosus	3	0
Postinfectious GN	2	100
Subacute bacterial endocarditis	2	100
Others	4	0
Total	100	21

*Modified from Fassett, R. G., et al., Lancet, *1*:1432, 1982.

†Patients with glomerular hematuria not accompanied by red-cell casts or proteinuria.

‡GN = glomerulonephritis.

measured. Additional screening laboratory tests include complete blood count, erythrocyte sedimentation rate, chest x-ray, and screening blood chemistries (SMA 20 or equivalent).

Since glomerular hematuria is a manifestation of a variety of glomerular abnormalities, additional studies are needed to establish the diagnosis. Such additional studies will clarify whether immune or nonimmune mechanisms are involved, a blood dyscrasia is present, or whether other causative factors are involved. Securing specimens of tissues such as skin and rectal mucosa is the appropriate procedure in some cases. In others, kidney biopsy may be required, especially if the definitive diagnosis and prognosis cannot be established otherwise and if it is likely that the management will be different as a result of the biopsy (Earle, 1982). It should be emphasized that kidney biopsies will be very informative if the tissue is studied by an experienced pathologist by light, immunofluorescent, and electron microscopy.

IGA NEPHROPATHY (BERGER'S DISEASE)

Recurrent gross hematuria after an upper respiratory tract infection or exercise is the typical presentation of IgA glomerulonephritis.

TABLE 60–2. Assessment of Glomerular and Nonglomerular Hematuria

Presentation	Studies	Diagnosis
Glomerular		
Dysmorphic erythrocytes and/or erythrocyte casts; ± proteinuria		
Infection?		
Recent upper respiratory or skin infection?	ASO titer Serum C_3 level	Poststreptococcal Gn
Multisystem diseases?		
Rash, arthritis?	C_3, C_4, ANA	Systemic lupus erythematosus nephritis
Hemoptysis?	Microcytic anemia	Goodpasture syndrome
Bleeding tendencies?		Henoch-Schönlein purpura
		Paraproteinemic disorders (e.g., multiple myeloma)
Hereditary?		
Glomerular	Urinalyses in family members	Familial hematuria
	Deafness? Audiogram	Familial (Alport) nephritis
Other glomerulopathies?	Serum creatinine; Creatinine clearance	Minimal change disease Focal glomerulosclerosis IgA nephropathy (Berger disease)
	Quantitative urine protein	Membranous glomerulopathy Proliferative glomerulonephritis
	ANA C_3, C_4 Hb, Hct Immunoglobulin level Cryoglobulins Skin, rectal, or renal biopsy	Hemolytic uremic syndrome
	Tests negative	Early glomerulonephritis Benign "idiopathic" hematuria
Nonglomerular		
Tubulointerstial, renovascular or systemic disorder		
Circular erythrocytes; no erythrocyte casts; ± proteinuria		
Exercise?		
Prolonged running?		Runner's hematuria
Systemic coagulation disturbance?		
Hematuria causing drug?		
Anticoagulant?	Stop drug	Drug-induced hematuria
Familial history of bleeding disorder?	Platelet values PT, PTT Bleeding time	Hemophilia Thrombocytopenia Disseminated intravascular coagulopathy
Hereditary?		
Parenchymal	IVU	Medullary sponge kidney Polycystic kidney
Papillary necrosis?		Papillary necrosis due to
Black?	Sickle cell screening	Sickle cell disease or trait
Analgesic abuse?	IVU	Analgesic nephropathy
Infection?	Culture; PPD skin test	Urinary tract infection, tuberculosis
Urinary tract abnormality?	IVU; cystoscopy	Tumor, obstructive or reflux nephropathy
Malignant hypertension?		Malignant hypertensive nephropathy
Vascular?		
Atrial fibrillaion?	IVU	
Recent myocardial infarct?	Renogram	Renal artery embolism and thrombosis
Umbilical catheter?	Renal angiography	
Trauma?		
Dehydration?	IVU CT scan	Renal vein thrombosis
Bruit?	Renal angiography	Arteriovenous fistula
Renal biopsy?		

ANA = antinuclear antibody titer
ASO = antistreptolysin O
C_3, C_4 = complement
CT = computerized tomography

GN = glomerulonephritis
IVU = intravenous urography
PPD = purified protein derivative
PT = prothrombin time
PTT = partial thromboplastin time

The condition is most common in children and young adults, with predominance in males. Back pain and renal colic due to clots in the urinary tract may be associated with the hematuria. Low-grade fever and an erythematous skin rash may also be present in some patients, although there are no systemic symptoms in the majority of cases. Hematuria may persist for days or weeks, or it may subside promptly to recur later. Between attacks, microscopic hematuria may be a constant finding in some patients. The course is chronic. Renal insufficiency develops in about 25 per cent of the patients. Old age at onset, heavy proteinuria, and hypertension are indicators of a poor prognosis.

The underlying pathology of IgA glomerulonephritis is limited to either some glomeruli or to lobular segments of a glomerulus. The changes are usually proliferative and confined mostly to mesangial cells. Deposits of IgA, IgG and β_1c globulin were first described by Berger in patients with gross hematuria and focal glomerulonephritis, hence the eponym Berger's disease (Berger and Hinglais, 1968). It should be noted, however, that IgA and IgG mesangial deposits are found in other forms of glomerulonephritis as well. Hence, the presence of IgA deposits is not truly pathognomonic of the disease. What role IgA plays is still unknown, though its deposits in mesangial cells may presumably trigger the glomerular reaction. Since gross hematuria frequently follows an upper respiratory tract infection, viral antigens have been implicated in some cases. Why hematuria is so prominent and why it so frequently follows exercise is yet to be clarified.

There is no evidence of any beneficial effect of therapy. However, since the clinical presentation of IgA glomerulonephritis may be alarming and similar to that of certain systemic diseases (e.g., Henoch-Schönlein purpura, systemic lupus erythematosus, hypersensitivity angiitis, bacterial endocarditis, Wegener's granulomatosis, Goodpasture's syndrome), careful clinical and laboratory evaluation is essential. The presence of red blood cell casts in the sediment confirms the renal origin of the hematuria. In the absence of such casts, urologic examination should be performed to exclude the urinary tract as the source of bleeding and to confirm that the hematuria is from both kidneys. Once these questions have been resolved, repeated urologic evaluation is not necessary with recurrent episodes of hematuria. Finally, the diagnosis should be validated by kidney biopsy and appropriate pathologic and immunofluorescent studies.

BENIGN IDIOPATHIC HEMATURIA

Benign idiopathic hematuria has been recognized by pediatricians for many years. Affected children have focal glomerulonephritis of unknown cause, with normal blood pressure and glomerular filtration rates (GFR). A similar syndrome appears to occur in adults and consists of recurrent or persistent gross or microscopic hematuria, normal blood pressure, normal serum creatinine level and creatinine clearance, and 24-hour urine protein excretion not exceeding 1 gm. In addition, known causes of glomerulonephritis or nonglomerular causes of hematuria are absent, and renal biopsy shows focal, local glomerular cellularity (Labovitz et al., 1972). Follow-up for 10 years after initial diagnosis in children and in adults usually shows no clinical progression of disease. The syndrome of idiopathic hematuria is best considered as multifactorial rather than a single disease, with varying underlying renal changes in which both immunologic and nonimmunologic mechanisms may be involved. Careful and extended follow-up of patients with idiopathic renal hematuria through several decades is required to determine the exact prognosis.

Nonglomerular Hematuria

Nonglomerular renal hematuria is associated with tubulointerstitial, renovascular, or systemic disorders (Table 60–2). A pattern of hematuria in relation to recent concomitant medications or exercise might suggest drug-induced or exercise-induced hematuria. Exercise-induced hematuria may be associated with stressful activities such as running or marching for an extended period of time. Young men and women who participate in such activities may present with gross or microscopic hematuria. If physical examination and initial screening laboratory tests are within normal limits, a more extensive evaluation may be avoided as long as subsequent urinalyses show no hematuria.

A family history of hematuria or bleeding tendency may suggest a blood dyscrasia detectable by appropriate hematologic studies. A family history of cystic renal disease should prompt radiologic evaluation for unsuspected medullary sponge or polycystic kidney disease. Papillary necrosis should be suspected in diabetic persons, blacks (owing to sickle cell disease or trait), and in compound analgesic abusers. Vascular abnormalities should be suspected if physical examination reveals severe or accelerated hypertension, atrial fibrillation, or flank bruit. Initial screening laboratory tests should include hematocrit, hemoglobin, erythrocyte sedimentation rate, serum creatinine, chest x-ray, and screening blood chemistries. Further studies to establish the diagnosis are listed in Table 60–2.

SICKLE CELL NEPHROPATHY

Sickle cell trait occurs in approximately 8 per cent of blacks, whereas sickle-cell disease affects approximately 1 in 600. Most of the symptoms of sickle-cell trait or disease are related to the presence of hemoglobin S. When sickle erythrocytes become physically trapped in smaller vessels, a vicious circle develops, leading to stasis, deoxygenation, decreased pH, increased sickling and thrombosis, and infarction. The major renal disturbances are hematuria, polyuria, renal failure, and thrombotic complications that may lead to the nephrotic syndrome (Strom et al., 1972) or priapism (Schmidt and Flocks, 1971). Although the true frequency of hematuria is not known, sickle-cell hemoglobinopathy accounts for approximately one third of cases of gross hematuria in blacks. Hematuria occurs more regularly in hemoglobin SS disease than in hemoglobin SA trait, but urologists more frequently see patients with hemoglobin SA trait because of the relative frequency of the two disorders. Although the mechanism of hematuria is not clear, it presumably results from increased sickling and sludging of blood in the medulla and papillae, leading to extravasation of red blood cells, ischemia, and papillary necrosis. Hemoglobin electrophoresis readily permits identification of sickle hemoglobin and differentiation of sickle-cell trait from sickle-cell disease. Cystoscopy and intravenous urography should be performed to localize the site of bleeding, which is usually from the left, and to rule out other disorders (Buckalew and Someren, 1974).

Treatment of hematuria should begin with rest and hydration. In addition, hematuria has been treated with a variety of techniques including intravenous distilled water, sodium bicarbonate, mannitol, and loop diuretics (Knochel, 1969; Vega et al., 1971). ε-Aminocaproic acid (which inhibits urokinase), administered intravenously in small doses of 1 gm at 4- to 6-hour intervals, appears to be effective and causes few or no side effects. However, this agent should be used only for severe and intractable bleeding, since clotting of the blood inhibits urokinase and can produce intrapelvic or ureteral clots. If life-threatening hematuria occurs and conservative treatment fails, arteriography with arterial embolization of selected vessels should be

considered. If this fails, pyeloscopy and segmental or total nephrectomy may be required. Recurrent episodes of hematuria may be diminished by regular administration of oral furosemide.

Papillary necrosis is a common complication of sickle-cell nephropathy but usually affects one papilla at a time and rarely results in serious deterioration of renal function. The loss of concentrating ability is perhaps the most characteristic renal functional lesion in individuals with hemoglobin S gene. Although the degree of concentration defect is not sufficient to cause symptoms under normal conditions, affected persons may develop manifestations of early sickle-cell crisis (malaise, anorexia, joint pain) with only moderate restriction of fluid intake.

RENAL ARTERY EMBOLISM AND THROMBOSIS

Thrombosis or embolism of the renal arterial vasculature can result in varied clinical, functional, and morphologic changes depending upon the size of vessels involved, rate and degree of development of obstruction, and extent of renal parenchymal involvement. Since intrarenal arteries are end arteries, complete occlusion of a main renal artery or one of its branches leads to wedge-shaped infarction with coagulation necrosis and extensive parenchymal damage.

Occlusion of the main renal arteries most commonly results from emboli associated with mitral stenosis and atrial fibrillation, artificial heart valves, subacute bacterial endocarditis, or mural thrombi associated with myocardial infarct. The most important noncardiac source of renal emboli is a ruptured aortic atheromatous plaque. Although spontaneous rupture is common, manipulation of vessels during arteriography or surgery is more frequently implicated. Thrombosis of major renal arteries is unusual, though it may occur following blunt abdominal trauma, manipulation of the aorta during angiography or surgery, or renal arterioplasty. Spontaneous thrombosis may occasionally occur in association with atherosclerotic or dissecting aneurysms of the aorta, or with inflammatory vascular disorders such as polyarteritis. Renal infarction occurs when a main or segmental renal artery is completely and suddenly occluded.

The clinical sequelae of major renal artery occlusion are extremely varied and may include sudden, sharp, persistent pain in the flank or upper abdomen, nausea, vomiting, and fever. However, most patients will be symptom free.

Urinary findings of microscopic or gross hematuria accompanied by mild proteinuria are present in only about half of the cases. Leukocytosis may be present. Renal infarction characteristically causes a rapid rise in serum glutamic-oxaloacetic transaminase, which returns to normal within 3 to 4 days followed by a striking elevation of lactate dehydrogenase, which remains elevated for as long as 2 weeks. Serum alkaline phosphatase may be slightly increased. If the contralateral kidney is normal, renal functional impairment may not be recognized. However, if preexisting renal functional impairment or a solitary kidney is present, marked or complete renal failure will occur. Partial thrombotic or embolic occlusion of the major renal artery may cause sudden development of hypertension due to activation of the renin-angiotensin system.

The key to diagnosis is a high index of suspicion in the proper setting. The first clue to renal infarction is usually provided by intravenous urography, which will show absence of visualization in all or part of the kidney. Radionuclide imaging demonstrating nonperfusion of the kidney and selective renal arteriography are required to confirm the diagnosis (Fig. 60–1). Early management of renal artery thromboembolism is determined by degree of renal involvement, duration of involvement, and cause of the occlusion. Early determination of complete oc-

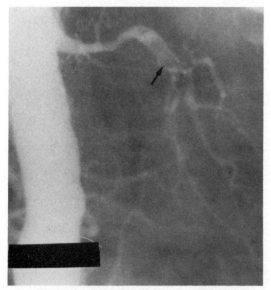

Figure 60–1. Renal artery embolus in a 68-year-old man with a history of atrial fibrillation, left flank pain, hematuria, and acute elevation in serum creatinine. Abdominal aortogram demonstrates conical tapering of the left main renal artery from atherosclerosis. There is a large intraluminal filling defect (arrow) in the main renal artery extending into the proximal interlobar arteries.

clusion of the main renal artery(ies) in patients with bilateral renal artery thrombi or unilateral renal artery thrombus of a single functioning kidney is best managed by surgical thrombectomy or embolectomy. The best results have been reported when surgery was performed a few hours after the occlusion, but significant return of renal function has been documented in patients operated on as long as 15 to 43 days following occlusion. This is probably because of the gradual development of collateral circulation prior to total occlusion (Besarab et al., 1976; Perkins et al., 1967). Unilateral thrombosis or embolism warrants a conservative approach, since the contralateral kidney will continue to function and recovery of function on the ischemic side has been reported. Treatment of embolic disease owing to a cardiac source is usually nonsurgical, since persons thus affected often have serious underlying cardiac disease and a high surgical mortality. Anticoagulants should be instituted promptly to prevent further propagation of the clot into the renal artery or embolization of other organs. Incomplete occlusion may lead to renal ischemia, increased renin production, and hypertension, which is best managed by nephrectomy.

ARTERIOVENOUS FISTULAS

Renal arteriovenous fistulas are described as either congenital or acquired, based on angiographic criteria. Congenital fistulas present as distinct, tortuous coiled vascular channels grouped in clusters, with multiple communications between arteries and veins. They are considered to be congenital, because the angiographic appearance is typical of other known congenital arteriovenous fistulas. These congenital fistulas account for approximately one quarter of all arteriovenous fistulas, are usually present in adults, and have an equal sex incidence (Messing et al., 1976). Acquired arteriovenous fistulas usually appear as solitary communications between artery and vein, account for almost three quarters of all renal arteriovenous fistulas, and are posttraumatic in origin. Percutaneous needle biopsy accounts for over 40 per cent of acquired fistulas, particularly in patients with nephrosclerosis and arterial hypertension (Wickre and Golper, 1982; O'Brien et al., 1974). Acquired renal arteriovenous fistulas also occur following penetrating or blunt abdominal trauma, partial nephrectomies, nephrolithotomies, or spontaneously, owing to tumor invasion into adjacent veins (Bosniak, 1965).

The clinical manifestations of renal arteriovenous fistulas depend primarily on their size and location. Although frequently silent, fistulas may be associated with hematuria, cardiac failure due to increased cardiac output, and hypertension due to renal ischemia distal to the fistula (Gomes and Bernatz, 1970). Almost three quarters of affected persons have a continuous abdominal or flank bruit. Intravenous urography shows no abnormalities in about one half of sufferers; the remainder manifest space-occupying lesions or nonvisualization of the kidney. Radionuclide angiography is a simple, noninvasive, and valuable screening test for arteriovenous fistulas (Lisbona et al., 1980). Although reliable when large arteriovenous communications are present, this technique may not detect small intraparenchymal fistulas such as those seen following renal biopsy. Contrast angiography remains the definitive diagnostic study for arteriovenous fistulas (Fig. 60–2). The arteriovenous communication usually shows as an immediate intense arterial blush, which disappears rapidly. Early visualization of the inferior vena cava is further evidence of shunting and is usually seen with high-flow shunts.

Management of arteriovenous fistulas should be based on the cause and associated symptoms. Most congenital fistulas are small, asymptomatic, and of little clinical importance. Spontaneous closure has been demonstrated

(Cho and Stanley, 1978). Similarly, approximately 95 per cent of postbiopsy arteriovenous fistulas heal spontaneously in 1 to 18 months (Iloreta and Blaufox, 1979). Surgical intervention is generally indicated in patients who have symptomatic fistulas not secondary to renal biopsy. Persistent microscopic or massive hematuria or frank rupture provide clear indications for therapeutic intervention, as do high-output cardiac failure and hypertension, which can frequently be controlled or cured once the fistula is removed.

Partial or total nephrectomy, as well as arterial reconstructive procedures, has been utilized traditionally to treat symptomatic renal arteriovenous fistulas (Nelson et al., 1973). Large congenital arteriovenous fistulas or tumors are best treated by nephrectomy; small congenital fistulas can be managed by partial nephrectomy. Acquired types of arteriovenous fistulas generally warrant a renal sparing procedure, traditionally by extrarenal or intrarenal vascular ligation or repair.

Recently, transcatheter arteriographically directed embolization has gained acceptance for both congenital and acquired arteriovenous fistulas (Clark et al., 1983; Cho and Stanley, 1978). Small arteriovenous fistulas may be managed

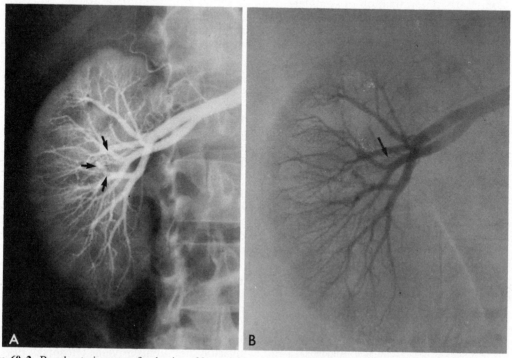

Figure 60–2. Renal arteriovenous fistulas in a 28-year-old woman with recurrent microscopic and gross hematuria. *A,* Selective right renal arteriography demonstrates a cluster of small abnormal vessels in the peripelvic region (arrows). *B,* Subtraction view demonstrates this abnormal collection of vessels as well as an early draining vein (arrow).

using autogenous clots, since lysis of this embolized material within a few hours may prevent renal infarction. If the fistulas are large, gelatin sponge emboli, coils, balloons, or bucrylate may be effective. Extensive embolization necessitating repeated catheterization may be required for arteriovenous malformations in which multiple vessels contribute to the lesion. Potential complications include remote venous embolization, hypertension secondary to renal ischemia, and renal infarction and refistulization in the infarcted areas.

RENAL VEIN THROMBOSIS

Renal vein thrombosis may occur in a variety of clinical conditions. Intralobular or arcuate vein thrombosis in infants may arise bilaterally in association with severe dehydration owing to diarrhea or vomiting or severe plasma hyperosmolarity in association with angiography (Arneil et al., 1973). In adults it is frequently unilateral and is usually associated with the nephrotic syndrome or invasion of renal veins by tumor or retroperitoneal disease. Whether renal vein thrombosis is the cause or consequence of the nephrotic syndrome is debatable. Increased renal venous pressure in association with congestive heart failure or after surgical ligation of the renal vein can produce proteinuria. However, animal experiments have shown that the contralateral kidney must be removed before the constriction leads to heavy proteinuria. In humans, obstruction of the vena cava above the renal veins or even renal vein thrombosis may not be associated with nephrotic syndrome. On the other hand, the nephrotic syndrome is a hypercoagulable state, and thrombotic events occur in various vessels. For example, pulmonary embolism with or without renal vein thrombosis is a relatively common complication. An increase in clotting factors and a decrease in antithrombin III, an inhibitor of coagulation, have been demonstrated. According to some investigators the incidence of renal vein thrombosis appears to be much higher (>30 per cent) in patients with nephrotic syndrome due to membranous glomerulonephritis than to other causes (Llach et al., 1980).

The clinical presentation and course of renal vein thrombosis are dependent upon degree of occlusion and rate at which it develops. Acute thrombosis occurs more often in young children and is associated with severe flank pain, hypertension, or shock. Kidney size is frequently increased, and renal blood flow may be decreased to 25 per cent. Gross hematuria due to focal renal infarction and reduced renal function is common. Progressive thrombosis of the renal vein occurs most often in adults and may present with flank pain, hematuria, and fever or as the nephrotic syndrome. Renal failure rarely develops if collateral venous drainage develops rapidly enough. Patients with acute or long-standing renal vein thrombosis may be asymptomatic or present with clinical manifestations due to other thrombolic events, the most serious of which is pulmonary embolism. Intravenous urography may show an enlarged kidney, which usually though not always excretes contrast material (Fig. 60–3). CAT scan has been used recently to demonstrate an enlarged kidney and thrombosis of the renal vein. The definitive diagnostic study, however, is renal venography. Care should be exercised in performing this study, since dislodgement and embolization may occur.

The management of renal vein thrombosis depends upon the age of the patient. In infancy, thrombosis associated with dehydration is frequently fatal, and the best results have been achieved with rehydration. Emergency thrombectomy has also been favorable (Thompson et al., 1975). In adults, anticoagulation should be initiated as soon as renal vein thrombosis has been diagnosed and if thromboembolic phenomena have been demonstrated. The role of prophylaxis with anticoagulation in patients with nephrotic syndrome and without renal vein thrombosis or other thromboembolic complications is not established. Surgical removal of the clots from the renal veins is not advisable or helpful, since thrombosis of intrarenal channels is most likely present.

PROTEINURIA

The qualitative detection of proteinuria, particularly in patients who appear to be healthy, always raises the question of renal disease. Proteinuria may be the first indication of an underlying renal glomerular, vascular, or tubulointerstitial disease or an early presentation of overflow of abnormal protein into the urine. However, proteinuria is also found in nonrenal disorders and various physiologic states.

Protein in Normal Urine

Healthy adults excrete approximately 80 to 150 mg of protein daily. The maximum level in small children is 140 mg/m^2 of body surface area

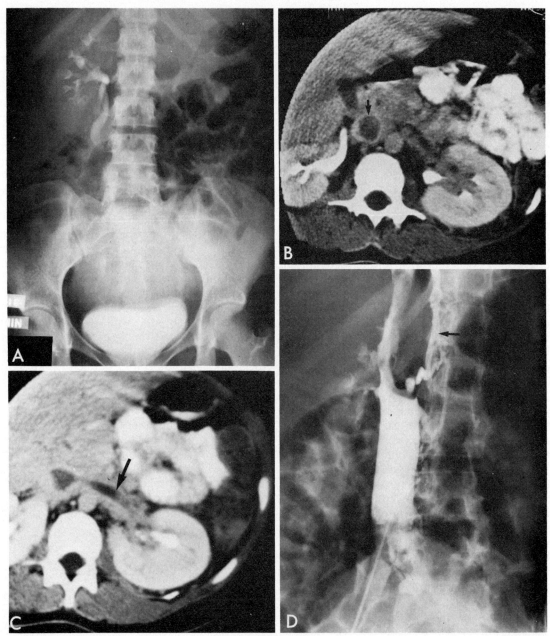

Figure 60–3. Renal vein thrombosis. A 40-year-old woman presented with pulmonary embolus, hematuria, and proteinuria. *A,* Intravenous urogram demonstrates a very poorly visualizing left kidney and no abnormality of the right kidney. Note contrast material in the distal left ureter. *B,* Computed tomography following an infusion of contrast material demonstrates a low-density area in the inferior vena cava (arrow) surrounded by a contrast-filled rim. *C,* Similar findings are noted in the left renal vein (large arrow). *D,* Inferior vena cavography demonstrates filling of the inferior vena cava below the level of the renal veins. A large intraluminal thrombus extends from the level of the renal veins to the diaphragm. A small amount of contrast traverses the thrombus and wall of the vena cava. There also is filling of lumbar veins (arrow), which serve as collateral channels.

per day. Protein excretion up to 300 mg per day occurs transiently following severe exercise and is generally found in adolescents between the ages of 10 and 18. For any given rate of protein excretion, the concentration of protein in a single voided sample of urine will vary inversely with urine flow. The concentration of protein in normal urine usually does not exceed 10 to 20 mg/dl, and thus higher concentrations imply the existence of proteinuria. However, in persons with dilute urine, significant proteinuria may be present with concentrations well below 20 mg/dl.

The normal composition of urine protein is about 30 to 40 per cent serum albumin, 30 per cent serum globulins, and 40 per cent tissue proteins (e.g., Tamm-Horsfall). This profile can be altered by both physiologic and pathologic conditions that affect filtration, reabsorption, or excretion of urine protein. It has been proposed that determination of the urine protein profile can assist in determining the source of proteinuria.

Detection of Proteinuria

Proteinuria can be detected by either turbidimetric (protein precipitation) or colorimetric (dipstick) methods. Turbidimetric methods rely on the detection of turbidity after proteins in solution have been precipitated by strong acids (e.g., 3 per cent sulfosalicylic). These methods are sensitive for total protein concentration as low as 10 mg/dl and react with all classes of proteins. The turbidimetric test has largely been replaced by the simpler colorimetric test. The dipstick consists of bibulous paper impregnated with tetrabromphenol blue, which changes color in the presence of albumin and to a lesser extent in the presence of other proteins. The intensity of the shade of green is proportional to the concentration of protein in the urine. The reagent strips are generally sensitive to total protein concentrations as low as 20 mg/dl. Because of difficulties in the discrimination of colors, the correlation between color change and actual protein concentrations may be only approximate (Rennie and Keen, 1967).

False-positive or false-negative test results can occur with either method. Highly concentrated urine in a dehydrated but otherwise healthy person may give a positive test result. In patients with gross hematuria, contamination of the urine with plasma proteins may cause false-positive proteinuria. However, rather massive bleeding is required to elevate the protein concentration into the 100 to 300 mg/dl (2+ to 3+ range) and to the values over 1.0 gm/24 hour commonly observed in patients with glomerular disease. Milder degrees of macroscopic or microscopic hematuria accompanied by heavy proteinuria (>300 mg/dl, or 3+) should always be assumed to have a glomerular or interstitial cause (Glassock, 1983). The other causes of false-positive reactions affect either the turbidimetric or colorimetric test but not both. Thus false-positive reactions are suggested by discrepancies between the two tests. False-positive turbidimetric reactions can be caused by the presence in the urine of radiographic contrast material, high concentrations of penicillin or cephalosporin analogs, or sulfonamide or tolbutamide metabolites. False-positive colorimetric tests can occur when urine is highly alkaline (pH >8) (e.g., as seen in urinary tract infections with urea-splitting bacteria) or following contamination with antiseptics such as chlorhexidine or benzalkonium chloride.

False-negative results may occur with dilute urine specimens, because even increased amounts of protein are diluted to below the level of detection of the method used. Highly buffered alkaline urine may give a false-negative turbidimetric test and so must be titered to a pH of between 5 and 6 before testing. Since the colorimetric strips react preferentially with albumin and are relatively insensitive to globulins and Bence Jones protein, urine that is sulfosalicylic acid positive and dipstick negative should be tested for light chains (Bence Jones proteinuria) to assess the patient for multiple myeloma.

Pathophysiology of Proteinuria

Proteins may enter the urine by filtration across the glomerular capillary membrane or by decreased tubular reabsorption of normally filtered protein. Increased plasma concentration of a protein with molecular features conducive to transglomerular passage (low molecular weight, cationic charge, and high deformability) will also cause proteinuria.

Glomerular proteinuria, the most common type of proteinuria, usually is caused by increased glomerular capillary permeability to proteins, especially albumin. Glomerular proteinuria may be due to any primary glomerular disease such as lipoid nephrosis as well as any glomerulopathy associated with a systemic illness such as systemic lupus erythematosus or diabetes mellitus. A transient increase in protein excretion may even occur in various physiologic settings in the absence of renal disease. For example, increased protein excretion such as may accompany standing or exercise in healthy subjects has been attributed to some alteration in renal hemodynamics plus simultaneous changes in filtration of normal protein. The likelihood of glomerular disease is high if protein excretion exceeds 1 to 2 gm/day, and proteinuria in excess of 3 to 5 gm/day (nephrotic range proteinuria) invariably indicates glomerular disease.

Tubular proteinuria is defined as the appearance in the urine of normally filtered protein as a result of impaired tubular reabsorption. Normally the majority of filtered proteins of low molecular weight (<40,000 Daltons) such as β_2-microglobulin, immunoglobulin light chains, zinc-binding protein, and lysozyme are reabsorbed by the proximal tubules, but in patients with interstitial or tubular disorders they escape tubular reabsorption. In tubular proteinuria, < 2 to 3 gm/day are excreted and low-molecular-weight proteins predominate over albumin. Examples of tubular proteinuria include Fanconi's syndrome and cadmium, lead, or mercury poisoning.

Overflow proteinuria occurs in the absence of any glomerular or tubular abnormality. Increased plasma concentrations of abnormal immunoproteins and other low-molecular-weight proteins with molecular features conducive to transglomerular passage lead to an excessive filtered load, which exceeds the reabsorptive capacity of the proximal tubules. Protein excretion may vary from 100 mg to 10 gm/day. The most common example of overflow proteinuria is seen in myeloma patients, who excrete immunoglobulin light chains (Bence Jones proteins). Other examples of overflow proteinuria include lysozymuria in patients with monocytic and monomyelocytic leukemia, hemoglobinuria, or myoglobinuria. Both hemoglobinuria and myoglobinuria will yield positive results for occult blood in the urine since both compounds contain a heme group. Hemoglobinuria is suspected when the urine is red or dark brown, the dipstick is positive for blood, but erythrocytes are not seen in the sediment. The plasma of patients with hemoglobinuria is reddish brown. Myoglobinuria in contrast is characterized by dark urine and normal-appearing plasma. Acute renal failure coinciding with overflow proteinuria has been well documented (Baker and Dodds, 1925; Rowland and Penn, 1972).

Evaluation of Proteinuria

Patients with a 1+ or greater dipstick test should have repeat dipstick and if possible turbidimetric tests on one or two additional urine samples. A large proportion of patients, as many as 100 per cent in some pediatric series (Randolph and Greenfield, 1967; Wagner et al., 1968), will have transient proteinuria that disappears within days of the initial positive specimen (King and Gronbeck, 1952; Larsen and Thysell, 1969). These patients and those with functional proteinuria associated with, for example, fever, exercise, emotional stress, or congestive heart failure require no further evaluation when urine protein excretion returns to normal. However, if repeat tests for protein remain positive, 24-hour urine protein should be determined.

The probability of an underlying renal disease may be predicted by the pattern and amount of proteinuria and identification of associated abnormalities. In general, persistent proteinuria is most likely to be associated with renal impairment than is intermittent proteinuria. Proteinuria that occurs only in the upright position (orthostatic) is usually less significant than constant proteinuria during both recumbency and quiet upright ambulation. The likelihood of renal disease is also high if quantitative determination of protein excretion exceeds 1 to 2 gm/day. Proteinuria in excess of 3 to 5 gm/day (nephrotic range proteinuria) almost invariably indicates a glomerular disease. Proteinuria due to overflow should be suspected if the proteins in the urine are not normal constituents of plasma but rather abnormal immunoproteins. The probability of underlying renal disease is also increased if proteinuria is associated with hypertension, diabetes mellitus, gout, elevated serum creatinine, or edema or other abnormalities of the urine sediment such as hematuria or casts. Conversely, when proteinuria is detected by chance in patients who have no evidence of systemic disease, renal functional impairment, or abnormal urine sediment, the probability of significant underlying renal disease is small.

Persistent Proteinuria

Persistent proteinuria is described as an increase in protein excretion above normal in all samples on repeated testing, regardless of the patient's posture. The most common causes of persistent proteinuria are listed in Table 60–3. The major renal causes of proteinuria without hematuria are diabetes mellitus, amyloidosis, multiple myeloma, arteriolar nephrosclerosis, pregnancy, and drug and heavy-metal intoxication. Patients with proteinuria and either gross or microscopic hematuria are likely to have a form of glomerulonephritis even if there is no renal functional impairment. These patients should be evaluated as noted in Table 60–2.

DIABETES MELLITUS

Proteinuria is the hallmark of diabetic nephropathy and may be the first manifestation of

TABLE 60–3. CAUSES OF PROTEINURIA

Primary glomerular disease
  Minimal change disease (lipoid nephrosis)
  Focal glomerulosclerosis
  Membranous glomerulopathy
  Proliferative glomerulonephritis

Infectious disease
  Poststreptococcal glomerulonephritis
  Infectious endocarditis
  Syphilis

Drugs and chemicals*
  Mercury
  Gold
  Penicillamine
  Probenecid
  Heroin

Neoplastic disease and paraproteinemia
  Multiple myeloma*
  Lymphoma and leukemia
  Carcinoma

Multisystem and connective tissue diseases
  Systemic lupus erythematosus
  Rheumatoid arthritis
  Amyloidosis*
  Scleroderma
  Polyarteritis
  Wegener's granulomatosis
  Cryoglobulinemia
  Goodpasture syndrome
  Sarcoidosis*
  Vasculitides

Metabolic disease
  Diabetes mellitus*

Heredofamilial diseases
  Alport syndrome
  Fabry's disease*
  Sickle cell disease

Miscellaneous
  Arteriolar nephrosclerosis*
  Pregnancy-associated*
  Renal vein thrombosis
  Reflux nephropathy
  Analgesic nephropathy

*Major causes of proteinuria without hematuria.

diabetes mellitus. Diabetic patients with proteinuria generally have a poorer prognosis than those without. In some patients the glomerular disease is severe enough that heavy proteinuria of >6 gm/24 hours and nephrotic syndrome result. Hypertension and decreased GFR are also usually present. Hematuria is usually absent in patients with diabetic nephropathy, and when hematuria is present other disorders such as papillary necrosis or immune complex glomerulonephritis should be considered.

MULTIPLE MYELOMA

Multiple myeloma is a neoplastic transformation of plasma cells leading to the production and secretion of abnormal and unique immunoglobulin proteins (paraproteins). This disorder is characterized clinically by bone pain, anemia, hypercalcemia, and renal failure. The renal dysfunction may take a variety of forms (acute renal failure, chronic renal failure, tubular disorders) related to the type of myeloma. IgG myeloma, which accounts for approximately 60 per cent of all myelomas, has the best prognosis. The IgA form causes 20 per cent of myelomas and is more likely to be associated with hypercalcemia and amyloidosis. Light chain disease (Bence Jones proteinuria) accounts for approximately 20 per cent of myeloma cases and has the highest frequency of renal involvement and the poorest prognosis. Renal tubular disorders are most common in this group due in part to the toxic effects of the light chains on tubular cells.

Acute renal failure occurs in 5 to 10 per cent of myeloma patients and is frequently associated with or precipitated by intravenous or retrograde urography, dehydration, hypercalcemia, hyperuricemia, or pyelonephritis. Regardless of the cause of the acute renal failure in myeloma patients, the prognosis is poor, with a 60 to 75 per cent mortality rate. Fluid restriction should be avoided in preparing patients with multiple myeloma for intravenous urography. Mild hypercalcemia (approximately 11 to 13 mg/dl) is a frequent complication in patients with multiple myeloma, and severe hypercalcemia (>13 mg/dl) is also encountered in as many as 25 per cent of patients. Prompt treatment by oral or parenteral hydration and diuretics, resulting in an output of at least 3 L/day, may be adequate to prevent renal failure. Hyperuricosemia is not uncommon in patients with multiple myeloma as a result of nucleic acid turnover, which arises spontaneously or following chemotherapy. Prevention of acute uric acid nephropathy should include reduction of uric acid production by allopurinol, a maintenance of the urine output of approximately 3 L/day, and maintenance of a urine pH of 6.0 or greater by administration of sodium bicarbonate. Multiple myeloma sufferers are also very susceptible to infections, and the most frequent portal of entry is the urinary tract. Instrumentation of the lower urinary tract should be avoided.

Chronic renal failure occurs in 40 to 50 per cent of myeloma patients and may be exacerbated by obstructive nephropathy due to ureteral amyloid deposits, nephrolithiasis, papillary necrosis, or proteinaceous renal pelvic cast formation. Both hemodialysis and renal transplantation have been performed successfully in patients with multiple myeloma.

INTERMITTENT OR ORTHOSTATIC PROTEINURIA

Most patients with intermittent proteinuria will be free of proteinuria after a few years (Larsen and Thysell, 1969). Those younger than 30 years have mortality rates similar to age-matched controls, and death due to renal disease is very uncommon. Intermittent proteinuria is less common after the age of 50, but when present is associated with an excess death rate that increases with age (Gajewski et al., 1976). When intermittent excretion exceeds 1 gm/day, blood pressure, urinalysis, and serum creatinine should be determined at 6 to 12-month intervals until the proteinuria disappears.

If an individual has evidence of orthostatic proteinuria that is transient, the likelihood of renal disease is rare. Patients with fixed ortho-static proteinuria rarely develop chronic renal disease, and a 10-year prognosis is excellent. Although renal biopsy is the only means of determining alterations in renal histology, it should be noted that the broad spectrum of histologic findings by light microscopy does not necessarily provide insight into the actual clinical significance or subsequent morbidity of the lesion. For these reasons, when proteinuria is <1 gm/day emphasis should be placed on follow-up, and biopsies should be deferred until there is evidence of progression of proteinuria, development of other abnormalities in the urine sediment, or other changes of the clinical course such as development of hypertension, impaired renal function, or an abnormal urine sediment. When proteinuria initially is >1 gm/day there is an increased merit to renal biopsy, and biopsy is almost surely indicated if the proteinuria is in the nephrotic range—that is, >3 gm/day.

ELEVATED OR RISING SERUM CREATININE

The creatinine clearance provides a simple and reliable means for estimating GFR and thus the status of renal function. Creatinine is produced at a constant rate by muscle cells from the breakdown of creatine at a rate of approximately 20 mg per kg per day. If lean body mass does not change appreciably, the plasma concentration and daily urine creatinine excretion remain relatively constant. When indicated, creatinine clearance should be performed to establish baseline data. Once the clearance has been determined, measurement of creatinine, which closely reflects creatinine clearance, is usually sufficient to monitor renal function serially. Fig-

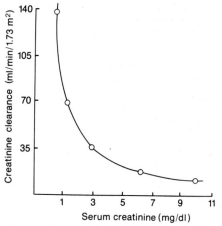

Figure 60–4. Relationship between creatinine clearance and serum creatinine. (From David P. Earle (Ed.): Manual of Clinical Nephrology. Philadelphia, W. B. Saunders Co., 1982, p. 29.)

ure 60–4 shows the relation between GFR and serum creatinine. For every 50 per cent reduction in GFR, the serum creatinine concentration approximately doubles. From this diagram it is apparent that in early stages of renal insufficiency, relatively large decreases in clearance are reflected by small changes in serum creatinine levels. In contrast, in advanced renal failure, relatively small changes in clearance result in large changes in the serum creatinine levels. Blood urea nitrogen is a less reliable indicator of renal function since factors other than the GFR such as protein intake, the degree of hydration, and anabolic or antianabolic agents (tetracycline and corticosteroids), fever, and infection all can cause changes in blood urea nitrogen in the absence of changes in renal function (Schrier, 1980).

An important consideration when evaluating renal function is the role of age. The mean serum creatinine gradually increases between the ages of 1 and 20 years. (Fig. 60–5). After the age of 50, the GFR gradually decreases in approximately half the population without hypertension or known renal disease (Fig. 60–6).

Impaired renal function as evidenced by abnormally elevated serum creatinine is usually associated with other features such as hematuria, shock, hypertension, obstructive nephropathy, infection, and nephrotoxins. Recent evidence has shown the important role played by atheromatous cholesterol emboli, analgesics, and x-ray contrast media in causing chronic and acute deterioration of renal function. A few comments about these causes of renal failure therefore seem to be appropriate.

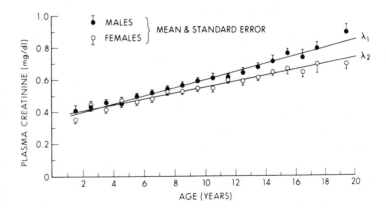

Figure 60–5. Mean plasma creatinine plotted against age for both sexes, with the regression lines derived from 1398 values (772 males, 626 females) superimposed. Standard error limits for estimate of the mean are shown. λ_1 (males): y = 0.35 + 0.025 x, r = 0.53, p<0.0001; λ_2 (females): y = 0.37 + 0.018 x, r = 0.49, p<0.0001. (From Schwartz, G. J., et al.: J. Pediatr., *88*:828, 1976.)

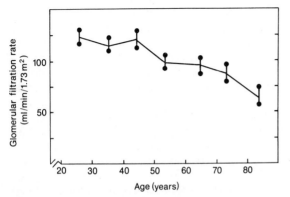

Figure 60–6. Age and glomerular filtration rate. − = mean values; $\updownarrow$ = standard deviation of the mean. (From David P. Earle (Ed.): Manual of Clinical Nephrology. Philadelphia, W. B. Saunders Co., 1982, p. 30.)

ATHEROEMBOLIC RENAL DISEASE

Atheromatous emboli of small arteries and arterioles should be suspected in patients 50 years of age and older with known atherosclerosis or abdominal aneurysms and unexplained renal failure. Atheromatous plaques on the wall of the abdominal aorta may spontaneously rupture or erode through, permitting their contents, including cholesterol crystals and amorphous debris, to occlude the lumina of multiple small renal arteries (arcuate, intralobular, terminal). Atheromatous emboli of the renal arteries have been identified in 15 to 30 per cent of patients with severe erosive atherosclerotic lesions of the aorta and 1 per cent of patients with slight to moderate erosions (Humphreys, 1981). Emboli also frequently follow aortic surgery, renal arteriography, and external cardiac massage. Spotty ischemic atrophy of the parenchyma in a wedge-shaped pattern predominates over acute infarction. Recanalization of the vessels may occur, or a fibrotic reaction may lead to reduc-

tion of renal function. The diagnosis is difficult since the clinical manifestations and signs are not dramatic. Hypertension or elevated serum creatinine levels may be the only clinical findings. Acute renal failure occurs rarely. Embolization of other organs occurs frequently and may lead to visual disturbances including sudden blindness (cholesterol retinal emboli), gastrointestinal bleeding, splenic infarcts, and livedo reticularis of the skin of the lower extremities or distal extremity gangrene. Laboratory findings are nonspecific. Proteinuria is usually mild, except in the presence of malignant hypertension, when heavy proteinuria may occur. Urinalysis may reveal hematuria or leukocyturia. The diagnosis can be established with certainty only by renal biopsy showing typical elongated clefts in the small intralobular and interlobular vessels. Cholesterol emboli can also be demonstrated in muscle biopsy of the lower extremities and occasionally can be seen by ophthalmoscopy. Renal angiography is not advisable, since the results are usually nonspecific and traumatic rupture of additional atheromatous plaques may occur.

Management of atheroembolic renal disease is difficult and usually unsatisfactory. No reported cases have regained normal renal function, and the mortality is very high as a consequence of associated widespread atheromatous disease and complicating events such as pancreatitis and gastrointestinal bleeding and uremia. The best treatment is prevention. Patients with widespread atheromatous disease of the aorta should not undergo angiography or be treated with anticoagulants if at all possible. During surgery the atheromatous aorta should be handled very carefully. Once the embolic event has occurred, there is no evidence that anticoagulation therapy is effective.

ANALGESIC NEPHROPATHY

Correlation between chronic analgesic abuse, interstitial nephritis, papillary necrosis, and chronic renal failure was noted more than 30 years ago in Switzerland and is now widely recognized. Analgesic nephropathy is the cause of chronic renal failure in 20 per cent of dialysis patients in Australia and in 3 to 7 per cent of those in Europe and the United States. Large doses of phenacetin and aspirin, especially in combination, may cause renal papillary necrosis and chronic interstitial nephritis. The total amount of analgesic consumed is directly related to the degree of renal function impairment. One gram of phenacetin per day in combination with other analgesics for 1 to 3 years or a total of 2 kg of phenacetin alone is considered the minimal amount that will cause nephropathy.

Analgesic nephropathy is predominantly seen in women between the ages of 30 and 50. The patient is typically depressed, complains of headaches and abdominal and musculoskeletal disorders, and gives a history of years of daily ingestion of analgesics containing caffeine, aspirin, and phenacetin. Alcoholism is common. Analgesic nephropathy is usually asymptomatic and does not manifest until an elevated serum creatinine is detected. The patient commonly presents with recurrent urinary tract infections. Proteinuria is usually <1 gm/day. Impaired urine concentrating ability also occurs early, and sterile pyuria is seen in more than half of the patients with papillary necrosis. Occasionally, sloughed renal papillary tissue will cause ureteral colic and microscopic or gross hematuria. Gastric ulcer and anemia associated with secondary gastrointestinal bleeding are frequent.

The diagnosis is based on history of significant analgesic abuse and the demonstration of renal papillary necrosis by intravenous urography or retrograde pyelography. Papillary necrosis is usually bilateral and involves all the calyceal groups. Effective treatment is not available. Affected individuals should be persuaded to avoid all nonsteroidal anti-inflammatory agents. Persons who continue to take even small amounts of analgesics will have progressive deterioration, and conversely more than 80 per cent of patients who stop abusing analgesics will frequently show an improvement or at least a slowing of deterioration in renal function. Fluid intake should be generous to maintain urine output of at least 2 L/day. The prognosis is poorest in patients who present with small kidneys or a GFR of <20 ml/minute, hypertension, or persistent proteinuria. The presence of hematuria should be carefully investigated and cytologic studies performed regularly because of an increased incidence of transitional cell carcinoma.

RADIOGRAPHIC CONTRAST NEPHROPATHY

Radiographic contrast nephropathy rarely occurs in individuals with normal renal function. Among hospitalized patients with normal renal function, the incidence of nephrotoxicity (defined as a rise in serum creatinine of >1 mg/dl) from intravenous pyelography is 0.6 per cent (Abraham et al., 1983) and 2 per cent following major angiography. The major predisposing factors to contrast nephropathy are preexisting renal insufficiency and diabetes mellitus. More than 50 per cent of patients with nondiabetic renal insufficiency (mean serum creatinine of 4 mg/dl) develop nephrotoxicity, and the risk of toxicity reaches 90 per cent in diabetic persons with serum creatinine of 5 mg/dl. Additional factors contributing to increased risk of contrast nephropathy are age (older than 55 years), dehydration, hypertension, atherosclerotic peripheral vascular disease, hyperuricemia, proteinuria, and recent nephrotoxic drug exposure. It is apparent therefore that many of the patients frequently evaluated for urologic disease are at high risk of developing contrast nephropathy.

The onset of renal failure is usually abrupt and may range in severity from transient undetected deterioration in renal function to acute renal failure requiring dialysis. The diagnosis is usually based on a thorough history of possible contributing events. The clinical diagnosis is supported by nonspecific findings of tubular epithelial casts and amorphous urates in the urine sediment and a persistent nephrogram on 24-hour delayed x-rays. The clinical course is characterized in 50 per cent of patients by oliguria, which begins shortly after the contrast injection and persists for 2 to 4 days. Diuretics and osmotic agents are not effective, and the severity of renal failure correlates with the severity of preexisting renal insufficiency. Although renal failure is reversible in most patients, dialysis may be required, and permanent renal failure may occur in some patients with severe preexisting renal insufficiency.

Contrast nephropathy can be reduced by the cautious use of contrast materials in patients at high risk. The use of ultrasonography, isotope renogram, or retrograde pyelography in lieu of intravenous contrast studies will prevent many episodes of acute contrast nephropathy. If contrast media must be utilized, the risk of nephrotoxicity may be reduced by avoiding dehydration and scheduling contrast studies at long intervals to avoid cumulative toxic effects. The dose of contrast material should be small, and diuretics plus osmotic agents should be administered before and after the study. The use of other potentially nephrotoxic drugs should be avoided (Schwartz et al., 1963; Byrd and Sherman, 1970; Teruel et al., 1981).

POLYURIA

Polyuria is generally defined as a urine volume of 2500 ml or more per day. It is invariably accompanied by nocturia. Polyuria can be caused by (1) compulsive water drinking due to psychogenic factors, (2) inadequate vasopressin secretion (neurogenic diabetes insipidus), (3) diminished response of the renal tubule to vasopressin (nephrogenic diabetes insipidus), or (4) osmotic diuresis owing to excessive endogenous or exogenous solute load. Since polyuria can lead to a negative water balance and polydipsia (increased water intake), the clinician is frequently presented with the dilemma of determining whether polyuria or polydipsia is the initial event. Patients with water diuresis (psychogenic polydipsia or neurogenic or nephrogenic diabetes insipidus) typically excrete hypotonic urine with a urine osmolality as low as 50 mOsm/kg of water. Patients with polyuria due to osmotic diuresis characteristically show isotonic or slightly hypertonic urine osmolality.

PSYCHOGENIC POLYDIPSIA

Affected individuals frequently are women with psychoneurotic disorders manifested by hypochondriac complaints and a pattern of a gradual onset of excessive daytime polydipsia. Urine osmolality is generally hypotonic to the plasma osmolality, which is usually normal. The plasma levels of antidiuretic hormone are undetectable. Management includes gradual reduction of fluid intake, which must proceed with care since the individual is unable to concentrate urine because of urea washout from the renal medulla.

NEUROGENIC DIABETES INSIPIDUS

Pituitary diabetes insipidus is sometimes seen as a consequence of brain tumor, after head trauma, or following pituitary ablation for acromegaly. The defect in antidiuretic hormone release is frequently transient, since only 10 per cent of normal hypothalamic nuclei, which produce antidiuretic hormone, are necessary to avoid diabetes insipidus. The disease usually starts abruptly with the sudden onset of polyuria and polydipsia. Nocturia is almost invariably present, as is continuous thirst. Since in these patients polyuria causes polydipsia, the plasma osmolality is in the high-normal range. The plasma levels of antidiuretic hormone are undetectable. The treatment of neurogenic diabetes insipidus is primary replacement therapy with exogenous antidiuretic hormone.

NEPHROGENIC DIABETES INSIPIDUS

Nephrogenic diabetes insipidus may be idiopathic or acquired. The idiopathic form is commonly genetic and more frequently affects males than females. During infancy the disorder may present with dehydration, vomiting, lethargy, fever, hypernatremia, and hypertonic urine. The hypernatremia may be severe enough to cause permanent brain damage and the associated mental retardation frequently seen in this disorder. Older children may present with enuresis. Intravenous urograms often show marked hydronephrosis, dilated ureters, and megacystis presumably secondary to increased urine flow rates (Ramsey et al., 1974). The plasma osmolality is usually high normal, and the plasma antidiuretic hormone level is greatly elevated. An acquired form of nephrogenic diabetes insipidus may be caused by a variety of conditions (e.g., obstructive uropathy, sickle-cell disease, potassium depletion, hypercalcemia, chronic pyelonephritis, analgesic nephritis) and drugs (e.g., lithium, amphotericin B).

Unexplained hypernatremia (hyperosmolality) is often an important clue that suggests nephrogenic diabetes insipidus. The diagnosis is established by demonstrating inability to concentrate urine despite an appropriate osmolalitic stimulus. In neurogenic diabetes insipidus, vasopressin administration corrects the concentrating defect, whereas in nephrogenic diabetes insipidus, vasopressin does not increase urine osmolality above 300 mOsm/kg (total unresponsiveness to antidiuretic hormone) or 800 mOsm/kg (partial nephrogenic diabetes insipidus).

Treatment consists of correcting the underlying cause if possible. The diuretic chlorothiazide coupled with a low-sodium diet (2 gm/day for an adult) has often been useful in reducing urine volume in patients with nephrogenic diabetes insipidus (Schotland et al., 1963). It acts by initially depleting total body sodium, which secondarily augments proximal tubular cellular reabsorption and presumably results in increased water reabsorption and reduced urine volume. Untreated nephrogenic diabetes insipidus can result in severe dehydration, especially in an infant who is unable to respond to thirst by increasing water intake. Correction of dehydration should be with 3 per cent dextrose in water, since 5 per cent dextrose alone or in saline solution may provoke an osmotic diuresis, increase water losses, and aggravate the condition. Partial nephrogenic diabetes insipidus, which is usually seen in females, may respond to chlorpropamide, which appears to sensitize the remaining functioning distal renal tubule to circulating endogenous vasopressin.

OSMOTIC DIURESIS

Increased solute excretion per nephron decreases urine osmolality irrespective of the presence or absence of antidiuretic hormone. Polyuria due to osmotic diuresis is seen in glycosuria associated with diabetes mellitus, after relief of obstructive uropathy, with high-protein feeding, and transiently with mannitol or radiographic contrast media infusion. Diuresis after relief of urinary tract obstruction may be due to physiologic excretion of excess salt and water or osmotic diuresis due to retained urea. In addition, inappropriate losses of sodium and water may be due to an intrinsic defect in tubular reabsorption of sodium or impaired renal concentrating capacity. Postobstructive diuresis may require intravenous fluid administration, but urinary losses should be replaced only to the extent necessary to prevent hypovolemia, hypotension, hyponatremia, and hypokalemia. Orthostatic hypotension and tachycardia are excellent indicators for fluid replacement. Daily weights and electrolyte and fluid balance should be monitored. In order to distinguish between inappropriate diuresis and appropriate excretion of retained fluids, the rate of intravenous fluid administration can be gradually reduced and a corresponding reduction in urine volume watched for.

RADIOLOGIC DIAGNOSES

Radiologic studies may reveal unsuspected nephrologic disorders that have acute or chronic urologic significance.

PAPILLARY NECROSIS

The renal medulla and papilla are particularly vulnerable to ischemic necrosis, owing to the peculiar arrangement of its blood supply and the hypertonic environment. Even when healthy, it exists in a state of relative hypoxia because of the slow rate of blood flow in the

vasa recta. Conditions that further reduce blood flow may therefore produce frank ischemic necrosis. The most common among these in adults are diabetes, with its associated vascular disease and infection; urinary obstruction, which may reduce blood flow within the kidney; pyelonephritis; and sickle-cell disease, in which sickling is intensified by the hypertonic and relatively hypoxic renal medulla. The high concentration of drugs such as phenacetin in these regions probably contributes to papillary necrosis characteristic of analgesic abuse.

Papillary necrosis is a pathologic description frequently diagnosed by radiologic criteria and is not a clinical entity, and therefore the clinical manifestations may be quite varied. It may present as an acute episode of severe sepsis associated with systemic toxicity and ureteral obstruction owing to a sloughed papilla. This form most frequently occurs in patients with diabetes and pyelonephritis. Patients may also present with colicky flank pain and hematuria. Latent papillary necrosis is diagnosed during pyelography and is probably the most common presentation of papillary necrosis. It should be expected in patients with sterile pyuria and impaired concentrating abilities. The calyceal deformities of renal papillary necrosis may be divided into two forms, medullary and papillary. In the medullary form there is central necrosis of the tip of the pyramid. Detachment of the necrotic papilla starts in the central region of the calyx, and a round or oval cavity occurs. In the papillary form, there is necrosis of the larger portion of the entire papilla. Detachment of the necrotic papilla usually begins in the region of the calyceal fornices, and the resulting defect is triangular in shape. Various stages of this process may be seen on the same radiographic examination. With poor renal function, retrograde pyelography may be required to demonstrate the calyceal changes.

Patients presenting with papillary slough and ureteral obstruction are probably best managed by ureteral catheterization or basket extraction if possible. Long-term remission may follow nephrectomy or partial nephrectomy since exacerbations are usually unilateral. As papillary necrosis proceeds, decreased GFR and kidney size may be minimized by careful management of infection, diabetes, and hydration.

MEDULLARY SPONGE KIDNEY

Medullary sponge kidney is characterized by dilatation of the collecting tubules, particularly in the papillary region. Intravenous urog-

TABLE 60–4. PEDIATRIC RENAL DISEASES OF
UROLOGIC SIGNIFICANCE

Hereditary nephritis and deafness (Alport syndrome)
Medullary cystic disease
Hemolytic uremic syndrome
Thrombotic thrombocytopenic purpura
Sickle cell nephropathy
Renal vein thrombosis

raphy characteristically demonstrates kidneys of normal size and shape, with ectatic distal collecting tubules containing clusters of calcifications. The calyceal blush may be distributed bilaterally or may involve only a few calyces. The medullary sponge kidney is asymptomatic, but it may be associated with nephrolithiasis or recurrent urinary tract infections. In the absence of complications, no therapy is required and the prognosis is excellent. Efforts to control the progression of nephrocalcinosis have not been assessed.

PEDIATRIC DISEASES OF UROLOGIC SIGNIFICANCE

The preceding discussion focused primarily on adult renal diseases of urologic significance. Renal disorders that are characteristically identified in a pediatric population are listed in Table 60–4.

References

Abraham, P., Harkmen, S., and Kjellstrand, C.: *In* Contrast nephropathy. Massry, S. G., and Glassock, R. J. (Eds.): Textbook of Nephrology. Baltimore, The Williams & Wilkins Co., 1983, p. 6.206.

Arneil, G. C., MacDonald, A. M., Murphy, A. V., and Sweet, E. M.: Renal venous thrombosis. Clin. Nephrol., *1*:119, 1973.

Baker, S. L., and Dodds, E. C. Obstruction of renal tubules during the excretion of haemoglobin. Br. J. Exp. Pathol., *6*:247, 1925.

Berger, J., and Hinglais, N.: Les dépots intercapillaires d'IgA–IgG. J. Urol. Nephrol. (Paris), *74*:694, 1968.

Besarab, A., Brown, R. S., Rubin, N. T., Salzman, E., Wirthlin, L., Steinman, T., Atlia, R. R., and Skillman, J. J.: Reversible renal failure following bilateral renal artery occlusive disease. Clinical features, pathology, and the role of surgical revascularization. JAMA, *235*:2838, 1976.

Bosniak, M. A.: Radiographic manifestations of massive arteriovenous fistula in renal carcinoma. Radiology, *85*:454, 1965.

Buckalew, V. M., and Someren, A.: Renal manifestations of sickle cell disease. Arch. Intern. Med., *133*:660, 1974.

Byrd, L., and Sherman, R. L.: Radiocontrast-induced acute renal failure: A clinical and pathophysiologic review. Medicine, *58*:270, 1970.

Cho, K. J., and Stanley, J. C.: Non-neoplastic congenital and acquired renal arteriovenous malformations and fistulas. Radiology, *129*:333, 1978.

Clark, R. A., Gallant, T. E., and Alexander, E. S.: Angiographic management of traumatic arteriovenous fistulas: Clinical results. Radiology, *147*:9, 1983.

Earle, D. P. (Ed.): Manual of Clinical Nephrology. Philadelphia, W. B. Saunders Co., 1982, pp. 29–30, 71–72.

Fassett, R. G., Horgan, B. A., and Mathew, T. H.: Detection of glomerular bleeding by phase-contrast microscopy. Lancet, *1*:1432, 1982.

Gajewski, J., Gonzales, C. I., and Rich, M.: Genitourinary diseases. *In* Singer, R. B., and Levinson, L. (Eds.): Medical Risks. Lexington, D. C. Heath and Co., 1976, pp. 151–156.

Glassock, R. J.: Hematuria and pigmenturia. *In* Massry, S. B., and Glassock, R. J. (Eds.): Textbook of Nephrology. Baltimore, The Williams & Wilkins Co., 1983, p. 414.

Gomes, M. M. R., and Bernatz, P.E.: Arteriovenous fistulas: A review and ten year experience at the Mayo Clinic. Mayo Clin. Proc., *45*:81, 1970.

Humphreys, M. H.: Thromboembolic disorders of the major renal vessels. *In* Brenner, B. M., and Rector, F. C. (Eds.): The Kidney. Philadelphia, W. B. Saunders Co., 1981, pp. 742–750.

Iloreta, A. T., and Blaufox, M. D.: Natural history of postbiopsy renal arteriovenous fistula: A 10-year follow-up. Nephron, *24*:250, 1979.

King, S. E., and Gronbeck, C.: Benign and pathological albuminuria: A study of 600 hospitalized cases. Ann. Intern. Med., *36*:765, 1952.

Knochel, J. P.: Hematuria in sickle trait: The effect of intravenous distilled water, urinary alkalinization, and diuresis. Arch. Intern. Med., *123*:160, 1969.

Labovitz, E. D., Steinmuller, S. R., Henderson, L. W., McCurdy, D. K., and Goldberg, M.: "Benign" hematuria with focal glomerulitis in adults. Ann. Intern. Med., *77*:723, 1972.

Larsen, S. O., and Thysell, H.: Four years follow-up of asymptomatic isolated proteinuria diagnosed in a general health survey. Acta Med. Scand., *186*:375, 1969.

Lisbona, R., Palayew, M. J., Satin, R., and Hyams, B. B.: Radionuclide detection of iatrogenic arteriovenous fistulas of the genitourinary system. Radiology, *134*:201, 1980.

Llach, F., Papper, S., and Massry, S. G.: The clinical spectrum of renal vein thrombosis: Acute and chronic. Am. J. Med., *69*:819, 1980.

Messing, E., Kessler, R., and Kavaney, P. B.: Renal arteriovenous fistulas. Urology, *8*:101, 1976.

Nelson, B. D., Brosman, S. A., and Goodwin, W. E.: Renal arteriovenous fistulas. J. Urol., *109*:779, 1973.

O'Brien, D. P., III, Parrott, T. S., Walton, K. N., and Lewis, E. L.: Renal arteriovenous fistulas. Surg. Gynecol. Obstet., *139*:739, 1974.

Perkins, R. P., Jacobsen, D. S., Feder, F. P., Lipchik, E. O., and Fine, P. H.: Return of renal function after late embolectomy. N. Engl. J. Med., *276*:1194, 1967.

Ramsey, E. W., Morrin, P. A. F., and Bruce, A. W.: Nephrogenic diabetes insipidus associated with massive hydronephrosis and bladder neck obstruction. J. Urol., *111*:225, 1974.

Randolph, M. F., and Greenfield, M.: Proteinuria: A six-year study of normal infants, preschool, and school-age populations previously screened for urinary tract diseases. Am. J. Dis. Child., *114*:631, 1967.

Rennie, I. D. B., and Keen, H.: Evaluation of clinical methods for detecting proteinuria. Lancet, 2:489, 1967.

Rowland, L. P., and Penn, A. S.: Myoglobinuria. Med. Clin. North Am., 56:1233, 1972.

Schmidt, J. D., and Flocks, R. H.: Urologic aspects of sickle-cell hemoglobin. J. Urol., 106:740, 1971.

Schotland, M. G., Grumbach, M. M., and Strauss, J.: The effects of chlorothiazides in nephrogenic diabetes insipidus. Pediatrics, 31:741, 1963.

Schrier, R. W. (Ed.): Renal and Electrolyte Disorders. 2nd ed. Boston, Little, Brown & Co., 1980, p. 417.

Schwartz, G. J., Haycock, G. B., and Spitzer, A.: Plasma creatinine and urea concentration in children: Normal values for age and sex. J. Pediatr., 88:828, 1976.

Schwartz, W. B., Hurwit, A., and Ettinger, A.: Intravenous urography in the patient with renal insufficiency. N. Engl. J. Med., 269:277, 1963.

Strom, T., Muehrcke, R. C., and Smith, R. D.: Sickle cell anemia with the nephrotic syndrome and renal vein obstruction. Arch. Intern. Med., 129:104, 1972.

Teruel, J. L., Marcen, R., Onaindia, J. M., Serrano, A., Quereda, C., and Ortuno, J.: Renal function impairment caused by intravenous urography, a prospective study. Arch. Intern. Med., 141:1271, 1981.

Thompson, I. M., Schneider, R., and Lababidi, Z.: Thrombectomy of neonatal renal vein thrombosis. J. Urol., 113:396, 1975.

Vega, R., Shanberg, A. M., and Malloy, T. R.: The use of epsilon-aminocaproic acid in sickle cell trait hematuria. J. Urol., 105:552, 1971.

Wagner, M. G., Smith, F. G., Jr., Tinglof, B. O., and Cornberg, E.: Epidemiology of proteinuria: A study of 4807 school children. J. Pediatr., 73:825, 1968.

Wickre, C. G., and Golper, T. A.: Complications of percutaneous needle biopsy of the kidney. Am. J. Nephrol., 2:173, 1982.

UROLOGIC SURGERY

CHAPTER 61

Perioperative Care

CHARLES B. BRENDLER, M.D.

INTRODUCTION

During the past decade there have been significant advances in perioperative care that have greatly facilitated the overall management of surgical patients. Urologists need to keep abreast of these developments, particularly since the scope of urologic surgery has expanded so dramatically in recent years. This chapter is intended to provide an update on the recent advances in perioperative care.

PERIOPERATIVE CARDIAC CARE

Preoperative Assessment and Management

CARDIAC RISK FACTORS

Goldman et al. have identified nine major perioperative cardiac risk factors (Table 61–1), and based on these factors they have developed a multifactorial index of cardiac risk (Table 61–2). (Goldman et al., 1977). Thirty-eight of the 53 risk points are derived directly from cardiac conditions, and 28 of the 53 points are reversible (Baesl and Buckley, 1983). Elective surgery thus should be postponed until the patient's cardiovascular status can be optimized. The assessment and management of specific cardiac problems are discussed in the following sections.

CONGESTIVE HEART FAILURE

Patients with clinical heart failure (New York Heart Classification III/IV) have little or no cardiac reserve and have a greater risk for cardiac morbidity and mortality. Goldman et al. (1977) studied 35 patients with either an S3 gallop or jugular venous distention who under-

went noncardiac surgical procedures. In this group, there was a 14 per cent incidence of cardiac complications and a 20 per cent incidence of cardiac mortalities. Conversely, patients with compensated congestive heart failure do not have an increased risk for surgically related cardiac complications. It is recommended, therefore, that patients with severe congestive heart failure undergo corrective treatment with digitalis, diuretics, and vasodilators prior to undergoing surgery.

The indications for preoperative administration of digitalis include (1) a prior history of congestive heart failure, (2) cardiac dysfunction with evidence of impaired ventricular perform-

TABLE 61–1. PERIOPERATIVE RISK FACTORS FOR CARDIAC MORBIDITY

1. S_3 gallop or jugular venous distention—11 points
2. Myocardial infarction in past 6 months—10 points
3. Arrhythmia other than premature atrial contractions—7 points
4. History at any time of > 5 PVCs per minute—7 points
5. Age > 70 years—5 points
6. Emergency operation—4 points
7. Intraperitoneal, intrathoracic, or aortic operation—3 points
8. Significant valvular aortic stenosis—3 points
9. Poor general condition—any one of factors below—3 points
   a. Po_2 < 60 mm Hg or Pco_2 > 50 mm Hg
   b. K < 3 mEq/L or HCO_3^- < 20 mEq/L
   c. BUN > 50 mg/dl or creatinine > 3 mg/dl
   d. Elevated SGOT
   e. Chronic liver disease
   f. Bedridden from noncardiac disease

Total possible: 53 points

(From Goldman, L., Caldera, D. L., Nussbaum, S. R., et al.: Multifactoral index of cardiac risk in noncardiac surgical procedures. N. Engl. J. Med., 297:845, 1977. Used with permission.)

TABLE 61–2. CARDIAC RISK INDEX

Class	Points	Life-Threatening Complications (%)	Deaths (%)
I	0 – 5	0.7	0.2
II	6 – 12	5	2
III	13 – 25	11	2
IV	26 – 53	22	56

(From Goldman, L., Caldera, D. L., Nussbaum, S. R., et al.: Multifactorial index of cardiac risk in noncardiac surgical procedures. N. Engl. J. Med., 297:845, 1977. Used with permission.)

ance, (3) nocturnal angina, (4) atrial fibrillation or flutter with a rapid ventricular response, and (5) frequent episodes of paroxysmal atrial or junctional tachycardia (Mason, 1974). Digitalis is not recommended on the basis of either advanced age or the presence of coronary artery disease alone. Digitalis should be started several days prior to surgery so that an adequate therapeutic level can be achieved.

Additional therapeutic measures that may be employed in patients with congestive heart failure include the administration of diuretics to decrease the ventricular fluid load and the use of cardiotonic and vasodilating agents, such as isoproterenol, dopamine, and nitroprusside, to improve myocardial function.

It was previously believed that propranolol and other beta-adrenergic blocking agents should be discontinued several days preoperatively because of possible myocardial depression (Viljoen et al., 1972). Recent studies have shown that there is no increased risk associated with continuing beta-blockers perioperatively (Slogoff et al., 1978), and that their withdrawal may precipitate serious myocardial ischemia (Miller et al., 1975). Furthermore, perioperative administration of these agents has beneficial antiarrhythmic effects and protects against myocardial ischemia. Therefore, beta-blockers should be continued until surgery and restarted immediately thereafter, administering them parenterally if necessary (Prys-Roberts et al., 1973).

MYOCARDIAL INFARCTION

Patients with a prior history of myocardial infarction have an increased risk of surgically related cardiac complications. Although the risk of surgically related myocardial infarction in patients without previous heart disease is less than 2 per cent, the infarction rate in patients who have sustained a previous myocardial infarction is between 6 and 8 per cent. (Goldman et al., 1977; Tarhan et al., 1972). Patients who undergo surgery within 3 months after a myocardial infarction have a 37 per cent incidence of reinfarction. This rate decreases to 16 per cent in the next 3 months, and stabilizes between 5 and 8 per cent 6 months after the original infarction (Steen et al., 1978; Tarhan et al., 1972). Perioperative myocardial infarction usually occurs in the first postoperative week and is not associated with chest pain in 50 per cent of patients (Goldman et al., 1978). Although the mortality rate from an initial myocardial infarction is about 20 to 30 per cent, the mortality rate from a recurrent myocardial infarction is between 50 and 80 per cent (Goldman et al., 1978; Plumlee and Boehner, 1972; Tarhan et al., 1972).

Because of the high mortality associated with a recurrent myocardial infarction, elective surgery should be postponed for at least 6 months after an infarction. Since about 50 per cent of recurrent myocardial infarctions are clinically silent, patients who have had a recent myocardial infarction and must undergo surgical procedures should be monitored closely in an intensive care unit for several days postoperatively. A continuous electrocardiogram, blood pressure monitoring with an arterial catheter, and evaluation of left ventricular function with a pulmonary arterial (Swan-Ganz) catheter may be required. Placement of an intra-aortic balloon pump may be necessary to provide optimal coronary blood flow. Hypoxia should be avoided, and electrolyte and acid-base disorders should be corrected promptly to decrease the incidence of arrhythmias. Arrhythmias should be treated with appropriate drugs, by the insertion of a cardiac pacemaker, or by the application of direct current countershock when necessary (Baesl and Buckley, 1983).

Local anesthesia can be administered during the first 6 months following a myocardial infarction (Backer et al., 1980), and cystoscopy can be performed safely under local anesthesia without cardiac complications (Fraser et al., 1967). It has been reported that transurethral resection of the prostate may be performed safely within the first 6 months following a myocardial infarction (Thompson et al., 1962), but it is prudent to postpone any elective surgery requiring general or regional anesthesia until 6 months have passed.

Patients with stable angina and without a prior history of myocardial infarction do not have an increased perioperative cardiac risk (Goldman et al., 1978). Patients with unstable angina have a markedly increased risk and should not undergo elective surgical procedures (Skinner and Pearce, 1964).

ARRHYTHMIAS

Preoperative. Patients with sinus bradycardia should be evaluated for a possible remedial problem, such as hypothyroidism or digitalis toxicity. If the cause cannot be determined, patients should undergo further evaluation, including exercise testing and the possible administration of atropine to determine if the heart rate can be elevated above 100 beats per minute. Patients with sick sinus syndrome should undergo placement of a temporary cardiac pacemaker preoperatively and should be scheduled for insertion of a permanent cardiac pacemaker after surgery (Rose et al., 1979).

Premature atrial contractions are usually benign, but they may reflect a decreased cardiac reserve, which may increase cardiac risk. Patients with ventricular arrhythmias are at increased risk when undergoing surgery, and patients with frequent premature ventricular contractions or potentially dangerous ventricular extra systoles (multifocal, salvos, or occurring on the preceding T wave) require preoperative treatment. The initial treatment is usually intravenous lidocaine given as a bolus of 50 to 100 mg, followed by a continuous infusion of 1 to 4 mg per minute (Rose et al., 1979).

Intraoperative. Premature ventricular contractions occur commonly during surgery and usually are of little clinical significance. They often are precipitated by inadequate ventilation and increased adrenergic stimulation and can be treated by decreasing the concentration of anesthetic agent, hyperventilation, decreased administration of catecholamines, and decreased manipulation of vital organs. Ventricular tachyarrhythmias should be treated with antiarrhythmic agents, since they may cause circulatory depression or ventricular fibrillation (Katz and Bigger, 1970).

Postoperative. Supraventricular tachycardia occurs in about 4 per cent of surgical patients postoperatively (Goldman et al., 1978). Atrial fibrillation is the most common supraventricular tachyarrhythmia and accounts for about half of the cases. Preoperative factors that are associated with the development of postoperative arrhythmias include age greater than 70 years; major thoracic, abdominal, or vascular operations; and the presence of pulmonary rales. Patients who develop postoperative arrhythmias frequently have one or more of the following associated problems: congestive heart failure, a history of a previous myocardial infarction, cardiac tamponade, a hematocrit of less than 30 per cent, hypotension, hypokalemia, metabolic acidosis, hypernatremia, hypoxia, or fever. Although the mortality associated with the arrhythmia alone is minimal, the overall mortality associated with these underlying conditions approaches 50 per cent (Goldman, 1978). A summary of antiarrhythmic therapy is provided in Table 61–3.

VALVULAR HEART DISEASE

Skinner and Pearce (1964) found that aortic stenosis and aortic insufficiency were the two valvular heart lesions associated with the greatest risk of cardiac complications in patients undergoing noncardiac surgery. Goldman et al. (1978) confirmed that aortic stenosis was associated with a 14-fold increase in cardiac death, but they found that a mitral regurgitation murmur greater than Grade II/VI was associated with the second greatest cardiac risk. Mitral regurgitation may be caused not only by mitral valvular disease but also by papillary muscle dysfunction resulting from ischemic heart disease.

Patients with serious cardiac murmurs, such as aortic stenosis or mitral regurgitation, should undergo corrective heart surgery prior to undergoing elective noncardiac surgery. All patients with valvular heart disease should receive antibacterial prophylaxis prior to undergoing any surgical procedure (see section on Infections and Antibiotic Therapy).

The perioperative management of patients with prosthetic heart valves receiving anticoagulation therapy is somewhat controversial. There is a high incidence of perioperative hemorrhage if anticoagulation is continued during surgery (Katholi et al., 1976). However, there is a significant risk of thromboembolic disease associated with cessation of anticoagulation therapy. This risk is greatest in patients with mitral valvular disease with associated left atrial enlargement and atrial fibrillation (Messmer et al., 1972). Currently, it is recommended that patients with a prosthetic aortic valve should discontinue anticoagulants 3 to 5 days preoperatively and should resume therapy 48 hours

TABLE 61–3. THERAPY OF ARRHYTHMIAS

Arrhythmias	Therapy (In Order of Preference)
Supraventricular	
Tachycardia	Verapamil, quinidine, procainamide
Atrial flutter	Cardioversion, digoxin
Atrial fibrillation	Cardioversion, quinidine, procainamide disopyramide (to maintain sinus rhythm); digoxin, propranolol (to control ventricular response)
Ventricular	
PVCs—emergency	Lidocaine, procainamide, bretylium
PVCs—chronic	Quinidine, procainamide, disopyramide, combinations (see below)
Tachycardia	Lidocaine, procainamide, bretylium, cardioversion
Combination therapy for suppression of ventricular ectopy	Quinidine—procainamide (for maximal quinidine—like effect at a lower dose for each agent)
	Quinidine or procainamide with propranolol in patients without congestive heart failure
	Quinidine—procainamide with lidocaine or diphenylhydantoin
Digitalis-induced arrhythmias	Lidocaine, diphenylhydantoin

(From Karliner, J., and Gregoratos, G. (Eds.): Coronary Care. New York, Churchill Livingstone, 1981. Used with permission.)

postoperatively. Patients with a prosthetic mitral valve should discontinue oral anticoagulants 24 hours preoperatively, and the prothrombin time should be normalized with fresh frozen plasma or vitamin K. Intravenous heparin is begun 12 hours after surgery and is continued for 3 days postoperatively, at which time anticoagulants are resumed. The use of intravenous heparin in the perioperative period has the advantages of a rapid onset of action and the potential for rapid reversibility if hemorrhage should develop (Katholi et al., 1978).

HYPERTENSION

Although it is desirable for patients to be normotensive prior to surgery, patients with diastolic blood pressures less than 120 mm Hg do not have an increased risk of cardiac complications (Goldman and Caldera, 1979). Patients with diastolic blood pressures greater than 120 mm Hg do have an increased risk at surgery, mainly because they may have wider and more frequent changes of blood pressure under anesthesia. Patients whose normal systolic blood pressure falls by more than one third for as little as 10 minutes during surgery have an increased incidence of cardiovascular complications (Goldman and Caldera, 1979; Mauney et al., 1970).

As with beta-adrenergic blockers, other antihypertensive agents should be continued until the time of surgery and should not be withdrawn preoperatively. Postoperatively, blood pressure should be regulated with parenteral agents until patients can restart their oral medications (Prys-Roberts et al., 1973). Clonidine, a central-acting antiadrenergic agent, deserves special mention, since abrupt cessation of this drug may precipitate severe hypertension. Patients receiving clonidine who will not be able to resume oral medications for several days postoperatively should discontinue clonidine 2 weeks preoperatively and start on alternative therapy (Blaschke and Melmon, 1980). Patients receiving diuretics should be evaluated preoperatively for possible hypokalemia and hypovolemia.

PACEMAKERS

Permanent pacemakers should be checked preoperatively to be sure they are capturing consistently and firing at the stated rate. Direct electromagnetic interference of a permanent demand pacemaker by the use of electrocautery during surgery may cause pacemaker inhibition. This is of particular concern in patients undergoing transurethral resection (Wojsycyuk et al., 1969), and certain precautions are necessary to protect patients in this situation. First, the pacemaker should be changed preoperatively from a demand to a fixed mode. Second, the diathermy plate should be positioned as far away from the pacemaker as possible, usually on the thigh or buttocks. Third, the duration of each cautery burst should be limited as much as possible. Fourth, a temporary pacemaker as well as antiarrhythmic agents should be available in the operating room in case a problem should develop (Simon, 1977).

Cardiovascular Effects of Anesthesia

All anesthetic agents produce some degree of myocardial depression, which may result in perioperative heart failure or cardiogenic shock (Kaplan and Dunbar, 1979). This depression may occur at levels that produce only light anesthesia. Halothane produces the greatest myocardial depression, and nitrous oxide produces the least (Price and Helrich, 1955). Narcotics have a variable effect on myocardial function. Morphine and fentanyl have minimal depressant activity, but meperidine has a marked depressant effect (Lee et al., 1976). Barbiturates produce vasodilatation and have little myocardial depressant action except in large doses (Eckstein et al., 1961). Valium is generally free of cardiovascular effects except when administered by rapid infusion (Stanley et al., 1976).

Anesthetic agents also may precipitate cardiac arrhythmias. Arrhythmias frequently occur during induction of anesthesia, intubation, and extubation because of associated blood pressure changes, hypoxia, hypercapnea, and endogenous catecholamine release (Katz and Bigger, 1970). The incidence of arrhythmias is greater in patients with a history of heart disease (Vanik and Davis, 1968).

Regional anesthesia is not necessarily safer than general anesthesia in terms of cardiac risk (Steen et al., 1978). Regional anesthesia has two potential disadvantages. First, it may produce hypotension by sympathetic blockade, and second, it is not as reversible as general anesthesia in case cardiac problems develop intraoperatively. Local anesthesia is usually safe, though local anesthetic agents may produce myocardial depression when administered in large amounts (Hughes et al., 1966).

Hemodynamic Monitoring

A variety of methods currently exist to monitor the cardiovascular status of the surgical patient. The purpose of this section is to review the indications, techniques, and complications of these methods.

ARTERIAL PRESSURE MONITORING

Indications. There are two major reasons to insert an arterial catheter. The first is to allow continuous blood pressure monitoring, which is desirable for surgical patients who are anticipated to lose large volumes of blood or for patients who can be expected to have rapid changes in blood pressure because of the nature of the surgical procedure (e.g., pheochromocytoma). Continuous blood pressure monitoring is required postoperatively for patients receiving intravenous infusions of vasopressor or vasodilating agents. The second reason to insert an arterial catheter is to facilitate repeated arterial blood sampling. Arterial puncture causes significant discomfort to patients, and percutaneous arterial samples may be inaccurate resulting from admixture of small amounts of venous blood (Sheldon and Leonard, 1983).

Techniques. The usual technique for the placement of an arterial catheter involves percutaneous insertion of a Teflon catheter over a thin needle into the radial artery. Alternatively, the catheter may be placed by a cutdown. Patency of the arterial catheter is maintained by a slow (3 ml per hour), continuous infusion of heparinized saline (5 U per ml). Continuous heparin infusion is preferable to intermittent flushing of the catheter with a bolus of heparin, because the latter technique is associated with an increased incidence of thromboembolic complications (Downs et al., 1974).

The risk of radial artery cannulation is related to the patency of the ulnar artery and the palmar arch. The palmar arch is interrupted in about 20 per cent of patients (Coleman and Anson, 1961). The Allen test should be performed whenever possible prior to radial artery cannulation (Allen, 1929). This test is done by occlusion of the radial and ulnar arteries and subsequent blanching of the hand by opening and closing the fist. The ulnar artery is then released, and the patency of the ulnar artery and palmar arch is assessed by the return of color to the hand.

Alternative sites of arterial cannulation should be considered if there is insufficiency of the ulnar artery or palmar arch. In adults and children, alternative sites include the brachial, femoral, and dorsalis pedis arteries, and in infants the umbilical and temporal arteries may be used.

Complications. Radial artery thrombosis occurs in 20 to 40 per cent of adults and in 50 per cent of children undergoing radial artery cannulation (Bedford and Wallinen, 1973; Evans and Kerr, 1975; Miyasaka et al., 1976). The risk of arterial thrombosis is related to several factors: (1) the duration of cannulation (Bedford and Wallinen, 1973; Evans and Kerr, 1975); (2) the size of the arterial cannula (Downs et al., 1973); (3) the age of the patient, the risk being increased in very young patients (Miyasaka et al., 1976); and (4) miscellaneous factors, including hypothermia, hypotension, the use of vasoconstrictor drugs, and the application of constrictive dressings over the cannulation site (Johnson et al., 1976). Arterial catheters should be removed as soon as they are no longer required and whenever thrombosis or ischemia is noted. Radial artery thrombosis may resolve and the artery may recannulize, but this may take as long as 75 days (Evans and Kerr, 1975).

Arteriography has demonstrated that arterial embolization occurs in 23 per cent of patients with arterial catheters (Downs et al., 1973). Cerebral embolism has resulted from the placement of temporal artery catheters in children, and several cases of hemiparesis in infants have been reported, most of which resolved spontaneously without serious sequelae (Browse et al., 1974; Simmons et al., 1978). The risk of arterial embolization can be reduced by using a continuous infusion rather than bolus administration of heparin to maintain catheter patency and by never irrigating the arterial cannula forcefully.

Heparin-induced thrombocytopenia may occur in patients with arterial catheters even with the small doses of heparin used for irrigation. Thrombocytopenia resolves after the heparin is discontinued (Sheldon and Leonard, 1983).

CENTRAL VENOUS PRESSURE MONITORING

Indications. The goals of cardiac monitoring are to ensure adequate perfusion of vital organs and to prevent cardiac decompensation and pulmonary congestion. The intravascular volume should be optimized to maximize arterial pressure and peripheral perfusion without exceeding left ventricular functional capacity. The most direct method of assessing circulatory volume and left ventricular function is by measurement of left atrial pressure via a left atrial catheter, which must be inserted at the time of open heart surgery. Alternatively, left ventricular end-diastolic pressure can be measured with a pulmonary arterial catheter inserted into the pulmonary arterial capillary bed (Swan and Ganz, 1975).

Central venous pressure measurements are unreliable in assessing intravascular volume and left ventricular function in patients with cardiorespiratory disease, in whom left ventricular and right ventricular function may differ significantly. Central venous pressure and left ventricular end-diastolic pressure may differ considerably in patients with coronary artery disease, valvular heart disease, and chronic obstructive pulmonary disease, and in patients with altered pulmonary vascular resistance resulting from sepsis or trauma (DeLaurentis et al., 1973; Russell et al., 1981). In the absence of cardiorespiratory disease, however, there is a close correlation between the two measurements (Civetta et al., 1972; Tousaint et al., 1964). Despite its limitations, the measurement of central venous pressure usually provides a useful first approximation of the adequacy of blood volume and ventricular function.

Techniques. Central venous pressure catheters are inserted via a percutaneous approach into the basilic, external jugular, internal jugular, or subclavian vein. Techniques of catheter insertion will be described briefly; the techniques are described in greater detail with accompanying diagrams in a recent publication. (Sheldon and Leonard, 1983).

The basilic vein can be cannulated safely by a percutaneous approach. The vein is punctured with a 14-gauge needle through which a 15-gauge Teflon catheter is advanced through the arm into the superior vena cava. The patient's head should be turned toward the side of catheterization to decrease the chance of advancing the catheter into the jugular vein.

The external jugular vein is cannulated by placing the patient in the Trendelenburg position and applying finger compression at the base of the neck to distend the vein. An 18-gauge catheter is inserted into the vein, and a guide wire is passed through the catheter and is used to negotiate the junction of the external and internal jugular veins. A 14- to 16-gauge catheter is threaded over the guide wire into the internal jugular vein.

Cannulation of the internal jugular vein provides direct access to the superior vena cava. The patient is placed in the Trendelenburg position, and the head is turned away from the side of cannulation. The needle is introduced 1 cm medial to the lateral edge of the sternocleidomastoid muscle and 5 cm above the clavicle. The needle is angled 30 degrees to the coronal plane and is advanced parallel to the anterior border of the sternocleidomastoid muscle. The internal jugular vein is punctured and cannulated, either with a catheter advanced over the needle or by inserting a guide wire and advancing the cannula over it.

Cannulation of the subclavian vein can be performed by a variety of techniques (Borja and Hinshaw, 1970). The risks associated with subclavian vein cannulation are greater than with any other technique, but the approach affords direct access to the superior vena cava. The patient is placed in the Trendelenburg position, and the vein is entered at the junction between the middle and medial thirds of the clavicle. The needle is directed either at or just above the sternal notch. The needle and syringe are kept against the chest wall so that the tip of the needle hugs the inferoposterior aspect of the clavicle to decrease the risk of pneumothorax. Maintenance of this angle is facilitated by the use of a small 3-ml syringe, which is kept against the anterior chest wall. Constant negative pressure is maintained on the syringe to identify when the vein is entered and to avoid piercing the subclavian artery.

Complications. The incidence of central venous catheter misplacement depends on the approach used. Catheter misplacement occurs in 30 per cent of patients undergoing basilic vein cannulation (Deitel and McIntyre, 1971) and in only 2 per cent of patients undergoing internal jugular vein cannulation (Eckstein et al., 1961). A chest roentgenogram must be obtained after insertion of a central venous pressure catheter to ascertain that the catheter is in correct position and that a pneumothorax does not exist. Misplacement of the catheter can be corrected either by repositioning the catheter over a guide wire or by passing a Fogarty catheter within the central venous pressure cannula; the balloon of the catheter is inflated and the cannula is flow-directed into correct position (Schaefer and Geelhoed, 1980).

Pneumothorax results in 1.4 to 6 per cent of patients undergoing subclavian vein cannulation (Guteen and Pollack, 1979; Herbst, 1978), but occurs only rarely with internal jugular cannulation (Brinkman and Costley, 1973). Hydrothorax may occur if the cannula tip is advanced accidentally into the mediastinum or the pleural space.

Erosion of the heart with resultant cardiac tamponade can occur if the catheter tip becomes lodged within the heart chambers (Nehma, 1980). This re-emphasizes the need for obtaining a chest roentgenogram following insertion of a central venous catheter and for periodic radiologic evaluation to monitor for possible catheter migration.

PULMONARY ARTERIAL PRESSURE MONITORING

Indications. Pulmonary arterial pressure monitoring is indicated in clinical situations in which there is a disparity between left ventricular and right ventricular function. In these conditions, central venous pressure measurements are unreliable, and measurements of pulmonary arterial and pulmonary wedge pressures must be relied upon to provide information about intravascular volume and left ventricular function. Changes in pulmonary arterial pressure accurately reflect changes in left atrial pressure (Jenkins et al., 1970), and there is a close correlation between an elevation in pulmonary wedge pressure above 18 to 20 mm Hg and radiologic evidence of pulmonary congestion (Del Guercio and Cohn, 1980).

Technique. A pulmonary arterial, or Swan-Ganz, catheter usually is inserted percutaneously via an internal jugular or subclavian approach. Once the catheter has been introduced, it is advanced under fluoroscopic guidance or by monitoring the pressure at the tip of the catheter to determine its position. Once the catheter enters the heart, the balloon at its end is inflated with air to facilitate flow guidance through the right ventricle and pulmonary artery. A typical pressure tracing obtained during placement of a Swan-Ganz catheter is shown in Figure 61–1. As the tip of the catheter enters the right ventricle, there is a sudden increase in pulse pressure with maintenance of a low diastolic pressure. Further advancement into the pulmonary artery is accompanied by a sudden rise in diastolic pressure with maintenance of a stable systolic pressure. As the catheter is advanced further, the balloon becomes wedged in the pulmonary capillary bed, which is accompanied by further dampening of the pulse pressure. The catheter is withdrawn slightly and is positioned so that wedging is achieved only upon full inflation of the balloon. Pulmonary wedge pressure normally varies between 5 and 12 mm Hg (Sheldon and Leonard, 1983).

Following insertion of a Swan-Ganz catheter, a chest roentgenogram should be obtained to check the position of the catheter tip, and daily chest films should be obtained to monitor for possible catheter migration. Patency of the

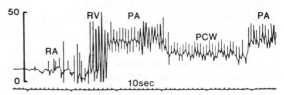

Figure 61–1. Pressure effects of the passage of a Swan-Ganz catheter tip. (RA, right atrium; RV, right ventricle; PA, pulmonary artery; PCW, pulmonary capillary wedge; PA, pulmonary artery pressure after deflation of the balloon.) (From Sheldon, C. A., and Leonard, A. S.: Hemodynamic monitoring. Urol. Clin. North Am. *10*:19, 1983. Used with permission.)

catheter is achieved by a continuous slow infusion of heparinized saline (Sheldon and Leonard, 1983).

Complications. The complications associated with pulmonary arterial catheters include technical problems such as catheter misplacement and pneumothorax. In addition, 80 per cent of patients undergoing insertion of a pulmonary arterial catheter will experience cardiac arrhythmias as the catheter is advanced through the right ventricle. These arrhythmias usually are self-limiting and resolve when the catheter passes into the pulmonary artery. It is important to monitor the electrocardiogram and to treat any serious arrhythmias promptly (Elliott et al., 1979).

Pulmonary infarction, arterial thrombosis, and arterial embolization have resulted from insertion of pulmonary arterial catheters (Foote et al., 1974). Perforation of the pulmonary artery also has been reported; it is a rare but devastating complication with a 50 per cent mortality (Barash et al., 1981). To minimize the risk of arterial perforation, the catheter balloon should never be inflated with fluid, the balloon should not be inflated too distally in the pulmonary capillary bed, and inflation of the balloon for measurement of pulmonary wedge pressure should be kept to a minimum (Kelley et al., 1981).

Damage to both the tricuspid and pulmonary valves has been reported from withdrawal of the catheter through the right heart chambers with the catheter balloon inflated (O'Toole et al., 1979; Smith et al., 1976). This re-emphasizes the importance of never inflating the catheter balloon with anything other than air.

CARDIAC OUTPUT AND MIXED VENOUS OXYGEN SATURATION

Placement of a pulmonary arterial catheter allows for direct measurement of cardiac output by a thermodilution technique. Measured cardiac output values are normalized by dividing the cardiac output by the body surface area and expressing the results in L per min per m.^{2} A normal cardiac index varies between 2.7 and 4.3 L per minute per m.^{2} Values between 2.2 and 2.7 L per minute per m^2 indicate subclinical myocardial depression; values between 1.8 and 2.2 L per minute per m^2 are associated with clinical myocardial depression; values less than 1.8 L per minute per m^2 reflect cardiac insufficiency (Forrester et al., 1976).

Placement of a pulmonary arterial catheter also makes possible the measurement of mixed venous oxygen saturation ($S\bar{v}O_2$), which is an additional parameter to assess the adequacy of peripheral perfusion. $S\bar{v}O_2$ is usually measured by blood sampling directly from the pulmonary arterial catheter. A newer technique uses an indwelling fiberoptic oxymeter on the pulmonary arterial catheter, which allows for a continuous digital readout of $S\bar{v}O_2$. The $S\bar{v}O_2$ correlates closely with cardiac output (De la Rocha et al., 1978). Values between 60 and 70 per cent are associated with adequate peripheral perfusion; values between 50 and 60 per cent suggest myocardial depression; values between 40 and 50 per cent reflect circulatory failure (Kazarian and Del Guercia, 1980).

PERIOPERATIVE PULMONARY CARE

Preoperative Assessment and Management

INITIAL EVALUATION

The initial evaluation of pulmonary status includes a history, physical examination, chest roentgenogram, and possibly an electrocardiogram. Important historical considerations include smoking, the presence of a productive cough or wheezing, exercise tolerance, previous exposure to general anesthesia, and the possibility of a recent upper respiratory tract infection. Significant physical findings include orthopnea or dyspnea at rest, pauses during speech caused by dyspnea, and wheezes with augmented breathing. The chest x-ray may not only reveal active pulmonary disease but may also detect distortion or deviation of the trachea, which may make intubation difficult (Harmon and Lillington, 1979).

Patients who have an increased risk of pulmonary complications may require further preoperative evaluation. Formal pulmonary function tests usually are unnecessary except in patients undergoing thoracic operations. Simple spirometry usually provides an accurate assessment of pulmonary reserve (Gilmour, 1983). Further testing is required only if the 1-second forced expiratory volume (FEV_1) is less than 15 ml per kg, the vital capacity is less than 1.5 L, or the maximum voluntary ventilation is less than 50 per cent (Hodgkin, 1979).

PULMONARY RISK FACTORS

Cigarette smokers and patients with chronic pulmonary disease have a three- to fourfold increased risk of postoperative pulmonary complications (Hedley-White et al., 1976). Patients with restrictive lung disease generally do better than patients with obstructive disease, because patients with restrictive disease maintain an adequate maximum expiratory flow rate, which allows a more effective cough with less retention of sputum (Malmberg et al., 1965). Patients with an acute or recent upper respiratory infection also have an increased risk of pulmonary complications (Steward and Sloane, 1969).

The site of the surgical incision also affects pulmonary risk. Except for thoracotomy incisions, upper abdominal incisions are associated with the highest incidence of atelectasis because of reduced diaphragmatic excursion and suppressed coughing and deep breathing due to incisional pain. Forthman found that 25 per cent of patients who had upper abdominal incisions developed pulmonary complications, whereas all patients who had pulmonary complications following lower abdominal incisions either had pre-existing lung disease or were cigarette smokers (Forthman and Shepard, 1969).

Age alone is not a risk factor for pulmonary complications, and older patients whose pulmonary function is comparable to younger patients do not experience increased pulmonary morbidity. (Boushy et al., 1971). Overall, there is a higher incidence of pulmonary complications in older patients because of the prevalence of pulmonary disease and associated abnormalities in pulmonary function (Grodsinsky et al., 1974).

Obesity is associated with a greatly increased incidence of pulmonary complications (Putnam et al., 1974). Obesity results in a decreased expiratory reserve volume, decreased functional reserve capacity, decreased Po_2, and increased breathing work. This results in earlier airway closure and ventilation-perfusion abnormalities (Strauss and Wise, 1978).

Anesthesia time in excess of 3 hours is associated with increased pulmonary complications (Wightman, 1968).

PREOPERATIVE MEASURES TO DECREASE PULMONARY RISK

In patients with pre-existing lung disease, cessation of smoking and the preoperative use of antibiotics and bronchodilators results in a significant reduction in postoperative pulmonary complications (Stein, 1970). Cigarettes should be discontinued at least 3 weeks prior to surgery (Hedley-White et al., 1976). Patients with acute respiratory infections should be treated with antibiotics, and elective surgery should be delayed until the infections are resolved. The use of preoperative antibiotics in patients with chronic bronchitis seems logical, but their efficacy has not been established in a controlled trial (Tisi, 1979). Bronchodilators are indicated for patients with obstructive pulmonary disease (Williams and Brenowitz, 1976).

Patients who require intensive care postoperatively benefit from preoperative psychological preparation and orientation to an intensive care environment. This results in decreased pain and narcotic usage postoperatively and may reduce the length of hospitalization (Egbert et al., 1964). Preoperative instruction in pulmonary therapy and deep breathing exercises also is beneficial. Thoren (1954) reported that only 12 per cent of patients who received preoperative instruction developed atelectasis postoperatively, compared with 27 per cent who received instructions postoperatively, and 42 per cent of an uninstructed control group.

Pulmonary Effects of Anesthesia and Surgery

In experimental studies, normal individuals given general anesthesia demonstrate impaired oxygenation and elimination of carbon dioxide, probably due to increased dead space ventilation, abnormalities of pulmonary ventilation and perfusion, and altered mechanics of chest wall and diaphragmatic motion (Rehder et al., 1975). During general anesthesia there is a progressive decrease in functional residual capacity (FRC), probably due to spontaneous atelectasis secondary to ventilation with decreased tidal volumes (Harman and Lillington, 1979). Barbiturates, halothane, and endotracheal intubation all interfere with mucociliary function and may cause retention of secretions and atelectasis (Gamsu et al., 1976).

It is often assumed that regional anesthesia is associated with a lower risk of pulmonary complications than is general anesthesia, but this has not been proved. General anesthesia has the advantage that it allows continuous control of the airway and pulmonary secretions (Hamilton and Sokoll, 1977). Furthermore, regional anesthesia may cause prolonged immobility in the supine position, with a resultant increase in pulmonary morbidity.

A number of physiologic changes occur postoperatively, which also contribute to the development of atelectasis and pulmonary morbidity. Tidal volume, FEV_1, and functional residual capacity are all decreased in the postoperative period (Meyers et al., 1975). These changes result from breathing in the supine position (Craig et al., 1971), postoperative pain, the administration of narcotics, and other factors that reduce diaphragmatic excursion, including abdominal distention, pneumoperitoneum, and constrictive bandages (Harman and Lillington, 1979). The normal pattern of ventilation is altered postoperatively, resulting in a decreased number of sigh breaths and an increased risk of atelectasis. Narcotics, atropine, and the use of increased inspired oxygen concentrations impair mucociliary function, resulting in retention of pulmonary secretions (Tisi, 1979).

Postoperative Pulmonary Care

The primary goal of postoperative respiratory therapy is to prevent atelectasis and subsequent pulmonary infection. The ideal maneuver to prevent atelectasis is sustained maximum inspiration with the glottis open or the so-called yawn maneuver (Bartlett et al., 1971). A variety of mechanical devices have been used to promote maximum inspiration. Regardless of the method employed, it must be repeated hourly to be effective, since alveoli will remain open for only 1 hour after inflation.

Positive pressure breathing initially was reported to be effective in achieving maximum inspiration and decreasing atelectasis (Anderson and Jensen, 1976), but subsequent studies have failed to demonstrate its efficacy (Baxter and Levine, 1969; Graham and Bradley, 1978). In order for positive pressure breathing to be effective, emphasis must be placed on the inflation volume achieved rather than the peak pressure obtained. Using peak pressure as a goal is ineffective, since postoperative atelectasis results in decreased pulmonary compliance; thus, a lower inspiratory volume is required to achieve a given pressure (Bartlett et al., 1973). Volume-oriented positive pressure breathing that achieves a tidal volume greater than 15 ml per kg may be beneficial (Welch et al., 1980). The use of blow bottles is variably effective. The main benefit is derived from the maximum inspiratory effort that precedes forced expiration (Iverson et al., 1978). The incentive spirometer is very effective in promoting maximum inspiration and preventing atelectasis. This device requires little instruction and can be left at the bedside for patients to use hourly.

Other measures may help prevent atelectasis. Early mobilization is desirable, since the supine position is associated with a decreased lung volume. Appropriate fluid management to avoid overhydration with subsequent pulmonary congestion or dehydration with drying of mucous secretions is important. Bronchodilators may be effective in reducing atelectasis, even in patients without airway disease (Gilmour, 1983). Antibiotics are indicated for patients with acute bronchitis or pneumonia (Hedley-White et al., 1976). Narcotics should be used cautiously to avoid respiratory depression (Egbert and Bendixen, 1974). Finally, patients with chronic pulmonary disease and a hypoxic respiratory drive should receive oxygen in low concentrations to avoid respiratory depression.

Mechanical Ventilation

INDICATIONS

The usual indication for positive pressure ventilation is acute respiratory failure manifested by a PCO_2 greater than 50 mm Hg and a blood pH less than 7.30, or by profound hypoxia with a PO_2 less than 60 mm Hg on an inspired oxygen concentration (F_IO_2) of greater than 60 per cent (Gilmour, 1983). Other parameters that may indicate a need for mechanical ventilation include a vital capacity of less than 15 ml per kg, an inspiratory force less than 25 cm H_2O, an alveolar-arterial oxygen gradient greater than 350 mm Hg, and a dead space:tidal volume ratio of greater than 0.6 (Pontoppidan et al., 1973).

The primary goal of mechanical ventilation is to achieve satisfactory blood oxygenation at the lowest possible F_IO_2. Ancillary goals include providing adequate airway humidification and removing pulmonary secretions.

PHYSIOLOGY

A spontaneously breathing person normally takes 10 to 15 sighs per hour to ventilate dependent lung tissue. Patients receiving fixed-volume positive pressure ventilation from a mechanical ventilator thus require larger tidal volumes to prevent atelectasis. The tidal volume in adults is set between 10 and 15 ml per kg and is delivered at a rate of 8 to 10 breaths per minute to achieve a minute volume between 8 and 15 L (Hedley-White et al., 1976; Shapiro, 1981). Children older than 10 years are managed similarly to adults, but infants and younger children need a higher minute volume and are ventilated at a rate between 20 and 25 breaths per minute (Downs and Raphaely, 1975).

The F_IO_2 is normally set to achieve a PO_2 between 60 and 90 mm Hg. An important exception is in patients with a hypoxic respiratory drive in whom a lower PO_2 may be desirable to avoid respiratory depression. Oxygen toxicity becomes a concern when an F_1O_2 of greater than 50 per cent is required to achieve an acceptable PO_2, and some form of continuous distending pressure is required to facilitate oxygen delivery without further increasing the F_1O_2 (Gilmour, 1983).

A mechanical ventilator usually should be used in the assist-control mode, and the sensitivity should be set so that the respirator is triggered easily by the patient's own inspiratory efforts. Patients should be able to take additional breaths with minimal effort to avoid psychological disturbance and because increased breathing efforts may result in atelectasis (Gilmour, 1983).

COMPLICATIONS

Mechanical ventilation may result in decreased cardiac output. Positive airway pressure increases intrathoracic pressure, thereby decreasing venous return and cardiac output (Morgan et al., 1966). Any maneuver that increases intrathoracic pressure, such as increasing tidal volume or applying continuous airway distending pressure, may result in a further decrease in cardiac output. Fortunately, the relationship between airway and intrathoracic pressures is modified by pulmonary compliance so that a stiff, noncompliant lung does not transmit pressure to the same degree as a healthy lung. Therefore, impairment of cardiac output is less severe in patients with respiratory disease, who may require increased intrathoracic pressure to achieve satisfactory oxygen delivery, than in patients with normal pulmonary function (Colgan et al., 1979).

A second major effect of mechanical ventilation is to disturb the normal pulmonary ventilation-perfusion relationship. Ventilation and perfusion are normally distributed primarily to dependent lung tissue. This is because of the effect of gravity on the blood and because the dependent sections of the lung are more compliant (Murray, 1976). Mechanical ventilation results in a disturbance of the ventilation-perfusion balance for a number of reasons. First, patients receiving positive pressure ventilation frequently have pulmonary disease. The dependent sections of the lung are usually the most diseased and have greater resistance to air flow as well as decreased compliance. Second, the supine position decreases the functional residual capacity and increases airway resistance principally in dependent lung tissue. Third, diaphragmatic excursion is reduced in patients receiving mechanical ventilation, and the weight of the abdominal contents may further impair the normal ventilation of dependent lung segments. These factors affect perfusion less than ventilation, and ventilation-perfusion imbalance therefore results. This imbalance can be overcome somewhat by periodically turning patients on mechanical ventilators to a prone position in order to improve ventilation of dependent lung segments (Douglas et al., 1977).

A third major complication of mechanical ventilation is barotrauma. This results either from mechanical trauma to the tracheobronchial tree or from overdistention of the lung. The risk of overdistention and subsequent pneumothorax is increased by the use of continuous airway distending pressure (Gilmour, 1983).

A fourth major complication of mechanical ventilation is acute respiratory alkalosis due to inappropriate hyperventilation. Respiratory alkalosis can result in decreased cardiac output, decreased cerebral blood flow, increased cardiac irritability, and a shift in the oxyhemoglobin curve to the left (Shapiro, 1981). The etiology of respiratory alkalosis can be either psychological, iatrogenic, or reflex. Psychological hyperventilation is managed by sedation, and iatrogenic hyperventilation can be corrected by adjusting the ventilatory rate. Reflex hyperventilation arises from either the lungs or the central nervous system and may be difficult to treat. Some patients may respond to increased tidal volume or positive end-expiratory pressure (PEEP), but usually some measure to increase alveolar ventilation is required. These measures include changing to intermittent mandatory ventilation (IMV) or lowering the ventilatory support rate, adding dead space to the respirator, or using muscle relaxants (Gilmour, 1983).

THE USE OF CONTINUOUS DISTENDING PRESSURE

Continuous distending pressure refers to the continuous elevation of transpulmonary pressure above baseline levels, and it is achieved by the techniques of PEEP and continuous positive airway pressure (CPAP). The goal of continuous distending pressure is to minimize abnormalities in the ventilation-perfusion balance and thus allow delivery of oxygen to the tissues at a lower F_1O_2. The increase in transpulmonary pressure results in an increased functional residual capacity, which allows recruitment of noncompliant lung units and prevents their collapse between breaths. Continuous distending pressure also splints small airways and inhibits atelectasis during ventilation (Falke et al., 1972; Pontoppidan et al., 1973).

Continuous distending pressure is associated with several complications. The further increase in transpulmonary pressure above that of mechanical ventilation alone results in a further decrease in venous return and cardiac output. Again, this effect may be less marked in patients with chronic pulmonary disease than in those with normal lungs because of the decreased compliance in diseased pulmonary tissue. Furthermore, decreased venous return may be desirable in patients with pulmonary congestion (Colgan et al., 1979).

Two other complications of continuous distending pressure result from overdistention of alveoli. The first is alveolar rupture. Second, overdistention of lung segments may cause compression of adjacent capillaries, which, through a Starling resistor effect, stimulates a redistribution of pulmonary blood flow. This may result in increased pulmonary vascular resistance and right ventricular failure (Pontoppidan et al., 1973).

Continuous distending pressure is usually employed with the goal of maintaining a PO_2 between 60 and 90 mm Hg with an F_IO_2 of less than 50 per cent. Alternatively, continuous distending pressure can be employed with the goal of maintaining a shunt fraction of less than 15 per cent. This may require continuous distending pressures in excess of 50 cm H_2O. This method requires more careful cardiovascular monitoring and is not recommended for the routine postoperative patient (Gilmour, 1983).

INTERMITTENT MANDATORY VENTILATION (IMV)

IMV was introduced about 10 years ago as an alternative to spontaneous respiration with a T-piece as a means of weaning patients from the respirator. With the T-piece, the patient ventilates on his own for increasing intervals of time, whereas with IMV the patient remains on the respirator, but provides an increasing fraction of his minute ventilation by spontaneous breaths.

IMV has several advantages over continuous mechanical ventilation. First, spontaneous breaths are achieved with a decrease in intrathoracic pressure, and, therefore, they promote venous return and cardiac output and allow higher levels of continuous distending pressure to be used (Downs et al., 1973). IMV also may result in decreased barotrauma, improved distribution of ventilation, and, by allowing the patient to breath on his own, better regulation of acid-base balance (Bistrian et al., 1975).

The technique of IMV usually involves maintaining a pH between 7.35 and 7.45 with a minute ventilation of less than 10 L and a respiratory rate of less than 30 per minute (Civetta, 1981). PO_2 is maintained between 60 and 90 mm Hg by altering the F_IO_2 and continuous distending pressure. The results of IMV are generally satisfactory, but it can result in increased respiratory work, which may delay weaning from the ventilator (Smith, 1981).

WEANING

Two tests correlate well with the ability of a patient to be weaned from the respirator: vital capacity (VC) and maximum inspiratory force (MIF) (Pontoppidan et al., 1977). A VC greater than 15 ml per kg and a MIF greater than -20 cm H_2O are acceptable values for weaning. It is inadvisable to wean patients with a VC less than 10 ml per kg, a respiratory rate greater than 30 per minute, or a minute volume greater than 10 L (Sahn and Lakshminarayan, 1973). Patients with an alveolar arterial oxygen gradient greater than 300 mm Hg on 100 per cent oxygen or with a dead space:tidal volume ratio of greater than 0.6 are also poor candidates for weaning (Pontoppidan et al., 1977). Adjunctive measures for successful weaning include adequate hydration, vigorous pulmonary therapy, and careful monitoring with periodic arterial blood gas determinations (Gilmour, 1983).

THROMBOEMBOLIC DISEASE

Incidence

Nearly all clinically significant pulmonary emboli arise in the deep veins of the legs (Hovig, 1977; Moser et al., 1977). It is difficult to estimate the incidence of deep venous thrombosis by physical examination, since at least 50 per cent of venous thrombi in the leg are clinically silent (Moser et al., 1977). A more accurate determination is achieved with either radioactive iodine-labeled fibrinogen scanning or venography. Using these techniques, the incidence of deep venous thrombosis in patients undergoing urologic surgery has been found to be between 30 and 60 per cent (Coe et al., 1978; Kutnowski, 1977). The incidence is highest in patients undergoing open prostatectomy, with estimates varying from 30 to 80 per cent (Coe et al., 1978; Collins et al., 1976). The incidence of deep venous thrombosis is considerably lower in patients undergoing transurethral prostatectomy but is still between 10 and 20 per cent (Mays et al., 1971).

The incidence of nonfatal pulmonary embolism in urologic patients also is underestimated by physical examination. Antila reported a 3 per cent incidence of clinically detectable pulmonary embolism following open prostatectomy (Antila et al., 1966), but Allgood observed a 22 per cent incidence of pulmonary embolism following urologic surgery when perfusion lung scans were routinely performed (Allgood et al., 1970). The incidence of fatal pulmonary embolism obviously is much lower than the incidence of nonfatal pulmonary embolism, but it has been reported to be as high as 1 to 2 per cent following open urologic procedures (Holbraad et al., 1976; Kakkar, 1975).

Risk Factors

The duration of anesthesia is a major risk factor contributing to thromboembolic disease, and the incidence of deep venous thrombosis increases markedly when anesthesia time is greater than 1 hour. This is in part due to venous stasis associated with the use of muscle relaxants (Kakkar, 1975). Other risk factors for thromboembolic disease include age greater than 60 years, the presence of malignant disease, the use of estrogens, and the period and degree of immobility following surgery (Gallus et al., 1973; Moser, 1983).

Diagnosis

The three principal tests used to diagnose deep venous thrombosis are radioactive iodine-labeled fibrinogen scanning, impedance plethysmography, and contrast venography. ^{125}I fibrinogen scanning is based on the principle that fibrinogen will be incorporated into an actively forming thrombus. The radiolabeled fibrinogen is injected intravenously, and the legs are scanned with a hand-held detector. Fibrinogen scanning is unreliable in detecting thrombi in the upper thigh because of the large pelvic blood pool (Moser, 1983). It is an extremely sensitive technique, however, for detecting thrombi in the calf and lower thigh (the locations at which the majority of thrombi form), and the results correlate well with venography (Kakkar, 1975). The technique is most reliable when the fibrinogen is injected while thrombi are actively forming, and false-negative results may be obtained with older thrombi that are no longer incorporating fibrinogen. Fibrinogen uptake may also be limited by previous treatment with heparin (Moser et al., 1977).

Impedance plethysmography is a reliable technique for detecting thrombi above the knee. It is performed easily at the bedside, and the results correlate well with venography. It is much less sensitive than radiolabeled fibrinogen scanning in detecting venous thrombi in the calf (Hull et al., 1977).

Contrast venography is the gold-standard method of diagnosis for deep venous thrombosis. It is an invasive technique, however, which may be difficult to perform and to interpret. Venography probably should be reserved for those cases when radiolabeled fibrinogen scanning and plethysmography are not available or when the results of these studies are equivocal (Moser, 1983).

The diagnosis of pulmonary embolism also may be difficult to establish on clinical grounds because many cases are clinically silent, and the signs and symptoms are often variable. The lung perfusion scan is a useful screening technique, and a normal scan rules out the possibility of pulmonary embolism. An abnormal scan, however, may not be diagnostic of pulmonary embolism, since many cardiopulmonary conditions can alter regional pulmonary blood flow and give rise to segmental perfusion defects (Moser et al., 1977).

The specificity of the perfusion scan can be enhanced by combining it with a ventilation scan. The patient inhales a radioactive labeled gas such as ^{133}X, and the pattern of distribution of the isotope on the ventilation (V) scan is compared with the pattern of distribution on the perfusion (Q) scan. In pulmonary embolism the V/Q scan reveals areas that are ventilated but not perfused, the so-called ventilation-perfusion mismatch (Alderson et al., 1979).

Ventilation-perfusion scans may be unreliable in diagnosing pulmonary embolism if the scan is abnormal only in areas in which the chest radiograph is also abnormal. This may occur with a pulmonary infiltrate or pleural effusion. In these cases one must rely on pulmonary angiography to establish the diagnosis with certainty (Moser, 1983).

Prophylaxis

SUBCUTANEOUS HEPARIN

There have been several prospective trials that have demonstrated that low-dose subcutaneous heparin decreases the incidence of deep venous thrombosis and pulmonary embolism associated with abdominal and thoracic surgery (Gallus et al., 1975; Kakkar, 1972; Lahnborg et al., 1974). Gallus et al. (1975) performed a double-blind study using radiolabeled fibrinogen leg scans in which patients treated with subcutaneous heparin for 1 week were compared with controls, and they found a significant decrease in the incidence of deep venous thrombosis in the heparin-treated group. In another double-blind study, Lahnborg et al. (1974) found that the incidence of postoperative pulmonary embolism determined by pulmonary perfusion scans was decreased from 35 to 14 per cent. The international multicentered trial performed in the 1970's concluded that prophylactic subcutaneous heparin was effective in reducing the incidence of fatal pulmonary embolism (Kakkar, 1975).

The efficacy of subcutaneous heparin in patients undergoing urologic surgery is somewhat controversial. Using radiolabeled fibrinogen leg scanning, Kakkar found that prophylactic heparin reduced the incidence of deep venous thrombosis in a large series of patients undergoing prostatectomy. Furthermore, there were two cases of fatal pulmonary embolism in the control group and none in the heparin-treated group (Kakkar, 1975). Two other studies of patients undergoing prostatectomy using fibrinogen leg scanning showed that heparin decreased the incidence of deep venous thrombosis from 28 to 0 per cent and from 42 to 6 per cent (Kutnowski et al., 1977; Nicolaides et al., 1972). Conversely, two other studies have concluded that prophylactic heparin does not reduce the incidence of deep venous thrombosis associated with prostatectomy (Coe et al., 1978; Rosenberg et al., 1975). Heparin may be more consistently effective in urologic procedures other than prostatectomy in preventing deep venous thrombosis (Sebeseri et al., 1975).

Prophylactic heparin has been associated with increased perioperative bleeding (Coe et al., 1978; Pachter and Riles, 1977), but most double-blind studies have demonstrated no difference in either blood loss or transfusion requirements in patients receiving heparin versus controls (Kakkar et al., 1972; Kiil et al., 1978). Although its use in urologic surgery remains controversial, the evidence suggests that prophylactic heparin should be considered in patients older than 40 years of age who undergo major surgical procedures, especially those with associated risk factors for venous thrombosis, such as malignant disease. Heparin usually is administered by giving 5000 U subcutaneously 2 hours preoperatively, and repeating this dose every 8 to 12 hours postoperatively. Although patients usually are treated for 1 week, there may be a significant incidence of venous thrombosis beyond this time, and it is important to continue heparin therapy until patients are fully ambulatory (Kakkar, 1975).

PROTHROMBINOPENIC AGENTS

Prothrombinopenic agents such as warfarin and dicumarol have not been used extensively in patients undergoing urologic surgery, and their value is uncertain. There have been two reports that suggest that the administration of prothrombinopenic agents simultaneously with epsilon aminocaproic acid (EACA) reduces the incidence of deep venous thrombosis and pulmonary embolism in patients undergoing open prostatectomy (Anderson and Jensen, 1966; Storm, 1967). Another study concluded that the administration of prothrombinopenic agents alone did not reduce the incidence of thromboembolic disease and was associated with increased perioperative bleeding (Holbraad et al., 1976). The risk of bleeding with warfarin and dicumarol may be greater than with heparin, since these agents are more difficult to reverse pharmacologically.

DEXTRAN

Dextran is a low molecular weight glucose polymer that has various effects on platelet function and coagulability (Rose, 1979). Two types are available, dextran 40 and dextran 70, and there does not appear to be any difference in their efficacy (Bergentz, 1978). Five hundred milliliters of dextran are administered intravenously during surgery, and this dose is repeated every other day postoperatively until the patient is ambulatory (Rose, 1979).

Most of the reported experience with dextran is contained in the orthopedic literature (Harris et al., 1977), and there have been no reports of its use in urologic patients. Although the literature suggests that dextran is effective in preventing thromboembolism (Bonnar and Walsh, 1972; Carter and Eban, 1973), it does not appear to be as effective as heparin (MacIntyre et al., 1974). In addition, dextran may be associated with significant complications, including anaphylaxis (Ring and Messmer, 1977), renal failure, fluid overload, and increased bleeding (Rose, 1979). Dextran is not recommended at present for use in urologic surgery.

ASPIRIN

Various agents that inhibit platelet aggregation have been used to prevent thromboembolic disease. There are no reports in the urologic literature, and the results with aspirin in the general surgical and orthopedic literature are controversial (Clagett et al., 1974; Hirsch, 1981; Hume et al., 1978). None of the studies has demonstrated that aspirin is more effective than low-dose heparin, and aspirin is not recommended as a means of prophylaxis.

PHYSICAL MEASURES

Early ambulation has been shown to decrease venous thrombosis after myocardial infarction (Miller et al., 1976). Although its efficacy has not been established by controlled trials, early ambulation likewise seems advantageous for surgical patients. For ambulation to be effective, the patient must either stand at the bedside or walk. Sitting in a chair or on the edge of the bed with the legs dangling serves only to promote venous stasis and increase the risk of venous thrombosis (Rose, 1979). Leg elevation and leg exercises in themselves appear to have little prophylactic benefit (Rosengarten and Laird, 1971).

Elastic compression stockings remain controversial. Initially they were reported to prevent venous thrombosis (Wilkins and Stanton, 1953), but subsequent studies showed them to be ineffective (Browse et al., 1974). Poorly fitting stockings may compress the popliteal area and thigh and promote venous stasis (Moser, 1983). A newer compression stocking that provides a pressure gradient to the leg, with the highest pressure in the ankle and the lowest pressure in the thigh, has been reported to be effective in increasing venous flow (Ishak and Morley, 1981; Scurr et al., 1977).

At the present time, the most effective mechanical agent to prevent venous thrombosis is the external pneumatic compression boot. This is a plastic sleeve that is applied around the calf and is used to apply intermittent external mechanical compression. The sleeve is inflated to between 40 and 50 mm Hg for 10 to 15 seconds every minute. Several studies have reported that the boot reduces deep venous thrombosis, including a study of urologic patients in which the device was found to be more effective than low-dose heparin (Coe et al., 1978; Hills et al., 1972; Skillman et al., 1978). The boot may be potentially uncomfortable when prolonged bed rest is required and may be difficult to apply over a leg cast, but the device seems to be otherwise free of complications.

SUMMARY

External pneumatic compression boots and early ambulation are the initial measures recommended to prevent venous thrombosis. Heparin seems to be the most effective pharmacologic agent, and it is associated with fewer complications than either thrombinopenic drugs or dextran. Heparin is recommended in all high-risk patients older than 40 years of age undergoing major urologic procedures, and it should be continued until the patient is fully ambulatory.

Treatment of Thromboembolism

The initial treatment of both deep venous thrombosis and pulmonary embolism is intravenous heparin, which is usually administered as a continuous infusion of 1000 U per hour. Alternatively, heparin may be given in boluses of either 5000 U every 4 hours, 7500 U every 6 hours, or 10,000 U every 8 hours. Although continuous infusion is the most popular method, it has not been shown to have any advantage in terms of efficacy or safety over bolus administration (Salzman et al., 1975). Intravenous heparin is continued for at least 7 days and longer in patients who remain immobilized or who have other associated risk factors. In the past it has been recommended that patients with pulmonary embolism receive an initial bolus of 15,000 to 20,000 U of heparin and that heparin be infused at an increased rate during the first 24 hours of therapy, but it is uncertain whether these additional measures are necessary (Moser, 1980).

The therapeutic effect of heparin is monitored by measurement of either the partial thromboplastin time (PTT) or the activated partial thromboplastin time (APTT), and they usually are maintained in the twice-normal range. It has been argued that measurement of PTT or APTT is unnecessary, because coagulation parameters may not reflect the efficacy of therapy and because the risk of bleeding with heparin is primarily related to other coexistent risk factors (Nelson et al., 1982).

Thrombolytic agents have been tried in the treatment of acute thromboembolic disease, but no clear benefit has resulted from their use (Sasahara and Dalen, 1980). Thrombolytic agents are contraindicated during the first 5 days following surgery because of the risk of increased bleeding (Moser, 1983).

Surgery is rarely indicated in the treatment of thromboembolic disease. Pulmonary embolectomy is performed only when there is massive pulmonary thromboembolism that has been documented by angiography and that is associated with profound hypotension. Surgical interruption of the vena cava or placement of a caval umbrella is indicated only when heparin cannot be used because of increased bleeding (Moser, 1983).

Following the treatment of acute postoperative thromboembolism, patients who have persistent risk factors should remain on anticoagulant therapy. Oral warfarin or low-dose subcutaneous heparin are the drugs commonly used. Warfarin is given in a dosage sufficient to maintain the prothrombin time (PT) at approximately one-and-a-half to two times control values (Hull et al., 1982). Heparin is administered in doses of 7500 to 10,000 U subcutaneously every 12 hours (Bynum and Wilson, 1979). How long patients should remain on anticoagulant therapy has not been resolved. Some feel that therapy should continue until all risk factors have resolved, whereas others treat empirically for 3 months to a year postoperatively (Moser, 1983).

PERIOPERATIVE MANAGEMENT OF PATIENTS WITH RENAL INSUFFICIENCY

This section deals with the preoperative evaluation of renal function and the perioperative management of patients with renal insufficiency. The evaluation and management of acute and chronic renal failure are discussed in Chapter 59.

Preoperative Assessment

EVALUATION OF RENAL FUNCTION

In patients with renal insufficiency the degree of reduction of the glomerular filtration rate (GFR) correlates with the surgical risk of postoperative renal failure and associated extrarenal morbidity. Therefore, it is important to assess the GFR preoperatively in patients with compromised renal function. Blood urea nitrogen (BUN) does not provide the best estimate of GFR. BUN lacks specificity because it is dependent on factors other than GFR, such as protein load and urinary flow rate. Patients with an increased dietary protein intake, hypercatabolism, or intestinal bleeding may have elevation of their BUN that is out of proportion to any decrease in the GFR. Conversely, patients with a decreased dietary protein intake, polyuria, or severe liver disease may have a decrease in their BUN that is unrelated to any increase in the GFR (Burke and Gulyassy, 1979).

Since serum creatinine is not dependent on either protein load or urinary flow rate, its measurement provides a more accurate estimation of GFR. Serum creatinine is dependent, however, on a patient's muscle mass. A serum creatinine of 1.5 mg per dl may reflect a normal GFR in a muscular young male but might be associated with as much as a 75 per cent reduction in the GFR in an older, malnourished patient with muscular wasting (Burke and Gulyassy, 1979).

The creatinine clearance correlates most closely with the GFR, but it is sometimes unreliable because of inaccuracy in obtaining a complete 24-hour urine collection. A 4-hour collection of urine is more easily obtained, and in a well-hydrated patient it provides a reasonable estimation of creatinine clearance. In situations in which timed collections of urine are not feasible, a rough estimation of creatinine clearance can be obtained by dividing the serum creatinine into 100. This simple calculation is more reliable in young patients, and a more accurate estimation in all patients is provided by the formula:

$$\text{Creatinine Clearance} = \frac{(140 - \text{age [years]}) \times (\text{body weight[kg]})}{72 \times \text{serum creatinine (mg per dl)}}$$

Adjustment for female equals 15 per cent less (Cockcroft and Gault, 1976).

RENAL INSUFFICIENCY AND SURGICAL RISK

Patients with mild renal insufficiency and a GFR between 50 and 75 ml per minute have an increased risk of developing perioperative renal failure. Patients with a moderate reduction in the GFR to between 25 and 50 ml per minute have an even greater risk and require close attention to perioperative fluid and electrolyte balance and may require adjustments in drug dosages. Patients with a GFR below 25 ml per minute have an increased risk of developing associated extrarenal complications such as increased bleeding (Kwaan and Connolly, 1980). Patients on chronic dialysis have a surgical mortality of between 2 and 4 per cent (Hampers et al., 1968; Hata et al., 1973), and a surgical morbidity of up to 60 per cent (Brenowitz et al., 1977).

Preoperative Management

FLUID AND ELECTROLYTES

Sodium and Water. Patients with renal insufficiency are usually able to maintain normal sodium and water balance until their renal function is severely reduced. As the GFR decreases, however, patients may lose the ability to respond to acute shifts in sodium and water (Depner and Gulyassy, 1979). They may not be able to handle the large amounts of sodium and water often administered during surgery and may have an increased risk of fluid overload and congestive heart failure in the perioperative period. Conversely, patients with salt-wasting nephropathy have an increased risk of perioperative volume depletion and may require increased amounts of intravenous saline to avoid dehydration and subsequent renal deterioration (Tasker et al., 1974).

Hyponatremia occurs commonly in patients with renal insufficiency and generally reflects an excess of free water rather than a deficiency of sodium. Hyponatremia becomes clinically significant when the serum sodium falls below 125 mEq per L because of the risk of cerebral edema. Prompt treatment is required with either diuretics and hypertonic saline or dialysis (Hantman et al., 1973). Hypernatremia is uncommon in renal insufficiency and usually reflects volume depletion (Burke and Gulyassy, 1979).

Potassium. Hyperkalemia is potentially a major problem in patients with renal insufficiency undergoing surgery. Although under normal conditions patients are able to maintain potassium balance until the GFR falls below 10 ml per minute, surgery increases the risk of hyperkalemia because of the increased endogenous and exogenous potassium load. Endogenous sources of potassium include rhabdomyolysis, surgical tissue trauma, and hemolysis. Exogenous sources include intravenously or orally administered potassium, total parenteral nutrition, and blood transfusions (Burke and Gulyassy, 1979). In addition, acidosis frequently occurs during the perioperative period, and this causes a rise in serum potassium of 0.6 mEq per L for every 0.1 U decrease in serum pH (Kunau and Stein, 1979).

The serum potassium should be normalized prior to surgery. Acute hyperkalemia may be precipitated by hypercapnea and acidosis associated with induction of anesthesia, and patients with pre-existing hyperkalemia have an increased risk for ventricular arrhythmias and cardiac death (Kasiske and Kjellstrand, 1983). Elective operations should be postponed if the serum potassium exceeds 5.5 mEq per L. Patients whose serum potassium exceeds 6.5 mEq per L require prompt treatment to prevent cardiac arrhythmias.

The treatment of hyperkalemia is outlined in Table 61–4. Calcium chloride antagonizes the effect of potassium on the myocardium, whereas the administration of sodium bicarbonate and insulin and glucose produce an intracellular shift of potassium. None of these agents has a lasting effect on serum potassium, and more permanent results can be achieved with either sodium-potassium exchange resins or dialysis (Kasiske and Kjellstrand, 1983).

Hypokalemia occurs commonly and most often results from diuretic therapy. Although renal failure is seldom the cause, hypokalemia should be corrected cautiously in patients with renal failure to avoid precipitating acute hyperkalemia and cardiac arrhythmias. Elective surgery should be postponed if the serum potassium

TABLE 61–4. TREATMENT OF HYPERKALEMIA

Agent	Mechanism	Route of Administration	Onset of Action	Comments
Calcium chloride	Antagonizes effect of potassium on myocardium	Intravenous bolus or drip	Immediate	Avoid in digitalized patients Give under EKG control
Sodium bicarbonate	Intracellular potassium shift	Intravenous bolus or drip	Immediate	May cause volume overload if used in large quantities
Insulin and glucose	Intracellular potassium shift	Intravenous bolus or drip; 1 U regular insulin for every 2 gm of glucose	Within minutes	
Sodium polystyrene (Kayexalate)	Removal of potassium	Oral: 30 gm Rectal: 60 gm Give with sorbitol	1 – 2 hr	
Hemodialysis and peritoneal dialysis	Removal of potassium		Immediate	Hemodialysis much faster

(From Kasiske, B., and Kjellstrand, C. M.: Perioperative management of patients with renal failure. Urol. Clin. North Am., *10*:35, 1983. Used with permission.)

is less than 3 mEq per L. Potassium should be replaced orally if possible, but it can be administered intravenously when necessary. It should not be replaced at a rate greater than 10 to 15 mEq per hour without careful electrocardiograph (EKG) monitoring. Hypokalemia in the postoperative period is usually due to the loss of potassium and hydrochloric acid from the gastrointestinal tract (Burke and Gulyassy, 1979).

Other Electrolytes. Hypocalcemia and hypophosphatemia occur commonly in patients with renal insufficiency and are generally well tolerated. Hypercalcemia occurs less frequently and is associated with secondary hyperparathyroidism. Hypermagnesemia also occurs commonly, especially in patients receiving antacids and cathartics. Serum magnesium levels greater than 3 mEq per L are associated with an increased risk of cardiac arrhythmias, respiratory paralysis, and prolonged muscle relaxation following anesthesia (Burke and Gulyassy, 1979).

ACID-BASE BALANCE

Patients with renal insufficiency frequently have a metabolic acidosis due to a decreased renal ability to excrete a normal acid load and to regenerate bicarbonate. Although metabolic alkalosis is seldom of renal origin, it occurs commonly in the postoperative period because of gastrointestinal losses. Metabolic alkalosis is usually corrected by the kidneys, and patients with renal insufficiency may be unable to compensate adequately (Burke and Gulyassy, 1979).

Both acidosis and alkalosis represent serious risks and should be corrected before elective surgery is undertaken. In addition, patients with metabolic acidosis due to renal insufficiency may compensate for this problem by chronic hyperventilation. If hyperventilation is not maintained during anesthesia, patients may develop a worsening metabolic acidosis, which in turn, may precipitate acute hyperkalemia and fatal cardiac complications (Goggin and Joekes, 1971).

HEMATOLOGIC CONSIDERATIONS

Anemia is common in patients with severe renal insufficiency primarily because of the decreased production and action of erythropoietin, but other factors include gastrointestinal bleeding, hemolysis, and deficiencies of iron and folate (Erslev and Shapiro, 1979). These patients usually are well adjusted to hematocrits between 18 and 24 per cent because of increased production of 2,3-diphosphoglycerate (2,3-DPG). 2,3-DPG causes a shift in the oxyhemoglobin dissociation curve to the right, facilitating oxygen delivery to the tissues (MacDonald, 1977). Preoperative transfusions are not usually required in these patients and may precipitate volume overload and congestive heart failure. Patients with lesser degrees of renal insufficiency or those whose renal failure is of short duration are more susceptible to complications from anemia, and these patients may require preoperative transfusions to a hematocrit above 30 per cent (Czer and Shoemaker, 1978).

Patients with moderate or severe renal insufficiency also are at risk for increased perioperative hemorrhage, primarily from abnormal platelet function. The best laboratory test to assess this risk is the bleeding time. The degree of abnormality of the bleeding time correlates closely with the degree of renal insufficiency, whereas the PT, PTT, and platelet count usually are normal. Patients with levels of blood urea nitrogen greater than 100 mg per dl should undergo dialysis prior to surgery to decrease the risk of perioperative hemorrhage (Kasiske and Kjellstrand, 1983). In some patients, dialysis will not be effective in normalizing the bleeding time, and these patients may respond to the administration of cryoprecipitate shortly before surgery. The mechanism of action of cryoprecipitate in these cases is not known (Janson et al., 1980).

DRUG THERAPY

The degree of renal insufficiency corrclates closely with the development of adverse drug reactions, and the administration of drugs in the perioperative period to patients with renal failure deserves careful consideration. Drug dosages must be decreased in accordance with the degree of renal impairment. This is particularly true for drugs that are normally excreted unchanged by the kidneys, but drugs that are not excreted by the kidneys must also be administered cautiously if the effects of these agents are synergistic with the effects of uremia. Such agents include anticoagulants, sedatives, analgesics, and tranquilizers (Burke and Gulyassy, 1979). Drug levels can be adjusted either by decreasing the drug dosage or by increasing the dose interval. Nomograms are available for many of the commonly used drugs, and serum levels should be followed when administering drugs with increased potential toxicity. Associated hepatic disease and congestive heart failure increase the risk of potential drug toxicity (Benet, 1976). A list of drugs commonly used in the perioperative period, with recommended dosage modifications for patients with renal failure, is shown in Table 61–5.

TABLE 61–5. MODIFICATIONS OF MAINTENANCE THERAPY IN RENAL FAILURE
FOR DRUGS OFTEN USED IN THE PERIOPERATIVE PERIOD *†

| Drug | Dosage Modification for Glomerular Filtration Rate‡ | | Remarks |
	10 – 15 ml/min	10 ml/min	
Digoxin	Minor	Moderate	Use 70% of normal loading dose
Magnesium or calcium antacids	Moderate	—	If CrCl§ < 25, check (Mg^{++}) or (Ca^{++}); do not use if CrCl < 10
Cimetadine	Minor	Moderate	If CrCl < 10 give no more than 300 mg q 12 h
Thiazides	—	—	Ineffective if CrCl < 30
Furosemide	None	None	Doses > 400 mg ineffective, potentially ototoxic
Triamterene, spironalactone	—	—	Avoid in patients with renal failure, may cause hyperkalemia
Barbiturates Narcotics Benzodiazepines Phenothiazines	None	Minor	In uremic patients use with caution—may cause excessive central nervous system depression
Succinylcholine	None	None	Increases (K^+) use with caution if (K^+) is elevated
Gallamine	—	—	Avoid if CrCl < 50
Penicillin G	Minor	< 3 million U/d	Potassium salt contains 1.7 mEq K/million units
Ampicillin	Minor	Moderate	
Nafcillin	None	Minor	
Carbenicillin	Minor	Moderate	Contains 4.7 mEq sodium/gm
Cephalothin	Minor	Moderate	
Cephalexin	Minor	Moderate	
Cephazolin	Moderate	Major	Consult available nomogram
Doxycycline	None	None	Avoid use of all other tetracyclines in patients with renal failure
Aminoglycosides	Moderate	Major	Consult available nomogram; measure blood levels

*Normal loading dose should be used, unless noted.
†Use of peritoneal or hemodialysis may require further adjustments.
‡Approximate adjustments are minor 0.5–0.75, moderate 0.25–0.5, major 0.1–0.25 of normal maintenance dosages.
§CrCl in ml/min.
(From Burke, G. R., and Gulyassy, P. F.: Surgery in the patient with renal disease and related electrolyte disorders. Med. Clin. North Am., *63*:1191, 1979. Used with permission.)

Aminoglycosides remain one of the major causes of acute renal insufficiency. Nephrotoxicity can be reduced by using nomograms to calculate proper loading and maintenance dosages and by following drug levels in the serum. The serum creatinine should be measured at least every other day while aminoglycosides are being administered and for 4 to 6 days after therapy. The creatinine clearance should be measured periodically in patients receiving prolonged aminoglycoside therapy (Burke and Gulyassy, 1976).

Radiocontrast agents have considerable nephrotoxic potential. In addition to renal insufficiency, factors that increase the risk of these agents are patient age greater than 60 years, diabetes, dehydration, and multiple myeloma (Byrd and Sherman, 1979). The risk of contrast-induced nephrotoxicity increases with progressive decline in renal function. In nondiabetic patients, there is a 31 per cent incidence of radiocontrast-induced renal failure when the serum creatinine is greater than 4.5 mg per dl (Van Zee et al., 1978), and the risk becomes even greater in diabetic patients with a creatinine above 2 mg per dl (Harkonen and Kjellstrand, 1977). The risk of contrast-induced nephrotoxicity can be greatly reduced by preventing or correcting dehydration prior to the administration of radiocontrast (Eisenberg et al., 1981; Rahimi et al., 1981). Patients at risk, particularly those with renal insufficiency or diabetes, should not have their fluids restricted prior to the administration of radiocontrast, and supplemental oral or intravenous fluids may be required. Cathartics and enemas should be kept to a minimum. Multiple radiologic studies should not be scheduled consecutively to prevent a cumulative effect on renal function.

Intraoperative Management

FLUIDS AND DIURETICS

Patients with renal insufficiency are more likely to develop fluid and electrolyte problems associated with surgery. Many patients have a diminished capacity to excrete free water. Since surgery and anesthesia cause the release of antidiuretic hormone, which further decreases the excretion of free water, these patients have an increased risk of fluid overload and congestive heart failure. Conversely, patients with severe renal insufficiency may have a decreased ability to concentrate their urine, and thus have an increased risk of volume depletion. It is essential, therefore, to monitor fluid and electrolytes closely in patients with renal impairment (Kasiske and Kjellstrand, 1983).

In the past, some have advocated routine preoperative salt-loading in patients with renal insufficiency to prevent further perioperative deterioration of renal function. Salt-loading is no longer routinely recommended, because it may result in fluid overload and congestive heart failure. Although all patients should be adequately hydrated at the time of surgery, the administration of supplemental intravenous saline is advisable only in those patients with salt-wasting nephropathy (Tasker et al., 1974).

Diuretics should be administered prophylactically during surgery to patients with renal insufficiency to increase the GFR and thereby decrease the risk of further renal deterioration (Kasiske and Kjellstrand, 1983). The evidence suggests that both mannitol and furosemide have a beneficial effect on renal function, and it has been recommended that patients with renal insufficiency receive a continuous intravenous infusion of these two diuretics during the perioperative period (Dawson, 1965; Nuuti-

nen et al., 1978). Five hundred milliliters of a 20 per cent mannitol solution is prepared to which is added 100 mg multiplied by the serum creatinine of furosemide (e.g., if the serum creatinine is 4 mg per dl, $100 \times 4 = 400$ mg of furosemide). The solution is infused at a rate of 20 ml per hour during surgery, and the rate is then tapered over the first 6 to 12 hours postoperatively. The infusion is slowed if excessive diuresis results. Urine volume is replaced with 0.45 per cent saline containing 20 to 40 mEq of potassium chloride per L. Serial serum and urine electrolytes are measured, and the sodium and potassium content of the replacement fluid is adjusted accordingly (Kasiske and Kjellstrand, 1983). The infusion is discontinued if the patient becomes anuric or oliguric because of potential mannitol toxicity (Borges et al., 1982).

ANESTHETIC AGENTS AND MUSCLE RELAXANTS

The use of inhalational agents in patients with renal insufficiency is generally safe, since excretion of these agents is independent of renal function. These drugs may produce a mild decrease in urine volume, free water clearance, and GFR, but these effects are transitory and usually of no clinical significance (Deutsch, 1975). Methoxyflurane is an exception; it is nephrotoxic and should not be used in patients with renal insufficiency (Kasiske and Kjellstrand, 1983). Preanesthetic agents such as morphine and meperidine may depress renal function slightly, but moderate doses can be given safely. Anticholinergics such as atropine have little effect on renal function and also are safe to use (Kasiske and Kjellstrand, 1983).

Muscle relaxants must be used cautiously in patients with renal insufficiency. The nondepolarizing agents *d*-tubocurarine and pancuronium are only partially dependent on renal excretion and can be administered safely in reduced doses. The depolarizing agent succinylcholine can be given safely during induction but should not be administered as a continuous infusion. It has active metabolites that are dependent on renal excretion, which may accumulate in patients with renal failure (Kasiske and Kjellstrand, 1983). Gallamine is excreted totally by the kidneys and is contraindicated in patients with renal failure (Sirotzky and Lewis, 1978).

Postoperative Management

The fluid and electrolyte balance of patients with renal insufficiency should be monitored carefully during the postoperative period. Volume assessment may necessitate placement of a central venous or Swan-Ganz catheter as well as measurement of daily patient weight and monitoring of fluid input and output. In patients with normal renal function, diuresis usually begins 24 to 48 hours postoperatively as patients regain the ability to excrete free water. In patients with renal insufficiency, this normal physiologic response must be distinguished from inappropriate fluid loss due to nephrogenic diabetes insipidus or renal salt wasting. These conditions can be differentiated by careful monitoring of intravascular volume and measurement of serum and urinary electrolytes (Vaughan and Gillenwater, 1973).

Patients with renal failure may have delayed wound healing, and skin sutures should be left in place a few extra days. Proper nutrition is important, not only to facilitate wound healing but also to reduce infections that occur more commonly in uremic patients. Nutrition preferably should be provided orally or via nasogastric tube feedings. If oral nutrition is not feasible, however, patients should be started promptly on parenteral nutrition, even if this necessitates dialysis to prevent fluid overload (Kasiske and Kjellstrand, 1983).

Surgery in Patients on Chronic Dialysis

Patients on chronic dialysis have an increased surgical risk, but with careful management the mortality in this group of patients can be reduced to between 1 and 3 per cent (Giacchino et al., 1981; Wiehle et al., 1981). Fluid and electrolyte problems must be corrected preoperatively in these patients. They should be dialyzed on the two consecutive days preceding surgery in order to optimize fluid status and to reduce the incidence of perioperative hemorrhage, hyperkalemia, hypotension, and acidosis. Blood transfusions, if necessary, are administered during the first dialysis so that hyperkalemia resulting from transfusion can be corrected during the second dialysis on the day before surgery. Since dialysis requires anticoagulation that may induce thrombocytopenia, minimal heparinization should be used during dialysis on the day preceding surgery and for all dialysis sessions required during the first week after surgery. Minimal heparinization is associated with fewer bleeding complications than the older technique of regional heparinization, which involved the simultaneous infusion of heparin and protamine (Swarts, 1981). Postoperatively, it is desirable to postpone dialysis for 48 hours because of the increased risk of bleeding and then to resume dialysis every 2 to 3 days as required (Kasiske and Kjellstrand, 1983).

Hyperkalemia is of particular concern in patients on chronic dialysis. The surgeon should attempt to minimize tissue trauma and to avoid blood transfusions. If transfusions are required, it is preferable to administer fresh blood to decrease the potassium load. It is important to monitor the serum pH as well as the serum potassium, since acidosis causes an extracellular shift of potassium.

Patients on dialysis often have associated hypertension. Hypertensive medications should be continued until the time of surgery and resumed immediately thereafter. When it is not possible to administer oral medications, blood pressure may be regulated with intravenous agents such as hydralazine and furosemide, which preserve renal blood flow. Hydralazine may cause tachycardia and should be administered cautiously in patients with coronary artery disease. Sodium nitroprusside may be given as a continuous infusion to control hypertension (Kasiske and Kjellstrand, 1983).

Patients on dialysis may develop pericarditis in the postoperative period, and preoperative dialysis may help prevent this complication. Heart auscultation should be performed daily during the postoperative period to detect a pericardial rub. If pericarditis is discovered, it should be treated by daily dialysis with minimal heparinization.

Finally, patients on dialysis have an increased risk of perioperative thrombosis of the hemodialysis access site, probably resulting from decreased blood flow and hypercoagulability associated with surgical stress. A blood pressure cuff should never be placed on the arm above the access site. Thrombosis of external shunts may be prevented by continuous infusion of heparin at a low rate into both limbs of the cannula (Kasiske and Kjellstrand, 1983).

HEMATOLOGIC CONSIDERATIONS IN UROLOGIC SURGERY

This section deals with three areas of hematology that are of particular concern to the urologist: anemia, transfusions, and coagulation disorders. Other hematologic disorders, such as white blood cell diseases, which are not commonly encountered by the urologist, are not discussed.

Anemia

EVALUATION

Mild to moderate degrees of anemia do not increase the risk of elective surgery, but an evaluation should be initiated to determine the etiology of the anemia. A careful history should be obtained with particular attention to a possible family history of anemia or other blood disorders, bleeding associated with previous dental or surgical procedures, and factors that might suggest chronic blood loss, such as heavy menstrual periods, fecal bleeding, and the use of drugs, most commonly aspirin and alcohol. Physical examination should include a fecal examination for occult blood. Other physical findings may include brittle nails, stomatitis, and a red and raw tongue associated with iron deficiency anemia; peripheral neuritis and a pale, smooth tongue seen in patients with vitamin B_{12} deficiency; and hepatomegaly, ascites, and spider angiomata seen in patients with chronic hepatic disease (Watson-Williams, 1979).

Anemias are classified on the basis of red cell morphology using the mean corpuscular volume (MCV) and mean corpuscular hemoglobin content (MCHC). The MCV normally varies between 82 and 100 fl per cell and the MCHC varies between 30 and 35 gm per dl of blood. The reticulocyte count is a measurement of the percentage of new blood cells seen in the peripheral smear and should be corrected for the degree of anemia to more accurately reflect the response of the bone marrow to anemia. The corrected reticulocyte percentage index (RPI) is calculated by multiplying the reticulocyte percentage by the hematocrit and dividing the product by 45. The RPI is normally between 1 and 2 per cent, but may be as high as 7 per cent in patients with severe hemolytic anemia (Watson-Williams, 1979).

IRON DEFICIENCY ANEMIA

Iron deficiency anemia is the most common cause of anemia in the United States. In this condition both the MCV and the MCHC are decreased, resulting in a microcytic hypochromic peripheral smear. The RPI is less than 1 per cent. Iron deficiency anemia is distinguished from other microcytic hypochromic anemias by the findings of decreased serum iron, increased total iron-binding capacity, and decreased serum ferritin. Since iron deficiency anemia usually reflects chronic blood loss, one should never simply treat the anemia without searching for the underlying cause. If iron deficiency anemia is associated with a positive stool guaiac test, elective surgical procedures should be postponed until the possibility of a gastrointestinal malignancy has been investigated.

Treatment of iron deficiency anemia is often required in the postoperative period. This is most commonly done by the administration of 300 mg of ferrous sulfate orally three times a day. Serum hemoglobin starts to rise about the seventh day of treatment and increases about 0.2 gm per dl every day thereafter. Iron dextran can be given parenterally but is seldom necessary (Watson-Williams, 1979).

FOLATE AND VITAMIN B_{12} DEFICIENCY

Serum folate or vitamin B_{12} deficiency is suggested by the finding of an increased MCV and is confirmed by the presence of hypersegmented neutrophils in the peripheral smear along with decreased serum levels of folate or vitamin B_{12}. Folic acid deficiency can be corrected by the oral administration of 1 mg of folate per day. Vitamin B_{12} is given intramuscularly in a dose of 1 mg every four weeks. The serum hemoglobin rises about 1 gm per dl for every week of therapy with either folate or vitamin B_{12}. Lifelong treatment may be required unless the underlying cause of the anemia is correctable (Watson-Williams, 1979).

HEMOLYTIC ANEMIA

Hemolytic anemia is suggested by the finding of an increased RPI without associated blood loss. Hemolytic anemias are classified as either immune or nonimmune on the basis of the Coombs' test, which tests for the presence of human globulin coating the red blood cells. A positive Coombs' test indicates an immune hemolytic anemia that may be due to autoimmune antibodies, drug-induced antibodies, or a transfusion reaction. Coombs' test-negative anemias can be classified further by testing of red blood cell fragility. Increased red blood cell fragility is associated with hereditary spherocytosis and elliptocytosis. Decreased red blood cell fragility is observed in abnormal hemoglobin disorders, such as sickle cell disease and thalassemia. Normal red blood cell fragility is seen in lead poisoning and alcoholism (Watson-Williams, 1979).

Transfusions

INDICATIONS

The optimum hematocrit for surgery is one that achieves a balance between increased oxygen transport and decreased blood viscosity and appears to be between 30 and 33 per cent (Czer and Shoemaker, 1978). There are two other factors, cardiac output and the oxygen dissociation curve, that affect oxygen delivery to the tissues and that should be considered in assessing the need for perioperative blood transfusions. Patients with a hemoglobin of 10 gm per dl must develop a cardiac output twice that of patients with a hemoglobin of 14 gm per dl in order to deliver the same amount of oxygen to the tissues. Patients with coronary artery disease who are unable to increase their cardiac output may require higher hemoglobin levels in order to withstand the stress of surgery. When transfusing such patients, it is advisable to administer packed red blood cells at a slow rate to avoid fluid overload and congestive heart failure (Lunsgaard-Hansen, 1975).

In patients with chronic anemia, there is a shift of the oxygen dissociation curve to the right, which facilitates the release of oxygen to the tissues. This shift is mediated by an increased amount of 2,3-DPG in the red blood cells. Patients with chronic anemia, therefore, may not require perioperative transfusion provided that their intravascular volume is normal and their cardiac function is not impaired (MacDonald, 1977).

Transfusion of stored whole blood or packed red blood cells does not immediately increase oxygen availability to the tissues to the extent indicated by a rising hemoglobin level (Bellingham and Grisus, 1973). This is because 2,3-DPG must be regenerated in the red blood cells following transfusion. There is about a 50 per cent recovery of 2,3-DPG within 4 hours, but normal oxygen delivery may not be achieved for 24 hours (Beutler and Wood, 1969). Furthermore, it requires 24 hours to readjust total blood volume and validate a successful increase in hemoglobin levels. Therefore, preoperative transfusions ideally should be completed 24 hours before surgery (Watson-Williams, 1979).

COMPLICATIONS

The incidence of adverse reactions occurring within the first 4 days following blood transfusion is approximately 5 per cent (Baker and Nyhus, 1970). Hemolytic reactions are classified as either immediate or delayed. Immediate reactions result from the transfusion of in-compatible blood and carry a mortality as high as 35 per cent (Walter, 1971). Immediate reactions usually result from physician error and are totally avoidable. Delayed hemolytic reactions occur several days to weeks following transfusion and are much milder, with an associated mortality of less than 2 per cent (Walter, 1971). Delayed reactions result from stimulation of a pre-existing antibody that was not detected at the time of compatibility testing and at present are not preventable (Solanki and McCurdy, 1978). The risk of delayed reactions is increased by previous blood transfusions and pregnancy.

Allergic reactions are most often caused by leukocyte antigens and occur in 2 to 3 per cent of patients receiving transfusions. Symptoms include fever less than 39 degrees C, erythema, and itching. Pyrogenic reactions are associated with a fever greater than 39 degrees C and have a bacterial or immunologic etiology. These reactions fortunately have become rare because of more careful storage and handling of blood (Collins, 1983).

Several complications are associated with large volume transfusions. Hypocalcemia may result from the increased citrate load, and supplemental intravenous calcium may be required in patients receiving multiple transfusions (Denlinger, 1978). Microembolization of blood particulate matter to the lungs may cause adult respiratory distress syndrome. The efficacy of transfusion microfilters in preventing this complication is controversial (Geelhoed, 1978). Multiple transfusions also result in depletion of platelets and coagulation factors, particularly factors V and VIII, which are labile in storage, and these patients may have an increased bleeding tendency (Sherman, 1978).

In spite of enhanced detection of donors carrying hepatitis B virus, hepatitis secondary to blood transfusion results in 3000 deaths per year in the United States (Watson-Williams, 1979). Most of these cases are caused by a virus other than hepatitis A or B, and the incubation period is between 14 and 140 days. Patients also may develop chronic active hepatitis following transfusion (Gradey, 1978). Other diseases, such as mononucleosis and cytomegalovirus infection, can be transmitted by transfusion (Lerner and Sampliner, 1977).

COAGULATION MECHANISMS

This section discusses the basic principles regarding the evaluation of hemostatic competence and the management of common coagulation disorders. A more detailed summary is provided in a recent review (Owen and Bowie, 1983).

NORMAL HEMOSTATIC MECHANISMS

Early Events. The early hemostatic events following vascular injury include constriction of bleeding vessels and formation of a platelet plug. Platelets adhere to exposed subendothelial tissue and aggregate within 2 to 3 minutes following injury. The platelet plug must be solidified by subsequent fibrin deposition or it will distintegrate spontaneously and bleeding will resume (Owen and Bowie, 1983).

Coagulation Mechanisms. Coagulation may be initiated by two mechanisms, the so-called intrinsic and extrinsic pathways. These pathways are initiated by different factors, but they ultimately merge into a final common pathway that results in the production of prothrombin, fibrinogen, and ultimately a fibrin clot. Figure 61–2 summarizes the coagulation pathways. The intrinsic pathway involves the interaction of platelet phospholipids with a number of plasma coagulation proteins and calcium. Four protein activation factors that are sequentially activated by the contact of plasma with a foreign surface are required to initiate the pathway. Following activation and interaction with platelets and calcium, factors VIII and IX initiate the final common pathway that ultimately results in the production of fibrin (Owen and Bowie, 1983).

The extrinsic pathway is so-called because it was believed originally that prothrombin could be converted into thrombin by the interaction of tissue juices (thromboplastin) and calcium alone. We now know that three other plasma proteins, factors V, VII, and X, are also required (Owen and Bowie, 1983).

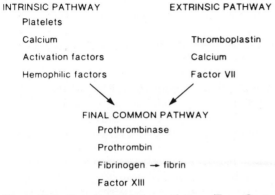

Figure 61–2. Overall coagulation pathways. (From Owen, C. A., Jr., and Walter Bowie, E. J.: Disorders of coagulation. Urol. Clin. North Am. *10*:77, 1983. Used with permission.)

EVALUATION OF HEMOSTATIC COMPETENCE

History and Physical Examination. A careful history is critical in order to assess hemostatic competence. The history may reveal the presence of a coagulation disorder that otherwise might be missed on routine laboratory screening. It is insufficient simply to inquire about easy bruising or bleeding because the patient may not be aware of these phenomena. Specific questions regarding family history, previous dental extractions and surgical procedures, nose bleeds, menstrual bleeding, and drug history must be asked. The physical examination also is important and may reveal fundal hemorrhages, petechiae and ecchymoses, and hematomas and hemarthroses (Watson-Williams, 1979).

Platelet Function. The adequacy of the number of platelets can be assessed from the peripheral blood smear, and a formal platelet count usually is unnecessary. Platelet function is assessed by the bleeding time, which is the time it takes for bleeding to stop after skin puncture and that correlates with the formation of a platelet plug. A normal bleeding time is between 2 and 3 minutes. The bleeding time is prolonged in patients with a deficient number of platelets, patients with an inherent abnormality in platelet function (e.g., patients with von Willebrand's disease), and in patients with an acquired abnormality of platelet function (e.g., patients with uremia or an abnormality from aspirin ingestion) (Owen and Bowie, 1983).

The intrinsic pathway of coagulation is evaluated by the PTT or by the APTT. Both tests measure the coagulation time when partial thromboplastin and calcium are added to the patient's plasma. They differ only in that in the APTT test activation is induced before the partial thromboplastin and calcium are added to the plasma, whereas in the PTT test the activation occurs after the partial thromboplastin is added. The PTT and APTT will be prolonged if there is a deficiency in one of the activation factors, factor VIII or factor IX, or if there is a deficiency in any of the factors in the final common pathway. The most common abnormality involving the intrinsic pathway is factor VIII deficiency (see further on). Factor IX deficiency, which produces Christmas disease, is the next most common abnormality and is much rarer (Owen and Bowie, 1983).

The extrinsic coagulation pathway is assessed by the PT, which is performed by adding a thromboplastic emulsion and calcium to plasma. The prothrombin time is prolonged by a deficiency of factor VII or by a deficiency of any of the factors in the final common pathway (Owen and Bowie, 1983).

The initial laboratory tests that should be obtained to screen for a coagulation disorder are a peripheral blood smear and either a PTT or an APTT. A formal platelet count is usually unnecessary, and since the only additional coagulation disorder that will be detected by the PT is a rare factor VII deficiency, a routine PT does not seem justified (Watson-Williams, 1979).

SPECIFIC COAGULOPATHIES

Inherited Diseases. Any of the coagulation factors may be lacking on an inherited basis. Factors VIII and IX are sex-linked; all the others have an autosomal mode of inheritance.

All the inherited coagulation disorders are rare except for classic hemophilia and von Willenbrand's disease. Both are related to a deficiency of a part of the factor VIII complex. Classic hemophilia is caused by a lack of the clotting portion of the complex (VIII:C), whereas von Willebrand's disease is caused by a deficiency of the high molecular weight carrier protein transhemophilin (VIII:T) (Owen, 1981). Transhemophilin has two important functions. First, it is necessary for platelet adherence, and patients with von Willebrand's disease have a prolonged bleeding time. Second, the liver will not release VIII:C unless VIII:T is present (Owen and Bowie, 1983). Classic hemophilia is inherited as a sex-linked recessive disease and occurs almost exclusively in men. von Willebrand's disease has an autosomal mode of inheritance. Both diseases are characterized by a normal prothrombin time and an abnormal PTT or APTT, but they can be distinguished from each other by the pattern of inheritance and the increased bleeding time associated with von Willebrand's disease.

Surgical management of patients with classic hemophilia and von Willenbrand's disease has changed dramatically since the introduction of factor VIII on a commercial basis in 1970. It is usually possible to administer a sufficient quantity of factor VIII so that patients with these diseases can undergo required surgical procedures. The risk of surgical bleeding and the need for factor VIII replacement are determined by the degree of factor VIII deficiency in the individual patient. Patients undergoing minor surgery usually require a level of factor VIII that is 40 per cent of normal, and patients undergoing major surgery require a level that is 80 per cent of normal (Manoa et al., 1970). Factor VIII is available as a concentrate, or it can be prepared from fresh plasma in the form of a cryoprecipitate. Factor VIII replacement is initiated 1 hour before surgery and is administered at regular intervals over the next 10 days. Patients with von Willenbrand's disease are somewhat easier to manage because the administration of cryoprecipitate results in a greater and more prolonged elevation of factor VIII (Gilchrist et al., 1980).

Unfortunately, about 5 to 10 per cent of patients with classic hemophilia will have an associated antibody to factor VIII. This is identified by measurement of factor VIII levels that are less than 1 per cent of normal and by the failure of fresh plasma added to the patient's serum to correct the PTT. Patients with antibodies to factor VIII have a severe hemorrhagic risk and usually are not candidates for any elective surgical procedure (Pintado et al., 1975).

Acquired Diseases. In contrast to inherited disorders, acquired coagulopathies usually are multifactorial in origin. Two specific entities, vitamin K deficiency and disseminated intravascular coagulation (DIC), will be discussed. Vitamin K is necessary for hepatic conversion of coagulation precursors to active factors VII, IX, X, and prothrombin. The most common abnormality related to vitamin K is not deficiency of the vitamin but pharmacologic blockade of its hepatic function caused by warfarin and other prothrombinopenic agents. These drugs prevent the liver from synthesizing active coagulation factors from their precursor forms (Owen and Bowie, 1983).

Hemorrhagic disease of the newborn results from a deficiency of vitamin K. Since vitamin K can be obtained only from its production by intestinal bacteria or by the ingestion of green leafy plants, vitamin K deficiency can occur in surgical patients whose diets have been restricted and who have received antibiotic bowel preparations in anticipation of intestinal surgery. Vitamin K deficiency also occurs in patients with biliary obstruction or fistulas (Owen and Bowie, 1983).

Patients with vitamin K deficiency will have prolongation of both their PT and their PTT. Vitamin K deficiency can be corrected preoperatively by the administration of 10 mg of vitamin K intravenously every 12 hours. Three doses usually will be sufficient (Watson-Williams, 1979).

DIC is a consumption coagulopathy manifested by spontaneous widespread thrombosis. The massive coagulation is followed by generalized fibrinolysis and increased bleeding, and a more appropriate name for this condition might be "intravascular clotting with fibrinolysis." (Owen and Bowie, 1983). Acute DIC may be precipitated by shock, septicemia, mismatched blood transfusions, amniotic fluid embolism, snake bite, and other unrelated conditions. A chronic, less severe form of DIC is seen in patients with large metastatic cancers (Sun et al., 1974).

In urologic patients, DIC usually occurs as a result of sepsis. The diagnosis should be suspected clinically in a patient with widespread purpura oozing from venipuncture sites and bleeding from mucous membranes. Associated laboratory findings include a decreased platelet count, elevation of both the PT and the PTT, and increased fibrin-split products resulting from fibrinolysis (Watson-Williams, 1979).

The treatment of DIC should be directed primarily at correcting the underlying cause of the condition. Administration of fresh plasma or cryoprecipitate may help restore clotting factors once the underlying problem has been corrected. The administration of heparin may be effective because fibrinolytic activity may diminish spontaneously once fibrin formation is blocked (Owen and Bowie, 1979). The administration of EACA (Amicar) is useful only in treating isolated fibrinolysis. Its administration to patients with DIC may lead to further widespread thrombosis (Naeye, 1962).

SICKLE CELL DISEASE

Although it is not strictly a coagulation disorder, sickle cell disease is commonly encountered by urologists in dealing with patients with papillary necrosis and priapism. Patients with sickle cell disease have an increased risk of perioperative thrombosis. This risk can be decreased by maintenance of adequate oxygenation, hydration, and normal body temperature. In addition, exchange transfusions are recommended for surgical patients with sickle cell disease to lower the percentage of abnormal cells to below 50 per cent (Morrison and Wiser, 1976). Sickle cell trait is not associated with increased surgical risk, and no special precautions are necessary (Sears, 1978).

ENDOCRINE CONSIDERATIONS

Diabetes Mellitus

Blood glucose levels should be well controlled prior to surgery; elective surgery in an uncontrolled diabetic patient is seldom justified. Blood glucose levels should be maintained between 125 and 250 mg per dl during the perioperative period to decrease the incidence of infections (Bagdade, 1976) and to facilitate wound healing (Goodsen and Hunt, 1977). To achieve this goal, a number of regimens for administering insulin during the perioperative period have been proposed (Shipp, 1968; Steinke, 1970; Taitelman et al., 1977). Regardless of the technique employed, therapy must reflect the fact that insulin requirements change frequently during the perioperative period. The stress of surgery may result in increased insulin requirements resulting from hyperglycemia caused by the release of epinephrine and cortisol (Baesl and Buckley, 1983). Conversely, insulin requirements may decrease following surgical treatment of an established infection, such as a perinephric abscess (White and Kumagai, 1979). Although it is desirable to control blood glucose levels within reasonable limits to reduce perioperative complications, overzealous regulation may result in fatal hypoglycemia.

During the past 10 years, I have had good success managing diabetic surgical patients with a protocol that recently has been recommended elsewhere (Backer et al., 1980). The patient receives one half of his usual morning insulin dose as NPH insulin at 7 A.M. on the morning of surgery. An intravenous infusion of a 5 per cent glucose solution is begun 2 hours preoperatively at a rate of 100 ml per hour. Blood glucose levels are checked every 4 to 6 hours. It is particularly important to follow blood glucose levels during prolonged surgery, since hypoglycemia is difficult to diagnose in the anesthetized patient. Hyperglycemia is managed by the supplemental administration of subcutaneous insulin as shown in Table 61–6. The time of peak effect of previously administered intermediate-acting insulin should be kept in mind when administering supplemental regular insulin.

TABLE 61 – 6. MANAGEMENT OF POSTOPERATIVE HYPERGLYCEMIA IN THE DIABETIC PATIENT

Blood Glucose (mg/dl)	Percentage of Normal Morning Insulin Dose (Subcutaneous)*
< 250	None
250 – 300	10
300 – 400	20
> 400	25

*Regular insulin dosage administered at 4- to 6-hr intervals according to serum glucose.
(From Izenstein, B., Dhuhy, R., and Williams, G.: Endocrinology. In Vandan L. (Ed.): To Make the Patient Ready for Anesthesia. Menlo Park, California, Addison-Wesley Co., 1980. Used with permission.)

The use of a sliding scale based on urinary glucose levels to determine supplemental insulin requirements has several disadvantages. First, voided urine specimens often are inaccurate because the urine may have been present in the bladder for several hours and does not reflect blood glucose levels. Catheterized urine specimens are more accurate but are associated with an increased risk of infection, particularly in the diabetic patient (White and Kumagai, 1979). Second, the threshold for glucose excretion may be elevated in diabetics with renal disease, and measurement of urinary glucose may lead to an underestimation of blood glucose (Backer et al., 1980). Third, many drugs interfere with both Clinitest and Tes-tape and cause them to be inaccurate (Feldman and Lebovitz, 1973).

During the early postoperative period when patients are unable to eat, an intravenous infusion that provides 50 to 100 gm of glucose per day should be continued. Blood glucose levels should be measured every 6 hours, and patients should receive regular insulin as required. Once insulin requirements have stabilized, blood glucose determinations may be necessary only in the early morning and in the midafternoon (Backer et al., 1980).

After the patient has resumed his preoperative diet, intravenous fluids may be discontinued, and the patient may be managed with an intermediate-acting insulin such as NPH, which is administered as a single dose in the morning. Blood glucose levels should be checked at 3 P.M., and adjustment of the morning insulin dose may be required as shown in Table 61–7.

Diabetic patients who are not insulin-dependent are easier to manage because they are not as likely to develop ketoacidosis or hyperosmolar dehydration. Patients on oral hypoglycemic agents should not be given their medication on the morning of surgery. An intravenous infusion containing 5 per cent glucose is begun 2 hours before surgery. Blood glucose levels should be measured in the recovery room and in the afternoon of surgery, and regular insulin should be administered as required to maintain blood glucose levels below 250 mg per dl. Patients who are able to eat following surgery usually do not require supplemental insulin, and they can resume their oral medication either on the evening following surgery or the next morning. Patients who are unable to eat for several days probably will require supplemental regular insulin. Diabetic patients who are managed by dietary restrictions alone usually do not require supplemental insulin during the perioperative period (Steinke, 1970).

Diabetic patients often have associated diseases that require attention during the perioperative period. They have a higher incidence of both coronary artery disease and congestive heart failure, and the risk of cardiovascular mortality is twofold greater in diabetic men and 4½ times greater in diabetic women than in nondiabetic patients (Garcia et al., 1974). Diabetic patients may have associated renal disease that will complicate perioperative fluid and electrolyte management (White and Kumagai, 1979). Diabetic patients with autonomic neuropathy may be particularly susceptible to respiratory depression and cardiopulmonary arrest associated with the use of certain drugs (Page and Watkins, 1978).

Adrenal Insufficiency

The normal response of the body to stress is to increase adrenal production of cortisol. Normally 15 to 25 mg of cortisol are produced by the adrenal glands daily, but under severe stress cortisol production may increase to between 250 and 300 mg daily (Backer et al., 1980). Adrenocortical insufficiency may develop not only in patients with primary adrenal or pituitary failure but also in patients who have received exogenous steroid therapy for the treatment of other diseases. Exogenous steroids suppress the pituitary-adrenal axis, and full recovery from steroid suppression may take as long as 1 year (White and Kumagai, 1979). Patients with steroid suppression are likely to develop acute adrenocortical insufficiency during the perioperative period unless they receive supplemental steroids.

The indications for supplemental perioperative steroid therapy are as follows: (1) chronic adrenal insufficiency, (2) continuous treatment

TABLE 61 – 7. Additional Morning Insulin Dose After Stabilization of Requirements

3 P.M. Blood Glucose (mg/dl)	Percentage of Morning Insulin Dose (Subcutaneous)
200 – 300	None
300 – 400	20 as intermediate insulin
> 400	20 as intermediate insulin and 20 as regular insulin

(From Izenstein, B., Dhuhy, R., and Williams, G.: Endocrinology. *In* Vandan, L. (Ed.): To Make the Patient Ready for Anesthesia. Menlo Park, California, Addison-Wesley Co., 1980. Used with permission.)

with topical steroids for greater than 1 month in the previous 6 months (Rabinowitz et al., 1977), (3) treatment with systemic steroids for greater than 1 week in the past 6 months (Gran and Pahle, 1978), (4) current steroid therapy, (5) anticipated bilateral adrenalectomy, and (6) anticipated unilateral adrenalectomy for a cortisol-producing tumor (Baesl and Buckley, 1983).

Patients with suspected steroid suppression should receive 100 mg of hydrocortisone intravenously at midnight and at 6 A.M. on the day of surgery and 100 mg every 6 hours for the first 24 hours postoperatively. Supplemental hydrocortisone is decreased to 50 mg every 6 hours for the next 24 hours, and is further decreased to 25 mg every 6 hours during the following 24 hours (Baesl and Buckley, 1983). Serum cortisol levels return to normal within 72 hours in control patients, and supplemental steroids in patients with steroid suppression usually are unnecessary after this time (Plumpton et al., 1969). Steroid supplementation should be continued, however, in patients with surgical complications, such as sepsis or ileus, which increase cortisol demand.

The relative anti-inflammatory and sodium-retaining properties of various glucocorticoids are shown in Table 61–8. Cortisone acetate is a poor choice for steroid replacement because it is rapidly metabolized to inactive hormones and is absorbed erratically following intramuscular administration (Kehlet et al., 1974).

NUTRITIONAL SUPPORT OF THE UROLOGIC PATIENT

About 50 per cent of patients undergoing major surgery are malnourished (Bistrian et al., 1974), and nutritional depletion is associated with increased surgical morbidity and mortality (Gibbons et al., 1976). Malnutrition results in delayed wound healing, increased frequency of wound infections, decreased vital organ func-

tion, decreased immunocompetence, increased sepsis, prolonged ileus, and more frequent respiratory infections and pulmonary insufficiency (Mullen, 1981; Pietsch and Meakins, 1977). These problems are related to a loss of body protein. Depletion of one quarter of the body's nitrogen content, which corresponds to a decrease of one third in body weight, is fatal. Nutritional problems are common in geriatric, renal failure, and cancer patients—groups of patients that the urologist deals with frequently. It is important, therefore, that the urologist be aware of nutritional requirements and be familiar with methods of nutritional evaluation and support.

Nutritional Requirements

CALORIES

An individual's daily caloric requirement is about 25 kcal per kg body weight (McDougal, 1983). The demands of surgery result in an increased caloric requirement to about 30 to 35 kcal per kg body weight, and severely burned or septic patients may require as many as 50 kcal per kg body weight (Teasley et al., 1983). Carbohydrates and protein both provide 4 kcal per gm, and fats provide 9 kcal per gm.

PROTEIN

Between 1.5 and 2 gm of protein per kg body weight are required daily to preserve lean body mass (Hensle, 1983). Protein consists of amino acids that are either nonessential or essential. The former can be manufactured by the body, whereas the latter cannot and must be supplied in the diet.

FATS

Fatty acids also can be classified as nonessential and essential. The three essential fatty acids are linoleic acid, arachidonic acid, and linolenic acid. Only linoleic acid is absolutely essential, since a fatty acid deficiency will not

TABLE 61 – 8. RELATIVE ANTI-INFLAMMATORY AND SODIUM-RETAINING POTENCIES OF GLUCOCORTICOIDS

Drugs	Potency	Sodium Retention
Cortisone acetate	0.8	0.8
Hydrocortisone	1	1
Prednisone	4	0.8
Prednisolone	4	0.8
Methylprednisolone	5	0.5
Dexamethasone	25	0

(From Baesl, T. J., and Buckley, J. J.: Preoperative assessment, preparation for operation, and postoperative care. Urol. Clin. North Am., *10*:3, 1983. Used with permission.)

develop if it alone is provided (McDougal, 1983).

Vitamins must be provided daily, particularly water-soluble vitamins because they are depleted rapidly. Minerals such as sodium, potassium, calcium, magnesium, and phosphate must be provided daily, and trace metals such as zinc, copper, magnesium, and iodine must be provided periodically (McDougal, 1983).

OVERALL NUTRITIONAL PLANNING

The goals of nutritional therapy are to protect body protein stores and to provide adequate calories. Although it is important to preserve body protein, excessive administration of protein should be avoided because it may result in an elevation of the BUN and altered hepatic and renal transport in critically ill patients (McDougal, 1983). Twenty-five kilocalories of carbohydrate or fat should be provided for each gram of protein administered, and it is important to supply a balance of both carbohydrate and fat to satisfy the body's energy demands (McDougal, 1983). Carbohydrate usually is administered as glucose, and though glucose provides only 4 kcal per gm, it has a protein-sparing effect. Supplying up to 700 calories per day as glucose provides maximal protection of body protein. A further increase in glucose does not increase protein-sparing, and it is impossible to maintain a positive nitrogen balance with glucose alone. Fats provide 9 kcal per gm, but they do not have as great a protein-sparing effect as do carbohydrates (McDougal, 1983).

Nutritional Evaluation

PREOPERATIVE EVALUATION

Preoperative evaluation of nutritional status is easy and inexpensive to accomplish and should be done in all patients who are undergoing major surgery. The basic evaluation includes only a determination of weight loss and measurements of the serum albumin and lymphocyte count. Additional tests are required only when uncertainty about nutritional status persists after these basic tests have been accomplished (McDougal, 1983).

Weight Loss. All patients should be asked about possible recent weight loss. Patients who have lost up to 10 lbs. in the preceding 3 months are assumed to be mildly malnourished. A weight loss of 10 to 20 lbs. reflects moderate malnutrition, and a weight loss greater than 20 lbs. indicates severe malnutrition. Absolute weight loss may underestimate the degree of malnutrition because there is an accumulation of extracellular fluid when body protein is metabolized that may offset total body weight loss. The use of a height-weight index may be helpful in assessing weight loss, but the index is often inaccurate in obese patients (McDougal, 1983).

Lymphocyte Count. The lymphocyte count reflects visceral protein status and is normally greater than 2000 per mm³. A value between 1200 and 2000 per mm³ reflects mild malnutrition, a value between 800 and 1200 per mm³ indicates moderate malnutrition, and a value less than 800 per mm³ is associated with severe malnutrition (McDougal, 1983).

Serum Albumin. Serum albumin also reflects visceral protein status and normally is greater than 3.5 gm per dl. A value between 3 and 3.5 gm per dl indicates mild malnutrition, a value between 2.5 and 3 gm per dl reflects moderate malnutrition, and a value less than 2.5 gm per dl is associated with severe malnutrition (McDougal, 1983).

Skin Test Antigens. The use of skin test antigens may be helpful when uncertainty about nutritional status exists after weight loss, serum albumin, and total lymphocyte counts have been assessed. Failure to respond to recall skin test antigens such as mumps, *Candida*, and streptokinase-streptodornase (SK-SD) indicates severe malnutrition (McDougal, 1983).

Other Tests. Serum transferrin is another measurement of visceral protein status. Normal values are in excess of 200 mg per dl. A value between 150 and 200 mg per dl reflects mild nutritional deficiency, a value between 100 and 150 mg per dl indicates moderate nutritional deficiency, and a value less than 100 mg per dl is associated with severe deficiency. Measurement of the midupper arm circumference and determination of the creatinine excretion index are tests used to evaluate lean body mass or muscle protein stores. The triceps skin fold thickness is used to assess fat stores (McDougal, 1983).

ASSESSING RESPONSE TO THERAPY

A response to therapy is indicated by weight gain and normalization of the lymphocyte count, serum albumin, and serum transferrin levels. It may take 2 to 3 weeks of therapy before an objective response is noted, and elective surgery should be postponed as long as necessary. About 50 per cent of cancer patients who are skin test–negative will convert to positive after nutritional repletion, and those patients who convert to a positive status respond better to surgery and chemotherapy (Daly et al., 1980).

Response to nutritional therapy can be assessed daily by determination of the body weight and nitrogen balance. Changes in body weight accurately reflect nutritional therapy provided that the patient is not overloaded with fluid. Nitrogen balance can be calculated readily. Eighty per cent of the nitrogen lost in the urine is excreted as urea, and about 1.25 gm of nitrogen are excreted per day in the feces and through the skin. The daily nitrogen loss can be calculated, therefore, by multiplying the amount of urea excreted in the urine in 24 hours by a factor of 1.25 and adding 1.25 gm to account for fecal and skin losses. The daily nitrogen intake can be calculated by the dietary service. Nitrogen balance is determined by subtracting the daily nitrogen loss from the daily nitrogen intake (McDougal, 1983).

Methods of Nutritional Support

ENTERAL NUTRITION

Enteral nutrition is associated with fewer complications and can provide a more balanced physiologic diet than intravenous nutrition. Enteral nutrition can be accomplished through a feeding tube, a gastrostomy, or a feeding jejunostomy. The newer small-caliber Silastic mercury-tipped feeding tubes are well tolerated by patients. There are a variety of commercially prepared solutions now available that provide about 1 kcal per ml and cause fewer gastrointestinal side effects than older preparations (Hensle, 1983).

Enteral diets are either nonelemental or elemental. Nonelemental diets consist of undigested and minimally digested protein hydrolysates, fat, and carbohydrates. Elemental diets consist of medium-chain triglycerides, glucose, and amino acids. Nonelemental preparations are cheaper and have a lower osmolality, and they are preferable to elemental preparations if the intestinal tract is not diseased. Elemental diets are bulk-free and are better tolerated in patients with gastrointestinal problems (Fairfull-Smith et al., 1980). Severely malnourished patients may have altered gastrointestinal absorption due to a decrease in the height of the mucosal brush border and a decrease in the height of the columnar epithelium, and they may have decreased gastrointestinal motility caused by overgrowth of anaerobic bacteria. These patients should be placed initially on an elemental diet until these changes associated with starvation have been reversed (Viteri and Schneider, 1974).

Enteral feedings are administered by continuous infusion. They are begun at a concentration of one-half strength at a rate of 50 to 75 ml per hour. The volume is increased as tolerated to provide 2000 to 3000 ml per day. The concentration or rate should be reduced if the patient develops abdominal cramps, diarrhea, or diaphoresis. Diarrhea also may be controlled by the administration of paregoric in doses of 5 ml (McDougal, 1983).

ISOSMOTIC INTRAVENOUS NUTRITION

Isosmotic intravenous nutrition is an ideal means of preserving normal metabolic function in short-term situations following trauma or surgery in which the gastrointestinal tract cannot be used. The advantages of using isosmotic solutions instead of hypertonic solutions are that they can be administered by peripheral vein and the rate of infusion may be adjusted rapidly without affecting serum osmolality. Isosmotic infusions may be temporarily discontinued so that colloids, medications, and blood may be administered as required. Unfortunately, a positive nitrogen balance cannot be achieved with isosmotic solutions alone, since the number of calories required would precipitate fluid overload. Therefore, long-term intravenous hyperalimentation requires the use of hypertonic solutions (McDougal, 1983).

A common solution used for isosmotic intravenous nutrition consists of a liter solution containing 500 ml of a 10 to 20 per cent dextrose solution and 500 ml of a 7 per cent amino acid solution. This balanced glucose and amino acid solution provides maximal protein-sparing while maintaining optimal hepatic, renal, and cardiac function. Additional calories are supplied through the administration of 500 ml of fat emulsions once or twice per day. Lipomal, a cotton-seed preparation that was formerly used as an intravenous fat emulsion, was associated with frequent febrile reactions, jaundice, and coagulative defects. Intralipid, which consists of soy bean oil emulsified with egg phospholipid, is the fat emulsion currently used, and it has none of the untoward effects observed with Lipomal (Hensle, 1983).

HYPEROSMOTIC INTRAVENOUS NUTRITION

Hyperosmotic intravenous nutrition was developed by Dudrick et al. in 1968. Standard solutions contain 1000 calories and 6 gm of nitrogen per L and are a mixture of 50 per cent dextrose and 7 per cent amino acid solutions. Electrolytes, trace elements, and vitamins are added to the solution as required. Essential fatty acids in the form of Intralipid are administered two or three times weekly.

Hyperosmotic intravenous solutions are about two osmolar and must be administered through a central venous catheter. A percutaneous subclavian or internal jugular catheter is sufficient for short-term use, but a Broviac or Hickman catheter is required for long-term hyperalimentation. These catheters are inserted into the superior vena cava and are tunneled across the anterior chest wall, exiting midway between the sternum and the nipple. These catheters have been maintained for as long as 14 months in children and 21 months in adults (McDougal, 1983). Central venous catheters must be inserted under strict aseptic conditions and must be kept sterile at all times. Blood, additional fluid, and medications cannot be given through a hyperalimentation catheter, and the line should never be used to measure central venous pressure.

Intravenous hyperalimentation is begun at a rate of 50 ml per hour. The rate is increased gradually to avoid hyperglycemia, and insulin is added to the solution as required to maintain a blood glucose level less than 200 mg per dl. Eventually, 3 to 4 L of solution may be infused per day, providing 3000 to 4000 kcal. When discontinuing hyperalimentation, the infusion rate should be tapered over 24 to 36 hours to avoid hypoglycemia (McDougal, 1983).

Patients receiving intravenous hyperalimentation must be followed carefully. Serum glucose and osmolality should be monitored closely, particularly when beginning therapy, to prevent hyperosmolar dehydration. Serum electrolytes, BUN, creatinine, calcium, and, phosphate levels should be assessed daily, and serum magnesium should be checked twice weekly.

The complications of hyperosmotic intravenous nutrition can be divided into three categories: technical, infectious, and metabolic. Technical complications are related to catheter insertion and include pneumothorax, hydrothorax, brachial plexus injury, arterial injury, venous thrombosis, and air embolism. The frequency of technical complications is inversely related to the experience of the person inserting the hyperalimentation catheter (Hensle, 1983).

Infectious complications occurred previously in 10 to 30 per cent of patients receiving intravenous hyperalimentation. With better techniques, the incidence of infectious complications has been lowered to between 1 and 3 per cent (Ryan et al., 1974).

The most serious metabolic complication of intravenous hyperalimentation is hyperosmolar nonketotic dehydration and coma, which occurs when blood glucose levels exceed 500 mg per dl. The mortality of this condition approaches 50 per cent, and it must be treated aggressively with large doses of insulin and fluid and by decreasing the rate of infusion (McDougal, 1983). Hyperalimentation also can cause alterations in amino acid metabolism, which result in hyperchloremic metabolic acidosis, azotemia, and hyperammonemia. A third metabolic complication may occur when excess calories are provided. This stimulates insulin release, which induces hepatic lipogenesis with subsequent fatty infiltration of the liver and colostatic jaundice. This complication may be avoided either by providing only the required number of calories in the infusion or by withholding glucose for an 8-hour period every day and infusing only amino acids and fat during this time (Maizels and Schaeffer, 1980). Other metabolic abnormalities result from improper amounts of nutrients in the intravenous solution, and these problems usually are minor and corrected easily. Vitamin, mineral, trace metal, and essential amino acid deficiencies all can occur and usually cause no clinical problems when corrected promptly.

Intravenous Nutrition and Renal Failure

ACUTE RENAL FAILURE

The mortality associated with acute renal failure can be reduced by 50 per cent by providing adequate calories and essential amino acids. Protein restriction and supplementation with essential amino acids result in a less rapid increase in BUN, which is associated with decreased catabolism, increased wound healing, and decreased duration of renal failure (Abel et al., 1973).

CHRONIC RENAL FAILURE

Surgical patients with chronic renal failure benefit from protein restriction and supplementation with essential amino acids. This therapy results in improvement in anemia associated with renal insufficiency, decreased BUN, and a positive nitrogen balance (Gilmour, 1983, Hu vannctti, 1966). It is not necessary to restrict

TABLE 61 – 9. DIETARY PROTEIN RESTRICTION IN RENAL FAILURE

GFR (ml/min)	Daily Protein Allowance (gm)
< 10	40
10 – 15	50
16 – 20	70
21 – 25	90

(From Hensle, T. W.: Nutritional support of the urologic patient. Curr. Trends Urol., *1*:157, 1981. Used with permission.)

protein until the GFR is less than 25 ml per minute. Recommended protein allowances for lower GFRs are shown in Table 61–9. Patients on dialysis must be allowed extra protein in their diet, since they lose between 6 and 10 gm of free amino acids during each hemodialysis and between 6 and 10 gm of protein during each peritoneal dialysis. Intravenous hyperalimentation is not a substitute for dialysis, but the combination of hyperalimentation and dialysis results in maximal protein synthesis, which may produce a positive nitrogen balance (Hensle, 1983).

INFECTIONS AND ANTIBIOTIC THERAPY

Urinary Tract Infections

PROPHYLAXIS

The majority of perioperative urinary tract infections are caused by bladder catheterization (Alexander, 1983). Between 0.5 and 2 per cent of patients will have bacteriuria following a single catheterization (Allo and Simmons, 1983). The risk of infection increases with the duration of catheterization, and even with the most careful management about 50 per cent of catheterized patients will have urinary tract infections after 10 days (Kunin and McCormack, 1966).

Preservation of a closed drainage system is the most effective means of reducing the risk of urinary tract infections in catheterized patients (Garibaldi et al., 1974). Closed drainage systems will not only delay urinary tract infections but also are effective in reducing the risk of cross-infection between catheterized patients (Pyrah, 1955).

Other measures to reduce the risk of urinary tract infections associated with catheterization have not been effective. Continuous bladder irrigation via a three-way catheter with either 0.25 per cent acetic acid or neomycin-polymyxin solutions may delay the onset of infections, but they risk selection of resistant organisms that may be more difficult to eradicate once the catheter is removed (Thornton et al., 1966). In addition, there is the risk of introducing infection into the catheter each time the empty irrigation containers are replaced. Application of antimicrobial agents at the urethral meatus has been similarly ineffective in reducing the risk of catheter-related infections. Application of povidone-iodine ointment to the urethral meatus does not reduce the risk of infection, and simple cleansing of the urethral meatus with soap and water is associated with an increased risk of infection, probably related to manipulation of the catheter and introduction of exogenous bacteria (Burke et al., 1981). Administration of systemic antibiotics may delay urinary tract infections by several days, but the antibiotics may select resistant organisms that ultimately may be more difficult to eradicate (Garibaldi et al., 1974).

There has been recent interest in the instillation of antiseptic solutions to the urinary drainage bag to reduce urinary tract infections. Addition of hydrogen peroxide to the drainage bag does delay the onset of bacteriuria in the bag itself (Maizels and Schaeffer, 1980). However, the drainage bag appears to be an infrequent source of urinary tract infection (Hartstein et al., 1981; Pien and Landers, 1983). Instillation of chlorhexidine into the urinary drainage bag has been ineffective in reducing the rate of urinary tract infection (Islam and Chapman, 1977). Thus, the addition of antiseptic agents to the urinary drainage bag does not appear effective in reducing urinary tract infections.

DIAGNOSIS

The diagnosis of urinary tract infection is made by obtaining a urine culture that grows greater than 100,000 colonies per ml of urine. Voided samples usually are accurate in men. In women, however, voided samples often are inaccurate because of perineal contamination, and catheterized specimens often are required to establish the diagnosis. A negative catheterized urine sample should contain less than 1000 colonies per ml; a greater number of organisms suggests the presence of infection. Hospital-acquired urinary tract infections usually are caused by gram-negative organisms (Alexander, 1983).

Urine dip sticks or Microstix are an effective means of screening for urinary tract infections. They are less expensive than routine cultures, costing about 60 cents each, and recent studies have demonstrated their accuracy. Patients with negative Microstix tests can be spared the cost of a formal urine culture (Craig et al., 1973; Pien and Landers, 1983).

TREATMENT

Asymptomatic bacteriuria should not be treated in a catheterized patient. Antibiotics should be reserved for those patients with symptomatic infections or bacteremia. A urine culture should be obtained prior to removal of the catheter, and infections should be treated after the catheter has been removed (Alexander, 1983).

Cystitis resulting from catheterization should be treated with a 3-day course of an appropriate antibiotic. Single dose antibiotic therapy may be appropriate in an outpatient setting but is not recommended for the treatment of hospital-acquired infections. A 3-day course of antibiotics is as effective as longer-term therapy and is associated with less alteration of the microbiologic intestinal and vaginal flora. Failure to eradicate infection with short-term therapy suggests the presence of a deep-seated parenchymal infection that requires more extended treatment (Kunin, 1981).

Wound Infections

PROPHYLAXIS

Preoperative shaving of the wound site should be accomplished with electric clippers; razor shaving is inadvisable, since it increases the risk of wound infections. Alternatively, a depilatory can be used to remove hair from the surgical site (Seropian and Reynolds, 1971). Preoperative skin preparation with an antiseptic agent reduces the risk of wound infection. Traditionally, a 10-minute scrub has been recommended, but shorter periods of time may suffice with the newer antiseptic agents, particularly when applied to smaller operative fields. Hexachlorophene, chlorhexidine, and povidone-iodine all have been used; of these, povidone-iodine is the most popular and hexachlorophene the least effective (Alexander, 1983).

Plastic skin drapes have not proved effective in reducing wound infections. Plastic drapes may shelter and allow bacteria to proliferate, and, thus, a larger bacterial inoculum is available to enter the wound when the drape is removed. Plastic drapes are recommended to exclude contaminated sites, such as a colostomy, from the operative field (Alexander, 1983).

Although surgical incisions are generally sealed after 48 hours, wound resistance to infection increases progressively until the fourth or fifth postoperative day. It is advisable, therefore, to maintain a sterile dressing over the wound site until that time. Wet dressings must be changed in a sterile manner, since they will promote bacterial proliferation. Once the surgical dressing has been removed, the dry wound coagulum should be left undisturbed, since it provides resistance to exogenous infection. Painting the incision with an antiseptic solution or application of an antibiotic ointment are contraindicated, since they may disrupt this defensive barrier (Alexander, 1983).

Contaminated wounds should be managed with delayed primary or secondary closure to reduce the risk of wound infection. A reactive vascular network develops along the wound edges, and this provides increasing resistance to infection, which becomes maximal about the fifth postoperative day. Delayed primary closure can be accomplished at this time without risking later infection (Edlich et al., 1969).

DIAGNOSIS

Wound infections usually occur between the 5th and 10th postoperative days. Infections that occur within 48 hours postoperatively are caused either by a hemolytic streptococcus or a clostridium (Allo and Simmons, 1983). Wound infections may cause pain and erythema over the surgical incision, but often the presentation is less obvious and is manifested by constitutional symptoms such as fever and tachycardia. The diagnosis is made by probing the wound; any purulent material should be cultured for both aerobic and anaerobic bacteria, and a gram stain should be obtained to guide immediate antibiotic therapy (Allo and Simmons, 1983).

TREATMENT

The treatment of superficial wound infections involves incision and drainage along with local wound care. The use of antibiotics in superficial wound infections remains controversial. Treatment of deeper wound infections involves administration of broad-spectrum antibiotics along with drainage of purulent material and debridement of devitalized tissue. Antibiotic therapy should be initiated before surgical manipulation of a wound because of the risk of bacteremia and septic shock. Initial antibiotic therapy usually should include an aminoglycoside to cover gram-negative organisms and clindamycin or a third-generation cephalosporin with broad anaerobic activity. Wound infections that occur within 48 hours postoperatively should be treated with penicillin to cover streptococci and clostridia (Allo and Simmons, 1983). Antibiotic therapy can be modified pending the results of the wound cultures.

Failure to eradicate an infection with drainage and antibiotic therapy suggests a deep-seated infection such as an abdominal or retroperitoneal abscess. Further tests including an ultrasound examination or a computerized tomography (CT) scan should be obtained to establish the diagnosis, and it may be possible to drain a deep abscess through a percutaneous catheter inserted under radiographic control (Van Sonnenberg et al., 1982).

Pulmonary Infections

PROPHYLAXIS

Lower respiratory tract infections account for about 15 per cent of all nosocomial infections and are particularly common following prolonged anesthesia. The risk of pulmonary infections can be reduced by employing aseptic technique during intubation and endotracheal suctioning and by maintaining sterile respiratory support equipment. Respiratory isolation procedures should be initiated in patients with pulmonary infections to prevent cross-infection of other patients (Alexander, 1983).

DIAGNOSIS

Pneumonia is usually readily diagnosed because it produces consolidation of pulmonary tissue on a chest roentgenogram. A tracheal aspirate should be obtained daily in all intubated patients and a gram stain should be performed. An early pneumonia may be detected when the gram stain findings change from scattered inflammatory cells to dense neutrophils and bacteria. Sputum cultures from nonintubated patients are usually worthless because of pharyngeal contamination. When pneumonia is suspected, a transtracheal aspiration should be performed to obtain a reliable culture. Renal transplant patients and other immunosuppressed patients are prone to develop nonbacterial pneumonias, and transbronchial or open pulmonary biopsies may be required to establish the diagnosis (Alexander, 1983).

TREATMENT

Pneumonias usually can be eradicated with pulmonary therapy and antibiotics. Empiric an-tibiotic therapy should include both gram-positive and gram-negative coverage. A more precise antibiotic regimen may be initiated when the results of the sputum cultures have been obtained (Alexander, 1983).

Other Considerations

PROSTATECTOMY

The use of perioperative antibiotics to decrease the risk of urinary tract infections in patients undergoing prostatectomy remains controversial. Some studies have shown a decrease in the rate of infection (Kudinoff et al., 1966; Morris et al., 1976), whereas others have found that antibiotics produce no difference in the infection rate (Gibbons et al., 1983; Holl and Rous, 1982). A recent study demonstrated that perioperative antibiotics administered 2 hours preoperatively and 12 hours postoperatively were effective in reducing the rate of urinary tract infections associated with prostatectomy. Short-term antibiotics were as effective as long-term antibiotics without the associated risk of selection of resistant organisms (Goldwasser et al., 1983).

Antibiotics are definitely indicated in patients undergoing prostatectomy whose urine is suspected or known to be infected. Such patients have a high risk of bacteremia associated with prostatectomy and should receive perioperative antibiotics (Cafferkey et al., 1982). Prostatectomy patients also should receive a single antibiotic dose prior to catheter removal, since catheter manipulation may also precipitate bacteremia (Murphy et al., 1983).

PROSTATIC NEEDLE BIOPSY

Transrectal needle biopsy of the prostate is associated with a high incidence of bacteremia. Patients undergoing this procedure should receive a preoperative enema and broad-spectrum antibiotics that provide gram-negative and anaerobic coverage. Perioperative antibiotics are not required in patients undergoing transperineal needle biopsy of the prostate unless their urine is infected (Packer et al., 1984).

SUBACUTE BACTERIAL ENDOCARDITIS

Patients who are at risk for bacterial endocarditis should receive prophylactic antibiotics prior to urologic instrumentation. Such patients include those with rheumatic heart disease, congenital heart disease, a prolapsing mitral valve, and idiopathic hypertrophic subaortic stenosis, and those with prosthetic heart valves. Enterococcus *(Streptococcus faecalis)* is the organism usually responsible for endocarditis after genitourinary surgery (American Heart Association, 1977).

Patients at risk for subacute bacterial endocarditis should receive ampicillin 1 gm (intravenously or intramuscularly) and gentamicin 1.5 mg per kg (intravenously or intramuscularly, not to exceed 80 mg) 30 to 60 minutes before any genitourinary procedure. Two additional doses of these antibiotics should be given at 8-hour intervals following the procedure. Since enterococcus is the organism most frequently responsible for bacterial endocarditis following urologic procedures, ampicillin is preferable to penicillin for prophylaxis. Patients allergic to penicillin should receive vancomycin 1 gm intravenously preoperatively and two doses at 8-hour intervals postoperatively (American Heart Association, 1977).

INTESTINAL SURGERY

Patients undergoing urologic procedures that involve entry into the intestinal tract, particularly the distal ileum or colon, should undergo bowel preparation. A recommended routine for bowel preparation is outlined in Table 61–10. Mechanical cleansing of the bowel should be accomplished mainly by dietary restriction and cathartics. Repeated enemas are not only unnecessary and uncomfortable to the patient but also risk introduction of resistant organisms into the gastrointestinal tract (Alexander, 1983). Oral antibiotics with little systemic absorption, such as neomycin and erythromycin base, have been shown to further reduce the incidence of postoperative infections and should be administered after mechanical cleansing is complete (Nichols, 1982). The issue of whether systemic antibiotics further reduce postoperative

infections is unresolved (Allo and Simmons, 1983).

Whole-gut lavage has been advocated as an alternative means of bowel preparation. This involves administration of 10 to 12 L of saline at a rate of 3 to 4 L per hour through a nasogastric or orogastric tube (Hewitt et al., 1973). Although whole-gut lavage may be less traumatic than the usual 3-day bowel preparation, the rapid administration of large volumes of saline risks fluid overload, pulmonary edema, and congestive heart failure, particularly in elderly patients with underlying cardiac and renal disease (Allo and Simmons, 1983). It is, therefore, not recommended for routine use in urologic patients.

Gram-Negative Bacteremia and Septic Shock

INCIDENCE

Gram-negative bacteremia occurs in more than 1 of every 100 hospital admissions in the United States (McCabe and Treadwell, 1983). It is a condition that urologists should recognize and treat promptly, since more than half of the cases result from urologic procedures (Hanno and Wein, 1981). Gram-negative bacteremia is one of the most frequent causes of hospital-acquired infection deaths. The mortality rate associated with bacteremia alone varies up to 40 per cent; septic shock is associated with a mortality rate of up to 80 per cent (Hanno and Wien, 1981).

ETIOLOGY

Gram-negative bacteremia accounts for about 70 per cent of septicemias. Mixed gram-

TABLE 61 – 10. Bowel Preparation for Elective Colorectal Operations

Preoperative day 3	Clear liquid or minimum residue diet, bisacodyl, 1 capsule orally at 6 P.M.
Preoperative day 2	Clear liquid or minimum residue diet; magnesium sulfate, 30 ml of 50 per cent solution (15 gm) orally at 10 A.M., 2 P.M., and 6 P.M.; saline enemas at bedtime until return is clear
Preoperative day 1	Clear liquid diet; magnesium sulfate (in dose above) at 10 A.M. and 2 P.M.; supplemental intravenous fluids as needed; no enemas; neomycin-erythromycin base, 1 gm orally at 1 P.M., 2 P.M., and 11 P.M.
Operative day	Rectum evacuated at 6:30 A.M.; operation at 8 A.M.

(From Nichols, R. L.: Prophylaxis for elective bowel surgery. *In* Wilson, S. E., Finegold, S. M., and Williams, R. A. (Eds.): Intra-abdominal Infection. New York, McGraw-Hill Book Co., 1982. Used with permission.)

positive and gram-negative infections account for another 10 to 20 per cent. Gram-positive bacteremia has become much less common with earlier recognition and treatment of gram-positive infections (Schwartz and Cerra, 1983). *Escherichia coli* is the single most common causative organism. It causes about 30 per cent of cases and is associated with the best prognosis (Hanno and Wein, 1981). The *Klebsiella-Enterobacter-Serratia* family is the next most common group of organisms, and accounts for about 20 per cent of cases (McCabe and Treadwell, 1983).

PATHOPHYSIOLOGY

The pathophysiology of gram-negative bacteremia is complicated and not completely understood. A brief discussion is included here, and for greater detail the reader is referred to the appropriate references (Hanno and Wien, 1981; McCabe and Treadwell, 1983; Schwartz and Cerra, 1983). The cell wall of gram-negative bacilli is composed of a lipid-carbohydrate complex termed lipopolysaccharide (LPS). This complex acts as an endotoxin, and considerable emphasis has been placed on this substance and its role in the pathophysiology of gram-negative bacteremia. More recent studies have indicated that this endotoxin is only partially responsible for the pathophysiologic changes that occur in this condition. Intact bacilli or endotoxin stimulate the complement system, resulting in the production of two vasoactive anaphylatoxins, C3a and C5a. These activated complement components stimulate the production of bradykinin, which produces the vasodilatation and increased vascular permeability observed in gram-negative bacteremia (Fearon et al., 1975; McCabe, 1973). Bradykinin also results in increased production of the prostaglandins PGE_2 and PGF_2. Prostaglandins and endorphins may contribute to the hypotension associated with this condition (Fletcher and Ramwell, 1977; Peters et al., 1981). Intact bacteria or endotoxin also may initiate the activation of Hageman factor, which, in turn, stimulates sequential activation of other components of the coagulation system, resulting in DIC and fibrinolysis (Mason et al., 1970).

The two major consequences of these complicated interactions are a reduction in vascular tone and a failure of oxygen extraction by the tissues. Gram-negative bacteremia thus is usually associated with an increased cardiac output and a decreased peripheral resistance (Schwartz and Cerra, 1983). In addition to cardiac failure, the hypoxia and altered vascular permeability results in a loss of the functional integrity of alveolar-capillary membranes in the lung. This may result in pulmonary edema and the adult respiratory distress syndrome, or "shock lung," which is one of the major causes of death in patients with bacteremia (Hanno and Wien, 1981).

DIAGNOSIS

The early symptoms of gram-negative bacteremia may be subtle and may include only fever, altered sensorium, or tachypnea. The astute clinician who is alerted by these early signs will act promptly and usually will be able to prevent the disastrous complications of septic shock. As bacteremia progresses, the patient will develop tachycardia and hypotension associated with an increased cardiac output and a decreased peripheral vascular resistance. Central venous pressure is usually normal or increased (Hanno and Wien, 1981).

Laboratory findings include changes in the white blood cell count, which is initially depressed and is then elevated. A coagulopathy is suggested by a decreased platelet count and is confirmed by a decrease in serum fibrinogen and an elevation in fibrin split products. Arterial blood gases demonstrate respiratory alkalosis initially and metabolic acidosis subsequently. Increasing levels of serum lactic acid are associated with a poor prognosis. Derangement of cellular function may give rise to hyperkalemia and hyponatremia (Hanno and Wien, 1981).

TREATMENT

Gram-negative bacteremia demands prompt, aggressive treatment to prevent septic shock. Blood, urine, and other appropriate cultures should be obtained, and broad-spectrum antibiotics should be administered immediately after obtaining these cultures. Antibiotics should include an aminoglycoside and a third-generation cephalosporin to provide maximal gram-negative as well as gram-positive and anaerobic bacterial coverage (McCabe and Treadwell, 1983).

Treatment of hypotension associated with bacteremia may require large volumes of crystalloid because of the decreased peripheral vascular resistance. Intravenous fluids must be administered judiciously, particularly in the elderly, to avoid fluid overload and congestive heart failure. A Swan-Ganz pulmonary arterial catheter may be invaluable in guiding fluid therapy (Hanno and Wien, 1981).

Patients with persistent hypotension following adequate volume replacement will require administration of vasoactive agents. Dopamine is the drug of first choice, since in low doses it increases renal blood flow and cardiac output without increasing heart rate or peripheral vascular resistance (Hanno and Wien, 1981).

Patients with hypoxemia may require supplemental oxygen, and mechanical ventilatory support may be necessary. Patients with adult respiratory distress syndrome may require large doses of PEEP to facilitate oxygen delivery (McCabe and Treadwell, 1983).

Other ancillary treatment measures include the administration of intravenous sodium bicarbonate to correct metabolic acidosis and the use of digitalis in patients with heart failure. Corticosteroids remain controversial in the treatment of septic shock. Their reported actions include vasodilatation with improved renal blood flow, a positive inotropic effect, decreased platelet aggregation, and stabilization of lysosomal membranes in the injured cell. Steroids appear to be more effective when they are administered early in the course of the disease (Hanno and Wien, 1981).

Once immediate therapeutic measures have been initiated, the cause of the bacteremia should be determined. If a focus of infection such as an abscess is identified, it should be drained as soon as possible following the initial resuscitation of the patient (Schwartz and Cerra, 1983).

UROLOGIC SURGERY IN PREGNANCY

Urologic surgery in pregnancy should be restricted to emergency procedures and generally is limited to the management of urinary tract calculi. The incidence of calculous disease is no greater during pregnancy (Coe et al., 1978), but the symptoms are often attributed to another cause, and the diagnosis frequently is not made until after delivery (Folger, 1955). A brief discussion of the diagnosis and management of urinary tract calculi in pregnancy is presented here.

Diagnosis

Radiographic evaluation of the urinary tract during pregnancy should be limited to emergency situations. When obstructive uropathy secondary to calculous disease is suspected, an intravenous pyelogram should be performed. The hazards of radiation exposure during pregnancy have been exaggerated, and the risk is far outweighed by the potential clinical benefits derived from a properly indicated examination.

The evidence suggests that harmful radiation effects to the fetus are associated with radiation exposure in excess of 50 rads. This is far in excess of the usual intravenous pyelogram, which has an associated radiation dosage of less than 1 rad (Swartz and Reichling, 1978). Although radiation is most hazardous to the fetus during the first trimester, a radiation dose of up to 5 rads that would result from an extensive radiologic procedure is still safely tolerated, and interruption of a pregnancy because of previous radiation exposure is seldom justified (Swartz and Reichling, 1978).

Although the risk of radiation is small, the radiation dose to the fetus incurred with an intravenous pyelogram can be reduced as much as 40-fold by careful radiographic technique (Bruwer, 1976). The number of films should be limited to a scout film, a 15-minute film, and a delayed film if necessary. This two- or three-film examination will demonstrate an obstructing calculus and will document the degree of obstruction. The x-ray beam should be collimated to the point of interest, and proper beam filtration should be used to limit radiation scatter. Placing the patient in the prone rather than the supine position further limits radiation exposure to the fetus because the roentgen rays are attenuated by the spine and the thick posterior abdominal wall. Application of compression bands around the maternal abdomen may further decrease fetal radiation exposure by decreasing the thickness of the maternal abdomen and will also result in less radiation scatter and an improved radiographic image. The use of fast films with short exposure times and high-speed radiographic screens will also decrease radiation exposure (Stern, 1982). Finally, the use of low kilovoltage of about 60 to 70 Kv affords better contrast and more detailed information than that obtained with a higher kilovoltage of about 120 Kv. Although the radiation dose to the skin is higher with lower kilovoltage, the radiation dose to deeper tissues and the fetus is no different (Fisher and Russell, 1975).

Alternative diagnostic modalities include ultrasound and radionuclide renography. Both techniques are less reliable than intravenous urography but are associated with less radiation exposure. Ultrasound is accurate in detecting renal calculi but is less reliable in detecting obstructing ureteral calculi. Furthermore, it may be difficult to distinguish physiologic hydronephrosis associated with pregnancy from pathologic hydronephrosis associated with an obstructing calculus (Freed, 1982). The radionuclide renogram is also somewhat less reliable than the intravenous pyelogram but can provide valuable information regarding renal function and the presence of obstruction. Renography is particularly accurate during the first and second trimesters of pregnancy. Physiologic obstruction may be confused with pathologic obstruction in about 10 to 20 per cent of cases during the third trimester (Wax, 1982).

Treatment

Although it is desirable to avoid surgery during pregnancy, obstructing urinary stones usually can be safely removed during any stage of pregnancy. The risk of spontaneous abortion associated with surgery is greatest during the first trimester. Surgery is most safely performed during the second trimester. During the third trimester, pelvic surgery for distal ureteral calculi can be very difficult because of the enlarged uterus and engorged vasculature (Freed, 1982).

There are several alternatives for management of obstructing urinary tract calculi that may obviate or delay the need for surgery during pregnancy. Most stones are small and should be given time to pass spontaneously as long as the clinical situation permits. Endoscopic basket extraction of distal ureteral calculi is possible during any phase of pregnancy. An obstructing distal ureteral stone may be milked into the bladder by transvaginal compression (Farkas and Firstater, 1979). It may be possible to push an obstructing calculus back into the renal pelvis or to bypass a stone with a Gibbons-type indwelling ureteral catheter that can be left in place for the duration of pregnancy (Freed, 1982). Large distal ureteral calculi that are too large to manipulate may be treated with percutaneous nephrostomy. This seems particularly advisable during the third trimester when pelvic surgery is particularly treacherous. We recently inserted a percutaneous nephrostomy into a woman in her third trimester with urinary obstruction and sepsis due to a large ureteral calculus. The catheter was left in place until the fetus was mature and a cesarean section was performed. The ureteral calculus subsequently was removed 1 week later with a successful outcome for both mother and child.

References

Abel, R. M., Beck, C. H., Jr., Abbott, W. M., et al: Improved survival from acute renal failure after treatment with intravenous essential L-amino acids and glucose. N. Engl. J. Med., 288:695, 1973.

Alderson, P. O., Lee, H., Summer, W. R., et al: Comparison of Xe-133 washout and single breath imaging for detection of ventilation abnormalities. J. Nucl. Med., 20:917, 1979.

Alexander, J. W.: Infection, host resistance, and antimicrobial agents. In Dudrick, S. J. et al., (Eds): Manual of Preoperative and Postoperative Care. Philadelphia, W. B. Saunders Co., 1983, p. 106.

Allen, E. V.: Thromboangitis obliterans: Methods of diagnosis of chronic occlusive arterial lesions distal to the wrist with illustrative cases. Am. J. Med. Sci., 178:237, 1929.

Allgood, R. J., Cook, J. H., Weedn, R. J., et al: Prospective analysis of pulmonary embolism in the postoperative patient. Surgery, 68:116, 1970.

Allo, M., and Simmons, R. L.: Surgical infectious disease and the urologist. Urol. Clin. North Am., 10:131, 1983.

American Heart Association Committee: Prevention of bacterial endocarditis. Circulation, 56:139A, 1977.

Anderson, R., and Jensen, P. B.: Prophylactic anticoagulant therapy in prostatic surgery. Acta. Chir. Scand., 132:144, 1966.

Anderson, W. H., Dorsett, B. E., and Hamilton, G. L.: Prevention of postoperative pulmonary complications. JAMA, 186:763, 1963.

Antila, L. E., Markkula, H., and Lisalo, E.: The years' experience of geriatric aspects in surgery of patients with benign prostatic hyperplasia. Acta Chir. Scand., (Suppl.) 357:95, 1966.

Backer, C. L., Tinker, J. H., Robertson, D. M., et al.: Myocardial infarction following local anesthesia for ophthalmic surgery. Anesth. Analg., 59:257, 1980.

Baesl, T. J., and Buckley, J. J.: Preoperative assessment, preparation, and routine postoperative care. Urol. Clin. North Am., 10:3, 1983.

Bagdade, J. D.: Phagocytic and microbial function in diabetes mellitus. J. Endocrinol., (Suppl.) 83(205):27, 1976.

Baker, R. J., and Nyhus, L. M.: Diagnosis and treatment of immediate transfusion reaction. Surg. Gynec. Obstet., 130:665, 1970.

Barash, P. G., Nardi, D., Hammond, G., et al.: Catheter induced pulmonary artery perforation. J. Thorac. Cardiovasc. Surg., 82:5, 1981.

Bartlett, R. H., Gazzaniga, A. B., and Geraghty, T. R.: The yawn maneuver: prevention and treatment of postoperative pulmonary complications. Surg. Forum, 22:196, 1971.

Bartlett, R. H., Gazzaniga, A. B., and Geraghty, T. R.: Respiratory maneuvers to prevent postoperative pulmonary complications. JAMA, 224:1017, 1973.

Baxter, W. D., and Levine, R. S.: An evaluation of intermittent positive pressure breathing in the prevention of postoperative pulmonary complications. Arch. Surg., 98:795, 1969.

Bedford, R. F., and Wallinen, H.: Complications of percutaneous radial-artery cannulation. Anesthesiology, 38:228, 1973.

Bellingham, A. J., and Grisus, A. J.: Red cell 2,3-diphosphoglycerate. Br. J. Haematol., 25:555, 1973.

Benet, L. (Ed): The Effect of Disease States on Drug Pharmacokinetics. Washington, D.C., Am. Pharmaceutical Assoc./Am. Pharmaceutical Sci., 1976.

Bergentz, S.: Dextran in the prophylaxis of pulmonary embolism. World J. Surg., *2*:19, 1978.

Beutler, E., and Wood, L.: The in vivo regeneration of red cell 2, 3 diphosphoglyceric acid (DPG) after transfusion of stored blood. J. Lab. Clin. Med., *74*:300, 1969.

Bistrian, B. R., Blackburn, G. L., Sherman, M., et al.: Therapeutic index of nutritional depletion in hospitalized patients. Surg. Gynecol. Obstet., *141*:512, 1975.

Blaschke, T. F., and Melmon, K. L.: Antihypertensive agents and the drug therapy of hypertension. *In* Goodman, A. G., Goodman, L. S., and Gilman, A. (Eds): Goodman and Gilman's Pharmacological Basis of Therapeutics. 6th ed. New York, Macmillan Publishing Co., 1980.

Bonnar, J., and Walsh, J.: Prevention of thrombosis after pelvic surgery by British dextran 70. Lancet, *1*:614, 1972.

Borges, H. F., Hocks, J., and Kjellstrand, C. M.: Mannitol intoxication in patients with renal failure. Arch. Intern. Med., *142*:63, 1982.

Borja, A. R., and Hinshaw, J. R.: A safe way to perform infraclavicular subclavian vein catheterization. Surg. Gynecol. Obstet., *130*:673, 1970.

Boushy, S., Billig, D. M., North, L., et al.: Clinical course related to preoperative and postoperative pulmonary function in patients with bronchogenic carcinoma. Chest, *59*:383, 1971.

Brenowitz, J. B., Williams, C. D., and Edwards, W. S.: Major surgery in patients with chronic renal failure. Am. J. Surg., *134*:765, 1977.

Brinkman, A. J., and Costley, D. O.: Internal jugular venipuncture. JAMA, *223*:182, 1973.

Browse, N. L., Jackson, B. T., Mayo, M. E., et al.: The value of mechanical methods of preventing postoperative calf vein thrombosis. Br. J. Surg., *61*:219, 1974.

Bruwer, A.: If you are pregnant, or if you think you might be . . . Editorial. Am. J. Roentgenol., *127*:696, 1976.

Bull, M. J., Schreiner, R. L., Gary, B. P., et al.: Neurologic complications following temporal artery catheterization. J. Pediatr., *96*:1071, 1980.

Burke, G. R., and Gulyassy, P. F.: Surgery in the patient with renal disease and related electrolyte disorders. Med. Clin. North Am., *63*:1191, 1979.

Burke, J. P., Garibaldi, R. A., Britt, M., et al.: Prevention of catheter-associated urinary tract infections: efficacy of daily meatal care regimens. Am. J. Med., *70*:655, 1981.

Bynum, L. J., and Wilson, J. E., III: Low dose heparin therapy in the long-term management of venous thromboembolism. Am. J. Med., *67*:553, 1979.

Byrd, L., and Sherman, R. L.: Radiocontrast-induced acute renal failure. A clinical and pathophysiological review. Medicine, *58*:270, 1979.

Cafferkey, M. T., Falkiner, F. R., Gillespie, W. A., et al.: DM: Antibiotics for the prevention of septicaemia in urology. J. Antimicrob. Chemother., *9*:471, 1982.

Carter, A. E., and Eban, R.: The prevention of postoperative deep venous thrombosis with dextran 70. Br. J. Surg. *60*:681, 1973.

Civetta, J. M., Gabel, J. C., and Gemer, M.: Internal-jugular-vein puncture with a margin of safety. Anesthesiology, *36*:622, 1972.

Civetta, J. M.: Goal directed respiratory therapy. ASA Refresher Course 110, 1981.

Clagett, G. P., Brier, D. F., Rosoff, C. B., et al.: Effect of aspirin on postoperative platelet kinetics and venous thrombosis. Surg. Forum, *25*:473, 1974.

Cockroft, D. W., and Gault, M. H.: Prediction of creatinine clearance from serum creatinine. Nephron, *10*:31, 1976.

Coe, F. L., Parks, J. H., and Lindheimer, M. D.: Neph-rolithiasis during pregnancy. N. Engl. J. Med., *298*:324, 1978.

Coe, N. D., Collins, R. E. C., Klein, L. A., et al.: Prevention of deep venous thrombosis in urologic patients: A controlled, randomized trial of low-dose heparin and external pneumatic compression boots. Surgery, *83*:230, 1978.

Coleman, S. S., and Anson, B. J.: Arterial patterns in the hand based upon a study of 650 specimens. Surg. Gynecol. Obstet., *113*:409, 1961.

Colgan, F. J., Barrow, R. E., and Fanning, G. L.: Continuous positive pressure breathing and cardiorespiratory function. Anesthesiology, *34*:145, 1979.

Collins, J. A.: Blood and blood products. *In* Dudrick, S. J. et al. (Eds.): Manual of Preoperative and Postoperative Care. Philadelphia, W. B. Saunders Co., 1983, p. 137.

Collins, R. E. C., Klein, L. A., Skillman, J. J., et al.: Thromboembolic problems in urologic surgery. Urol. Clin. North Am., *3*:393, 1976.

Craig, D. B., Wahba, W. M., Don, H. F., et al.: Closing volume and its relationship to gas exchange in the seated and supine positions. J. Appl. Physiol., *31*:717, 1971.

Craig, W. A., Kunin, C. M., and DeGroot, J.: Evaluation of new urinary tract infection screening devices. Appl. Microbiol., *26*:196, 1973.

Czer, L. S. C., and Shoemaker, W. C.: Optimal hematocrit value in critically ill postoperative patients. Surg. Gynecol. Obstet., *147*:363, 1978.

Daly, J. M., Dudrich, S. J., and Copeland, E. M.: Intravenous hyperalimentation: effect in delayed cutaneous hypersensitivity in cancer patients. Ann. Surg., *192*:587, 1980.

Dawson, J. L.: Post-operative renal function in obstructive jaundice: Effect of a mannitol diuresis. Br. Med. J., *1*:82, 1965.

Deitel, M., and McIntyre, J. A.: Radiographic conformation of site of central venous pressure catheters. Can. J. Surg., *14*:42, 1971.

De la Rocha, A. G., Edmonds, J. F., Williams, W. G., et al.: Importance of mixed venous oxygen saturation in the care of critically ill patients. Can. J. Surg., *21*:227, 1978.

DeLaurentis, D. A., Hayes, M., Matsumato, T., et al.: Does central venous pressure accurately reflect hemodynamic and fluid volume patterns in the critical surgical patient? Am. J. Surg., *126*:415, 1973.

Del Guercio, L. R. M., and Cohn, J. D.: Monitoring operative risk in the elderly. JAMA, *243*:1350, 1980.

Denlinger, J. K.: Calcium metabolism during blood transfusion and citrate toxicity. *In* Brzica, S. M., Jr. (Ed.): Blood Transfusion Dilemmas. Washington, D.C., American Association of Blood Banks, 1978, p. 45.

Depner, T. A., and Gulyassy, P. F.: Chronic renal failure. *In* Earley, L. E., and Gottschalk, C. W. (Eds.): Strauss and Welt's Diseases of the Kidney. Boston, Little, Brown & Co., 1979.

Deutsch, S.: Effects of anesthetics on the kidney. Surg. Clin. North Am., *55*:775, 1975.

Douglas, W. W., Rehder, K., Beynen, F. M., et al.: Improved oxygenation in patients with acute respiratory failure. The prone position. Am. Rev. Resp. Dis., *115*:559, 1977.

Downs, J. B., and Raphaely, R. C.: Pediatric intensive care. Anesthesiology, *43*:238, 1975.

Downs, J. B., Chapman, R. L., and Hawkins, I. F.: Prolonged radial artery catheterization: An evaluation of heparinized catheters and continuous irrigation. Arch. Surg., *108*:671, 1974.

Downs, J. B., Perkins, H. M., and Modell, J. H.: IMV: An evaluation. Arch. Surg., *109*:519, 1974.

Downs, J. B., Rackstein, A. D., Klein, E. F., et al.: Hazards of radial-artery catheterization. Anesthesiology, *38*:283, 1973.

Dudrick, S. J., Wilmore, D. W., Vars, H. M., et al.: Long-term parenteral nutrition with growth development and positive nitrogen balance. Surgery, *64*:135, 1968.

Dunbar, R. D., Mitchell, R., and Lavine, M.: Aberrant locations of central venous catheters. Lancet, *1*:711, 1981.

Eckstein, J. W., Hamilton, W. K., and McCammond, J. M.: The effect of thiopental on peripheral venous tone. Anesthesiology, *22*:525, 1961.

Edlich, R. F., Rodgers, W., Kasper, G., et al.: Studies in the management of the contaminated wound. Am. J. Surg., *117*:323, 1969.

Egbert, L. D., and Bendixen, H. H.: Effect of morphine on breathing patterns. JAMA, *188*:485, 1964.

Egbert, L. D., Battit, G. E., Welch, C. E., et al.: Reduction of postoperative pain by encouragement and instruction of patients. N. Engl. J. Med., *270*:825, 1964.

Eisenberg, R. L., Bank, W. O., and Hedgock, M. W.: Renal failure after major angiography can be avoided with hydration. AJR, *136*:859, 1981.

Elliott, C. G., Zimmerman, G. A., and Clemmen, T. P.: Complications of pulmonary artery catheterization in the care of the critically ill patient. Chest, *76*:647, 1979.

Erslev, A., and Shapiro, S.: Hematologic aspects of renal failure. *In* Earley, L. E. and Gottschalk, C. W. (Eds.): Strauss and Welt's Diseases of the Kidney. Boston, Little, Brown & Co., 1979.

Evans, P. J. D., and Kerr, J. H.: Arterial occlusion after cannulation. Br. Med. J., *3*:197, 1975.

Fairfull-Smith, R., Abunassar, R., Freeman, J. B., et al.: Rational use of elemental and nonelemental diets in hospitalized patients. Ann. Surg., *192*:600, 1980.

Falke, K. J., Pontoppidan, H., Kumar, A., et al.: Ventilation with end inspiratory pressure in acute lung disease. J. Clin. Invest., *51*:2315, 1972.

Farkas, A., and Firstater, M.: Transvaginal milking of lower ureteric stones into the bladder. Br. J. Urol., *51*:193, 1979.

Fearon, D. R., Ruddy, S., Schur, P. H., et al: Activation of the properdin pathway of complement in patients with gram-negative bacteremia. N. Engl. J. Med., *292*:937, 1975.

Feldman, J. M., and Lebovitz, F. L.: Tests for glucosuria: An analysis of factors that causes misleading results. Diabetes, *22*:115, 1973.

Fisher, A. S., and Russell, J. G. B.: Radiography in Obstetrics. London, Butterworth & Co., 1975.

Fletcher, J. R., and Ramwell, P. W.: Modification by aspirin and indomethacin of the haemodynamic and prostaglandin releasing effects of E. coli endotoxin in the dog. Br. J. Pharmacol., *61*:175, 1977.

Folger, G. K.: Pain and pregnancy. Treatment of painful states complicating pregnancy, with particular emphasis on urinary calculi. Obstet. Gynecol., *5*:515, 1955.

Foote, G. A., Schabel, S. I., and Hodges, M.: Pulmonary complications of the flow-directed balloon-tipped catheter. N. Engl. J. Med., *290*:927, 1974.

Forrester, J. S., Diamond, G., Chatterjee, K., et al: Medical therapy of acute myocardial infarction by application of hemodynamic subsets. N. Engl. J. Med., *295*:1356, 1976.

Forthman, H. J., and Shepard, A.: Postoperative pulmonary complications. South. Med. J., *62*:1198, 1969.

Fraser, J. G., Ramachandran, P. R., and Davis, H. S.: Anesthesia and recent myocardial infarction. JAMA, *199*:318, 1967.

Freed, S. Z.: Urinary tract calculi in pregnancy. *In* Freed, S. Z., and Herzig, N. (Eds.): Urology in Pregnancy. Baltimore, Williams & Wilkins, 1982, p. 135.

Gallus, A. S., Hirsh, J., Tuttle, R. J., et al.: Small subcutaneous doses of heparin in prevention of venous thrombosis. N. Engl. J. Med., *288*:545, 1973.

Gallus, A. S., Hirsh, J., Tuttle, R. J., et al.: Prevention of venous thrombosis with small subcutaneous doses of heparin. JAMA, *235*:1980, 1975.

Gamsu, G., Singer, M. M., Vincent, H. H., et al.: Postoperative impairment of mucous transport in the lung. Am. Rev., *114*:673, 1976.

Garcia, M. J., McNamara, P. M., Gordon, T., et al.: Morbidity and mortality in diabetics in the Framingham population. Sixteen year follow-up study. Diabetes, *23*:105, 1974.

Garibaldi, R. A., Burke, J. P., Dickman, M. L., et al.: Factors predisposing to bacteriuria during indwelling urethral catheterization. N. Engl. J. Med., *291*:215, 1974.

Geelhoed, G. W.: Microembolization in blood transfusion. A nondisease for which we have a cure. *In* Brzica, S. M., Jr.: Blood Transfusion Dilemmas. Washington, D.C., American Association of Blood Banks, 1978, p. 35.

Giacchino, J. L., Geis, W. P., Wittenstein, B. H., et al.: Surgery, nutritional support, and survival in patients with end-stage renal disease. Arch. Surg., *116*:634, 1981.

Gibbons, G. W., Blackburn, G. L., Hasken, D. E., et al.: Pre- and postoperative hyperalimentation in the treatment of cardiac cachexia. J. Surg. Res., *20*:439, 1976.

Gibbons, R. P., Stark, R. A., Correa, R. J., Jr., et al.: The prophylactic use—or misuse—of antibiotics in transurethral prostatectomy. J. Urol., *119*:381, 1978.

Gilchrist, G. S., Hagedorn, A. B., Owen, C. A., Jr., et al.: Management of patients with von Willebrand's disease undergoing surgical procedures. *In* Mamen, E. F., Barnhart, M. I., Lusher, J. M., and Walshe, R. T. (Eds.): Review of Hematology. Vol. I. Treatment of Bleeding Disorders with Blood Components. Westbury, New York, P.J.D. Publications, 1980, p. 83.

Gilmour, I. J.: Perioperative respiratory care. Urol. Clin. North Am., *10*:65, 1983.

Giordano, C.: Use of exogenous and endogenous urea for protein synthesis in normal and uremic patients. J. Lab. Clin. Med., *62*:231, 1963.

Giovannetti, S.: Diet in chronic uremia. Proc. 3rd Int. Cong. Nephrol., *3*:230, 1966.

Goggin, M. J., and Joekes, A. M.: I. Dangers of hyperkalemia during anesthesia. Br. Med. J., *2*:244, 1971.

Goldman, L.: Supraventricular tachyarrhythmias in hospitalized adults after surgery. Chest, *73*:4, 1978.

Goldman, L., and Caldera, D.: Risks of general anesthesia and elective operation in the hypertensive patient. Anesthesiology, *50*:285, 1979.

Goldman, L., Caldera, D. L., Nussbaum, S. R., et al.: Multifactoral index of cardiac risk in noncardiac surgical procedures. N. Engl. J. Med., *297*:845, 1977.

Goldman, L., Caldera, D. L., Southwick, F. S., et al.: Cardiac risk factors and complications in noncardiac surgery. Medicine, *57*:357, 1978.

Goldwasser, B., Bogokowsky, B., Nativ, O., et al.: Prophylactic antimicrobial treatment in transurethral prostatectomy—how long should it be instituted? Urology, *22*:136, 1983.

Goodsen, W. H., and Hunt, T. K.: Studies on wound

healing in experimental diabetes mellitus. J. Surg. Res., 22:221, 1977.

Gradey, C. F.: Transfusion and hepatitis update in '78 (editorial). New Engl. J. Med., 298:1413, 1978.

Graham, W., and Bradley, D.: Efficacy of chest physiotherapy and intermittent positive pressure breathing in the resolution of pneumonia. New Engl. J. Med., 299:624, 1978.

Gran, L., and Pahle, J. A.: Rational substitution therapy for steroid-treated patients. Anaesthesia, 33:59, 1978.

Grodsinsky, C., Brush, B. E., and Ponka, J. L.: Postoperative pulmonary complications in the geriatric age group. J. Am. Geriatr., 22:407, 1974.

Gutzen, L. C., and Pollack, E. W.: Short-term femoral vein catheterization: A safe alternative venous access? Am. J. Surg., 138:875, 1979.

Hamilton, W. K., and Sokoll, M. D.: Choice of anesthetic techniques in patients with acute pulmonary disease. JAMA, 197:789, 1977.

Hampers, C. L., Bailey, G. L., Hager, E. B., et al.: Major surgery in patients on maintenance hemodialysis. Am. J. Surg., 115:747, 1968.

Hanno, P. M., and Wien, A. J.: Management of septic shock. American Urological Association Update Series, 1:3, 1981.

Hantman, D., Rossier, B., Zohlman, R., et al.: Rapid correction of hyponatremia in the syndrome of inappropriate secretion of antidiuretic hormone: an alternative treatment to hypertonic saline. Ann. Intern. Med., 78:870, 1973.

Harkonen, S., and Kjellstrand, C. M.: Exacerbation of diabetic renal failure following intravenous pyelography. Am. J. Med., 63:939, 1977.

Harman, E., and Lillington, G.: Pulmonary risk factors in surgery. Med. Clin. North Am., 63:1289, 1979.

Harris, W. H., Salzman, E. W., Athanasoulis, C., et al.: Aspirin prophylaxis of venous thromboembolism after total hip replacement. New Engl. J. Med., 297:1246, 1977.

Hartstein, A. I., Garber, S. B., Ward, T. T., et al.: Nosocomial urinary tract infection: a prospective evaluation of 108 catheterized patients. Infect. Control, 2:380, 1981.

Hata, M., Remmers, A. R., Lindley, J. D., et al.: Surgical management of the dialysis patient. Ann. Surg., 178:134, 1973.

Hedley-Whyte, J., Burgess, G. E., Feeley, T. W., et al.: Applied physiology of respiratory care. Boston, Little, Brown & Co., 1976.

Hensle, T. W.: Nutritional support of the surgical patient. Urol. Clin. North Am., 10:109, 1983.

Herbst, C. A.: Indications, management and complications of percutaneous subclavian catheters. Arch. Surg., 113:1421, 1978.

Hewitt, J., Reeve, J., Rigby, J., et al.: Whole-gut irrigation in preparation for large-bowel surgery. Lancet, 2:337, 1973.

Hills, N. H., Pflug, J. J., Jeyasingh, K., et al.: Prevention of deep vein thrombosis by intermittent pneumatic compression of the calf. Br. Med. J., 1:131, 1972.

Hirsh, J.: Choosing the best of old and new ways to prevent venous thrombosis. J. Cardiovasc. Med., 6:691, 1981.

Hodgkin, J. E.: Preoperative evaluation of pulmonary function. Am. J. Surg., 138:355, 1979.

Holbraad, L., Thybo, E., and VeNits, H.: A controlled investigation of the value of anticoagulant therapy in cases of prostatectomy. Scand. J. Urol. Nephrol., 10:39, 1976.

Holl, W. H., and Rous, S. N.: Is antibiotic prophylaxis worthwhile in patients with transurethral resection of prostate? Urology, 19:43, 1982.

Hovig, O.: Source of pulmonary emboli. Acta Chir. Scand. (Suppl.) 478:42, 1977.

Hughes, C. L., Leach, J. K., Allen, R. E., et al.: Cardiac arrhythmias during oral surgery with local anesthetic. J. Am. Dent. Assoc., 73:1095, 1966.

Hull, R., Delmore, T., Carter, C., et al.: Adjusted subcutaneous heparin versus warfarin sodium in the long-term treatment of venous thrombosis., N. Engl. J. Med., 306:189, 1982.

Hull, R., Hirsh, J., Sackett, D. L., et al.: The combined use of leg scanning and impedance plethysmography in suspected venous thrombosis: An alternative to venography. N. Engl. J. Med., 296:1497, 1977.

Hume, M., Donaldson, W. R., and Suprenant, J.: Sex, aspirin, and venous thrombosis. Orthop. Clin. North Am., 9:761, 1978.

Ishak, M. A., and Morley, K. D.: Deep venous thrombosis after total hip arthroplasty: A prospective controlled study to determine the prophylactic effect of graded pressure stockings. Br. J. Surg., 68:429, 1981.

Islam, A. K. M. S., and Chapman, J.: Closed catheter drainage and urinary infection—a comparison of two methods of catheter drainage. Br. J. Urol., 49:215, 1977.

Iverson, L. I. G., Ecker, R. R., Fox, H. E., et al.: A comparative study of IPPB, the incentive spirometer and blow bottles: the prevention of atelectasis following cardiac surgery. Ann. Thorac. Surg., 25:197, 1978.

Janson, P. A., Jubelirer, S. J., Weinstein, M. J., et al.: Treatment of the bleeding tendency in uremia with cryoprecipitate. N. Engl. J. Med., 303:1318, 1980.

Jenkins, B. S., Bradley, R. D., and Braithwaite, M. A.: Evaluation of pulmonary arterial end-diastolic pressure as an indirect estimate of left atrial mean pressure. Circulation, 42:75, 1970.

Johnson, F. E., Summer, D. S., and Standness, D.: Extremity necrosis caused by indwelling arterial catheters. Am. J. Surg., 131:375, 1976.

Kakkar, V. V.: The diagnosis of deep vein thrombosis using the ^{125}I-fibrinogen test. Arch. Surg., 104:152, 1972.

Kakkar, V. V.: International multicentre trial-prevention of fatal post-operative embolism by low doses of heparin. Lancet, 2:45, 1975.

Kakkar, V. V., Spindler, J., Flute, P. T., et al.: Efficacy of low doses of heparin in prevention of deep-vein thrombosis after major surgery: A double-blind randomized trial. Lancet, 2:101, 1972.

Kaplan, J. A., and Dunbar, R. W.: Anesthesia for noncardiac surgery in patients with cardiac disease. In Kaplan, J. A. (Ed.): Cardiac Anesthesia. New York, Grune and Stratton, 1979, p. 377.

Kasiske, B. L., and Kjellstrand, C. M.: Perioperative management of patients with chronic renal failure and postoperative acute renal failure. Urol. Clin. North Am., 10:35, 1983.

Katholi, R. E., Nolan, S. P., and McGuire, L. B.: Living with prosthetic heart valves. Am. Heart J., 92:162, 1976.

Katholi, R. E., Nolan, S. P., and McGuire, L. B.: The management of anticoagulation during noncardiac operations in patients with prosthetic heart valves. Am. Heart J., 96:163, 1978.

Katz, R. L., and Bigger, J. T., Jr.: Cardiac arrhythmias during anesthesia and operation. Anesthesiology, 33:193, 1970.

Kazarian, K. K., and Del Guercia, L. R. M.: The use of mixed venous blood gas determinations in traumatic shock. Ann. Emerg. Med., *9*:179, 1980.

Kehlet, H., Nistrup-Madsen, S., and Binder, C.: Cortisol and cortisone acetate in parenteral glucocorticoid therapy? Acta Med. Scand., *195*:421, 1974.

Kelley, T. F., Morris, G. C., Crawford, E. S., et al: Perforation of the pulmonary artery with Swan-Ganz catheters. Ann. Surg., *193*:686, 1981.

Kiil, J., Axelsen, F., et al.: Prophylaxis against postoperative pulmonary embolism and deep-vein thrombosis by low-dose heparin. Lancet, *1*:1115, 1978.

Kudinoff, Z., Finegold, S. M., Kalmanson, G. M., et al.: Use of kanamycin or urinary acidification for prophylactic chemotherapy in transurethral prostatectomy. Am. J. Med. Sci., *251*:70, 1966.

Kunau, R. T., and Stein, J. H.: Disorders of potassium metabolism. *In* Earley, L. E., and Gottschalk, C. W. (Eds.): Strauss and Welt's Diseases of the Kidney. 3rd ed. Boston, Little, Brown & Co., 1979.

Kunin, C. M.: Duration of treatment of urinary tract infections. Am. J. Med., *71*:849, 1981.

Kunin, C. M., and McCormack, R. G.: Prevention of catheter-induced urinary tract infections by sterile closed drainage. N. Engl. J. Med., *274*:1155, 1966.

Kutnowski, M., Vandendris, M., Steinberger, R., et al.: Prevention of postoperative deep-vein thrombosis by low-dose heparin in urological surgery. A double blind randomized study. Urol. Res., *5*:123, 1977.

Kwaan, J. H. M., and Connolly, J. E.: Renal failure complicating aortoiliofemoral reconstructive procedure. Am. Surg., *295*, May, 1980.

Lahnborg, G., Friman, L., Bergstrom, K., et al.: Effect of low-dose heparin on incidence of postoperative pulmonary embolism detected by photoscanning. Lancet, *1*:329, 1974.

Lee, G., DeMaria, N. A., Amsterdam, E. A., et al: Comparative effects of morphine, meperidine and pentazocine on cardio-circulatory dynamics in patients with acute myocardial infarction. Am. J. Med., *60*:949, 1976.

Lerner, P. I., and Sampliner, J. E.: Transfusion-associated cystomegalovirus mononucleosis. Ann. Surg., *185*:406, 1977.

Lundsgaard-Hansen, P.: Blood transfusion and a capillary function. *In* Ikkala, E., and Nykanen, A. (Eds.): Transfusion and Immunology. Helsinki, Int. Soc. of Blood Transfusions, 1975, p. 121.

MacDonald, R.: Red cell 2,3-diphosphoglycerate and oxygen affinity. Anaesthesia, *32*:544, 1977.

MacIntyre, I. M. C., Vasilescu; C., Jones, D. R. B., et al.: Heparin versus dextran in the prevention of deep vein thrombosis: a multi-unit controlled trial. Lancet, *2*:118, 1974.

Maini, B., Blackburn, G. L., Bistrian, B. R., et al.: Cyclic hyperalimentation: An optimal technique for preservation of visceral protein. J. Surg. Res., *20*:515, 1976.

Maizels, M., and Schaeffer, A. J.: Decreased incidence of bacteriuria associated with periodic instillations of hydrogen peroxide into the urethral catheter drainage bag. J. Urol., *123*:841, 1980.

Malmberg, R., Dottori, O., Berglund, E., et al.: Preoperative spirometry in thoracic surgery. Acta Anesthesiol. Scand., *9*:57, 1965.

Mason, D. T.: Cardiovascular management. *In* Mason, D. T. (Ed.): Essays in Medicine. New York, Medcom Publishers, 1974.

Mason, J. W., Kleeberg, U., Dolan, P., et al.: Plasma kallikrein and Hageman factor in gram-negative bacteremia. Ann. Intern. Med., *73*:545, 1970.

Mauney, F. M., Jr., Ebert, P. A., and Sabiston, D. C., Jr.: Postoperative myocardial infarction: A study of predisposing factors, diagnosis and mortality in a high risk group of surgical patients. Ann. Surg., *172*:497, 1970.

Mayo, M. E., Halil, T., and Browse, N. L.: The incidence of deep vein thrombosis after prostatectomy. Br. J. Urol., *43*:738, 1971.

Mazza, J. J., Bowie, E. J. W., Hagedorn, A. B., et al.: Antihemophilic factor VIII in hemophilia: Use of concentrates to permit major surgery. JAMA, *211*:1818, 1970.

McCabe, W. R.: Serum complement levels in bacteremia due to gram-negative organisms. N. Engl. J. Med., *288*:21, 1973.

McCabe, W. R., and Treadwell, T. L.: Gram-negative bacteremia. Monographs in Urology *4*:193, 1983.

McDougal, W. S.: Surgical nutrition. American Urological Association Update Series, *2*:16, 1983.

Messmer, B. J., Okies, J. E., Hallman, G. L., et al.: Early and late thromboembolic complications after mitral valve replacement. J. Cardiovasc. Surg., *13*:281, 1972.

Meyers, J. R., Lembeck, L., O'Kane, H., et al.: Changes in functional residual capacity of the lung after operation. Arch. Surg., *110*:576, 1975.

Miller, R. R., Lies, J. E., and Carretta, R. F.: Prevention of lower extremity venous thrombosis by early mobilization. Ann. Intern. Med., *84*:700, 1976.

Miller, R. R., Olson, H. G., Amsterdam, E. A., et al.: Propranolol-withdrawal rebound phenomenon: Exacerbation of coronary events after abrupt cessation of anti-anginal therapy. N. Engl. J. Med., *293*:416, 1975.

Miyasaka, K., Edmonds, J. F., and Conn, A. W.: Complications of radial artery lines in the pediatric patient. Can. Anesthesiol. Soc. J., *23*:9, 1976.

Morgan, B. C., Martin, W. E., Hornbein, T. F., et al.: Hemodynamic effects of intermittent positive pressure respiration. Anesthesiology, *27*:584, 1966.

Morris, M. J., Golovsky, D., Guinness, M. D. G., et al.: The value of prophylactic antibiotics in transurethral prostatic resection: a controlled trial with observation on the origin of postoperative infections. Br. J. Urol., *48*:479, 1976.

Morrison, J. C., and Wiser, W. L.: The use of prophylactic partial exchange transfusion in pregnancies associated with sickle cell hemoglobinopathy. Obstet. Gynecol., *48*:516, 1976.

Moser, K. M.: Pulmonary thromboembolism. *In* Isselbacher, K. J., et al. (Eds.): Harrison's Principles of Internal Medicine. 9th ed. New York, McGraw-Hill Book Co., 1980.

Moser, K. M.: Thromboembolic disease in the patient undergoing urologic surgery. Urol. Clin. North Am., *10*:101, 1983.

Moser, K. M., Brach, B., and Dolan, G. F.: Clinically suspected deep venous thrombosis of the lower extremities. JAMA, *237*:2195, 1977.

Mullen, J. L.: Consequences of malnutrition in the surgical patient. Surg. Clin. North Am., *61*:465, 1981.

Murphy, D. M., Falkiner, F. R., Carr, M., et al.: Septicemia after transurethral prostatectomy. Urology, *22*:133, 1983.

Murray, J. F.: The Normal Lung. Philadelphia, W. B. Saunders Co., 1976.

Naeye, R. L.: Thrombotic state after a hemorrhagic diathesis, a possible complication of therapy with epsilon-aminocaproic acid. Blood, *19*:694, 1962.

Nehma, A. E.: Swan-Ganz catheter: Comparison of insertion techniques. Arch. Surg., *115*:1194, 1980.

Nelson, P. H., Moser, K. M., Stoner, C., et al.: Risk of

complications during intravenous heparin therapy. West. J. Med., *136*:189, 1982.

Nichols, R. L.: Prophylaxis for elective bowel surgery. *In* Wilson, S. W., Finegold, S. M., and Williams, R. A. (Eds.): Intra-abdominal Infection. New York, Mc-Graw-Hill Book Co., 1982.

Nicolaides, A. N., Field, E. S., Kakkar, V. V., et al.: Prostatectomy and deep-vein thrombosis. Br. J. Surg., *59*:487, 1972.

Nuutinen, L. S., Kairaluoma, M., Tuononen, S., et al.: The effect of furosemide on renal function in open heart surgery. J. Cardiovasc. Surg., *19*:471, 1978.

O'Toole, J. D., Wurtzbacher, J. J., Wearner, N. E., et al.: Pulmonary-valve injury and insufficiency during pulmonary artery catheterization. N. Engl. J. Med., *301*:1167, 1979.

Owen, C. A., Jr.: Factor VIII terminology (letter to the editor). Lancet, *2*:359, 1981.

Owen, C. A., Jr., and Walter Bowie, E. J.: Disorders of coagulation. Urol. Clin. North Am., *10*:77, 1983.

Pachter, H. L., and Riles, T. S.: Low dose heparin: bleeding and wound complications in the surgical patient: a prospective randomized study. Ann. Surg., *186*:669, 1977.

Packer, M. G., Russo, P., and Fair, W. R.: Prophylactic antibiotics and Foley catheter use in transperineal needle biopsy of the prostate. J. Urol., *131*:687, 1984.

Page, M. McB., and Watkins, P. J.: Radiorespiratory arrest and diabetic autonomic neuropathy. Lancet, *1*:14, 1978.

Peters, W. P., Johnson, M. W., Friedman, P. A., et al.: Pressor effect of naloxone in septic shock. Lancet, *1*:529, 1981.

Pien, F. D., and Landers, J. Q.: Indwelling urinary catheter infections in small community hospital. Role of urinary drainage bag. Urology, *22*:255, 1983.

Pietsch, J. B., and Meakins, J. L.: The delayed hypersensitivity response: Clinical application in surgery (1976 Davis and Geck Surgical Essay). Can. J. Surg., *20*:15, 1977.

Pintado, T., Taswell, H. F., and Bowie, E. J. W.: Treatment of life-threatening hemorrhage due to acquired factor VIII inhibitor. Blood, *46*:535, 1975.

Plumlee, J. E., and Boehner, R. B.: Myocardial infarction during and following anesthesia and operation. South. Med. J., *65*:886, 1972.

Plumpton, F. S., Besser, G. M., and Cole, P. V.: Corticosteroid treatment and surgery. Anaesthesia, *24*:12, 1969.

Pontoppidan, H., Geffin, B., and Lowenstein, E.: Acute Respiratory Failure in the Adult. Boston, Little, Brown & Co., 1973.

Pontoppidan, H., Wilson, R. S., Rite, M. A., et al.: Respiratory intensive care. Anesthesiology, *47*:96, 1977.

Price, H. L., and Helrich, M.: The effect of cyclopropane, diethyl ether, nitrous oxide, thiopental and hydrogen ion concentration on the myocardial function of the dog heart-lung preparation. J. Pharmacol. Exp. Ther., *115*:206, 1955.

Prys-Roberts, C., Foex, P., and Biro, G. P.: Studies of anaesthesia in relation to hypertension. V. Adrenergic-beta-receptor blockade. Br. J. Anaesthesiol., *45*:671, 1973.

Putnam, L., Jenicek, J., Allen, C., et al.: Anesthesia in the morbidly obese patient. South. Med. J., *67*:1411, 1974.

Pyrah, L. M.: Control of pseudomonas infection in a urology ward. Lancet, *2*:314, 1955.

Raahave, D.: Effect of plastic skin and wound drapes on the density of bacteria in operative wound. Br. J. Surg., *64*:421, 1976.

Rabinowitz, I. N., Watson, W., and Farber, E. M.: Topical steroid depression of the hypothalamic-pituitary-adrenal axis in psoriasis vulgaris. Dermatologica, *154*:321, 1977.

Rahimi, A., Edmondson, P. S., and Jones, N. F.: Effect of radio-contrast mediums on kidneys of patients with renal disease. Br. Med. J., *282*:1194, 1981.

Rehder, K., Jessler, A., and Marsh, H. M.: General anesthesia and the lung. Am. Rev. Resp. Dis., *112*:541, 1975.

Ring, J., and Messmer, K.: Incidence and severity of anaphylactoid reactions to colloid volume substitutes. Lancet, *1*:466, 1977.

Rose, S. D.: Prophylaxis of thromboembolic disease. Med. Clin. North Am., *63*:1205, 1979.

Rose, S. D., Gorman, L. C., and Mason, D. T.: Cardiac risk factors in patients undergoing noncardiac surgery. Med. Clin. North Am., *63*:1271, 1979.

Rosenberg, I. L., Evans, M., and Pollack, A. V.: Prophylaxis of postoperative leg vein thrombosis by low-dose subcutaneous heparin or preoperative calf muscle stimulation: a controlled clinical trial. Br. Med. J., *1*:649, 1975.

Rosengarten, D. S., and Laird, J.: The effect of leg elevation on the incidence of deep vein thrombosis after operation. Br. J. Surg., *58*:182, 1971.

Russell, R. D., Mantel, J. A., Rogers, W. J., et al.: Current status of hemodynamic monitoring: Indications, diagnosis, complications. Cardiovasc. Clin., *2*:1, 1981.

Ryan, J. A., Jr., Abel, R. M., Abbott, W. M., et al.: Catheter complications in total parenteral nutrition: A prospective study of 200 consecutive patients. N. Engl. J. Med., *290*:757, 1974.

Sahn, S. A., and Lakshminarayan, S.: Bedside criteria for discontinuation of mechanical ventilation. Chest, *63*:1002, 1973.

Salzman, E. D. W., Deykin, D., Sharpiro, R. M., et al.: Management of heparin therapy: Controlled prospective trial. N. Engl. J. Med., *292*:1046, 1975.

Sasahara, A. H., and Dalen, J. E.: Controversy: Should fibrinolytic drugs be used to treat acute pulmonary embolism? J. Cardiovasc. Med., *5*:793, 1980.

Schaefer, C. F., and Geelhoed, G. W.: Redirection of misplaced central venous catheters. Arch. Surg., *115*:789, 1980.

Schwartz, R. A., and Cerra, F. B.: Shock: a practical approach. Urol. Clin. North Am., *10*:89, 1983.

Scurr, J. H., Ibrahim, S. Z., Faber, R. G., et al.: The efficacy of graduated compression stockings in the prevention of deep vein thrombosis. Br. J. Surg., *64*:371, 1977.

Sears, D. A.: The morbidity of sickle cell trait: A review of the literature. Am. J. Med., *64*:1021, 1978.

Sebeseri, O., Kummer, H., and Zingg, E.: Controlled prevention of post-operative thrombosis in urological disease with depot heparin. Eur. Urol., *1*:229, 1975.

Seropian, R., and Reynolds, B. M.: Wound infections after postoperative depilatory versus razor preparation. Am. J. Surg., *121*:251, 1971.

Shapiro, B. A.: Airway pressure therapy for acute restrictive pulmonary pathology. *In* Critical Care: State of the Art 1981. Fullerton, Calif., Society for Critical Care Medicine, 1981.

Sheldon, C. A., and Leonard, A. S.: Hemodynamic monitoring. Urol. Clin. North Am., *10*:19, 1983.

Sherman, L. A.: Alterations in hemostasis during massive transfusion. *In* Nusbacher, J. (Ed.): Massive Transfusion. Washington, D.C., American Association of Blood Banks, 1978, p. 53.

Shipp, J. C.: Diabetes mellitus, anesthesia and surgery. Int. Anesthes. Clin., 6:189, 1968.

Simmons, M. A., Lavine, R. L., Lubschenco, L. I., et al.: Warning: Serious sequelae of temporal artery catheterization. J. Pediatr., 92:284, 1978.

Simon, A. B.: Perioperative management of the pacemaker patient. Anesthesiology, 46:127, 1977.

Sirotzky, L., and Lewis, E. J.: Anesthesia related muscle paralysis in renal failure. Clin. Nephrol., 10:38, 1978.

Skillman, J. J., Collins, R. E. C., Coe, N. P., et al.: Prevention of deep vein thrombosis in neurosurgical patients: a controlled, randomized trial of external pneumatic compression boots. Surgery, 83:354, 1978.

Skinner, J. F., and Pearce, M. L.: Surgical risk in the cardiac patient. J. Chron. Dis., 17:57, 1964.

Slogoff, S., Keats, A. S., and Ott, E.: Preoperative propranolol therapy, and aorto-coronary bypass operation. JAMA, 240:1487, 1978.

Smith, R. A.: Respiratory care. In Miller, R. D. (Ed.): Anesthesia. New York, Churchill Livingstone, 1981.

Smith, W. R., Glauser, F. L., and Jamison, P.: Ruptured chordae of the tricuspid valve: The consequence of flow-directed Swan-Ganz catheterization. Chest, 70: 790, 1976.

Solanki, D., and McCurdy, P. R.: Delayed hemolytic transfusion reactions: An often missed entity. JAMA, 239:729, 1978.

Stanley, T. H., Bennett, G. M., Lorser, E. A., et al.: Cardiovascular effects of diazepam and droperidol during morphine anesthesia. Anesthesiology, 44:255, 1976.

Steen, P. A., Tinker, J. H., and Tarhan, S.: Myocardial reinfarction after anesthesia and surgery. JAMA, 239:2566, 1978.

Stein, M. A.: Preoperative pulmonary function evaluation and therapy for surgical patients. JAMA, 211:787, 1970.

Steinke, J.: Management of diabetes mellitus and surgery. N. Engl. J. Med., 282:1472, 1970.

Stern, W. Z.: Diagnostic imaging of the urinary tract in pregnancy. In Freed, S. Z., and Herzig, N. (Eds.): Urology in Pregnancy, Baltimore, Williams & Wilkins, 1982, p. 48.

Steward, D. J., and Sloan, I. A. J.: Recent upper respiratory infections and pulmonary artery clamping in the etiology of postoperative respiratory complications. Can. Anaesth. Soc. J., 16:57, 1969.

Storm, O.: Suprapubic prostatectomy with pre-operative dicumarol and epsilon-aminocaproic prophylaxis. Scand. J. Urol. Nephrol., 1:1, 1967.

Strauss, R. J., and Wise, L.: Operative risks of obesity. Surg. Gynec. Obstet., 146:286, 1978.

Sun, N. C. J., Bowie, E. J. W., Kazmier, F. J., et al.: Blood coagulation studies in patients with cancer. Mayo Clin. Proc., 49:636, 1974.

Swan, H. J. C., and Ganz, W.: Use of a balloon flotation catheter in critically ill patients. Surg. Clin. North Am., 55:501, 1975.

Swarts, R. D.: Hemorrhage during high-risk hemodialysis using controlled heparinization. Nephron, 28:65, 1981.

Swartz, H. M., and Reichling, B. A.: Hazards of radiation exposure for pregnant women. JAMA, 239:1907, 1978.

Taitelman, U., Reece, E. A., and Bessman, A. N.: Insulin in the management of the diabetic surgical patient. JAMA, 237:658, 1977.

Tarhan, S., Moffitt, E. A., Taylor, W. F., et al.: Myocardial infarction after general anesthesia. JAMA, 220:1451, 1972.

Tasker, P. R. W., MacGregor, G. A., and deWardener, H. E.: Prophylactic use of intravenous saline in patients with chronic renal failure undergoing major surgery. Lancet, 2:911, 1974.

Teasley, K. M., Lysne, J., Nuwer, N., et al.: Nutrition and metabolic support of the surgical patient. Urol. Clin. North Am., 10:119, 1983.

Thompson, G. J., Panayotic, P. K., and Connolly, D. C.: Transurethral prostatic resection after myocardial infarction. JAMA, 182:908, 1962.

Thoren, L.: Postoperative pulmonary complications: observations on their prevention by means of physiotherapy. Acta Chir. Scand., 107:193, 1954.

Thornton, G. E., Lytton, B., and Andtiole, V. T.: Bacteriuria following indwelling catheter drainage—effect of constant bladder rinse. JAMA, 195:179, 1966.

Tisi, G. M.: Preoperative evaluation of pulmonary function. Am. Rev. Resp. Dis., 119:293, 1979.

Tousaint, G. P. M., Burgess, J. H, and Hampson, L. G.: Central venous pressure and pulmonary wedge pressure in critical surgical illness: A comparison. Arch. Surg., 109:265, 1974.

Vanik, P. E., and Davis, H. S.: Cardiac arrhythmias during halothane anesthesia. Anesth. Analg., 47:299, 1968.

VanSonnenberg, E. F., Ferrucci, J. T., Mueller, P. R., et al.: Percutaneous radiographically guided catheter drainage of abdominal abscesses. JAMA, 247:190, 1982.

VanZee, B. E., Hoy, W. E., Talley, T., et al.: Renal injury associated with intravenous pyelography in nondiabetic and diabetic patients. Ann. Intern. Med., 89:51, 1978.

Vaughan, E. D., and Gillenwater, J. Y.: Diagnosis characterization and management of post-obstructive diuresis. J. Urol., 109:286, 1973.

Viljoen, J. F., Estafanous, G., and Kellner, G. A.: Propranolol and cardiac surgery. J. Thorac. Cardiovasc. Surg., 64:826, 1972.

Viteri, F. E., and Schneider, R. E.: Gastrointestinal alterations in protein-calorie malnutrition. Med. Clin. North Am., 58:1487, 1974.

Walter, C. W.: Blood donors, blood and transfusion. In Kinney, J. M., et al. (Eds.): Manual of Preoperative and Postoperative Care. Philadelphia, W. B. Saunders Co., 1971, p. 139.

Watson-Williams, E. J.: Hematologic and hemostatic considerations before surgery. Med. Clin. North Am., 63:1165, 1979.

Wax, S. H.: The use of the radioisotope renogram in pregnancy. In Freed, S. Z., and Herzig, N.: Urology In Pregnancy. Baltimore, Williams & Wilkins, 1982, p. 64.

Welch, M. A., Jr., Shapiro, B. J., Mercurio, P., et al.: Methods of IPPB. Chest, 78:463, 1980.

White, V. A., and Kumagai, L. F.: Preoperative endocrine and metabolic considerations. Med. Clin. North Am., 63:1321, 1979.

Wiehle, S. P., Banowsky, L. H., Nicastro-Lutton, J. J., et al.: Pretransplant bilateral nephrectomy and adjuvant operations. Urology, 18:349, 1981.

Wightman, J. A. K.: A prospective survey of the incidence of postoperative pulmonary complications. Br. J. Surg., 55:85, 1968.

Wilkins, R. W., and Stanton, J. R.: Elastic stockings in the prevention of pulmonary embolism. II. A Progress Report. N. Engl. J. Med., 248:1087, 1953.

Williams, C. D., and Brenowitz, J. B.: "Prohibitive" lung function and major surgical procedures. Am. J. Surg., 132:763, 1976.

Wojsycyuk, W. J., Mowry, F. M., and Dugan, N. L.: Deactivation of a demand pacemaker by transurethral electrocautery. N. Engl. J. Med., 280:34, 1969.

CHAPTER 62

Surgery of the Kidney

BERNARD LYTTON, M.B., F.R.C.S.

The first nephrectomies were probably performed serendipitously. Early reports of removal of large and extensive ovarian tumors state that the surgeon was sometimes surprised to find the kidney included in the surgical specimen.

Definitive renal surgery was probably first performed in 1869 by Gustav Simon, who carried out a planned nephrectomy on Frau Kolb for treatment of a ureterovaginal fistula. The operation was preceded by extensive experimental investigation of uninephrectomy in dogs to demonstrate that they could survive normally with only one kidney. This application of an experimental model to a clinical problem was the forerunner of the method by which many current surgical procedures were developed. Renal transplantation is one of the recent examples. During the 100 or more years since the first planned nephrectomy, renal surgery has reflected the dramatic progress that has taken place in the whole field of surgical science. Much of the present scope and extent of the procedures performed has been made possible by the advances in our understanding of the basic physiologic, biochemical, and immunologic mechanisms together with the corresponding progress in anesthesia and pharmacology. Anticipation, control, and correction of the serious disturbances of these functions, which can occur during or after surgery, are as important in achieving a good result and in reducing morbidity as are the care and skill with which the procedure is performed.

PREOPERATIVE PREPARATION

This is of particular importance in individuals undergoing renal surgery because of the special positions in which the patient may have to be placed and the serious systemic disturbances that may occur secondary to renal infections and impairment of renal function.

Cardiorespiratory function is evaluated by eliciting any history of heart disease, chest pain, or respiratory distress on exertion. Smoking habits should be discussed. An electrocardiogram, chest x-ray, and complete blood count should be carried out on all patients. The flank position with lateral flexion of the spine is known to cause embarrassment of ventilatory capacity and the venous return may be significantly diminished in this position, resulting in severe hypotension. Therefore, alternatives to the flank approach should be used, whenever possible, in patients with a decreased pulmonary reserve. Pulmonary function studies and blood gas analysis in patients suspected of having impairment of respiratory function can be helpful in planning the surgical approach. The decision to approach the kidney anteriorly with a patient in the supine position is often predicated on the results of these tests. Respiration may be seriously impaired postoperatively, as incisions are made in the upper abdomen, muscles are transected, and frequently one of the lower ribs is removed or the intercostal muscles are divided. Moreover, the upper poles of the kidneys encroach on the undersurface of the diaphragm, and the removal of a large upper pole renal mass often interferes temporarily with its function. Preoperative breathing exercises, alleviation of bronchospasm, cessation of smoking, and evaluation of cardiopulmonary function are helpful in improving respiratory function and in anticipating and preventing postoperative atelectasis and cardiorespiratory difficulties. A review of 347 patients who underwent nephrectomy showed that cardiovascular and pulmonary complications occurred in 10 per cent of those in whom the operation was done through a flank incision, whereas such complications occurred in only 5 per cent when an anterior approach was used.

Bleeding tendencies should be assessed by examination of platelet function and coagulation factors. Patients should be questioned about excess alcohol intake and ingestion of drugs, such as aspirin, that might influence blood clotting.

Complete examination of the urinary tract should be made in all patients undergoing renal surgery. This should include urinalysis and excretory urography together with cystoscopy, retrograde pyelography, and cystourethrography when indicated.

Renal function is evaluated by estimation of serum creatinine levels, endogenous creatinine clearance, and tubular concentrating ability. Radioisotopic methods using I-131 hippuran or technetium-99 (^{99}Tc) chelated with either DTPA or DMSA are quicker and can provide information on differential renal function. I-131 hippuran is cleared rapidly by both glomeruli and tubules and is most useful for measuring the degree of impairment on one side when overall renal function is normal. ^{99}Tc-DTPA is filtered only by the glomeruli; thus it is better concentrated and provides a better demonstration of the kidneys when there is some impairment of renal function. Both these isotopes are excreted in the urine; therefore, in the presence of obstruction, parenchymal concentration is obscured by the high concentration of the isotope in the accumulated urine. ^{99}Tc-DMSA, on the other hand, is taken up by the tubular cells; so that it provides a mode of evaluating the renal parenchyma, particularly in the presence of obstruction, but gives little information on excretory function. Ureteral catheterization to determine the function of each kidney may sometimes be necessary, particularly in patients with bilateral stone disease. Information about renal function may help in deciding between a reparative procedure and nephrectomy. Excretory urography no longer provides a satisfactory measure of renal function. The newer contrast agents are given in large amounts, are rapidly filtered, and produce good anatomic definition of the urinary tract, even in patients with some impairment of function.

Computerized axial tomography (CAT) scanning is a good noninvasive method for the detection and differential diagnosis of renal masses, for better definition of the extent of renal injuries, and for the evaluation of any local extension of renal tumors.

Renal ultrasound scanning will differentiate between cystic and solid lesions and will detect the presence of nonradiopaque stones. It is also helpful for detecting tumor thrombus in the vena cava.

Renal angiography to define the arterial anatomy is particularly helpful in patients undergoing surgery for renal injuries; for stone disease, especially when they have had previous surgery; and for renal anomalies. It may also greatly facilitate nephrectomy in patients with large renal tumors, in whom early ligation of the arterial supply is important. Subtraction angiography following the intravenous injection of a large bolus of contrast material will visualize the anatomy of the larger renal vessels and provides an alternative to an intra-arterial injection.

Patients with infections of both kidney and the lower urinary tract should receive adequate and appropriate antibiotic therapy, based on sensitivity studies, for at least 48 hours preoperatively. Severe bacteremia can occur during operations on an infected kidney, and it has been found that there is a significant increase in mortality for nephrectomy associated with infections.

Embolization of the kidney by a percutaneous technique is done either for definitive treatment of a vascular lesion or to reduce the vascularity of a large renal cancer. The renal artery is catheterized under radiographic control by the Seldinger method used for selective renal angiography. Several methods for occluding the vascular supply have been employed. The blood supply can be decreased before surgery by a 7 F double-lumen balloon catheter that is passed a few hours preoperatively and inflated in the proximal portion of the renal artery. This, however, does not always completely occlude the blood flow, and it may slip out of the renal artery. Embolization can be accomplished by the placement of a Santurco coil in the renal artery, on which a clot forms and occludes the vessel. Migration of a coil into the contralateral renal artery or to a femoral artery has been reported. Other methods include the injection of preformed clot, thrombin, Gelfoam, or minced muscle directly into the renal artery 12 to 24 hours preoperatively, the latter two materials being the most popular. The use of preformed clot has the disadvantage that emboli may enter the venous side of the circulation through arteriovenous shunts in the tumor and lodge in the lungs. Recently, 95 per cent ethanol injected directly into the renal artery or into the main tumor vessel has proved to be a satisfactory method of infarcting a kidney or renal tumor. Patients have experienced severe pain and sometimes fever after renal embolization or infarction.

Patients are often concerned about how the removal of a kidney may affect their renal function, and it is surprising how many will ask about dialysis when told they need a nephrectomy. Some patients are concerned about loss of body image. Reassurance and a full explanation of the procedure should be given to all patients to promote confidence in the surgeon and to alleviate their anxiety. There is a compensatory increase in size of the nephrons with an increase in renal mass in the remaining kidney following nephrectomy. A marked diminution in this response occurs after the age of 40 years. More importantly, there is a marked adaptive increase in function of the remaining kidney depending on the mass of renal tissue removed. Within 24 hours after nephrectomy there is an approximate 50 per cent increase in GFR and renal blood flow in the remaining kidney.

BASIC PRINCIPLES OF SURGICAL PROCEDURES

Adherence to basic surgical principles is the key to the successful performance of any operative procedure. They apply, with suitable modifications, to surgery of the kidney.

The incision should be planned in relation to the anatomy of the individual patient and the nature of his disease. Examination of the urogram to define the relationship of the kidney to the lower ribs will enable the surgeon to decide at which level to make the flank incision, remembering that the level of exposure must be projected to the midaxillary line (see Fig. 62–2). An anterior retroperitoneal approach to the kidney might be ideal for a patient with a wide subcostal angle who requires an open biopsy or a simple nephrectomy for hypertension but is unsuitable for a pyelolithotomy, in which a flank incision provides better access to the posteriorly placed pelvis. The choice of incision is discussed further under each procedure.

Exposure must be adequate to perform the procedure and to deal with any possible complications. This is particularly important in renal surgery, as the kidney is deeply placed in the retroperitoneum in the upper part of the abdominal cavity. Access is limited by the lower ribs and by the liver and spleen. Injuries to large renal vessels are difficult to control or repair through small incisions, particularly in the pres-

ence of a large tumor or when there are inflammatory changes in the perinephric tissues. Poor exposure, apart from making the surgical procedure unnecessarily difficult, also leads to excessive retraction, with bruising of the muscles and possible injury to the intercostal nerves, which may cause more postoperative pain.

Control of the vascular pedicle is particularly important when operating for renal tumor or renal injury and should be accomplished before exposing the kidney. The renal pedicles are in the midline at the level of the first or second lumbar vertebra, and an anterior approach is necessary to do this. Preoperative arteriography is helpful not only to define the renal pathology but also to delineate the vascular anatomy.

Familiarity with the anatomy is necessary. A three-dimensional concept of the anatomy enables the surgeon to dissect out the structures in the correct tissue planes and avoid excessive bleeding and inadvertent injury to the kidney, blood vessels, and ureter. Anatomic landmarks are particularly helpful during dissections in the presence of scarring due to previous surgery, infection, or injury.

Good hemostasis, maintenance of an adequate blood supply, and avoidance of tension are the best prescriptions for good wound healing. Attention to these factors, approximation of the correct layers, and reliance on the stronger fascial layers rather than friable muscle to hold the sutures are more likely to result in a strong, well-healed wound than the choice of suture materials and whether the sutures are placed in an interrupted or a continuous fashion. Sutures should be used to approximate tissues and not to constrict them. Individual surgeons favor different types of suture materials, and usually the choice is based on long-term use and experience that results in a personal preference. Electrocoagulation or 000 plain catgut is used for ligation of small bleeding points. This author prefers 00 and 0 catgut or polyglycolic sutures for most renal wounds that are likely to be contaminated with urine. These are inserted as running sutures, and the external fascial layers are reinforced with interrupted sutures. Tension sutures of 0 nylon are passed through all layers of the wound, and 30-gauge wire is used to close the fascial layers when there are metabolic deficiencies, such as are present in patients with chronic renal failure and malignant disease. This applies particularly to the closure of abdominal and thoracoabdominal incisions, in which dehiscence is more likely to occur than with flank incisions.

SURGICAL APPROACH

The kidney may be approached by four principal routes:
1. Flank approach—extraperitoneal:
   a. Transcostal incision, with or without rib resection.
   b. Intercostal incision.
   c. Subcostal incision (osteoplastic flap extension).
2. Abdominal approach—transperitoneal or extraperitoneal:
   a. Midline or paramedian incision.
   b. Anterior subcostal incision.
   c. Chevron incision.
3. Lumbar approach (Gil-Vernet, Lurz).
4. Thoracoabdominal approach—transpleural or extrapleural:
   a. Transcostal incision.
   b. Intercostal incision.

The urologist should be familiar with each of these approaches, as there are indications and advantages for each one. The choice of any one approach depends largely on the patient's anatomy and disease entity. Each approach is discussed separately, together with indications, contraindications, advantages, disadvantages, postoperative care, and complications specifically related to the particular incision.

Flank Approach

This approach provides good access to the renal parenchyma and collecting system. It is the most direct route to the kidney and involves the least disturbance to other viscera. Contamination of the peritoneal cavity is avoided, and drainage of the perinephric space is easily and effectively established. A sound closure of the wound can be achieved, and the incidence of incisional hernia is less than that which occurs with abdominal incisions. The approach does not provide for early control of the renal pedicle, which is desirable in patients with tumors or injuries of the kidney. The lateral position is sometimes poorly tolerated in patients with cardiorespiratory problems.

The approach through the bed of the twelfth or eleventh rib or through the tenth or eleventh intercostal space is most commonly used for the flank approach to the kidney. The choice of rib depends on the position of the kidney and on whether the upper or lower pole is the site of disease. This incision is somewhat easier to make and to close than is the subcostal incision, and it provides wider access to the

kidney. It can be made between the neurovascular bundles so that these do not limit the extent of the incision. This incision should be used if the kidney has been operated on previously through a subcostal incision. It is advocated for removal of stones from the kidney and pelvis, ureteropelvic junction repairs, partial nephrectomy, and late explorations for certain cases of renal trauma when the primary problem is urinary extravasation.

The subcostal incision is advocated for the establishment of nephrostomy drainage, drainage of a perinephric abscess, and removal of stones from the upper ureter. It has the disadvantage of being rather low in relation to the usual position of the kidney, unless the twelfth rib is rudimentary and the incision is made under the eleventh rib. This makes access to the pedicle and renal pelvis more difficult and requires extensive mobilization of the kidney before access can be accomplished. Exposure may be hampered by the iliac crest and subcostal nerve. The subcostal incision does not have this disadvantage in children, in whom it provides good access to the kidney, as the lower ribs are soft and easily displaced upward.

Positioning in the Flank Approach. The patient is placed in the lateral position after being anesthetized and having an endotracheal tube inserted. The back should be placed fairly close to the edge of the operating table to ensure unimpeded access by the surgeon, and the patient should be positioned so that the tip of the twelfth rib is over the kidney rest. The bottom leg is flexed to 90 degrees, with the top leg straight to maintain stability. A pillow is placed between the knees, and a sponge rubber pad is placed under the axilla to prevent compression of the axillary vessels and nerves. The patient is secured in this position with a 3-inch adhesive tape passed over the greater trochanter and attached to the movable portion of the table (Fig. 62–1). The extended upper arm may be supported on a padded Mayo stand that can be adjusted to the appropriate height to maintain the arm in a horizontal position with the shoulder rotated slightly forward.

Flexion of the table and elevation of the kidney rest should be performed slowly and may be delayed until the surgeon is ready to make the skin incision in order to minimize the time spent in this position. The flexion increases the space between the costal margin and iliac crest and puts the flank muscles and skin on tension. Care must be taken with patients who have stiff spines to ensure that their extremities remain in contact with the table, as their range of lateral

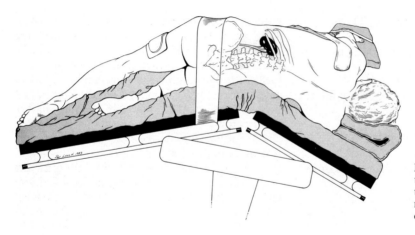

Figure 62–1. Position of the patient for the flank approach. Note the axillary pad. The kidney rest may be elevated if further lateral extension is needed.

flexion is limited. The position is not well tolerated in elderly patients or in those with some impairment of cardiopulmonary function, as it results in a decreased venous return caused by compression of the inferior vena cava and the dependent position of the legs. It also limits aeration of the lung on the dependent side. It is important to determine the patient's blood pressure after he has been turned on his side and again after the table has been flexed and the kidney rest elevated. The rest may have to be lowered and the table unflexed if hypotension persists. Another approach should be utilized if the patient is unable to tolerate the position.

It must be understood that in a flank incision the midportion of the wound and the site of maximum exposure are in the midaxillary line. Access in the posterior part, at the neck of the rib, is limited by the sacrospinalis muscle. The level of the incision may therefore best be determined by drawing a horizontal line on the urogram from the hilum of the kidney to the most lateral rib that it intersects (Fig. 62–2).

When access to the upper pole is primarily required, the rib or costal space above is selected (Fig. 62–3).

TRANSCOSTAL FLANK INCISION

Transcostal flank incisions are made directly over the appropriate rib, beginning at the lateral border of the sacrospinalis muscle (Fig. 62–4). After dividing the external oblique latissimus dorsi and slips of the underlying serratus posterior inferior muscles (Fig. 62–5), the surgeon incises the periosteum over the rib with a scalpel or by diathermy. The flat periosteal elevator is used to reflect the periosteum off the rib (Fig. 62–6). The intercostal muscles are directed downward and forward between the ribs, so that the leading edge of the elevator is moved from behind forward to separate the periosteum from the superior border of the rib, and from in front backward to separate it from the inferior border. In this way the elevator is inserted into the acute angle made between the muscle fibers and the rib and is directed down

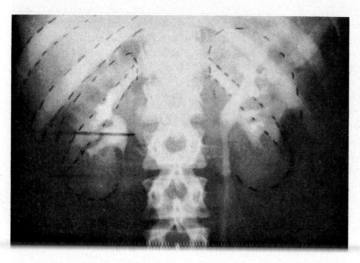

Figure 62–2. The right kidney is traversed at its midpoint by the twelfth rib. The ideal incision is chosen by drawing a horizontal line from the hilum to the lateral rib cage. Exposure of this kidney would best be accomplished by resection of the twelfth and, on the left, of the eleventh rib. (From Smith, D. R. et al.: *In* Campbell, M. F., and Harrison, J. H.: Urology. Vol. 3, 3rd ed. Philadelphia, W. B. Saunders Co., 1970.)

Figure 62–3. Carcinoma of the kidney. A horizontal line drawn from the hilum of the kidney shows that the long tenth and eleventh ribs would make exposure difficult, even with resection of the eleventh rib. The ideal incision would be a thoracoabdominal approach through the bed of the tenth rib or interspace. (From Smith, D. R. et al.: *In* Campbell, M. F., and Harrison, J. H.: Urology. Vol. 3, 3rd ed. Philadelphia, W. B. Saunders Co., 1970.)

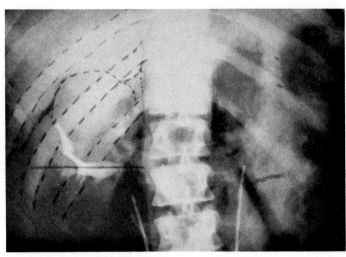

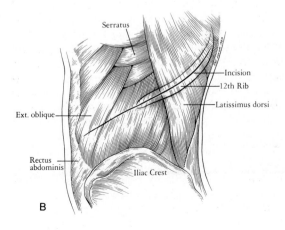

A

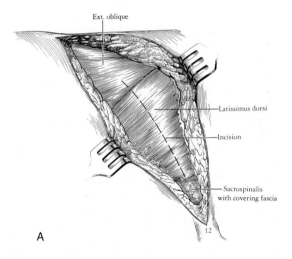

B

Figure 62–4. *A,* Left transcostal incision. Anterior edge of the latissimus dorsi muscle overlies the posterior edge of the external oblique muscle; *B,* Left transcostal incision showing the relationship of the twelfth rib to the overlying muscles.

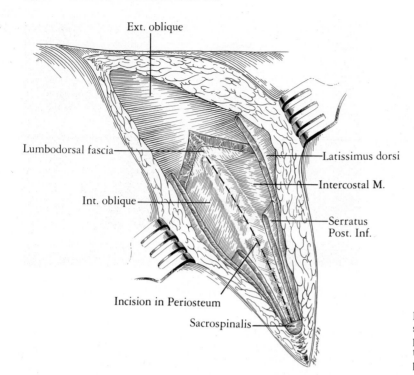

Ext. oblique

Lumbodorsal fascia

Int. oblique

Incision in Periosteum

Sacrospinalis

Latissimus dorsi

Intercostal M.

Serratus
Post. Inf.

Figure 62–5. Left transcostal incision. The muscles in the posterior part of the wound have been divided to expose the rib for incision of the periosteum.

onto the bone. The lateral border of the sacrospinalis is retracted, so that the dissection can be carried down to the angle of the rib where it articulates with the transverse process of the vertebra. It is generally unnecessary to resect the rib, as adequate exposure can be obtained by reflecting the periosteum off the upper or lower border (preferably the upper) and the posterior surface of the rib as far back as the transverse process of the vertebra.

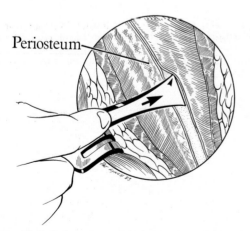

Periosteum

Figure 62–6. Left transcostal incision. The periosteum is reflected off the upper surface of the rib. Note that the periosteal elevator is moved distally or downward on the upper edge of the rib against the direction of the intercostal muscle fibers.

An incision is now made through the periosteal bed of the rib, care being taken to avoid the pleural reflection in the posterior part of the wound. The fascial attachments of the pleura to the diaphragm should be divided sharply to enable the pleura to be reflected upward. The lower slips of the diaphragm are then divided close to their origin from the ribs to avoid injury to the pleura and to expose Gerota's fascia (Fig. 62–7). The incision is completed anteriorly by incising the lumbar fascia at the tip of the rib and inserting two fingers into the perinephric space to push the underlying peritoneum forward. The lateral peritoneal reflection is peeled off the undersurface of the anterior abdominal wall and transversalis fascia by sweeping it forward with the fingers. The external and internal oblique muscles are now divided, and this may be done by incising them sharply or with electrocautery while they are tented up over the two fingers insinuated below the transversus muscle (Fig. 62–8). A little upward pressure will control bleeding from severed vessels, allowing them to be clamped by the assistant. This should expose the intercostal neurovascular bundle as it courses forward and downward between the internal oblique and transversus muscles (Fig. 62–7A). The transverse fibers of the transversus muscle may be split by blunt dissection below the nerve, allowing it to fall away with the upper margin of the incision. A Finochietto retractor is used to maintain the exposure, which can be

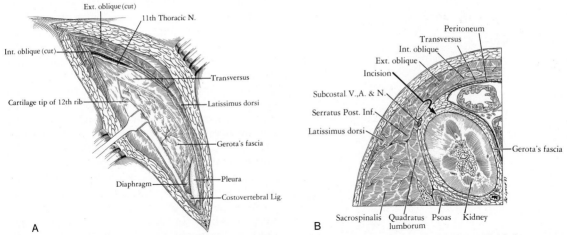

Figure 62–7. *A,* Left transcostal incision. The periosteal bed of the rib and transversus muscle have been divided to expose Gerota's fascia. Slips of the diaphragm should be divided close to their insertion into the ribs to avoid injury to the pleura. *B,* Transverse section at level of the midportion of the twelfth rib.

improved further by dividing the costotransverse ligament posteriorly to displace the rib. Care should be taken to avoid the underlying vessels. The blades of the retractor should be placed anteriorly over moistened gauze sponges, preferably on the soft tissues, to avoid breaking the rib. Should breakage occur, the distal portion of the rib is removed. The retractor should be released periodically if the procedure is prolonged.

If resection of the rib is needed for wider exposure or following previous surgery, the elevation of the periosteum is completed by separating it from the inner aspect of the rib, using a Doyen periosteal elevator (Fig. 62–9). The proximal end of the rib is then transected as far back as possible with the guillotine rib resector. The retracted muscle mass is allowed to fall back over the sharp cut edge, protecting the operator from injury. The rib is grasped with a Kocher clamp and is separated from the muscles attached anteriorly by sharp dissection to complete its removal (Fig. 62–10). Following resection of the eleventh rib, the pleural reflection, which crosses its lower border at the junction of the anterior and middle thirds, occupies the posterior part of the wound as it lies on the

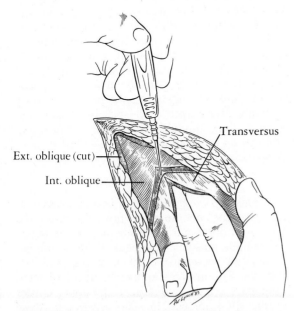

Figure 62–8. Left transcostal incision. Two fingers are insinuated into the incision in the posterior part of the transversus muscle to sweep the peritoneal reflection forward and divide the anterior abdominal muscles.

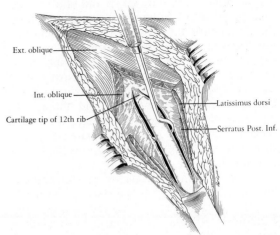

Figure 62–9. Left transcostal incision. The periosteum is dissected off the rib, using a Doyen's periosteal elevator, prior to resection of the rib.

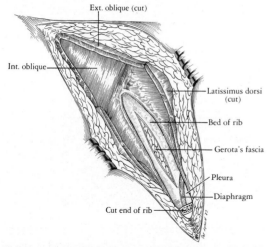

Figure 62–10. Left transcostal incision. The rib has been resected, exposing the diaphragm and pleura in the posterior part of the wound. The slips of the diaphragm inserting into the rib have been divided according to the pleura to be displaced upwards.

lower fibers of the diaphragm. It may be reflected upward by sharply dividing the fascial attachments to the diaphragm. Alternatively, the lower fibers of the diaphragm are detached from their insertion into the posterior inner aspect of the twelfth rib. This allows the lower diaphragm and pleura to be retracted upward, out of the wound. The incision is made transpleurally when the pleural reflection is unusually low or when the approach is through the tenth rib.

To expose the kidney an incision is now made in Gerota's fascia posteriorly to avoid injury to the peritoneum. The perinephric space is entered, and the perinephric fat is dissected off the renal capsule by sharp and blunt dissection. Small vessels are present that pass through the perinephric fat between the fascia and kidney capsule. These may become enlarged in order to provide a collateral blood supply in the presence of tumor, infection, or obstruction of the renal vein. Care should be taken to avoid injury to the iliohypogastric and ilioinguinal nerves as they emerge from behind the lateral border of the psoas muscle and pass down over the anterior surface of the quadratus lumborum in the renal fossa.

The incision is closed by careful approximation of the corresponding muscle and fascial layers. The kidney rest is lowered, and the table is returned to the horizontal position to facilitate this. Injection of 0.5 per cent Marcaine into the fascial sheath around the intercostal nerves as they emerge from the intervertebral foramina is helpful in diminishing postoperative pain and involuntary splinting of the lower chest. It is best to begin the closure from each end of the incision and sew toward the middle. Anteriorly the transversus and internal oblique muscles are closed in separate layers with a running 0 polyglycolic suture. Sutures are placed in the fascial covering of the muscles rather than in the fleshy part. Care must be taken to avoid inclusion of any intercostal nerves or branches during closure of the transversus muscle. Posteriorly the sacrospinalis muscle is retracted, and the reflected edge of the periosteum is sutured to the periosteum and intercostal muscles on the anterior surface of the rib using a 0 polyglycolic suture. When the rib has been resected, the reflected periosteum and intercostal muscles above and below are sutured together; the subcostal neurovascular bundle should be visualized to avoid including it in the suture. The lumbodorsal fascia is closed separately with interrupted 0 polyglycolic sutures. The external oblique and latissimus dorsi muscles are then closed with running 0 polyglycolic sutures; here again, the sutures should be placed in the fascial layers that cover these muscles. Two or three interrupted sutures are placed in the last muscle layer to reinforce the closure.

It should be remembered that because of the obliquity of the incision a shear tends to develop, so that the corresponding muscle and fascial layers may not lie opposite each other. This can be corrected by first approximating the posterior border of the external oblique muscle and the anterior border of the latissimus dorsi to bring these two severed muscles into correct alignment. The subcutaneous fascia is approximated with interrupted 000 plain catgut, and the skin is closed with 000 nylon or staples. Drains are usually brought out posteriorly through a separate stab incision below the wound. They should be positioned to facilitate application of an adhesive drainage bag if there is excessive drainage.

INTERCOSTAL INCISION

This approach, first described by Pressman, has recently become more popular. After the latissimus dorsi and posterior part of the external oblique muscles have been divided, a finger is inserted between the costal margin and diaphragm. The intercostal muscles in the selected interspace are divided close to the upper border of the rib (Fig. 62–11). The incision must be kept close to the upper border of the rib to avoid injury to the intercostal nerve and vessels lying on the undersurface of the rib above. The

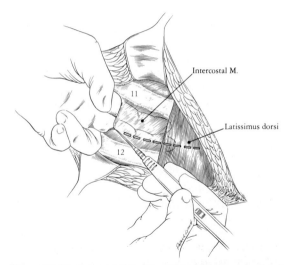

Figure 62–11. Intercostal incision. Two fingers are inserted between the intercostal muscles and the diaphragm so that they may be divided without injury to the underlying pleura. Note that the incision is made closer to the upper border of the rib below to avoid injury to the intercostal nerve.

diaphragm is incised back as far as the quadratus lumborum, which allows the lung and pleura to be elevated upward. The costotransverse ligament, which anchors the neck of the rib to the transverse process of the corresponding vertebra, is divided to allow the rib to be hinged upward.

Turner-Warwick (1965) advocates a supracostal incision. The intercostal muscles are detached from the upper border of the rib. The diaphragmatic attachments are divided, and the rib is dislocated downward. The extrapleural dissection is then continued in the manner described following resection of the eleventh rib. The intercostal wound is closed either by suturing the superficial intercostal muscles and overlying fascia to the periosteum on the anterior surface of the rib or, more simply, by approximating the rib above and below with three 0 chromic or polyglycolic sutures. These are passed around the rib, using a tapered needle that skims the periosteum to avoid injury to the intercostal nerves and vessels.

SUBCOSTAL FLANK INCISION

This incision is begun at the subcostal angle at the lateral border of the sacrospinalis muscle where it crosses the inferior edge of the twelfth rib, and is carried forward, about a finger-breadth below the lower border of the last rib onto the anterior abdominal wall. The medial end of the incision is curved slightly downward as it passes the midaxillary line to avoid the subcostal nerve and may be extended as far as the lateral border of the rectus abdominis muscle.

The extent of the incision is modified, depending on the location of the kidney and the nature of the disease. When the twelfth rib is rudimentary, the incision is made along the lower border of the eleventh rib and passes between the eleventh and twelfth subcostal nerves and vessels. The latissimus dorsi muscle, passing upward from the lumbodorsal fascia over the chest wall to be inserted into the humerus, is first divided in the posterior part of the wound. This exposes the posterior edge of the external oblique muscle in the anterior part of the wound (Fig. 62–12). Exposure of the muscle layers can be facilitated by the use of rake retractors to hold back the cut edges. The serratus posterior inferior muscles, arising from the lumbar fascia and inserting into the lower four ribs, are divided in the posterior portion of the wound. The fused layers of the lumbodorsal fascia are now exposed, as they give origin to the internal oblique and transversus muscles. The subcostal neurovascular bundle can sometimes be seen crossing deep to the glistening white transverse fibers before traversing the fascia to lie on the transversus muscle. After the internal oblique muscle is divided, the transversus is separated bluntly either above or below the subcostal nerve depending on the course of the nerve in relation to the incision (Fig. 62–13).

The subcostal nerve can be further mobilized, if necessary, by incising the fascial sheath that encloses the neurovascular bundle on the undersurface of the rib, so that it can then be displaced downward. Every effort should be

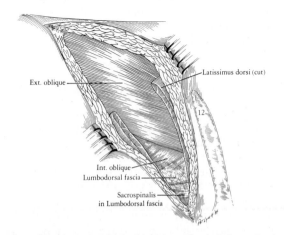

Figure 62–12. Left subcostal incision. The latissimus dorsi muscle has been divided to expose the lumbodorsal fascia and posterior aspects of the abdominal muscles.

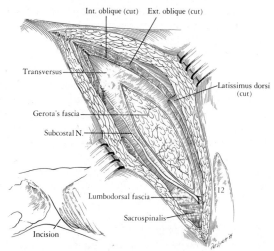

Figure 62–13. Subcostal incision. The lumbodorsal fascia and transversus muscles have been divided to expose Gerota's fascia. The subcostal nerve and vessels pierce the lumbodorsal fascia posteriorly and course forward on the transversus muscle.

made to avoid injury to the intercostal nerves, as this may cause persistent postoperative pain or bulging in the flank due to paresis of the denervated muscle. Good exposure can be maintained by the use of a Finochietto self-retaining retractor placed in the wound, with the ratchet positioned posteriorly, the edges being protected with moistened gauze sponges. This should be relaxed periodically if the procedure is prolonged.

The lumbar fascia and the lateral border of the sacrospinalis may need to be incised to improve the exposure in the posterior part of the wound. There is usually a large vessel coursing along the lateral edge of the muscle under the fascia that needs to be ligated. Division of the costotransverse ligament, as it passes up to the neck of the twelfth rib, will allow the rib to be retracted upward to further improve the exposure. The closure is as described for the other flank incisions.

OSTEOPLASTIC FLAP INCISION

Further access may be obtained with this incision by raising the posterior part of the lower rib cage as an extrapleural flap, as described by Nagamatsu (1950) (Fig. 62–14). This may be necessary when the kidney is high or when wider exposure of the upper pole or suprarenal gland is needed. The skin incision is extended upward along the lateral border of the sacrospinalis muscle to the ninth interspace. The tendinous insertions of the sacrospinalis muscle into the medial aspect of the lower three ribs are divided.

Short segments (2 cm) of the lower two or three ribs are resected subperiosteally just medial to their angles. Division of the lumbocostal ligament at its attachment to the twelfth rib, together with the lateral lumbocostal arch (arcuate ligament) of the diaphragm, allows the diaphragm and pleura to be swung upward, together with the flap (Fig. 62–15). The lumbocostal ligament is sutured when the wound is closed.

SECONDARY FLANK INCISION

If the patient has undergone previous renal surgery, the secondary incision should be approached with caution. The new incision should not necessarily be made through the bed of the old scar. Study of the position of the kidney in relation to the ribs may dictate a higher approach (e.g., resection of the eleventh rib), and this is then the preferred approach. The incision should first be developed, when possible, through recognizable anatomic structures, usually found above or below the kidney. The peritoneum will often be found lying more laterally than usual and is normally adherent to the kidney. The kidney may lie directly under the wound and be inadvertently incised. As a general principle, it is best to work from the more dissectible area to the more difficult.

Abdominal Approach

This approach is advocated when early access to the renal pedicle is required, as in the case of renal trauma or tumors of the kidney. The choice between a vertical or transverse type of incision is in part dictated by the patient's anatomy and disease entity.

A vertical incision is easier and quicker to perform and repair, as it involves only division of the linea alba or the anterior and posterior layers of the rectus sheath rather than several muscle layers. It is therefore subject to a somewhat higher incidence of wound dehiscence and hernia than is the transverse incision. The vertical incision is favored in patients with a narrow subcostal angle, as the subcostal incision in this case provides little advantage in access because of the extreme obliquity of the incision. It is also preferred in patients with renal injury, as it allows better access for the inspection of the remainder of the abdominal contents for associated injuries. The vertical incision allows equal access to both kidneys when performing bilateral nephrectomy in preparation for renal transplantation. In the case of polycystic disease the

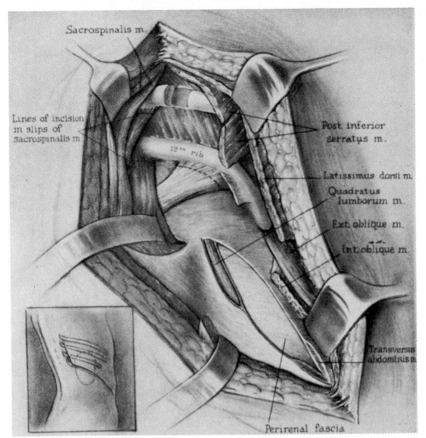

Figure 62–14. Nagamatsu incision. Inset shows line of skin incision. Latissimus dorsi and underlying posterior inferior serratus muscles are divided. Tendinous slips of sacrospinalis inserting on lower three ribs are incised. Subperiosteal resection of 2.5 cm of lower two or three ribs is done just posterior to rib angles. Anterior portion of wound is developed. Lumbocostal ligament and lumbocostal arch of diaphragm are divided, allowing mobilization of lower rib cage, including diaphragm and pleura. (From Smith, D. R. et al.: *In* Campbell, M. F., and Harrison, J. H.: Urology. Vol. 3, 3rd ed. Philadelphia, W. B. Saunders Co., 1970.)

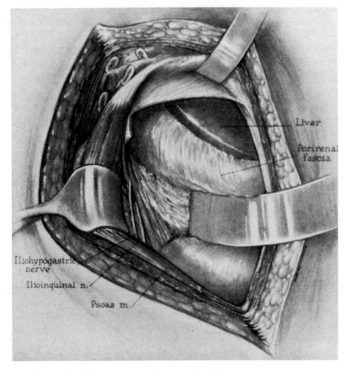

Figure 62–15. Osteoplastic flap of lower rib cage reflected upward, affording wide and high exposure. (From Smith, D. R. et al.: *In* Campbell, M. F., and Harrison, J. H.: Urology. Vol. 3, 3rd ed. Philadelphia, W. B. Saunders Co., 1970.)

vertical incision has the advantage of allowing easy extension downward to deliver the lower poles, which may extend into the pelvis.

Transverse incisions are preferred for patients with wide subcostal angles and for the exploration of renal mass lesions. This incision allows better visualization and access to the kidney, especially when mobilization is difficult because of adhesions or collateral vessels, as in patients with renal tumor. A unilateral subcostal incision can be extended across the midline as a chevron incision to provide further access, as when a renal mass extends across the midline or for the correction of a horseshoe kidney.

A chevron incision provides excellent access to both kidneys for procedures involving bilateral tumors, anterior exploration of the adrenal glands, or bilateral renal artery repair.

MIDLINE INCISION

The patient is placed supine on the operating table with a small sponge rubber pad positioned under the flank on the side of the lesion to extend the lumbodorsal spine and force the kidney and its pedicle into a more anterior position. It is helpful to tilt the table with the patient's feet down 10 degrees and to the opposite side 5 degrees to allow the abdominal contents to fall away from the kidney.

The incision should extend from the xiphoid-costal angle on the side of the lesion to just above the umbilicus. The linea alba is identified by scraping away the subcutaneous fat to reveal the decussation of the tendinous fibers of the anterior rectus sheath in the midline. This is divided to expose the extraperitoneal fat and peritoneum.

Exposure of the rectus muscle indicates deviation from the midline, which should be corrected. The incision of the linea alba necessarily deviates to one side at the upper end of the wound in the xiphisternocostal angle, where the anterior rectus sheath should be divided as far up as possible. The upper part of the muscle is retracted laterally, and the posterior sheath is divided between clamps and suture ligated, as there is usually a short terminal branch of the internal mammary artery at this point that can cause troublesome bleeding. High division of the rectus sheath facilitates retraction of the upper part of the abdominal wall and improves the access to the origin of the renal artery at the level of the epigastrium between the first and second lumbar vertebrae (Fig. 62–16). The peritoneum should first be incised in the upper part of the wound, as the underlying liver prevents any bowel from adhering to the anterior

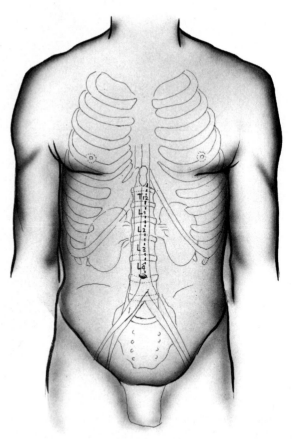

Figure 62–16. Upper midline incision extends from costo-xiphisternal angle to umbilicus. Note that renal hilus is in upper part of the incision.

peritoneum. The inner aspect of the peritoneum in the lower part of the wound can then be palpated to ensure that there is no adherent bowel in the line of the incision. The abdomen should be explored at this stage to detect any other intra-abdominal disease or extension of the renal disease.

The renal pedicle may be approached either directly through the posterior parietal peritoneum or after medial reflection of the colon. The former approach allows only limited access because of the colonic vessels; it is recommended when it is inadvisable to enter the retroperitoneal space before obtaining control of the renal artery, as in the case of renal injuries or a large vascular tumor, or if nephrectomy is performed for small contracted kidneys, when it is often unnecessary to reflect the colon to remove them. As a rule, it is better to reflect the colon prior to dissection of the renal pedicle, as this provides wider access for the dissection and identification of the main artery and any accessory vessels. The colon has to be reflected in any event to expose the kidney (see page 2408).

PARAMEDIAN INCISION

A paramedian incision may be preferred, as the separate closure of the two layers of the rectus sheath with the rectus muscle between makes the wound more secure. The incision is made about 3 cm lateral to the midline to provide an adequate margin of rectus sheath medially (Fig. 61–17). The anterior sheath is divided and reflected medially off the underlying muscle by sharp division of the tendinous intersections. The free medial edge of the muscle is retracted laterally to allow the posterior rectus sheath and peritoneum to be incised (Fig. 62–18).

An extraperitoneal approach to the kidney may be made through a paramedian incision by carefully reflecting the peritoneum off the posterior rectus sheath after it has been divided. This is best initiated in the lower part of the incision, where the peritoneum is less closely adherent to the posterior rectus sheath and abdominal wall. It is necessary to incise the transversalis fascia over its lower lateral aspect, where it covers the anterior parietal peritoneum, so that the peritoneal envelope can be reflected upward and medially (Fig. 62–18). The extraperitoneal approach has been recommended for extensive exposures of the ureter and for nephroureterectomy, which necessitates an extension of the incision well into the lower abdomen in order to gain sufficient access to the lower ureter and bladder. It would seem preferable to

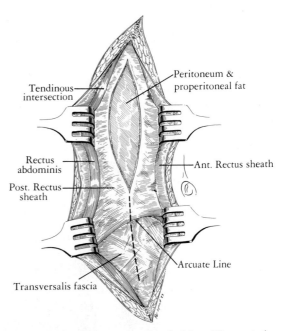

Figure 62–18. Right paramedian incision. The posterior rectus sheath and transversalis fascia must be incised to expose properitoneal space. The peritoneum may then be reflected medially to expose the kidney and ureter extraperitoneally.

utilize two smaller, less extensive incisions for nephroureterectomy, an upper abdominal incision for the nephrectomy and a Pfannenstiel incision that provides the ideal exposure for excision of the lower ureter and cuff of bladder.

ANTERIOR SUBCOSTAL INCISION

The incision extends from a point in the midline, one third of the way from the xiphisternum to the umbilicus, to the tip of the lowermost palpable rib in the anterior axillary line. It is curved slightly downward, so as to avoid making the incision over the costal margin (Fig. 62–19). The anterior rectus sheath and external oblique muscles are divided in the line of the incision. The rectus muscle is transected, and the superior epigastric artery is clamped and divided as it lies in the substance of the muscle posteriorly. The posterior rectus sheath, internal oblique muscle, and transversus muscle and fascia, together with the underlying peritoneum adherent to them, are then divided. The approach to the renal pedicle and kidney is the same as the midline approach just described.

An *extraperitoneal anterior subcostal approach* is particularly useful when there is a possibility that the patient may require peritoneal dialysis postoperatively or when there has been a previous intra-abdominal procedure. It

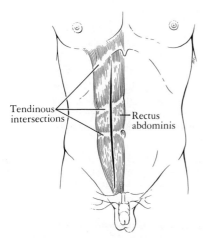

Figure 62–17. Right paramedian incision. The incision is made 3 cm lateral to the midline, and after incision of the anterior rectus sheath, the tendinous intersections are divided sharply to allow the medial border of the rectus abdominis muscle to be retracted.

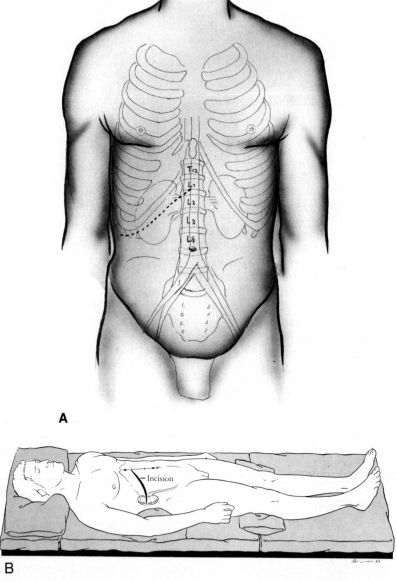

A

B

Figure 62–19. *A,* The anterior subcostal incision extends from a point in the midline, one third of the way from the xiphisternum to the umbilicus, to the tip of the lowermost palpable rib. *B,* Position of patient for subcostal incision. A small pad is placed under the loin, and the table is placed feet down at an angle of 20 degrees and tilted slightly to the opposite side. The table may also be extended to increase the exposure, if necessary.

is a good approach for the exploration of a lower pole renal mass or for an open renal biopsy, particularly in children. The extraperitoneal approach is recommended for the nephrectomy portion of a total nephroureterectomy, with a second lower abdominal incision being made for the lower ureter. An added advantage of this approach is that the abdominal contents can be readily retracted in their peritoneal envelope, thus minimizing postoperative ileus and the chances of intra-abdominal complications. Reflection of the peritoneum off the anterior abdominal wall may at times be difficult, and access to the renal pedicle is sometimes less satisfactory than with the transperitoneal approach.

The incision is subcostal, and following division of the rectus and external oblique muscles (Fig. 62–20), the fibers of the internal oblique and transversus muscles are separated by blunt dissection as far laterally as possible, at which point the underlying peritoneum is not very adherent (Fig. 62–21). The extraperitoneal space is entered, and the peritoneum is stripped medially from the overlying muscles by dissection with the fingers.

The incision is now extended through the muscles at the site where the peritoneum has been reflected from them. The peritoneum is most adherent to the abdominal wall at the lateral border of the posterior rectus sheath,

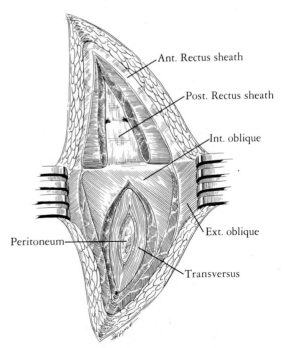

Figure 62–21. Anterior subcostal incision. The rectus and external oblique muscles and superior epigastric artery have been divided. The fibers of the internal oblique and transversus muscle have been separated laterally to expose the peritoneum.

where it fuses with the oblique muscles (linea semilunaris), and this is the point at which it is usually torn. The peritoneum here is reflected by grasping the divided edges of the transversalis muscle with Allis forceps and dividing the fascial attachments to the muscle with scissors. The separation can now be completed behind the posterior rectus sheath to the midline, using a cotton dissector, and the sheath can be divided (Fig. 62–22). The peritoneum should be freed from the abdominal wall for about 6 to 8 cm on either side of the wound to enable it to be retracted freely. It is now swept off the lateral abdominal wall to expose Gerota's fascia. The fascia is incised over the lateral aspect of the kidney to avoid injury to the peritoneum (Fig. 62–23). The anterior layer of Gerota's fascia, together with the posterior parietal peritoneum, can now be reflected medially and the duodenum mobilized to expose the kidney and renal pedicle (Fig. 62–24).

TRANSVERSE CHEVRON INCISION

This transverse upper abdominal incision was recommended by Chute and his associates (1967) for procedures on both kidneys, bilateral renal artery reconstruction, bilateral adrenalectomy, and retroperitoneal node dissection. It

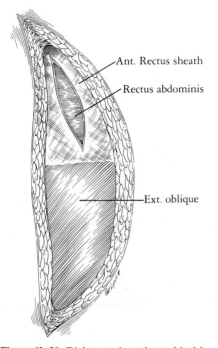

Figure 62–20. Right anterior subcostal incision.

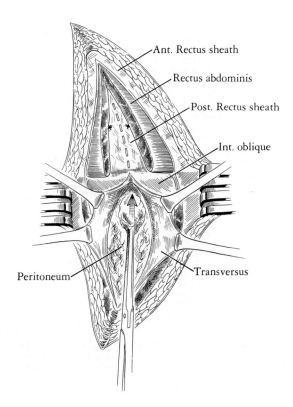

Ant. Rectus sheath

Rectus abdominis

Post. Rectus sheath

Int. oblique

Peritoneum

Transversus

Figure 62–22. Anterior subcostal incision. The peritoneum is reflected from the posterior surface of the transversus muscle as it joins the posterior rectus sheath, where it is most adherent, by careful blunt and sharp dissection.

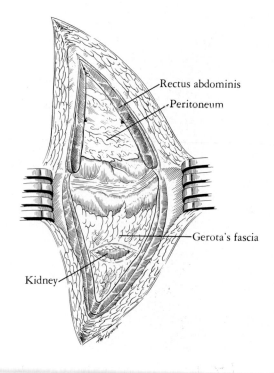

Rectus abdominis

Peritoneum

Gerota's fascia

Kidney

Figure 62–23. Anterior subcostal incision. Gerota's fascia is incised and the anterior layer is reflected off the kidney with the colon and mesocolon. A plane can be established between the mesocolon and Gerota's fascia if it is adherent or needs to be removed with the kidney.

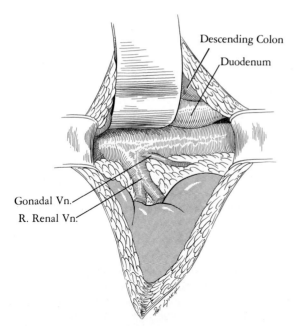

Figure 62–24. Anterior subcostal incision. The duodenum has been mobilized and reflected off the renal hilum to expose the inferior vena cava and renal vessels.

Lumbar Approach—Posterior Lumbotomy

This is a useful approach for removal of a small kidney, for bilateral nephrectomy in patients with chronic renal failure, for pyeloplasty, for pyelolithotomy when a stone fills the pelvis and is not able to migrate, or for an upper ureterolithotomy when the stone is firmly impacted. It provides for a very direct approach to the renal hilum and avoids division of muscles, which decreases postoperative pain and disability and makes for a strong wound closure. It has an advantage over the flank incision in that there is a significant reduction in postoperative pain and a more rapid return to normal activity. An average of only 4.2 injections of analgesic per patient were required following lumbotomy as compared with 6.3 following a flank incision. Recovery of full mobility occurred in an average of 3.3 days versus 4.3 days for the flank approach (Gardiner et al., 1979). The major disadvantage of the lumbar approach is the limited access to the kidney, which can be a serious problem if there are intraoperative complications, such as migration of a calculus or injury to the renal pedicle or accessory vessels with bleeding. However, the incision can be readily enlarged in the form of a T by making a subcostal incision or even resecting the twelfth rib, should the need arise.

The patient is placed in the lateral position and rotated anteriorly about 30 degrees, with the tip of the twelfth rib over the break in the table (Fig. 62–25). A sandbag is placed between the abdomen and the table for support and helps to push the kidney posteriorly. The table is slightly flexed. When access to both kidneys is required, the patient may be placed prone

probably provides a better exposure of both kidneys than a midline incision in obese patients with a wide subcostal angle. The major disadvantage is that it involves extensive transection of the abdominal wall musculature.

The patient is placed in the supine position and slightly hyperextended. The incision is the same as a subcostal incision performed bilaterally. The round ligament is ligated and divided in the midline to allow the liver to be retracted more easily. Closure may be facilitated by flexing the patient.

Figure 62–25. Posterior lumbotomy incision. The patient is placed in the lateral position with the table slightly flexed to widen the space between the twelfth rib and the iliac crest. The incision curves forward toward the anterior iliac spine, as the longitudinal incisions frequently result in an unsatisfactory scar.

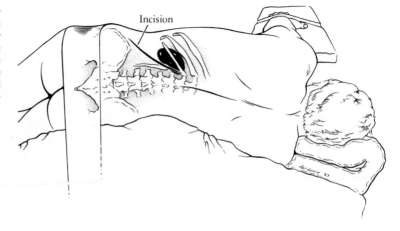

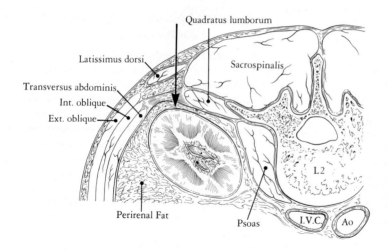

Figure 62–26. Posterior lumbotomy incision. The fused layers of the lumbar fascia at the lateral border of the sacrospinalis muscle are incised to enter the perirenal space.

and slightly flexed to increase the space between the twelfth rib and iliac crest. When patients are placed prone, it is important that they be supported over the sternum and pubis so that there is free excursion of the anterior abdominal wall to prevent embarrassment of respiration and venous return.

Essentially, the approach involves dividing the fused layers of the lumbar fascia at the lateral border of the sacrospinalis and quadratus lumborum muscles to expose the renal fossa (Fig. 62–26). The approach was first described by Gustave Simon in 1870, who performed the first elective nephrectomy. Two variations of the incision were later popularized by Gil-Vernet (1965) and Lurz (1969).

The incision is made from the costovertebral angle, where the lateral border of the sacrospinalis muscle crosses the lower border of the twelfth rib, and is curved downward and laterally along the edge of the muscle toward

the anterior superior iliac spine (Fig. 62–25). A vertical incision frequently results in an ugly scar with a tendency to keloid formation. The latissimus dorsi muscle and its aponeurosis are incised along the lateral border of the sacrospinalis muscle (Fig. 62–27), and the lowest slip of the serratus posterior inferior muscle is divided in the upper part of the wound as it inserts into the twelfth rib underneath the latissimus dorsi muscle (Fig. 62–28). The lateral edges of the cut aponeurosis and muscle are elevated with Allis clamps, and the lateral edge of the sacrospinalis muscle is identified by palpation to find the fused posterior middle and anterior lamellae of the lumbar fascia, which envelop the sacrospinalis and quadratus lumborum muscles and give origin to the internal oblique and transversus abdominis muscles. This is incised longitudinally along the lateral border of the sacrospinalis muscle to expose the quadratus lumborum, which is retracted medially to expose the peri-

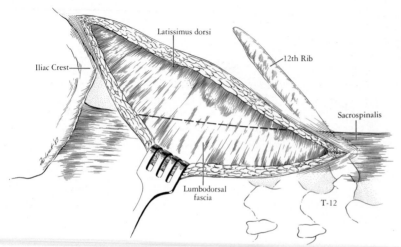

Figure 62–27. Posterior lumbotomy incision. The latissimus dorsi muscle and lumbodorsal fascia are incised over the lateral border of the sacrospinalis muscle.

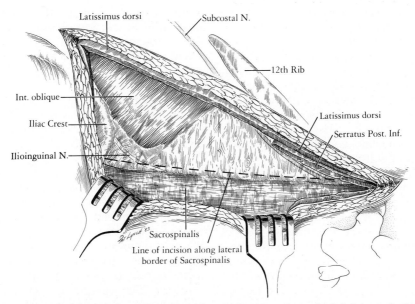

Figure 62–28. Posterior lumbotomy incision. The latissimus dorsi and serratus posterior inferior muscles have been divided. The fused layers of the lumbodorsal fascia are incised along the lateral border of the sacrospinalis muscle. The ilioinguinal nerve, which lies deep to the fascia, should be identified to avoid injury.

nephric space (Fig. 62–29). The incision should be begun in the middle part of the wound to make sure that it is in the right place, as it is not uncommon to be too far medial. Once the lateral edge of the quadratus lumborum muscle and perinephric space are identified, the incision in the lumbar fascia is extended with scissors upward to the lower border of the twelfth rib and downward to the iliac crest. The subcostal nerve should be identified and preserved as it courses forward in the upper part of the incision and runs downward on the undersurface of the lateral flap of the cut lumbar fascia and anterior abdominal wall muscles. The iliohypogastric branch of the first lumbar nerve is usually seen on the medial side of the lower end of the

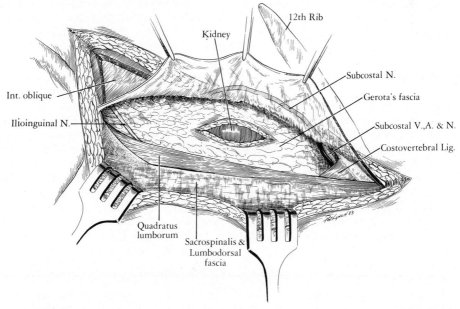

Figure 62–29. Posterior lumbotomy incision. The lumbodorsal fascia has been divided to expose Gerota's fascia and the kidney.

wound as it emerges from the edge of the quadratus lumborum muscle and runs downward and forward into the pelvis. Greater access can be obtained by incising the costovertebral ligament in the upper part of the wound (Fig. 62–29), but care must be taken to avoid injury to the subcostal nerve and vessels that lie immediately below or anterior to this ligament. Once the ligament has been divided, the rib can be dislocated cephalad. Exposure can best be maintained with a self-retaining retractor of the ratchet type. Gerota's fascia is incised, and dissection of the kidney can be facilitated by abdominal compression to push it into the wound.

The wound is closed by suturing the cut edges of the lumbar fascia with a continuous 0 polyglycolic suture. It is best to begin the closure at each end of the wound and work toward the middle to ensure adequate access. The lumbar fascia and latissimus dorsi muscle are approximated in the same way.

Posterior Lumbotomy for Nephroscopy. An abbreviated version of this incision has been advocated (Gittes and Belldegrun, 1983) for stone surgery with nephroscopy, as an alternative to percutaneous nephrostomy. The advantage over this standard endourologic approach is that a direct visual approach to the pelvis or upper ureter avoids all the difficulties of needling a nondilated collecting system, including peri- and intrarenal bleeding, radiation exposure of patient and operative team, and the need for a large hole in the cortex with its concomitant nephron loss. The disadvantage is that this procedure does still require general anesthesia and a surgical incision.

Thoracoabdominal Approach

This approach provides wide access to the kidney, renal vessels, abdominal aorta, and vena cava and combines some of the advantages of both the flank and the abdominal approaches. It is the preferred approach for radical nephrectomy for renal cancer and is usually the incision of choice for partial nephrectomy for tumor in a solitary kidney. It is also useful for repair of renal artery lesions, when the vessels have a high origin, and for excision of large suprarenal tumors.

The incision may be intrapleural or extrapleural, depending on which rib or intercostal space is selected. This again depends on the position of the kidney and the nature, site, and size of the lesion. Resection of the ninth or tenth rib or incision of the tenth intercostal space will involve the pleura, whereas an incision through the bed of the eleventh rib or intercostal space may be performed extrapleurally unless the pleural reflection is particularly low.

The patient is placed on the operating table with a large towel or sandbag positioned under the back, so as to elevate and tilt the patient away from the operative side. The lower leg is flexed and the upper one extended with a pillow between the legs. The pelvis assumes a more horizontal position, being tilted only about 10 to 15 degrees, which allows free access to the anterior abdominal wall. The patient is secured to the table with adhesive tape attached over the pelvis, and the table is adjusted so that the patient's back assumes an angle of 45 degrees to the horizontal plane with a 10 degree downward tilt. The uppermost arm is swung across and supported on a Mayo table to maintain the position (Figs. 62–30 and 62–31).

The incision is usually made over the ninth or tenth rib, depending on the position of the kidney. After division of the latissimus dorsi and external oblique muscles, the distal two thirds of the rib is resected (Fig. 62–32). The incision is extended forward and slightly downward onto the abdominal wall through the costal margin to avoid injury to the intercostal vessels and nerves. The external oblique, internal oblique, and transversus muscles are divided in the line of the incision (Fig. 62–33).

Rib resection is advocated, as it provides for a somewhat wider exposure than an incision through the intercostal space. However, many surgeons prefer the latter method, as it does provide good exposure if the incision is carried far enough posteriorly. It is important to keep close to the upper border of the rib below when making an intercostal incision, so as to avoid injury to the neurovascular bundle. Another alternative that is employed to avoid rib resection is to reflect the periosteum from the upper surface and posterior aspect of the rib and make the incision through the bed of the rib, leaving it in situ. This maneuver avoids cutting the intercostal muscles, while preserving the rib, and seems to provide for a more satisfactory closure.

Sometimes the incision can be made through the bed of the eleventh rib and the pleura can often be dissected off the lateral aspect of the diaphragm, first by sharply incising the fascial attachments at the pleural edge and then by completing the reflection by blunt dissection. This exposes the upper lateral aspect of

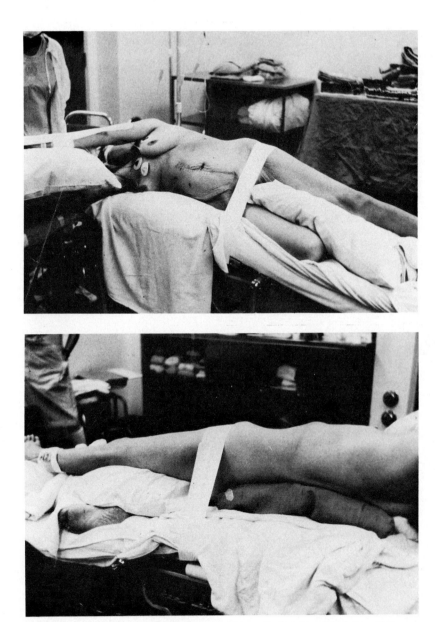

Figures 62–30 and 62–31. Thoracoabdominal approach to left kidney. Patient is positioned at 45 degrees on the operating table with a downward tilt of 10 degrees. Lower leg is flexed to 90 degrees and upper leg is straight, with a pillow between them. A sandbag behind the back and adhesive tape maintain the position. The upper arm is supported on a pillow placed on a Mayo stand. Note that the pelvis is rotated to assume a more horizontal position.

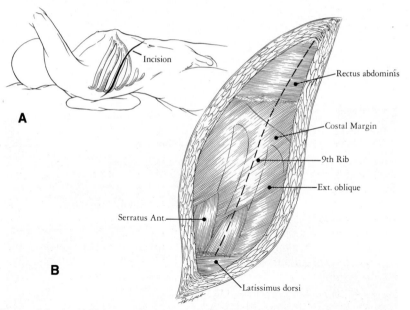

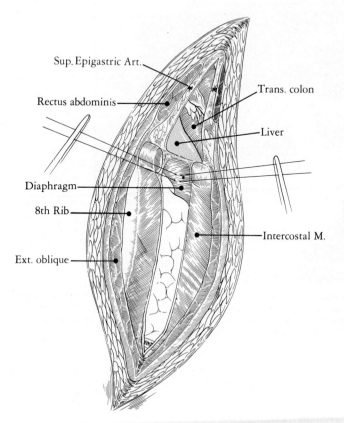

Figure 62–32. Thoracoabdominal incision. *A,* Showing the position of the incision. *B,* Superficial muscles to be divided.

Figure 62–33. Thoracoabdominal incision. The ninth rib has been resected and the pleural cavity entered.

the diaphragm overlying the liver or spleen, which can then be incised or detached from the inner aspect of the ribs without opening the pleural cavity. When the incision is transpleural, the lower edge of the lung must be protected while the diaphragmatic pleura and diaphragm are incised. The incision in the diaphragm is continued downward and laterally as far as the peritoneal reflection on the lateral side of the colon. It is helpful to mark the anterior cut edges of the diaphragm at the costal margin with silk sutures to facilitate their accurate reapproximation (Fig. 62–34). The incision is extended forward as far medially as is necessary to obtain adequate exposure, usually to the lateral border of the rectus abdominis muscle. This may be extended further by dividing the rectus muscle and its sheath and, if necessary, continuing down the midline. A self-retaining retractor (a Finochietto is ideal) is now placed in the posterior part of the wound, which is protected with moistened laparotomy pads. The retractor is spread as widely as possible to maintain the exposure, and because of the patient's position, the abdominal contents tend to fall away from the kidney. The remainder of the operation is described under each specific procedure.

At the completion of the procedure, the abdominal viscera are replaced in their anatomic position. Closure of the lateral paracolic incisions is unnecessary. The omentum should be pulled down over the loops of intestine, whenever possible, to prevent their adherence to the wound. The peritoneum is closed with a continuous 00 chromic catgut suture, and the diaphragm is repaired with interrupted mattress sutures of 00 silk with the knots tied on the undersurface. When only the lower fibers have been detached, repair is unnecessary. When the rib has been removed, suture of the periosteum with a running 0 polyglycolic suture effectively approximates the chest wall. Care must be taken to avoid including the neurovascular bundle in the suture, which runs in its sheath under the lower leaf of the periosteum.

Intercostal incisions are closed by suturing the superficial muscle layers and overlying fascia to the periosteum over the upper and outer surface of the rib or by passing three 0 polyglycolic sutures around the ribs above and below to approximate the chest wall. These sutures should be passed on a tapered needle to avoid cutting any vessels, and the needles should closely hug the surface of the rib to avoid the neurovascular bundle. The internal and external

Figure 62–34. Right thoracoabdominal incision. The diaphragm has been incised to expose the right lobe of the liver. Stay sutures mark the anterior margin of the diaphragm to facilitate accurate reapproximation.

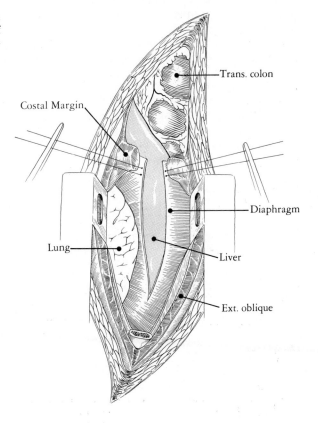

oblique muscle layers are then approximated separately, using 0 polyglycolic sutures. A nonabsorbable suture, such as 00 silk, Tevdek, or No. 28 stainless steel wire, may be preferred for repair of the external oblique and latissimus dorsi muscles and fascia. This is recommended in debilitated or elderly patients suspected of being in negative nitrogen balance.

The pleura is closed, together with the closure of the rib bed. A 20 F multi-eye tygon chest tube is placed in the pleural cavity through a separate stab wound in the posterior axillary line, usually in the tenth or eleventh interspace, so that the patient does not lie on it. It is connected to an underwater drain and should be anchored to the skin with a braided silk suture. The chest tube is usually removed after 24 hours if there is no persistent leakage of air and if a chest x-ray shows satisfactory expansion of the lung.

Small inadvertent openings in the pleura can be closed with a continuous 000 chromic catgut suture. The anesthesiologist is asked to inflate the lung maximally to expel the air from the pleural cavity as the final loop of the suture is drawn tight to close the defect. A chest tube is not usually required. A radiograph of the chest should always be taken in the recovery room to see if there is a significant pneumothorax causing either respiratory embarrassment or collapse of the lung. This is managed by the insertion of a 14 F catheter through the second or third intercostal space anteriorly by means of a trochar and cannula. The catheter is then connected to an underwater drain.

Drainage of the nephrectomy site is not always carried out but is advisable if there is an unusual amount of oozing or if there is evidence of infection. A Penrose drain is placed retroperitoneally and is usually brought out through a separate stab incision below the wound.

COMPLICATIONS OF RENAL SURGERY

There are systemic complications that may occur after any surgical procedure. These include cerebrovascular accidents, myocardial infarction, congestive heart failure, pulmonary embolism, atelectasis, pneumonia, and thrombophlebitis. The complication rate appears to have some relationship to the type of surgical approach. Among 347 patients who underwent nephrectomy between 1964 and 1975 by a variety of approaches, the flank incision had a 25 per cent complication rate compared with 14.7 per cent for other incisions. This difference persisted even when infectious complications were excluded, even though most patients with renal infections and stone disease were operated on through a flank incision. It is of interest that the fewest complications occurred when the anterior extraperitoneal approach was used, the rate being only 7 per cent in 44 patients (Table 62–1).

The incidence of these problems can be reduced by adequate preoperative preparation, avoidance of prolonged periods of hypotension intraoperatively, appropriate blood and fluid replacement, postoperative breathing exercises, early mobilization, and elastic support of the legs both during and after surgery. It is our practice to administer subcutaneous heparin, 5000 units every 8 hours, immediately preoperatively and for 7 days postoperatively in older patients and in those in whom an increased risk of venous thrombosis and pulmonary embolism is thought likely.

A number of other complications are specifically associated with renal surgery, and these may be immediate or late.

Immediate Complications

Secondary hemorrhage is manifested by pain, a profuse blood loss from the drain site, signs of shock, or the development of a flank mass. Bleeding may be from the kidney or renal pedicle but is sometimes from an unrecognized injury to a neighboring structure, such as the spleen, liver, or a mesenteric vessel. Patients should be given blood replacement if possible, but Ringer's lactate solution and fresh frozen

TABLE 62–1. COMPLICATIONS FOR NEPHRECTOMIES PERFORMED 1964–1973 (YNHH)

Approach	No. of Patients	Pulmonary	CV*	GI*	Infectious	Total (%)
Flank	225	15	11	8	23	25%
Transperitoneal	68	4	1	4	4	19%
Anterior Retroperitoneal	44	–	1	–	1	7%
Thoracoabdominal	10	–	1	–	1	20%
Total	347	5.4%	4%	3.4%	8.6%	22%

*CV = cardiovascular; GI = gastrointestinal.

plasma may be used as temporary substitutes if necessary. In most cases it is best to reopen the wound as soon as possible, evacuate the hematoma, and secure the bleeding point. When bleeding is diffuse, a clotting disorder, such as follows a mismatched blood transfusion, must be considered. In such cases, it may be necessary to apply Gelfoam to the bleeding site and temporarily pack the wound with gauze, which can then be gradually removed after the first 24 hours.

Pneumothorax may occur during flank or thoracoabdominal incisions. The intraoperative and postoperative management of this complication is described in the sections dealing with these procedures.

Gastrointestinal injuries should always be checked for during the procedure, and lacerations should be repaired and drained. Tears of the liver may be repaired with mattress sutures. Splenic injuries are usually treated by splenectomy, although small lacerations, especially in children, may be managed by application of Avitene and tamponaded with omentum held in place by sutures. This procedure preserves the spleen for its protective effect against septicemia. Injuries to the tail of the pancreas, which may occur with operations on the left kidney, are best managed by partial amputation.

LATE COMPLICATIONS

Infection is the most common complication encountered later in the postoperative period. Superficial wound infections are best managed by removal of skin sutures to allow for drainage. Deeper infections must be treated by the establishment of adequate drainage and the administration of the appropriate antibiotics when there are systemic manifestations of the infection. If the drainage is persistent and profuse, the possibility of a retained foreign body or a fistulous communication with the intestine should be considered.

It should be remembered that patients with diabetes may develop an exacerbation of this disorder in the presence of severe infection with polyuria and ketoacidosis. This may sometimes occur in patients not previously suspected of having the disease, and failure to recognize this problem can lead to serious consequences. Accumulations of lymph or serous fluid in the renal fossa or pleura are best managed expectantly, unless they are causing respiratory embarrassment. Such accumulations may become infected or may be complicated by bleeding if treated by needle aspiration.

Gastrointestinal problems are usually due to a generalized ileus or a functional obstruction caused by a localized ileus of the colon overlying the operated kidney. Oral feeding should not be allowed until adequate bowel sounds are present and the patient has passed flatus. Nasogastric suction is used in the more severe cases.

Unrecognized injuries of the bowel or pancreas with fistula formation will require drainage and sometimes hyperalimentation and secondary surgical procedures. When a prolonged period of ileus is anticipated or if the patient is in a poor nutritional state, parenteral hyperalimentation should be instituted preoperatively. Establishment of an intraoperative gastrostomy should also be considered in these patients as well as in those with a pulmonary problem that may be aggravated by the prolonged presence of a nasogastric tube.

Wound dehiscence is uncommon with flank incisions. Bulging of the flank in these patients is more common and is usually due to muscular weakness secondary to intercostal nerve injury, rather than to disruption of the wound. Evisceration following abdominal incisions is usually heralded by a sudden discharge of serosanguineous fluid from the wound on the fifth to seventh postoperative day. This is best treated by prompt secondary suturing, using No. 2 nylon tension sutures passed through the entire thickness of the abdominal wall. Sutures should not pass through the peritoneal cavity, if this can be avoided, as they may occasionally erode through distended loops of bowel if there is prolonged ileus.

Intercostal neuralgia may be severe and can be controlled temporarily in the early postoperative period by injection of a long-acting local anesthetic into the posterior intercostal space. Persistent pain after the immediate postoperative period should be managed by the administration of mild analgesics and diazepam (Valium) and the injection of the appropriate intercostal nerve with 2 ml of local anesthetic together with 40 mg of hydrocortisone. The majority of patients improve after several months, and every effort should be made to avoid more active treatment. If incapacitating symptoms persist, percutaneous radiofrequency neurolysis under local anesthesia may be helpful. Crushing or sectioning the nerve should be avoided, as this frequently leads to phantom pain.

Mortality of Renal Surgery. The mortality following nephrectomy in 347 patients at Yale–New Haven Medical Center was 1.4 per cent (Schiff and Glazier, 1977), corresponding closely to the 1.35 per cent mortality that followed 814 renal procedures reported from Duke

University (Gonzalez-Serva et al., 1977). The most important factors associated with increased mortality are cancer, infections, and azotemia. The mortality in patients undergoing nephrectomy in the absence of these problems was 0.4 per cent and 0.63 per cent, respectively, in the two studies. The mortality after simple nephrectomy in other series was higher. For example, there was a 3.3 per cent mortality following nephrectomy for hypertension reported by the Cooperative Study Group on Renal Vascular Hypertension (Franklin et al., 1975), and a 1.58 per cent mortality has been reported after renal cyst exploration. However, in a review of 3873 live-donor nephrectomies for renal transplantation, there were only three deaths.

It is encouraging that the most recent reports indicate that surgical procedures on the kidney have become progressively safer. However, the surgeon should be aware of the greatly increased risks of operation in patients with infections, azotemia, and cancer.

SIMPLE NEPHRECTOMY

Indications

Infections. Pyonephrosis, chronic pyelonephritis with severe parenchymal destruction, carbuncle of the kidney, or severe pyelonephritis that cannot be controlled by appropriate antibiotic therapy are indications for simple nephrectomy. The last-named disorder is usually due to multiple small pyemic abscesses and occurs most commonly in diabetic patients. Patients with xanthogranulomatous pyelonephritis and occasionally those with renal tuberculosis may also require nephrectomy.

Trauma. Severe parenchymal or pedicle injuries in which a reparative procedure is not feasible or is contraindicated because of the patient's general condition are indications for nephrectomy. Other candidates include patients with a ureteral injury with good contralateral renal function, in whom ureteral repair is contraindicated because of age or general condition or in whom local conditions, such as previous irradiation or chronic infection, make repair unlikely to succeed. This is particularly so when preliminary nephrostomy drainage is required, necessitating two or more operative procedures to accomplish the repair.

Symptomatic Hydronephrosis. Symptomatic hydronephrosis with marked parenchymal loss is an additional indication. The decision to perform nephrectomy for hydronephrosis in children is particularly difficult, as remarkable degrees of recovery can occur after drainage, even with severe hydronephrosis and poor radiographic visualization. If there is doubt, a repair should be attempted.

Hypertension. Unilateral parenchymal diseases due to arteriosclerosis, pyelonephritis, extensive scarring following trauma, or congenital dysplasia (Aske-Upmark kidney) are the usual indications for nephrectomy. Renovascular disease that is not amenable to reconstructive procedures, or that occurring in older, poor-risk patients whose hypertension cannot be controlled by drug therapy, is best treated by nephrectomy. It is important to establish that the vasculature of the contralateral kidney is not compromised.

Measurement of renal vein renin levels, which should show at least a 2:1 ratio between the affected and the unaffected sides, is valuable in predicting a successful result from nephrectomy. Although nephrectomy will cure hypertension in only 60 per cent of patients, it will frequently make the disease much easier to control by antihypertensive drugs in most of the remainder. Patients with chronic renal failure who have severe hypertension and elevation of peripheral vein renin levels will benefit from bilateral nephrectomy. It should be remembered that the mortality from nephrectomy for hypertension has been reported by some to be as high as 5 per cent, although others have found it to be only 1 per cent. Death occurs primarily from cardiovascular complications related to the generalized vascular disease in many of these patients. The procedure should, therefore, not be undertaken without careful preoperative evaluation and preparation.

Surgical Approach

The surgical approach is predicated on the nature of the problem and the patient's anatomy, as has been outlined on page 2408. Generally, a flank incision is used for hydronephrosis or infectious problems in order to avoid contamination of the peritoneal cavity. The transabdominal incision is preferred for hypertension or acute trauma, as it provides for early access to the pedicle, and it is also used in patients who have difficulty tolerating the lateral position. Secondary operations for trauma, however, particularly in the presence of gross urinary extravasation or infection, are probably best dealt with through a retroperitoneal flank incision. A posterior lumbotomy, which minimizes injury to the abdominal wall, lessens postoperative respiratory embarrassment, and is followed by a more rapid recovery, is a good approach for the removal of a contracted kidney causing hypertension.

FLANK APPROACH

Once the perinephric space is entered, access to the kidney is obtained by incising Gerota's fascia on the lateral aspect of the kidney to avoid injury to the overlying peritoneum. The plane of cleavage between the perinephric fat and the renal capsule is usually developed easily, unless there has been a perinephritis. Blunt dissection should be performed gently; sharp dissection should be used if there is any resistance, as attempts to tear the more dense adhesions between the fascia and the renal capsule, particularly if they are secondary to inflammation, may result in tearing of the renal capsule and cause troublesome bleeding from the raw surface of the kidney. There may be large collateral veins if there is any obstruction to the renal vein or severe inflammation. The lower pole is mobilized, and the ureter is identified as it lies on the psoas muscle, enveloped in the retroperitoneal fat in the less well-defined inferior part of Gerota's fascia below the kidney. The gonadal vein is seen lying medially, and on occasion these two structures have been confused.

The ureter is freed by dissection of the loose fascial layer surrounding it, and a small Penrose drain is passed around it to facilitate retraction and further dissection. It is preferable to divide the ureter after ligation of the pedicle to avoid congestion of the kidney. The kidney is now pulled downward, and the upper pole is dissected free. Accessory vessels to the upper pole, especially veins, should be looked for. Bleeding from such veins may be difficult to control if they are inadvertently torn, as they tend to retract into the perinephric fat under the diaphragm. There is normally a separate compartment in Gerota's fascia for the suprarenal gland, which enables it to be readily separated from the upper pole. Sometimes, however, the suprarenal gland adheres to the capsule of the upper pole, and the surgeon should be on the lookout for the characteristic butter-yellow tissue that can be fairly easily distinguished from the surrounding fat. The adrenal gland is friable and tears easily, so it may be the cause of persistent bleeding from the renal fossa.

The kidney can now be pulled laterally, and Gerota's fascia together with the overlying parietal peritoneum or duodenum can be reflected off the anterior aspect of the renal vessels. There is a definite plane between the perinephric and perihilar fat that should be identified to avoid dissecting the vessels in the renal hilum, which could cause troublesome bleeding. Whenever possible, it is preferable to secure the vessels individually away from the hilum, and the artery should always be ligated first. The vein is usually visualized easily, and if the fascial layer over it is incised in the line of the vessel, in most cases the periadventitial space is entered easily to provide a natural cleavage plane. Dissection of the artery generally requires retraction of the vein, which usually overlies it (Fig. 62–35). On the left side this can be facilitated by ligation and division of the

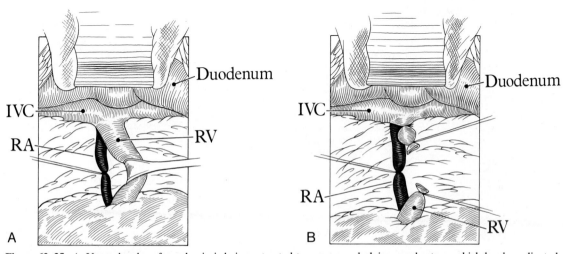

Figure 62–35. *A*, Upper border of renal vein is being retracted to expose underlying renal artery, which has been ligated. *B*, Vein has been doubly ligated proximally to leave a cuff of 3 to 4 mm after it is divided. This provides access to the artery, which has already been ligated.

gonadal and adrenal veins to improve the mobility of the vein. Sometimes it is easier to approach the artery posteriorly by mobilizing the kidney and retracting it up into the wound. The artery is surrounded by a dense fascial layer, containing a network of sympathetic nerves and lymphatics, which needs to be dissected off to enter the periadventitial layer. This is best done by a combination of sharp scissors dissection and blunt dissection with a Kotner sponge.

When there is a great deal of perihilar inflammatory reaction, it may be easier to approach the right renal artery between the vena cava and aorta, the vena cava being mobilized and retracted laterally to expose it (Fig. 62–36). The artery is ligated with 0 silk sutures, and, if possible, two sutures are placed proximally. When only one suture can be placed proximally, a right-angle clamp should be placed on the proximal side, and another ligature should be applied after division of the artery. Once the artery has been ligated, division of the artery may be more easily accomplished after the vein has been divided.

The vein is then similarly ligated in continuity and divided (Fig. 62–35). It is not uncommon for a large lumbar vein to enter the posterior aspect of the renal vein, and, if present, it must be carefully dissected out and ligated separately. A lumbar vein can cause serious bleeding, which may be difficult to control if it is inadvertently torn or divided. When it is not feasible to dissect out the vessels individually

because of severe perihilar inflammation, the kidney is mobilized and the pedicle is isolated. It is ligated as far proximally as possible, after being divided into two or three sections. Clamps are applied distal to the ligatures, and the pedicle is divided close to the renal hilum distal to the clamps, to leave as much of a stump as possible. The pedicle is again ligated, with removal of the clamps.

When severe hemorrhage occurs that necessitates prompt and early clamping of the pedicle, it is best to use a large vascular clamp, closing it only one or two notches for temporary control of bleeding. The vessels can then be either dissected out individually or ligated en masse under controlled conditions and direct visualization. The use of a vascular clamp helps to avoid tearing of friable vessels and minimizes any injury to other structures, such as the duodenum, which might be inadvertently included when clamping the pedicle in an emergency situation.

The ureter is now clamped and divided, and the distal end is transfixed and ligated with 0 chromic catgut. The kidney is usually still tethered medially by sympathetic nerves and fascia, and care must be taken to identify any secondary renal vessels when these are being divided.

A Penrose drain is placed in the wound if there is bacterial contamination or excessive oozing. This may be brought out through the wound or via a separate stab incision.

Sometimes, when the kidney has been the

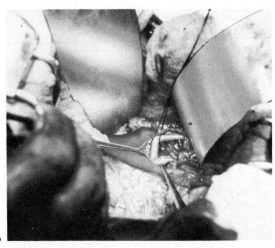

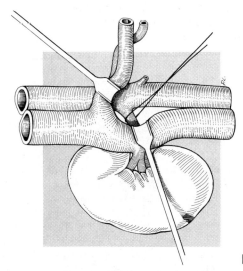

A   B

Figure 62–36. *A,* Right renal artery ligated on medial side of inferior vena cava. Junction of left renal vein and vena cava is retracted to expose the artery as it arises from the aorta. *B,* Diagrammatic representation of ligation of right renal artery between the vena cava and aorta.

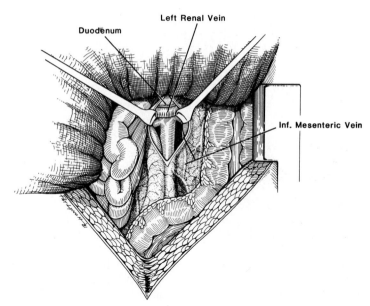

Figure 62–37. Exposure of the renal arteries through a vertical incision in the posterior parietal peritoneum.

site of severe inflammatory disease so that it becomes densely adherent to the surrounding fat and fascia, it may be necessary to include some of the perinephric fat and fascia or to perform a subcapsular removal of the kidney.

Subcapsular nephrectomy is carried out by incising the capsule on the lateral border of the kidney and stripping it digitally from the renal parenchyma. This usually separates easily as far as the hilum, where the vessels lie in a separate plane. The reflected capsule is now incised to expose the pedicle, which must be freed for ligation. The perinephritis may make it impossible to dissect out enough to divide the pedicle between ligatures. It is sufficient to doubly ligate the pedicle and divide the vessels right in the hilum of the kidney.

TRANSABDOMINAL APPROACH

This is used when the renal vessels need to be secured first. They may be approached by incising the posterior parietal peritoneum or by reflecting the left colon or the right colon and duodenum. It is particularly important to obtain control of the renal vessels first in patients with renal trauma in order to prevent further hemorrhage when Gerota's fascia is opened to expose the kidney and the tamponade effect is lost. The renal artery can be temporarily occluded by a balloon catheter passed percutaneously during arteriography. This will control the bleeding to allow a more planned approach to nephrectomy or a repair with less blood loss.

The approach to the left renal artery through the posterior parietal peritoneum is by a vertical incision in the peritoneum over the aorta just below the duodenojejunal flexure, which is retracted medially (Fig. 62–37). The left renal vein will be seen in front of the aorta and should be dissected free, so that it can be elevated with a vein retractor to expose the artery, which usually lies behind and slightly superiorly, as it comes off the lateral side of the aorta. The right renal pedicle is approached by making an incision over the inferior vena cava, so that the vein can be moved either medially or laterally to expose the artery. It is usually advisable to secure the right renal artery on the medial side of the vena cava in this situation, as the right renal vein is usually short and access may be limited on the lateral side.

The second and third parts of the duodenum must be freed laterally by sharp dissection and reflected medially to expose the renal pedicle. Care must be taken to avoid injury to the lumbar veins, as bleeding from torn veins can be difficult to control. If a branch of the inferior vena cava is inadvertently avulsed from the main vessel, or if there is a tear of the vena cava, bleeding is best controlled by digital pressure and application of an Allis clamp to grasp the tear, after which it can be repaired with a 0000 Tevdek or Prolene suture (Fig. 62–38).

Reflection of the colon is effected by dividing the lateral peritoneal reflection along the avascular white line representing the site of fusion between the mesocolon and the posterior parietal peritoneum. Dissection should be carried around the splenic or hepatic flexure to ensure adequate mobilization. The colon and

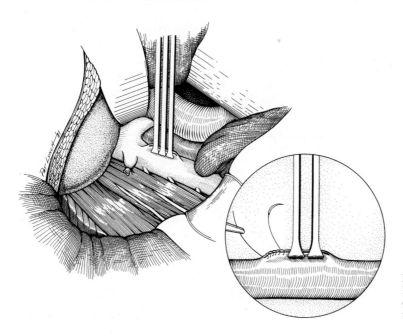

Figure 62–38. Injury of the vena cava. Bleeding is controlled by application of Allis clamps to enable the laceration to be sutured.

mesenteric vessels can now be separated easily from Gerota's fascia in a natural cleavage plane.

The renal pedicle is exposed by a vertical incision in the anterior leaf of Gerota's fascia medially and by separation of the retroperitoneal fat transversely in the line of the vessels. The left renal vein is generally seen first. The gonadal vein, which enters the inferior border of the renal vein, and the suprarenal vein, which enters superiorly and more proximally, should be identified. Lumbar veins join the posterior aspect of the main renal vein in about 30 per cent of patients and should be looked for to avoid injury during dissection and division of the renal vein. The renal vein is retracted to expose the underlying artery, which can be identified by palpation if it is not readily visualized. This may be facilitated by division of the suprarenal and gonadal veins, which increases the mobility of the renal vein.

On the right side, the duodenum is reflected medially by dividing the avascular fascia on the lateral side (Kocher maneuver) to expose the renal pedicle.

The right renal artery may be exposed on the medial side of the inferior vena cava (Fig. 62–36). This approach to the artery is particularly useful when there is a large renal tumor or hematoma present that obscures the hilum. It should be emphasized that whenever possible the renal artery should be ligated prior to ligating the vein to prevent venous congestion, which causes undue bleeding and swelling of the kidney. Usually it is easier just to ligate the artery

prior to division of the vein, as the exposure is limited (Fig. 62–35). After the vein has been divided, the artery can be dissected further to provide an adequate pedicle. The right renal vein is ligated flush with the vena cava, and the left renal vein is ligated as it crosses the aorta. The vessels should be doubly ligated proximally and divided between ligatures, leaving a cuff of at least 2 to 3 mm. When the distance between the ligatures is limited, the vessel should be held up with a right-angled clamp and transected with a small knife. Clamping the vessels is avoided if possible, as there is less chance of accidental tearing, and it avoids having to rely on an assistant to remove the clamps correctly.

When a renal tumor is present, once the renal vessels have been divided, the kidney, with the perinephric fat and Gerota's fascia, is mobilized by blunt dissection. This is done by dividing the loose areolar tissue between the fascia and the posterior abdominal muscles, and the kidney is delivered into the wound. The suprarenal gland is removed with the kidney in a radical procedure for tumor. The suprarenal vein on the right side is divided between ligatures or hemoclips as it enters the inferior vena cava behind the posterior aspect of the right lobe of the liver, which must be retracted upward to expose the vein. On the left side the suprarenal vein is included by division of the renal vein medially, or it may be ligated and divided separately. The ureter is clamped and divided at a convenient site to finally free the kidney, and the distal stump is transfixed and ligated with a 0 chromic catgut suture. Accessory vessels, more frequently encountered at the upper pole, should be looked for. When it is not necessary to remove Gerota's fascia, the kidney is dissected from the perinephric fat and the suprarenal gland is preserved, as it lies in a separate compartment of Gerota's fascia.

The drain may be brought out retroperitoneally through a separate stab incision in the flank, but this is necessary only when infection is present or when there is concern over hemostasis. The colon is replaced and quickly becomes adherent, so that it is not necessary to suture the peritoneum in the paracolic gutter. The omental apron should be freed and pulled down over the small intestines to interpose it between the bowel and the abdominal wound. The peritoneum is closed with a running suture of 00 chromic catgut, and the rectus sheath is approximated with a nonabsorbable suture, either 0 Prolene or 28-gauge wire. These may be placed as two running sutures, beginning at either end of the wound and tying them in the middle, or as interrupted sutures. It is important that the suture incorporate both the anterior and the posterior layers of the rectus sheath, if the incision has deviated from the midline, to ensure a firm closure. Subcutaneous tissues are approximated with interrupted 000 plain catgut sutures and the skin with 0000 nylon sutures or staples.

RADICAL NEPHRECTOMY

This is the procedure of choice for the treatment of renal carcinoma, as there is evidence to suggest that radical surgery improves the prognosis. It is, however, the extent of the local spread of the tumor that exerts the greatest influence on survival (Robson, 1963). Preoperative preparation should include a bone scan, using technetium-99m phosphate, and chest x-rays with tomograms to exclude the presence of any metastatic lesions that would contraindicate a radical procedure.

Renal arteriography is performed for diagnosing the tumor in most cases and should define the vascular anatomy. The study may show evidence of extrarenal spread of the tumor, indicating that complete removal of the neoplasm may not be possible. The arteriographic appearance, however, is not always a reliable indicator of operability. CAT scanning is valuable for determining the extent of the tumor and for detecting involvement of the vena cava. A venacavogram is necessary to define the ex-

tent of the venous involvement. Both these studies will probably be replaced by magnetic resonance imaging, which provides better definition of local spread and venous involvement.

The operation involves an en bloc removal of the kidney and suprarenal gland together with the perirenal fat and Gerota's fascia. An abdominal lymphadenectomy is performed from the diaphragmatic hiatus to the origin of the inferior mesenteric artery. This provides for more accurate staging of the disease, but its therapeutic value remains controversial. The tumor has been found to extend outside the capsule in 25 per cent of patients, and unsuspected lymph node metastases are found in about 15 per cent of patients.

The optimal approach is through a thoracoabdominal incision (as described earlier), which combines some of the advantages of both the flank and the abdominal incisions and provides wide access to the renal pedicle, aorta, and vena cava. The procedure differs somewhat on each side after the incision has been made in the chest wall and abdomen, and each is therefore described separately. It is advisable to develop the upper part of the abdominal incision first to palpate the tumor. Thus one can determine whether it is removable and detect the presence of any metastases that would preclude a radical procedure.

Surgical Approach—Left Side

The descending colon and the splenic flexure are seen in the midportion of the wound. The incision in the subdiaphragmatic peritoneum is continued up and down along the lateral peritoneal reflection, which is seen as a thickened white line, in the paracolic gutter. This enables the colon and splenic flexure, together with the mesentery and vessels, to be reflected medially off Gerota's fascia, as far as the anterior aspect of the aorta. The inferior mesenteric vein is usually easily identified at this stage, as it courses up on the left side of the aorta to join the splenic vein (Fig. 62–39). The origin of the superior mesenteric artery is found just medial to this vein and should be identified, as it has on occasion been ligated mistakenly in place of the left renal artery. The thin anterior layer of Gerota's fascia, which extends over the front of the great vessels to the other side, is now incised to expose the left renal vein as it crosses the front of the aorta. It is mobilized by entering the periadventitial plane by sharp dissection with scissors. The suprarenal and gonadal veins

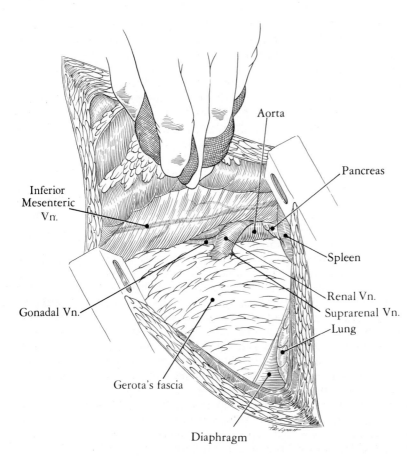

Aorta

Pancreas

Inferior
Mesenteric
Vn.

Spleen

Renal Vn.

Suprarenal Vn.

Gonadal Vn.

Lung

Gerota's fascia

Diaphragm

Figure 62–39. Left thoracoabdominal approach. The left colon has been reflected, and the inferior mesenteric vein can be seen coursing up in the reflected mesentery to join the splenic vein. The spleen and tail of the pancreas are seen in the upper part of the wound.

should both be identified as they enter the renal vein near the lateral border of the aorta, and these are ligated with 000 silk ligatures and divided to allow for greater mobility of the vein and to prevent bleeding from an accidental tear.

The renal artery should now be localized by referring to the arteriogram and by palpation. It usually lies behind the upper border of the vein, which is gently retracted downward to expose the artery at its origin. The artery is freed from the surrounding fascia, lymphatics, and nerve fibers by sharp and blunt dissection. A right-angle Mixter clamp is passed around the artery as close to its origin as possible, and a 0 silk ligature is drawn through and tied. Once this is accomplished, there is a noticeable diminution in size and vascularity of the kidney and tumor, which facilitates further dissection. Any secondary renal arteries should be identified, ligated, and divided at this point.

The renal vein is now ligated over the aorta. Two 0 silk ligatures are placed distally on the caval side and one proximally, making sure that there is an adequate bridge of tissue for division of the vein between the ligatures. This provides for much better access to the artery. It is not

uncommon for a lumbar vein, often of considerable size, to join the posterior aspect of the renal vein near the hilum, and this should be looked for so that it can be individually ligated. Inadvertent injury of such a lumbar vein may cause considerable bleeding that can be difficult to identify and control, as it is often profuse and as the severed vessel may retract behind the psoas muscle or aorta. Other venous anomalies are fairly common on the left side, such as duplication of the renal vein, with one of these vessels draining into a lumbar vein or into the hemiazygos vein.

A second ligature is now placed proximally on the renal artery, and another is placed sufficiently far distally so that an adequate cuff of 2 to 3 mm of artery remains after the vessel is divided. This may often be done more easily by supporting the artery with a right-angled clamp and dividing it with a knife, if the bridge is short. Such a procedure helps avoid inadvertent injury to an underlying vessel or branch or to an oblique division of the vessel, resulting in one of the ligatures slipping off or being cut posteriorly. When the renal artery divides proximally, it is best to ligate each branch separately to prevent the ligatures from slipping closer together and to ensure a good cuff beyond the proximal ligatures. It is preferable to use this method of ligation in continuity prior to division, as it obviates having to rely on the assistant to remove the clamp correctly or incurring any loss of control due to accidental tearing of the vessel by the clamp or breakage of the ligature.

The dissection should be continued up along the lateral side of the aorta, dividing any accessory vessels and the arterial supply to the suprarenal gland, which is derived directly from the aorta and the musculophrenic artery as well as the renal artery. These vessels may be easily controlled by the application of surgical clips.

The hand can now be passed lateral to the renal mass; the posterior layer of Gerota's fascia is separated from the lateral and posterior abdominal wall muscles by blunt and sharp dissection using hemoclips to control small transected blood vessels. It may be necessary to ligate and divide numerous collateral veins between the tumor and the abdominal wall. These are usually thin-walled and friable. Particularly large and distended collateral veins may be secondary to obstruction of the main renal vein by tumor. Superiorly there may be accessory renal veins that must be ligated.

The fascial attachments to the undersurface of the diaphragm and peritoneum over the inferior border of the spleen are often quite strong and require careful, sharp dissection to avoid injury to the spleen. Splenic injury is particularly liable to occur if blunt dissection in this area is pursued too vigorously. Any structures or bands that provide a little extra resistance should always be visualized and divided with scissors between ligatures or clamps.

The lower pole is now mobilized, and the ureter is identified as it emerges from the lower, less well-defined region of Gerota's fascia. It is clamped and divided a little above the pelvic brim, and the distal end is transfixed and ligated with a 0 chromic catgut suture. The gonadal vein may be involved in the mass and may receive collateral vessels from the tumor. It is divided at the site of transection of the ureter and is removed with the specimen.

The dissection can now be continued along the medial border of the kidney by retracting the renal mass laterally to aid in the identification of the numerous fascial attachments and autonomic nerves that need to be divided to remove the kidney. The spleen should be removed if it is adherent to the tumor or if its capsule is inadvertently torn during the dissection. The main splenic vessels are usually easily

identified at the upper border of the pancreas and are ligated just distal to the tail of the pancreas and divided. The left gastroepiploic artery and short gastric vessels running in the gastrosplenic ligament between the fundus of the stomach and the splenic hilum should be ligated and divided individually, as they tear easily and tend to slip out of mass ligatures.

Surgical Approach—Right Side

The right lobe of the liver must be retracted upward, and this is best accomplished with a wide Deaver retractor, using a large moistened sponge to protect the liver from injury. The exposure may be improved by division of the triangular ligament (Fig. 62–40). The hepatic flexure and ascending colon are mobilized by incising the lateral peritoneal reflection to expose the anterior layer of Gerota's fascia and the duodenum, which overlies the renal hilum. The avascular fascial attachment on the lateral side of the duodenum is divided sharply, which enables it to be reflected medially (Kocher maneuver). The underlying fascia is incised to expose the short right renal vein as it enters the vena cava. This is dissected free, and the renal artery is located, usually behind the vein. Retraction of the vein may enable the underlying artery to be dissected out and ligated. Frequently, however, it is easier to expose the artery by dissecting between the aorta and vena cava and retracting the left border of the vena cava just below the origin of the left renal vein. The artery is then readily ligated at its origin (Fig. 62–36). This is a particularly useful maneuver when the renal mass is large and overlies the great vessels. Care must be taken not to mistake the hepatic or pancreaticoduodenal artery for the renal artery.

The renal vein is now ligated and divided to provide better access for division of the artery. The dissection is continued superiorly along the lateral border of the vena cava to find the adrenal vein as it enters the vena cava behind the right lobe of the liver. This usually needs to be retracted upward to expose the vein, which is now ligated or occluded with a hemoclip and divided. Should the tumor be adherent to the vena cava, a portion of its wall may be resected, together with the tumor, after application of a Satinsky clamp. It is advisable to pass tapes around the vena cava above and below the site of resection to provide for better control of the vessel. The defect is repaired with a running 5-0 Prolene suture. The remainder of

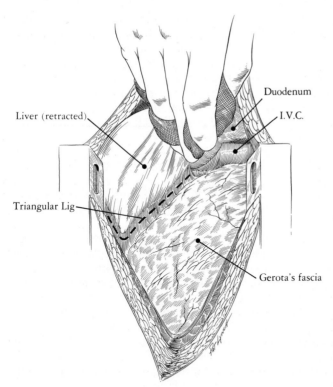

Figure 62–40. Right thoracoabdominal approach. The right lobe of the liver has been retracted to expose the lateral part of the triangular ligament, which may be divided to mobilize the right lobe so that it can be retracted medially. The duodenum has been reflected to expose the inferior vena cava.

the nephrectomy is then carried out as previously described for the left side.

When the operation is performed for transitional cell carcinoma, the incision may be extended down along the rectus sheath to remove the distal ureter and an adjoining cuff of bladder. The author prefers to divide the ureter at the pelvic brim, fulgurate the cut ends, and remove the distal ureter and bladder cuff through a separate transverse suprapubic incision. This is a less extensive incision with less mutilation of the muscles of the abdominal wall, and it provides the best access to the lower ureter and bladder. Alternatively, the distal ureter may be removed endoscopically after inverting it into the bladder with a ureteral catheter that has been tied to it with an intraabdominal ligature.

It is our practice now to perform a regional lymphadenectomy, unless the patient's age or general condition is a contraindication to the procedure. It provides for a more accurate prognosis, and there is some evidence, although controversial, to suggest that it improves survival. The dissection is begun at the crura of the diaphragm just below the origin of the superior mesenteric artery. There is a readily definable periadventitial plane close to the aorta that can be entered so that the dissection can be carried

along the aorta and onto the origin of the major vessels to remove all the periaortic glands and lymphatic channels. Care must be taken to avoid injury to the origins of the celiac axis and superior mesenteric artery superiorly as they arise from the anterior surface of the aorta and pass into the root of the mesentery.

The dissection of the periaortic fat and fascia containing the lymph nodes is now carried downward en bloc, exposing the origins of the right and left renal arteries, and is continued to the origin of the inferior mesenteric artery at about the level of the third lumbar vertebra. The sympathetic ganglia and nerves are removed together with the lymphatic tissue. The cisterna chyli should be identified medial to the right crus behind the origin of the right renal artery. The entering lymph vessels and any other transected lymphatics should be occluded with hemoclips to prevent the possible development of chylous ascites. Careful dissection between the great vessels can accomplish removal of all the lymph nodes without injury to the underlying lumbar vessels. Hemoclips are particularly useful for controlling the small vessels arising from the aorta and the lumbar arteries, which if inadvertently divided may bleed vigorously. This can be a troublesome problem caused by retraction of severed vessels into the paravertebral muscles. Bleeding can usually be controlled by the application of Allis clamps and oversewing with an atraumatic suture.

Involvement of the Vena Cava. Inferior vena cava involvement occurs in about 5 per cent of patients, usually with right-sided tumors; one third have evidence of distant metastases. Ultrasound identifies a solid mass within the cava, and CAT scanning should confirm this finding and demonstrate the presence and extent of any perivascular or local perinephric extension of tumor. Venacavography is then carried out to delineate the extent of involvement. Occasionally, tumor vessels are seen within the vena cava during arteriography. When secondary thrombosis of the vena cava occurs, the patient frequently presents with swelling of the legs and proteinuria. Venacavography by both the femoral and the superior vena caval routes is then needed for adequate visualization.

The tumor embolus can usually be extracted from the vena cava, as it rarely invades the vessel wall. Removal requires adequate exposure to control the vena cava and its major branches above and below the thrombus. The upper end is exposed by dividing the triangular ligaments of the liver posteriorly so that the right lobe can be rotated forward (Fig. 62–40).

The lower hepatic veins are divided between ligatures so that a small Penrose drain can be passed around the upper end of the vena cava and used as a Rummel ligature to occlude it at the appropriate time (Fig. 62–41). The cava is clamped below, and vascular tapes are passed as double throws around the major branches, the smaller ones being occluded with surgical clips. A vertical venotomy is made just medial to the entrance of the right renal vein, and the tumor thrombus is milked out. It may be necessary to separate it from the vessel by blunt dissection with the tip of a clamp or digitally.

When the embolus is more extensive, a 12 F Foley catheter may be passed up the vein next to the thrombus into the right atrium. The balloon is inflated and the catheter then withdrawn slowly to deliver the thrombus. Positive intrathoracic pressure should be applied during this maneuver to assist in expulsion of the thrombus and to minimize aspiration of fragments. The Rummel ligature above is tightened as the catheter is pulled out. The vein is flushed out with heparinized saline and allowed to fill with blood from below to avoid air embolus formation; a large Satinsky clamp is then placed on the side of the vena cava medial to the venotomy. The clamps on the vena cava and its

Figure 62–41. Right thoracoabdominal approach. The right lobe of the liver has been retracted after division of the triangular ligament to expose the upper part of the inferior vena cava. The lower hepatic veins have been divided to improve the access, and a Rummel type tourniquet has been passed around the vena cava just below the diaphragmatic hiatus to provide for occlusion of the vessel above when venotomy is required to remove a tumor thrombus.

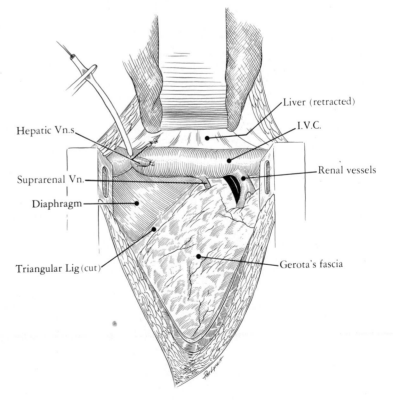

Hepatic Vn.s

Suprarenal Vn.

Diaphragm

Triangular Lig (cut)

Liver (retracted)

I.V.C.

Renal vessels

Gerota's fascia

branches are removed to restore blood flow. The venotomy is now carried posteriorly to divide the right renal vein so that the kidney and tumor thrombus can be removed. When the tumor is large, it may be easier to complete the nephrectomy prior to the cavotomy. The opening in the vena cava is closed with a running 5-0 Prolene suture.

Vena caval involvement may be associated with a very poor prognosis, but the composite results reported by seven groups seem to justify an aggressive surgical attack on this problem. Nine (18 per cent) of 49 patients with vena caval involvement, without demonstrable metastases, lived 5 years or more. Another 15, or 30 per cent, lived 1 to 5 years, for an average of 28 months (Skinner et al., 1972).

Complete resection can be undertaken if there is thrombosis of the vena cava or invasion of the wall by tumor, which fortunately is uncommon. This requires ligation of the left renal vein at its origin for right-sided tumors, with reliance on the collateral circulation through the adrenal, gonadal, and ureteral veins for venous return. The problem is more difficult in the 10 per cent to 20 per cent of patients who have left-sided tumors. The right renal vein may be anastomosed to the side of the portal vein, or a small portion of the vena cava may be preserved and tubularized to provide a venous return for the right kidney. A significant degree of morbidity, composed of proteinuria, renal impairment sometimes requiring temporary dialysis, and lower limb swelling, occurs in about 50 per cent of the patients undergoing vena caval resection. Unfortunately, the prognosis in these patients is poor, and all those reported to date have died of metastatic disease within 1 to 2 years. Vena caval resection is probably a procedure that has been developed before its time, and it will not achieve its true place in the treatment of renal cancer until a satisfactory adjunctive chemotherapeutic agent is available to control the disseminated micrometastases that seem to be already present in these patients.

Extension of the intravascular tumor embolus above the hepatic veins into the right atrium requires a much more extensive exposure, either through a thoracoabdominal incision at the level of the fifth rib or via a midline abdominal incision with median sternotomy and reflection of the liver by division of the coronary ligaments. Clamps are applied to the abdominal aorta and porta hepatis (Pringle maneuver) to control bleeding, and the inferior vena cava is controlled above in its intrapericardial portion. Cardiopulmonary bypass with deep hypother-mia, cardiac arrest, and temporary exsanguination has been instituted in some patients to create a bloodless field. A Foley catheter placed in the vena cava with inflation of the balloon can temporarily control bleeding from the hepatic veins. Again, the long-term results in these patients are disappointing; nevertheless, at the present time, removal of all local tumor tissue, in the absence of distant metastases, offers the best chance of prolonging survival.

PARTIAL NEPHRECTOMY

Indications

1. Hydronephrosis with parenchymal atrophy or atrophic pyelonephritis in a duplicated segment.
2. Calculous disease with obstruction of the lower pole calyx or segmental parenchymal disease with impaired drainage.
3. Tumor in a solitary kidney.
4. Segmental parenchymal scarring secondary to injury or vascular disease causing hypertension.

Preoperative renal angiography should be performed to delineate the blood supply to the segment to be resected.

Surgical Approach

Partial nephrectomy is usually best accomplished through a flank incision, as the procedure is most commonly performed for stone disease or for abnormalities of the collecting system. This allows for good visualization of the renal parenchyma and exposure of the pedicle and renal pelvis. A thoracoabdominal incision is preferred for tumors in a solitary kidney.

The kidney should be completely mobilized from the surrounding fat and fascia except when the resection is being performed for tumor, when Gerota's fascia around the tumor is left intact. The renal artery is dissected out, and a vascular tape is passed around it to facilitate application of an occlusive clamp. An incision is made in the capsule over the convex outer border of the pole of the kidney to be resected, and the capsule is peeled back to approximately the line of resection. The resection should be started near the renal hilum. The major branches of the renal artery are traced into the kidney by blunt dissection of the parenchyma, and, if possible, the segmental arteries to the portion to be resected are ligated. This results in demarcation of the parenchyma, which may be further clarified by injecting 20 ml of methylene blue intravenously to stain the remaining vascularized portion of the kidney. The main renal artery is occluded at this stage after injection of 100 ml of 10 per cent mannitol and will sustain the blue coloration of the kidney. Sometimes the vessels supplying the part to be resected are numerous and are not all identified until the medial portion of the parenchyma has been divided. It should be emphasized that the renal vein is not clamped.

The parenchyma at the site of demarcation is divided bluntly, and the infundibulum of the calyx or calyces to be removed is identified and transected. The defects in the collecting system are closed with a running 00000 chromic catgut suture. The cut ends of the vessels are then oversewn with figure-of-eight 0000 chromic catgut sutures. The arterial clamp may be intermittently released to demonstrate any vessels that have not been secured. It is important to resect most or all the parenchyma draining into the resected portion of the collecting system and to avoid leaving a partially resected calyx, as this can cause a persistent urinary fistula postoperatively. When possible, the line of resection should be wedge-shaped to facilitate closure and hemostasis.

The edges of the resection are approximated by passing interrupted mattress sutures of atraumatic 00 chromic catcut through the renal capsule and parenchyma at the cut edges. These sutures should be placed carefully and tied without tension to avoid laceration of the kidney. They will become tight when the kidney swells after restoration of arterial flow. The redundant capsule is embraced over the raw area to improve hemostasis (Fig. 62–42). A piece of perinephric fat on a pedicle may be included in the "vest-over-pants" closure of the capsule to provide extra tamponade to the cut surface of the kidney.

Williams et al. (1967) have advocated a guillotine type of amputation, in which a 0 chromic catgut ligature is placed around the pole to be resected. The ligature is gradually pulled tight so that it cuts through the soft parenchyma and occludes the vascular supply. The redundant parenchyma is then excised, leaving a 1-cm cuff of tissue distal to the ligature. This method, although expeditious, allows for less precise division and closure of the calyceal system.

When resection is being performed for tumor in a solitary kidney or when resection and repair are to take more than 20 to 30 minutes,

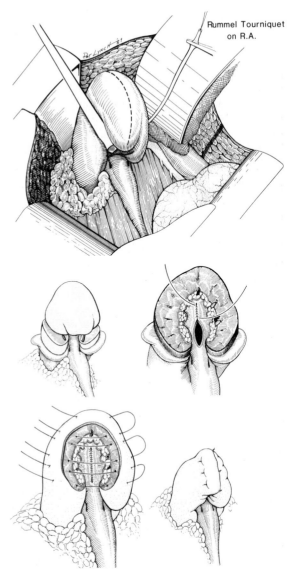

Figure 62–42. Lower pole partial nephrectomy. The renal artery is occluded with a Rummel type tourniquet for hemostasis. The renal capsule is reflected to the line of resection. The dissection is begun in the hilum to secure the large branch vessels and infundibulum of the collecting system to be removed. The collecting system is closed with continuous 00000 chromic catgut. Hemostasis is secured by oversewing the larger vessels with individual sutures and occluding the cut surfaces with mattress sutures. The redundant capsule is then embraced over the suture line.

it is advisable to cool the kidney after occlusion of the main renal artery. The kidney is surrounded by a rubber dam, and iced saline slush is poured over it. Satisfactory cooling can be achieved in 8 to 10 minutes, which will prolong the time of safe ischemia for as much as 60 to 90 minutes, depending on how quickly the kidney warms up.

For resection of tumors, no separate incision is made in the capsule, which is incised 1 cm proximal to the edge of the tumor. The parenchyma is again separated by blunt dissection, which helps keep the line of resection outside the pseudocapsule of the tumor. The resected portion of the kidney should be removed together with the surrounding portion of Gerota's fascia. The collecting system is repaired with 00000 chromic catgut sutures, and bleeding is controlled as previously described. Fixation of the kidney is important after partial nephrectomy, as the kidney sometimes has a tendency to rotate and occlude its blood supply. This is best done by replacing the kidney in Gerota's fascia and securing this to the fascia of the posterior abdominal wall with several 00 chromic sutures. The sutures should include a small amount of renal capsule for better fixation. Care should be taken not to cause partial occlusion of the ureter during this procedure. The perinephric space should always be drained, as there is often a temporary leakage of urine.

SURGERY FOR RENAL CYSTS

Simple Cysts

These usually present as mass lesions in the kidney and are often detected during routine pyelographic examination. They must be differentiated from renal tumors as described in Chapter 29. A small number of patients will still require exploration to distinguish between a cyst and an atypical tumor mass.

An anterior extraperitoneal approach is ideal for lower pole cysts. Upper pole lesions are probably best approached through a flank incision or an anterior retroperitoneal incision. Gerota's fascia is opened, and the mass is inspected. Needle aspiration of an intrarenal lesion may be helpful to localize a cyst and confirm the presence of fluid. When the cyst is superficial, the extrarenal portion of the wall is excised and the renal portion of the lining is inspected and biopsy performed if any suspicious areas are seen. The cut edges of the renal parenchyma are oversewn with a continuous 00 chromic catgut suture for hemostasis. Intrarenal cysts may be partially marsupialized, depending upon their location. Cauterization of the remaining wall is unnecessary. Drainage is not required unless the cyst is infected.

Polycystic Kidney Disease

Both kidneys are removed in patients with end-stage renal failure who are being prepared for renal transplantation. This is best performed through an anterior midline incision that can be easily extended to deliver the lower poles, which may extend deep into the pelvis. Care should be taken not to remove the adrenal glands, which may be stretched out and quite adherent to the upper poles of the kidneys, particularly if there has been previous inflammation in the kidney.

Sometimes unilateral nephrectomy is required before the patient develops end-stage renal failure when the polycystic kidney is a site of complications, such as infection, severe pain due to bleeding or obstruction, or development of a tumor. Sometimes infection of cysts can be controlled with prompt administration of antibiotics supplemented, if necessary, with cyst drainage, thus obviating the need for nephrectomy. Again, the adrenal gland may be inadvertently removed if it has become adherent to the upper pole. Surprisingly, there is sometimes little deterioration in renal function after uninephrectomy in patients with polycystic kidney disease because of the functional adaptive increase in filtration in the remaining kidney following removal of renal mass.

Cyst puncture and unroofing of cysts may be helpful when they obstruct the collecting system. The obstruction may present as flank pain (Lue et al., 1966).

Multiple cyst punctures and deroofing of cysts (Rovsing's operation), does not appear to improve renal function or prevent further deterioration and is not recommended for this purpose (Milam et al., 1963). Peripelvic cysts may require decompression and partial excision if they produce obstruction of the pelvis or upper ureter. They may be exposed at the renal hilum by developing a plane between the collecting system and the renal parenchyma. Portions of the cyst wall can then be excised to marsupialize these cysts.

Calyceal Diverticula

These are cavities in the renal parenchyma that are lined by transitional epithelium and that communicate with a calyx. This communication may not always be patent. Calyceal diverticula may be asymptomatic and may be visualized as an incidental finding on excretory urography.

They may be a source of chronic infection associated with acute episodes, or they may be the site of stone formation. Under these circumstances the diverticula will require surgical treatment.

They should be well localized preoperatively with oblique and lateral films. The kidney is exposed through a flank incision. Localization of the diverticulum may be difficult, and intraoperative ultrasound scanning may be of great help in determining its position and depth from the surface of the kidney. Marsupialization is usually sufficient. The communication with calyx should be oversewn, if visualized. Sometimes, when the diverticulum is large and there is scarring and inflammation of the surrounding parenchyma, a partial nephrectomy may be performed.

Parasitic Cysts

Echinococcal infestation is uncommon but should be suspected whenever a calcified cystic lesion is seen on urography. The Casoni skin test is usually positive, and the patient may have an eosinophilia. Nephrectomy is usually required. Occasionally a partial nephrectomy can be carried out with excision of the cyst. Care must be taken not to spill the contents to avoid implantation of daughter cysts.

CAVERNOTOMY

This procedure, now rarely performed, is used for drainage of a localized chronic suppurative process of the renal parenchyma, usually tuberculosis. A calyx is frequently involved. The kidney should be exposed retroperitoneally through a flank incision. The contents of the abscess cavity are first aspirated, if possible, through a wide-bore needle. The outer wall of the cavity is then removed, and the cut edge is oversewn with a running 00 catgut suture for hemostasis. This process has the potential for producing a urinary fistula. It is important to ensure that the neck of an exposed calyx is completely occluded by the inflammatory process, and, if not, the neck should be circumcised and closed with sutures.

NEPHROSTOMY

This form of high urinary diversion may be performed intraoperatively at the time of a reparative procedure such as a pyeloplasty or as an emergency procedure for drainage of a pyonephrosis, for the relief of bilateral ureteral obstruction due to injury or disease, or for obstruction of a solitary kidney. The primary surgical procedure has largely been supplanted by the percutaneous placement of a nephrostomy tube under radiographic or ultrasound control. This technique is now well developed and is preferable to an open operation, especially in a seriously ill patient. It should generally be used only as a temporary method of urinary diversion, but occasionally it is required as a permanent diversion. Some form of tubeless diversion, such as an ileal conduit, should be substituted whenever possible because of the numerous problems associated with long-term nephrostomy drainage, namely infection, stone formation, bleeding, and accidental dislodgment of the tube.

The establishment of nephrostomy drainage in patients with bilateral ureteral obstruction due to malignant disease is to be discouraged. It has been found that 50 per cent of these patients die within 3 months and 80 per cent die within 6 months after diversion. Moreover, they are susceptible to a high incidence of serious complications, frequently require secondary operations, and spend an average of 65 per cent of their remaining life in the hospital. The exceptions are patients with cancer of the prostate, as their disease does not progress as rapidly and appears to respond favorably to hormonal and radiation therapy, with survival for 1 to 2 years after diversion (Brin et al., 1975). The use of indwelling ureteral catheters is preferable in patients with malignant disease, as it does not involve a surgical procedure. Specially designed double-pigtail catheters to keep them in place are available, and they are introduced over a guide wire passed either through a cystoscope or percutaneously from above through the renal collecting system.

When nephrostomy is performed as an emergency, it is often a difficult and hazardous procedure because the patient is usually in poor condition as a result of sepsis or uremia with fluid and electrolyte imbalance. The flank position is poorly tolerated and the kidney and surrounding tissues are vascular and friable because of venous congestion and edema, but these problems are again best overcome by the use of percutaneous nephrostomy placement, whenever possible. Should the procedure fail or should there be complications such as bleeding or extravasation due to misplacement of the catheter, surgical drainage with insertion of a nephrostomy tube is required. Preoperative peritoneal dialysis should be considered in uremic patients with serious cardiorespiratory problems if a temporary period of ureteral catheter drainage cannot be established.

Surgical Approach

A flank approach is used, either subcostally or with resection of the distal portion of the twelfth rib. The lower pole of the kidney is exposed by incising Gerota's fascia and carefully dissecting off the perinephric fat. The lower pole can then be retracted upward and forward by placing a small sponge around it as a sling. The dilated proximal ureter is dissected out of the edematous retroperitoneal fat on the posterior abdominal wall at the level of the lower pole of the kidney. It is traced upward to the renal pelvis, which is exposed by blunt dissection of the perihilar fat, with care taken to avoid tearing the numerous small distended veins in the fat. Two 0000 chromic catgut stay sutures are placed in the inferior aspect of the renal pelvis, which is incised. A suitably curved instrument, such as a small curved clamp, Randall stone forceps, or nephrostomy hook, is introduced through the pelviotomy into a dependent calyx having the least amount of overlying parenchyma, and the tip is pushed through. It is important to ensure that the nephrostomy is made near the convex border of the kidney and not in the anterior or posterior surface, as this allows for a better lay of the tube and minimizes the risk of injury to the larger intrarenal vessels.

The tip of the catheter is grasped, stretched to flatten out the wings, and carefully guided through the renal parenchyma into the calyx, using the instrument as much for a guide as for traction. Sometimes, when the overlying parenchyma is thick, it may be easier to use the forceps to grasp the tip of another curved clamp and guide the tip of this back out through the pyelotomy. The narrow proximal end of the nephrostomy tube can then be grasped and pulled back through the kidney (Fig. 62–43).

When the parenchyma is thin and the collecting system distended, it may be possible to push the nephrostomy tube, stretched out over an introducer such as a tonsil clamp, directly into the renal collecting system without performing a pyelotomy. A two-wing Malecot catheter, 24 or 26 F, is preferred, as the flaps are soft and accommodate to the renal pelvis. A Foley catheter occupies more space because of

the retention balloon, which is rigid and unyielding, and its lumen is necessarily compromised by the conduit for the balloon. Spontaneous rupture of the balloon may result in loss of the tube and possibly in retention of a small piece of rubber. Occasionally Foley balloons do not deflate, and such a situation in the kidney could cause a serious problem. A straight tube with a rounded end may be used but has the disadvantage of being more easily dislodged, especially before a track is formed. The tube should irrigate freely and drain by gravity, if properly positioned. It is important to ensure that this is the case before the tube is brought out through the abdominal wall, so that the position of the tube can be readjusted with ease. It should be emphasized that in emergency situations the kidney and pelvis may be unduly friable, and that unless the procedure is performed gently and the curves of the instruments are followed in their withdrawal, serious laceration of the lower pole of the kidney may occur.

Once the tube is well positioned, the kidney should be replaced in Gerota's fascia and the tube brought out through the wound or through a separate stab incision at the site where the nephrotomy is closest to the abdominal wall. As soon as the tube is correctly positioned so that its intra-abdominal course is not kinked or under tension, it should be secured with strong silk ligatures passed through the skin and tied around the tube. Securing of the nephrostomy tube to the renal capsule and fixation of the nephrotomy site to the abdominal wall are advocated by some surgeons. However, this has been found to be unnecessary if the tube is properly positioned. It has the disadvantage of causing bleeding on occasion if the friable capsule and parenchyma are lacerated by the sutures.

The pyelotomy is now closed with a running 0000 chromic catgut suture. A Penrose drain should be placed behind the kidney down to the pyelotomy site and brought out posteriorly.

Complications

Hemorrhage. There is nearly always some fresh bleeding following nephrostomy, but this usually subsides fairly quickly once the tube is in position. It may, however, be significant and persistent if one of the interlobar vessels has been injured. This can usually be controlled with a mattress suture of 0 chromic catgut placed through the renal parenchyma transversely around or alongside the tube. Secondary hem-

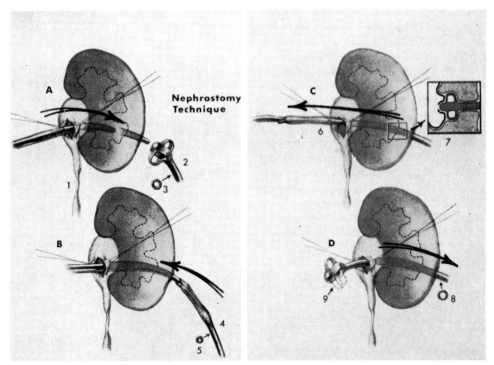

Figure 62–43. *A,* A Malecot catheter is preferred. A curved clamp is passed through the pyelostomy and previously operated calyx, then slowly "worked" through the renal parenchyma. *B,* The clamp is securely clamped to the cloth-reinforced tip of the Malecot catheter. With the clamp firmly held, the Malecot catheter is stretched sufficiently to substantially reduce its diameter. *C,* With an assistant holding the kidney firmly, the Malecot catheter, in its taut state, is brought through the newly formed parenchymal fistula. The head of the catheter is always brought out through the pyelotomy before the traction is released. This assures us that the head of the catheter will not be trapped beneath the calyceal mucosa in a totally obstructed position. *D,* With the tension released, the catheter will immediately return to its normal diameter and exert effective hemostatic pressure throughout the length of the new parenchymal fistula. There is also the added advantage of a "snug fit," which helps keep the catheter in its proper place. One or two wings of a four-wing catheter may be removed to assure better placement and drainage when the nephrostomy tube has been withdrawn to its proper position in the pelvis. Such an alteration will not affect the self-retaining qualities of this type of head. (From Smith, D. R. et al.: *In* Campbell, M. F., and Harrison, J. H.: Urology. Vol. 3, 3rd ed. Philadelphia, W. B. Saunders Co., 1970.)

orrhage may occur following lysis of clots, infection, or erosion of a vessel by the tube and may pose a difficult problem. Replacement of the tube with a larger one, if there is a well-formed track, may help to tamponade the bleeding.

Selective injection of the appropriate renal branch artery with vasopressin under radiographic control should be considered in patients in whom reoperation constitutes a serious risk. If this fails, embolization of the branch vessel with Gelfoam is usually effective. Reoperation with insertion of mattress sutures or occasionally amputation of the bleeding lower pole may be required to control severe hemorrhage. Formation of an intrarenal false aneurysm has been reported and has been successfully managed by ligation and excision of the injured vessel. Angiographic infarction is proving to be as effective in thrombosing the aneurysm in some cases.

Displacement of the Tube. If drainage should suddenly decrease or cease or if the tube cannot be easily irrigated, prompt radiologic evaluation is indicated to check the position. A few hours' delay can make the difference between successfully replacing the tube and being unable to re-establish satisfactory drainage. Radiographic screening by image intensification has greatly facilitated the prompt diagnosis and repositioning of displaced nephrostomy tubes.

If the track has become constricted, an attempt should be made to dilate it gently with serial gum elastic bougies or uterine sounds. Care should be taken not to pass these instruments farther than the depth to which the original tube had been inserted. This can be readily estimated by examination of the old tube, which becomes discolored up to the point at which it exits from the skin. A smaller tube may have to be placed initially, but this can sometimes be replaced with progressively larger ones at intervals of a few days. The constricted track may be distended with lubricant and an 8 F ureteral catheter passed as a guide, over which a larger catheter can be passed to re-establish drainage. It is important to take oblique as well as anteroposterior views to verify the position of the tube in relation to the calyceal system.

Stone Formation. This occurs more often in some patients than in others. Tubes are usually changed every 6 to 8 weeks, but this may have to be done more frequently if rapid encrustation occurs. The use of Silastic catheters will decrease the rate of encrustation. Stone formation is enhanced by the presence of urea-splitting organisms. Acidification of the urine by dietary means, large doses of ascorbic acid or cranberry juice, and frequent irrigation with Suby G solution may be helpful. Stones can generally be irrigated out, but with larger aggregations, continuous irrigations with Suby G solution or hemiacidrin may be required to produce sufficient dissolution to enable them to be removed. Small stones can sometimes be visualized through a nephroscope or panendoscope inserted directly into the sinus and can be removed with forceps under direct vision.

Persistent Fistula. A fistula that remains after removal of the tube usually indicates a persistent obstruction. As a rule, this will not close until the obstruction is relieved.

U-Tube Nephrostomy

Several modifications of this method, first introduced by Tressider (1957), have been described. Essentially, a tube with apertures in the central portion is positioned in the renal pelvis, with its two ends exiting separately through the skin (Fig. 62–44). The tube is changed by railroading another tube behind the one to be removed. The point to which it is to be inserted must be measured beforehand (Fig. 62–45). This type of nephrostomy procedure theoretically provides for better drainage and facilitates irrigation and changing. The tube is often troublesome to maintain in the correct position, however, because of problems in attaching it securely to the skin. Leakage occurs around the tube if one of the drainage holes moves outside the renal collecting system.

Percutaneous Nephrostomy

This form of nephrostomy, utilizing the insertion of a flexible catheter along a guide

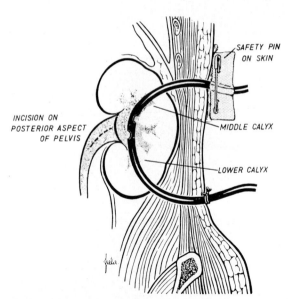

Figure 62–44. U-tube nephrostomy. Kidney is completely mobilized. Curved clamp enters middle calyx through pyelotomy and is pushed through parenchyma. Latex tubing (24 to 30 F.) 18 inches long is drawn through pyelotomy. With finger or clamp in lower calyx, a clamp is advanced through the parenchyma from without inward. End of tube is grasped and drawn through kidney. Two to four holes are made in portion of tube that will drain kidney. Upper end of tube is brought out through stab wound above posterior portion of wound. Lower end is brought out below anterior portion of wound and stitched to the skin. Upper end of tube is tied off, fixed in position, and redundant portion excised. Lower end can later be taped to skin over nephrostomy tube disc. (From Tresidder, G. C.: Br. J. Urol., *29*:130, 1957.)

wire, has largely replaced the surgical placement of a nephrostomy tube over the past few years (see Chapter 51 for details).

SURGERY FOR RENAL ANOMALIES

Horseshoe Kidney

This developmental anomaly occurs in about 1 in 700 individuals and is frequently associated with other genitourinary anomalies, particularly hypospadias. The isthmus that joins the kidneys usually lies anterior to the great vessels, but on rare occasions it may lie behind one or both of them. Ureteral obstruction with hydronephrosis, stone formation, or infection is the most common problem associated with this abnormality. This may require surgical correction of the anomaly as well as treatment for the specific complications. Abdominal pain in the absence of any demonstrable renal symptomatology is rarely due to the presence of polar fusion alone.

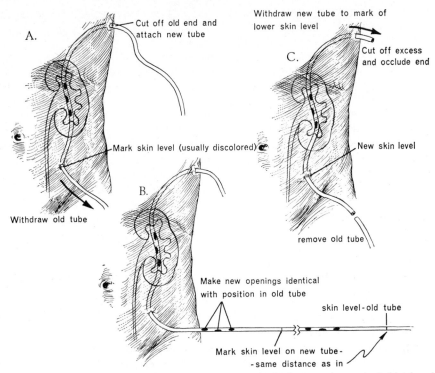

Figure 62–45. Method of changing U-tube. *A,* New 18-inch length of tube is sutured to end of old tube. At skin level at lower end of tube, a tie is placed about the tube. *B,* Most of new tube is pulled out through lower stoma. New drainage holes are placed as shown. *C,* New tube is then pulled back into kidney until marked point of "skin level" becomes flush with skin. (From Weyrauch, H. M., and Rouse, S. N.: J. Urol., 97:225, 1967.)

Prior to surgery relating to a horseshoe kidney, it is mandatory to perform aortography to demonstrate the vascular supply, which is frequently abnormal. The main blood supply may be derived from the aorta below the isthmus, and occasionally one side may be supplied by an artery crossing the isthmus from the contralateral side.

In patients with ureteral or ureteropelvic junction obstruction, division of the isthmus alone is insufficient, and appropriate correction of the obstruction is usually required. Similarly, removal of calculi requires correction of any obstruction in the collecting system, together with division of the isthmus.

SURGICAL APPROACH

An anterior subcostal retroperitoneal approach is preferred. The patient is placed supine on the operating table with a pad under the affected flank and a slight tilt of the table 10 degrees to the opposite side. This provides good access to the kidney and particularly to the isthmus, as it overlies the third lumbar vertebra.

The incision can be extended across the midline if access to the opposite side is needed.

Alternatively, a midline or paramedian transperitoneal incision may be made with reflection of the appropriate segment of colon to expose the kidney. The pelvis and ureter are rotated anteriorly and are therefore best approached from the front for removal of calculi or performance of pyeloplasty. There is usually a groove that demarcates the site of union. The isthmus may be fibrous but often consists of parenchymal tissue.

Division is performed by mobilizing the isthmus from the great vessels, being careful to avoid injury to any anomalous vessels, and placing mattress sutures of 0 chromic catgut through the parenchyma about 1 cm on either side of the line of section in order to control the bleeding. The divided ends can subsequently be further oversewn with sutures passed through the capsule of the cut edges. Two or three sutures through the divided isthmus and into the fascia overlying the muscles of the posterior abdominal wall are used to fix the lower pole, which is rotated outward to allow room for the ureter to lie on the posterior abdominal wall.

Heminephrectomy is performed by ligating and dividing the renal vessels first to demarcate the line of fusion. The isthmus is then divided by placing the mattress sutures through the line of demarcation and dividing it 1 cm distal to the sutures.

The isthmus of a horseshoe kidney may occasionally be an unexpected finding during resection of an abdominal aortic aneurysm. It is again important to define the renal blood supply prior to division of the isthmus and resection of the aneurysm. Intraoperative angiography should be considered if the anatomy is not readily apparent.

Pelvic Kidney

Surgery is usually required for an obstructive problem. There may be unilateral renal ectopia or a fused renal ectopia, the so-called pancake kidney, when this is the only renal tissue present. The best approach is through a transabdominal lower midline incision. The patient is placed in a slight Trendelenburg position, and the abdominal contents are packed into the upper abdomen before incising the peritoneum over the kidney. Identification of the ureter and vessels may be difficult because of malrotation and anatomic abnormalities. In women of childbearing age, an attempt should be made to transpose the kidney above the pelvic brim after reconstructive surgery. The ability to do this will depend on the anatomy of the renal vasculature. Exploring a kidney solely for this purpose is inadvisable, as it is frequently not possible to accomplish transposition because of the vascular anatomy. Pregnancy in women with pelvic kidneys is best concluded by cesarean section.

PEDIATRIC RENAL SURGERY

Surgery in children, particularly infants, should not be considered merely as procedures performed on small adults. There are particular anesthetic problems, and it should be remembered that relatively small amounts of blood loss represent significant proportions of a child's total blood volume. The blood volume of a 2-year-old child who weighs 10 kg is only 900 ml. All surgical procedures should be performed with great gentleness and by sharp dissection, as the tissues are well defined but fragile. Sutures should be fine and meticulously placed, as the margin for error, particularly in anastomoses, is much smaller.

Postoperatively, fluid and electrolyte replacement based on drainage, temperature, and metabolic needs must be carefully controlled. A moisturized tent with controlled delivery of oxygen is desirable in the early postoperative period after major surgical procedures in infants. All sponges should be weighed routinely and blood loss accurately replaced. It is important that the child's temperature be well controlled throughout the surgical procedure. A thermal blanket under the patient and careful monitoring with a rectal thermal probe are used to effect this. Rapid, serious heat loss can occur when the abdomen is opened for prolonged periods of time or when cold irrigants are used during endoscopic procedures.

Surgical Approach

The kidney is generally approached transperitoneally for nephrectomy, which is most often performed after exploration for a renal mass. When this proves to be a tumor, early control of the pedicle is desirable and is facilitated by the transabdominal incision. An anterior subcostal incision is preferred, as it provides good access to the pedicle and affords inspection of the contralateral kidney and the kidney mass. It also can be extended across the midline to improve the exposure, if required. The supine position also allows for the most efficient use of the thermal blanket. A small pad may be placed under the flank to push the kidney forward.

When hydronephrosis is suspected, a flank approach is recommended. A reconstruction of the ureteropelvic junction should be attempted in most cases, as even severely hydronephrotic kidneys in children, which visualize only poorly on excretory urography, are capable of remarkable degrees of recovery. A kidney with marked thinning of the parenchyma that is merely a hydronephrotic sac, however, should not be preserved.

Pyeloplasty, nephrostomy, anterior pyelostomy, high cutaneous ureterostomy, and removal of stones are best performed through a subcostal flank incision. Rib resection is rarely necessary in infants, as the lower ribs are very flexible and can be easily retracted or dislocated upward to improve the exposure. In older children the incision should be made through the appropriate rib bed or intercostal space. Adequate lateral flexion can usually be achieved by a small rolled towel placed under the dependent flank.

CUTANEOUS PYELOSTOMY

This is usually the preferred method of high urinary diversion when the renal pelvis is large and there is an impairment of renal function or some other condition that precludes a primary correction of the obstruction. A small flank incision is made, and the anterior surface of the renal pelvis is exposed by reflection of the overlying colon and posterior parietal peritoneum. The enlarged pelvis usually displaces the renal vessels cephalad. Two 5-0 chromic catgut sutures are inserted over a suitable site in the pelvis that is to be anastomosed to the edges of the anterior part of the incision. Care should be taken to avoid the area of the ureteropelvic junction. A 1.0 to 1.5 cm incision is made in the pelvis in the line of the wound, and the edges are approximated to the overlying skin edges with interrupted 4-0 chromic catgut sutures. Slight eversion of the edges of the pelvic incision is effected by passing the suture into the wall of the pelvis 2 to 3 mm from the edge of the opening and then through the cut edge of the pelvis. The muscle layers and skin are then closed around the stoma on each side, using 000 chromic catgut sutures.

Tubeless drainage of the kidney by pyelostomy or high ureterostomy is preferred to nephrostomy drainage whenever possible. A tube is often not well tolerated by the child, has a tendency to be pulled out, and in some cases may lead to ureteropelvic junction stenosis with complete obstruction.

NEPHROSTOMY

The kidney is exposed through a flank incision. A small pyelotomy is made posteriorly, and the kidney is gently explored with a curved clamp, such as a right-angled Mixter clamp. A dependent calyx with a minimal amount of overlying parenchyma is located, and the tip of the clamp is pushed through. This is grasped by another similar clamp that is pulled back into the renal pelvis. The smaller distal end of the nephrostomy tube can now be grasped and pulled through the lower pole of the kidney. A 16 or 18 F two-wing Malecot type catheter is used and preferably is positioned in one of the calyces. It has been found that a Foley type of balloon catheter usually occupies too much space to be positioned optimally.

The tube should now be brought out through the abdominal wall opposite the exit wound from the kidney, which is usually a little below the incision. It should be positioned so that it lies without kinking and should be secured to the skin with two 00 silk ligatures. Tubes secured on only one side sometimes slip out, particularly in young children.

The pyelotomy is closed with interrupted 00000 chromic catgut sutures, and a small Penrose drain is placed down to the site of the closure and brought out through the posterior part of the wound. The wound is now closed in layers, using 00 chromic catgut sutures. The skin is closed with 0000 monofilament nylon sutures, as these seem to produce less cutaneous irritation in the presence of urine than other suture materials.

References

Adams, A. W.: The moveable kidney syndrome. A successful nephropexy: Historical survey and current assessment. Br. J. Surg., *48*:319, 1960.

Andaloro, V. A., and Lilien, O. M.: Posterior approach to the kidney. Urology, *5*:600, 1975.

Barry, J. M., and Hodges, C. V.: The supracostal approach for live-donor nephrectomy. Arch. Surg., *109*:448, 1974.

Bensimon, H.: Muscle protective incisions in renal surgery. Urology, *4*:476, 1974.

Bensimon, H., Bresett, J. F., Maxted, W. C., Ceplenski, P. J., and Dougherty, W. E.: Misconceptions about posterior approach for renoureteral surgery. Urology, *19*:462, 1982.

Blandy, J. P., and Tresidder, G. C.: Extender pyelolithotomy for renal calculi. Br. J. Urol., *39*:121, 1967.

Bodner, H., and Briskin, H. L.: Subdiaphragmatic renal exposure by resection of the eleventh rib. Urol. Cutan. Rev., *54*:272, 1950.

Bolich, P. R., and Crummy, A. B.: Extravascular use of angiographic techniques to establish drainage. JAMA, *227*:655, 1974.

Boyce, W. H., and Smith, M. G. U.: Anatrophic nephrotomy and plastic calyrrhaphy. Trans. Am. Assoc. Genitourin. Surg., *59*:18, 1967.

Brin, E. N., Schiff, M., Jr., and Weiss, R. M.: Palliative urinary diversion for pelvic malignancy. J. Urol., *113*:619, 1975.

Burnett, L. L., Correa, R. J., Jr., and Bush, W. H., Jr.: A new method for percutaneous nephrostomy. Radiology, *120*:557, 1976.

Chute, R., Baron, J. A., Jr., and Olsson, C. A.: The transverse upper abdominal "chevron" incision in urological surgery. Trans. Am. Assoc. Genitourin. Surg., *59*:15, 1967.

Chute, R., Soutter, T., and Kerr, W.: The value of thoracoabdominal incision in the removal of kidney tumors. N. Engl. J. Med., *241*:951, 1956.

Cinqualbre, J., and Bollack, C.: Renal cell carcinoma extending into the inferior vena cava. Technical problems. Prog. Clin. Biol. Res., *100*:529–531, 1982.

Clarke, B. G., Rudy, H. A., and Leadbetter, W. F.: Thoracoabdominal incision for surgery of renal, adrenal and testicular neoplasms. Surg. Gynecol. Obstet., *106*:363, 1958.

Comarr, A. E.: An improved U-tube catheter. J. Urol., 92:78, 1964.

Culp, O. S.: Heminephrol-ureterectomy: Comparison of one-stage and two-stage operations. J. Urol., 83:369, 1960.

Culp, O. S., and Winterringen, J. R.: Surgical treatment of horseshoe kidney: Comparison of results after various type of operations. J. Urol., 73:747, 1955.

Cumming, K. B., Li, W.-I., Ryan, J. A., et al.: Intraoperative management of renal cell carcinoma with supra-diaphragmatic caval extension. J. Urol., 112:829, 1979.

Dick, V. S.: Technique of nephro-ureterectomy. Surg. Clin. North Am., 40:771, 1960.

Franklin, S. S., Young, J. D., Jr., Maxwell, M. H., et al.: Operative morbidity and mortality in renovascular disease. JAMA, 231:1148, 1975.

Freed, S. Z., and Gleidman, M. L.: The removal of renal carcinoma thrombus extending into the right atrium. J. Urol., 113:163, 1975.

Freiha, F., and Zeineh, S.: Dorsal approach to upper urinary tract. Urology, 11:15, 1983.

Gardiner, R. A., Naunton-Morgan, T. C., Whitefield, H. N., et al.: The modified lumbotomy versus the oblique loin incision for renal surgery. Br. J. Urol., 51:256, 1979.

Gibbons, R. P.: Experience with indwelling Silastic catheters. J. Urol., 115:22, 1976.

Gibson, T. E.: Ureteral splint: Its value in surgery of renal calculi. J. Urol., 42:1169, 1939.

Gil-Vernet, J.: New surgical concepts in removing renal calculi. Urol. Int., 20:255, 1965.

Gittes, R. F.: Locally extensive renal cell carcinoma—current surgical management of invasion of vena cava, liver, or bowel. Prog. Clin. Biol. Res., 100:497, 1982.

Gittes, R. F., and Belldegrun, A.: Posterior lumbotomy: Surgery for upper tract calculi. Urol. Clin. North Am., 10:625, 1983.

Goldstein, A. E.: Secondary renal operations. Am. J. Surg., 80:405, 1950.

Gonzalez-Serva, L., Weinerth, J. S., and Glenn, J. F.: The minimal mortality of renal surgery. Urology, 9:523, 1977.

Goodwin, W. E., Casey, W. C., and Woolf, W.: Percutaneous trocar (needle) nephrostomy in hydronephrosis. JAMA, 157:891, 1955.

Graves, F. T.: The anatomy of the intrarenal arteries and its application to segmental resection of the kidney. Br. J. Surg., 42:132, 1954.

Hanley, L. G.: Recent Advances in Urology. Boston, Little, Brown & Co., 1957, pp. 79–81.

Hess, E.: Resection of the rib in renal operations. J. Urol., 42:943, 1939.

Hinman, F., Jr.: Ballottement of peripelvic cyst for operative diagnosis and localization. J. Urol., 97:7, 1967.

Hinman, R.: Nephrectomy. Surg. Gynecol. Obstet., 45:347, 1927.

Hudson, P. B.: Extrapleural thoracolumbar surgical approach for adrenalectomy and for radical retroperitoneal dissection. Ann. Surg., 139:44, 1954.

Hughes, F. A.: Resection of the twelfth rib in surgical approach to the renal fossa. J. Urol., 61:159, 1949.

Johanson, K. E., Plaine, L., Farcon, E., and Morales, P.: Management of intrarenal peripelvic cysts. Urology, 4:514, 1974.

Johnson, D. E.: Radical nephrectomies. Urol. Rounds, 1:5, 1980.

Kearney, G. P., Waters, W. B., Klein, L. A., Richie, J. P., and Gittes, R. F.: Results of inferior vena cava resection for renal cell carcinoma. J. Urol., 125:769, 1981.

Kerr, W. K., Kyle, V. N., Keresteci, A. G., and Smythe, C. A.: Renal hypothermia. J. Urol., 84:236, 1960.

Khoury, E. N.: Thoraco-abdominal approach in lesions of kidney, adrenal and testis; morbidity studies. J. Urol., 96:631, 1966.

Kimbrough, J. C., and Morse, W. H.: Subcapsular nephrectomy. Surg. Gynecol. Obstet., 96:235, 1953.

Kittredge, W. E., and Fridge, J. C.: Subcapsular nephrectomy. JAMA, 168:758, 1958.

Landes, R. R., McCauley, R. T., and Stoneburner, J. M.: A technique for securing the difficult renal pedicle. J. Urol., 88:9, 1962.

Levitt, S. B., Delph, W. I., Kogan, S. J., Hanna, M. K., and Hardy, M. A.: The posterior approach for bilateral nephrectomies in children with end-stage renal failure. J. Pediatr. Surg., 16:677, 1981.

Lue, Y. B., Anderson, E. E., and Harrison, J. H.: The surgical management of polycystic renal disease. Surg. Gynecol. Obstet., 122:45, 1966.

Lurz, L., and Lurz, H.: Tratato de technica operatoria general y especial. Spain Editorial Labor S. A., 1969, p. 105.

Lyon, R. P.: An anterior extraperitoneal incision for kidney surgery. J. Urol., 79:383, 1958.

Lytton, B.: Current problems in compensatory renal growth. Bull. N.Y. Acad. Med., 50:1147, 1974.

Lytton, B.: Renal surgery. Monogr. Urol., 3:35, 1982.

Malatinsky, J., and Kadlic, T.: Inferior vena caval occlusion in the left lateral position. Br. J. Anaesth., 46:165, 1960.

Marshall, F. F., Reitz, B. A., and Diamond, D. A.: A new technique for management of renal cell carcinoma involving atrium: Hypothermia and cardiac arrest. J. Urol., 131:103, 1984.

Marshall, M., Jr., and Johnson, S. H. III: A simple, direct approach to the renal pedicle. J. Urol., 84:24, 1960.

Marshall, V. F., Whitsell, J., McGovern, J. H., and Miscall, B. G.: The practicality of renal autotransplantation in humans. JAMA, 196:1154, 1966.

Mathes, G. L., and Terry, J. W., Jr.: Non-suture closure of nephrotomy. J. Urol., 89:122, 1963.

McCullough, D. L., and Gittes, R. F.: Vena cava resection for renal cell carcinoma. J. Urol., 112:162, 1974.

McKeil, C. F., Graf, E. C., and Callahan, D. H.: Renal artery aneurysms: A report of 16 cases. J. Urol., 96:593, 1966.

Mee, A. D., and Heap, S. W.: Pre-operative balloon occlusion of the renal artery for radical nephrectomy. J. Urol., 50:153, 1978.

Milam, J. H., Magee, J. H., and Bunts, R. C.: Evaluation of surgical decompression of polycystic kidneys by differential renal clearances. J. Urol., 90:144, 1963.

Mortensen, B.: Transthoracic nephrectomy. J. Urol., 60:855, 1948.

Murphy, J. J., Glantz, W., and Schoenberg, H. W.: The healing of renal wounds. III. A comparison of electrocoagulation and suture ligation for hemostasis in partial nephrectomy. J. Urol., 85:882, 1961.

Nagamatsu, G. R.: Dorsolumbar approach to the kidney and adrenal with osteoplastic flap. J. Urol., 63:569, 1950.

Noller, D. W., Gillenwater, J. Y., Howards, S. S., et al.: Intercostal nerve block with flank incision. J. Urol., 117:759, 1977.

Novier, A. C.: Posterior surgical approach to the kidney and ureter. J. Urol., 124:192, 1980.

Opit, L. J., McKenna, K. P., and Nairn, D. E.: Closed renal injury. Br. J. Surg., 48:240, 1960.

Pansadoro, V.: The posterior lumbotomy. Urol. Clin. North Am., 10:573, 1983.

Presman, D.: An evaluation of the eleventh intercostal space incision for renal surgery. J. Urol., *82*:18, 1959.

Rabinovitch, H. H.: Renal operation in children via a posterior approach. J. Urol., *125*:61, 1981.

Reservitz, G. B.: A historic review of nephro-ureterectomy. Surg. Gynecol. Obstet., *125*:853, 1967.

Roberts, J. B. M.: Conservative renal surgery—an anatomical basis. Br. J. Surg., *48*:1, 1960.

Robson, C. J.: Radical nephrectomy for renal cell carcinoma. J. Urol., *89*:37, 1963.

Robson, C. J., Churchill, B. M., and Anderson, W.: The results of radical nephrectomy for renal cell carcinoma. J. Urol., *101*:297, 1969.

Sames, C. P.: Kidney exposure through the twelfth rib. Lancet, *258*:303, 1950.

Schiff, M., Jr., and Glazier, W. B.: Nephrectomy: Indications and complications in 347 patients. J. Urol., *118*:930, 1977.

Schiff, M., Jr., Bagley, D. H., and Lytton, B.: Treatment of solitary and bilateral renal carcinomas. J. Urol., *121*:581, 1979.

Schiff, M., Jr., Lytton, B., and Card, D. J.: Nephrectomy in impaired renal function. Urology, *3*:404, 1974.

Scott, H. W., Jr., Cantrell, J. R., and Bunce, P. L.: The principle of aortic compression in the management of massive hemorrhage from the renal pedicle after nephrectomy. J. Urol., *69*:579, 1952.

Scott, R. F., Jr.: Transperitoneal approach to renal pedicle. Urology, *4*:223, 1974.

Scott, R. F., Jr., and Selzman, H. M.: Complications of nephrectomy: Review of 450 patients and a description of a modification of the transperitoneal approach. J. Urol., *95*:307, 1966.

Siegelman, S. S., and Caplan, L. H.: Acute segmental renal artery embolism: A distinctive urographic and arteriographic complex. Radiology, *88*:509, 1967.

Silverblatt, S. P.: Postnephrectomy arteriovenous fistula. JAMA, *202*:501, 1967.

Simon, G.: Extirpation einer niere am menschen. Deutsch. Klin., *22*:137, 1870.

Skinner, D. G., Pfister, R. F., and Colvin, R.: Extension of renal cell carcinoma into the vena cava: The rationale for aggressive surgical management. J. Urol., *107*:711, 1972.

Spence, H. M.: Nephro-ureterectomy and heminephroureterectomy in infancy and childhood. J. Urol., *71*:171, 1954.

Tessler, A. N., Yuvienco, F., and Farcon, E.: Paramedian extraperitoneal incision for total nephroureterectomy. Urology, *5*:397, 1975.

Thomas, D.: A case of ruptured aneurysm of the renal artery. Aust. N.Z. J. Surg., *36*:36, 1966.

Thompson, I. A., and Hooks, C. A.: Nephrostomy: A new method. Obstet. Gynecol., *9*:307, 1957.

Tresidder, G. C.: Nephrostomy. Br. J. Urol., *29*:130, 1957.

Turner-Warwick, R. T.: The supracostal approach to the renal area. Br. J. Urol., *37*:671, 1965.

Verhagen, A. D., Hamilton, J. P., and Genel, M.: Renal vein thrombosis in infants. Arch. Dis. Child., *40*:214, 1965.

Waters, E. B., Hershman, M., and Klein, L. A.: Management of infected polycystic kidneys. J. Urol., *122*:383, 1979.

Weyrauch, H. M., and Rous, S. N.: U-tube nephrostomy. J. Urol., *97*:225, 1967.

Williams, D. F., Schapiro, A. E., Arconti, J. S., and Goodwin, W. E.: A new technique of partial nephrectomy. J. Urol., *97*:955, 1967.

Woodruff, L. M.: Eleventh rib, extrapleural approach to the kidney. J. Urol., *73*:183, 1955.

Yoho, A. V., Drach, G., Koletsky, S., and Persky, L.: Experimental evaluation of tissue adhesive in urogenital surgery. J. Urol., *92*:56, 1964.

Zimmerman, S. J., and Radding, R. S.: Hypertension due to trauma of the kidney. N. Engl. J. Med., *26*:238, 1961.

CHAPTER 63

Partial Nephrectomy: In Situ or Extracorporeal

RUBEN F. GITTES, M.D.

INTRODUCTION

This chapter attempts to present in detail the applications and techniques of partial nephrectomy, whether performed in situ or with extracorporeal dissection of the kidney and autotransplantation. Partial nephrectomy in situ has been practiced for many decades, although its popularity has varied considerably between institutions and between generations of urologists. Following work by Seldinger in the Scandinavian countries, the use of renal angiography—especially selective studies—became increasingly widespread. Taking advantage of this technique, other pioneers in the field, such as Semb (1955) in Norway and Puigvert (1966) in Spain, went on to clarify selection factors and potential benefits of segmental nephrectomy.

Making a second important contribution to modern surgical capabilities was the cumulative work of many excellent urologic surgeons in the area of renal transplantation. Although autotransplantation with vascular anastomoses dates back nearly a century to the work of Alexis Carrel (1906), it was the practical application of those techniques in immunosuppressed transplant recipients that emboldened urologic surgeons to combine meticulous partial nephrectomy with autotransplantation and what has been commonly labeled as renal "bench" surgery or extracorporeal surgery. The autotransplantation of the whole kidney to circumvent ureteral or vascular pathology was introduced by bold surgical innovators such as Campos-Freire of Brazil, Hardy (1963) of the United States, and Serrallach-Mira (1965) of Spain. But the use of bench surgery to extend the limits of partial nephrectomy, especially in difficult cases

of tumor of the solitary kidney, was first explored by Gelin et al. (1971) in Sweden and Roy Calne (1971) in England. Others familiar with transplantation techniques followed their lead and brought bench surgery to many centers (Ota et al., 1967; Gil-Vernet et al., 1969, 1975; Kaufman et al., 1969; Dettmar, 1970; Lawson et al., 1972; Martinez-Pineiro and Sicilia, 1972; Orcutt et al., 1974; Gittes and McCullough, 1975).

INDICATIONS FOR PARTIAL NEPHRECTOMY

Renal Calculi

The initial enthusiasm for partial nephrectomy in stone disease after the pioneering efforts of Stewart (1952), Puigvert (1966), and others (Poutasse, 1962; Papathanassiadis and Swinney, 1966) about 20 years ago has generally much dissipated, but strong indications for partial nephrectomy in certain patients with stone disease still exist (Benchekroun et al., 1978; Bates et al., 1981; Coleman and Witherington, 1979; Gonzalez-Castillo et al., 1982; Redman, 1983).

The popularity of the procedure at one time was based on the hypothesis that the lower pole of the kidney tended to trap calculi and that it served as the focus of origin for recurrent calculi and for the development of stones into staghorn calculi. Retrospective statistics were collected to demonstrate the relative predilection for stones to form in the lower calyx. These studies showed a decreased rate of true stone recurrence when a patient was subjected to amputation of the lower pole with its contained stone.

In addition, "lithogenic foci" could be demonstrated histologically in the renal tissue surrounding such a stone. Based on that reasoning, lower pole partial nephrectomy was carried out even when patients had only a solitary kidney (Puigvert and Gittes, 1968). It was clear that in many of these cases a significant amount of functioning renal tissue was being sacrificed, but the benefits were thought to offset this loss. Urologists may also have been attracted to the facility with which an otherwise elusive calyceal stone, especially one that might be associated with infection, could be removed, together with its envelope of tissue. Alternatives such as operative nephroscopy, good-quality intraoperative x-ray, ultrasound procedures, and endourologic manipulation were not available. In any case, the lack of controlled series to prove the value of the procedure, as well as suggestions that partial nephrectomy certainly did not prevent the formation of new stones in metabolic stone-formers, led to a turning away from routine performance of that operation in most centers (see Chapter 64).

In some isolated cases, however, a stone implanted in the lower infundibulum has led to atrophy and a shell-like scarring of the lower pole. When it is undeniable that saving the parenchyma would save very little, if any, renal function, and when it is clear that the stagnant cavity left by removal of only the stone would be a likely place for infectious debris or stone formation to persist, partial nephrectomy may be indicated (Fig. 63–1).

Stone surgery is obviously in a state of flux at this time; it is quite possible that even these "obvious" candidates for partial nephrectomy might be treated with extracorporeal shock waves or endourologic disintegration. If, in the near future, such stones can be turned to powder, the powder passed spontaneously, and the patient then monitored with stone-preventing medication, open surgery will be avoided and an era will have come to an end.

Congenital Anomalies

In this category are the cases of *duplication* with obstructive atrophy behind an ectopic ureterocele or ectopic ureter with incontinence. In such duplicated systems, the division between the diseased kidney and the healthy portion to be preserved is usually quite clear; separation of the tissue is carried out in a nearly avascular plane (see further on).

Calyceal diverticulum complicated by infection or stones, or both, is often an indication for partial nephrectomy, either polar or cuneiform (Mangin et al., 1980).

Occasionally, a grapelike cluster of cysts or a *multilocular cyst* essentially replaces the upper or lower pole of a kidney. We have seen these present with spontaneous rupture and bleeding. Others present as an indeterminate polar mass, raising the question of cystic tumor (see further on). Such cases have been well treated by excisional partial nephrectomy, in both children (Fobi et al., 1979) and adults (Geller et al., 1979).

Less common instances of congenital anomaly as an indication for partial nephrectomy are *horseshoe kidney* or crossed renal ectopia in which there is secondary inflammatory damage or tumor in the fused kidney. Such cases are managed individually according to the vascular supply as delineated by angiography.

Granulomatous Disease

Chronic medical therapy is effective in most granulomatous diseases. Tuberculosis, however, has a tendency to secondary atresia by scar tissue and can, in some cases, lead to an expanding polar kidney. Either "cavernotomy" or limited partial nephrectomy has been used effectively (Puigvert and Gittes, 1968). Hypertension may be cured in the process (Studer and Weidmann, 1981). Xanthogranulomatous pyelonephritis can appear as a polar mass, and if caught early, the preferred treatment is excisional partial nephrectomy (Elder and Marshall, 1980) with precautions at dissection as if it were a tumor (see further on). We have done such a procedure on a solitary kidney with upper pole xanthogranulomatous pyelonephritis.

Renal Hypertension

Unusual cases of severe renovascular hypertension result from segmental renal vascular ischemia of a kidney. In these rare instances, angiography shows the main renal artery to be normal, but a relatively hypovascular, hypotrophic portion of the renal cortex is the source of renin causing the hypertension (Aoi et al., 1981). We have seen such occurrences in all age groups; some cases in childhood may be due to trauma. More commonly, the condition results from the presence of an easily occluded separate polar vessel in early atherosclerosis.

The diagnostic indication for partial ne-

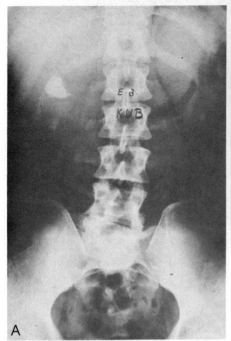

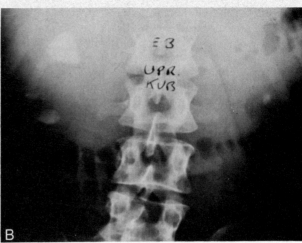

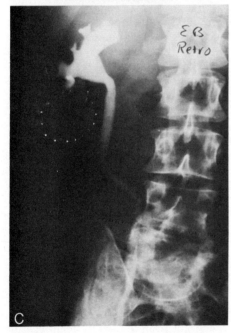

Figure 63–1. Renal calculus with "milk of calcium" in lower pole cavity of right kidney. *A* and *B,* Supine and upright plain films show layering of granular calcified debris in the cavity. *C,* Retrograde study. Lower pole partial nephrectomy is the treatment of choice in the presence of sacculation and loss of cortex, as in this patient. (From Gittes, R. F.: *In* Libertino, E. J., and Zinman, L. A. (Eds.): Reconstructive Urologic Surgery: Pediatric and Adult. Baltimore, The Williams & Wilkins Co., 1977.)

phrectomy is generally a radiologic clue, usually a relative reduction in the thickness of the parenchyma, combined, if possible, with direct documentation of an elevated renin concentration in the segmental vein (Schambelan et al., 1974; Lee and Drach, 1980; Parrott et al., 1984).

In some cases, a combined lesion of the main renal artery and branch arteries may require a partial nephrectomy in conjunction with repair or bypass of the main renal artery lesion.

Such a case is shown in Figure 63–2; here a fibromuscular main renal artery lesion was associated with a branch lesion that included a small aneurysm of an upper pole vessel in a 16-year-old boy. Other cases, which might have extensive involvement of the branches, might once have been treated with nephrectomy. However, with the development of microsurgery with magnification and cooling, these branch lesions can now be successfully repaired. A

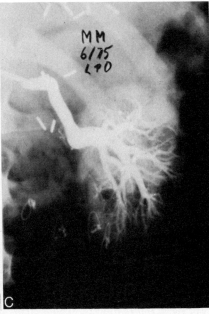

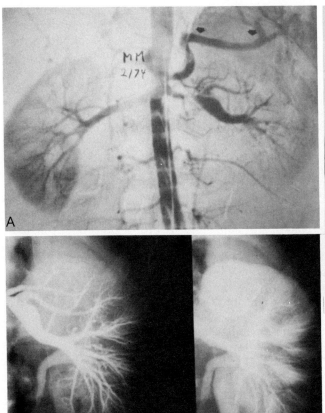

Figure 63–2. Partial nephrectomy with repair of main renal artery. Angiogram of a 16-year-old boy with severe hypertension. *A,* Stenotic segment just proximal to upper pole branch. *B,* Selective view reveals an aneurysm at the takeoff of a second polar branch. A segment of splenic artery was inserted to replace the excised stenotic segment. The upper pole was removed along with its abnormal branch vessels. *C,* Postoperative angiogram reveals the absence of the upper pole. The patient is normotensive. (From Gittes, R. F.: *In* Libertino, E. J., and Zinman, L. A. (Eds.): Reconstructive Urologic Surgery: Pediatric and Adult. Baltimore, The Williams & Wilkins Co., 1977.)

number of branch-lesion cases in solitary kidneys have been described; the use of bench surgery in such cases is appropriate and successful (Belzer et al., 1970, 1975; Lawson and Hodges, 1974; Novick et al., 1980). The vascular surgery involved in these cases and the choice of autotransplantation are discussed by Kaufman in Chapter 67.

Segmental renal vein renins are used in the rare cases of benign *renin-secreting tumors,* which can then be cured by partial nephrectomy. Such tumors are small and may be missed by angiography. But the selective renins are decisive and dictate exploration and curative partial nephrectomy (Valdes et al., 1980).

Trauma

During renal exploration for trauma, whether early or late, partial nephrectomy may be indicated to remove infarcted renal parenchyma and to permit the salvage of renal function, avoiding urinary fistulae and nephrectomy. Prior angiography is useful and usually available. Initial isolation and control of the renal pedicle are important (McAninch and Carroll, 1982; Gibson et al., 1982).

Unilateral Essential Hematuria

Essential hematuria is the term used to describe the unusual cases in which the cause of episodic or continuous gross hematuria cannot be determined by the usual radiologic and hematologic criteria. Such cases usually occur in young or middle-aged adults of either sex. The work-up must include urinary cytology, skin tests and urine cultures for tuberculosis, hemoglobin electrophoresis for sickle cell anemia trait, cystoscopy during bleeding to confirm the site of origin, retrograde pyelograms to rule out ureteral varices or tumors, and selective arteriography.

When all these diagnostic procedures are negative, one can be fairly certain that the gross hematuria is coming from a small mucosal hemangioma, usually in a renal calyx or papilla. By definition these sites are small, are nonmalignant, and have a good prognosis. As concluded in some retrospective studies, a number of them stop spontaneously (Lano et al., 1979; Gittes and Varady, 1981). In this day and age, there is increased pressure on the urologist to bring about an end to the bleeding. Patients may need to pass a physical examination for school athletics, a new job, or life insurance coverage. Some patients are troubled by intermittent clot colic. A few lose enough blood to require iron therapy or even a transfusion.

Some urologists have had limited success in stopping the bleeding through retrograde instillations of a sclerosing solution, such as silver nitrate. Ulceration of the transitional epithelium over the bleeding microhemangioma may conceivably provide a selective portal for the sclerosing solution to denature the exposed bleeding tissue and thus stop the bleeding without significant damage to the rest of the collecting system and kidney. However, plain films taken after silver nitrate retrograde instillations occasionally show deposits of radiopaque silver throughout the collecting system. In addition, the long-term effect on renal function has not been studied.

Another conservative measure with which we have experimented successfully is treatment with epsilon-amino-caproic acid (EACA). If the patient is a young adult (decreasing the possibility of a tumor) and meets the diagnostic criteria described previously, EACA can be used. Its mechanism of action is to initiate a surface clot on the bleeding that will be resistant to urokinase-induced fibrinolysis. Such a clot is thought to stay in place long enough to develop subjacent organization and scarring that will thicken the exposed wall of the hemangioma, allow the epithelium to regenerate, and prevent bleeding. The procedure involves placing the patient on strict bed rest until the urine clears, starting EACA with an oral loading dose of 2 gm, and then following it up with 0.5 gm four times a day. This very small dose is essentially free of complications. The urine continues to be kept clear by strict bed rest for 2 to 3 days. The patient may then resume normal physical activity but continues on the EACA for at least 1 month and preferably 2 months. This routine allows the bleeding area to heal and recover

completely. We have only recently evolved this more protracted therapy, and our experience with it is unpublished. Treatment of upper tract bleeding with EACA when there was no clot formation, especially in patients with sickle cell trait, has been used for years without complication, although usually with only very brief success. More prolonged treatment seems to ensure some lasting cures of unilateral essential hematuria.

Patients who fail to respond to conservative measures and who have a strong psychologic or practical motivation for eliminating the source of their continuous gross hematuria have been subjected to open renal exploration and operative nephroscopy. Proper precautions should be taken to facilitate continued bleeding during the exploration; these precautions include immediate cystoscopy, overhydration and avoidance of hypotension, minimal handling of the renal pedicle or dissection of the kidney from its bed, and minimal trauma to the renal pelvis while opening a small window for the nephroscope to enter. Venous bleeding in such cases usually occurs when there is no added pressure from the irrigation inflow fluid. Consequently, it is best to turn off the irrigation and watch for the appearance of blood from the affected calyx; one guides the nephroscope into that calyx and, with on-off irrigation, can completely visualize the source of the bleeding and ascertain that there is no tumor (Fig. 63–3).

When the source of the bleeding has been visualized, one has the choice of trying to fulgurate the bleeding under direct vision or doing a small partial nephrectomy to remove that calyx. In our earlier experience (Gittes and Elliott, 1973), we invariably carried out partial nephrectomy because we failed in attempts to lead a fulgurating electrode to the bleeding point through the rigid nephroscope. The problem usually stemmed from parallax, requiring withdrawal of the tip of the scope to see the tip of the electrode. The resultant collapse or flexion of the infundibulum prevented accurate fulguration with the electrode tip. By resorting to partial nephrectomy, we ascertained the removal of the source of the bleeding, eliminated the possibility of a malignant tumor left behind, and allowed the histologic determination of the nature of the pathologic process. It should be stressed that the actual bleeding point in relation to the other gross features of the papilla and calyx must be noted carefully so that when the small specimen is removed, immediate dissection can lead the surgeon to the same site of bleeding, which can then be isolated for serial

Figure 63–3. Endoscopic photographs of a papilla in the upper pole calyx of a young woman with essential hematuria. *A,* With the water inflow turned on, there is a subtle dark area at the tip of the papilla (arrow). *B,* With the water inflow shut off, venous blood floods out and obscures the field. The gross specimen excised is shown in Figure 63–4, and the histologic findings are shown in Figure 63–5*B.* (From Gittes, R. F.: Urol. Clin. North Am., *6*:55, 1979.)

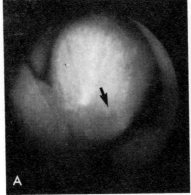
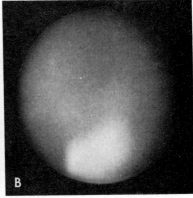

sections (Figs. 63–4 and 63–5). Failure to do so or disorientation regarding the source of the bleeding seen under the nephroscope has often led to fruitless histologic processing of the bleeding specimen. Other centers have reported similar results (Beurton et al., 1980; Chabrel et al., 1982; Michel et al., 1983).

Recently, we were able to cure one such case with direct visual fulguration. Improvement in the instrumentation in terms of its flexibility and its miniaturization may soon make it possible to fulgurate in more cases and perform less open surgery.

Transitional Cell Tumors of the Kidney

There is very little indication for partial nephrectomy in transitional cell tumors of the kidney unless the kidney happens to be solitary or is paired with a diseased kidney. As discussed in Chapter 30, the likelihood of an ipsilateral field defect with abnormal urothelium, and the increased difficulty and risk of a partial procedure and of any necessary subsequent surgery, add up to an indication for nephroureterectomy rather than partial nephrectomy. This is un-

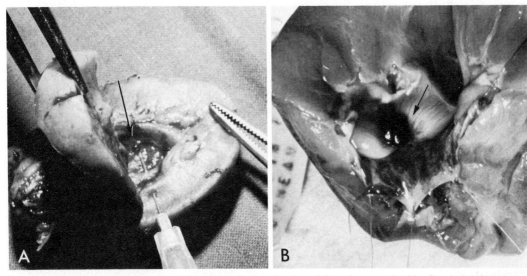

Figure 63–4. Globular blood clots (arrows) are attached to the site of the microvascular bleeding lesion in two patients with essential hematuria. Nephroscopy located the source, and partial nephrectomy cured the long-standing hematuria. The lesion in *A* was in the lower pole of a kidney with megacalyces; its histology is shown in Figure 63–5*C.* The lesion in *B* was that photographed in Figure 63–3; its histology is shown in Figure 63–5*B.* (From Gittes, R. F.: Urol. Clin. North Am., *6*:555, 1977.)

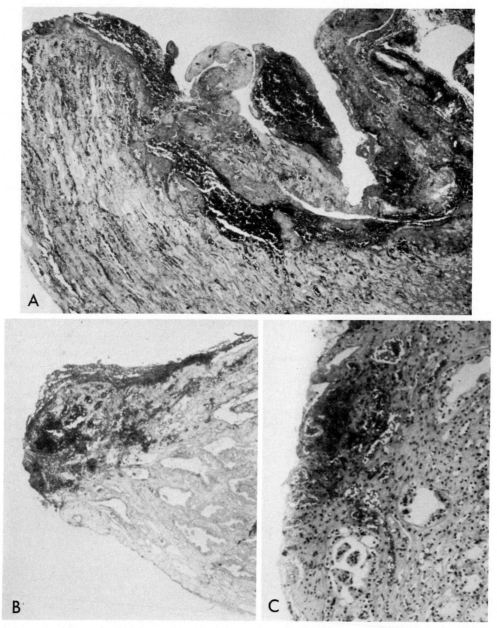

Figure 63–5. *A* to *C*, Microvascular lesions are shown on the surface of the renal papilla in three different patients with essential hematuria. All have large capillary lakes with erosion into the lumen of the calyx (see Figs. 63–3 and 63–4). (From Gittes, R. F.: Urol. Clin. North Am., 6:55, 1979.)

doubtedly true for any tumor with positive exfoliative cytology, which is usually a high-grade, high-stage tumor. Conversely, if the patient has an obvious low-grade tumor in either the ureter or the pelvis, or in a superior or inferior pole calyx that could be easily removed, consideration must be given to conservative surgery as a calculated risk (Gittes, 1980).

In a solitary kidney with a transitional cell carcinoma, partial nephrectomy is indicated in two very different situations. The first situation, in which a lesion has negative cytology and, if possible, a positive histologic biopsy, may call for partial nephrectomy after the involved portion of the collecting system is sealed off and the remainder of the collecting system is thoroughly examined with operative nephroscopy. Special precautions are to be used to avoid tumor seeding during nephroscopy (Gittes, 1979, 1984; Tomera et al., 1982). In the second situation, in which a solitary kidney is found to contain an invasive tumor with proven spread to lymph nodes or distal sites but with salvageable renal tissue, partial nephrectomy may avoid the necessity for hemodialysis. Although a patient with metastases will not be cured, the quality of remaining life may be improved by retention of a functioning portion of the residual kidney.

Indeterminate Polar Mass

When a mass in the upper or lower pole of the kidney is ill defined by currently available imaging techniques (including CT scan and angiography), one may reasonably expect that it may consist of a multilocular cyst, with or without calcification; an avascular papillary adenocarcinoma; an oncocytoma; or an angiomyolipoma. A tentative in situ partial nephrectomy is indicated, thus permitting an excisional biopsy of the affected kidney tissue with its surrounding fat and allowing the pathologist to make a frozen-section diagnosis to determine whether the rest of the kidney is left in place or taken as an additional specimen. Imaging techniques are not *absolute* indicators of the nature of any of the parenchymal tumors that might fit this situation. Thus, angiographic findings of oncocytoma or CT scan and ultrasound findings of angiomyolipoma (Bosniak, 1981) occasionally occur in renal cell carcinoma as well. Because of the overwhelming abundance of renal cell carcinoma compared with the rare benign lesions, even a small incidence of suggestive imaging findings means that a given patient with such findings is very likely to have the malignant tumor instead of the hoped-for benign tumor.

Renal Cell Carcinoma

Renal cell carcinoma in a solitary kidney is clearly an indication for partial nephrectomy, either in situ or, as discussed further on, at bench surgery. In a nonsolitary kidney, a non-controversial mass that fulfills the imaging criteria for renal cell carcinoma, and one large enough or central enough to preclude a very simple excisional biopsy (as discussed earlier), should receive the benefit of optimal surgery in the form of a radical en bloc nephrectomy without violation of Gerota's fascia or the peri-nephric fat. In the few instances we have made exceptions, we have locally excised lesions in patients with some abnormality of the opposite kidney, with mild overall renal failure, or with the suspicion that the lesion was metastatic.

Bilateral renal cell carcinoma, or the belated appearance of another tumor in a residual kidney after nephrectomy for renal cell carcinoma, occasionally occurs. Some controversy exists as to whether these growths are to be considered metastases or coincidental, independently arising tumors. Bilaterality is much more common in families with a tendency to develop renal cell carcinoma (Berg et al., 1981) and in patients with von Hippel–Lindau disease (Pearson et al., 1980) in the absence of distant metastases; this fact suggests that the determining factor is the tumor diathesis, or previous disposition of those kidney cells to be transformed into a tumor. The rarity of bilaterality in other situations or in the presence of demonstrable metastatic disease from one side attests to the fact that the kidney is not a particularly fertile bed for metastases of a renal cell carcinoma. Indeed, many recent reports on bilateral renal adenocarcinoma stress that the prognosis is dependent on the *local* stage of the lesions, negating the dismal prognosis that would pertain if metastases were usually already present (Beraha et al., 1976; Berg et al., 1981; de Voogt, 1983; Garrett and Donohue, 1978; Gislason et al., 1981; Gittes and McCullough, 1975; Jacobs et al., 1980; Marberger et al., 1981; Palmer, 1983; Schiff et al., 1979; Smith et al., 1984; Zincke and Swanson, 1982). The point to be made is that patients with bilateral tumors or subsequent tumors in the residual kidney should be considered as especially susceptible to further tumors after partial nephrectomy; it is also likely that these subsequent tumors will be independent entities, unrelated to cells left behind or to inadequate surgery.

RENAL PROTECTION TECHNIQUES IN PARTIAL NEPHRECTOMY

Reviewed here are various preoperative and intraoperative maneuvers that have been developed to protect renal function from ischemic damage. Of primary importance are not only preventing unnecessary ischemic damage during controlled clamping or division of the renal vessels but also avoiding inadvertent damage to walls of the renal vessels, with secondary thrombosis.

Preoperative Preparation

In addition to the usual preoperative care, a patient about to undergo partial nephrectomy should receive hydration with overnight intravenous fluids; this routine has been demonstrated to improve the immediate function of transplant donor kidneys. We recommend infusion with 5 per cent dextrose and half normal saline at a rate between 100 and 200 ml per hour the night before surgery and up to the induction of anesthesia. After anesthesia is induced, a Foley catheter is routinely placed to avoid overdistending the bladder and to prevent back-pressure in repairing of the collecting system.

Intraoperative Protection Against Ischemia

The blood pressure of the patient should be well maintained, thus continuing optimal perfusion of the renal capillary bed. Hypovolemia or hypotension seem to potentiate the development of renal artery spasm consequent to the dissection of a kidney; this is particularly evident following the isolation of the renal pedicle prior to intentional application of vascular clamps. If the kidney feels relatively soft or looks less than hyperemic, the anesthetist should bring up the pressure, without using any catecholamines. Local anesthetic to the renal pedicle is also considered: It may be sprayed on the pedicle with a blunt needle or a syringe without a needle so as to avoid any puncture injuries.

The anticoagulation agent heparin (usually 50 mg or 5000 units as an intravenous bolus) is routinely administered prior to clamping of the pedicle. Although this precaution is unnecessary in most cases, it should prevent the occasional disaster of intravascular thrombosis following inadvertent intimal injury after the clamps are removed, particularly if there are periods of limited run-off or venous congestion. The usual plan is not to reverse the heparinization from this single dose but to let it carry through the rest of the operation. This may well account for some unnecessary bleeding and may require the use of an additional unit of blood during reconstruction and closure, but we consider that to be an acceptable cost/benefit tradeoff in older patients. We omit the heparin in children and young adults.

A diuretic is used intraoperatively in most cases. We use mannitol, 12.5 gm as a bolus in a 10 per cent solution. Much work was done in the years past to demonstrate the protective effect of mannitol against the acute tubular necrosis of ischemia and of pigment nephritis. Preoperative overhydration with glucose solution may possibly preclude any added benefit from mannitol in this situation. However, this moderate dose adds no significant risk, and its effects of increased renal plasma flow, reduced interstitial edema after clamping, and possible protection against intratubular protein-plugging make it a desirable adjunct. The alternative use of a nephrotoxic diuretic, such as furosemide, is more controversial; we avoid routine use of this type of diuretic.

CLAMPING OF THE RENAL PEDICLE

Clamping of the pedicle or the renal artery alone is not used in every case of partial nephrectomy. The kidney must always be freed up sufficiently to permit immediate access to the pedicle, manual compression of it, and then control by a vascular clamp, if needed. But shutting off the circulation to the entire kidney is neither necessary nor reasonable if the tissue transected is very peripheral, such as the tip of the upper or lower pole.

When the artery must be temporarily clamped, whether in extensive partial nephrectomy, vascular surgery, or stone surgery with kidney-cooling, the surgeon must be very careful not to injure the arterial wall, particularly the intima. The appropriate vascular clamp must not crush the intima or tear it over a pre-existing plaque. Either a long bulldog clamp with "vascular" teeth or a full-length vascular clamp of the Satinsky variety is recommended. The surgeon should test the clamp first by clamping across his own thenar web between thumb and index finger. If the clamp causes pain when closed, it is too tight for the renal artery. Two gentle bulldog clamps in series are better than one single clamp applied too tightly. Either a rubber-cushioned Fogarty occlusion clamp or a silicone rubber vessel loop, or "noodle," double-circled around the vessels and held tightly by a hemoclip, is a safe alternative. The artery must be palpated at the clamping site to avoid the compression of hard plaques that will crack the intima. The renal vein is often clamped with the renal artery both to minimize risk of dissection of the artery and to cushion the jaws of the vascular clamp.

COOLING OF THE IN SITU KIDNEY

Optimal protection from ischemia always requires cooling the kidney. In situ cooling is done selectively, whenever the ischemic period is likely to exceed 15 minutes. Cooling the kidney without clamping the pedicle is worthless—it probably does nothing except cool the surface of the organ and risk dangerous systemic hypothermia. External application of sterile crushed saline ice, or "slush," after clamping the pedicle causes the core temperature of the kidney to drop rapidly to below 10°C. This low temperature permits a safe occlusion period of at least 2 hours without risking renal failure, even in a patient with a healthy contralateral kidney.

For topical cooling, we use frozen Ringer's lactate "slush." Various techniques can be used to make and dispense sterile slush. Wide-mouth pour bottles kept in the freezer overnight and held ready in a salted ice or alcohol-ice tub will yield adequate slush.

Packing the in situ kidney with slush must be achieved without unnecessary loss of melted fluid into the patient. An impermeable material, such as a plastic bag or a thin rubber dam, is used to wall off the melting slush from the bowel, diaphragm, liver, and pericardium. Dangerous arrhythmias can result either from sudden cooling of a venous return or from transmural direct cooling of the heart across the pericardium. We use a Lahey bag, a clear plastic bag normally used to contain the small intestine in prolonged transabdominal surgery. The bag is cut open opposite its usual pursestring opening. The kidney is fitted through the pursestring opening, and the drawstring is carefully tightened around the dissected pedicle without occluding the vessels. The circular wall of the bag drapes over the self-retaining retractor blades on either side of the wound to form a receptable surrounding the kidney. The artery or entire pedicle is clamped (as described earlier), and the slush is poured in around the kidney. A suction tip draws off melted slush from inside the bag as well as any fluid that slips out through the tightened drawstring into the operative field.

TECHNIQUES

Partial Nephrectomy for a Polar Tumor

In polar mass lesions that are so peripheral they fail to involve the collecting system, it is best to simply perform a guillotine-like amputation across the normal parenchyma about 2 cm proximal to the palpable edge of the lesion. These lesions may be of undetermined nature until examined by the pathologist. When the nature of the lesions is unknown, the first objective of the operation is their excisional biopsy, en bloc, with all adjacent perirenal fat plus a rim of normal cortex.

In preparation for the guillotine incision, the whole kidney is freed along the plane outside Gerota's fascia as if for a radical nephrectomy. For a lower pole lesion, the upper pole is separated from the adrenal gland, leaving the adrenal in its fatty bed. For an upper pole lesion, the peripheral margin must not be compromised by an effort to save one adrenal gland. The *adrenal status* of the patient should be considered and determined preoperatively. In practice, one can assume a normal opposite adrenal is present *unless* the patient has had a contralateral nephrectomy for cancer.

The ureter is visualized and bluntly retracted medially away from the lower pole. With the kidney and the perinephric fat freed up, Gerota's fascial envelope is bivalved over the pole *opposite* the lesion; the fat is then dissected off the normal capsule and rolled back, like a banana peel, toward the lesion.

The capsule is divided where it is clearly normal and well exposed and where the underlying normal cortex is at least 1 cm away from the edge of the mass. Completing the superficial incision all around the kidney then allows the capsule to be rolled back another 1 cm or so. It is often convenient to double-check the location of the guillotine incision by bluntly working a finger tip into the renal sinus between the renal pelvis and the hilar edge of the parenchyma. The finger can be insinuated slowly and gives a three-dimensional grasp of the extent of the sinus. If the guillotine incision is close to the sinus, we will certainly proceed to clamp the pedicle (see earlier) and then insinuate the finger into the sinus to protect the vessels from the subsequent transverse incision. If a distinct polar vessel is present, it is ligated separately and injected distally with a dilute solution of indigo carmine or methylene blue dye. This maneuver reduces the amount of bleeding and defines any avascular tissue that may be left behind.

The cortex is transected in a full circle with the knife. Once close to the sinus area, we prefer blunt dissection with the handle of the knife and then scissors to define any vessels or wall of the collecting system that can be safely spared.

During this procedure, an assistant holding the kidney with broad pressure between the thumb and fingers achieves the best hemostasis. After the specimen is removed, the pressure is intermittently released and the slightly concave surface is examined for pulsating small vessels, usually at the corticomedullary junction; these are controlled with shallow figure-of-eight sutures of 4-0 catgut (Fig. 63–6). Open veins require minimal suturing as long as the pedicle is not twisted or obstructed.

If the collecting system has been opened, it is closed separately with 5-0 catgut sutures. The renal pelvis is then injected with dilute solution of blue dye to confirm that it is watertight.

The method used to cover the amputated surface depends upon the extent of tissue removed, the consistency of the kidney, and the availability of a capsule. When the capsule has been rolled back, the previously peeled-back edge of the capsule is rolled forward over the cut edge, providing healthy tissue in an overlapping flap to cover the collecting system. The capsular coverings are held in place with separate horizontal mattress sutures of 2-0 or 3-0 chromic catgut. If there is enough capsular tissue, each horizontal mattress suture punctures the capsular covering eight times before it is tied (Fig. 63–7). The suture catches the corner of the parenchyma only superficially with shallow bites. No significant amount of tissue is sacrificed, and hematoma formation is avoided.

When the capsule is not available and the kidney tissue is broad and stiff, we usually turn

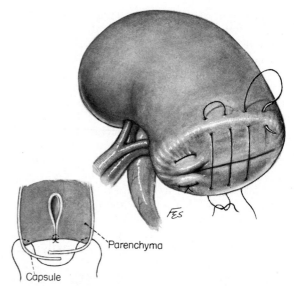

Figure 63–7. Closure of capsular layer over cut edge of renal parenchyma. Horizontal mattress sutures of 3-0 catgut catch the free edges of capsule (inset) after arterial hemostasis has been completed and after the collecting system has been closed. Gentle compression of these sutures and apposition of the capsular tissue against the cut parenchyma complete hemostasis and prevent postoperative fistula formation. (From Gittes, R. F.: *In* Libertino, E. J., and Zinman, L. A. (Eds.): Reconstructive Urologic Surgery: Pediatric and Adult. Baltimore, The Williams & Wilkins Co., 1977.)

to a free patch of peritoneum or of transversalis fascia. This is tacked down across the raw surface with individual mattress sutures around the edge; no attempt is made to squeeze the amputated parenchyma together across its center. If there is persistent venous oozing of the surface before we apply the patch, we apply a thin layer of oxycellulose or other topical absorbable hemostatic material and cover it with the free patch.

If the polar nephrectomy is for malignant tumor, a few lymph nodes along the aorta or vena cava at the level of the renal pedicle are removed for prognostic purposes.

Midportion Partial Nephrectomy

This unusual, more demanding technique removes the full girth of the midportion of the kidney while preserving both upper pole and lower pole collecting systems. The author has performed it only six times: four for hemangioma with essential hematuria (Fig. 63–8), once for transitional cell carcinoma of the middle calyx, and once for renal cell carcinoma in a solitary kidney (with bench surgery).

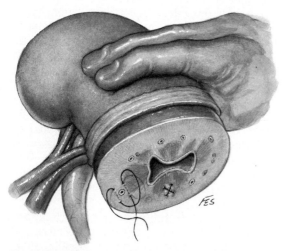

Figure 63–6. Hemostasis of the cut surface is achieved with figure-of-eight shallow sutures. Manual pressure by the assistant controls loss of blood. Intermittent release of pressure identifies pulsatile open vessels for ligation by suture. Note open collecting system and rolled-back cuff of capsular layer. (From Gittes, R. F.: *In* Libertino, E. J., and Zinman, L. A. (Eds.): Reconstructive Urologic Surgery: Pediatric and Adult. Baltimore, The Williams & Wilkins Co., 1977.)

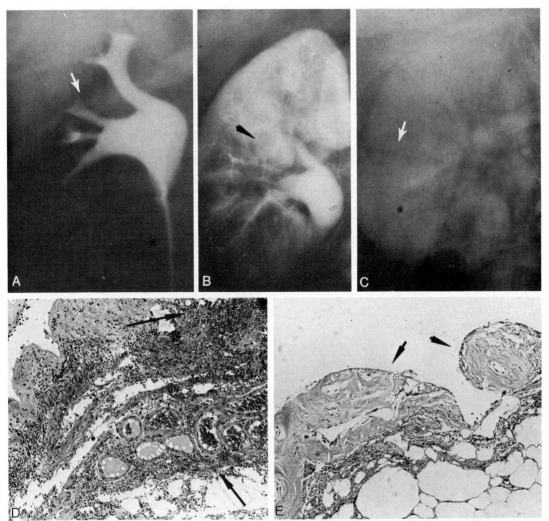

Figure 63–8. *A,* IVP demonstrates location of bleeding calyx. *B,* Nephrogram phase of arteriogram shows adjacent inferior calyx. *C,* Nephrogram phase (15 seconds) of IVP 3 months after midkidney partial nephrectomy (see Fig. 63–9). Seam between two approximated polar masses is seen (arrow). *D,* Cluster of microvascular channels (lower arrow) similar to microhemangiomas, with organized clot breaking into calyceal lumen (upper arrow). *E,* Hyalinized microscopic vessels (arrows) lying on surface of calyx adjacent to cortical rest. (From Gittes, R. F., and Elliott, M. L.: J. Urol., *109*:14, 1973.)

Painstaking selective arteriography is essential; oblique views clarify the anterior/posterior arrangement of all arterial branches and their cortical distribution. The surgical procedure itself was developed in Scandinavia by Semb (1955) shortly after techniques of selective arteriography were perfected (Fig. 63–9). With adenocarcinoma in the midportion of a solitary kidney, venography is often added because of the likelihood of venous invasion from that location.

A bloodless field, achieved either by in situ clamping and cooling (see earlier) or with bench surgery (see further on), is eventually required.

First, however, all the sinus structures are dissected out and identified. This process is best accomplished by opening the renal sinus with palpebral or vein retractors (Gil-Vernet), identifying the arterial branches, dissecting out the hilar fat bluntly with vascular forceps, isolating the surface of the renal pelvis and the neck of each infundibulum, and protecting the main hilar veins from dissection injury. Loose traction loops of silicone or silk are placed around the isolated structures.

To minimize the amount of ischemic tissue to be left behind, one of the two secondary arterial branches presumed to supply the area

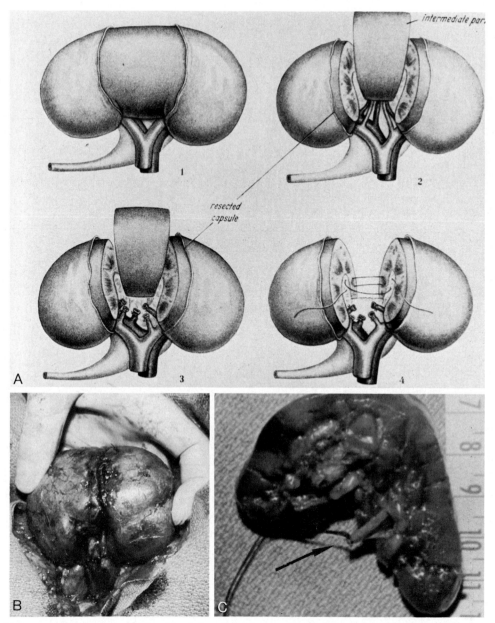

Figure 63–9. *A,* Technique for midkidney partial nephrectomy as described by Semb (1955). *B,* View of completed procedure in case shown in Figure 63–8. *C,* Specimen in same case with ligated calyx (arrow) leading into wedge of cortex containing cortical rest and microvascular pathology seen in Figure 63–8*D.* (From Gittes, R. F., and Elliott, M. L.: J. Urol., *109*:14, 1973.)

to be removed is tied off with fine silk following the dissection. The lumen is then injected distally with a diluted solution of blue dye (indigo carmine or methylene blue). If the blue parenchyma thus demarcated corresponds to that seen on the arteriogram, the vascular tagging is correct and the secondary arterial branches can be divided. This division protects the primary arterial branches by allowing them to be retracted

from the central target tissue. The venous branches similarly are double-tied and divided. The calyceal infundibulum involved is then tied and transected. In cases of benign hemangioma or collecting system tumor, the capsule is peeled back on each side to expose the wedge of demarcated central parenchyma (Fig. 63–10). The pedicle is then clamped and the kidney cooled (see earlier). With a fingertip in the

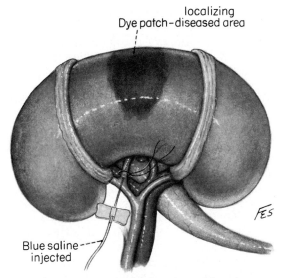

localizing
Dye patch-diseased area

Blue saline
injected

FES

Figure 63–10. Dissection technique in partial nephrectomy of the midsection. Tertiary arterial branches are dissected gently in the renal sinus, aided by palpebral retractors of the Gil-Vernet type. Identification of a small blood vessel, such as one that supplies part of the diseased parenchyma, is achieved by injecting a diluted solution of indigo carmine dye into the lumen with a scalp-vein needle and correlating the region stained with that seen angiographically. (From Gittes, R. F.: *In* Libertino, E. J., and Zinman, L. A. (Eds.): Reconstructive Urologic Surgery: Pediatric and Adult. Baltimore, The Williams & Wilkins Co., 1977.)

dissected sinus for guidance, the surgeon excises a full-thickness wedge of cortex with a scalpel and scissors. The bloodless field permits ligature of any residual arterial or venous twigs tethering the specimen to the hilar vessels. Obvious open arcuate vessels on the cut surfaces at the corticomedullary junctions are suture ligated with shallow figure-of-eight 4-0 catgut sutures. The arterial pedicle clamp is then released, and any further arterial bleeding is controlled.

The collecting system is tested for inadvertent openings by distending it with a blue saline solution. The capsular apron is draped over the cut edges, and the two remaining kidney sections are approximated with horizontal mattress sutures (Fig. 63–11).

Heminephrectomy in Duplicated Collecting Systems

Because the indications for partial nephrectomies are usually hydronephroses and parenchymal atrophy of one of the two segments, the demarcation of the tissue to be removed is usually clear-cut. In addition, there is often a dual blood supply, with separate pedicles to the upper third and lower two thirds of the renal cortex. The atrophic parenchyma lining the dilated system can be nicely outlined by blue pyelotubular backflow if the ureter is ligated and the affected collecting system distended by blue dye under pressure. If the tissue is cut along the blue/pink demarcation, the residual surface will not contain open calyces or major bleeding vessels and added coverage with the capsule is not needed.

The management of the lower collecting system in these cases is fully discussed in Section XIII, Pediatric Urology.

Bench Surgery and Autotransplantation

CASE SELECTION

Bench surgery and autotransplantation have been used for indications that include tumors, vascular lesions, trauma, and even stone disease (Olsson, 1979; Novick et al., 1981). We now stress that it should be considered only in solitary kidneys for (1) large, centrally located cortical tumors or some cases of multicentric tumors (Gittes, 1982); and (2) complex and peripheral vascular lesions (Belzer et al., 1975; Lawson and Hodges, 1974).

Caution against the unnecessary use of bench surgery when in situ cooling and partial nephrectomy can do as well has been widely advised in the past decade (Wickham, 1975; Gibbons et al., 1976; Palmer, 1983; Olsson, 1979; Novick et al., 1977; Smith et al., 1984).

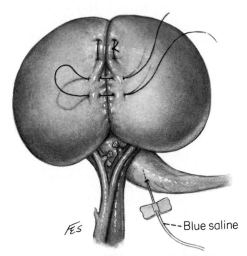

FES

Blue saline

Figure 63–11. Polar remnants are rejoined after releasing the arterial clamp and achieving hemostasis. Closure of the collecting system is tested with blue saline solution. (From Gittes, R. F.: *In* Libertino, E. J., and Zinman, L. A. (Eds.): Reconstructive Urologic Surgery: Pediatric and Adult. Baltimore, The Williams & Wilkins Co., 1977.)

PREOPERATIVE STUDIES

In addition to tumor-staging studies and careful CT scanning of the kidney, selective arteriography should be performed, with oblique views to define anterior and posterior distribution of both normal vessels and tumor mass. In central tumors, renal venography is advised to detect the unexpected invasion of venous channels.

Vascular disease of the internal iliac artery is common in older patients with renal tumors. Pelvic arteriography is useful if included in the flush aortogram. The surgeon can then elect beforehand to implant the renal artery end-to-side into the common iliac artery.

PERFUSION TECHNIQUE

A small, adjustable-height instrument stand (Mayo stand) is the "bench." It attaches to the edge of the incision after the kidney has been dissected completely except for its vessels and ureter (see further on). We use several towel clips to secure the watertight drape of the Mayo stand to the wound's edge (Fig. 63–12).

Sterile tubing for perfusion and multiple bottles of precooled sterile renal preservation solution must be readily at hand. We use a Collins-type high-potassium solution which, in theory, would permit overnight storage of the kidney if the patient had sudden unforeseen surgical anesthetic complications, forcing rapid termination of the procedure (Collins et al., 1969; Sacks et al., 1973). Alternatively, irrigation with cold Ringer's plasma solution can be planned if an oxygenated perfusion pump is available for emergency storage (Fig. 63–13). A recirculating pump should be used only after the tumor is excised from the kidney to avoid seeding the renal remnant with tumor cells (Gittes and McCullough, 1975).

A soft-tipped arterial cannula must be pre-selected to connect the perfusion tubing to the cut artery. We use the type available for the perfusion of cadaver kidneys, but any variant will suffice if the surgeon is familiar with it and knows how to ligate it into the renal artery without damage to the arterial wall. The vein is not cannulated; instead, an intestinal suction catheter is placed under sterile towels covering the waterproof Mayo stand cover to remove irrigation and perfusion fluid.

In the case of surgery for defects of branches of the renal artery, some groups have used pulsatile continuous perfusion, as with the Waters pump (Fig. 63–13). Such cases may require venous cannulation and distal arterial branch cannulation as well (Belzer et al., 1970, 1975).

DISSECTION OF THE KIDNEY AND URETER FOR EXTRACORPOREAL SURGERY

For tumors or complex vascular lesions that are likely to require extracorporeal surgery and

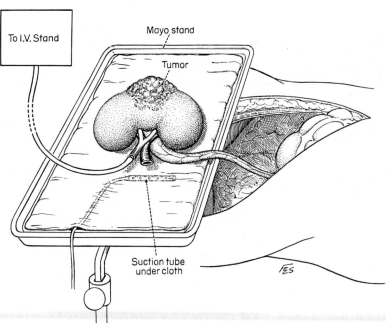

Figure 63–12. Bench technique with the ureter still attached to the bladder. The kidney is cooled by flushing as described in the text. The ureter and pelvis are nourished by retrograde blood flow, permitting full dissection into the renal hilus without risk to the blood supply of the ureter. Autotransplantation to the ipsilateral iliac vessels is accomplished with the flip-over maneuver shown in Figure 63–15. (From Gittes, R. F.: *In* Libertino, E. J., and Zinman, L. A. (Eds.): Reconstructive Urologic Surgery: Pediatric and Adult. Baltimore, The Williams & Wilkins Co., 1977.)

To I.V. Stand

Mayo stand

Tumor

Suction tube under cloth

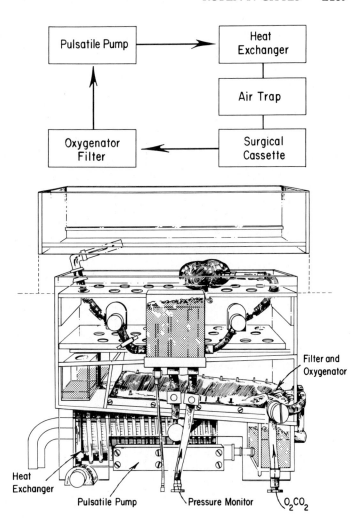

Figure 63–13. Extracorporeal perfusion device (Waters Instruments, Rochester, Minn.) showing position of kidney on a specially designed surgical cassette, allowing free access to the perfused organ during extracorporeal surgery. The upper portion of the illustration describes perfusate flow. From the surgical cassette, venous perfusate effluent is collected into an oxygenator-filter and transmitted to a pulsatile pump. The perfusate is then pumped through a heat exchanger, and the pulsatile flow is transmitted back to the surgical cassette for arterial perfusion of the excised kidney. Excess oxygen bubbles are removed from the system just prior to organ perfusion by means of an air trap. (From Transactions of The American Society for Artificial Internal Organs, with the permission of Columbia-Planograph Company, Washington, D.C.)

autotransplantation, we position the patient in the thoracoabdominal position; that is, the chest and shoulder are rotated up 30 degrees on a roll, the hips are supine, and the table is antiflexed behind the costal margin. The incision is thoraco-midabdominal: The thorax is opened in the ninth or tenth interspace, and the incision is taken diagonally across to the midline of the abdomen. There it is extended as needed downward to permit easier exposure of the ipsilateral pelvic brim vessels, for autotransplantation.

The dissection of the kidney in tumor cases is comparable to that of a radical nephrectomy, *except* (1) that the vessels are not divided but are skeletonized at their origins next to the aorta and vena cava, and (2), that the ureter is not divided. The ureter is carefully freed up, perserving all of its longitudinal blood supply down to a point well below the pelvic brim. The ureter is left attached to the bladder and to the retrovesical vessels, which will nourish it retro-

grade should the extracorporeal dissection in the renal sinus damage the antegrade blood supply derived from the renal artery. This precaution is important to prevent acute ischemic death of the renal pelvis and ureter in midkidney tumors and in vascular repairs in the renal sinus.

When the kidney enclosed in its perinephric fat is left attached to the patient only by the artery, vein, and distal ureter, the "bench" is approximated to the open wound and secured with towel clips, binding the sterile covers of the Mayo stand to the skin of the incision at the level of the iliac crest. The bottle of cold perfusate solution is taken from the ice bath (0 to 4°C) and suspended about 1 meter above the "bench." Sterile IV tubing tipped by the arterial cannula is plugged into the cold bottle, cleared of air bubbles, and secured at the ready on the "bench." The intestinal suction tube, which is under the sterile towels but outside the sterile plastic cover of the Mayo instrument stand, is placed on vacuum suction. The surgeon checks the perfusion setup and then proceeds to lift the kidney, clamp and divide the vein and artery at their caval and aortic origins, and move the kidney out of the patient and onto the "bench," with the ureter still in continuity, gently stretched over the wound's edge.

The renal artery is tied onto the cannula with silk, avoiding unnecessary intimal damage and tying on only the tip of the arterial stump. The tied-on arterial wall will be cut off the cannula later so as to not use the silk-crushed artery for the reanastomosis. The kidney is flushed clear by the gravity drip of the cold solution, and a slower cold drip is continued throughout the extracorporeal dissection and repair. The perfusate simply trickles out of the vein and is drawn off by the suction.

The surgery required, whether tumor or vascular, is now done with optimal exposure, in an unhurried manner, and with the added advantage of risk-free confirmation of the adequacy of the excision and reconstruction (Fig. 63–14). Thus, in cases of tumor the closest margins are checked by frozen section, and more tissue is resected if the margin is positive or doubtful. The vein can be gently back-flushed to check for tears. In vascular cases the anastomoses are checked for leaks of irrigant, and arteriography can be done with dilute contrast. Arteriography in a hypothermic kidney can be dangerous. Iothalamate should be used, *not diatrizoate*, because diatrizoate can crystallize at

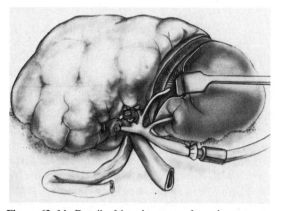

Figure 63–14. Detail of bench surgery for a large tumor, illustrating the sparing of dissected hilar vessels to the renal remnant of the lower pole and the arterial cannula for cold nonpulsatile perfusion. However, the illustrated division of the ureter is of controversial value at best—the renal pelvis and upper ureter may be infarcted by the hilar dissection and the deprivation from retrograde blood flow. (From Montie, J.: *In* Javadpour, N. (Ed.): Principles and Management of Urologic Cancer. 2nd ed. Baltimore, The Williams & Wilkins Co., 1983.)

low temperatures and has led to renal loss (Corman et al., 1973). The collecting system is back-filled with dilute blue saline to check for inadvertent or inadequately repaired openings.

The reconstruction of the kidney on the bench makes use of the various techniques already described under partial nephrectomy in situ.

AUTOTRANSPLANTATION TECHNIQUE

The vascular anastomoses for renal autotransplantation are the same as those in allotransplantation (see Chapter 66) and customarily join the kidney to the iliac vessels at the pelvic brim. When clinical autotransplantation was first done (Hardy, 1963), it was the length of the ureter that was critical, and hence transposing the kidney close to the bladder was important. But it must be remembered that other large vessels will do as well. Thus, Carrel placed kidneys in the neck of dogs (Carrel and Guthrie, 1906). Also, the aorta and the cava are used for renal transplants into babies (see Chapter 66). Therefore, in bench surgery in older patients in whom the iliac vessels are severely atherosclerotic, the surgeon may replace the kidney into the aorta and cava as long as the length of the ureter is not a problem.

In one case of a 74-year-old diabetic man, we noted diseased iliac vessels but a wide and very long renal artery on the arteriogram done for tumor of his solitary kidney. We used the renal artery stump for reanastomosis, without technical difficulty, and the cava for the vein.

In the usual case with ipsilateral iliac vessel anastomoses, we flip over the kidney, end-over-end, to get the vessels to lie posteriorly against the iliac vessels on the pelvic brim. This allows the renal pelvis to be free anteriorly and to aim the proximal ureter *cephalad* into a gentle hairpin curve to avoid kinking of the full-length ureter (Fig. 63–15).

In unusual circumstances a pyelovesical anastomosis can be used to drain the kidney. The feasibility and stability of this drainage technique were first demonstrated in renal allotransplantation cases, in which the ureter and pelvis were rejected or sloughed out and a secondary pyelovesical reconstruction saved the kidney's function. Olsson (1979) has used it intentionally in a few cases of multiple recurrent stone formation to permit free passage of stones (Fig. 63–16). In tumors of the ureter and renal pelvis in a solitary kidney, a technique of total ureterectomy and subtotal resection of the renal pelvis followed by such an autotransplantation and pyelovesicostomy is one alternative to be

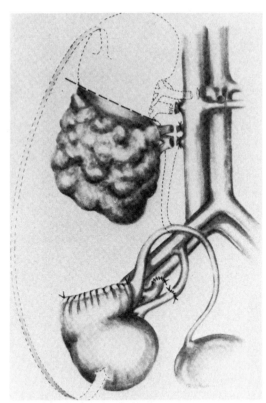

Figure 63–15. Flip-over maneuver for ipsilateral autotransplantation of renal remnant after bench surgery with maintenance of ureteral continuity. The renal vessels are turned posteriorly against the recipient vessels, and the pelvis and ureter course unimpeded anteriorly. (From Gittes, R. F., and McCullough, D. L.: J. Urol., *113*:12, 1975.)

considered; it permits transvesical nephroscopy to be done for follow-up. We have so far preferred to use an ileal ureter in such cases.

Repeated surgery for tumor in the solitary kidney has been required when new tumors appeared in the residual cortex. One of our patients, now alive and well, received two separate bench procedures and one added in situ partial nephrectomy in a span of 7 years (Gittes and Blute, 1982) (Fig. 63–17).

COMPLICATIONS OF PARTIAL NEPHRECTOMY

Impaired Renal Function

Every kidney subjected to partial nephrectomy has some temporary decrease of renal function associated with parenchymal swelling after ischemia, hilar dissection, and hemostatic parenchymal sutures. Solitary kidneys subjected to simple polar nephrectomy, even without clamping of the pedicle, are always associated with mild azotemia that peaks on the second or third postoperative day.

Paired kidneys have more severe impairment of function from the same surgical insult, and early tests of relative function, such as an IVP or a nuclear scan in the first week postoperatively, give unduly pessimistic reports. If all is going well, it is better to wait a month before ordering such tests, and then do them as outpatient procedures.

Acute tubular necrosis (ATN) can occur from extended warm ischemia. In patients with solitary kidneys, dialysis may be required. We have had to use dialysis support for several days to 3 weeks in three patients aften bench surgery for tumor. Their serum creatinine returned to normal levels eventually. As in the case of ATN in renal allografts, *isotope renograms* are very reassuring in such cases, showing good parenchymal uptake, which rules out vascular catastrophe.

Vascular thrombosis of the renal pedicle may occur in the first few hours after surgery. We believe that there are two major causes. After in situ surgery, it represents damage from clamping the pedicle and injuring the intima of the artery. We prevent that both by pretesting the clamps on our own hand (see earlier) and by giving a single dose of heparin IV before clamping, *without* reversal by protamine. After *autotransplantation*, thrombosis can occur from technical error at the arterial suture line, venous obstruction at the venous anastomosis, or injury to a previously diseased internal iliac artery. The last includes crush injury from clamping across an atherosclerotic plaque, or kinking the lumen of a diseased internal iliac artery while rotating it up to the renal artery at the pelvic brim.

Urinary Fistula

Nephrocutaneous urinary fistula is rare after simple polar nephrectomy because the unobstructed residual collecting system heals well. As Stewart (1952) pointed out, however, the surgeon must inspect the cut surface of the kidney to ensure that he is not leaving exposed a papilla with no other drainage than to the perinephric space. When seen, such papillary tissue without a closable calyx and infundibulum must be shaved off sharply, or fistula may result.

Fistula is more common after extensive resection for tumor, especially after excavation of large masses that leave the collecting system

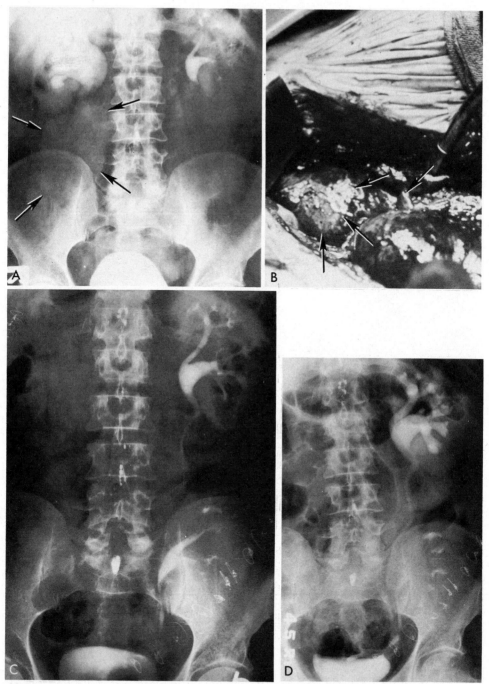

Figure 63–16. *A,* A patient with recurrent ureteral calculi requiring bilateral operative removal developed an upper right ureteral stone that was removed surgically. Preautotransplant intravenous pyelography demonstrates large urinoma cavity (arrows) situated just below the proximal 1 inch of ureter. Five separate operative procedures were carried out to repair this problem, resulting in loss of the entire ureter down to the bladder. *B,* The kidney was excised and autotransplanted to the contralateral groin. The ureteral stump (single arrow) was freed from dense fibrotic tissue but would not extend to the bladder (arrows to left), necessitating a Boari flap interposition between the bladder and the autotransplanted kidney ureter. *C,* Postautotransplant intravenous pyelography demonstrates excellent drainage of the pelvic kidney through the Boari bladder tube. *D,* Intravenous pyelogram performed 1 year later, at which time the patient developed another ureteral stone in the orthotopic kidney. It can be seen that the orthotopic kidney is hydronephrotic. If the previously autotransplanted kidney had simply been excised, one would have been faced with the difficult management of an obstructing ureteral calculus in a patient with a solitary kidney. (Courtesy of Dr. C. A. Olsson.)

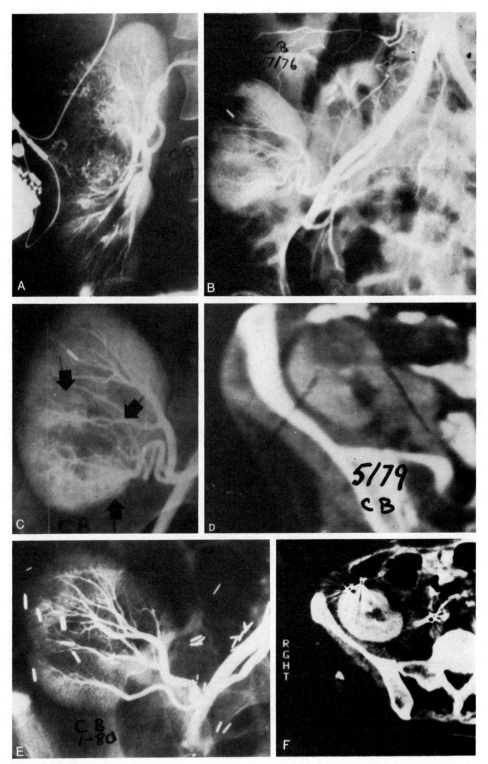

Figure 63–17. Repeat surgery for three sequential tumors. *A,* Angiogram made in 1975 of solitary kidney shows large vascular tumor. Note cardiac pacemaker previously placed subcutaneously in right upper quadrant. Bench surgery and autotransplantation were done. *B,* Angiogram made in July 1976 after first bench surgery demonstrates renal remnant free of vascular tumor. *C* and *D,* Angiogram and CT scan in 1979 demonstrate extent and anterior location of a new tumor in the autotransplanted remnant. *E* and *F,* Angiogram and CT in 1980 after second bench surgery. Patient is free of tumor.

Illustration continued on following page

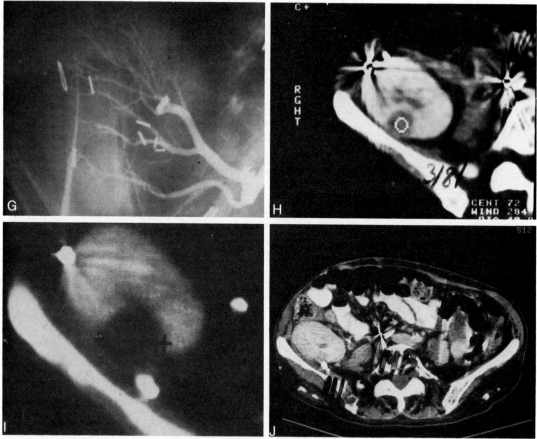

Figure 63–17 *Continued. G* and *H,* Angiogram and CT in March 1981. Angiogram was negative, but a new posterior tumor was clearly seen on CT. The tumor was removed in situ with cooling. *I* and *J,* CT scans July 1981 and November 1983, after removal of the third tumor, demonstrate the shrinking cavity filled with fat on the posterior surface of the kidney. In 1985, 10 years after removal of her first tumor, the patient is tumor-free and well with a serum creatinine of 2 mg/dl and no proteinuria.

in the renal sinus exposed, sutured-closed, and perhaps with impaired local blood supply. A patch of peritoneum and a wad of fat or of oxycellulose gauze are poor protection against fistula in such cases. Treatment is the placement of an internal double J stent and bladder catheter for a few days. Intraoperative placement of an 8.5 F ureteral stent is indicated in some cases, even if back-filling with blue saline shows no immediate leak. Delayed cystoscopic stent placement is used when the fistula persists over 48 hours after a Foley catheter is placed in the bladder. If no new intrarenal obstruction is present, the nephrocutaneous fistula will close eventually. We have seen it take 5 weeks, in the days before internal stents were used. Further surgery may be required in some cases (Pompeo et al., 1979).

Bleeding

Arterial and significant venous bleeding from the cut parenchymal surface is usually controlled at surgery. However, early postoperative bleeding may occur. This usually takes the form of parenchymal bleeding through the cut surface to the perinephric space. Unfortunately, the drains that we leave in place, even ones with gentle suction, do not drain this clotted blood readily, and a hematoma may accumulate that will dissolve slowly and drain out. Severe, life-threatening bleeding should be controlled by re-exploration in the immediate postoperative period. Embolization techniques are not realistic in this distorted anatomy and in a situation in which previous damage to the renal vessels may be compounded by the catheter techniques. In addition, venous bleeding, which may be increased by relative venous compression from the extrarenal hematoma already present, is not controlled unless severe renal parenchymal infarction is carried out by angiography. We think that is counterproductive and against the best interests of the patient who has had his renal tissue carefully saved by accurate surgery.

Hypertension

Transient, mild hypertension is occasionally seen after partial nephrectomy; it reflects the closure of the capsule over the cut surface and the ischemic tension of the parenchyma under that while there is postoperative tissue swelling. In particular, when partial nephrectomy has been done for renal hypertension (see earlier), this temporary complication can be disconcerting. Nuclear scan can give reassurance that there is perfusion of the tissue, and time can be taken to await the passage of the postoperative swelling.

Ureteral Obstruction

Ureteral obstruction is likely after partial nephrectomy in two situations. The first is the presence of some postoperative bleeding into the collecting system that leads to clot obstruction of the ureter and pelvis. This block will often lead to temporary extravasation of urine, but it is best left to clear itself spontaneously rather than risk new instrumentation and infection. We have encountered the second situation after "bench" surgery, when the redundant ureter in the retroperitoneum is kinked or damaged. We anticipate that possibility now, and if there is any damage or questionable area of poor perfusion in the long ureter, we proceed to drain the kidney through the ureter to the bladder with a double J stent placed intraoperatively. This stent is soft enough to accept the curvature of the retroperitoneal redundance and avoids kinking. In one early case, we were forced to re-explore and to carry out a ureteropyeloplasty because of loss of viability and fibrosis of the ureter between the renal pelvis and the middle third. Because of the preserved retrograde vascularization from the bladder, the repair worked very well.

References

Aoi, W., Akahoshi, M., Seto, S., Doi, Y., Suzuki, S., Matsumoto, Y., Kuramochi, M., Hashiba, K., and Tsuda, N.: Correction of hypertension by partial nephrectomy in segmental renal artery stenosis and electron microscopic studies of renin. Jpn. Heart J., *22*:686, 1981.

Bates, R. J., Heaney, J. A., and Kerr, W. S., Jr.: Segmental calculus disease: potential of partial nephrectomy. Urology, *17*:409, 1981.

Belzer, F. O., Keaveny, T. V., Reed, T. E., and Pryor, J. P.: A new method of renal artery reconstruction. Surgery, *68*:619, 1970.

Belzer, F. O., Salvatierra, O., Palubinskas, A., and Stoney, R. J.: Ex vivo renal artery reconstruction. Ann. Surg., *182*:456, 1975.

Benchekroun, A., Meziane, M., Lakrissa, A., Benosman, A., Ghazi, D., Tazi, A., and Mikou, M.: Partial nephrectomy in the treatment of kidney calculi (apropos of 54 cases). Maroc Med., *1*, 41, 1978.

Bennett, A. H., Lempert, N., Rivard, D. J., and Harrison, J. H.: Surgical options in solitary and bilateral renal carcinoma. A report of 7 cases. Br. J. Urol., *54*:480, 1982.

Beraha, D., Block, N. L., and Politano, V. A.: Simultaneous surgical management of bilateral hypernephroma: an alternative therapy. J. Urol., *115*:648, 1976.

Berg, S., Jacobs, S. C., Cohen, A. J., Li, F., Marchetto, D., and Brown, R. S.: The surgical management of hereditary multifocal renal carcinoma. J. Urol., *126*:313, 1981.

Beurton, D., Pascal, B., Moreau, J. F., Michel, J. R., and Cukier, J.: Haematuria as the presentation of a vascular abnormality of the kidney or its excretory system. J. Urol. (Paris), *86*:173, 1980.

Bosniak, M. A.: Angiomyolipoma (hamartoma) of the kidney; a preoperative diagnosis is possible in virtually every case. Urol. Radiol., *3*:135, 1981.

Brannen, G. E., Correa, R. J., Jr., and Gibbons, R. P.: Renal cell carcinoma in solitary kidneys. J. Urol., *129*:130, 1983.

Calne, R. Y.: Tumor in a single kidney: nephrectomy, excision and autotransplantation. Lancet, *2*:761, 1971.

Carrel, A., and Guthrie, C. C: Successful transplantation of both kidneys from a dog into a bitch with removal of both normal kidneys from the latter. Science, *23*:394, 1906.

Chabrel, C. M., Hickey, B. B., and Parkinson, C.: Pericaliceal haemangioma—a cause of papillary necrosis? Case report and review of 7 similar vascular lesions. Br. J. Urol., *54*:334, 1982.

Clunie, G. J. A., Hartley, C. J., Collins, G. M., and Gordon, R. D.: Renovascular hypertension: The place of renal autotransplantation. Br. J. Surg., *60*:562, 1973.

Coleman, C. H., and Witherington, R.: A review of 117 partial nephrectomies. J. Urol., *122*:11, 1979.

Collins, G. M., Bravo-Shugarman, M., and Terasaki, P. I.: Kidney preservation for transportation. Initial perfusion and 30 hours' ice storage. Lancet, *2*:1219, 1969.

Corman, J. L., Girard, R., Fiala, M., et al.: Arteriography during ex vivo renal perfusion. Urology, *2*:222, 1973.

Dettmar, H.: Autotransplantation der Niere als operative Behandlung des renovascularen Hochdrucks bei der Nierenarterienstenose. Urologe, *9*:277, 1970.

deVoogt, H. J.: Bilateral renal adenocarcinoma. Urol. Int., *38*:378, 1983.

Elder, J. S., and Marshall, F. F.: Focal xanthogranulomatous pyelonephritis in adulthood. Johns Hopkins Med. J., *146*:141, 1980.

Fobi, M., Mahour, G. H., and Isaacs, H., Jr.: Multilocular cyst of the kidney. J. Pediatr. Surg., *14*:282, 1979.

Garrett, R. A., and Donohue, J. P.: Bilateral Wilms tumors. J. Urol., *120*:586, 1978.

Gelin, L. E., Claes, G., Gustafsson, A., and Storm, B.: Total bloodlessness for extracorporeal renal organ repair. Rev. Surg., *28*:305, 1971.

Geller, R. A., Pataki, K. I., and Finegold, R. A.: Bilateral multilocular renal cysts with recurrence. J. Urol., *121*:808, 1979.

Gibbons, R. P., Correa, R. J., Cummings, K. B., and Mason, J. T.: Surgical management of renal lesions using *in situ* hypothermia and ischemia. J. Urol., *115*:12, 1976.

Gibson, S., Kuzmarov, I. W., McClure, D. R., and Morehouse, D. D.: Blunt renal trauma: the value of a conservative approach to major injuries in clinically stable patients. Can. J. Surg., *25*:25, 1982.

Gil-Vernet, J. M., Caralps, A., Revert, L., Andreu, J., Carretero, P., and Figuls, J.: Extracorporeal renal surgery. Urology, *5*:444, 1975.

Gil-Vernet, J. M., Caralps, A., Revert, L., Vidal, M. T., and Carretero, P.: Auto-transplantation du rein pour hypertension arterielle de cause vasculaire. J. Urol. Nephrol. (Suppl.), *75*:469, 1969.

Gislason, T., Purcell, M. H., Hawatmeh, I. S., and Gregory, J. G.: Aggressive management of bilateral renal cell carcinoma. J. Urol., *126*:686, 1981.

Gittes, R. F.: Partial nephrectomy and bench surgery: Techniques and applications. *In* Libertino, E. J., and Zinman, L. A. (Eds.): Reconstructive Urologic Surgery: Pediatric and Adult. Baltimore, The Williams & Wilkins Co., 1977.

Gittes, R. F.: Nephroscopy. Urol. Clin. North Am., *6*:555, 1979.

Gittes, R. F.: Management of transitional cell carcinoma of the upper tract: Case for conservative local excision. Urol. Clin. North Am., *7*:559, 1980.

Gittes, R. F.: Bench surgery. *In* Kuss, R., Murphy, G. P., Khoury, S., and Karr, J. P. (Eds.): Renal Tumors. First International Symposium on Kidney Tumors—PCBR. New York, Alan R. Liss, 1982.

Gittes, R. F.: Retrograde brushing and nephroscopy in the diagnosis of upper-tract urothelial cancer. Urol. Clin. North Am., *11*:617, 1984.

Gittes, R. F., and Blute, R. D., Jr.: Repeat bench surgery on a solitary kidney. J. Urol., *127*:530, 1982.

Gittes, R. F., and Elliott, M. L.: Renal cortical rest and chronic hematuria: a syndrome treated by mid-kidney partial nephrectomy. J. Urol., *109*:14, 1973.

Gittes, R. F., and McCullough, D. L.: Bench surgery for tumor in a solitary kidney. J. Urol., *113*:12, 1975.

Gittes, R. F., and Varady, S.: Nephroscopy in chronic unilateral hematuria. J. Urol., *126*:297, 1981.

Gonzales-Castillo, P., Diaz-Gonzalez, R., Paniagua-Andres, P., Usera-Sarraga, L., Mayor-Sanchez, J., Amo-Garcia, J. A., and Borobia-Lopez, V.: Partial nephrectomy for renal lithiasis: lithogenic foci. Acta Urol. Esp., *6*:323, 1982.

Graham, S. D., and Glenn, J. F.: Enucleative surgery for renal malignancy. J. Urol., *122*:546, 1979.

Hardy, J. D.: High ureteral injuries—management by autotransplantation of the kidney. JAMA, *184*:97, 1963.

Harris, A. P., Chamberlain, N. O., and Porch, P. P.: Conservative surgical management of benign hematuria. J. Urol., *86*:504, 1961.

Jacobs, S. C., Berg, S. I., and Lawson, R. K.: Synchronous bilateral renal cell carcinoma: Total surgical excision. Cancer, *46*:2341, 1980.

Kaufman, J. J., Alferez, C., and Navarrete, R. V.: Autotransplantation of a solitary functioning kidney for renovascular hypertension. J. Urol., *102*:146, 1969.

Lano, M. D., Wagoner, R. D., and Leary, F. J.: Unilateral essential hematuria. Mayo Clin. Proc., *54*:88, 1979.

Lawson, R. K., and Hodges, C. V.: Extracorporeal renal artery repair and autotransplantation. Urology, *4*:532, 1974.

Lawson, R. K., Hodges, C. V., and Pitre, T. M.: Nephrectomy, microvascular repair, and autotransplantation. Surg. Forum, *23*:539, 1972.

Leach, G. E., and Kieber, M. M.: Partial nephrectomy: Mayo Clinic experience 1957–1977. Urology, *15*:219, 1980.

Lee, S. M., and Drach, G. W.: Renovascular hypertension from segmental renal artery stenosis: importance of segmental renal vein renin sampling. J. Urol., *124*:704, 1980.

Mangin, P., Mitre, A., Pascal, B., and Cukier, J.: Calyceal diverticula: review of 80 diverticula in 70 patients. J. Urol. (Paris), *86*:653, 1980.

Marberger, M., Pugh, R. C. B., Auvert, J., Bertermann, H., Costantini, A., Gammelgaard, P. A., Petterson, S., and Wickham, J. E. A.: Conservative surgery of renal carcinoma: the EIRSS experience. Br. J. Urol., *53*:528, 1981.

Marshall, F. F., and Walsh, P. C.: *In situ* management of renal tumors: renal cell carcinoma and transitional cell carcinoma. J. Urol., *131*:1045, 1984.

Martinez-Pineiro, J. A., and Sicilia, L. S.: Kidney autotransplantation for the treatment of renal artery stenosis: report of two cases. J. Urol., *108*:35, 1972.

McAninch, J. W., and Carroll, P. R.: Renal trauma: kidney preservation through improved vascular control—a refined approach. J. Trauma, *22*:285, 1982.

Michel, F., Gattegno, B., Valade, S., and Thibault, P.: Renal haemangioma: emergency partial nephrectomy. Br. J. Urol., *55*:336, 1983.

Mitchell, A., Fellows, G. J., and Smith, J. C.: Partial nephrectomy for renal haemangioma. J. R. Soc. Med., *75*:766, 1982.

Mitty, H. A., Dan, S. J., Goldman, H. J., and Glickman, S. I.: Urinary fistulas after partial nephrectomy: treatment by segmental renal embolization. Am. J. Roentgenol., *141*:101, 1983.

Novick, A. C., Stewart, B. H., and Straffon, R. A.: Extracorporeal renal surgery and autotransplantation: indications, techniques and results. J. Urol., *123*:806, 1980.

Novick, A. C., Stewart, B. H., Straffon, R. A., and Banowsky, L. H.: Partial nephrectomy in the treatment of renal adenocarcinoma. J. Urol., *118*:932, 1977.

Novick, A. C., Straffon, R. A., and Stewart, B. H.: Experience with extracorporeal renal operations and autotransplantation in the management of complicated urologic disorders. Surg. Gynecol. Obstet., *153*:10, 1981.

Olsson, C. A.: Extracorporeal renal surgery. *In* Harrison, J. H., Gittes, R. F., Perlmutter, A. D., Stamey, T. A., and Walsh, P. C. (Eds.): Campbell's Urology. Philadelphia, W. B. Saunders Co., 1979.

Orcutt, T. W., Foster, J. H., Richie, R. E., Wilson, J. P., and Warner, H. E.: Bilateral *ex vivo* renal artery reconstruction with autotransplantation. JAMA, *228*:493, 1974.

Ota, K., Mori, S., Awane, Y., and Ueno, A.: *Ex situ* repair of renal artery for renovascular hypertension. Arch. Surg., *94*:370, 1967.

Palmer, J. M.: Role of partial nephrectomy in solitary or bilateral renal tumors. JAMA, *249*:2357, 1983.

Papathanassiadis, S., and Swinney, J.: Results of partial nephrectomy compared with pyelolithotomy and nephrolithotomy. Br. J. Urol., *38*:403, 1966.

Parrott, T. S., Woodard, J. R., Trulock, T. S., and Glenn, J. F.: Segmental renal vein renins and partial nephrectomy for hypertension in children. J. Urol., *131*:736, 1984.

Pearson, C., Weiss, J., and Tanagho, E. A.: Plea for conservation of kidney in renal adenocarcinoma associated with von Hippel–Lindau disease. J. Urol., *123*:910, 1980.

Pompeo, A. C., Wroclawsky, E. R., Lucon, A. M., Freire, G. C., Borrelli, M., and de Goes, G. M.: Partial nephrectomy in urinary fistula following a kidney transplant. Rev. Hosp. Clin. Fac. Med. Sao Paulo, *34*:232, 1979.

Poutasse, E. F.: Partial nephrectomy: new techniques, approach, operative indications and review of 51 cases. J. Urol., *88*:153, 1962.

Puigvert, A.: Partial nephrectomy for renal lithiasis. Experience with 208 cases. Int. Surg., *461*:555, 1966.

Puigvert, A., and Gittes, R. F.: Partial nephrectomy in the solitary kidney. I. Results in 10 cases of renal lithiasis. J. Urol., *100*:243, 1968.

Redman, J. F.:Partial nephrectomy. Urol. Clin. North Am., *10*:677, 1983.

Sacks, S. A., Petritsch, P. H., and Kaufman, J. J.: Canine kidney preservation using a new perfusate. Lancet, *1*:1024, 1973.

Schambelan, M., Glickman, M., Stockigt, J. R., et al.: Selective renal-vein renin sampling in hypertensive pa-

tients with segmental renal lesions. N. Engl. J. Med., *290*:1153, 1974.

Schiff, M., Jr., Bagley, D. H., and Lytton, B.: Treatment of solitary and bilateral renal carcinomas. J. Urol., *121*:581, 1979.

Semb, C.: Partial resection of the kidney; operative technique. Acta Chir. Scand., *109*:360, 1955.

Serrallach-Mila, N., Paravisini, J., Mayol-Valls, P., Alberti, J., Casellas, A., and Nolla-Panades, J.: Renal autotransplantation. Lancet, *2*:1130, 1965.

Smith, R. B., DeKernion, J. B., Ehrlich, R. M., Skinner, D. G., and Kaufman, J. J.: Bilateral renal cell carcinoma and renal cell carcinoma in the solitary kidney. J. Urol., *132*:450, 1984.

Stewart, H. H.: Partial nephrectomy in the treatment of renal calculi: Hunterian lecture. Ann. R. Coll. Surg., *11*:32, 1952.

Studer, U., and Weidmann, P.: Cause and therapeutic consequence of arterial hypertension and kidney tuberculosis. Helv. Chir. Acta, *48*:411, 1981.

Tomera, K. M., Leary, F. J., and Zincke, H.: Pyeloscopy in urothelial tumors. J. Urol., *127*:1008, 1982.

Topley, M., Novick, A. C., and Montie, J. E.: Long-term results following partial nephrectomy for localized renal adenocarcinoma. J. Urol., *131*:1050, 1984.

Valdes, G., Lopez, J. M., Martinez, P., Rosenberg, H., Barriga, P., Rodrigues, J. A., and Otipka, N.: Renin-secreting tumor. Case report. Hypertension, *2*:714, 1980.

Wickham, J. E. A.: Conservative renal surgery for adenocarcinoma: the place of bench surgery. Br. J. Urol., *47*:25, 1975.

Zincke, H., and Swanson, S. K.: Bilateral renal cell carcinoma: influence of synchronous and asynchronous occurrence on patient survival. J. Urol., *128*:913, 1982.

CHAPTER 64

Surgery for Calculus Disease of the Urinary Tract

RALPH A. STRAFFON, M.D.

INTRODUCTION

Any calculus within the urinary tract places the kidney in some danger. Calculi are often associated with obstruction or infection, which may lead to renal damage. Surgical removal may be difficult, and incomplete removal or early recurrence is possible. This is particularly true for staghorn or branched calculi. In each individual case a decision must be made as to whether the stone should be removed. Once it is decided to remove the calculus, the choice of surgical technique becomes important. The most commonly used and reliable of these surgical procedures to remove calculi from the upper urinary tract will be described in this chapter.

HISTORIC ASPECTS OF SURGERY FOR CALCULI

Hippocrates (460–373 B.C.) described four diseases of the kidneys, one of which was stone disease. He recognized the signs and symptoms of perinephric abscesses and incised and drained these, noting that urinary fistulas were sometimes produced. It is likely that some of these perinephric abscesses were pyohydronephrotic kidneys, and calculi were probably extracted through these incisions or were passed spontaneously.

There are numerous accounts from the eleventh through the seventeenth centuries, both in Europe and in the Middle East, of extraction of renal calculi from palpably distended kidneys or through draining flank incisions. During the eighteenth century a great deal of knowledge regarding the pathophysiology of renal calculus disease was gained from autopsy studies. Various European surgeons reported experiences using renal parenchymal incisions to remove renal calculi. Most agreed that nephrotomies should be used only when the kidneys were pyohydronephrotic. They advised complete drainage of the kidney, either removing the stones at the time of drainage or leaving them to be expelled spontaneously. Though success was not frequent, many patients were relieved of their pain by these procedures.

In 1880, Henry Morris, an English surgeon, performed the first nephrolithotomy on an otherwise healthy kidney. He later reported his experiences with nephrolithotomy on 34 patients with only a single death. He accurately defined the terms nephrolithiasis, nephrolithotomy, nephrectomy, and nephrotomy. Czerny, in 1887, was the first surgeon to reapproximate the nephrotomy incision with catgut sutures.

Discovery of the roentgen ray in 1895 led to improvement in the diagnosis and treatment of renal calculus disease. In 1899 both Albarran and Abbe reported radiographic demonstration of renal calculi.

Because of the severe hemorrhage often following a nephrolithotomy, surgeons began employing a posterior pyelotomy incision to remove renal calculi. Lower, in 1913, advocated pyelotomy as a procedure of choice for stones that could be reached by this approach. In 1915 Howard Kelly extended the pyelotomy incision obliquely upward through relatively avascular parenchyma to allow removal of large renal stones.

The first surgeons to address the problem of removing staghorn calculi were Cullen and Derge (1911). Using Brodel's (1901) observation of the intrarenal arterial distribution, they performed a nephrotomy using a thin silver wire that was passed between the arterial blood supply from within outward in an attempt to gain wider exposure and avoid severe hemorrhage. These authors recommended an L-shaped incision on the posterior surface of the kidney. The lower limb of the L avoided the blood supply to the posterior and basilar segment of the kidney, and the upper limit was positioned in the avascular plane between the posterior and anterior segments of the kidney. This approach is very similar to the incision used for anatrophic nephrolithotomy today.

During the decade from 1920 to 1930, various techniques were developed to minimize further parenchymal damage during the various lithotomy procedures. In addition, techniques for the closure of nephrotomy incisions were developed using interrupted mattress sutures or continuous Lembert sutures. In 1926 Carson and Goldstein performed a number of nephrotomies in dogs; these were closed by interrupted catgut sutures through the renal capsule. This technique produced less renal damage than was seen with either the Lembert suture or the interrupted mattress suture. Smith and Boyce (1967) noted that careful reconstruction of the calyces and renal pelvis combined with a continuous capsular closure produced an excellent repair of the nephrotomy incision.

Robson (1898) was the first to suggest the use of x-rays to localize stones in the kidney at the time of surgery. Braasch and Carman (1919) used intraoperative fluoroscopy to identify residual stone fragments in the kidney. In 1925 Quinby described the use of a static x-ray cassette to obtain intraoperative films to detect renal calculi.

Since that time, development of new techniques as well as refinement of previous procedures has given the urologic surgeon a number of methods for removing stones from the urinary tract. These methods will be described as they are applied today in the surgical removal of calculi.

OPERATION VERSUS CONSERVATIVE MANAGEMENT OF CALCULUS DISEASE OF THE UPPER URINARY TRACT

Each patient merits special consideration regarding the need to remove a calculus versus conservative management. If a patient is elderly and is a poor surgical risk, conservative management may be the treatment of choice. This is particularly true if the stone is small and asymptomatic, is not producing obstruction, and is not associated with a chronic urinary tract infection. Patients with this type of stone disease may be placed on a good medical program and simply checked at periodic intervals with an x-ray of the renal area, a urinalysis, urine culture, and renal function studies.

Conservative management may also be the procedure of choice for patients in whom multiple operations to remove calculi from the urinary tract and to clear an associated urinary tract infection have failed. For these patients surgical intervention is required if renal function continues to deteriorate or the patient develops an obstructed kidney associated with infection or persistent pain. Blandy and Singh (1976) have presented clinical evidence that surgical removal of a staghorn calculus is more likely to preserve renal function and the clinical well-being of the patient than does leaving the stone in the urinary tract. It is only after the removal of all renal calculi that a coexisting urinary tract infection can be effectively treated.

Factors That May Delay Surgical Intervention

All patients with renal calculi should undergo careful evaluation to attempt to determine the cause of the stone disease. Findings obtained from this metabolic evaluation may delay surgical removal of the stone. However, if there exists obstruction associated with sepsis, immediate surgical removal may be necessary.

If the patient is found to have primary hyperparathyroidism, surgical exploration of the neck should be performed to remove a parathyroid adenoma. This is best done prior to the surgical removal of renal calculi, since the operative procedure could produce a parathyroid crisis or the calculi may recur during the postoperative convalescence.

There are certain types of stones that may be dissolved by appropriate medical therapy. This is particularly true of pure uric acid calculi, which respond to a program of forcing fluids, administration of allopurinol, and alkalinization of the urine (pH 6.5 to 7.0). This may save patients a surgical procedure and, if they continue on the program, prevent the formation of additional stones in the future.

Selected cystine calculi, those not calcified, will often respond to a medical program of forcing fluids, alkalinization of the urine (pH > 7.5) and the use of D-penicillamine. Impacted ones may be bypassed by a catheter and dissolved with retrograde or antegrade alkaline irrigants (Crissey and Gittes, 1979; Dretler et al., 1984).

Other correctable metabolic problems may be indentified, such as vitamin D intoxication, renal tubular acidosis, and hypercalcemia produced by coexisting medical problems such as sarcoidosis or neoplasm. In the case of calcified stones, it is unlikely that the identification of the underlying cause of stones will allow dissolution of the existing calculi, but once the urinary tract is cleared of stones it is important to initiate treatment that will prevent recurrence. This is covered in much more detail in Chapter 25.

Factors That May Influence Immediate Operation for Removal of Calculi

The presence of a concretion of any size or shape places the involved renal unit at risk. Small calculi within the parenchyma (nephrocalcinosis) or in a minor calyx, without coexisting infection or obstruction, can be safely followed for many years.

There are certain indications, however, for urgent removal of calculi in the urinary tract. Since the endourologic approach to stones is discussed in Chapter 8, these remarks will be directed toward the operative removal of renal calculi.

Obstruction. Pre-existing obstruction to the kidney (e.g., ureteropelvic junction obstruction) may predispose to stone formation. On the other hand, the calculus may produce obstruction to a renal unit, resulting in progressive renal damage. Persistent obstruction by a calculus too large to pass spontaneously or by a small calculus that could pass but does not is an indication for the operative removal of the stone.

Infection. The presence of a urinary tract infection associated with a calculus is usually an indication for surgical removal of the stone and vigorous treatment of the associated infection. It is virtually impossible to eradicate a urinary tract infection in the presence of calculi, because bacteria lodge in the interstices of the calculus. If neither the stone nor the infection is treated, renal damage ultimately results.

The combination of obstruction and infection associated with a stone is particularly dangerous. The risk of renal damage is increased, as is the risk of developing bacteremia or septicemia. Immediate therapy is often indicated when these entities occur together.

Pain. Severe colic may be caused by a renal or ureteral calculus, and if relief is not achieved with analgesics, operative removal is indicated. In general, renal stones smaller than 0.5 cm will frequently pass spontaneously. A calculus between 0.5 to 1.0 cm in diameter may pass spontaneously but frequently requires operative removal. Stones larger than 1 cm will seldom if ever pass spontaneously.

Progressive Renal Failure. Renal failure may be present and may be accentuated by an obstructing calculus. Prompt removal may be indicated, particularly in an individual with a solitary kidney.

Hematuria. A renal calculus seldom produces significant bleeding. Microscopic hematuria is nearly always present, but massive gross hematuria is seldom produced by a renal calculus. Therefore hematuria is an infrequent indication for immediate removal of the stone.

PREOPERATIVE PREPARATION OF THE PATIENT

General Medical Evaluation. Every patient requires a general medical evaluation to determine the presence of any underlying medical problem that might influence the operative procedure or the postoperative recovery. Appropriate medical consultation may be required to aid in preparing patients for the operative procedure.

Metabolic Evaluation. All patients with renal calculi should have a basic metabolic evaluation. This should include several serum calcium determinations and the collection of 24-hour urine specimens to measure the excretion of calcium, uric acid, and creatinine (to check the accuracy of the urine collection). In selected patients, oxalate or cystine excretion studies or both should also be obtained.

Patients with "active" stone disease deserve a more extensive investigation, as outlined in Chapter 25.

A stone that has passed spontaneously or was previously removed should be analyzed to determine the composition of its nidus and layers. This will provide useful information for the postoperative management of the patient.

Radiographic Studies. An intravenous pyelogram with delayed and oblique films should be obtained to identify the position of the calculus, to be sure it is within the urinary tract and to evaluate the degree of obstruction.

For certain patients, a voiding cystourerogram may be advisable to demonstrate the presence or absence of reflux.

Renal angiography is sometimes necessary to define the position and number of renal arteries supplying each kidney. Oblique views should be obtained to identify the anterior and posterior blood supply to the kidney. These studies will aid in planning an anatrophic nephrolithotomy.

Evaluation of Renal Function. Assessment of renal function is an important aspect of the preoperative preparation of the patient. This may be done in a number of ways depending on the clinical problem encountered. Serum creatinine and creatinine clearance determinations should be obtained for nearly all patients. For selected patients, additional information regarding renal function can be obtained by the following procedures: (1) an I-131 iodohippurate or technetium 99-DTPA radionuclide scan; (2) an I-125 iothalamate determination of glomerular filtration rate; (3) a CT scan utilizing contrast material, to determine the thickness of the renal cortex; and (4) a selective renal angiography to evaluate the renal cortical tissue. For more detailed information about renal function evaluation, see Chapter 2.

Control of Infection. A urine culture and sensitivity study will identify the presence of specific bacteria in the urine and aid in selecting appropriate antimicrobial therapy. The antibiotics should be started at least 48 hours prior to the planned surgical intervention in patients with urinary tract infection, to achieve adequate parenchymal and urine levels of the drug of choice. In many cases the bacteria present may be sensitive only to drugs that can be given by the parenteral route. This therapy is continued during the operative procedure and the postoperative period to try to eradicate a coexisting urinary tract infection, which may be an important factor in stone recurrence. It will also lessen the incidence of serious bacteremia.

Cystoscopy and Retrograde Pyelograms. These studies may be required for certain patients, particularly when the ureter cannot be visualized, even on delayed films, below the obstructing calculus. The procedure is best performed just before operative intervention.

RENAL ANATOMY

A detailed description of the anatomy of the kidney is presented in Chapter 1. It is worthwhile, however, to briefly review the surgical anatomy of the kidney as it relates to the removal of renal calculi.

Renal Arteries. There are four surgical segments of the kidney: (1) apical, (2) basilar, (3) anterior (superior and inferior), and (4) posterior. The anterior division of the renal artery supplies apical, basilar, and anterior segments as shown in Figure 64–1. The posterior division of the renal artery supplies the posterior segments of the kidney (Fig. 64–2). It is important to identify the junction of the blood supply of the anterior and posterior segments on the posterior surface of the kidney. This junction is about two thirds of the distance from the hilum to the lateral border of the kidney.

Each segmental branch divides into interlobar (paracalyceal) arteries. These originate as pairs near the base of each major calyx, from which point the two members of the pair separate to course toward the papillae along opposite margins of the major calyces. These vessels then become transmedullary arteries, which pass

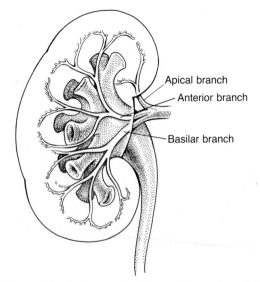

Figure 64–1. Arterial supply to the anterior surface of the right kidney, showing the segmental branches.

- Apical branch
- Anterior branch
- Basilar branch

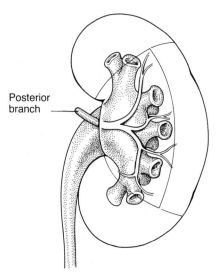

Figure 64–2. Arterial supply to the posterior surface of the right kidney, showing the distribution of the posterior division of the renal artery and its relationship to the anterior segmental vessels.

through the medulla of the kidney and end in arcuate arteries at the corticomedullary junction.

Selective renal angiography will identify vessels to the arcuate and subarcuate levels, and with anterior-posterior and oblique films a surgeon can identify the various branches of the renal arteries. There are variations of this vasculature in about 20 per cent of patients.

Renal Calyces. There are eight to ten major calyces that open into the renal pelvis (Fig. 64–3). The apical segment has one major calyx,

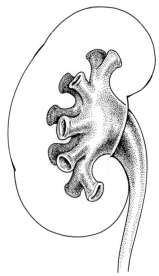

Figure 64–3. Anatomic arrangement of the major calyces and their relationship to the segments of the kidney and to the renal pelvis.

which lies in the midfrontal plane and usually receives two minor calyces (medial and lateral). The basilar segment has a single major calyx in the median plane and receives two minor calyces (anterior and posterior).

There are usually three major calyces in the anterior segment that enter the renal pelvis at about a 20 degree angle to the midfrontal plane. The posterior segment also has these major calyces joining the renal pelvis at a 75 degree angle with the midfrontal plane.

Urographic studies, with both oblique and lateral views, will identify the calyces and the position of the calculus in the collecting system. With this information a surgeon can plan the operative procedure best suited for the removal of the stones.

PYELOLITHOTOMY

Pyelolithotomy is a procedure of choice for most stones in the renal pelvis when they are too large to pass spontaneously and surgical removal is indicated. Stones that extend into minor calyces, particularly if the infundibulum is not dilated, are difficult to remove through a standard pyelolithotomy, as are isolated stones in minor calyces.

Surgical Incisions
(see also Chapter 62)

The Twelfth Rib Flank Incision. The standard approach to renal calculi is through a flank incision in which the twelfth rib is resected. The incision is then made through the bed of the twelfth rib and extended forward from this area as shown in Figure 64–4. The patient is placed in the lateral position, with the operating table flexed and the kidney rest elevated. The center of the kidney rest should be just below the twelfth rib. The incision begins over the twelfth rib and extends forward and medial to the lateral border of the rectus muscle. The anterior portion of the latissimus dorsi muscle is divided. Beneath the latissimus dorsi muscle posterior lies the posterior inferior serratus muscle, which is usually not divided in this approach to the kidney. The periosteum over the rib is incised and stripped from the rib using a periosteal elevator. By following the old adage "up on the downside and down on the upside," the periosteum can be stripped away from the rib. A Doyen rib elevator is used on the posterior side of the rib, and, when the periosteum is

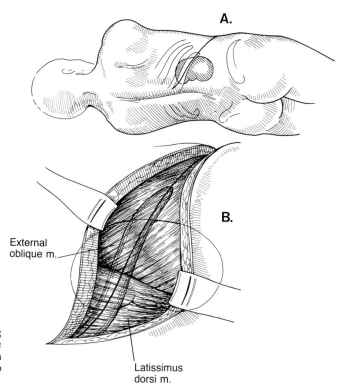

A.

B.

External
oblique m.

Latissimus
dorsi m.

Figure 64–4. Twelfth rib flank incision, showing positioning of the patient for this incision. The incision is begun near the angle of the twelfth rib and is carried off the tip of the twelfth rib anterior to a point above the umbilicus.

completely freed from the length of the rib to be removed, the rib can be cut with a rib cutter and removed. The rough edges of the cut rib are then smoothed with bone rongeurs.

The external abdominal oblique and internal abdominal oblique muscles are divided in line with the incision. The aponeurosis of the transversus abdominis muscle (formed by the fusion of the anterior and posterior layers of the thoracolumbar fascia) is exposed, and the retroperitoneal space can be entered posteriorly through the bed of the twelfth rib and the thoracolumbar fascia. Care must be taken to avoid injury to the pleura and damage to the subcostal neurovascular bundle. The incision can be easily extended forward by splitting the fibers of the transversus abdominis muscles, pushing the peritoneum out of the way. Good exposure can be maintained using a Finochietto self-retaining retractor. There are numerous other flank approaches to the kidney, but this has the advantage of giving good exposure as well as avoiding injury to the subcostal nerve. If the kidney is unusually high, a similar approach can be made through the bed of the eleventh rib, but here one must be careful to avoid entering the pleural cavity. Gerota's fascia can be opened, giving access to the kidney, renal pelvis, and upper ureter.

Posterior Vertical Lumbotomy Incision.
This is an excellent approach for a calculus in the renal pelvis or upper third of the ureter. Neither muscles nor nerves should be divided with this incision; hence the postoperative convalescence is relatively free of incisional pain and the patient can frequently be discharged from the hospital in 3 or 4 days (Gittes and Belldegrun, 1983).

The patient is placed in the lateral position with the knees flexed toward the abdomen to prevent lumbar lordosis. The patient may also be placed in a prone or intermediate position, particularly if both kidneys or ureters are going to be approached simultaneously.

The vertical incision extends from the twelfth rib to the iliac crest, as shown in Figure 64–5A, and is made directly over the midportion of the lumbosacral muscle mass. The posterior layer of the thoracolumbar fascia overlying this muscle mass is divided and detached from the lateral margin of the muscle until contact is made with the transverse process of the lumbar vertebrae. Here one encounters the anterior layer of the thoracolumbar fascia, which lies directly over the quadratus lumborum muscle (Fig. 64–5B). This aponeurosis is incised vertically near its attachment to the transverse processes of the lumbar vertebrae. Care must be

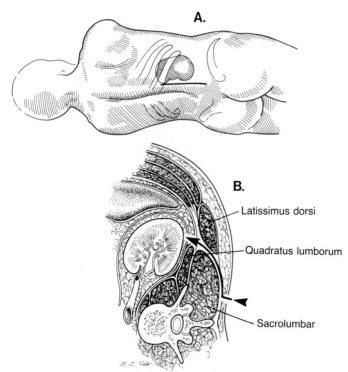

A.

B.

Latissimus dorsi

Quadratus lumborum

Sacrolumbar

Figure 64–5. *A,* The patient is placed in the lateral position without flexing the table to a marked degree. The incision is made vertically from the twelfth rib to the iliac crest on the posterior surface of the lumbosacral muscles. *B,* The anatomic approach used for the posterior lumbotomy incision through the anterior and posterior layer of the lumbodorsal fascia, retracting the lumbosacral muscle mass and quadratus lumborum muscle medially.

taken to avoid injury to subcostal, ilioinguinal, and iliohypogastric nerves. At the upper level of the incision, the anterior layer of thoracolumbar fascia is dissected off the quadratus lumborum muscle until reaching the lateral edge of this muscle, which can be retracted medially. This procedure is carried out throughout the entire length of the vertical incision. A self-retaining retractor can then be placed in the incision, and dissection of the ureter and renal pelvis is carried out to gain exposure for removal of the calculus.

Subcostal Incision. This incision can be used for selected patients who have had previous flank incisions. It should be reserved for simple stones in the renal pelvis, when mobilization of the entire kidney is not required. The standard subcostal transperitoneal approach to the kidney is shown in Figure 64–6. The right kidney is exposed by freeing up the hepatic flexure and using the Kocher maneuver on the duodenum (Fig. 64–6*A*). The left kidney is exposed by mobilizing the splenic flexure, taking care to avoid injury to the spleen by dividing the splenocolic ligament (Fig. 64–6*B*).

An extraperitoneal anterior approach can also be used on either side to gain access to the renal pelvis anteriorly. After dividing the external and internal abdominal oblique muscle, the transversus abdominis muscle is separated as far

laterally as possible. The underlying peritoneum is pushed medially as the transverse abdominis muscle is bluntly divided to gain access to the retroperitoneum and the kidney. The rectus muscle may need to be divided to gain adequate exposure. As the renal pelvis is approached, care must be taken to avoid injury to the renal artery and vein. This approach is best used for patients with an extrarenal pelvis.

Standard Pyelolithotomy. For most patients the twelfth rib flank incision is used to approach the kidney, as this provides good access to the posterior side of the renal pelvis yet allows access to the renovascular supply if necessary. Gerota's fascia is opened posteriorly, and the ureter is identified below the renal pelvis. A vessel loop is placed around the ureter, and traction can be applied to this as an aid in dissecting the ureter and renal pelvis free from surrounding tissue. For certain patients a posterior lumbotomy or subcostal incision may be used.

Excessive mobilization of the kidney is usually not required for a simple pyelolithotomy. The kidney is pushed forward, in the incision, and the upper ureter and renal pelvis are dissected from surrounding tissue. It is best to start the dissection at the level of the normal ureter, near the ureteropelvic junction. Once the ureter is identified, dissection can be carried upward

TABLE 64–2. Constituents Used in Coagulum Pyelolithotomy Related to Measured Volume of Renal Collecting System*

Measured Capacity of Renal Pelvis (ml)	Volume of Cryoprecipitate (ml)	Calcium Chloride (100 mg/ml)	Thrombin (100 U/ml)
10	9	9 (0.10 ml)	18 (0.20 ml)
15	14	14 (0.15 ml)	28 (0.30 ml)
20	19	19 (0.20 ml)	38 (0.40 ml)
25	24	24 (0.25 ml)	48 (0.50 ml)
30	28	28 (0.30 ml)	56 (0.55 ml)
35	33	33 (0.35 ml)	66 (0.65 ml)
40	38	38 (0.40 ml)	76 (0.75 ml)
45	43	43 (0.45 ml)	86 (0.85 ml)
50	48	48 (0.50 ml)	96 (1.00 ml)
		(qs with normal saline to make 1, 2, or 3 ml)	

*Ratio of 1 ml cryoprecipitate to 2 U thrombin to 1 mg calcium chloride is maintained regardless of the volume required to fill the collecting system.

From Fischer, C. P., Sonda, L. P., III, and Diokno, A. C.: Urology, *15*:6, 1980.

determine the amount of coagulum to be injected according to the formula shown in Table 64–2. The bulldog clamp is removed to allow complete drainage of the renal pelvis, and the angiocatheter is simply left in place.

The correct amount of coagulum is then prepared by placing the cryoprecipitate in a large syringe. The required amounts of thrombin and calcium chloride are combined in a second syringe.

The bulldog clamp is again applied to the ureter. The thrombin and calcium chloride are then added to the syringe containing the cryoprecipitated plasma and immediately injected through the angiocatheter into the renal pelvis. Although my preference is injection through a single angiocatheter, two angiocatheters can be placed in the renal pelvis, injecting the cryoprecipitate through one and the thrombin and calcium chloride solution through the other. Gentle distention of the renal pelvis must be obtained, and if the capacity was accurately measured, this is usually achieved by injecting the predetermined volume.

The coagulum is allowed to remain in place for 7 to 8 minutes. Then a transverse pyelotomy incision is made; this may be extended upward into a major calyx as well as downward to create a semicircular flap (Fig. 64–9B).

The coagulum is then gently teased from the renal pelvis. When successful, a mold of the entire collecting system should be obtained, with the small stone fragments trapped within the coagulum. An intraoperative x-ray should al-

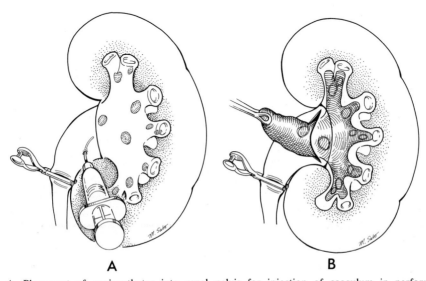

A　　　　　　**B**

Figure 64–9. *A,* Placement of angiocatheter into renal pelvis for injection of coagulum in performing coagulum pyelolithotomy. *B,* Transverse pyelotomy with removal of coagulum and entrapped calculi.

ways be obtained to be sure all stone fragments are removed.

A small catheter is then passed down the ureter into the bladder, and the renal collecting system is irrigated thoroughly with saline. Should residual calculi remain, the fiberoptic nephroscope is ideal to localize the calculus and either flush it out of the minor calyx or grasp it with a special grasping forceps, which may be passed through the nephroscope. For some patients a small radial nephrotomy may be required to remove a retained calculus.

Coagulum inadvertently left in the collecting system will dissolve in 24 hours or less. Pence et al. (1981) reported a fatal intraoperative pulmonary embolus, which they believed was due to overdistention of the renal pelvis and the use of a high concentration of thrombin in the coagulum.

Extended Pyelolithotomy. In 1965 Gil-Vernet described the extended pyelolithotomy. He advocated the intrasinus approach to the major calyces and the use of a transverse pyelotomy and longitudinal calycotomy. This procedure is particularly useful if the patient has an intrarenal pelvis containing a large calculus that extends into minor calyces. I have not used it for staghorn calculi in which the stone in the minor calyx is much larger than the infundibulum draining the calyx. In addition we have frequently combined this approach with clamping of the renal artery and cooling of the kidney, allowing additional exposure of the intrasinus area of the kidney. This procedure can be combined with radial nephrotomies for certain patients with staghorn calculi.

ANATOMIC CONSIDERATIONS FOR THE EXTENDED PYELOLITHOTOMY. The term intrarenal sinus was introduced by Henle in 1866. It is a rectangular cavity filled by the intrarenal portion of the renal pelvis, calyces, renal vessels, nerves, and lymphatics. The space between these structures is filled with fatty tissue, which allows distention and contraction of the calyces in the renal pelvis.

The intrarenal sinus is entered posteriorly at the junction of the hilar edge of the parenchyma with the renal pelvis (Fig. 64–10). Once this space is opened, care should be taken to stay close to the renal pelvis. The posterior division of the renal artery supplying the posterior midportion of the kidney may pass along the hilar area from above downward. Although it is usually buried in renal parenchyma, it is sometimes outside the parenchyma, particularly at the upper end of the opening into the renal sinus. Care must be taken to elevate this vessel with the hilar portion of the renal parenchyma.

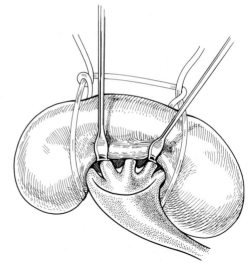

Figure 64–10. Gil-Vernet approach to the kidney by development of the intrarenal sinus area for stone removal.

Once the intrasinus area is entered, it may be developed by blunt dissection into a space limited by the medullary portion of the renal parenchyma laterally and the renal pelvis medially. Additional exposure to the major calyces can be obtained by clamping the renal artery and cooling the kidney. This softens the renal parenchyma and allows greater retraction for exposure of the intrarenal collecting system. Elevation of the renal parenchyma of the renal pelvis is facilitated by the use of Gil-Vernet sinus retractors of various sizes (Fig. 64–11).

The transverse pyelotomy incision is started in the renal pelvis and extended in a curvilinear

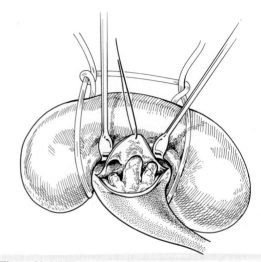

Figure 64–11. Transverse pyelotomy with extension into the superior and inferior major calyces for removal of a large pelvic stone.

fashion into the major calyces of the upper and lower poles of the kidney. This creates a flap of renal pelvis, allowing greater access to the collecting system for the removal of a large calculus that is located in the renal pelvis and extends into the minor calyces. Often the infundibulum to the calyx can be dilated, and the extension of a branched calculus can be teased out of a minor calyx.

Once all calculi are removed, a catheter is passed down the ureter into the bladder and the collecting system is thoroughly irrigated. The Water-Pik, a commercially available irrigator for dental hygiene (Gibbons et al., 1974), is useful for irrigating minor calyces free of debris and small stone fragments. The operative nephroscope may also be used to inspect minor calyces for retained calculi. An intraoperative x-ray should always be obtained to be certain all calculi are removed. If a minor calyx retains a calculus that cannot be removed through the infundibulum, a radial nephrotomy may be required.

A double J Silastic internal stent is frequently placed in the ureter from the renal pelvis to the bladder to ensure good drainage. This is placed prior to closing the pyelotomy incision. The pyelotomy is then closed with fine suture material, as previously described, to secure a watertight closure. A drain is placed in the retroperitoneal space, behind the kidney, and brought out through a stab wound below the incision. The incision is then closed in layers.

NEPHROLITHOTOMY

Anatrophic Nephrolithotomy. This is the surgical procedure described by Smith and Boyce in 1967. It is the procedure of choice for removing most branched calculi, particularly in patients with an intrarenal pelvis or patients who have had one or more pyelolithotomies and now have a staghorn calculus.

In Situ Renal Preservation. Cooling of cells and organs to 4 to 10°C markedly decreases their metabolic activity and physiologic function. Oxygen requirements are reduced, rendering the organ more resistant to ischemic damage. The sodium-potassium metabolic pump is inactivated by hypothermia, leading to influx of sodium into the cell and potassium outward. This results in cell damage, which can be prevented by the infusion of hyperosmotic solutions with ionic concentration more similar to the intracellular levels, such as Collins solution (1971).

Clamping the renal artery causes a very rapid drop in the level of adenosine triphosphate (ATP) in the renal cortex, to less than 50 per cent of normal within 1 minute. Renal hypothermia will significantly retard the high degradation rate of ATP that occurs when the kidney is ischemic. Since the kidney is entirely dependent on endogenous ATP as its energy source, during the period of renal ischemia it is most important to have rapid cooling within a short period from the time the renal artery is clamped.

Temporary in situ clamping of the renal artery is required for procedures such as partial nephrectomy, nephrolithotomy, and anatrophic nephrolithotomy. The temporary clamping limits intraoperative arterial bleeding and, by reducing tissue turgor, improves access to the intrarenal structures. Prior to clamping the renal artery, the patient should be well hydrated and given intravenous mannitol to ensure good diuresis.

The simplest and most commonly used technique for achieving in situ hypothermia is surface cooling. It has been shown both experimentally and clinically that, with the renal artery occluded and using surface cooling, renal core temperature of 15 to 20°C can be easily achieved. This will allow preservation of renal function during the ischemic period if it does not exceed 3 hours.

The technique for surface cooling is to mobilize the entire kidney, leaving the renal pedicle and ureter intact (Fig. 64–12). The renal artery is dissected from surrounding tissue, and the branch to the posterior renal segment is identified. A rubber dam or plastic sheet is wrapped around the kidney, and the renal artery is clamped with a vascular clamp. This clamp should be carefully selected (e.g., by clamping the surgeon's thenar web) to produce occlusion of the artery without damaging the wall of the vessel. The kidney is then packed in ice slush. Renal core temperature will reach 15 to 20°C in 15 to 20 minutes. Ice slush is best produced with a special refrigerating unit produced by the Taylor Freezer Company.★ The solution is simply placed in a sterile container and continuously stirred, rapidly forming ice slush. The advantage of this technique is that a sufficient supply of slush is always available during the operative procedure; the slush is homogeneous, providing for better surface cooling.

There are other techniques for surface cooling using various devices to deliver a coolant to the kidney. They are cumbersome and require

★Taylor Freezer Company, Rockton, Ill.

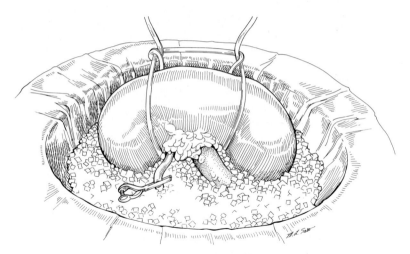

Figure 64–12. Cooling the kidney with ice slush.

intermittent reapplication of the device, since the operation cannot be performed with the cooling device in place.

Intrarenal perfusion can be accomplished by way of the renal artery, vein, or renal pelvis. Arterial perfusion is the most effective route and can be achieved by direct needle puncture of the renal artery or transfemoral placement of a balloon catheter into the renal artery prior to the operation. If a small amount of normokalemic perfusate is used, this can go back into the systemic circulation. When using larger amounts of cold physiologic solution or a hyperkalemic perfusate (e.g., Collins solution), one must clamp the renal vein and create a venotomy to allow exodus of the perfusate. A fatal cardiac arrhythmia may result if the high potassium of the perfusate reaches the heart. A simple arterial flush of 200 ml of Collins solution at 4°C will give excellent protection against renal ischemia.

There are a variety of drugs that will give pharmacologic protection to the kidney against ischemia in addition to intravenous mannitol. Experimental studies with inosine have suggested that this drug can protect the kidney against damage produced by warm ischemia. A variety of other agents have been tested in our laboratory, including phenoxybenzamine, α-methyldopa, timolol, propranolol, captopril, pranolium chloride, angiotensin II, sodium nitroprusside, and calcium channel blockers. The most effective drugs have been the D-isomer of propranolol and one of its analogs, pranolium chloride. The mechanism by which D-propranolol is effective does not appear to be through the β-adrenergic blockage of renin release but rather through its membrane-stabilizing or local anesthetic properties. In situ pharmacologic pre-vention of postischemic renal failure remains an area of intensive investigative study with promising clinical application.

SURGICAL PROCEDURE. The surgical approach for an anatrophic nephrolithotomy is the standard twelfth rib flank incision previously described. The incision should be carried anteriorly to the lateral border of the rectus muscle. This will allow the kidney, when dissected free from surrounding tissue, to be pushed forward, giving good exposure to the posterior surface.

Once the incision is completed, the ureter is identified and dissection is carried upward to expose the renal pelvis. The entire kidney is then mobilized, using both sharp and blunt dissection, around its periphery. Once the kidney has been completely mobilized leaving only the renal pedicle and ureter intact, a surgical tape can be placed around each end of the kidney and used as a sling to facilitate handling of the kidney (Fig. 64–13).

The kidney is then retracted medially, and the main renal artery, identified by palpation, can be dissected free from surrounding tissue. This will allow subsequent placement of a vascular clamp on the renal artery. The anterior and posterior divisions of the renal artery can be identified by dissecting laterally along the main renal artery. A selective renal angiogram, obtained during the preoperative period, is a useful "road map" to guide this dissection.

A priming dose of 12.5 gm of mannitol is given intravenously prior to occluding the renal artery. It is suggested that mannitol may increase the osmolarity of the glomerular filtrate, reducing the hazard of ice crystallization in renal tissue during the cooling process. It also ensures diuresis both prior to clamping the renal artery and after removing the clamp.

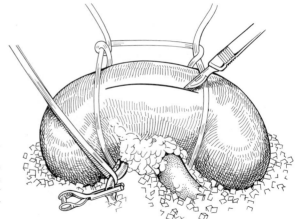

Figure 64–13. Complete dissection of the kidney from surrounding tissue except for the renal pedicle and ureter. The renal artery is then exposed and a sling fashioned to manipulate the kidney. This shows the position for the capsular incision on the posterior surface of the kidney between the junction of the blood supply to the anterior and posterior segments of the kidney.

With the kidney suspended by a surgical tape, a plastic dam is wrapped around the renal pedicle to create a reservoir around the kidney for ice slush. Preparation of the ice slush and the advantages of hypothermia during this period of renal ischemia have already been discussed. The renal artery is clamped with an adjustable vascular clamp, and the kidney is immediately packed in ice slush. The objective of the cooling process is to obtain a renal core temperature of 10 to 15°C, which usually takes about 15 minutes.

Even as the kidney is cooling, an incision is made in the capsule on the posterior surface of the kidney, at the junction of the blood supply to the anterior and posterior segments of the kidney (Fig. 64–13). This is a longitudinal incision that should not extend into the apical or basilar segments of the kidney.

The correct position for this incision can be identified by placing a vascular clamp on the anterior division of the renal artery and leaving the posterior division patent. The anesthesiologist then injects a bolus of 20 ml of methylene blue intravenously. The posterior segment of the renal parenchyma will stain blue, and the junction between the anterior and posterior segment is easily identified. The dye may cause hypotension, and so many surgeons use palpation of the softened segment. Other segments of the kidney can be identified by dissecting out additional branches of the anterior division of the renal artery (e.g., apical and basilar) and selectively clamping these segmental vessels.

The capsular incision for the anatrophic nephrolithotomy is seldom a straight line as depicted in the drawing (Fig. 64–13). Once the capsule has been sharply incised, the blunt end of the knife is an excellent instrument for sep-

aration of the renal parenchyma, along the line of demarcation between anterior and posterior arterial segments.

It is very important to approach the posterior calyces in the proper plane, as shown in Figure 64–14. Dissecting too far forward, which is the natural tendency of the surgeon, can expose the peripelvic venous plexus and cause excessive postclamping bleeding. If the dissection continues too far posteriorly, the blood supply to the posterior segment of the kidney will be damaged. The correct plane is nearly avascular and should lead the surgeon to the

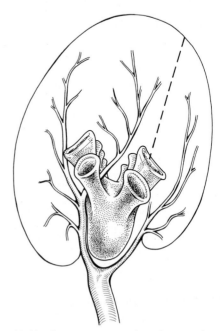

Figure 64–14. The proper approach to the posterior calyces of the kidney between the segmental blood supply of the anterior and posterior portions of the kidney.

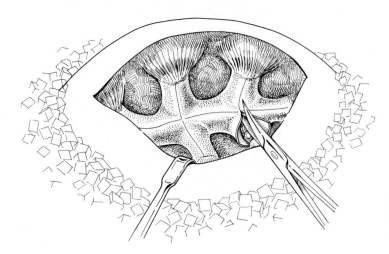

Figure 64–15. The incision on the anterior surface of a posterior major calyx. This incision can then be extended into the renal pelvis.

anterior surface of one of the major calyces draining the posterior segment of the kidney. Small venous and arterial potential bleeders can be suture ligated with 4–0 or 5–0 chromic sutures.

In instances when the staghorn calculus does not completely fill the collecting system, one can inject the collecting system with methylene blue–stained coagulum. This is prepared as previously described in performing a coagulum pyelolithotomy and will complete the filling of the collecting system, making identification of minor calyces much easier.

A posterior calyx containing a branched calculus is identified by palpation and is opened on its anterior surface (Fig. 64–15). This incision can then be extended into the renal pelvis and from there into all posterior calyces containing extensions of the staghorn calculus by incision along the anterior margin of the calyx. The incision can be extended from the renal pelvis into the anterior segmental calyces by incision on the posterior surface of the calyx, staying in the midline. Thus one gradually exposes the entire staghorn calculus (Fig. 64–16).

Malleable brain retractors and nerve hooks are useful instruments for obtaining exposure and identifying calyces. Surgical loupes and microsurgical instruments designed for intrarenal surgery are very useful in the operation.

When the collecting system is adequately exposed, the staghorn calculus can sometimes be removed intact but more often is removed in large segments. Before removing the calculus, a bulldog clamp should be placed across the ureter at the ureteropelvic junction to prevent any free stone fragments from passing down the ureter. A very hard staghorn calculus is much easier to remove than the softer stones, which tend to fragment. Sometimes stones are composed of very soft matrix-like material.

Occasionally the extension of calculus into a major or minor calyx will break off, and the fragment will have to be removed separately. The infundibulum leading to the calyx should be incised, opening the calyx and allowing the

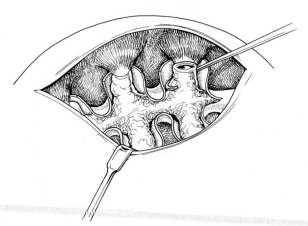

Figure 64–16. Exposure of a staghorn calculus obtained through a posterior longitudinal nephrotomy.

stone fragments to be easily removed. It is imperative to inspect each calyx carefully to be sure all stones and stone fragments are removed. The entire area can then be thoroughly lavaged. A Water-Pik is particularly useful in lavaging the minor calyces and renal pelvis. A small catheter is usually passed down the ureter to the bladder and left in place while flushing the collecting system.

An intraoperative roentgenogram of the kidney is always obtained to ensure that all calculi are removed. Occasionally, small fragments will remain in a minor calyx that has a very narrow infundibulum. If a retained fragment is identified, the renal pelvis should be searched carefully, using a nerve hook to try to identify the infundibulum leading to the retained calculus. Sometimes the fragment can be palpated through the parenchyma of the kidney and removed by a separate, radial nephrotomy.

The use of a small, ophthalmic B-scan, ultrasonic probe may aid in the localization of intrarenal calculi that cannot be identified. Some experience is required to recognize the characteristic ultrasonic images and shadows produced by stones. I have not used this modality.

Internal reconstruction of the collecting system is a most important part of this operative procedure. It would be ideal if the surgeon could reorganize the collecting system into a single large renal pelvis. Whenever possible, the adjacent margins of major calyces are sutured together using either interrupted or running 5-0 chromic sutures (Fig. 64–17). This approximation is carried outward to the level of the renal papillae, as shown in Figure 64–18.

An individual calyx with a narrow infundibulum can be widened by calicorrhaphy. The longitudinal incision in the wall of the calyx is closed transversely, approximating the minor calyx toward the renal pelvis. This in effect shortens the calyx but widens the infundibulum, providing better drainage for the calyx.

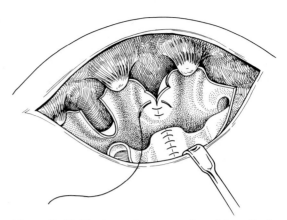

Figure 64–17. The internal reconstruction of the collecting system after removal of a staghorn calculus.

Adjacent minor calyces can be opened to provide better drainage by calicoplasty, as shown in Figure 64–18. The adjacent infundibular walls are incised from their pelvic origin into the minor calyces (Fig. 64–18A). The intervening peripelvic tissue is separated by blunt dissection (Fig. 64–18B). The V shape that is produced is then closed in a transverse manner (Fig. 64–18C), thus producing improved drainage to each of the adjacent minor calyces.

When the internal reconstruction of the calyces and renal pelvis has been completed (Fig. 64–19), a double J internal Silastic stent is passed down the ureter into the bladder, and the upper end is placed in the lower pole major calyx. To ensure that migration does not occur, it is fixed in position by 5–0 chromic suture to the superficial epithelium of the renal pelvis. This suture is easily pulled out when the stent is removed. Some surgeons leave an 8 French nephrostomy tube to allow irrigation of residual fragments with hemiacidrin (Jacobs and Gittes, 1976).

The longitudinal nephrotomy is closed with 4–0 chromic sutures, as shown in Figure 64–20.

Figure 64–18. Calicoplasty. *A*, Incision between two adjacent minor calcyes. *B*, The intervening peripelvic tissue is then separated by blunt dissection. *C*, Closure of the incision to open up the infundibular area of two adjacent minor calyces.

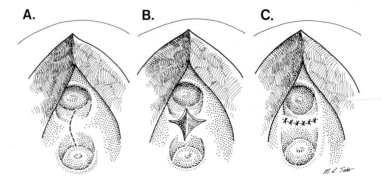

A.   **B.**   **C.**

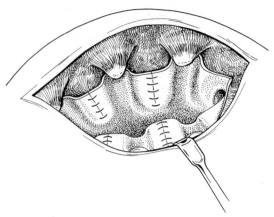

Figure 64–19. The completed internal reconstruction of the renal pelvis.

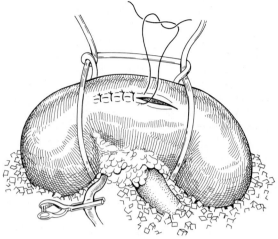

Figure 64–21. Closure of the renal capsule with either running or interrupted sutures.

Running sutures are initially used in each end of the collecting system, but in the central portion interrupted sutures are placed but not tied until all are in proper position. This facilitates accurate placement of these sutures, which can then be tied to complete the closure of the collecting system. Closure of the nephrotomy is completed with interrupted or running 3–0 chromic sutures in the renal capsule, as shown in Figure 64–21.

All anatrophic nephrolithotomies require good hemostasis. When the dissection is performed in the proper plane, one encounters only a few veins and no significant arterial bleeders that require suture ligatures. The vascular clamp can be removed just before closing the nephrotomy, to identify any major bleeders

and to be sure hemostasis is obtained. With secure closure of both the collecting system and the renal capsule, venous bleeding is tamponaded between the surfaces of the approximated nephrotomy and is seldom a problem. Once the capsular closure is completed, the renovascular clamp is removed and the kidney is warmed with irrigating solution.

A Penrose drain is placed in the retroperitoneal space and brought out through a stab wound below the incision, where it is sutured in place. The incision is closed in layers. There is usually no urine leakage, and the internal silastic stent can be removed at the same time the sutures and drain are removed. This is easily accomplished by cystoscopy under local anesthesia.

Nephrotomies. In the management of certain patients with calculi, single or multiple nephrotomies may be required to remove calculi in minor calyces. When the renal cortex is scarred and very thin over the calculus, placement of the nephrotomy incision is of little importance. However, when the renal parenchyma is in good condition, the proper placement of the nephrotomy in the renal cortex is very important to avoid damage to the blood supply. Certain rules should be adhered to in the placement of these nephrotomies: (1) The incision should be limited to one segment of the kidney; (2) the incision should be in a straight line; (3) the incision should be placed so as to do as little damage to the arterial supply of the renal segment as possible; and (4) the renal artery should nearly always be clamped and the kidney cooled prior to making the nephrotomy. All nephrotomies in the posterior segment

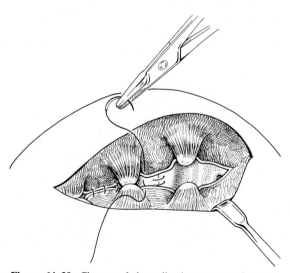

Figure 64–20. Closure of the collecting system after performance of an anatrophic nephrolithotomy.

of the kidney should be placed along the line of the incision used for the anatrophic nephrolithotomy, which gives easy access to any of the major calyces draining the posterior segment of the kidney. A nephrotomy in the anterior and apical segment of the kidney should be radial and parallel to the renal arteries in these segments. A sterile, ultrasonic Doppler probe is invaluable in identifying segmental arteries when placed directly on the surface of the kidney.

A pyelotomy can be extended into the renal parenchyma posteriorly between the junction of the posterior and basilar segments of the kidney (Fig. 64–22). This will allow removal of a branched calculus filling the renal pelvis and extending into the calyces draining the basilar segment of the kidney.

In making a nephrotomy, the capsule is sharply incised and the parenchyma separated with blunt dissection down to the calyx containing the calculus. The calyx is then opened with a knife and the stone removed. If the infundibulum is narrowed, calicorrhaphy should be performed if possible, after thoroughly lavaging the minor calyx. The nephrotomy is then closed in two layers, after hemostasis is secured. If the parenchyma is thin over the calyx, a single layer closure may be used.

PARTIAL NEPHRECTOMY

It is quite easy to combine a lower pole partial nephrectomy with a pyelocalycotomy to remove a staghorn calculus. Proponents of partial nephrectomy believe that removal of the scarred lower pole of the kidney, with its dependent collecting system, will decrease the incidence of recurrent calculi in this kidney. The disadvantage of the procedure is that viable renal tissue is often lost. The most important factor in preventing recurrent calculi is a good stone management program accompanied by eradication of any coexisting urinary tract infection.

In some patients the parenchyma of the basilar segment of the kidney may be very thin and scarred from a calculus associated with chronic pyelonephritis. For these patients partial nephrectomy with removal of the entire basilar segment and associated calculus is the procedure of choice.

The basilar branch of the renal artery is identified and dissected free from surrounding tissue. Methylene blue is then injected directly into the artery to stain the renal parenchyma supplied by this vessel. The artery is then ligated and divided (Fig. 64–23A). The capsule of the lower pole is incised and stripped back from the basilar segment (Fig. 64–23B).

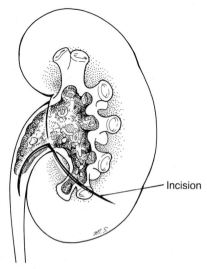

Figure 64–22. Extension of a pyelolithotomy into the lower pole calyces by an incision into the parenchyma between the junction of the posterior and basilar segments.

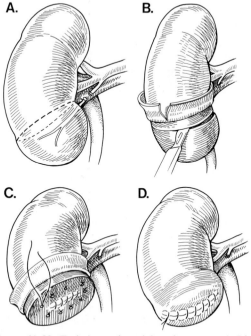

Figure 64–23. Technique of partial nephrectomy. *A,* Ligation of the basilar segmental branch of the renal artery. *B,* Stripping of the renal capsule back from the parenchyma that is to be resected. *C,* Resection of the renal segment and suture ligature of arteries and veins and closure of the collecting system. *D,* Closure of the capsule over the exposed surface of the kidney.

An amputation of the basilar segment is carried out along the lines of demarcation produced by the methylene blue injection. The collecting system is opened as necessary to remove the calculus, and it is then thoroughly lavaged. A small catheter should be passed down the ureter to be sure it is patent, and after this a double J Silastic stent can be placed to ensure good drainage.

Hemostasis is secured with suture ligature of renal arteries and veins using 4–0 or 5–0 chromic suture. The collecting system is closed with a running suture of 4–0 chromic to effect a watertight closure (Fig. 64–23C). The capsule is then closed over the lower pole of the kidney as shown in Fig. 64–23D.

NEPHRECTOMY

A calculus associated with long-standing infection may severely damage the kidney, and, in selected patients, nephrectomy may be the procedure of choice, removing both stones and kidney. The decision to perform a nephrectomy can usually be made preoperatively by assessment of renal function with one of the techniques previously described. An effort should be made to conserve renal tissue whenever possible. A simple flank nephrectomy is usually used, but sometimes great difficulty is encountered because of the inflammatory reaction around the kidney. A subcapsular nephrectomy is sometimes required to remove such a kidney.

URETEROLITHOTOMY

The clinical management of ureteral calculi requires consideration of a number of factors. The surgeon must decide when a calculus can be managed by watchful expectancy, hoping the stone will pass spontaneously. If it fails to pass, then intervention is required and a decision must be made as to whether the calculus can be removed with an endourologic procedure or whether ureterolithotomy will be required.

Although dogmatic statements regarding the need for ureterolithotomy cannot be made, there are a number of relative indications for this operative procedure: (1) calculi > 0.5 cm in diameter that fail to move down the ureter during a period of observation not to exceed 4 to 6 weeks in the absence of significant obstruction or infection; (2) impacted ureteral calculi that are producing obstruction associated with sepsis and cannot be bypassed by ureteral cath-

eter; (3) calculi producing frequent, recurrent, renal colic; (4) calculi producing significant obstruction, particularly when the opposite kidney has pre-existing damage; (5) calculi < 0.5 cm in diameter that fail to move after a reasonable period of observation; and (6) calculi that fail to be removed by endourologic procedures.

In determining the operative procedure to be used, one must know the functional status of both kidneys. If there has been long-standing obstruction due to a ureteral calculus and there is little or no functioning renal parenchyma remaining, the preferred operation may be nephrectomy or nephroureterectomy, particularly if the contralateral kidney is normal. In addition it is important to know if there are other calcifications in the renal collecting system. It may be necessary to remove these stones, if possible, at the time of the ureterolithotomy, to prevent them from dropping into the ureter and obstructing it in the postoperative period.

If ureterolithotomy is planned, it is important to be sure the calcific density is actually in the ureter. Usually this information can be obtained with an intravenous pyelogram with delays and then an oblique film obtained when the contrast material is in the area of the calcific density. The surgeon should also be sure the ureter below the level of the calculus is normal. If this information cannot be obtained by an intravenous pyelogram, then cystoscopy and retade pyelography are indicated, immediately prior to ureterolithotomy. If cystoscopy and retrograde pyelogram are not required, a flat plate of the abdomen should always be obtained before ureterolithotomy, to check the position of the calculus at the time of the operation.

Operative Removal of Calculi in the Upper Third of the Ureter. The standard flank incision through the bed of the twelfth rib is the usual incision used for removal of stones in the upper third of the ureter. Some surgeons will use the posterior lumbotomy to reduce morbidity. The ureter is identified, and control is obtained above and below the calculus by vessel loops. Care must be taken not to allow the stone to migrate upward into the renal collecting system. A longitudinal incision is made in the wall of the ureter directly over the calculus, and the stone is removed (Fig. 64–24). A small catheter is then passed down the ureter into the bladder, to be sure there is no obstruction below, and then upward into the renal pelvis, which is irrigated thoroughly.

The ureterolithotomy is usually closed with either interrupted or continuous 5–0 chromic

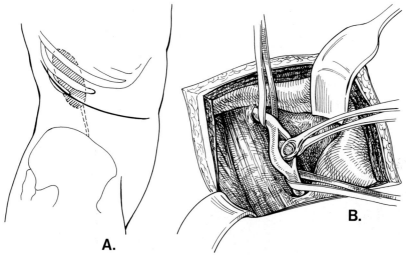

Figure 64–24. Removal of a calculus from the upper third of the ureter through the twelfth rib flank incision. *A,* Position of incision. *B,* Exposure of ureter with removal of ureteral calculus.

sutures, attempting to produce a watertight closure. The ureter is then surrounded by periureteral fatty tissue, if this is available, and a Penrose drain is placed behind the ureter and brought to the exterior through a stab wound below the flank incision, where it is sutured to the skin. The incision is then closed in layers.

If additional calculi are present in the kidney, an attempt should be made to remove these at the time of ureterolithotomy. If for various reasons this is not possible, it is wise to place an internal double J stent within the ureter before closing the ureterolithotomy. This will prevent a stone in the kidney from dropping into the ureter, producing obstruction during the postoperative period. The internal stent can easily be removed by cystoscopy under local anesthesia prior to discharge.

Operative Removal of Calculi in the Middle Third of the Ureter. The surgical approach to the middle third of the ureter may be made through a flank incision. Certain patients, provided they are not extremely obese, may be placed in the supine position and a roll placed beneath the shoulder and buttock to elevate the side to some degree (Fig. 64–25*A*). An extraperitoneal approach to the ureter can then be achieved by a muscle-splitting incision (Figs. 64–25*B* and *C*), or the muscle layers can be divided for better exposure. The ureter is identified, and control is gained with vessel loops placed above and below the calculus, taking great care not to dislodge the stone. A longitudinal incision is made in the ureteral wall over the calculus, which is then removed (Fig. 64–25*D*). A small catheter is passed both down and

up the ureter, as described above, to be sure it is patent. The incision is closed with sutures to obtain a watertight closure. A Penrose drain is placed near the ureter and brought out through a separate stab wound below the incision. When muscle-splitting incisions are used, they are easily closed, and these patients tend to have minimal postoperative pain associated with their incision.

Operative Removal of Calculi in the Lower Third of the Ureter. The patient is placed in the supine position, and a modified Gibson incision is used to approach the calculus in the lower third of the ureter (Fig. 64–26*A*). The external abdominal oblique muscle and fascia are divided, and an incision is made in the internal abdominal oblique and transverse abdominis muscles (Fig. 64–26*B*). The rectus muscle can be treated one of three ways (Fig. 64–26*C*): (1) it can simply be retracted medially; (2) it can be incised at its lateral border to give more exposure; or (3) its insertion into the symphysis pubis can be completely divided to give greater exposure.

An extraperitoneal approach is then made to identify the ureter and obtain control, initially above the calculus, and to prevent upward migration (Fig. 64–26*D*). The ureter is opened directly over the calculus, and the stone is removed. Patency of the ureter into the bladder and upward is established, and the ureter is closed and drained as previously described.

Operative Removal of a Calculus in the Intramural Portion of the Ureter. Calculi near the ureterovesical junction and in the intramural portion of the ureter are frequently quite diffi-

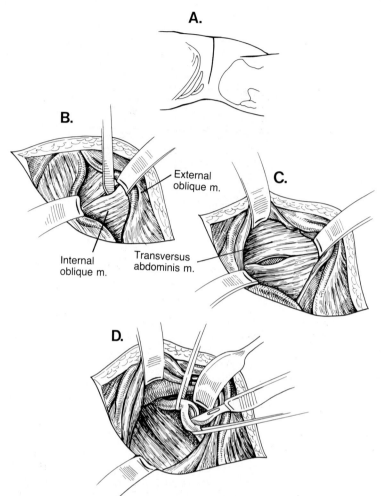

A.

B.

External oblique m.

C.

Internal oblique m.

Transversus abdominis m.

D.

Figure 64–25. Removal of a calculus in the middle third of the ureter. *A,* Site of the incision for the anterior extraperitoneal approach to the ureter. *B,* Muscle-splitting incision to approach the ureter. *C,* Separation of the remaining muscles with retraction of the peritoneum for exposure of the ureter. *D,* Removal of the calculus in the ureter through a longitudinal ureterotomy.

cult to remove surgically. There are several alternative approaches to manage calculi located in these positions.

Ureteroneocystostomy. If the ureteral calculus is impacted in the lower third of the ureter near the ureterovesical junction, it is often difficult if not impossible to identify the calculus, particularly if there is any periureteral inflammation. An easy method to manage this problem is simply to bypass the calculus by doing a simple ureteroneocystostomy. The stone can sometimes be removed or may be simply left in place and the ureter ligated. This has been an excellent method to manage what can be a very difficult surgical problem. The retained stone does not cause problems as long as the ureter below the stone is patent into the bladder.

Transvesical Ureterolithotomy. The transvesical approach may be used if a stone is impacted in the intramural portion of the ureter and cannot be removed with cystoscopic manip-

ulation. The modified Gibson incision is used and should be extended across the midline. The rectus muscle on the side involved is divided at its insertion into the symphysis pubis, and the inferior epigastric artery and vein must be ligated and divided to give access to the area. The bladder is opened, and the ureteric orifice on the side containing the calculus is identified. If the stone can be palpated, which is often the case, an incision is made in the vesical mucosa directly over the calculus (Fig. 64–27). The calculus is extracted, and a 5 French ureteral catheter is passed up the ureter. The incision can then be closed over the ureteral catheter with interrupted 5–0 chromic catgut sutures.

If there has been considerable damage to the intramural portion of the ureter, a double J internal Silastic stent can be passed up the ureter to the renal pelvis and left in place for 5 to 7 days while the suture line heals. It can later be easily removed cystoscopically.

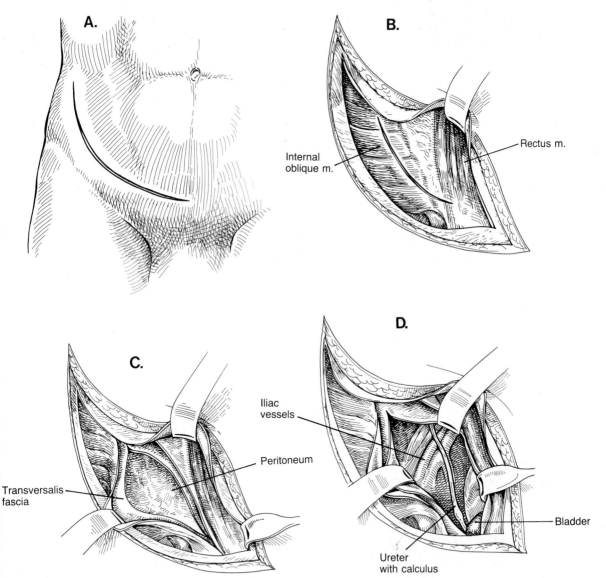

Figure 64–26. Surgical removal of a calculus in the lower third of the ureter. *A*, Modified Gibson incision. *B*, Division of the external abdominal oblique muscle and extraperitoneal approach to the lower third of the ureter. *C*, Approach to rectus muscle. *D*, Exposure of the ureter with a longitudinal ureterotomy and removal of the calculus.

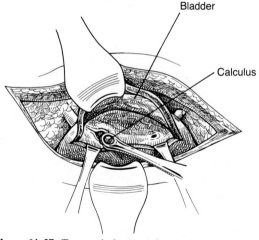

Bladder

Calculus

Figure 64–27. Transvesical approach to a ureteral calculus in the intramural portion of the ureter.

Vaginal Ureterolithotomy. In females a calculus in the distal 5 to 6 cm of the ureter may be palpated on vaginal examination. A simple approach to the calculus may be made through an incision in the anterior vaginal wall, directly over the calculus, as shown in Figure 64–27. In experienced hands, the incidence of postoperative complications is minimal, although a ureterovaginal fistula may develop.

Operative Removal of Calculi in Both the Upper and Lower Regions of the Ureter. Patients may present with multiple stones impacted in the ureter as well as stones in the renal pelvis. The best surgical approach to this problem is the modified flank incision with downward extension (Fig. 64–28*A*). This incision will give exposure to the kidney as well as to most of the ureter, as shown in Figure 64–28*B*.

A.

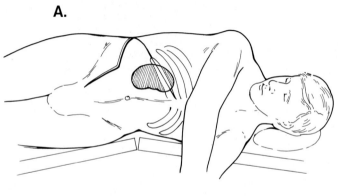

Figure 64–28. Extended flank incision. *A*, Position of the modified twelfth rib flank incision with downward extension. *B*, Exposure of the kidney and ureter through this incision.

B.

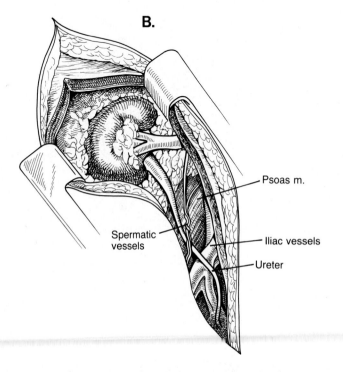

Psoas m.

Spermatic vessels

Iliac vessels

Ureter

If the patient has stones in the upper and lower ureter but not in the renal pelvis, one can use a paramedian incision to approach the ureter on the side involved. The right ureter is approached by mobilizing the hepatic flexure, ascending colon, and cecum medially. The left ureter is approached by mobilizing the splenic flexure and the descending and sigmoid colon medially (Fig. 64–29). Appropriate ureterotomies are made over the various calculi, and the stones are removed. The patency of the ureter is tested in both directions, and the ureterotomies are closed. The area is drained extraperitoneally through stab wounds in the flank, and the colon is reapproximated to its peritoneal attachments.

Operative Removal of Bilateral Ureteral Calculi. When both ureters are obstructed by calculi, they can be approached quite easily through a midline incision (Fig. 64–29). The ureters on either side are approached as described above, and the calculi are removed.

POSTOPERATIVE CARE

Preservation of Renal Function. After the removal of a difficult staghorn calculus that requires renal artery clamping and hypothermia, it is important to maintain good urine output after releasing the vascular clamp. The use of intravenous furosemide (20 to 40 mg intravenously) at periodic intervals is an excellent method to achieve good diuresis. If the central venous pressure is not being monitored, the use of furosemide, particularly in elderly patients, may be associated with a drop in blood pressure. This is usually the result of volume depletion produced by the diuretic, and it can easily be treated with additional intravenous fluids. Central venous pressure monitoring can prevent this problem. Intravenous mannitol (12.5 gm) can also be used to maintain good diuresis in the postoperative period.

Treatment of Associated Urinary Tract Infection. If a patient has a calculus and an

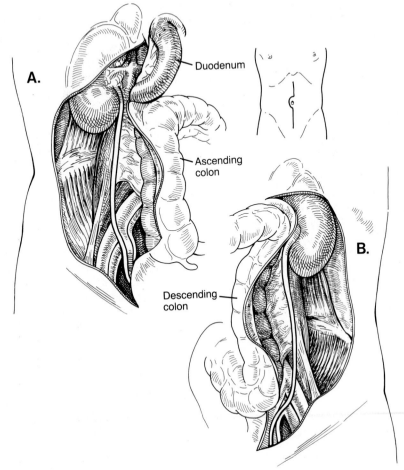

Figure 64–29. The anterior approach to ureteral calculi using a midline incision. *A,* Exposure of the right ureter. *B,* Exposure of the left ureter.

Duodenum

A.

Ascending colon

B.

Descending colon

associated urinary tract infection, parenteral therapy with the antibiotic of choice is usually started 24 to 48 hours before the operation. This is then continued postoperatively for 4 to 5 days or until the patient can be switched to an effective oral antibiotic if one is available. Long-term suppressive therapy is always used with periodic urine cultures obtained to be sure the urine remains sterile.

General Care of the Incision and Drain Site. Since skin clips are usually used, most surgical dressings are removed from the incision after 24 hours, and a dressing remains on only the drain site. If excessive drainage of urine occurs from the Penrose drain site, the enterostomal therapist can easily place a postoperative appliance over this to help keep the patient dry and comfortable.

General Care of the Patient. Intravenous fluids are maintained until the patient has good bowel sounds and is passing gas per rectum. Early ambulation is encouraged, as well as deep breathing and coughing to prevent pulmonary atelectasis. Incentive spirometry as well as chest physiotherapy may be used for patients who have difficulty with their pulmonary secretions.

Prevention of Recurrent Calculi. Once the urinary tract is free of stones, an attempt should be made to prevent any further stone formation. All patients should be on a stone prevention program based on the preoperative metabolic evaluation and analysis of the calculi removed. Increased fluid intake is the cornerstone of all therapy to prevent recurrent calculi. Most patients are instructed in maintaining a diet restricted to 600 mg of calcium. Additional medication is added to the basic program, depending on the cause of the calculus. If an infection was present, long-term suppressive medication is used to try to prevent recurrent infection.

The follow-up program is important. Patients are initially seen 4 to 6 weeks postoperatively to check the incision, obtain a urine culture, and obtain necessary blood studies (e.g., hemoglobin, creatinine).

At 6 months a return visit is scheduled for an intravenous pyelogram, urine culture, and blood chemistries as indicated. Repeat urinary excretion studies may also be obtained. The long-term management program is then determined on the basis of these studies. Periodic surveillance from this time on depends on the needs of the patient.

COMPLICATIONS

Urinary Tract Fistulas. A watertight closure combined with good internal drainage of urine is the goal of every operation in which a calculus is removed from the urinary tract. External drainage in case there is urine leakage must be provided by a Penrose drain. Internal drainage can be provided in several ways, such as by an intact, unobstructed ureter, or by a double J internal Silastic stent in selected patients.

The Penrose drain, if properly positioned, should allow any urine leakage through the suture line to escape to the outside. If this does not occur, the urine will pool in the retroperitoneal space and produce a urinoma, which may become an abscess. A prolonged ileus usually results when this occurs. Incision and drainage of the urinary abscess may then be required.

A urinary fistula can occur in spite of the above described measures and may be handled in a number of ways. An intravenous pyelogram with delayed and oblique films will usually indicate the area of the fistula and also determine the presence or absence of obstruction, which might be produced by a retained stone fragment.

If an internal stent was not used, cystoscopy and passage of a ureteral catheter (size 6 or 7 French) into the renal pelvis should be performed. The ureteral catheter is fixed in position by tying it to an indwelling urethral catheter. If a retained stone fragment is in the ureter, it may be dislodged or bypassed by the ureteral catheter, which will allow the urinary fistula then to close. The stone may pass spontaneously or may require subsequent operative removal.

If the ureteral catheter cannot be introduced beyond a retained stone fragment, surgical removal of the calculus may be required to allow the urinary fistula to close. At the time of removing the calculus an internal stent should be placed in the ureter to promote closure of the fistula.

When a urinary fistula persists in spite of these measures, surgical closure may occasionally be necessary. At the time of closure it is important to provide good external and internal drainage. An attempt should be made to cover the repair with surrounding fatty tissue.

Postoperative Bleeding. Bleeding during the postoperative period may be either internal (manifested by hematuria) or external (manifested by a mass in the retroperitoneal area), usually associated with bloody drainage through the Penrose drain site.

Hematuria nearly always occurs after a nephrolithotomy, but it is usually not severe and is of short duration. Significant bleeding that persists after the operation or occurs as a secondary event may necessitate blood transfusion and ultimately some type of intervention.

The procedure of choice is selective renal angiography, which may demonstrate an actively bleeding vessel within the kidney. This specific vessel can then be occluded by embolization with Gelfoam or an autologous blood clot. Some loss of renal parenchyma may result, but the bleeding is usually controlled. The procedure can be repeated if the first attempt is not successful. Surgical exploration is seldom required unless the bleeding is from some area other than the renal parenchyma.

Persistent Urinary Tract Infection. Inability to eradicate a urinary tract infection during the postoperative period will necessitate further investigation. An intravenous pyelogram should be obtained, with delayed and oblique films to look for retained calculi or obstruction. If either is present, it may be impossible to completely clear the urinary tract infection and the likelihood that more calculi will form is great.

When investigation discloses neither a calculus nor an obstruction, a repeat urine culture and sensitivity study are obtained and the drug therapy altered in an attempt to eradicate the infection. Once the urine is sterile, long-term chemotherapy with periodic urine cultures to monitor the effectiveness of the therapy is essential.

Retained Calculus. A retained calculus is a stone not removed at the time of the operative procedure. If intraoperative roentgenograms are used, the surgeon should be aware of any stones that are left behind at the time of the operation. If a thorough search for retained calculi has been carried out, with inspection of all identified calyces either visually or with a nephroscope, one can assume the stone may be in a minor calyx with a stenosed infundibulum. There is little to be gained by leaving a nephrostomy tube in place to irrigate the collecting system postoperatively, because the stenotic infundibulum will prevent the irrigating fluid from reaching and dissolving the calculus.

Recurrent Calculi. Recurrent calculi are usually the result of persistent urinary tract infections that cannot be eradicated. In some patients without infections, recurrent calculi may be due to either an underlying metabolic disorder that has not been treated (e.g., hyperparathyroidism) or the failure of the patient to follow the stone prevention program.

Prior to undergoing another operative procedure, the patient should be thoroughly evaluated to try to define the cause of the recurrent calculus. In most cases it is due to persistent chronic urinary tract infection. The surgeon must then decide whether further operation with removal of calculi is worthwhile.

RESULTS

Long-term success in the treatment of urinary tract calculi requires (1) complete removal of all calculi, (2) eradication of coexisting urinary tract infections, and (3) a good medical program to prevent further stone formation. Lifelong follow-up must be stressed for patients who are recurrent stone formers.

References

Abbe, R.: Observations on the detection of small renal calculi by the roentgen rays. Ann. Surg., *30*:178, 1899.

Albarran, J.: Radiographic des calculs du rein. A. Franc. d'Urol., *4*:569, 1899.

Bergman, A.: The Ureter. New York, Springer-Verlag, 1981, pp. 265–268.

Blandy, J. P., and Singh, M.: The case for a more aggressive approach to staghorn stones. J. Urol., *115*:505, 1976.

Braasch, W. F., and Carman, R. D.: Renal fluoroscopy at the operating table. JAMA, *73*:1751, 1919.

Brodel, M.: The intrinsic blood vessels of the kidney and their significance in nephrotomy. Bull. Johns Hopkins Hosp., *12*:10, 1901.

Carson, W. J.: Experimental nephrotomies. Surg. Gynecol. Obstet., *42*:53, 1926.

Carson, W. J., and Goldstein, A. E.: Experimental nephrotomies. III. Nephrotomies without sutures in dogs with single kidneys. J. Urol., *15*:505, 1926.

Collins, G. M., Bravo-Shugarman, M., and Terasacki, P. I.: Kidney preservation for transplantation. Lancet, 2:1219, 1971.

Crissey, M. M., and Gittes, R. F.: Dissolution of cystine ureteral calculus by irrigation with tromethamine. J. Urol., *121*:811, 1979.

Cullen, E. K, and Derge, H. F.: The use of silver wire in opening the kidney. Surg. Gynecol. Obstet., *13*:365, 1911.

Czerny, V.: Veber Nierenextripation. Zentralbl. Chir., *6*:737, 1897.

Dees, J. E.: The use of intrapelvic coagulum in pyelolithotomy. South. Med. J., *36*:167, 1943.

Dees, J. E.: The use of fibrinogen coagulum in pyelolithotomy. J. Urol., *56*:271, 1946.

Deming, C. L.: Suture of kidney wounds—experimental. N. Engl. J. Med., *201*:924, 1929.

Drach, G. W.: Urolithiasis. *In* Conn, H. F. (Ed.): Current Therapy. Philadelphia, W. B. Saunders Co., 1976, p. 552.

Dretler, S. P., Pfister, R. C., et al.: Percutaneous catheter dissolution of cystine calculi. J. Urol., *101*:126, 1984.

Fischer, C. P., Sonda, L. P., III, and Diokno, A. C.: Use of cryoprecipitate coagulum in extracting renal calculi. Urology, *15*:6, 1980.

Gibbons, R. P., Correa, R. J., Jr., Cummings, K. B., and Mason, J. T.: Use of the Water-Pik and nephroscope. Urology, *4*:605, 1974.

Gil-Vernet, J.: New surgical concepts in removing renal calculi. Urol. Int., *20*:255, 1965.

Gil-Vernet, J.: Las voies d'abord du bassinet de des calices dans la chirurgie de la lithiese renale. Progrés de la médicine. Paris, 479 Editions Médicales, Flammarion, 1967.

Gittes, R. F., and Belldegrun, A.: Posterior lumbotomy: Surgery for upper tract calculi. Urol. Clin. North Am., *10*:625, 1983.

Glenn, J. F.: Urologic Surgery. Philadelphia, J. B. Lippincott Co., 1983, pp. 181–194.

Graves, F. T.: The anatomy of the intrarenal arteries and its application to segmental resection of the kidney. Br. J. Surg., *42*:132, 1954.

Graves, F. T.: The anatomy of the intrarenal arteries in health and disease. Br. J. Surg., *43*:605, 1956.

Harrison, J. H., Gittes, R. F., Perlmutter, A. D., Stamey, T. A., and Walsh, P. C. (Eds.): Campbell's Urology. 4th ed. Philadelphia, W. B. Saunders Co., 1979, pp. 2033–2042.

Harrison, L. H., and Nordan, J. M.: Anatrophic nephrotomy for the removal of renal calculi. Urol. Clin. North Am., *1*:333, 1974.

Hevan, P.: Recherches historiques et critiques sur la nephrotomie ou taille du rein. Mem. Acad. R. Chir., *3*:238, 1778.

Hippocrates, quoted by Murphy, L. J. T.: The History of Urology. Springfield, Ill., Charles C Thomas, 1972, p. 72.

Jacobs, S. C., and Gittes, R. F.: Dissolution of residual renal calculi with Remiacidrin. J. Urol., *115*:2, 1976.

Kaufman, J. J., and Woo, Y.: Further studies of renal preservation: Protection of the ischemic kidney with inosine. Trans. Am. Assoc. G.U. Surg., *69*:131, 1978.

Kelly, H. A.: Diseases of the kidney, ureter, and bladder. Vol. I. London, Appleton Publisher, 1915.

Lower, W. E.: Conservative surgical methods in operating for stone in the kidney. Cleve. Med. J., *12*:260, 1913.

Marberger, M., et al.: Simultaneous balloon occlusion of the renal artery and hypothermia perfusion in in-situ surgery of the kidney. J. Urol., *119*:453, 1978.

Marshall, S., Lyon, R. P., and Scott, M. P., Jr.: Further simplications for coagulum pyelolithotomy. J. Urol., *119*:588, 1978.

McDonald, J. E., and Henneman, P. H.: Stone dissolution in-vivo and control of cystinuria with D-penicillamine. N. Engl. J. Med., *273*:578, 1965.

Morris, H.: A case of nephrolithotomy or the extraction of a calculus from an undilated kidney. Trans. Clin. Soc. (London), *14*:31, 1881.

Novick, A. C., and Straffon, R. A.: Vascular Problems in Urologic Surgery. Philadelphia, W. B. Saunders Co., 1982.

Patel, V. J.: The coagulum pyelolithotomy. Br. J. Surg., *60*:230, 1973.

Pence, J. R., II, Airhart, R. A., and Novicki, D. E.: Coagulum pyelolithotomy. Letter. J. Urol., *125*:134, 1981.

Quinby, W. C.: A note on localization of renal calculi by the aid of x-ray film made during operation. J. Urol., *13*:59, 1925.

Reid, F., and Finlayson, B.: Anatrophic nephrolithotomy. Letter. J. Urol., *22*:428, 1979.

Robson, A. W. M.: A method of operating on the kidney without division of muscles, vessels, or nerves. Lancet, *1*:1315, 1898.

Roth, R. A., and Finlayson, B.: Stones: Clinical Management of Urolithiasis. Baltimore, The Williams & Wilkins Co., 1983.

Smith, M. J. V., and Boyce, W. H.: Anatrophic nephrolithotomy and plastic calyorrhaphy. Trans. Am. Assoc. G.U. Surg. *59*:18, 1967.

Stewart, B. H.: Operative Urology: The Kidneys, Adrenal Glands, and Retroperitoneum. Baltimore, The Williams & Wilkins Co., 1975.

Stowe, N., et al.: Protective effects of propranolol in the treatment of ischemically damaged canine kidneys prior to transplantation. Surgery, *84*:265, 1978.

Stueber, P., et al.: Regional renal hypothermia. Surgery, *44*:77, 1958.

Thomas, W. C., Jr.: Clinical concepts of renal calculus disease. J. Urol., *113*:423, 1975.

CHAPTER 65

Surgical Management of Ureteropelvic Junction Obstruction

ANTHONY J. SCHAEFFER, M.D.
JOHN T. GRAYHACK, M.D.

INTRODUCTION

Dilatation of the renal pelvis and calyces, commonly called hydronephrosis, may be caused by a variety of pathologic, anatomic, and physiologic conditions. However, obstruction to the flow of urine is the most common cause. The designation "ureteropelvic junction obstruction" indicates the site of obstruction and is usually reserved for causes that are not related to calculus. Traditionally, the diagnosis of hydronephrosis due to ureteropelvic junction obstruction has been based on functional and anatomic observations on intravenous and retrograde urography. Recognition and assessment of ureteropelvic junction obstruction are achieved by a combination of objective and subjective indicators. Symptoms of flank pain associated with progressive renal pelvic dilatation, deterioration of renal function, and signs of significant renal stasis, such as stone and infection, are accepted as indicators of clinically significant ureteropelvic junction obstruction that warrants serious consideration for surgical correction. Unfortunately, the presence and clinical significance of ureteral obstruction are often difficult to establish. Anatomic renal changes resembling hydronephrosis can occur without true obstruction. For example, dilatation of the renal pelvis, or pyelectasis, may be a functionally insignificant variation of normal. Calycectasis may be due to chronic inflammatory disease or a nonobstructive congenital enlargement (megacalycosis) due to a malformation of the renal papillae (Gittes and Talner, 1972). Conversely, obstruction of the uretero-pelvic junction may be present but of no clinical significance, or only intermittently so. On the other hand, minimal anatomic obstruction that is clinically significant can be very difficult to detect in its early stages. It is hoped that new diagnostic modalities, such as nephroscopy and retrograde ureteropyeloscopy, will provide opportunities to assess trabeculation and other physiologic responses to true obstruction. Such direct techniques are expected to complement the radiologic and physiologic studies that are currently used to diagnose ureteropelvic junction obstruction.

PATHOGENESIS OF URETEROPELVIC JUNCTION OBSTRUCTION

Most upper ureteral lesions that produce hydronephrosis are incomplete obstructions and vary widely in genesis and anatomy. They may be either congenital or acquired obstructions and can be classified as follows:

Congenital:
1. Segmental dysfunction
2. Intrinsic ureteral stricture
3. Kinks, adhesions, bands, or valves
4. Ureterovascular tangle
5. Obstructive high insertion

Acquired:
1. Postinflammation or ischemic scarring or fixation
2. Kinking or fixation due to ureterovesical reflux
3. Tumors

Segmental dysfunction, intrinsic ureteral strictures, and ureteral kinks are the most common causes of ureteropelvic junction obstruction in children (McMartin et al., 1957). Other causes, such as high insertion of the ureter, ureterovascular tangle, or acquired stricture secondary to inflammation or ischemia, are more common in adults (Persky and Tynberg, 1973).

Congenital Obstructions

Segmental Dysfunction. An adynamic segment in the lumbar or proximal ureter produces a functional obstruction that may be indistinguishable by x-ray from a mechanical obstruction. The obstruction appears to be initiated by a congenital, segmental lack or anatomic distortion of the ureteral muscle that adversely affects normal peristalsis (Foote et al., 1970; Allen, 1970). The degree of interference with normal peristaltic urine transport will determine the ultimate extent and progression of the obstruction (Foote, 1970). At the time of surgery an adynamic segment may be difficult to identify and appears as a grossly normal ureter with calibration of 14 to 16 French. The lesion may be bilateral but unrecognizable as such until, after contralateral nephrectomy, a full water load is placed on the now inadequate system. Peripelvic and periureteral fibrosis and scarring may be superimposed secondarily on the obstruction by the mechanical trauma of intermittent pelvic distention.

Intrinsic Ureteral Stricture. Most congenital ureteral strictures occur at the ureteropelvic junction, although they may develop at any point along the lumbar ureter. Strictures usually measure 1 to 2 mm in length; however, some may be fusiform and 1 to 3 cm long. They characteristically produce incomplete obstructions that may lead to secondary kinking. This type of obstruction is present in a high percentage of hydronephrotic ectopic and anomalous kidneys. Failure to recognize multiple obstructed sites will result in treatment failure. Electron microscopy has demonstrated excessive collagen fibers between and around muscle cells at the obstruction and in compromised muscle cells proximal to the collagenous segment (Hanna, 1976). This produces an inelastic stenotic collar that impedes urine flow and causes obstructive changes in the proximal kidney tissues.

Kinks, Adhesions, Bands, or Valves. Retention of congenital and developmental kinks or valves commonly found in the lumbar ure-

teral segment of developing fetuses has been postulated to play a part in subsequent intrinsic ureteral obstruction (Ostling, 1942). The most common obstructions found in infants and children are folds and stenosis at or just below the ureteropelvic junction (Johnston et al., 1977). Congenital kinks and angulation account for approximately two thirds of ureteropelvic junction obstructions in children.

Ureterovascular Tangle. So-called aberrant renal vessels have been associated with approximately one third of ureterovesical junction obstructions. Whether the vessel, ureter, or bulging pelvis is the primary obstruction has been controversial. The term "aberrant" favors the vessel as the primary cause, although this term is a misnomer (Stephens, 1982). A lower hilar segmental vessel may arise from any point along the course of the main renal artery or from the aorta, and all such variants are normal. An artery that enters the lower pole directly has been termed an accessory or aberrant vessel. However, Graves (1971) found that these vessels were the main segmental vessels to the lower pole and therefore were neither accessory nor aberrant. In a study of hydronephrosis caused by ureteropelvic obstruction and accompanied by a ureterovascular tangle, the vessel implicated was the lower anterior hilar segmental artery, which forms before or during rotation of the kidney and gains entrance into the hilus across the ureteropelvic junction anterior to the pelvis. This vessel is not obstructing if normal rotation of the kidney occurs. However, if rotation is arrested, as with the horseshoe kidney, or is retarded or incomplete, the pelvis remains fixed in its anterior orientation with respect to the renal vessels, and the ureteropelvic junction is vulnerable to compression by the lower segmental branch (Fig. 65–1). This anterior pelvis bulges between the middle and lower vessels and hooks up and angulates the ureter over the artery, causing ureteropelvic obstruction (Stephens, 1982). Although anterior orientation of the pelvis occurs early in development of the embryo, the obstruction induced by the vessel is only partial initially; serious obstructive crises usually develop only when sufficient time has elapsed to permit severe pelvic ballooning. Hence, the onset of the symptoms of pain indicating intermittent obstructive crisis may be delayed until school age or even later.

Obstructive High Insertion. Obstructive high pelvic insertion of the ureter is a distinctive type of deformity (Fig. 65–2). Whether the high insertion of the ureter is actually primary or is a secondary phenomenon associated with peri-

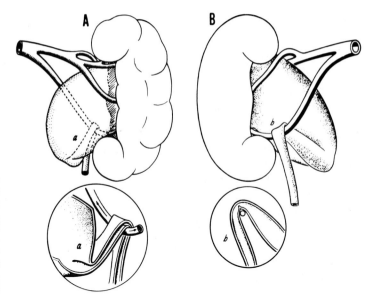

Figure 65–1. Ureterovascular hydrone-phrosis. *A*, Anterior view. *B*, Posterior view. Pelvis protrudes anteriorly between the middle and lower segmental vessels, angulating the ureteropelvic junction and hooking the upper ureter over vessel. Insets show flattening and obstructive mechanisms at ureteropelvic junction and upper ureter. (From Barnett, J. S., and Stephens, F. D.: Aust. N.Z. J. Surg., *31*:201, 1962.)

pelvic fibrosis, due to infection or ureterovesical reflux and progressive asymmetric pelvic dilatation with relative superior migration of the ureteropelvic junction, is controversial. Once the defect is established, it becomes irreversible and is functionally obstructive even without stenosis. This lesion is infrequently diagnosed in children and is nearly always associated with renal ectopia or fusion (Zincke et al., 1974).

Acquired Obstructions

Postinflammation or Ischemic Scarring or Fixation. Ureteropelvic junction obstruction

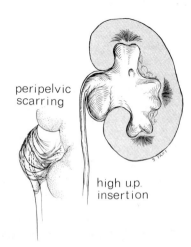

peripelvic scarring

high u.p. insertion

Figure 65–2. Obstructive high pelvic insertion combined with progressive pelvic distention may be congenital or acquired as the result of infection or ureterovesical reflux.

may be acquired following injury or inflammation owing to stones or prior surgical intervention and has been reported secondary to ischemia. Friedland et al. (1974) reported a 74-year-old woman who developed a narrow stricture due to fibrosis in the submucosa and muscle at the ureteropelvic junction 3 years after a radiologic study suggesting spasm in the same area. The histologic picture was similar to that seen in myocardial and colonic ischemia. The prevalence of ischemic ureteral stricture in acquired ureteropelvic junction obstruction is unknown.

Kinking or Fixation Due to Ureterovesical Reflux. Ureterovesical reflux may produce ureteral kinking, periureteral fibrosis, and fixation, causing ureteropelvic junction obstruction. High insertion of the ureter into the renal pelvis is frequently an associated factor.

Tumors. Benign tumors, such as polyps, as well as malignant neoplasms can produce obstruction at the ureteropelvic junction. The malignancy can be a primary urothelial tumor, an extrinsic primary tumor, or an intrinsic or extrinsic metastatic lesion.

Bilaterality and Associated Genitourinary Anomalies

Whatever the cause of congenital ureteropelvic junction obstruction, there is a definite tendency toward bilateral involvement. The incidence ranges from 15 to 40 per cent (Drake et al., 1978; Roth and Gonzales, 1983; Perlmutter et al., 1980) and is highest in patients younger than 1 year. In many cases the dilatation of the renal pelvis is more pronounced on one side than the other. Asynchronous presentation of bilateral ureteropelvic junction obstruction has also been reported with as long as a 9-year interval between manifestations of obstruction of the two sides (Michigan et al., 1978; Williams et al., 1966).

Associated genitourinary anomalies are frequently encountered in children with ureteropelvic junction obstruction. Duplex pelvis, vesicoureteral reflux, and contralateral absent or dysplastic kidney are most frequently encountered (Johnston et al., 1977; Drake et al., 1978). In infants, the contralateral kidney frequently manifests multicystic dysplasia, a diagnosis that becomes increasingly likely in the absence of function on urography (Zincke et al., 1974).

CLINICAL PRESENTATION

The age distribution of patients presenting with ureteropelvic junction obstruction is surprisingly relatively uniform from infancy through old age (Koff, 1982; Culp, 1967; Roberts and Slade, 1964). Ureteropelvic junction obstruction is more common in male than in female children at a ratio of approximately 2:1, in particular in children younger than 1 year (Johnston et al., 1977; Zincke et al., 1974; Williams and Karlaftis, 1966). In adults it is evenly distributed between the sexes (Roberts and Slade, 1964).

Hydronephrosis is a relatively common renal problem that is usually, but not always, straightforward in its presentation. In newborns and infants, the most common finding is a palpable abdominal mass in the flank, frequently in association with abnormal urinary sediment. Azotemia due to bilateral hydronephrosis is also not uncommon. The palpable mass is typically huge, often extends beyond the midline, and can be transilluminated (Perlmutter et al., 1980). A history suggestive of urinary tract infection or failure to thrive is another common presenting clinical feature (Johnston et al., 1977; Drake et al., 1978). In a recent report, approximately 12 per cent of ureteropelvic junction obstructions in infants were found during contrast studies to evaluate other anomalies such as congenital heart disease (Roth and Gonzales, 1983). In older children the early symptom is usually vague, intermittent abdominal pain that is notorious for mimicking gastrointestinal disorders (Kelalis et al., 1971). Episodic flank or back pain or discomfort that is at times associated with nausea and vomiting is common. Spontaneous or post-traumatic hematuria should also raise suspicion of hydronephrosis.

The majority of affected adults will give a history of symptoms that have existed for many years. The most common may be complaints of vague back pain of varying degrees of severity, often exacerbated by diuresis after excessive fluid intake. A history of recurrent urinary tract infection or observation of persistent pyuria may signal the presence of ureteropelvic junction obstruction (Nesbitt et al., 1964; Roberts and Slade, 1964). Hematuria, particularly following trauma, is another presenting symptom. Ureteropelvic junction obstruction should always be suspected in patients who present with renal pelvic calculi. Renal obstruction, even unilateral, may present with a clinical picture suggestive of renal vascular hypertension (Riehle and Vaughan, 1981).

DIAGNOSTIC STUDIES

Intravenous Urography, Ultrasonography, CAT Scan. In patients with suspected ureteral obstruction, the goal of a diagnostic evaluation is to demonstrate its presence, site, and functional significance. In most persons, the initial evidence for a ureteropelvic junction obstruction is provided by intravenous urography (Fig. 65–3). The affected renal unit may show findings ranging from complete nonvisualization to a typical hydronephrosis to a promptly visualized, anatomically normal collecting system. Delayed films for 24 hours or more are useful and may be necessary to demonstrate the secondary anatomic changes resulting from the probable site of the obstruction. Hydration or drug-induced diuresis may accentuate the effects of an obstructing or potentially obstructing lesion and may facilitate the diagnosis. At times, as in some patients with intermittent hydronephrosis, satisfactory demonstration of the obstruction is possible only when the patient is symptomatic with flank pain (Bourne, 1966). Both ultrasonography and CAT scan may be useful to demonstrate that the nonfunctional status of a kidney on intravenous urography is associated with hydronephrosis rather than some other cause. However, aside from the demonstration of the presence of a nonopaque stone or a mass lesion, these techniques do not usually demonstrate the site or the probable cause of a ureteropelvic junction obstruction.

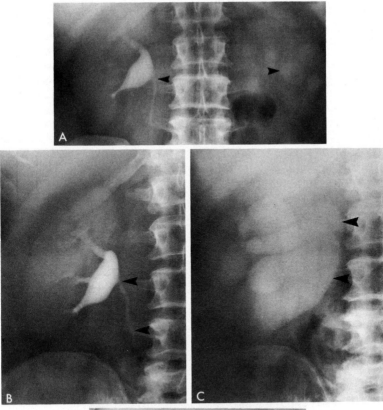

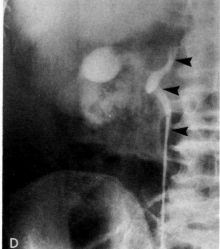

Figure 65–3. *Unexpected acquired marked hydronephrosis following contralateral nephrectomy. A,* Intravenous urogram of a 49-year-old male (October 1968) shows left hydronephrosis secondary to papillary carcinoma of renal pelvis. Patient had left flank pain and total gross hematuria. Radical left nephrectomy and total ureterectomy with bladder cuff was performed. Note "normal-appearing" right kidney with some suggestion of unobstructed high ureteropelvic placement. Patient had no previous history of renal problems. Note the normal ureteral caliber.

B, Closer look at insidious congenital right ureteropelvic junction defect and normal lumbar ureter (this was a 15-minute film of the original intravenous urogram). At this point the kidney was considered well compensated, and there was little x-ray evidence to indicate the drastic subsequent results of increased water load.

C, Patient was not seen for 7 years (until April 1975, at the age of 56). Since the left nephrectomy performed in 1968 he had been asymptomatic except for gradual onset of general malaise (uremia) of 3 to 4 months' duration. His creatinine level was 5.2; blood urea nitrogen was 71; and there was marked anemia. There was no right flank pain at any time. On intravenous (high-dose) urography a 6-hour delayed film shows massive right hydronephrosis secondary to incomplete ureteropelvic obstruction. Urine was sterile.

D, Ureteropyelogram obtained just before surgery shows a flap valve type obstructive high insertion of ureter in the renal pelvis. There is distortion and compression of the proximal lumbar ureter with adherence to the dilated pelvis by acquired dense enveloping layers of peripelvic and periureteral fibrous tissue. (Note the distorted course of the ureter between markers.)

All of these findings were verified during dismembered Foley Y-plasty repair, resection of redundant pelvis and ureter with stenting, and nephrostomy diversion. The obstruction was primarily an adynamic segment with secondary fibrous angulation and compression. The ureteral caliber was normal. (Compare these changes in relationship of the pelvis and upper lumbar ureter with those in *B.*)

Retrograde or Antegrade Pyelography.
Retrograde pyelography is the procedure of choice for demonstrating the site and the nature of a ureteropelvic junction abnormality. It has the advantage of being independent of function and, of significant importance, permitting visualization of the ureter distal to the recognized obstructing site. The disadvantages of this procedure are (1) the necessity for cystoscopy, making it difficult and possibly hazardous in infants; and (2) the risk of introduction of infection at the time of ureteral catheterization and retrograde instillation of contrast medium. The risk of infection can be managed by meticulous attention to sterile technique; instillation of an antibiotic, such as neomycin, with the contrast medium; and performance of the retrograde study just before the planned surgical procedure, if possible. In infants, percutaneous antegrade pyelography can be used to achieve excellent visualization of the urinary tract proximal to the obstruction, but, unfortunately, the distal ureter may be difficult to visualize adequately with this technique. The percutaneous catheter can be left in place to provide drainage and allow limited preoperative assessment of renal function. The placement and retention of percutaneous catheters may produce bleeding and an inflammatory reaction that will complicate the surgical repair. In general, the limited risks involved in achieving an accurate preoperative assessment of the site and degree of obstruction are justified, as are studies of the urinary tract distal to the obstruction.

Cystography. The importance of evaluating a patient for vesicoureteral reflux warrants consideration routinely. Although reflux is rarely associated with ureteropelvic junction obstruction (Johnston et. al., 1977; Zincke et al., 1974), its recognition, if it is present, is important. Reflux may produce the appearance of an obstruction of the ureteropelvic junction. Furthermore, Shopfner (1966) has suggested that long-standing vesicoureteral reflux and concomitant infection eventually may produce secondary changes of the ureteropelvic junction and permanent ureteropelvic junction obstruction. If vesicoureteral reflux and equivocal ureteropelvic junction obstruction are identified, a trial of continuous bladder drainage should be instituted. If definite improvement of the hydronephrosis with satisfactory emptying is demonstrated on repeat intravenous urogram or furosemide renogram, then ureteropelvic junction obstruction is probably secondary to vesicoureteral reflux.

Renal Isotope Studies. Renal isotope studies are particularly useful in studying the non- or poorly functioning kidney and in assessing the significance of pyelectasis and calycectasis. Technetium-99m dimercaptosuccinic acid (DMSA), a renal cortical labeling agent, is distributed to each kidney in proportion to the relative functioning tubular mass. This allows evaluation of the relative function of the renal mass present in each kidney at a given time. It does not allow the effect of relief of obstruction on this assessed renal function to be evaluated, however. The response of accumulated technetium-99m diethylenetriaminepenta acetic acid (DTPA) to administration of a diuretic is useful to differentiate the obstructed dilated upper urinary tract from the nonobstructed dilated upper urinary tract (Stage and Lewis, 1981; Thrall et al., 1981). This procedure is based on the hypothesis that prolonged retention of the isotope in a nonobstructed dilated system is due to a reservoir effect that can be diminished by the washout effect of increased urine flow after diuretic administration. Conversely, in the dilated obstructed system, retention of isotope proximal to the obstruction should persist even after administration of a diuretic. Normally, a prompt uptake of radionuclide in the first 1 to 5 minutes of the study is followed by a spontaneous washout of the radionuclide even before the furosemide is administered (Fig. 65–4). In the presence of obstruction, an initial slow excretion is followed by prolonged accumulation of radioactivity in the dilated system. The curve may plateau or continue to increase progres-

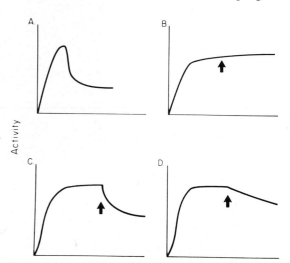

Figure 65–4. Schematic representation of response categories observed with diuretic radionuclide renogram. *A,* Normal pattern. *B,* Obstructed pattern. *C,* Dilated nonobstructed pattern. *D,* Equivocal pattern. Arrows indicate time of furosemide administration. (From Weiss, R. M.: Am. J. Kidney Dis., *11:*409, 1983.)

sively. Intravenous administration of a diuretic does not effect a significant washout of the radioactivity. In the dilated but unobstructed system, the initial portion of the renogram curve is similar to that observed with obstruction, with a slow uptake and gradual accumulation of radioactivity in the dilated system. However, in contrast to the pattern observed with obstruction, administration of an intravenous diuretic is followed by a prompt and effective washout of the radionuclide. Thus, the hallmark of significant obstruction is a failure of renal radioactivity to decrease after diuretic administration. An equivocal pattern, with accumulation and minimal or moderate washout of radionuclide after administration of a diuretic, may be present if a limited obstruction exists or a reduced diuresis results. Misleading results may be due to radioactivity in an overdistended bladder or because of reflux of radioactive urine.

Perfusion Studies. Antegrade perfusion studies eliminate reliance on renal function to achieve high fluid flow rates and allow a direct assessment of upper tract pressures in an attempt to differentiate dilated systems that are obstructed from those that are not (Whitaker, 1973, 1978). The technique requires percutaneous puncture of the upper urinary tract to place a catheter in the renal pelvis. Pressures are monitored while the upper urinary tract is perfused at 10 ml per minute. The bladder is continuously drained to eliminate its effect on urine transport. Evidence suggests that the upper urinary tract can transport 10 ml per minute without a significant increase in pressure (12 to 15 cm of water). A minor degree of obstruction that can handle this rate of flow need not be repaired, since, it is assumed, the pressure in the system is not sufficient to produce renal deterioration. Pressures above 12 to 15 cm of water are considered to indicate significant obstruction and correlate with deterioration of renal function. The Whitaker test is based on the assumption that high intrapelvic pressure causes nephron damage. There is limited evidence to suggest that low pressures do not affect renal function or that the presence of high pressures is associated with a clinically significant lesion. When properly performed, the Whitaker test provides information that is particularly useful as part of an overall assessment of a questionable or apparent ureteropelvic junction obstruction. This approach to evaluation of a possible ureteral obstruction has some disadvantages that should be considered. These include the fact that it is invasive, is difficult to repeat for follow-up studies, and shows overlap between partially obstructed and nonobstructed systems.

Differential Diagnosis

As noted by O'Conor (1955), it is "often difficult to distinguish between the large normal pelvis and early hydronephrosis. In the former, the minor calyces are not flattened, clubbed, or dilated, whereas the early hydronephrotic calyces always showed distortion from the usual umbilicated outline." Demonstration of delayed emptying of the renal pelvis also provides a good differential diagnostic point and furthermore suggests that early hydronephrosis is present. Some calyceal deformities seen on x-ray may be attributable to congenital megacalyces that mimic hydronephrotic calyceal changes. Congenital megacalyces, or megacalycosis, is a nonobstructive enlargement of the calyces due to malformation of the renal papillae. Despite the calyceal deformity, the infundibula are normal or widened and the renal pelvis shows no dilatation, shows no smooth muscle hypertrophy of its wall, and has a well-funneled outlet into a ureter of normal caliber. The kidney is normal-sized to slightly enlarged, with a smooth surface. The renal cortex is grossly and histologically normal (Gittes and Talner, 1972).

The possibility of unrecognized ureteropelvic junction obstruction warrants serious consideration in patients with pelvic stones or urinary tract infection. The relationship of these conditions is well recognized, and effective management demands correction of all the abnormalities present. Ureteropelvic junction obstruction may also be caused by a polyp or tumor within the ureteropelvic junction.

INDICATIONS FOR TREATMENT

Obstruction producing functional impairment or symptoms or leading to chronic infection or stone is usually considered an indication for treatment of ureteropelvic junction obstruction. The goals of therapy are to preserve or improve renal function, relieve the patient's symptoms, eliminate infection, and, if possible, restore anatomic normality. Reproducible objective evidence of the presence and significance of ureteral obstruction with regard to symptoms, infection, and impaired renal function is obviously a prerequisite for treatment. Once the need for and goals of therapy are established, certain factors warrant consideration in selection of the type of treatment. Both the decision to undertake surgical repair and the selection of the type of procedure are influenced by the age of the patient. Infants, children, and young adults are particularly appropriate candidates for surgical intervention attempting to conserve renal function, particularly when the disease is bilateral or involves a solitary kidney. Likewise, correction of progressive or symptomatic unilateral obstruction of an apparently salvageable kidney should be seriously considered for patients of all ages. Circumstances in which the likelihood of a successful surgical procedure is compromised, such as unusual or complicated congenital anomalies or a kidney with long-standing infection, should be recognized. It is important to assess the probability of and need for successfully correcting the obstruction and achieving the goals of pyeloureteroplasty. In elderly or chronically ill individuals with unilateral disease, reparative surgery may not be indicated. Minimal asymptomatic, uninfected ureteropelvic junction obstruction in middle-aged adults or older individuals warrants consideration for nonoperative management and periodic evaluation. If preoperative evaluation indicates nonfunction with significantly compromised renal parenchyma and if intraoperative evaluation demonstrates minimal, scarred renal parenchyma, nephrectomy rather than surgical reconstruction is appropriate.

The choice of surgical procedure is also influenced by the probable cause of the ureteropelvic junction obstruction and the status of the opposite kidney and lower urinary tract. Recognition of bilateral disease is important in assessing management options. For example, uninfected hydronephrosis of an equal degree may be repaired sequentially or, particularly in neonates or infants, simultaneously. If both kidneys are considered salvageable but are unequally affected, the more severely damaged kidney should generally be operated on first unless the contralateral side is more symptomatic. When the more obstructed kidney is repaired, the less obstructed kidney may remain unchanged and well compensated for years. If the better of the two kidneys is infected, it should be repaired first, after the infection has been controlled. The poor side should be repaired as soon as is practicable in order to obtain the maximal salvage of renal function. Similarly, when calculi are present in one kidney, that kidney should be repaired first. If bilateral stones are present, the size, number, configuration, and composition of the stones are im-

portant considerations in assessing the likelihood of their producing ureteral obstruction and of their being completely removed. Finally, when there is little evidence of function on one side and significant hydronephrosis on the other, the better kidney should be repaired initially. When adequate function has been achieved, the contralateral, severely obstructed, poorly functioning kidney can be removed or reconstruction can be attempted, depending on the accumulated preoperative and operative observations. If contralateral surgery is delayed, evidence that maximum benefit from the initial surgery has been achieved should be obtained.

When ureteropelvic junction obstruction coexists with vesicoureteral reflux, the ureteropelvic junction obstruction should be repaired first. A nondismembered type of pyeloureteroplasty warrants primary consideration in an effort to preserve as much ureteral arterial blood supply as possible. Vesicoureteroplasty should not be performed until there is satisfactory evidence of a successful pyeloureteroplasty. With chronic infection, stones, or extensive upper tract damage, placement and retention of a nephrostomy tube will assure adequate drainage of the pelvis until the vesicoureteral repair is performed.

MANAGEMENT ALTERNATIVES

Continued Observation. Asymptomatic patients with minimal radiographic evidence of ureteropelvic junction obstruction can be observed without intervention. These obstructions usually are discovered incidentally on excretory urography, ultrasonography, or CAT scan carried out to seek other abdominal pathologic conditions. The recommendation to observe a patient is based on the premise that ureteropelvic junction obstruction will be stable or, if it does progress, that it will do so gradually. Experience such as that reported by Nesbitt et al. (1964), who monitored 24 patients with ureteropelvic junction obstruction for 14 months to 9 years without finding evidence of symptomatic or radiologic progression, justifies the practice of observing rather than operating on selected patients. However, this approach is not without risk. A rapid increase of ureteropelvic junction obstruction has been observed in some children and adults (Hinman et al., 1983; McAlister et al., 1980). Furthermore, although this change in status is often symptomatic, obstruction causing a nonfunctioning kidney can develop without warning. Patients with a box pelvis laid down without a tapering outlet (Hinman et al., 1983) and those with repetitive episodes of diuresis are at significant risk of accelerated obstruction. During the crest of the diuretic phase, the marginal ureteropelvic junction cannot transport the volume it receives, and thus the pelvis decompensates further. Contralateral renal failure also increases the excretory load, resulting in progression of hydronephrosis in the remaining kidney (Jacobs et al., 1979; Michigan et al., 1978).

Nephrectomy. Preservation of functioning renal tissue is a primary consideration in advising treatment of ureteropelvic junction obstruction. Nevertheless, nephrectomy is the treatment of choice for some patients, because of the high probability that useful function cannot be salvaged, because of the improbability of a successful surgical outcome, or because of a patient's general status and life expectancy. The status of the contralateral kidney is always a major consideration in the decision to recommend removal of a kidney. In general, nephrectomy is indicated in the following circumstances: (1) The kidney is nonfunctioning on both radionuclide and radiographic studies and shows a hydronephrotic shell on intravenous urography; (2) the kidney is hypoplastic or dysplastic and is associated with obstructive symptoms; and (3) the obstruction has resulted in significant circulatory problems or extensive stone disease and infection as well as significant functional impairment in an adult with a normal contralateral kidney. For patients who have had repeated failed pyeloureteroplasties, technical considerations may lead to a decision to remove the kidney. In individuals with a long life expectancy, however, pyeloureteroplasty or a variety of more complex reconstructive procedures warrant serious consideration and may be justified even if the chance of satisfactory postsurgical status is limited.

Nephrostomy. Formal isolated operative nephrostomy is rarely indicated in the management of ureteropelvic junction obstruction. It may be necessary to decompress the obstructed kidney in an acutely infected symptomatic patient. If a ureteral catheter or stent or percutaneous nephrostomy tube cannot be inserted or does not function satisfactorily, nephrostomy drainage is occasionally employed to achieve maximal renal functional improvement in patients with bilateral obstruction or obstruction of a solitary kidney. It may also be instituted to assess achievable functional return in unilateral obstruction. Nephrostomy is a useful procedure to relieve obstruction resulting from complications following pyeloureteroplasty. Unquestionably, the use of percutaneous nephrostomy is increasingly replacing formal operative nephrostomy in our practice. The reluctance to carry out transcutaneous renal drainage prior to pyeloureteroplasty is based on the concern that these procedures may produce changes in the kidney and renal area ranging from hematuria and scarring to infection that will compromise the planned surgical attempt to correct the existing obstruction.

Pyeloureteroplasty. Pyeloureteroplasty is the procedure of choice when the kidney is judged to have significant salvageable function on the basis of preoperative evaluation. The status of the contralateral kidney is a major factor in considering treatment alternatives for a patient with ureteropelvic junction obstruction. Preservation of functioning renal tissue is of particular concern in patients with long life expectancy.

GENERAL PRINCIPLES OF TREATMENT

Incision. Adequate exposure is essential for performance of a pyeloureteroplasty. Although an abdominal transperitoneal approach is used by some, our prejudice is that ureteropelvic junction repair in adults is technically easier and adequate drainage is more certain with a flank incision. The flank incision should be made either just below or through the bed of the eleventh or twelfth rib. The transperitoneal approach may be satisfactory in thin individuals but is difficult in obese patients and those with peritoneal adhesions associated with previous operations. In young children and infants, a transperitoneal or extraperitoneal approach to the kidney may be obtained through a high transverse, anterolateral abdominal incision. This approach is preferable in an infant or a small child presenting with a large low-lying kidney, particularly when the diagnosis remains uncertain. In young children with bilateral hydronephrosis, simultaneous transperitoneal or extraperitoneal pyeloureteroplasties can be accomplished with excellent results (Perlmutter et al., 1980; Drake et al., 1978).

Extraperitoneal exposure of a horseshoe kidney can be accomplished readily through a flank incision if it is placed low and extended medially rather than into the costovertebral angle. If both pelves require repair in conjunction with horseshoe abnormality, exposure is best accomplished through a midline transperitoneal incision.

Ureteral Stent. The ureteral stent, once considered an integral part of ureteropelvic reconstruction, is now used infrequently and selectively by most urologists (Hamm and Weinberg, 1955). The tubeless technique has been adopted by many in an attempt to reduce the risk of postoperative infection and iatrogenic ureteral injury. Stenting is used selectively with varying frequency to reduce the risk of disruption of suture lines with urinary extravasation, to ensure maintenance of proper alignment of the ureter, and to facilitate and direct ureteral regeneration. Stents are employed commonly in complicated repairs when the conditions are not optimal. Their use warrants serious consideration in patients with scarring from previous surgical procedures, chronic renal infections, or extensive stone disease. They are also often employed if the anastomosis of the ureter and pelvis is technically compromised.

Although the incidence of stricture due to stenting is not established, concern that the stent may contribute to, rather than reduce, fibrosis and scarring has been a major limitation of its use. The lumbar ureteral lumen may normally vary in its internal caliber (Ostling, 1942). If areas of relative narrowing are unrecognized, ureteral stents may produce ureteral ischemia and partial necrosis leading to stricture formation. This is especially true for small ureters in infants and children.

Ureteral Calibration. The diagnosis of ureteral stricture is best made radiographically (especially with cineradiography) before surgery. The preoperative assessment can be verified at surgery by noting the relative thickness of the muscle above and below the obstructive site and by observing pelvic and ureteral peristalsis. To facilitate the latter, the pelvis is filled via a small needle. Obstruction will be demonstrated by ineffective, interrupted peristalsis. Calibration is difficult to perform and evaluate and should be used only to confirm the radiographic impression.

Stent Technique. The ureteral stent should be placed through the reconstructed ureteropelvic anastomosis from the opened pelvis. A pliable, inert, lubricated stent should be small enough so that it passes readily through the ureter. Silicone, Silastic, or other inert pliable tubing of appropriate size can be used. The proper catheter will slip easily into the normal ureter. Although the end of the stent is commonly placed in the ureter, we prefer to place the end of the catheter in the bladder to prevent mucosal erosion of the ureter by the tip. A catheter that fits snugly is too large. Several

small holes can be made in the portion of the stent that will lie within the renal pelvis. These holes will allow the urine to pass to the bladder or the exterior if the nephrostomy tube fails to function properly. If the stent is to be exteriorized, as is usually the case, it should be brought through a calyx that will allow it to be positioned so it will not distort or put tension on the anastomotic site. If a nephrostomy tube is used, the stent may or may not be placed through the same calyx. Anchoring the stent with a chromic catgut suture at the renal capsule will ensure maintenance of its position. A nephrostomy tube with a stenting tail is rarely, if ever, used. Not all surgeons exteriorize stents. Stents placed into the bladder may be anchored with catgut to the pelvis or with a pull-out suture to the ureter. If internal stenting is used, free retrograde flow of urine on suction will indicate that the lower end of the catheter is in the bladder. Our general practice in these circumstances is to visualize the catheter end cystoscopically at the completion of the surgical procedure to assure its proper bladder placement.

Nephrostomy. Nephrostomy drainage has also changed from a routine to a selective procedure in pyeloureteroplasty repairs. Performance of nephrostomy provides adequate renal drainage while the ureteropelvic operative site heals and regains function. It reduces the risk of renal damage from back-pressure and infection as well as the risk of systemic reaction to uncontrolled infection. The nonobstructed, resting pelvis is judged by some to provide an optimal opportunity for noncicatricial healing. The nephrostomy tube provides access for introduction of fluid to measure pelvic pressures and visualize the reconstructed ureteropelvic junction radiographically. One other advantage is that the nephrostomy site can be used to allow percutaneous access to the kidney to remove retained stones and to carry out other intrarenal inspections and manipulations. The disadvantages of nephrostomy drainage include the possibility of occasional technical problems such as bleeding in placement of the tube and the risk of introduction of bacterial infection. The catheter is thought by many to produce a significant tissue reaction, often in the region of the reconstructed pelvic outlet, compromising rather than facilitating healing. These aspects of concomitant nephrostomy drainage warrant consideration in selecting patients for whom the procedure seems appropriate. We tend to use nephrostomy drainage in a solitary or principal functioning kidney, in the presence of infection or complicated stones, in repeat pyeloureteroplasties, or in technically complex procedures when the probability of prompt function of the reconstructed ureteropelvic junction seems small. Every attempt is made to avoid placing the nephrostomy tube in the area of the new pelvic outlet.

NEPHROSTOMY TECHNIQUE. Figure 65–5 illustrates a detailed technique for nephrostomy tube placement in the renal pelvis. A four-winged Malecot is an ideal catheter. Adults usually tolerate a 24 to 30 French size. Smaller catheters are available for children and adults with intrarenal pelves. A large tube will hold the kidney at any desired level without nephropexy. By using the lower, middle, or upper major calyx, the relative position of the kidney may be varied by as much as 5 to 7 cm. This is

NEPHROSTOMY PLACEMENT TECHNIQUE

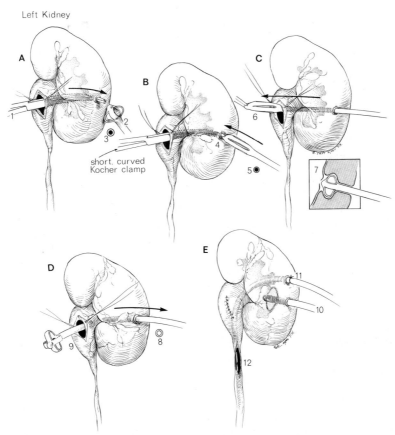

Figure 65–5. *A,* (1) Short curved Kocher clamp is passed through pyelostomy and previously selected calyx, then slowly "worked" through renal parenchyma. (2) Correct-size nephrostomy tube, previously checked, to fit and drain the renal pelvis adequately. (3) Normal diameter of Malecot catheter.

B, (4) Kohler clamp is securely clamped to cloth-reinforced tip of Malecot catheter. With clamp firmly held in palm of hand, catheter is stretched sufficiently to substantially reduce its diameter. (5) Note decrease in diameter of catheter under tension (up to 50 per cent) when compared with (3).

C, (6) With assistant holding kidney firmly, the Malecot catheter in its taut state is brought through newly formed parenchymal fistula. Head of catheter is always brought out through pyelotomy before traction is released. (7) Thus, head of catheter will not be trapped beneath calyceal mucosa in a totally obstructed position.

D, (8) With tension released, catheter will immediately return to its normal diameter and exert effective hemostatic pressure throughout length of new parenchymal fistula. As an added advantage, the "snug fit" keeps the catheter in its proper place and also makes it a more efficient nephropexy device. (9) At times, depending on the contour and size of the pelvis, one wing of the catheter head may be removed to ensure better placement and drainage when the nephrostomy tube has been withdrawn to its proper position in the pelvis. Such an alteration will not affect the self-retaining qualities of this type of head. If the right-angle catheter is used, be certain it is either the anterior or the posterior wing that is removed.

E, (10) Ideal position of nephrostomy tube for satisfactory pelvic urinary diversion. (11) Ureteral stent (silicone-coated red rubber Robinson catheter) is in place. Orientation tie (00 cotton or silk) marks level of renal capsule. (This orientation point is desirable to determine if there has been any displacement of the stent at the end of the operation.) (12) Stenting catheter traverses anterior ureterotomy and extends far enough down the ureter to stabilize itself.

helpful when a high renal position will eliminate ureteral redundancy or when a low position will relieve undesirable stress on a suture line. Before placing the nephrostomy tube, one should consider the calyceal site for the nephrostomy so that effective drainage and satisfactory kidney function will be achieved without interfering with either the ureteral stent or subsequent pelvic wall closure. Both nephrostomy tube and ureteral stents can be maintained in position with 2–0 or 1–0 chromic catgut sutures placed in the renal capsule and snugged around the tubes. This suture may incorporate renal tissue as necessary for control of bleeding. The nephrostomy tube can be irrigated with saline solution after the pelvis is closed. The nephrostomy and stent catheters are brought through stab wounds on a straight tract that facilitates replacement, and they are then sutured to the skin.

Pyelostomy. Pyelostomy offers an alternative approach to nephrostomy tube placement. Since this technique does not traumatize the renal parenchyma, the risk of bleeding is markedly reduced. However, since pyelostomy tubes are not only difficult to maintain in position but also prone to malfunction and are almost impossible to replace, most urologists prefer a nephrostomy tube if assurance of renal drainage is the goal.

Drainage and Fixation of the Kidney. Some type of satisfactory drainage of the kidney or the renal fossa is essential to prevent disruption of the suture lines, perirenal urinoma and inflammatory reaction, infection, and severe obstruction. The advantages and disadvantages of formal drainage of the kidney by ureteral stent, nephrostomy tube, or pyelostomy have been described. The tendency has nevertheless been to avoid tube drainage, if possible. Our practice and that of others is to make a superficial pyelotomy incision away from the suture line to allow drainage from the kidney if obstruction is persistent. If the pyelotomy is made within the hilum and if a drain is anchored near this site, adequate opportunity for drainage is provided without an intrarenal tube and without bathing the suture line with extravasated urine. An increasing number of urologists are forgoing any type of venting of the kidney and simply draining the perirenal area after attempting a watertight closure. Although our experience does not support this approach, the results of these efforts seem satisfactory.

In addition to adequate drainage, some type of fixation of the kidney to assist in maintaining a dependent, unkinked ureteropelvic junction deserves consideration in most pyeloureteroplasties. If the mobilization of the kidney has been limited, this may be unnecessary. At times, the nephrostomy-splint drainage will serve to maintain a satisfactory position of the kidney. At other times, limited suture fixation of a portion of the kidney to the posterior abdominal wall is indicated. At any rate, the position of the kidney and its potential for displacement should be considered prior to beginning closure of the wound.

Adequate drainage of the wound is essential to prevent accumulation of urine. Penrose or suction (e.g., Jackson-Pratt or Heyer-Schulte) drains can be used. One or two drains should be in close proximity to, but not in contact with, the ureteropelvic suture line. Drains should not be in direct contact with the ureter. One technique that allows accurate placement and control of the drain is as follows: The free end of a 0 chromic suture ligature is tied to the end of a Penrose drain, and the needle is passed through tissue (e.g., psoas muscle) adjacent to the drainage site. The drain is pulled down and maintained in position by tension on the suture as it exits with the drain. Precise, gradual removal of the drain is accomplished by releasing tension on the suture. In general, drains should exit through a stab wound rather than through the operative wound.

Perioperative Antimicrobial Therapy. The urine should be sterile prior to ureteropelvic junction surgery. If an infection is suspected, urine cultures should be obtained and the patient started on specific antimicrobial therapy as indicated by the antimicrobial sensitivity testing. A repeat urine culture should be obtained to verify that the antimicrobial agent is effective. A patient who presents with a urinary tract infection should be maintained on appropriate antimicrobial therapy throughout the postoperative period. If a nephrostomy tube or stent is left indwelling, there is a risk of acquiring resistant bacteria. Therefore, cultures should be obtained periodically while the tubes are in place and before their removal so that adjustments in antimicrobial drugs can be made. If a patient does not have a urinary tract infection prior to surgery, the use of perioperative antimicrobial therapy is not clearly indicated. However, the edematous ureteropelvic junction with adjacent drains may make the urinary tract more susceptible to infection from blood-borne bacteria or those that may infect the urinary tract in a retrograde fashion via the bladder, ureter, or nephrostomy tube. Since the complications of infection can be very severe, in most instances we favor short-term perioperative antimicrobial therapy with extended-spectrum cephalosporins or aminoglycosides.

The risk of retrograde spread of bacteria from the nephrostomy drainage bag to the kidney can be minimized by periodic instillations of 30 ml of hydrogen peroxide into the drainage bag each time it is emptied. It is important that the drainage bag have an antireflux valve to prevent inadvertent passage of hydrogen peroxide from the bag to the kidney through the renal pelvis.

TECHNIQUES FOR
URETEROPELVIC JUNCTION
REPAIR

A variety of techniques have been designed to relieve hydronephrosis by removing or correcting the ureteropelvic junction obstruction, whether it be mechanical, physiologic, or both. Normal peristalsis moves the urine through a conical or funnel-shaped pelvis that is in unobstructed continuity with the dependent ureter. When ureteropelvic junction obstruction and hydronephrosis occur, one or more of these features may be lost. If successful, the operations designed to correct these deficiencies and provide a dependent ureteropelvic segment that is funnel-shaped and of adequate caliber will allow peristaltic activity to effectively transport the pelvic urine into the ureter.

Preoperative assessment should determine both the location and the length of ureteral obstruction. The status of the distal ureter and the lower urinary tract should be established prior to surgical repair.

Owing to the complexity and variety of lesions causing obstructions, numerous methods for correction of ureteropelvic junction obstructions have been proposed. No single procedure is satisfactory for all cases. Consequently, familiarity with a variety of techniques is essential in order to select the best approach for a specific type of ureteropelvic junction obstruction. Pyeloureteroplasties have been classified into six basic types (Devine et al., 1970): (1) Lateral anastomosis of pelvis and ureter (Trendelenburg, 1890). This technique may not produce satisfactory funneling of the pelvis. (2) Resection of the ureter and reimplantation into the dependent portion of the renal pelvis (Küster, 1892). This technique is prone to produce a recurrent stricture at the site of anastomosis. (3) The Heineke-Mikulicz method of longitudinal incision with transverse closure (Fenger,

1894). This technique often produces shortening of the suture line on one side of the ureteropelvic junction, causing buckling and kinking with recurrent obstruction. (4) Flap procedures with sutured pyeloureteroplasty, including a Y flap (Foley, 1937). The Foley operation, consisting of flap procedure with sutured pyeloureteroplasty, introduced an entirely new and successful concept. Because it is not applicable to the obstructed ureteropelvic junction that already occupies a dependent position, several modifications of the flap procedure have evolved and have gained wide acceptance since its introduction. These include the spiral flap (Culp and DeWeerd, 1951) and vertical flap (Scardino and Prince, 1953). (5) Incision and intubation with no sutures (Davis, 1943). This technique consists of a simple longitudinal incision of the strictured area with intubation without sutures. The ease of this operation has led to great popularity, but there are certain hazards associated with prolonged intubation. It is particularly suited for long or multiple ureteral strictures below the ureteropelvic junction. (6) Elliptical anastomosis (pelvic cuff) (Nesbit, 1949). This is an important modification of Küster's operation of resection and anastomosis. Nesbit demonstrated that a broad, spatulated anastomosis of ureter to pelvis limited the likelihood of circumferential stricture at the anastomotic site. Anderson and Hynes (1949) modified this by leaving a projection at the lower end of the pelvis as the redundant portion is resected; this projection is anastomosed with continuous suture to the spatulated ureter, giving a long, watertight elliptical anastomosis.

The last three techniques are most frequently applied in urology today. Additional procedures, such as those designed for elimination of pure extrinsic obstruction (e.g., nephropexy or pelvioureterolysis) and those designed for repair of obstruction in anomalous kidneys, are required in special situations and are also described.

Sutures and Instruments. Meticulous care is needed in handling the tissues during pyeloureteroplasty. Small, sharp scissors should be used to provide straight, clean margins. Fine vascular forceps will minimize crushing damage to the tissues. Most ureteral and pelvic margin bleeding will stop spontaneously. If persistent bleeding occurs, delicate point clamping with mosquito forceps and 4-0 absorbable (chromic catgut or polyglycolic acid) suture tie will suffice. Electrocoagulation of the pelvis or ureter seems inadvisable. Tissues should be accurately approximated with interrupted sutures of fine 4-0 or 5–0 absorbable material. Sutures can be placed at intervals of 3 to 6 mm, and the knots should be tied without tension on the exterior surface. Some surgeons prefer a fine running suture for rapid closure of residual pelvic defects.

Pelvic Flap Operations

Foley Y-Plasty. The Foley Y-plasty (Foley, 1937) was specifically designed for, and should be restricted to, the correction of an obstructive high insertion of the ureter into the pelvis (Figure 65–6). For these conditions, no other operation preserves ureteropelvic continuity and produces as effective funneling of the pelvis into a dependent ureteropelvic segment. The Y principle uses minimal incisions for maximal alteration of contour with less resultant distortion than any other operation.

The kidney should be exposed in order to obtain free access to the entire renal pelvis and upper ureter. In most cases of high ureteropelvic insertion, the upper ureteral segment is tightly bound to the renal pelvis by layers of dense

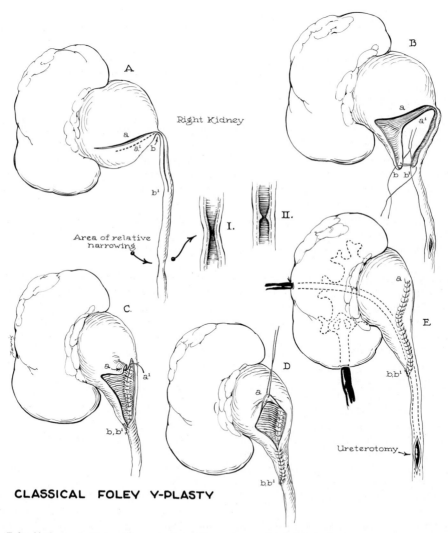

CLASSICAL FOLEY Y-PLASTY

Figure 65–6. *Foley Y-plasty. A,* Note placement of anterior and posterior pelvic incisions. The ureterotomy (shown here for clarity) is placed along the lateral aspect of the ureter. *B,* The two sutures (b, b′) are important for proper placement of the flap tip into the lower end of the ureterotomy. *C* and *D,* The closure is started at (b, b′) and extended upward to (a) and (a′), thus ensuring a smooth suture line. With pelvic closure a "dog ear" or pucker may form at point (a). This need not cause concern, as it will be eradicated by tissue resilience. I and II illustrate two types of nonobstructive segments exhibiting relative narrowing in the lumbar ureter. *E,* Such segments, if not relieved by ureterotomy, may produce obstructive strictures when stented.

fibrous tissue that require careful but complete dissection. When the pelvis and ureter are free, the length and size of the pelvic flap needed for adequate dependency of the ureteropelvic segment should be planned. The anterior pelvic incision is started just beneath the ureteropelvic junction and extended downward and laterally in the anterior wall of the pelvis toward the hilum of the kidney. The posterior incision is made in a similar fashion, producing a generous V-shaped pelvic flap with a wide base. These incisions to construct the flap are most easily made with small plastic scissors to assure sharp, clean margins. The stem of the Y incision is made down the lateral aspect of the ureter, long enough to extend well below the floor of the renal pelvis to assure dependent drainage of the proposed new ureteropelvic segment. If these three incisions are made correctly, the pelvic flap will easily fall into its proper position for a V-type closure without angulation or kinking (Fig. 65–6B to E). The sharp tip of the flap should be rounded to assure better marginal blood supply at this critical junction. The distal end of the pelvic flap should be sutured into the lower angle of the ureterotomy.

The anastomosis is performed with absorbable sutures of 4–0 or 5–0 chromic or polyglycolic acid on atraumatic needles. The first sutures are placed in both sides of the pelvic flap near its tip, approximating it snugly into the lower angle of the ureteral incision (Fig. 65–6B). This step should proceed very carefully, since these sutures are critical to proper approximation of the flap and the ureterotomy. Sutures at the tip of the apex are undesirable because they may compromise blood supply.

The posterior margin of the ureteral incision is sutured to the posterior margin in the pelvic flap with interrupted 4–0 or 5–0 absorbable suture placed approximately 2 to 4 mm apart. Careful placement to avoid interference with the blood supply of the flap is important. The sutures should be tied just firmly enough to approximate the tissue, and the knots should be on the outside. Closure of the remaining defect in the anterior pelvis is then accomplished in a similar fashion. Any discrepancy in the length of the edges can be adjusted by positioning the sutures. Excision of pelvic tissue may be hazardous because of risk of compromising the blood supply to the tissues at the anastomotic site and should be avoided in general. If the surgeon believes that the size of the pelvis must be reduced, a procedure other than the Foley Y-plasty is usually preferable. Prior to closing the pelvis, the patency of the anastomosis should be confirmed by passing a catheter or an instrument through it. If desired, the anastomosis may be left stented.

In unusually long lumbar ureteral constrictions associated with high ureteropelvic insertion, this technique may be combined with the Davis intubated ureterotomy, thus assuring a dependent ureteropelvic segment with funneling and an adequate ureteral caliber throughout the remainder of the involved segment.

Culp-DeWeerd, Scardino-Prince, and Patel Pyeloureteroplasties. The basic idea of fashioning a pelvic flap that is turned down and incorporated into the adjacent ureter is common to these procedures. The major difference is that Culp and DeWeerd (1951) (Fig. 65–7) and Patel (1982) use a spiral type of flap and Scardino and Prince (1953) (Fig. 65–8) employ a vertical flap. The Patel technique provides a flap of pelvic tissue of adequate length to bridge unusually long segments of narrowed upper ureter. The advantage of the spiral flap operation is that a longer flap may be secured from the pelvis because it follows the longest axis of the pelvis. The Scardino-Prince vertical flap operation cannot be classically applied unless there is an adequate pelvic wall between the ureteropelvic juncture and the renal hilus. It is well suited for the box-shaped pelvis with a ureteropelvic angle that approximates 90 degrees. These techniques are not applicable to a high insertion of the ureter or small intrarenal pelvis.

Two further comments on the spiral versus the vertical flap procedure are appropriate. Figures 65–7 and 65–8 show two types of hydronephrotic pelves with dependent ureteropelvic junction obstructions, both of which are amenable to pelvic flap correction. The primary difference is that in Figure 65–7A the long axis of the ureter and the floor of the extrarenal pelvis form an obtuse angle, and in Figure 65–8A these structures form a right angle. The pelvic flap must hinge or swing on its base so that it parallels the course of the ureter without twisting. The angle of the base of the flap in these two types of pelves depends entirely on the angle taken by the floor of the pelvis (between the ureteropelvic junction and the renal hilum) and the long axis of the ureter. The angle should be determined with the pelvis normally distended and the kidney lying in its normal position. To bring the pelvic flap down parallel to the ureteral axis (Figs. 65–7C and 65–8C) it is necessary to fashion the flaps differently. For example, if a vertical flap were used in the pelvis shown in Figure 65–7, the difference in the

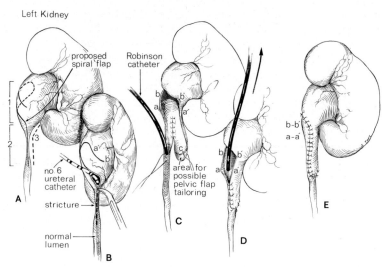

Figure 65–7. *Technique of Culp-DeWeerd spiral flap pyeloureteroplasty. A,* If the ureteropelvic angle is oblique (greater than 90 degrees), a spiral flap will produce an acceptable ureteropelvic funnel. (1) and (2) designate the estimated equal lengths for pelvic flap and corrective ureterotomy. This method also produces a longer flap than the vertical flap operation. The spiral flap technique gives a very good approximation of flap to the ureter without folding or kinking at its base.

B, Care should be taken to make the *initial pyelotomy incision* along the *proposed pelvic flap incision.* Any indiscriminate placement of pyelotomy incision at this point could jeopardize the formation of an effective pelvic flap. In a collapsed pelvis, strict attention to relative orientation has to be maintained while cutting the flap. When unsure of yourself, use orientation sutures or surgical marking pencil with the pelvis just moderately distended. An angle and ratio in length to width of 2 or 3 to 1 must be observed. Detailed data on the production of the flap and ureterotomy are the same as those described in Figure 65–8*B* (vertical flap). Procuring an adequate flap is the most tedious part of this operation.

C, Note the orientation points a-a' and b-b' and how they relate to proper closure. Closure should start as indicated and proceed down the posterior wall. The rounded tip of the flap is folded into the lower ureteropelvic angle over a catheter. The catheter should distend the ureter to its normal caliber to prevent sewing in a stenosis (if the ureteral musculature is in spasm).

D, Anterior margins are closed with 0000 interrupted chromic or polyglycolic acid sutures at 2-mm intervals. The entire closure is not unlike a "zipper" with careful equal margin suturing and gentle tissue approximation without kinks or folds.

length of the medial and lateral margins would deflect the flap at almost a right angle to the renal pelvis. However, the spiral flap is designed so that it may be turned down along the course of the ureter for effective closure without kinks or folds.

When a spiral flap has been turned down and the posterior suture line has been completed (Fig. 65–7*C*), point (a'), on the lateral margin of the flap, and point (a) are at an equal distance from the lower angle of the ureterotomy. When the anterior suture line is closed, (a) and (a') are in approximation at the level of the new ureteropelvic segment (Fig. 65–7*E*). The part of the flap margin above this point is incorporated into the pelvic wall closure. This detail is stressed to prevent attempting to suture the entire lateral margin on the flap from point (b') to the medial margin of the ureter (a), which would result in marked folding and kinking. However, in the vertical flap closure (Fig. 65–8*A*), points (a) and (a') are both situated on the margins of the pelvic wall at the base of the flap

and fall into perfect approximation when the entire lengths of both flap margins are sutured to the spatulated ureter (Fig. 65–8*D*).

TECHNIQUE. After adequate exposure of the pelvis and lumbar ureter, the pyelotomy incision should be made only along the medial border of the proposed flap (Figs. 65–7*B* and 65–8*B*). With the ureter stabilized, the tip of the number 12 hooked-blade knife (Bard-Parker) or the right-angle tenotomy or vascular scissors is used to extend the pyelotomy incision downward through the ureteropelvic junction, through the obstructed ureteral segment, and about 1 to 2 cm distally into the section of the ureter with normal caliber (Fig. 65–8*A*). A 4–0 atraumatic suture is passed through all layers of the ureteral wall at the distal angle of the incision (Fig. 65–8*C*).

The dimensions of the flap are determined by the required length of the ureterotomy. Because of subsequent tissue contraction, the pelvic flap should be made a little longer than the ureterotomy. Any excess flap may be tailored

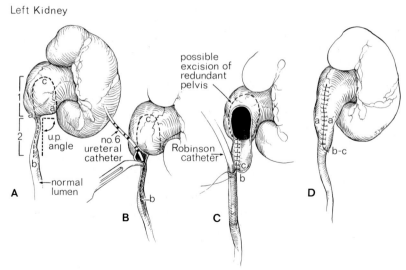

Figure 65–8. *Technique of Scardino-Prince vertical flap pyeloureteroplasty. A,* This technique is used when the ureteropelvic angle is approximately 90 degrees. (1) Length of proposed pelvic flap should adequately traverse (2) the segment of ureteral obstruction. The medial and lateral margins at the base of the pelvic flap are (a-a'); (b) is lower angle of ureterotomy; (c) is rounded tip of pelvic flap.

B, A pyelotomy incision is made in the lower pelvis along the medial border of the proposed pelvic flap incision. A No. 6 ureteral catheter is passed down the ureter. The tip of a hooked blade knife is buried in its wall and, using the catheter as a sliding guide, a clean, precise ureterotomy incision is made. If the stenotic ureteral segment is longer than the available pelvic flap, a Davis intubated ureterotomy operation may be combined with this procedure. If stenting and diversion are required, their selection and placement should be made at this time.

C, A 0000 fixation and retention suture is placed well within the ureteral wall at the lower angle of the ureterotomy. A wide-based pelvic flap is fashioned with sharp plastic scissors, taking care not to "saw tooth" its margins. Tip of flap (c) should be rounded to ensure a good blood supply. If necessary, take a somewhat larger flap than needed (wider base). It can always be tailored for excellent approximation. At the time of incision, a 0000 orientation and traction suture is placed deeply in the tissue at the tip of flap (c). This ensures accurate subsequent orientation. At times the tip can become distorted by irregular tissue contraction. Equal-margin, interrupted 0000 Dexon suturing is started at the base of the medial margin of the flap and the lateral ureteral margin and continued down to approximate points (b) and (c). When suturing the pelvic flap to the spatulated ureteral ribbon, an assistant should gently wipe the surface so the mucosal margins can be clearly seen for accurate approximation. (It is difficult to determine the margins of blood-stained mucosa.)

The ureter is distended to its normal caliber with a Robinson catheter. The tip of the flap is now carefully folded and fitted into the lower angle of the ureterotomy. This is the most vital part of the funnel. At this point, the surgeon should be certain that he engages the ureteral mucosa with the needle. When working around a catheter this vital layer of the ureteral wall can be easily missed and the tip of the flap may be inadvertently sutured to the outer layers of the ureter.

D, Any redundant pelvis may be excised. The anterior margins are closed, approximating b-c and a-a'. The pelvis and new ureteropelvic funnel are reconstituted.

for satisfactory anastomosis. If the pelvis is asymmetric, the body and the tip of the flap should be constructed from the largest portions. When accessory vessels cross anteriorly, the base of the flap should be on the posterior surface so that when the revision is completed, the vessels will cross the intact pelvic wall rather than the suture lines. The base of the flap should be wide enough to assure adequate blood supply to all margins. The ratio of length to width can be from 2:1 to 3:1. The end of the flap should be rounded to avoid the increased risk of necrosis occasioned by a sharp, angular tip.

When properly fashioned, the flap should fit the ureteral defect exactly. Tension must be avoided and excess length trimmed away to prevent the formation of redundant folds. Clo-

sure may be accomplished by initially suturing the tip of the flap to the apex of the ureteral incision with 4–0 chromic catgut placed 1 mm to each side of the center of the rounded flap tip. A stent may facilitate the placement of sutures in this area. Conversely, the closure may be performed by starting at the base of the flap and proceeding to its tip. This technique, which is our preference, allows the greatest control of the critical approximation of the ureter and flap at the pelvic outlet. The lateral border of the ureterotomy and the medial margin of the flap are approximated with interrupted 4–0 or 5–0 sutures on an atraumatic needle and placed 2 to 4 mm apart with the knots on the outside (Figs. 65–7C and D and 65–8C). Next, the lateral margin of the flap is sutured to the medial border of the ureteral incision. If further reduction of pelvic size is desired, resection of the pelvic wall should be made in such a manner that there is no twisting or folding of the newly formed ureteropelvic segment. In general, however, reduction of pelvic size is unnecessary. If a ureteral stent has been used, it may be removed or brought through the renal parenchyma with a nephrostomy tube, as outlined earlier, after the dependent portion of the anastomosis is completed. If no stent has been used, the anastomotic site should be calibrated before closure of the pelvis is completed.

Dismembered Pyeloureteroplasty. The operation utilizes excision of the obstructed ureteropelvic junction. Dismembered pyeloureteroplasty may be used in almost any circumstance in which a ureter of normal caliber can be brought without tension to a level at least 1 cm above the lower aspect of the pelvis. A high insertion or redundancy or tortuosity of the upper part of the ureter is ideal for this procedure. This technique facilitates placement of a new ureteropelvic funnel anterior to obstructing lower pole renal vessels, if present; excision of redundant pelvis as required; and elimination of excessive ureteral length with establishment of a straight ureter. A small intrarenal or extrarenal pelvis makes the procedure difficult to perform satisfactorily. In addition, the operation is not suited for lengthy upper ureteral strictures.

The dismembered Foley Y-plasty (Smart, 1979) and Anderson-Hynes pyeloureteroplasty (Anderson and Hynes, 1949) both achieve an interdigitating anastomosis by employing a tongue-like dependent pelvic flap fitted into a lateral ureterotomy incision. They differ in that Foley proposed interrupted 4–0 sutures about 2 mm apart for accurate tissue approximation and minimal interference with wound margin blood supply and diverted closure, whereas Anderson-Hynes used a continuous 4–0 suture for watertight, nondiverted closure.

TECHNIQUE. Preliminary exposure and mobilization of the kidney and pelvis are performed as outlined previously. The redundant portion of the pelvis is excised along a projected line that leaves an adequate margin for closure without tension (Fig. 65–9). The ureter is transected immediately below the stricture site and spatulated on its lateral margin for approximately 1 cm. An orientation and retraction suture should be positioned at the medial margin of the ureter to prevent any subsequent twisting.

The formation of the dependent V-pelvic flap may start at the ureteropelvic junction

opening or at any point that will produce a flap of adequate length with a wide base in order to assure good blood supply. The V-pelvic flap is fitted into the spatulated ureter. A limited lateral distal longitudinal ureterotomy facilitates this planned approximation and allows a satisfactory anastomosis. Usually, the posterior margins are approximated first, starting at a point about 1 cm proximal to the distal end of the flap and the lower angle of the ureterotomy. Placement of a ureteral stent before the anastomosis is begun may aid accurate identification of the lumen. Next, the distal anastomosis is completed with interrupted 4–0 or 5–0 absorbable sutures. Additional sutures secure the margin of the ureter to the pelvis, and the pelvic margins are sutured to complete the closure. Toward the end of the closure the pelvis should be flushed of debris and clots. If no stent has been used, the anastomotic site is calibrated. The closure is completed, and the kidney is returned to and anchored in the renal fossa in a position that does not produce tension on the suture lines or kink or distort the course of the ureter. Drainage and wound closure are the same as described previously.

For a kidney with a small hilum but an adequate intrarenal pelvis (Fig. 65–10), a wedge of renal parenchyma may be resected, if necessary, to expose a section of pelvic wall sufficient for fashioning a flap large enough to permit satisfactory corrective dismembered Y-plasty. In children with moderate pyelectasis, simple ureteropyelostomy without pelvic reduction may be adequate (Zincke et al., 1974).

Anderson and Hynes (1949) stressed the watertight anastomosis and the value of primary closure without the use of nephrostomy and stenting (Fig. 65–11). Drake et al. (1978) reported excellent results in a series of 88 pediatric patients, chiefly using the Anderson-Hynes technique with a transperitoneal approach. Johnston et al. (1977), Perlmutter et al. (1980), and Williams and Kenawi (1976) have modified the Anderson-Hynes concept by the addition of stenting and diversion. This combination has also given excellent clinical results. As stated, we prefer, in general, to use an intrahilar vent without a stent.

Ureterocalyceal Anastomosis

Ureterocalyceal anastomosis should be used only when circumstances demand that a kidney be saved despite ureteropelvic damage and advanced intrarenal hydronephrosis. Con-

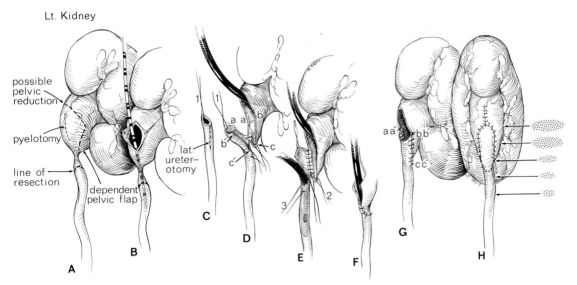

Figure 65–9. *Dismembered Foley Y-Plasty.* This operation is designed to correct successfully most obstructive situations in the ureteropelvic area. It combines elimination of the defective ureteral segment and resection of the redundant pelvis, and forms a dependent ureteropelvic funnel with adequate ureteral caliber.

A, This situation is amenable to dismembered Y-plasty.

B, Whistle-tip ureteral catheter is passed through medial pyelotomy and down the ureter. (1) Orientation 0000 suture is placed through medial side of ureter; this ensures correct lateral ureterotomy placement and eliminates unrecognized twisting of ureter after division. During formation of the dependent pelvic flap an orientation and traction suture will be placed deeply in the rounded tip; this will provide orientation during subsequent suturing, as pelvic tissue can become distorted by muscle contraction and the original tip may not be recognizable.

C, If stenting and diversion are to be used, the stent and nephrostomy tube should be put in place at this time before the ureteropelvic anastomosis is started. The defective ureteral segment is excised. The lateral ureterotomy should be of such length that, when sutured to the dependent flap, a satisfactory funnel will be formed. The traction suture is placed in the lower angle of the ureterotomy.

D, Start suturing on posterior margins about 1 cm proximal to the tip of the flap and 1 cm above the dependent angle of the ureterotomy. Work superiorly with equal-margin suturing to secure the ureter to the pelvis. This is the most difficult segment to approximate. Keep well oriented. It may be difficult at this point to visualize how a well-formed, dependent funnel will emerge.

E, Use traction sutures 1, 2, and 3 to approximate wound margins for suturing. Gentle tissue handling is important. Spatulated ureter is anastomosed to the posterior edge of the pelvic flap with 0000 absorbable interrupted sutures about 2 mm apart. This stabilizes the ureter to the pelvis.

F, The tip of the flap is now folded into the lower angle of the ureterotomy; this is a critical area of tissue suturing. Margins should be firmly but gently held in approximation. The stent is in place during this phase to ensure an adequate caliber of ureter. It also stabilizes the tissue margins.

G, With the funnel completed, any redundant pelvis can now be resected. The stent may be removed or put in position down the lumbar ureter, depending on the technique used. If primary closure is accomplished with continuous suture and without stenting or diversion, the technique is basically that of Anderson-Hynes (1949).

H, The pelvis is reconstituted. If a nephrostomy tube is in place, the pelvis should be distended and any gross leaks reinforced. Note the progression of internal caliber discs 1 through 5.

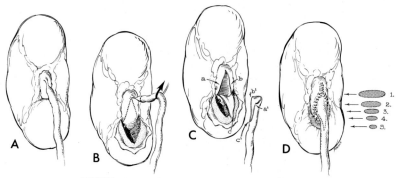

DIFFICULT HIGH INSERTION REPAIR

Figure 65–10. Variation of dismembered Foley Y-plasty technique for high insertion of a small stenotic ureter in a large but intrarenal pelvis. *A,* A small renal hilum but large intrarenal pelvis with ureteral stenosis that requires resection. (In cases of extreme ureteral stenosis, it is often not practical to maintain ureteropelvic continuity.) *B,* Resection of renal parenchyma to expose sufficient pelvis for flap. Ureter severed distal to stenosis. *C,* Formation of pelvic flap. Resection of stenotic ureteral segment with spatulation of ureter. Approximate a-a', b-b', and c-c' to produce a satisfactory dependent, funneled ureteropelvic segment. *D,* Anastomosis completed. Numbers 1 to 5 illustrate the progressive caliber of the lumen from the pelvis to the ureter through the newly formed ureteropelvic segment.

sideration of this procedure is usually limited to individuals with advanced bilateral disease or a solitary hydronephrotic kidney in whom previous ureteropelvic junction surgery has failed. The ureterocalyceal anastomosis can be expected to yield a greater percentage of operative failures or poorly draining kidneys than do other corrective procedures. This surgery is advisable for previous operative failures when the extra-

renal pelvis and a significant segment of ureter are damaged beyond repair (Wesolowski, 1975). Preventing postoperative stricture or kinking of the anastomosis is a formidable problem; most failures occur at this juncture. The larger the caliber of the available ureter at the level of the lower pole of the kidney, the better the chances of success. An area of thin renal parenchyma is an advantage in obtaining a patent anastomosis

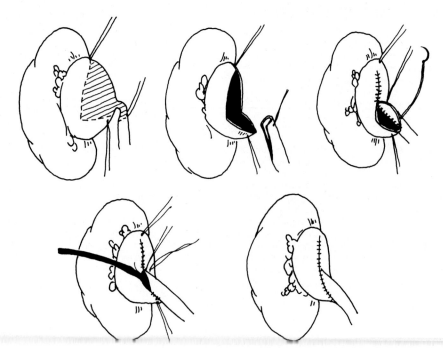

Figure 65–11. *The Anderson-Hynes renal plastic operation.* The ureteric catheter is inserted while the lower angle is negotiated in order to prevent both walls being picked up by the needle. (From Anderson, J. C.: Hydronephrosis. Springfield, Ill., Charles C Thomas, Publishers, 1963, p. 55.)

(Fig. 65–12) (Hawthorne et al., 1976). Resecting the renal parenchyma so that the ureteral calyceal anastomosis is outside and free of surrounding kidney tissue is an essential step to reduce the risk of stricture and to maintain an open ureteral funnel.

A nephrostomy tube and stent are usually indicated in these complicated procedures and are placed before the closure. The stent is usually left in place for 3 to 4 weeks if extensive fibrosis is present. Following removal of the stent, the patency of the anastomosis can be checked via the nephrostomy tube; if the anastomosis is successful, the nephrostomy tube can be removed several days later.

Enlargement of Ureteral Caliber (Davis Intubated Ureterotomy)

The Davis intubated ureterotomy is used much less often now than it was in the past. Nevertheless, it is a highly successful method of correcting strictures of the lumbar ureter when there is inadequate ureteral length for primary resection and anastomosis. This procedure should be a part of the surgical armamentarium of every urologist. The operation is usually performed under adverse conditions (Davis, 1943) and requires strict attention to detail (Fig. 65–13). Incorrect stenting and inadequate urinary diversion are the two most common iatrogenic causes of failure. In his initial effort, Davis (1943) used only an anterior ureterotomy. This technique is still applicable for patients with long ureteral strictures or for those with small ureters in whom an additional posterior ureter-

otomy could impair the blood supply or weaken the tissue "bridge." There are two basic requirements for successful completion of this procedure: an adequate-sized stent through the involved segment during the healing period of 3 to 8 weeks and a complete and satisfactory urinary diversion via the nephrostomy for this entire period.

Technique. To expose the ureter, Gerota's fascia is opened posterolaterally. It is important not to disturb any fat that may be lying between the ureter and psoas muscle, since the fat assures postoperative mobility of the ureter. The pelvis and ureteropelvic junction are visualized after the removal of redundant perirenal fat and areolar tissue; at times this may be quite fibrous and adherent, since many of these patients are previous surgical failures with dense scar formation and probably impaired circulation. As a rule, the obstructed segment can be seen easily at this time.

As it is exposed, the ureter should be dissected minimally from its bed. If it must be removed from the bed, the investing periureteral tissues carrying the blood vessels that supply the ureter should be preserved as much as possible. The ureter is exposed to well below the obstructed site previously identified by radiographic studies. The obstructed area should be evident on inspection. The ureter above it should be dilated and thickened. Often, erratic peristaltic activity will be evident on stimulation.

A pyelotomy should be made between stay sutures placed in the pelvic wall to permit excison of redundant tissue, if necessary. An anterior ureterotomy is made in the thickened

Figure 65–12. Representation of method of ureterocalicostomy. *A,* Lower pole cortex is removed to expose inferior calyx and to free anastomotic site. *B,* Ureter is sectioned obliquely and spatulated. *C,* Anastomosis is performed over stenting catheter. (From Hawthorne, N. J., et al.: J. Urol., *115*:583, 1976.)

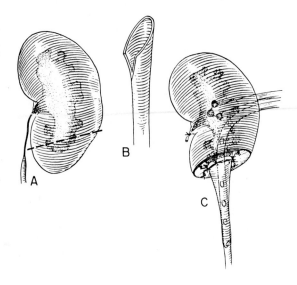

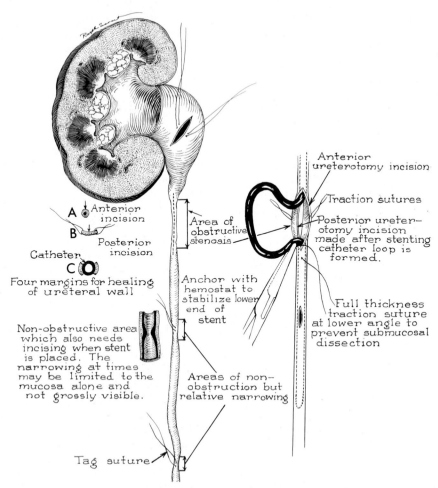

Figure 65–13. *Modified Davis intubated ureterotomy technique.* Nonobstructed areas of "relative stenosis" in the lumbar ureter. A simple method of making the posterior ureterotomy. (From Smart, W. R.: J. Urol., *85*:512, 1961.)

dilated ureter above the obstructed segment, avoiding any obvious ureteral vessels. Using either small right-angle tenotomy or vascular scissors or the size 12 hooked-blade knife, the entire stricture segment is incised longitudinally through all layers, starting 1 cm above the level of stricture and extending 1 cm below. This effectively opens the ureter, with segments of normal caliber above and below the stricture. A 4–0 atraumatic stay suture placed through all layers of the ureteral wall at the lower angle of the anterior ureterotomy will help to prevent submucosal dissection during stent placement. Stay sutures are placed in the midportion of both edges of the ureterotomy margins. Calibration of the distal ureter may be attempted if radiographic studies indicated questionable areas or if there is concern about the extent of incision relative to the strictured area. However, interpretation of these efforts is often difficult.

The ureterotomy should clearly extend into the normal ureter. A pliable, inert, well-lubricated catheter that passes without resistance and fills the normal distal ureter without tension should be inserted as a stent. The stent may be brought through the renal parenchyma, may be anchored in the ureter, or may be of the self-retaining internal type, depending on the site of the ureteral stricture and the exposure used. In the previous edition of this book, Dr. Smart (1979) discussed the use of a second posterior ureterotomy if an adequate "ribbon" of ureter existed. The current authors have no experience with this procedure. The length of time the stenting ureteral catheter should be left in place is uncertain. Davis et al. (1948) recommended 4 to 6 weeks. Shorter periods have become common practice with experience. However, the use of self-retaining, internal stents has been associated with a return to longer stenting periods.

Elimination of Pure Extrinsic Obstruction

Management of Accessory Blood Vessels.
Accessory blood vessels to the lower aspect of the renal pelvis are frequently found in close proximity to the ureteropelvic junction or the ureter. As noted previously (Stephens, 1982), these arteries enter the lower pole directly and, in fact, are segmental vessels to the lower pole and therefore are neither accessory nor aberrant. Because the segmental arteries are end-arteries, the lower segmental vessel should not be divided as a means of relieving the ureteropelvic junction obstruction. The Anderson-Hynes dismembered pyeloureteroplasty permits trimming of the ureteropelvic redundancy, elimination of any suspected intrinsic stenosis, and preservation of the viability of the lower pole while repositioning the segmental vessels posterior to the reconstructed ureteropelvic junction. Pelvic flap reconstruction procedures (described earlier) will also usually relocate the ureteropelvic junction caudal to the lower pole segmental vessels and thus neutralize any possible compression effect they may have. Aberrant veins may be divided with relative impunity. Graves's studies of the renal vascular system showed that veins do not follow a segmental

arrangement and in fact have an extensive collateral network (Graves, 1969).

The Hellström procedure is a simple and unique method of transplanting obstructive aberrant vessels to a nonobstructive position without interference with renal blood flow (Fig. 65–14). This operation should be used only in cases of proven purely extrinsic "aberrant" vessel obstruction—for example, the true vessel obstruction that produces intermittent hydronephrosis with almost normal-appearing ureterograms between the episodes of pain. In most circumstances, the possible coexistence of an intrinsic and an extrinsic obstruction makes the use of a simple vascular relocation procedure hazardous. We have not used this procedure in our practice.

Although fixation of the kidney to assure maintenance of a satisfactory relationship of the reconstructed ureter and pelvis often warrants consideration in pyeloplasty procedures, nephroptosis causing significant hydronephrosis requiring nephropexy is rarely identified. If it is, multiple subcapsular sutures of 0 or 2–0 chromic catgut or other suitable absorbable suture may be employed to anchor the kidney in the desired position to posterior abdominal wall musculature, permitting the ureter to lie in a straight line without tension. Subcapsular su-

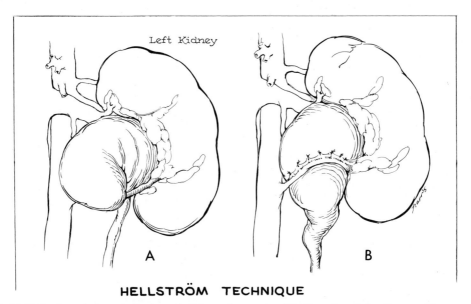

HELLSTRÖM TECHNIQUE

Figure 65–14. *Hellström technique.* A simple method for replacement and fixation of an obstructive vessel to a nonobstructive position. If an associated intrinsic ureteral obstruction is demonstrated, this transplantation technique may be combined with another appropriate corrective procedure.

A, The anterior herniation of the renal pelvis over the aberrant vessel, producing progressive ureteral obstruction.

B, Fixation of the vessel in this position will relieve *extrinsic* obstruction only.

The perivascular tissue may be insufficient for proper fixation. If so, a tunnel may be fashioned by folding the pliable pelvic wall around the vessel and suturing the wall to itself. Take care not to occlude the artery. (From Hanley, H. G.: Recent Advances in Urology. Boston, Little, Brown & Co., 1957.)

tures should be placed in parallel rows about 1 to 2 cm apart across the posterior surface of the kidney and into the appropriate muscle mass, going from the medial to the lateral surface. With the assistant holding the kidney in place, all sutures are drawn just tight enough to secure the best fixation and then are tied.

Pelvioureterolysis. Pelvioureterolysis is successful in relieving hydronephrosis when the acquired obstruction proves to be a purely extrinsic disorder from upper ureteral kinking, angulation, or compression. Examples include retroperitoneal fibrosis, previous vascular surgery, extrarenal masses, adhesions, previous stone surgery, certain pyeloureteroplasty failures, and retroperitoneal neoplasms. These obstructions are rarely congenital. One must beware of misinterpreting a few periureteral adhesions or a small lower pole vessel as a cause of primary obstruction to an obviously hydronephrotic kidney. Although lysis alone may suffice to correct such obstructions, the possibility of obstructing intrinsic factors despite the apparently normal appearance of the ureter or ureteropelvic junction usually requires reconstruction of the ureteropelvic junction.

REPAIR OF OBSTRUCTIONS IN ANOMALOUS KIDNEYS

Pyelopyelostomy. Pyelopyelostomy is appropriate when hydronephrosis occurs in a kidney with duplication of the pelvis and ureteropelvic juncture. In most cases the upper segment is hydronephrotic because of a ureteral stricture or lower ureteral obstruction secondary to ureterocele or ectopia. If the upper segment has no function or very compromised function, the treatment of choice is a partial nephrectomy. In most instances in which the upper segment has functional renal tissue, pyelopyelostomy may be performed. The adjoining surfaces of the dilated and normal pelvis are incised, and the margins are joined with interrupted sutures of 4–0 or 5–0 chromic catgut to create a permanent window between the two. Management of the ureter to the upper segment depends on the nature of the obstructing lesion, but resection of at least a portion of the ureter is usually carried out.

Dismembered Ureteropelvioplasty. Dismembered ureteropelvioplasty is appropriate if hydronephrosis is encountered in both segments of a reduplicated system. The proximal ends of the ureters are spatulated, joined to form a single unit, and sutured to the pelvis.

Horseshoe Kidney. Hydronephrosis from ureteropelvic junction obstruction is the most common problem in patients with horseshoe kidney. In a series of 106 patients with true horseshoe kidney reviewed by Culp and Winterringer (1955), males predominated over females by 4 to 1; more than 50 per cent presented in the third and fourth decades of life; and 85 per cent had stones or hydronephrosis, or both. In more than 50 per cent of the corrective operations, the isthmus was left intact. In most instances the isthmus is at the level of the third lumbar interspace. The midline transperitoneal approach provides excellent exposure for surgery of the horseshoe kidney with bilateral disease. Unilateral disease can be managed through an anterior flank incision.

Pyeloureteroplasty of the hydronephrotic horseshoe kidney may include division of the isthmus, with lateral displacement of the lower pole and medial rotation of the renal masses. A more normal medial course of the ureter, which is free of compression obstruction over the lower pole renal parenchyma, results. If symphysiotomy is being considered, the blood supply to the isthmus should be determined by selective renal arteriography. In newborns and infants, the renal scan will easily detect the thick isthmus of functional renal tissue. In some cases, symphysiotomy involves a simple incision. In most cases, however, rows of vertical mattress sutures of 0 chromic catgut should be used to provide a narrow avascular plane through which the incision can be made. Residual bleeding points can then be suture-ligated with 4–0 chromic. In cases in which division of the isthmus is impractical because of multiple short renal arteries or a thick vascular isthmus, the steps illustrated in Figure 65–15 may decrease iatrogenic failures.

The ureteropelvic junction is reconstructed according to the principles previously outlined. The anterior pelvis may be further distorted by the extrarenal extension of the thick, finger-like infundibula that arise from shallow calyces and fuse to form the pelvis. When the dependent funnel is created, care should be exercised not to inadvertently narrow or kink one of these extrarenal infundibula. In some instances, surgical fusion of two or more of the infundibula may be useful.

Pelvic Kidneys and Other Ectopic Kidneys. The incision to approach ectopic kidneys that are below the aortic bifurcation should be planned on the basis of preoperative knowledge of the blood supply and the ureteropelvic pathology to provide adequate exposure while minimizing risk of vascular compromise. Pelvic

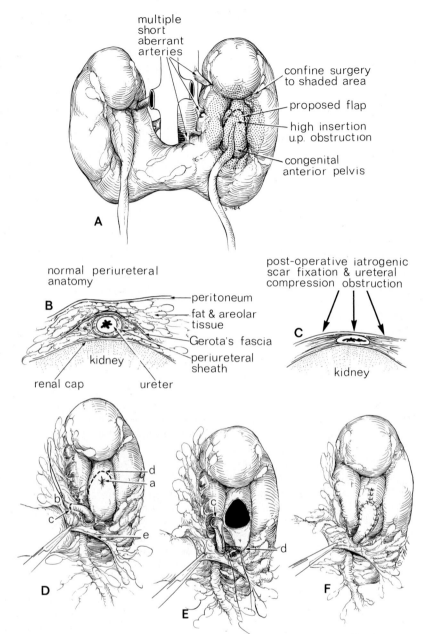

Figure 65–15. *Horseshoe Kidney Problems. A,* Horseshoe kidney with left obstruction from high ureteropelvic insertion. Cluster of arteries at lower pole produces vascular renal fixation. Proposed operation is now restricted to the shaded area.

B, Cross section of normal anatomy of lower lumbar ureter as it traverses the anterior surface of lower pole renal parenchyma.

C, Cross section of postoperative fibrous compression obstruction of an identical ureteral segment. During surgery the segment was stripped from its bed and divested of its protective sheaths, retroperitoneal fat, and areolar tissue. Such extensive surgical dissection may evoke intense fibrosis in the healing phase, trapping the ureter between the overlying peritoneum and the renal capsule. Such a compression obstruction can produce a surgical failure. This technique may prevent such problems.

D, The following steps may be taken to preserve the anatomic ureteral status quo as noted in *B*. 1, Enter Gerota's fascia along lateral border of kidney and carefully reflect it medially to expose pelvis. 2, Dissect ureter only in area of renal hilus. 3, Leave lower lumbar ureter as intact as possible, including its investing fat structures.

a, The ureter is divided at the ureteropelvic junction. If the stenotic ureteropelvic junction lies within the border of the proposed pelvic flap, close it with a small fine mattress suture. *b,* Preserve as much ureteral length as possible, as the vascular fixation of the kidney precludes mobilization. *c,* The obstructive segment may be resected. *d,* Proposed pelvic flap outline. It should be as high in the pelvis as practical. The lower limits of the proposed funnel should, if at all possible, lie in the renal hilus area to prevent compression obstruction in the healing phase. *e,* Cut edge of intact Gerota's fascia reflected medially.

E, Spatulated end of ureter (c) is now folded into (d) dependent pelvic flap to form adequate funnel.

F, Completed anastomosis which will be covered by Gerota's fascia and protective fat.

These steps may also serve well in pyeloplasty repair of other restrictive ectopic situations with vascular fixation of the renal mass—crossed fused ectopy, pelvic kidney, or sacral pancake kidney.

kidneys often present with short ureters of normal caliber but with high insertion, causing ureteropelvic obstruction. Classic Foley Y-plasty with primary closure is an excellent procedure in these instances. Because these kidneys may be placed deep in the true pelvis between the iliac vessels, effective drainage may require ingenuity and the use of a combination of drainage techniques.

SECONDARY PROCEDURES

Secondary operative procedures for management of failed previous surgical attempts to repair ureteropelvic junction obstruction represent a major challenge. If the contralateral kidney is normal, a nephrectomy may be the procedure of choice. If there is evidence of significant residual functional tissue or if a solitary kidney or bilateral disease is present, then further reconstructive efforts are probably indicated. A 3- to 6-month period of preliminary nephrostomy drainage should be allowed to permit maximum resolution of perirenal fibrosis. Control of urinary tract infection during this period is important.

Preoperative evaluation should include radionuclide renography to assess renal function and antegrade pyelography and retrograde ureterography to determine the distance between normal pelvis and ureter. Review of the previous operative report may provide important information about the type of previous repair and the amount of renal pelvic tissue that has been excised. Catheter or digital subtraction angiography is very useful to define the renal blood supply. Ureteral catheters placed cystoscopically immediately before the operation facilitate identification of the ureter.

Although a flap ureteropelvioplasty can be utilized if there is sufficient residual pelvic tissue to bridge the gap between the pelvis and viable distal ureter, dismembered pyeloureteroplasty is usually the procedure of choice. If a long vascular pedicle is present, the kidney may be mobilized to facilitate downward displacement. If the kidney still will not reach the ureter without undue tension, anastomosis of the ureter to the lower pole calyx should be considered (Wesolowski, 1975). Diversion of a portion or all of the blood supply to the kidney with reanastomosis to allow inferior displacement has been described. Use of the renal capsule has been reported to correct defects in the upper ureter and pelvis. A broad pedicle flap of the capsule that is hinged at the renal sinus can be turned down to reconstitute the ureteropelvic junction (Thompson et al., 1969). The authors have had no experience with this procedure. Although direct suture anastomosis is preferred currently, the Davis intubated ureterotomy as described has been used frequently in the past to attempt correction of postoperative ureteropelvic junction obstruction, and it remains a procedure that warrants consideration. Nephrostomy drainage and ureteral stenting should be used in all secondary procedures.

In some situations, procedures such as pelvioileovesicostomy (ileal ureteral replacement) or autotransplantation and ureteral neocystostomy or pyelocysostomy may be required to preserve renal function and avoid permanent nephrostomy drainage.

POSTOPERATIVE MANAGEMENT AND COMPLICATIONS

Removal of Drains. Many iatrogenic pyeloureteroplasty problems result from premature or inadvertent removal of the drains, stents, or nephrostomy tubes. Penrose drains are usually removed approximately 24 hours after the drainage ceases. This usually occurs on the third to the fifth or sixth day. The drainage site should be probed to maintain its patency for 2 or more days after drain removal. If a nephrostomy tube and ureteral stent have been used, the ureteral stent is removed on the seventh to the tenth postoperative day if the procedure and the postoperative course are uneventful. The stent should be left in longer if the procedure is a secondary operation, if a urinary tract infection has been present, or if prolonged extravasation or infection has been noted postoperatively. If a Davis intubated ureterostomy has been performed, 3- to 8-week periods of drainage have commonly been allowed. When the nephrostomy tube is to be removed, the urine should be sterilized and a gravity nephrostogram carried out. If this is satisfactory, the tube can be clamped. If there is no leakage around the tube and no pain and if unclamping demonstrates minimal backflow, the tube may be removed. Prompt cessation of urine drainage within 24 hours after removal of the tube is an additional important indicator of good function.

Complications. Complications of surgical procedures to correct ureteropelvic junction obstruction include (1) hemorrhage, (2) urinoma, (3) accidental dislodgment of the drains or tubes, and (4) infection. Hemorrhage is associated with renal parenchymal manipulation and is usually self-limited. Extensive clots may cause obstruction, dilatation of the pelvis, and disruption of the suture line. Spontaneous or induced diuresis will frequently minimize clot formation. Gentle irrigation of the nephrostomy tube, if one is in place, may be required to remove clots. Approximately 2 to 5 ml of sterile saline should be instilled, and essentially all the irrigated solution should be returned before further irrigation is initiated.

A collection of urine outside the kidney or ureter may occur early in the postoperative period. If this does not drain, a pseudocapsule of fibrous tissue adjacent to viscera and retroperitoneal structures will encapsulate the urine, forming a urinoma. Such a mass may be associated with accidental or premature dislodgment of the nephrostomy tube or drains. Gentle attempts to re-establish drainage may be successful, but this is often difficult. Ultrasonography may identify the urinoma, and percutaneous placement of a second drain can provide adequate drainage. Insertion of retrograde ureteral catheters may be difficult and more hazardous but necessary if adequate perirenal drainage cannot be established.

Infections associated with drains, nephrostomy tubes, and stents or indwelling ureteral or Foley catheters are common. Short-term prophylactic antimicrobial therapy may effectively reduce the incidence of bacterial colonization. Prolonged therapy frequently leads to development of resistant bacterial strains. An awareness of the possibility of an infection, its probable causes, and procedures to prevent it or control its clinical significance are important to maximize the probability of a satisfactory surgical result in reconstructive surgery of the upper urinary tract.

Late complications, such as strictures of the ureteropelvic anastomosis, are often associated with ischemia and necrosis of the tissue or with peripelvic or periureteral accumulations of serum, blood, or urine. The resulting persistent obstruction can be associated with persistent hydronephrosis and chronic infection. Calculus formation and further deterioration of renal function are frequent consequences of this series of events.

FOLLOW-UP EVALUATION

Follow-up should include urinalysis and possibly culture at 2- to 3-week intervals postoperatively. Evaluation of the upper tract by intravenous urography, renography, or ultrasonography should be considered in the early postoperative period if the clinical course appears less than satisfactory. Ordinarily, we obtain a urogram or radionuclide study at approximately 6 months postoperatively. It is generally recognized that dramatic improvement in the anatomic (radiographic) appearance of kidneys may be anticipated in infants and children, but that in older individuals the probability of restoration of normal or nearly normal appearance postoperatively is limited. Results of the intravenous urogram also should be evaluated in conjunction with the initial pathology. When intrarenal hydronephrosis and cortical atrophy are present initially, the calyceal residual urine and dilatation may persist despite satisfactory clinical recovery. In reviews of large series of pyeloplasty procedures in children, Williams and Kenawi (1976) and Zincke and coworkers (1974) showed that good clinical results were compatible with persistent calycectasis, suggesting that improved calyceal appearance need not be obtained and is not an essential ingredient of a successful operation. Cherrie and Kaufman (1983) reported that 91 per cent of 52 patients who had undergone pyeloureteroplasty for ureteropelvic junction obstruction had satisfactory clinical results manifested by relief of symptoms, stabilization or improvement of function, and absence of infection. The calyceal appearance on the postoperative excretory urogram showed diminution of calycectasis in 65 per cent, was unchanged in 30 per cent, and deteriorated in 5 per cent. Earlier appearance of contrast medium in the upper ureter on the postoperative excretory urogram was seen in all patients who had a satisfactory clinical result. Deterioration of calyceal grade or delayed appearance of contrast medium in the ureter in the postoperative excretory urogram was always associated with a poor clinical result and further parenchymal loss. Serial radionuclide renography is particularly useful to assess changes in renal function.

In summary, a variety of anatomic and possibly functional causes for obstruction of the ureteropelvic junction of the kidney exist. Careful preoperative evaluation of each patient will permit recognition of the presence and nature of the obstructive lesion in almost all instances. The appropriate surgical procedure to correct the obstructing abnormality should be selected from the group of techniques described, based on the preoperative evaluation and the operative findings. In addition to technical skill in performing the appropriate surgical procedure, control of infection and assurance of adequate drainage during the healing process are essential to obtain the satisfactory result that is usually achieved.

References

Allen, T. D.: Congenital ureteral strictures. J. Urol., *104*:196, 1970.

Anderson, J. C.: Hydronephrosis. Springfield, Ill., Charles C Thomas, 1963, p. 55.

Anderson, J. C., and Hynes, W.: Retrocaval ureter; case diagnosed and treated successfully by a plastic operation. Br. J. Urol., 21: 209, 1949.

Barnett, J. S., and Stephens, F. D.: The role of the lower segmental vessel in the etiology of hydronephrosis. Aust. N.Z. J. Surg., *31*:201, 1962.

Bourne, R. B.: Intermittent hydronephrosis as a cause of abdominal pain. JAMA, *198*:1218, 1966.

Cherrie, R. J., and Kaufman, J. J.: Pyeloplasty for ureteropelvic junction obstruction in adults: Correlation of radiographic and clinical results. J. Urol., *129*:711, 1983.

Culp, O. S.: Management of ureteropelvic obstruction. Bull. N.Y. Acad. Sci., *43*:355, 1967.

Culp, O. S., and DeWeerd, J. H.: Pelvic flap operation for certain types of ureteropelvic junction obstruction: Preliminary report. Proc. Staff Meet. Mayo Clin., *26*:483, 1951.

Culp, O. S., and Winterringer, J. R.: Surgical treatment of horseshoe kidney: Comparison of results after various types of operations. J. Urol., *73*:747, 1955.

Davis, D. M.: Intubated ureterotomy; a new operation for ureteral and ureteropelvic stricture. Surg. Gynecol. Obstet., *76*:513, 1943.

Davis, D. M., Strong, G. H., and Drake, W. M.: Intubated ureterotomy: Experimental work and clinical results. J. Urol., *59*:851, 1948.

Devine, C. J., Jr., Devine, P. C., and Prizzi, A. R.: Advancing V-flap modification for the dismembered pyeloplasty. J. Urol., *104*:810, 1970.

Drake, D. P., Stevens, P. S., and Eckstein, H. B.: Hydronephrosis secondary to ureteropelvic obstruction in children: A review of 14 years of experience. J. Urol., *119*:649, 1978.

Fenger, C.: Operation for the relief of valve formation and stricture of the ureter in hydro- or pyonephrosis. JAMA, *22*:335, 1894.

Foley, F. E. B.: A new plastic operation for stricture at the ureteropelvic junction; report of 20 operations. J. Urol., *38*:643, 1937.

Foote, J. W., Blennerhassett, J. B., Wigglesworth, F. W., and MacKinnon, K. J.: Observations on the ureteropelvic junction. J. Urol., *104*:252, 1970.

Friedland, G. W., Droller, M. J., and Stamey, T. A.: Obstruction of ischemic ureteropelvic junction. Urology, *4*:439, 1974.

Gittes, R. F., and Talner, L. B.: Congenital megacalices versus obstructive hydronephrosis. J. Urol., *108*:833, 1972.

Graves, F. T.: The arterial anatomy of the congenitally abnormal kidney. Br. J. Surg., *56*:533, 1969.

Graves, F. T.: The Arterial Anatomy of the Kidney. The Basis of Surgical Technique. Baltimore, The Williams & Wilkins Co., 1971.

Hamm, F. C., and Weinberg, S. R.: Renal and ureteral surgery without intubation. J. Urol., *73*:475, 1955.

Hanley, H. G.: Recent Advances in Urology. Boston, Little, Brown & Co., 1957.

Hanna, M. K., Jeffs, R. D., Sturgess, J. M. and Barkin, M.: Ureteral structure and ultrastructure. II. Congenital ureteropelvic junction obstruction and primary obstructive megaureter. J. Urol., *116*:725, 1976.

Hawthorne, N. J., Zincke, H., and Kelalis, P. P.: Ureterocalicostomy: An alternative to nephrectomy. J. Urol., *115*:583, 1976.

Hinman, F., Jr., Oppenheimer, R. O., and Katz, I. L.: Accelerated obstruction at the ureteropelvic junction in adults. J. Urol., *129*:812, 1983.

Jacobs, J. A., Berger, B. W., Goldman, S. M., Robbins, M. A., and Young, J. D., Jr.: Ureteropelvic obstruction in adults with previously normal pyelograms: A report of 5 cases. J. Urol., *121*:242, 1979.

Johnston, J. H., Evans, J. P., Glassberg, K. I., and Shapiro, S. R.: Pelvic hydronephrosis in children: A review of 219 personal cases. J. Urol., *117*:97, 1977.

Kelalis, P. P., Culp, O. S., Stickler, G. B., and Burke, E. C.: Ureteropelvic junction obstruction in children: Experiences with 109 cases. J. Urol., *106*:418, 1971.

Koff, S. A.: Ureteropelvic junction obstruction: Role of newer diagnostic methods. J. Urol., *127*:898, 1982.

Küster: Ein Fall von Resection des Ureter. Arch. Klin. Chir., *44*:850, 1892.

McAlister, W. H., Manley, C. B., and Siegel, M. J.: Asymptomatic progression of partial ureteropelvic obstruction in children. J. Urol., *123*:267, 1980.

McMartin, W. J., Culp, O. S., Flocks, R. H., Foley, F. E. B., Gibson, T. E., and Moore, T. D.: Panel discussion on hydronephrosis. Urol. Surv., *7*:91, 1957.

Michigan, S., Whelton, P. K., and Walsh, P. C.: Forgotten kidney: Asynchronous bilateral ureteropelvic junction obstruction. Urology, *12*:565, 1978.

Nesbit, R. M.: Elliptical anastomosis in urologic surgery. Ann. Surg., *130*:796, 1949.

Nesbitt, T. E., McClellen, R. E., Tudor, J. M., and Carter, O. W.: Experiences with congenital hydronephrosis. South. Med. J., *57*:189, 1964.

O'Conor, V. J.: Diagnosis and treatment of hydronephrosis. J. Urol., *73*:451, 1955.

Ostling, K.: The genesis of hydronephrosis. Acta Chir. Scand. (Suppl.), *72*:86, 1942.

Patel, V. J.: A new spiral-flap pyeloplasty for short, long and very long ureteral stenosis. Presented at the 77th Annual Meeting of the American Urological Association, May 16–20, 1982, Kansas City, Mo.

Perlmutter, A. D., Kroovand, R. L., and Lai, Y. W.: Management of ureteropelvic obstruction in the first year of life. J. Urol., *123*:535, 1980.

Persky, L., and Tynberg, P.: Unsplintered, unstinted pyeloplasty. Urology, *1*:32, 1973.

Riehle, R. A., Jr., and Vaughan, E. D., Jr.: Renin participation in hypertension associated with unilateral hydronephrosis. J. Urol., *126*:243, 1981.

Roberts, J. B. M., and Slade, N.: The natural history of primary pelvic hydronephrosis. Br. J. Surg., *51*:759, 1964.

Roth, D. R., and Gonzales, E. T., Jr.: Management of ureteropelvic junction obstruction in infants. J. Urol., *129*:108, 1983.

Scardino, P. L., and Prince, C. L.: Vertical flap ureteropelvioplasty; preliminary report. South. Med. J., *46*:325, 1953.

Shopfner, C. E.: Ureteropelvic junction obstruction. Am. J. Roentgenol. Radium Ther. Nucl. Med., *98*:148, 1966.

Smart, W. R.: An evaluation of intubation ureterotomy

with a description of surgical technique. J. Urol., *85*:512, 1961.

Smart, W. R.: Surgical correction of hydronephrosis. *In* Harrison, J. H., Gittes, R. F., Perlmutter, A. D., Stamey, T. A., and Walsh, P. C. (Eds.): Campbell's Urology. 4th ed. Vol. III. Philadelphia, W. B. Saunders Co., 1979, p. 2047.

Stage, K. H., and Lewis, S.: Use of the radionuclide washout test in evaluation of suspected upper urinary tract obstruction. J. Urol., *125*:379, 1981.

Stephens, F. D.: Ureterovascular hydronephrosis and the "aberrant" renal vessels. J. Urol., *128*:984, 1982.

Thompson, I. M., Baker, J., Robards, V. L., Jr., Kovaci, L., and Ross, G., Jr.: Clinical experience with renal capsule flap pyeloplasty. J. Urol., *101*:487, 1969.

Thrall, J. H., Koff, S. A., and Keyes, J. W.: Diuretic radionuclide renography and scintigraphy in the differential diagnosis of hydroureteronephrosis. Semin. Nucl. Med., *10*:89, 1981.

Trendelenburg, F.: Uber Blasenscheidenfisteloperationen and über Beckenhochlagerung bei Operationen in der Bauchhöhle. Samml. Klin. Vortr. Chir., *109*:3373, 1890.

Weiss, R. M.: Clinical correlations of ureteral physiology. Am. J. Kidney Dis., *11*:409, 1983.

Wesolowski, S.: Uretero-calicostomy. Eur. Urol., *1*:18, 1975.

Whitaker, R. H.: Methods of assessing obstruction in dilated ureters. Br. J. Urol., *45*:15, 1973.

Whitaker, R. H.: Clinical assessment of pelvic and ureteral function. Urology, *12*:146, 1978.

Williams, D. I., and Karlaftis, C. M.: Hydronephrosis due to pelviureteric obstruction in the newborn. Br. J. Urol., *38*:138, 1966.

Williams, D. I., and Kenawi, M. M.: The prognosis of pelviureteric obstruction in childhood: A review of 190 cases. Eur. Urol., *2*:57, 1976.

Zincke, H., Kelalis, P. P., and Culp, O. S.: Ureteropelvic obstruction in children. Surg. Gynecol. Obstet., *139*:873, 1974.

CHAPTER 66

Renal Transplantation

OSCAR SALVATIERRA JR., M.D.

The development of human renal transplantation can be characterized as one of the truly outstanding medical achievements of this century. The field of renal transplantation encompasses a unique integration of surgical, medical, and immunologic disciplines that can now result in total rehabilitation and normal lives for most patients undergoing this therapy. Prior to the emergence of renal transplantation and dialysis therapy, all patients with end-stage organ failure succumbed to their illness. Although long-term hemodialysis can prolong survival and provide partial rehabilitation for many individuals with end-stage renal disease, only renal transplantation can currently restore normal life.

The history of renal transplantation began in about 1905 with the experiments of Carrel, who developed the techniques of vascular anastomoses that are still in use. However, the principal historical impediment to the successful transplantation of a human kidney has been that most transplant procedures necessitate transplantation of an organ between a donor and a recipient who are genetically dissimilar, although of the same species (an allograft). The possibility of transplantation between a donor and a recipient who are genetically perfectly identical, such as transplantation between monozygotic twins (an isograft), is very rare. The transplantation of an organ from a donor to a recipient of a different species (a xenograft) has never been successful experimentally or clinically.

The immunologic barriers that needed to be overcome were clearly demonstrated in the classic experiments of Medawar in the mid-1940's when he characterized the rejection of skin allografts in an outbred population of rabbits. That renal transplantation was feasible, however, was shown in 1954, when a Harvard University team performed the first successful kidney transplantation between identical twins. The next phase in human renal transplantation was an era when various procedures, such as irradiation, were attempted in order to abrogate the host reaction against a nonidentical twin allograft. It was not until the early 1960's that reasonable and successful immunosuppression was employed, with the advent of the drug azathioprine (Imuran) and its concomitant use with prednisone. The dramatic success with this double-drug therapy led to a period of great enthusiasm and greater utilization of kidney transplantation in patients other than those with an identical twin donor.

Later significant developments include refinement of surgical procedures, optimal utilization of both living related and cadaver donor organs, and dramatic improvements in immunosuppression regimens. This has resulted in the performance of over 6000 transplants in 1983 in the United States, of which approximately 30 per cent were from living related donors and 70 per cent from cadavers. These transplants were performed with remarkable graft and patient survival rates when compared with the results being achieved just two decades earlier.

The distribution of renal diseases leading to renal failure currently treated by transplantation is as follows: (1) chronic glomerulonephritis, 55 per cent; (2) diabetic nephropathy, 20 per cent; (3) chronic pyelonephritis, 8 per cent; (4) malignant nephrosclerosis, 6 per cent; (5) polycystic kidney disease, 5 per cent; and (6) other renal disease, 6 per cent.

In patients with end-stage renal disease who are 10 years of age and under, the incidence of glomerulonephritis is lower (30 per cent), with congenital nonobstructive and obstructive uropathies occurring more frequently (20 per cent) than in older groups.

PATIENT SELECTION—PREOPERATIVE TRANSPLANTATION STRATEGY

Histocompatibility Testing

The immune response of the recipient to the kidney graft histocompatibility antigens is the major barrier to the successful transplantation of organs. A single chromosomal complex of closely linked genes makes up the code for the major histocompatibility antigens. The major histocompatibility complex (MHC) in humans is called the HLA system (originally for human leukocyte antigen) and occupies a considerable segment of the short arm of the sixth human chromosome. The HLA system is known to include five histocompatibility loci within the MHC: HLA-A, HLA-B, HLA-C, HLA-D, and HLA-DR. Each HLA gene locus is highly polymorphic, so that approximately 8 to 35 separate antigens are controlled by each of these loci. Incompatibility with these histocompatibility antigens constitutes the immunologic barrier to organ transplantation.

When donor and recipient are identical twins, there is no antigenic difference whatsoever, and grafts are accepted without immunosuppressive therapy; such transplants are rare, however. Grafts from HLA-identical siblings give the next best results and constitute what is regarded as the most common immunologically privileged situation in transplantation (Fig. 66–1). Nevertheless, even though there may be perfect matching for the major histocompatibility antigens in an HLA- identical sibling match, immunosuppression is required because of incompatibilities at minor histocompatibility loci. Parents, offspring, and half of siblings will share one HLA haplotype plus many minor antigens and thus inherit the same single chromosome.

The HLA chromosomal complex, including HLA-A, HLA-B, HLA-C, HLA-D, and HLA-DR antigens, is termed a haplotype, which refers to that portion of a phenotype determined by closely linked genes of a single chromosome inherited from one parent. HLA histocompatibility testing is primarily of value in the search for HLA-identical siblings. HLA testing has not proved to be of significant worth in choosing between parents, offspring, or HLA-nonidentical siblings as donors, except to identify the zero-haplotype match sibling. Since cadaver transplantation represents the use of an organ from an unrelated individual, it is not surprising that many authorities question the value of HLA matching for cadaver kidney transplantation. Since the HLA system is the most polymorphic genetic system known, it is all but impossible to find perfectly matched cadaver kidney donors for prospective recipients.

Regardless of tissue-typing and antigen-matching results, it is essential to determine whether a recipient has preformed antibodies against antigens on the tissue of a potential donor, since the presence of such antibodies would result in immediate (hyperacute) rejection of the graft following implantation. These antibodies can be identified by crossmatch testing of the patient's serum against the donor lymphocytes prior to transplantation. The presence of these antibodies can usually be attributed to prior exposure to foreign histocompatibility antigens, as by blood transfusion, pregnancy, or previous transplantation.

Despite the emphasis on histocompatibility and crossmatch testing as described, it is important to recognize that an absolute prerequisite for transplantation of any organ is the presence of ABO blood group compatibility.

Living Related Donor Transplantation

The superior results in both patient and graft survival after living related donor transplantation suggest that this method be considered initially. As previously indicated, an HLA-identical sibling match is the optimal immunologic situation. However, only a few prospective transplant recipients have an ideally compatible related donor with good graft survival expectation so that, until recently, a potential organ recipient had to rely primarily on cadaver transplantation.

DONOR-SPECIFIC BLOOD TRANSFUSIONS (DST) IN HLA-MISMATCHED DONOR-RECIPIENT COMBINATIONS

The DST protocol was introduced at the University of California, San Francisco (UCSF), in 1978 in order to select one haplotype–related donor-recipient pairs to achieve better graft survival and, in addition, to alter the recipient immune response. Since blood transfusions from the prospective kidney donor to the potential recipient before renal allografting may result in sensitization to the donor and subsequent hyperacute rejection, clinicians had previously hesitated to employ this technique in human renal transplantation. The rationale for the UCSF trial was based on multiple factors, both experimental and clinical. With confirmed suc-

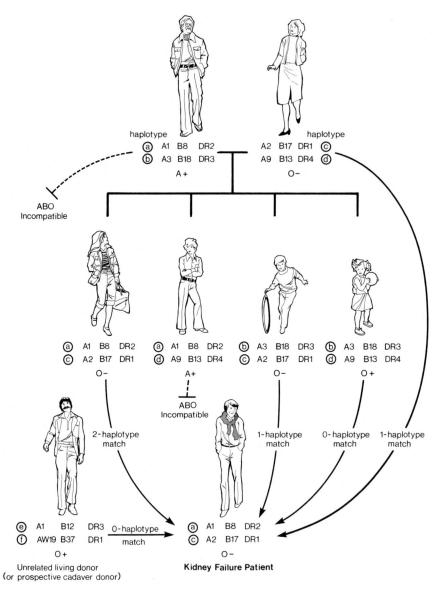

Figure 66–1. The inheritance of haplotypes and the influence of ABO blood group compatibility and HLA antigens in selecting potential donors for renal transplantation.

cess, candidates for the DST protocol now include non–HLA identical donor-recipient pairs, whether one- or zero-haplotype matched. The DST procedure involves the administration of approximately 200 ml of fresh whole blood or packed cell equivalent on three separate occasions at 2-week intervals. Until transplantation is performed, the potential recipient's sensitization against a blood donor is closely monitored by crossmatch testing of the recipient's sera obtained during and after the blood transfusions. The criterion for proceeding with transplantation has been a negative T-warm and B-

warm donor-specific crossmatch; recently, however, by utilizing flow cytometry, the majority of patients with a positive B-warm crossmatch can be safely transplanted.

Graft survival in the post-transplant course of DST recipients, without any exclusions, has been essentially the same as that in the concurrently transplanted HLA-identical sibling group—the immunologically privileged grade in renal transplantation. Graft survival, however, was markedly better than in the non–DST treated one-haplotype group (p <0.0005). These results have now been confirmed by a large variety of reports worldwide. Earlier it was feared that the DST effect might dissipate with time, but an analysis of graft survival in consecutive nondiabetic DST recipients with more than a 3-month follow-up shows that the transfusion effect persists for at least 5 years, with a 5-year graft survival of 88 per cent, slightly better than the graft survival in the HLA-identical group. The immunosuppressive protocol for the DST and the HLA-identical groups has been the same, with emphasis on a strict ceiling on immunosuppressive medication administered so as to minimize complications and enhance patient survival.

The results with the DST protocol continue to indicate that the process in itself does not jeopardize the potential recipient, even those in whom a positive crossmatch to their potential related donor develops. In the group that did become sensitized to the DST, the sensitization usually has been narrow, as would be expected from exposure to a limited number of transplantation antigens. A substantial number of these sensitized patients have now received transplants from a donor other than the transfusion donor, most often a cadaver graft, which would have been the transplant of choice in any case before the DST protocol was introduced.

For the potential kidney donors in the DST protocol, the process of preliminary blood donation has been harmless and has spared many donors the possibility of donating a kidney that would probably later be rejected. The potential donor who has a positive donor-specific crossmatch has experienced increased self-esteem in actively participating with the family member in the identification of a compatible kidney. For the blood transfusion donor who eventually undergoes an operation, the process of renal donation is being accomplished with excellent prospects of success, and the donor is able to approach the surgical procedure with more confidence and less anxiety.

The mechanism of action of the donor-specific blood transfusions is not fully understood. There is the process of selection, as the DST protocol segregates responders from non-responders by means of the careful monitoring of the specific antibody response to the blood donor. The DST protocol thus appears to eliminate donor-recipient pairs destined for certain graft loss by specific advance testing. However, the excellent graft survival and generally benign post-transplant course achieved in many patients who eventually receive a kidney from their crossmatch-negative donor demands other explanations. Because immunogenic exposure has

involved repetitive transfusion of donor-specific antigens in modest doses, the induction of some degree of specific unresponsiveness to these same antigens on the subsequently transplanted kidney can be theorized. The post-transplant, donor-specific transfusion effect probably encompasses a complex of various mechanisms, and it may be that suppressor cells and anti-idiotypic antibodies play an important role in this induction. Because of the shortage of cadaver donor organs and the potential of DST for excellent results, the possibility of routinely extending the procedure to zero haplotype match–related and unrelated donor-recipient pairs is being explored. In addition, the prospective study assessing the efficacy of the DST protocol and the new immunosuppressive agent cyclosporine in one haplotype–matched donor-recipient pairs needs to be assessed.

Cadaver Transplantation

For patients with no potentially compatible living donor, cadaver transplantation has been a viable alternative despite an inferior success rate compared with living related transplantation. Recently, with the advent of cyclosporine immunosuppression, cadaver graft survival rates have shown an approximate 20 per cent improvement in comparison with survival rates for conventional immunosuppressive therapy. Immunologic factors that may influence cadaver graft survival, such as pretransplant third-party blood transfusions and HLA match grade, must be considered separately under the immunosuppressive therapy utilized.

With conventional immunosuppressive therapy, third-party blood transfusions before first cadaver kidney transplants have a significantly beneficial effect on graft survival. The principal problem with larger numbers of pretransplant transfusions from multiple donors is the risk of hepatitis as well as the greater likelihood of achieving sensitization from exposure to a large variety of foreign histocompatibility antigens. The latter could reduce the possibility of readily identifying a compatible cadaver kidney by direct crossmatch testing, although the presence of preformed lymphocytotoxic antibodies has not in itself impaired graft success. The superior graft survival rates achieved with cyclosporine immunosuppression do not appear to be significantly influenced by pretransplant blood transfusions. Thus, there is no compelling reason to intentionally transfuse potential cadaver graft recipients with cyclosporine therapy. This obviates the risk of these transfusions, particularly the risk of increased sensitization to a variety of histocompatibility antigens, which could markedly delay the identification of a crossmatch-negative compatible cadaver graft. Nevertheless, the lack of significant efficacy of pretransplant blood transfusions with cyclosporine therapy awaits further study to confirm the initial impression.

The degree of HLA matched grade at the A, B, and C loci appears to have no bearing on eventual graft outcome. However, whether matching at the DR locus improves cadaver graft survival under conventional immunosuppression is still controversial. Under cyclosporine therapy, the improved graft survival rate appears to override any possible influence of HLA matching. Because of the extreme polymorphism of the histocompatibility system, complete HLA-identical matches of recipients with cadaver grafts are extremely rare.

MANAGEMENT OF PRE-EXISTING UROLOGIC DISEASE PRIOR TO TRANSPLANTATION

Preliminary Bilateral Nephrectomy

Approximately 90 per cent of all patients now receive kidney transplants with their native kidneys left in situ. The indications for preliminary nephrectomy prior to transplantation, described in order of frequency of performance, are as follows:

1. *Anatomic abnormalities of the urinary tract with or without infection*, as with hydronephrosis or moderately severe ureteral reflux. In patients with moderately severe reflux or ureteral abnormalities, nephroureterectomy should be performed with removal of the ureter close to the ureterovesical junction. Mild or fleeting reflux has not proved to be an absolute indication for preliminary bilateral nephroureterectomy prior to transplantation. In fact, mild or fleeting reflux is rarely a cause of end-stage kidney disease, it is most likely to be a finding associated with some other primary etiologic mechanism. Reflux as an actual cause of end-stage kidney disease is almost always at least moderately severe. It is worth noting that in cases of moderately severe or severe reflux, successful antireflux operation during a time when only minimal impairment of renal function existed has frequently resulted in a noninfected and nondilated urinary tract that has obviated the need for preliminary nephrectomy. In pa-

tients with successful antireflux surgery in whom a nondilated urinary tract exists but persistent renal infection has continued to occur, only the kidneys themselves need to be removed, without total ureterectomy.

2. *Some cases of polycystic renal disease.* If the patient has a history of renal infection or significant hematuria requiring repeated transfusions, preparation by nephrectomy is a prerequisite to transplantation. If the history is negative, transplantation without nephrectomy is preferred and has proved to be safe. The size of the polycystic kidney has not been an indication for preliminary nephrectomy in the UCSF series.

3. *Severe hypertension uncontrolled by medication or dialysis.* This is now a very rare indication for nephrectomy prior to transplantation. If severe hypertension persists as a problem following transplantation, the patient then is a much better candidate for bilateral nephrectomy of the usually small kidneys. This can easily be accomplished through a bilateral posterior lombotomy approach utilizing two small incisions. One is then assured that the kidneys are being removed only after it is established that the transplant kidney is providing good renal function.

The advantages of leaving native kidneys in situ relate primarily to the pretransplant period and also to those instances in which the kidney graft is lost and the patient is returned to dialysis. Reasons for avoiding preliminary pretransplant nephrectomy except when absolutely indicated are as follows:

1. Many patients maintain a moderate urinary output, even after the initiation of maintenance dialysis, which reduces the need for fluid restriction and allows greater freedom during dialysis therapy.

2. The anemia of uremia is less severe with native kidneys in situ, particularly in patients with polycystic kidney disease, in whom a relative erythrocythemia seems to prevail. Even without the erythrocythemia that is seen in polycystic kidney disease, patients with renal failure from other causes can often be maintained at a stable, relatively low hematocrit without the need for third-party blood transfusions. These third-party blood transfusions hold a certain risk of hepatitis and the development of lymphocytotoxic antibodies, which may make it difficult to find a negative cross-match–compatible cadaver graft and, at times, even a living related donor graft. One of the most distressing conditions following transplantation occurs in those patients who lose their

kidney graft and are left without native in situ kidneys. In these patients, dialysis management is extremely difficult and the transfusion requirement excessive. Despite transfusion in some cases, the hematocrit level remains quite low, and the patient's level of activity is severely compromised compared with his prenephrectomy status.

3. A major surgical procedure is avoided. This is particularly the case in patients with large polycystic kidneys if absolute indications for the procedure are nonexistent.

SURGICAL APPROACHES FOR PRELIMINARY NEPHRECTOMY

When polycystic kidneys are to be removed or a bilateral nephroureterectomy is to be performed, surgery can best be accomplished through a midline abdominal incision from the xyphoid to near the symphysis pubis. When small kidneys are to be removed, as for hypertension, end-stage atrophic kidneys with hydronephrosis but without hydroureter, and recurrent pyelonephritis without significant ureteral dilatation (e.g., after earlier successful surgical correction of reflux), a bilateral posterior lombotomy approach or the use of small flank incisions is most appropriate. These approaches eliminate the need to enter the abdominal cavity, thus obviating the minimal risk of intestinal obstruction in the post-transplant period. Management of intestinal obstruction post transplantation, while the patient is on immunosuppression medication, can be a very difficult problem. It should be underscored that the end-stage kidney is usually a small kidney and a flank or posterior lombotomy incision can certainly be limited in extent.

The most important considerations regarding preliminary bilateral nephrectomy prior to transplantation relate to the uremic state, the need for postoperative dialysis, and the awareness and avoidance of hyperkalemia postoperatively. Because of coagulation abnormalities associated with uremia, surgery in the uremic patient mandates meticulous and thorough hemostasis. This is of extreme importance when one realizes that the patient will require dialysis during the postoperative period. The practice at UCSF is to have the patient undergo extended hemodialysis the afternoon before the day of surgery, so that dialysis postoperatively can be withheld until the second or, if possible, the third postoperative day. Even then, heparinization must be minimal and controlled by regular and repetitive serial clotting times. The need for meticulous hemostasis is also important

in that blood transfusions should be avoided as much as possible. Blood transfusions in the postoperative uremic anephric patient can easily increase the risk of postoperative hyperkalemia.

Another important consideration for preliminary nephrectomy in the uremic patient relates to the need for a meticulous and strong wound closure. A patient undergoing preliminary nephrectomy prior to transplantation is a patient with long-standing chronic illness and uremia with secondary impaired wound healing.

The Long-Term Defunctionalized Urinary Bladder

Since obstructive uropathy and primary vesical ureteral reflux with significant hydroureteronephrosis can result in end-stage renal failure, potential transplant recipients are often evaluated following multiple reconstructive urologic procedures and urinary diversion. Not infrequently there has been long-term defunctionalization of the urinary bladder. A major question regarding the patients is whether the native urinary bladder can serve as a satisfactory receptacle for the transplant ureter. If not, it is necessary to create an ileal loop for anastomosis of the transplant ureter or renal pelvis.

The approach at UCSF has been to provide maximal rehabilitation for the patient with the renal transplant, including avoidance of ileal loop urinary diversion for the transplanted kidney. In the UCSF series of over 2300 renal transplants, ileal loop diversion was utilized in only five. With this experience as substantiation, it appears that the only absolute indication for ileal loop diversion may be a true neurogenic bladder or absence of a urinary bladder from previous surgery. Most patients presenting with renal failure and urinary diversion have primarily obstruction or severe reflux as causes for their hydroureteronephrosis. In patients with diverted severe reflux, the urinary bladder should be perfectly acceptable. In those with outlet obstruction, usually of posterior urethral valves, correction of the obstruction should also make these bladders satisfactory receptacles for the transplant ureter.

The assessment of these patients includes a history and physical examination that evaluates for the absence of fecal incontinence, the absence of somatic neurologic deficits, and the presence of good anal sphincter tone and volitional contraction. The urologic assessment consists primarily of cystoscopy and retrograde cystography. Urinary continence and voiding potential are verified and the postvoid residual assessed. Since these bladders often have been defunctionalized for long periods (as much as 18 years in the UCSF series), complete emptying of the bladder is not often possible with this evaluation. In addition, urodynamic studies have not been helpful and are not utilized at present. Figure 66–2 is an example of a patient with a 15-ml capacity bladder preoperatively; Figure 66–3 represents a 3-month post transplant IVP showing an already enlarging bladder capacity in the same patient. At 6 months post transplantation, bladder capacity had increased to approximately 350 ml.

TRANSPLANTATION SURGERY

Cadaver Donor Nephrectomy

Because a medically and immunologically suitable living related donor is not always available for a transplant recipient, approximately 70 per cent of transplant recipients must currently rely on cadaver grafts. Transplantation of cadaver grafts of the highest quality is of extreme importance in achieving maximal effectiveness with the lowest possible patient morbidity and mortality. Strict adherence to technical details during donor nephrectomy is therefore of utmost importance.

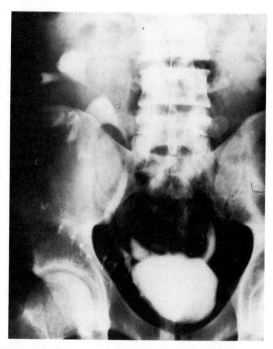

Figure 66–3. Intravenous pyelogram post transplant in the same patient shown in Figure 66–2. It demonstrates a well-functioning transplant kidney with a nondilated collecting system and, most important, a urinary bladder of increased capacity. The previously demonstrated dilated distal ureteral segments are now seen as small remnants on the superior aspect of the bladder, indicating that the increased capacity was attributable, in part, to an expanded trigonal area.

There are various ways to perform cadaver donor nephrectomy; as the need for extrarenal organs increases, surgeons responsible for the procurement of kidneys will find themselves more frequently involved with teams removing other organs, such as the heart and liver. In general, the kidneys can be removed in a heart-beating or non–heart beating cadaver. In this era of multiple organ donation, the nephrectomy surgeons must coordinate their organ removal with that of those performing a cardiectomy, hepatectomy, or pancreatectomy.

At UCSF, donor nephrectomy generally has been performed in non–heart beating cadavers, although most centers use heart-beating cadavers, which are essential when extrarenal organs are being removed. A non–heart beating cadaver provides an essentially bloodless field, permits quick removal, and allows efficient removal of the kidneys as part of multiple organ donation, such as after cardiectomy, which in itself eliminates further renal perfusion. With hepatectomy, en bloc concomitant infusion of kidneys is accomplished with that of the liver, and then the kidneys are removed after hepatectomy.

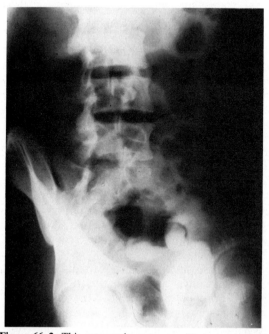

Figure 66–2. This retrograde cystogram illustrates a 15-ml capacity bladder that had been defunctionalized for approximately 18 years. The distal ureteral stumps are seen superiorly, and the dilated prostatic urethra is seen inferiorly.

Cadaver donor nephrectomy is described herein as it is performed at UCSF and can easily be modified so as to ensure maximal protection of the heart or liver in multiple organ donation. Generally, cadaver donors are systemically heparinized with 20,000 units of intravenous aqueous heparin prior to the cessation of assisted respiratory support of the brain-dead donor. Phenoxybenzamine is a potent alpha-blocking agent that is given to cadaver donors, in a dose of 100 mg intravenously for adults, approximately 20 minutes prior to nephrectomy. The UCSF experience supports the previously reported role of phenoxybenzamine in preventing agonal renal vasospasm. Once renal vasospasm is established, it usually persists during preservation, resulting in inadequate tissue perfusion and organ damage.

Except for pediatric donors and in instances of bilateral multiple arteries, when the kidneys are removed en bloc with the aorta, individual nephrectomy is usually performed for organ procurement. Laparotomy is performed through a midline abdominal incision from xyphoid to symphysis pubis. Bilateral transverse extensions of this incision toward each flank facilitate exposure. In situ aortic flushing of the kidneys with cold lactated Ringer's solution is instituted after freeing up of the left ureter so as not to injure it. Rapid access to the distal aorta for cannulation is accomplished by incising the left lateral peritoneal reflection and retracting the sigmoid colon medially. The left ureter is then easily identified and meticulously dissected free with adequate surrounding tissue from just above the bladder, where it is divided, to well above the bifurcation of the aorta so as to not to traumatize it during aortic cannulation. The latter is accomplished by encircling the lower portion of the aorta with two umbilical tapes just above the bifurcation. The aorta is then opened between the tapes, and the modified Foley catheter is inserted into the aortotomy and advanced so that the balloon comes to lie above the renal arteries, at which point it is inflated to occlude the aorta. The catheter has been modified by occlusion of its normal distal opening with Silastic glue and construction of a new opening into the lumen proximal to the balloon. In situ perfusion of the isolated aortic segment and renal arteries can thus be performed easily, achieving rapid cooling of the kidneys, which affords additional time if donor nephrectomy proves to be difficult because of multiple vessels.

Next, the gonadal and the adrenal tributaries of the left renal vein are ligated and divided, and the left renal vein itself is divided close to the junction with the vena cava. The anterior surface of the aorta is now easily dissected, allowing a search for multiple renal arteries on both sides. Division of the crus of the diaphragm enveloping the aorta allows easy superior access to that portion of the aorta where a superior polar artery may originate. If a single renal artery to the left kidney is found, it is divided and the left donor nephrectomy completed.

One should avoid manipulating the kidneys during dissection or placing traction on the kidneys prior to dividing the vessels. The latter is emphasized in order to avoid an intimal arterial tear, which would predispose to thrombosis after revascularization of the graft.

If a single renal artery is found to the right kidney, that kidney is removed in identical fashion to the left, after medial reflection of the cecum and ascending colon. If multiple arteries are found to either kidney, that particular kidney is removed en bloc with the aorta so that washout and perfusion can be performed through the aorta, and the kidney subsequently can be transplanted with a Carrel patch encompassing the multiple vessels. If bilateral multiple renal arteries are present, the kidneys are both removed en bloc with the aorta.

Donor nephrectomy must be accomplished in a manner that consistently preserves the blood supply to the ureter from the renal vessels. Interruption of the venous circulation of the ureter can be as lethal as interruption of the arterial blood supply. Although blood supply to the ureter has multiple origins, with free anastomoses in the ureteral adventitia, the ureter of the transplanted kidney receives its blood supply only from the renal vessel branches that course in the hilar and upper periureteral tissues. Small aberrant renal vessels can easily be overlooked, and a divided vessel to the lower pole of the kidney may provide the major ureteral blood supply. Because the ureteral blood supply courses in the adventitia, the ureter must be meticulously removed with adequate surrounding tissue. A sufficient length of ureter also must be obtained to prevent tension at the ureterovesical anastomoses during and after implantation into the recipient. No dissection should be performed in the area of the renal pelvis or hilus of the kidney. For maximal assurance of preservation of ureteral blood supply, a large conical mass of hilar and periureteral fatty tissue should be removed en bloc with the kidneys and ureter (Fig. 66–4).

The potentially lethal dangers of ureteral urinary extravasation in the immunosuppressed

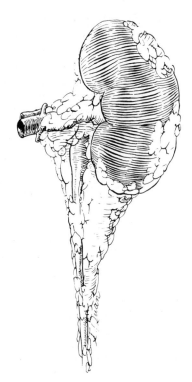

Figure 66–4. Diagrammatic representation of the left kidney with a large conical mass of hilar and periureteral fatty tissue. (From Salvatierra, O., Kountz, F., and Belzer, F.: J. Urol., *112*:445, 1974.)

transplant recipient with impaired healing and resistance to infection cannot be overemphasized. Vascular insufficiency is probably the fundamental cause of ureteral necrosis with subsequent urinary extravasation. The very low rate of ureteral leak noted in the UCSF series is believed to be directly related to strict adherence to detail in organ procurement and strict attention to the management of the ureter and multiple arteries.

CADAVER ORGAN PRESERVATION

Preservation of the cadaver kidney prior to transplantation can be accomplished in two basic ways: by simple hypothermic storage or by perfusion preservation. In simple hypothermic storage, the kidneys are removed from a heart-beating cadaver donor and then are rapidly cooled, usually by a combination of a flush-out solution, such as Collins, and external cooling to reduce the renal core temperature. The kidneys are then stored in a plastic container and immersed in another container packed with crushed ice. The principal disadvantage of this method is that the period of preservation when good early renal function might be expected after implantation is limited to about 24 to 30

hours. There are reports of extended preservation times following cold storage, but they are accompanied by an extremely high incidence of acute tubular necrosis postoperatively. The latter may potentiate the risk of nephrotoxicity from the immunosuppressive agent cyclosporine and may additionally require a long period of costly postoperative dialysis.

A variety of perfusates have been used over the years for perfusion preservation, with current perfusates being modified albumin solutions. The major advantage of continuous perfusion preservation is that there is a low incidence of postoperative acute tubular necrosis, with extended storage up to nearly 3 days. There are some additional advantages. No kidneys need be discarded because of time limitations of the storage method, and a sudden influx of several cadaver organs to a single transplant center can be satisfactorily transplanted by a small team. Perfusion preservation also allows removal of kidneys after a period of warm ischemia (less than 1 hour) and utilization of donors with elevated serum creatinine values (but less than twice normal at the time of nephrectomy). However, to ensure viability of the organ and to minimize the need for postoperative hemodialysis for acute tubular necrosis, it is important that perfusion preservation be started immediately after donor nephrectomy. Utilizing perfusion preservation, the postoperative dialysis rate following transplantation at UCSF is currently less than 30 per cent, regardless of the time of preservation.

The most recent report of the Human Renal Transplant Registry and other studies have shown that the choice between perfusion preservation and cold storage probably has no ultimate influence on long-term survival of cadaver grafts. In fact, a majority of centers currently utilize cold storage, and good results can be expected from either method. Whatever the storage method selected, it must be utilized within its limitations. If the transplant center is utilizing cyclosporine immunosuppressive therapy, the major emphasis should be on minimizing the post-transplant acute tubular necrosis rate so as to minimize the risk of nephrotoxicity from this agent.

Living Related Donor Nephrectomy

Living related donor nephrectomy is best accomplished through the standard flank approach, with or without removal of the distal eleventh and twelfth ribs (see Chapter 63). The principles of nephrectomy described for cadaver donor nephrectomy also apply in the case of a living related donor. The donor nephrectomy must be performed in such a way that the blood supply to the ureter from the renal vessels is preserved. Since all living related donors have preoperative arteriograms, the presence of multiple arteries is determined prior to transplantation. Most donors have a single renal artery to at least one of their kidneys. Sometimes a related donor kidney with multiple arteries must be used, but without a Carrel patch, because removal of a portion of the donor aorta would involve increased donor risk. In cases of multiple arteries, these vessels are implanted separately or an ex vivo renal artery reconstruction is performed prior to kidney reimplantation.

Multiple renal veins may often be encountered on the right side, but the right renal vein can safely be taken with a small cuff of donor vena cava. The vena cava is then oversewn with a running 5-0 cardiovascular suture following nephrectomy.

There are other considerations that apply to a living related donor. Anesthesia is not started in the donor until intravenous hydration has resulted in excellent diuresis. If anesthesia is induced prior to diuresis, the ADH effect will make it difficult to later obtain diuresis. In related donor nephrectomy, it is also important to avoid traction on the pedicle and to frequently feel the kidney to assure that it is well perfused. It is stimulation of the nerve supply to the kidney during dissection that probably produces vasospasm and causes the kidney to become soft, with no urine production. If the kidney becomes soft, dissection should be discontinued until the kidney has again become firm. Mannitol is given in divided doses during dissection of the renal pedicle, not only to maintain diuresis but also to prevent the cell swelling that occurs with ischemic injury of the kidney. It is imperative that the kidney be firm and that urine be spurting from the ureter prior to final division of the renal vessels for completion of the nephrectomy. By using this approach for donor nephrectomy, postoperative dialysis should rarely be necessary in living related donor transplants.

The procedure of living related donor nephrectomy can best be placed in perspective by realizing that kidney extirpation is not being carried out for disease, but that the kidney is being removed in a way that ensures the same function and anatomic integrity in the recipient as was present in the donor.

Graft Implantation

Transplantation of a kidney graft in the renal failure patient requires precision and careful surgical technique. There is no other operation that is routinely performed under the same high-risk constraints attended with uremia and immunosuppression, which conditions give no latitude for surgical error. It is also important that the prospective transplant recipient be in optimal metabolic and electrolyte balance so as to avoid difficult operative hemostasis associated with inadequate dialysis. Inadequate dialysis preoperatively can also result in postoperative hyperkalemia, which would necessitate early postoperative dialysis and heparinization, with their risks during this period.

INCISION AND PREPARATION OF THE ILIAC FOSSA

A gentle curvilinear incision is made in either the right or the left lower quadrant, extending from near the symphysis pubis to approximately 1.5 cm medial to the anterior superior iliac spine and up to approximately 2 cm below the lower thoracic cage (Fig. 66–5A). The upper four fifths of the incision is extended through the external oblique, internal oblique, and transversus abdominis muscle; the lower one fifth of the incision usually requires partial division of the lower rectus. The inferior epigastric vessels are identified and skeletonized as they pass across the line of the incision, and then they are divided and ligated. There is an anterior extraperitoneal thin fascial layer that is divided in the direction of the incision, permitting entry into the extraperitoneal space and easy development of an essentially avascular plane immediately adjacent to the peritoneum.

The peritoneum is then retracted medially, at which time the spermatic cord in the male or the round ligament in the female is easily identified. In the male patient, the connective tissue around the cord is freed to permit easier retraction of the cord so that a self-retaining retractor can be inserted easily. Cord ligation should be avoided to prevent post-transplantation testicular atrophy or hydrocele formation. In the female patient, the round ligament is divided and ligated. Once the self-retaining retractor is in place, the extraperitoneal space can further be developed with exposure of the distal common and external iliac arteries.

The dissection and skeletonization of the iliac vessels must be performed in a manner that allows secure ligation of the divided lymphatics passing over these vessels. This is best accom-

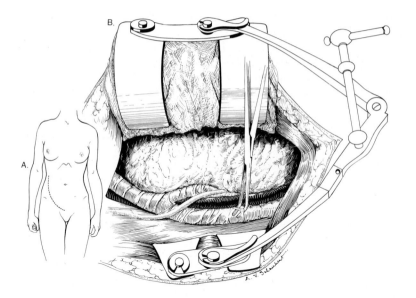

Figure 66–5. *A,* The incision for the transplant procedure is indicated for the right abdomen. However, the transplant itself can be performed on either the right or the left side. *B,* The iliac fossa is exposed with a self-retaining retractor, following which segmental separation, ligature, and division of perivascular tissue containing lymphatics are carried out. (From Salvatierra, O.: *In* Glenn, J. F. (Ed.): Urologic Surgery. Philadelphia, J. B. Lippincott Co., 1983.)

plished by the use of a fine right angle forceps to develop the plane of Leriche over the external and distal common iliac arteries (Fig. 66–5*B*). The tissue overlying the arteries and containing the lymphatics is segmentally separated in sequential fashion so that the tissue can be doubly ligated with 4-0 suture and divided. This maneuver greatly reduces the incidence of lymphocele, which can occur in the postoperative period from lymphatic leakage secondary to free draining transected lymphatic vessels. Following this procedure, the iliac artery can be skeletonized and freed up from adjacent tissue by sharp scissor dissection. Palpation of the common iliac bifurcation and internal iliac artery will determine whether the internal iliac artery should also be skeletonized in preparation for an end-to-end anastomosis with the graft renal artery. If there is moderate atherosclerosis extending into the bifurcation, an end-to-side anastomosis with the external iliac artery is preferable. However, if endarterectomy can be safely performed or if there is no evidence of atherosclerosis in the internal iliac vessel, skeletonization of this vessel can also be accomplished. Again, before skeletonization is begun, the traversing logitudinal lymphatics on the medial aspect of the iliac bifurcation should be doubly ligated and divided. If the internal iliac artery is to be used, it can be clamped proximally with a Wylie hypogastric artery clamp and divided distally with appropriate ligation of the distal stump. The freed internal iliac artery should be irrigated with heparinized saline solution.

Skeletonization of the iliac vein can now be accomplished, but with the same segmental ligature and division of anterior lymphatic-containing tissue as was done with the arterial dissection. Posterior venous tributaries are often encountered and must be divided if maximal anterior mobility of the iliac vein is desired. It is important to doubly ligate these posterior tributaries with 2-0 or 3-0 suture prior to actual division, because the double-clamping maneuver may sometimes result in injury or avulsion of the delicate distal stump during ligature. Hemostasis then can be achieved only with great difficulty and with risk of obturator nerve injury.

VASCULAR ANASTOMOSES

The iliac vein is prepared for the end-to-side renal vein anastomosis by placement of vascular clamps proximal and distal to the proposed venotomy for the anastomoses. The venotomy is fashioned to accommodate the caliber of the renal vein and can best be accomplished with curved endarterectomy scissors that permit removal of a smooth ellipse of vein. The isolated segment of the iliac vein can then be irrigated with heparinized saline. Following this, four 5-0 or 6-0 cardiovascular sutures can be placed at the superior and inferior apices of the venotomy and at the midpoints of the medial and lateral margins of the venotomy. The sutures will later be passed through corresponding points on the renal vein for a four-quadrant end-to-side attachment of the renal vein to the iliac vein.

If a cadaver kidney is being used, the graft is removed from either cold storage or perfusion preservation. With living related donor transplantation, the graft is obtained from the live donor in an adjacent operating room and is placed in a container with cold Ringer's lactated solution. The renal artery is additionally flushed with cold heparinized Ringer's lactate.

To facilitate implantation, the kidney is secured in a sling and held in position for the vascular anastomoses by the assistant. A clamp is used to secure the sling to prevent the assistant from holding the kidney in position with his hands, which might accelerate warming of the kidney during the period of vascular anastomosis.

The previously placed four sutures through the iliac vein are now passed through the corresponding points of the renal vein, which, when secured, bring the renal vein into juxtaposition with the iliac venotomy (Fig. 66–6A). The medial and lateral sutures are retracted with mosquito clamps, which separate the venotomy opening to facilitate rapid anastomoses without inadvertent suture of the back wall. The superior suture is used as a running suture down one side of the renal vein, and the inferior suture is used as a running suture up the other side of the renal vein.

If the internal iliac artery is to be used for the arterial anastomoses, and end-to-end anastomosis is performed with the renal artery (Fig. 66–6B). The two vessels are positioned so as to allow a gentle upward curve from the iliac

bifurcation to the kidney by fixation of the superior and inferior arterial apices with interrupted 5-0 or 6-0 cardiovascular sutures. The anastomosis can be completed with either running or interrupted sutures, but the latter is preferred. Interrupted sutures absolutely avoid any pursestring effect, as might occur from a running suture, and allow better accommodation of the two vessels to each other even when a size discrepancy exists. With the use of interrupted anastomoses, there was less than a 1 per cent incidence of subsequent renal artery stenosis in the UCSF series.

As for the technique used in the interrupted anastomosis, the initial interrupted suture is placed midway between the apical sutures on the anterior vessel walls facing the operator, thus allowing optimal approximation of the opposing arterial margins, particularly when discrepancy in vessel size exists. The remaining interrupted sutures are placed to approximate each anterior quadrant. Following this, the previously placed apical sutures are used to rotate the arteries, so that the posterior vessel walls will now face the operator for further suture placement. Just as before, a suture is put midway between the apical sutures, which divides the rotated posterior vessel walls into quadrants for subsequent interrupted suture placement.

Figure 66–6. *A,* The renal vein is brought into exact juxtaposition with the iliac vein venotomy by the previously placed four quadrant sutures, following which a running suture anastomosis is accomplished. *B,* The renal artery is seen positioned for an end-to-end anastomosis with the internal iliac artery following the placement of superior and inferior apical sutures. *C,* The completed venous and arterial anastomoses are demonstrated. (From Salvatierra, O.: *In* Glenn, J. F. (Ed.): Urologic Surgery. Philadelphia, J. B. Lippincott Co., 1983.)

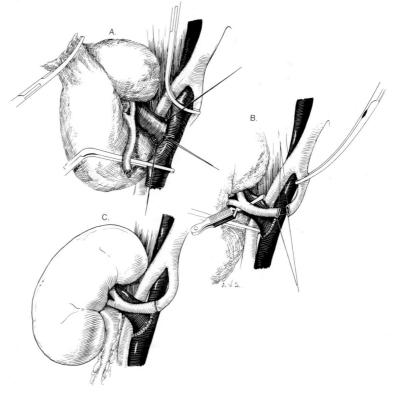

The completed venous and arterial anastomoses are shown in Figure 66–6C.

If extensive arteriosclerotic plaques extend into the bifurcation of the common iliac artery, an end-to-side anastomosis of the renal artery to the external or common iliac artery is preferred. Usually this anastomosis is performed superior to the level of the venous anastomosis. Appropriate vascular clamps are placed superior and inferior to the proposed location of the iliac arteriotomy. The location of the clamps must be carefully selected so as not to injure or disrupt any existing arteriosclerotic plaques. The longitudinal incision is then made on the anterior or anterolateral portion of the iliac arterial segment with a No. 11 blade knife. Following incision, regional heparinization of the lower extremity is accomplished by instilling approximately 50 ml of heparinized saline (500 units/dl) into the distal iliac artery. Systemic heparinization is not necessary during the procedure. Following regional heparinization, ellipses of arterial wall are removed on each side with a curved DeBakey endarterectomy scissors, which allows a smooth, oval arteriotomy to accommodate the end of the renal artery. This anastomosis is also performed with interrupted 5-0 or 6-0 cardiovascular sutures after initial fixation of the ends of the renal artery to the apices of the arteriotomy with superior and inferior sutures. The intervening interrupted sutures may then be placed according to the operator's preference.

The previously placed sling around the kidney can be removed at this time. It is extremely important to have obtained preoperative assessment of the recipient for existing cold agglutinins, because moderate to high titers of these agglutinins will require some warming of the kidney before re-establishment of circulation. The vascular clamps can then be released, with the venous clamps removed before the arterial clamps.

MULTIPLE RENAL VESSELS

A cadaver kidney with multiple renal arteries perfused with the aorta is best transplanted with an end-to-side anastomosis with a Carrel patch encompassing the multiple arteries (Fig. 66–7). If the vessels are in close proximity to each other, a single Carrel patch will suffice. If the vessels are some distance apart, two Carrel patches, or some other modification as will be described for the living donor kidney, can be used. The Carrel patch of the donor aorta is fashioned to accommodate the multiple vessels, and its anastomosis to the common or external

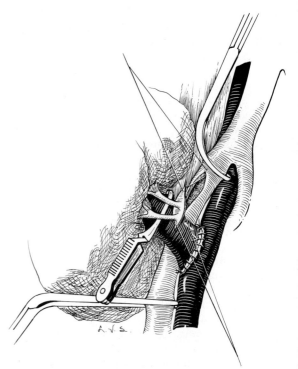

Figure 66–7. A donor aorta Carrel patch encompassing two renal arteries is positioned to an iliac arteriotomy by apical sutures. The arteriotomy was fashioned to accommodate the configuration of the Carrel patch. (From Salvatierra, O.: *In* Glenn, J. F. (Ed.): Urologic Surgery. Philadelphia, J. B. Lippincott Co., 1983.)

iliac artery is performed after an arteriotomy that accommodates the length and width of the Carrel patch. This anastomosis is best performed by fixing the patch at the superior and inferior apices of the arteriotomy with 5-0 cardiovascular suture. The superior suture is then used as a running suture down one side of the arterial anastomosis, and the inferior suture is used as a running suture up the opposite side of the arterial anastomosis.

The presence of multiple arteries in living related donor transplantation is known in advance, because all live related donors have preoperative arteriograms. Most donors have at least a single artery to one of their kidneys, but at times, a donor kidney with double arteries or triple arteries must be used. However, these arteries cannot be taken with a Carrel patch because of the risk to the live donor. In these instances, there are various alternatives that can be tailored to the size and length of the vessels and the capability of the vessels to be anastomosed without tension. These alternatives include double end-to-side renal arteries to iliac artery, and end-to-end superior renal artery to internal iliac artery, with end-to-side inferior renal artery to external iliac artery. Small polar vessels can perhaps best be sutured to the side of the main renal artery with interrupted 6-0 or 7-0 cardiovascular suture after an appropriate oval arteriotomy is created in the main stem renal artery. The larger renal artery can then be anastomosed to the internal, external, or common iliac artery. If there are multiple small renal arteries, it is usually easier to remove the internal iliac artery and its branches from the recipient and to separately perform the anastomoses of the multiple renal arteries to the internal iliac artery or its branches as an ex vivo procedure. This technique will allow precise anastomosis of each of the small vessels while the kidney is preserved in an ice bath. Alternatively, this could also be done with perfusion preservation on the table. These small anastomoses are best accomplished using 6-0 or 7-0 cardiovascular suture. The distal end of the internal iliac artery can then be anastomosed in end-to-side fashion to the common or external iliac artery in the recipient.

If there are two renal arteries of equal size that are long enough and close enough together, they can be spatulated on their adjacent sides and the spatulated ends of the arteries then approximated to each other so as to create a single lumen. These spatulated vessels can best be brought together by beginning the anastomosis with a single double-armed 6-0 or 7-0 cardiovascular suture joining the apices. Each end of the suture is run down each side of the vessels toward the newly created common lumen. The common vessel can then be anastomosed to the recipient artery of preference just as if the kidney had a single renal artery.

URETERONEOCYSTOSTOMY

A modified Politano-Leadbetter submucosal tunnel technique is used for the ureteral implantation and is performed through an anterior cystotomy incision. Previous filling of the bladder following anesthetic induction facilitates a longitudinal anterior cystotomy incision at this time, with minimal handling of the bladder wall. A submucosal tunnel is fashioned near the bladder floor, where angulation of the ureter upon vesical distention is avoided. The tunnel is constructed between two transverse mucosal incisions about 2 cm to 2.5 cm apart, with the distal aspect of the tunnel in close proximity to the trigone (Fig. 66–8A).

A small 8 F Robinson catheter is then passed through the tunnel in a retrograde manner. Following this, a muscular ureteral hiatus

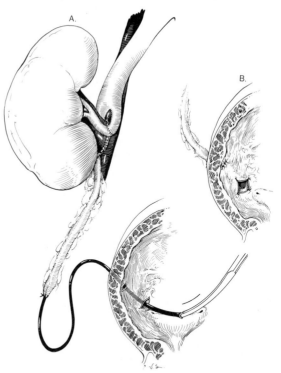

Figure 66–8. Steps in the performance of the ureteroneocystostomy. *A,* Following the creation of the submucosal tunnel, a small Robinson catheter is brought through the tunnel and through the bladder wall hiatus. Attachment is then made to the distal segment of the transplanted ureter. Subsequently, the ureter will be brought into position in the bladder by gentle inferior traction on this catheter. *B,* The completed transplant ureteroneocystostomy with a spatulated ureteral orifice is demonstrated. (From Salvatierra, O.: *In* Glenn, J. F. (Ed.): Urologic Surgery. Philadelphia, J. B. Lippincott Co., 1983.)

is obtained with the right angle forceps adjacent to the superior aspect of the submucosal tunnel and the previously placed Robinson catheter is then brought out into the extravesical space. The end of the catheter is secured to the end of the ureter, and the ureter is brought down and into position inside the bladder by gentle traction on the catheter. This maneuver avoids any handling of the ureter, which is important because the ureter of the transplanted kidney receives its blood supply exclusively from the renal vessel branches that course in its adventitia. In the male patient, it is important to pass the ureter below the spermatic cord. Within the bladder, the ureter is divided transversely approximately 1 cm distal to its exit from the submucosal tunnel. The remaining distal intravesical portion of the ureter is spatulated anteriorly and then secured to the adjacent mucosa and muscularis of the bladder with three interrupted sutures of 5-0 chromic catgut that incorporate the corners of the spatulation and the distal midportion of the ureter. An additional 5-0 chromic catgut suture approximates the proximal apex of the spatulation to the distal margin of the submucosal tunnel (Fig. 66–8B). The superior mucosal opening is then approximated with two or three interrupted sutures of 5-0 chromic catgut. The ureter is not stented postoperatively.

The following are important principles in obtaining a successful transplant ureteroneocystostomy:

1. A "no-touch" technique is essential so as to avoid vascular insufficiency (and subsequent ureteral necrosis and urinary extravasation) from injury to the adventitial anastomotic network of the ureter.

2. The submucosal tunnel and muscle hiatus must accommodate the ureter comfortably to avoid postoperative obstruction from edema, especially since no stent is used.

3. Care must be taken to avoid making the muscle hiatus directly beneath and at a right angle to the superior end of the tunnel because angulation of the ureter may result. This is an important consideration, since the ureter of a transplanted kidney has a more direct upward course than does the native ureter, and it crosses the iliac vessels in a much more caudal position because of the location of the transplanted kidney in the iliac fossa.

4. A little redundancy of the ureter is established above the bladder to ensure that the ureteroneocystostomy is performed without tension.

Following the ureteroneocystostomy, patency is confirmed by gently passing a No. 8 soft Robinson catheter toward the renal pelvis.

Kidneys with a double ureter can also be successfully transplanted by strict adherence to the principles enumerated. However, double ureters cannot be used unless they have been dissected en bloc with their common adventitial sheath and periureteral fat, so as to protect the ureteral blood supply. For the ureteroneocystostomy the ureters are brought through together, side by side, in a generous submucosal tunnel. The distal end of each ureter is spatulated, and the adjacent margins are approximated with 5-0 chromic catgut. The distal midportion of each ureter, the corners of the spatulation, and the proximal apices of each spatulation are managed in the same manner as for a single ureter.

To ensure a watertight closure that does not break down in patients with an impaired healing process, the cystotomy incision is closed in three layers (Fig. 66–9). The author's preference is for the long-lasting absorbable PDS suture. The first layer is closed with a continuous 4-0 PDS for the mucosa; the second layer of the closure is with a continuous 3-0 PDS for the muscularis; and the third layer of the closure is with an interrupted 3-0 PDS that includes the adventitia and muscularis with minimal inversion. The ends of the second and third layers should overlap the immediately underlying layer

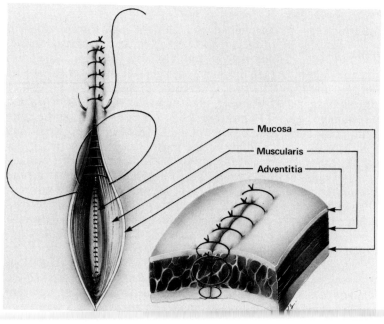

Figure 66–9. Anterior and cross-sectional views of the three-layer bladder closure described in the text. (From Salvatierra O., Olcott, C., Amend, W. J. C., et al.: J. Urol., *117*:421, 1977.)

Mucosa

Muscularis

Adventitia

by about 0.5 cm so as to avoid urinary extravasation at these two points.

Pediatric Cadaver Kidneys

It has been shown previously that it is not necessary to transplant both kidneys from young children en bloc, but that each kidney can be used for a different recipient as with adult cadaver donors. All pediatric kidneys at UCSF have been transplanted as single units, with the arterial anastomosis performed by using a Carrel patch of donor aorta and, whenever possible, a Carrel patch of vena cava for the venous anastomosis (Fig. 66–10). A Carrel patch is mandatory for the arterial anastomosis because direct implantation of a small artery into a much larger vessel may result in actual thrombosis or produce functional stenosis concomitant with graft hypertrophy. If a Carrel patch of vena cava cannot be used, the venous anastomosis should be performed with interrupted sutures. The arterial and venous anastomoses are usually carried out on the iliac vessels, with the aorta and vena cava used only in small pediatric recipients. Pediatric cadaver kidneys have proved to be excellent donor grafts in both adults and children, with considerable early hypertrophy occurring in the immediate post-

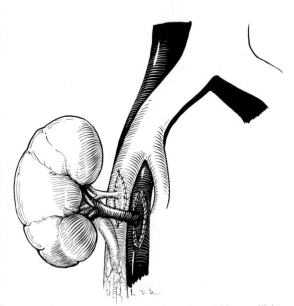

Figure 66–10. Implanted pediatric cadaver kidney utilizing Carrel patches of donor aorta and vena cava encompassing the smaller renal vessels. The Carrel patches have been anastomosed to the larger recipient iliac vessels with running cardiovascular suture. (From Salvatierra, O.: *In* Glenn, J. F. (Ed.): Urologic Surgery. Philadelphia, J. B. Lippincott Co., 1983.)

transplant period. At UCSF, pediatric cadaver kidneys transplanted as single units have provided good renal function to more than 100 recipients whose ages range from 18 months to 53 years. The youngest pediatric cadaver kidney utilized was 10 months of age, although, in general, pediatric donors 2 years of age or older are preferable. At 6 months post transplantation, the recipients of pediatric grafts have graft survival and serum creatinine levels equivalent to those obtained following adult cadaver kidney transplantation.

Transplantation in Pediatric Recipients

In small children, the iliac fossa is not large enough to accommodate a kidney from an adult donor, which is what one would encounter with living related donor, and frequently with cadaver, transplantation in these cases. In addition, the pelvic vessels in young children are so small that the disparity in size between the adult donor renal vessels and the recipient vessels rules out use of the technique described for adults. Thus in small children, graft implantation must use the recipient aorta and vena cava, access to which is best accomplished through a midline abdominal incision; this provides ready exposure to the great vessels as well as to the urinary bladder (Fig. 66–11). After the lateral posterior parietal peritoneum is incised, the right colon is reflected medially and the right kidney is usually removed. The vena cava is then freed from the level of the right renal vein to the iliac bifurcation. Posterior lumbar veins are doubly ligated with 5-0 silk and divided. Mobilization of the vena cava is important to facilitate an end-to-side anastomosis of the renal vein, which is performed with running 6-0 cardiovascular sutures as described for the adult. It is preferable to perform the venous anastomosis superiorly so as to facilitate end-to-side anastomosis of the renal artery to the inferior abdominal aorta. Aortic mobilization should be limited to its distal portion from the level of the inferior mesenteric artery superiorly to (and including) both proximal iliac arteries inferiorly. The segment of the aorta to be used for the end-to-side renal artery anastomosis can be isolated by a superior pediatric vascular clamp and by two inferior clamps on the common iliac arteries. A slightly oval aortotomy is done on the anterior lateral surface of the aorta. The subsequent end-to-side anastomosis is usually performed with interrupted 6-0 cardiovascular sutures.

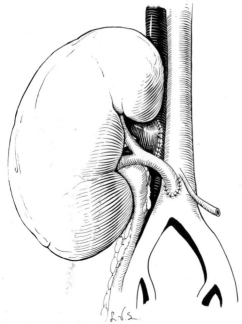

Figure 66–11. Anatomic relationships of an adult donor kidney in a small child with renal vessel anastomoses to the inferior vena cava and the aorta below the inferior mesenteric artery. (From Salvatierra, O.: *In* Glenn, J. F. (Ed.): Urologic Surgery. Philadelphia, J. B. Lippincott Co., 1983.)

There are important considerations in the revascularization of an adult kidney in a small child. Of utmost importance is the realization that vascular clamp release will result in immediate renal consumption of several hundred milliliters of the child's effective blood volume. It is desirable to initiate blood transfusion prior to beginning the vascular anastomoses so as to avoid hypotension after release of the vascular clamp. When the vascular anastomoses are completed, the superior aortic clamp must be kept loosely in place until it is determined that hypotension is not a problem. Immediately after establishing circulation in the graft, the anesthesiologist must continuously monitor the blood pressure until stabilization is ensured.

The ureteral implantation in the small child is carried out as previously described for the adult, except that the ureter must be passed retroperitoneally behind the intact inferior peritoneum. Following ureteral implantation, the graft and superior ureter are reperitonealized by developing and freeing up the lateral peritoneal margin. The lateral peritoneal margin is then approximated to the medial peritoneal margin adjacent to the mobilized colon with a running suture, thus ensuring a retroperitoneal position for the kidney and ureter. The midline abdominal incision can be closed according to the operator's preference.

OTHER CONSIDERATIONS

The ureter of the transplanted kidney is not stented, and the space of Retzius and the iliac fossa are not drained. If good hemostasis has been obtained, and if the principles of implantation as outlined have been followed, there will be no need whatsoever for postoperative drainage other than a urethral catheter. The length of Foley catheter drainage is debatable. In the UCSF series, bladder decompression has been maintained for approximately 1 week, and this practice appears to account, in part, for the low incidence of urinary vesical extravasation, even in insulin-dependent juvenile diabetics with "sensory-loss" bladders.

IMMUNOLOGIC CONSIDERATIONS OF GRAFT REJECTION

The host response against HLA antigens is the principal barrier to successful renal transplantation. Recently, histocompatibility antigens have been classified by immunologists according to their function and biochemistry as Class I (antigens at the A, B, and C loci) and Class II (antigens at the D and DR loci). Class I antigens are composed of a 44,000 dalton heavy chain carrying the alloantigenic specificity and a 12,000 dalton light chain identified to beta 2-microglobulin. Class II antigens are composed of a 33,000 dalton alpha chain and a 28,000 dalton beta chain that carries the HLA specificities. Although both Class I and Class II antigens can elicit an immunologic response, Class I antigens act as targets of cytotoxic T cells, and Class II antigens have an important function in antigen presentation in vivo and in stimulation in vitro of the proliferative response of the mixed lymphocyte culture. Class I and Class II antigens are also distributed differently on cells. Class I antigens are present on virtually all nucleated cells in the body, including T- and B-lymphocytes and platelets; Class II antigens are expressed only on B-lymphocytes, monocytes, macrophages, some types of endothelial cells, and activated T-lymphocytes and are not expressed on platelets or unstimulated T-cells. In the kidney, the Class I antigens have a general distribution on the glomeruli, the vasculature, and the tubules. In contrast, the Class II antigens appear to be primarily distributed on interstitial dendritic cells.

Lymphocytes can be categorized into T- and B-cells. The cellular response that is directed against mismatched HLA antigens is T cell–dependent. Functional T-cell subsets can again be generally divided into (1) helper T-lymphocytes, which are programmed to preferentially recognize Class II HLA antigens; (2) cytotoxic T-lymphocytes, which preferentially recognize Class I antigens; and (3) suppressor cells, which act favorably to enhance graft survival. Allograft rejection is a complex event that results from the cytodestructive effects of activated helper T-cells, cytotoxic T-cells, B-lymphocytes, and activated macrophages. The activation sequence leading to the proliferation of alloreactive T-cells and the production of lymphokines, such as interleukin-1 and interleukin-2, as well as antibody formation, is illustrated in Figure 66–12. Activation of helper T-cells by Class II antigens results in stimulation of the release of various factors, including interleukin-2 and macrophage-stimulating lymphokine.

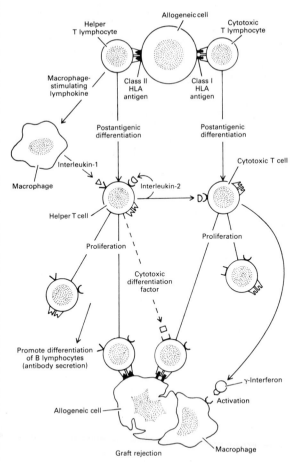

Figure 66–12. Diagrammatic representation of the activation sequence leading to the proliferation of alloreactive cells and secretory factors responsible for allograft rejection. (From Strom, T. B.: Kidney Int., *26*:353, 1984.)

Cytotoxic T-lymphocytes stimulated by Class I HLA antigens develop interleukin-2 receptors. Subsequently, stimulated macrophages and other accessory cells release interleukin-1, which, in turn, also influences the release of interleukin-2. Interleukin-2 then interacts with specific interleukin-2 receptors expressed on activated helper and cytotoxic T-cells. This interaction stimulates the initiation of DNA synthesis and eventual clonal proliferation of receptor-bearing cells. In addition, the continued viability of activated T-cell clones is interleukin-2–dependent. In essence, the activation of helper T-cells by alloantigens and interleukin-1 stimulates the release of a variety of lymphokines from helper T-cells that, in turn, activate macrophages, cytotoxic T-cells, and antibody-releasing B-cells. Rejection is thus a complex consequence that results from the cytodestructive effects caused by the cytotoxic T-cells, activated macrophages, and antibodies. Although cytotoxic T-cells are the dominant cell type that infiltrates the allograft during rejection episodes, helper T-cells are most important in the initiation of the process.

The humoral response is also extremely important, especially in Class I antigens. Recipients who mount a primary immune response against Class I antigens, which is detectable by the presence of cytotoxic antibody in the serum, can produce an overwhelming secondary antibody response upon re-exposure to the same antigens. The existence of cytotoxic anti-HLA antibody in a recipient at the time of transplantation, with a graft bearing antigens to which these antibodies may be directed, results in an immediate graft-destructive hyperacute rejection due to fixation of antibody to the donor vascular endothelium, with formation of platelet and fibrin plugs and ischemic necrosis of the organ. In practice, this is avoided by performance of a complement-mediated cytotoxic cross-match with pretransplant recipient sera against T-lymphocytes from the potential donor prior to transplantation.

Postoperative Immunosuppressive Medication

The principal historical impediment to the successful transplantation of the human kidney has been that most transplant procedures require transplantation of an organ between a donor and a recipient who are genetically dissimilar. It was not until the early 1960's that reasonable and successful immunosuppression was employed, with the advent of the drug azathioprine and its concomitant use with prednisone. The dramatic success with this double-drug therapy led to a period of great enthusiasm and to greater utilization of kidney transplantation in patients other than those with an identical twin donor. During the ensuing years, there have been a number of significant developments in immunosuppression agents and regimens. These developments have resulted in the performance, for the first time, of over 6000 transplants in a single year (1983) in the United States. Most important, however, these transplants were performed with remarkable graft and patient survival rates compared with the results achieved just a few years earlier. The principal immunosuppressive agents utilized in transplantation will be briefly described.

AZATHIOPRINE

Azathioprine is an imidazole derivative of 6-mercaptopurine. Azathioprine is used primarily as maintenance therapy together with prednisone. Metabolites of azathioprine are incorporated into cellular DNA, inhibit purine nucleotide synthesis and metabolism, and alter the synthesis and function of RNA. Since lymphocyte DNA and RNA synthesis and subsequent proliferation result from antigenic stimulation, azathioprine acts at an early step in either T- or B-lymphocyte activation during the proliferative phase of the effector response. This drug is never given in increased doses during an acute rejection episode. The administration of this medication is primarily monitored by the white cell count in order to avoid leukopenia.

CORTICOSTEROIDS

Corticosteroids are almost always used with azathioprine and, more recently, with cyclosporine. High doses of corticosteroids are used to treat an acute rejection episode. However, the dosages must be regulated carefully so as to prevent complications such as infection and the development of cushingoid features. Corticosteroids exert their effect by preventing monocytes from releasing interleukin-1, thereby blocking interleukin-1–dependent release of interleukin-2 from antigen-activated T-cells. Thus, they deny activated T-cells an essential trophic factor.

CYCLOSPORINE

Cyclosporine is a new, potent immunosuppressive agent that has been shown in both animal and human studies to improve allograft survival when compared with results obtained by conventional double-drug therapy of azathioprine and corticosteroids. Cyclosporine is a cyclic endecapeptide whose mechanism of action appears to be selective, with preferential suppression of certain T-lymphocytes without attendant myelosuppression. Cyclosporine differs from corticosteroids in that it does not inhibit the capacity of most accessory cells to release interleukin-1. Cyclosporine's principal mechanism of action is to block interleukin-2 release from activated helper T-lymphocytes. The expression of interleukin-2 receptors and the responsiveness of activated T-lymphocytes to lymphokines are not blocked. Most important is another sparing action of this drug—cyclosporine does not interfere with the activation of suppressor T-cells, which are important in enhancing graft survival. In general, cyclosporine can be considered to modify and redirect the immunologic response to the more beneficial suppressor mode. The most effective use of cyclosporine in clinical renal transplantation has been in conjunction with corticosteroids because of the ability of both agents to abrogate interleukin-2 release through different sites of action. Cyclosporine blocks interleukin-2 release from helper T-cells, whereas corticosteroids inhibit the secretion of interleukin-1 from accessory cells.

The principal problem with cyclosporine relates to its potential nephrotoxicity. This was underscored in a recent report showing impaired renal function in cardiac allograft recipients who were treated with cyclosporine (Myers et al., 1984). However, this report deals with an early experience with this drug, when most centers were in a learning phase concerning proper dosage regimens. Marked improvement of graft survival not only of kidney allografts but also of heart, liver, and heart-lung transplants has been seen through 2 years of follow-up. However, long-term follow-up studies are needed to better evaluate any possible nephrotoxic detrimental effect on graft survival following 5 or more years of graft function. It is probable that, as has been the case with most immunosuppressive agents, cyclosporine dosage protocols will be developed such that early noted side effects can be controlled and prove not to be significant risk factors.

ANTILYMPHOCYTE GLOBULIN

Heterologous antithymocyte antibodies have been used with moderate success in the treatment of acute rejection episodes and also routinely at some centers during the first 2 weeks following transplantation. The primary advantage of these antibodies is their ability to spare the patient exposure to higher doses of corticosteroids. The principal disadvantage is that these are polyclonal antibodies that can vary from lot to lot with respect to both the antibody content of the preparation desired and the presence of unwanted antibodies. The future of this type of therapy probably lies with monoclonal antibodies, which would be directed against specific T-cell differentiation antigens instead of the spectrum of T-cells involved in the immune response, whether destructive or beneficial.

MONOCLONAL ANTIBODIES

The technique of hybridoma formation has allowed immunologists to prepare virtually unlimited quantities of antibodies that are chemically, physically, and immunologically completely homogeneous. These molecules are therefore unencumbered by nonspecificity and cross reactivity. Hybridomas or somatic cell hybrids can be formed readily by fusing a single-cell suspension of splenocytes or lymphocytes from immunized mice or rats to cells of continuously replicating tumor cells, for example, myelomas or lymphomas.

Clinical trials aimed at treating acute cellular rejection have been carried out with at least three monoclonal antibodies against T-cell surface antigens present on cells infiltrating the allografts. These monoclonal antibodies have been used with some encouraging results. Ideally, one would like to be able to treat rejection episodes with monoclonal antibodies directed selectively against the specific cell subsets involved in the process of graft destruction, while leaving intact those cells that suppress the immunologic response. The future of monoclonal antibody therapy will depend on the development of newer antibodies that will be able to distinguish between helper cells and inducers of suppressor cells or between cytotoxic and suppressor cells. Such antibodies might be able to selectively eliminate the cells responsible for allograft destruction while leaving intact the cells (suppressor cells) that suppress the immunologic response.

TECHNICAL COMPLICATIONS OF RENAL TRANSPLANTATION

Vascular Complications

The principal vascular complications are renal artery thrombosis and stenosis. Thrombosis is an early complication, whereas stenosis is a late complication post transplant. Renal artery thrombosis usually is related to technical causes, such as intimal injury from excessive traction of the kidney during donor nephrectomy or poor alignment of the intima at the anastomosis, particularly with disparity in vessel size; at times, it is secondary to excessive length of the two vessels being joined, particularly in end-to-end anastomoses. The diagnosis of renal artery thrombosis should be suspected in any patient who suddenly becomes anuric or severely oliguric during the immediate post transplant period. Even though other causes of acute renal failure, such as rejection or tubular necrosis, are likely at this time, a misdiagnosis of renal artery thrombosis will always result in loss of the graft if surgical intervention is not carried out early. It is the practice at UCSF in such a case to alert the operating room for the possible emergency exploration and to have a 99-Tc renal scan performed. If there is no flow, the patient is taken directly to the operating room. Renal artery thrombosis should be a rare complication. In the UCSF experience of over 2300 transplants performed, the incidence of this complication is 0.2 per cent.

Renal artery stenosis should also be an uncommon complication. In the UCSF experience, the incidence is 0.6 per cent. This low incidence is primarily attributable to the manner in which the renal vessels are handled and the attempt to avoid suture line stenosis by the use of interrupted sutures in all arterial anastomoses, except those in which a Carrel patch is utilized. The stenotic lesions are generally of two types: suture line stenosis and stenosis distal to the suture line, which is oftentimes smooth and tubular.

The diagnosis of renal artery stenosis should be considered in any patient with moderately severe hypertension or hypertension associated with a decline in renal function, especially if there is an arterial bruit over the renal allograft or over the femoral artery in the area of the inguinal ligament. There is no diagnostic test for the lesion other than renal angiography. This should be performed when there is strong suspicion of the presence of renal artery stenosis. The renal angiogram is also important because it will define the status of the peripheral arteries of the kidney, where the presence of multiple stenotic lesions would be consistent with chronic rejection. Chronic rejection can produce severe hypertension, and its existence often contraindicates any surgical intervention for stenosis of the main renal artery. Otherwise, surgical correction of the stenotic lesion is important. Transluminal angioplasty is an alternative but probably holds much higher risk than in the non–transplant recipient who has native renal artery stenosis. In a transplant recipient there is often a significant degree of cicatricial reaction around the renal artery, which is a part of the allograft reaction. Because of this, transluminal angioplasty can result in injury to the artery with subsequent thrombosis or bleeding.

Urologic Complications

Urologic complications following transplantation, particularly those associated with urinary extravasation, can be particularly morbid events. Urologic complications can be minimized by strict adherence to certain principles in donor nephrectomy, management of multiple and small arteries, and the technique of graft implantation, including ureteroneocystostomy and cystotomy closure. In addition, when a urologic complication does occur, prompt recognition and surgical management will provide a high rate of graft salvage and a low incidence of sepsis without patient mortality.

URINARY EXTRAVASATION

The most common cause of ureteral urinary extravasation or fistula is ureteral ischemic necrosis from injury to the ureteral blood supply during the donor nephrectomy. The incidence of primary ureteral leak in the UCSF series is 0.5 per cent.

Urinary extravasation or fistula from the urinary bladder is often due to inadequate closure of the cystotomy incision; it may also be related to pre-existing bladder abnormalities when the initial voiding process results in unsatisfactory bladder emptying. Those who are at higher risk for a urinary bladder leak are insulin-dependent juvenile diabetics with "sensory-loss" bladders and sometimes inadequate emptying and patients with small contracted defunctionalized bladders, most often after multiple urologic procedures and later urinary diversion.

URETERAL OBSTRUCTION

Ureteral obstruction is generally an infrequent complication. Early ureteral obstruction is most often secondary to a tight submucosal tunnel or opening in the bladder wall, or torsion of the ureter. Late ureteral obstruction is a more common complication. Late obstruction is most frequently due to ureteral ischemia, usually secondary to an inadequate blood supply to

the distal ureter. As previously indicated, although the blood supply to the in situ ureter has multiple origins, with numerous collaterals in the ureteral adventitia, the ureter of the transplanted kidney receives its blood supply exclusively from the renal vessel branches that course in the hilar and upper periureteral tissues. Lymphocele is an extrinsic cause of ureteral obstruction and is discussed later.

MANAGEMENT OF UROLOGIC COMPLICATIONS

The two basic principles for control of urologic complications are (1) prompt recognition and treatment; and (2) avoidance of misdiagnosing a urologic complication as a rejection eposide. Each of the urologic complications discussed earlier can result in an elevation of serum creatinine similar to that seen in a rejection episode. Precise distinction between these two processes is absolutely essential, since increased steroid therapy for a misdiagnosed rejection episode predisposes to sepsis, graft loss, and patient mortality. On the other hand, urinary extravasation or infection associated with ureteral obstruction demands reduction of immunosuppressive therapy to the lowest possible levels until the complication has been resolved.

Diagnosis of bladder or ureteral urinary extravasation after the appearance of a cutaneous urinary fistula probably occurs too late for successful management of the complication, and secondary infection is likely. Radioisotope renal scans and ultrasonography should be employed when any elevation of serum creatinine occurs or when there is concern about a possible urologic complication. These studies cause no patient discomfort or morbidity, are simple to perform, and provide means for good anatomic visualization even in uremia, which may exist after transplantation with rejection or resolving acute tubular necrosis. Postvoid scintiphotographs are included with radioisotope renal scans because a small bladder extravasation may not be manifest except by the increased intravesical pressure of voiding. Furthermore, a lower ureteral leak may not be recognized until after evacuation of the isotope from the bladder demonstrates retained isotope in an extravesical location.

With ureteral obstruction, ultrasonography is extremely helpful. Isotope renal scans are also helpful except in patients with mild obstruction. Severe ureteral obstruction can be identified easily by the presence of a large hilar defect in the graft, corresponding to the absence of radioisotope in an enlarged renal pelvis. Moderate ureteral obstruction can be differentiated from rejection by the accumulation and persistence of radioisotope in an enlarged renal pelvis.

Surgical Management. Ureteral necrosis with urinary extravasation and ureteral obstruction require some urinary reconstruction. Resection of the distal ureter and ureteroneocystostomy are possible with distal pathology. Otherwise, the native ureter can be utilized and anastomosed to the transplant ureter or renal pelvis, utilizing a ureteroureterostomy or a pyeloureterostomy. If there is an inadequate native ureter as a result of previous native nephroureterectomy, a Boari flap of bladder can be anastomosed to the renal pelvis. In cases of disruption of the cystotomy closure, it is best to take down the entire anastomoses and resect any necrotic tissue at the cystotomy edge. A three-layer closure can then be accomplished as previously described.

LYMPHOCELE

Lymphoceles represent an extraperitoneal fluid collection in the transplant fossa from leak of lymphatic fluid in the post-transplant period. This is most often a consequence of inadequate ligature of divided lymphatics when the iliac vessels were skeletonized for the graft implantation. Clinically, lymphoceles may compress the transplanted ureter or the iliac vein with expected secondary manifestations, such as ureteral obstruction and edema of the ipsilateral lower extremity. Diagnosis of a lymphocele can be confirmed by ultrasonography. Treatment involves surgical intervention, with drainage of fluid and internal marsupialization of the lymphocele cavity into the peritoneal cavity by excision of peritoneum to create a peritoneal window for subsequent internal drainage of the fluid. External drainage can only lead to secondary infection and should not be carried out except in instances of established infection. Accuracy in the method of drainage to be employed can easily be achieved with an emergency Gram stain of the lymphocele fluid on initially entering the lymphocele cavity.

CURRENT TRANSPLANTATION EXPECTATIONS

Loss of kidney grafts from rejection is most likely to occur during the first 3 months following transplantation. With increasing time, there is a decreasing risk of rejection and graft loss. At 2 years, there is generally good stabilization of the graft so that graft survival rates after this time show minimal attrition secondary to graft loss from rejection. Patient survival is closely related to the amount of immunosuppression required in the post-transplant period. The risk of infection and other complications and possibly death is greatest in those transplant recipients treated for multiple rejections with high dosages of antirejection drugs.

Currently, with the procedures previously described, living related donor transplantation can be performed with an expected graft survival of 90 per cent or better at 2 years, regardless of whether an HLA-identical sibling is used or whether one prepares the potential recipient with donor-specific blood transfusions. In addition, there is limited experience with cyclosporine immunosuppressive therapy in one haplotype–mismatched living related donor–recipient pairs with early good results. Long-term results are awaited, however, to determine whether a drug nephrotoxic influence might result in impaired graft survival. Results in zero haplotype–matched related and unrelated donor–recipient pairs after DST appear to have the same early graft survival rates as in DST-prepared one haplotype–matched donor-recipient pairs. Concomitant with these excellent results now achieved in living related and nonrelated transplantation, patient survival is also excellent. At 2 years, patient survival rates are expected to be 95 per cent or better.

One of the greatest recent improvements obtained in renal transplantation is in cadaver transplantation, in which the usually expected 50 to 55 per cent graft survival at 2 years has been improved to 75 to 80 per cent with the use of cyclosporine immunosuppression. The major side effect of cyclosporine is the potential nephrotoxicity that may develop in patients using this medication. As with the initiation of any drug therapy, there is a learning phase, and the early experience with this drug has identified the major risk factors leading to nephrotoxicity. Recent experience with this drug has resulted in a decreased incidence and earlier recognition and correction of nephrotoxicity when it occurs. In addition to improved graft survival rates with cyclosporine, the major benefit of this medication has been the decrease in the incidence and severity of complications that were associated with previous conventional immunosuppression—complications primarily derived from high dosages of corticosteroids. Cyclosporine also decreases the length of hospital stays following transplantation, because of decreased complications. Another advantage is the degree and facility of rehabilitation of patients receiving cyclosporine when compared with patients under alternative therapies, such as cadaver transplantation with conventional immunosuppression and dialysis therapy. Almost 90 per cent of patients with functioning grafts under cyclosporine are fully rehabilitated. As can be expected with the improved results achieved in cadaver renal transplantation, patient survival rates are also high—greater than 90 per cent at 2 years.

In summary, patients with end-stage renal disease and their physicians have never been so encouraged and optimistic about the current status and the future of renal transplantation. The patient with end-stage renal disease now has the best opportunity ever for achieving a normal life. It is truly a new era for transplantation, and the preliminary results of current research efforts in transplantation immunology and renal preservation are extremely encouraging for even greater improvement.

References

Anderson, C., Sicard, G., and Etheredge, E.: Pretreatment of renal allograft recipients with azathioprine and donor-specific blood products. Surgery, 92:315, 1982.

Belzer, F. O.: Renal preservation, current concepts. N. Engl. J. Med., 291:402, 1974.

Belzer, F. O., Kountz, S. L., and Perkins, H. A.: Red cell cold autoagglutinins as a cause of failure of renal allotransplantation. Transplantation, 11:422, 1971.

Belzer, F. O., Salvatierra, O., Schweizer, R., et al.: Prevention of wound infections by topical antibiotics in high risk patients. Am. J. Surg., 126:180, 1973.

Borel, J., Feurer, C., Magnee, C., et al.: Effects of the new anti-lymphocyte peptide cyclosporin A in animals. Immunology, 32:1017, 1977.

Calne, R., White, D., Thiru, S., et al.: Cyclosporin A in patients receiving renal allografts from cadaver donors. Lancet, 2:1323, 1978.

The Canadian Multicentre Transplant Study Group: A randomized clinical trial of cyclosporine in cadaveric renal transplantation. N. Engl. J. Med., 309:809, 1983.

Cohen, D., Loertscher, R., Rubin, M., et al.: Cyclosporine: A new immunosuppressive agent for organ transplantation. Ann. Intern. Med., 101:667, 1984.

Cosimi, A., Burton, R., Colvin, R., et al.: Treatment of acute renal allograft rejection with OKT3 monoclonal antibody. Transplantation, 32:535, 1981.

European Multicentre Trial Group: Cyclosporine in cadaveric renal transplantation: one-year follow-up of a multicentre trial. Lancet, 2:986, 1983.

Flechner, S., Payne, W., Van Buren, C., et al.: The effect of cyclosporine on early graft function in human renal transplantation. Transplantation, 36:268, 1983.

Hess, A., Tutschka, P., and Santos, G.: Effect of cyclosporin A on human lymphocyte growth factors in secondary mixed lymphocyte responses in vitro. III. CsA inhibits the production of T lymphocyte growth factors in secondary mixed lymphocyte responses but does not inhibit the response of primed lymphocytes to TCGF. J. Immunol., 128:355, 1982.

Hutchinson, I., Shadur, C., Duarte, J., et al.: Cyclosporin A selectively spares lymphocytes with donor-specific suppressor characteristics. Transplantation, 32:210, 1981.

Kirkman, R., Araujo, J., Busch, G., et al.: Treatment of acute renal allograft rejection with monoclonal anti-T12 antibody. Transplantation, 36:620, 1983.

Mendez, R., Iwaki, Y., Mendez, R., et al.: Seventeen consecutive successful one-haplotype matched living related first renal transplants using donor-specific blood transfusions. Transplantation, 33:621, 1982.

Merion, R., White, D., Thiru, S., et al.: Cyclosporine: five years experience in cadaveric renal transplantation. N. Engl. J. Med., 310:148, 1984.

Muraguchi, A., Butler, J., Kehrl, J., et al.: Selective suppression of an early step in human B cell activation by cyclosporine A. J. Exp. Med., 158:690, 1983.

Myers, B., Ross, J., Newton, L., et al.: Cyclosporine-associated chronic nephropathy. N. Engl. J. Med., 311:699, 1984.

Najarian, J., Ferguson, R., Sutherland, D., et al.: A prospective trial of the efficacy of cyclosporine in renal transplantation at the University of Minnesota. Transplant Proc. 15:438, 1983.

Opelz, G., and Terasaki, P.: Dominant effect of transfusions on kidney graft survival. Transplantation, 29:153, 1980.

Salvatierra, O.: Renal transplantation. In Glenn, J. F., (Ed.): Urologic Surgery. Philadelphia, J. B. Lippincott Co., 1983, pp. 359–367.

Salvatierra, O., and Belzer, F.: Pediatric cadaver kidneys: their use in renal transplantation. Arch. Surg., 110:181, 1975.

Salvatierra, O., and Tanagho, E. A.: Reflux as a cause of end stage kidney disease: report of 32 cases. J. Urol., 117:441, 1977.

Salvatierra, O., Iwaki, Y., Vincenti, F., et al.: Incidence, characteristics, and outcome of recipients sensitized after donor-specific blood transfusions. Transplantation, 32:528, 1981.

Salvatierra, O., Kountz, S., and Belzer, F.: Prevention of ureteral fistula after renal transplantation. J. Urol., 112:445, 1974.

Salvatierra, O., Olcott, C., Amend, W. J. C., et al.: Urological complications of renal transplantation can be prevented or controlled. J. Urol., 117:421, 1977.

Salvatierra, O., Olcott, C., Cochrum, K., et al.: Procurement of cadaver kidneys. Urol. Clin. North Am., 3:457, 1976a.

Salvatierra, O., Potter, D., Cochrum, K., et al.: Improved patient survival in renal transplantation. Surgery, 79:166, 1976b.

Salvatierra, O., Powell, M., Price, D., et al.: The advantages of 131-I-orthoiodohippurate scintiphotography in the management of patients after renal transplantation. Ann. Surg., 180:336, 1974.

Salvatierra, O., Vincenti, F., Amend, W. J. C., et al.: Four year experience with donor-specific blood transfusions. Transplant. Proc., 15:924, 1983.

Salvatierra, O., Vincenti, F., Amend, W. J. C., et al.: Deliberate donor-specific blood transfusions prior to living related transplantation: a new approach. Ann. Surg., 192:543, 1980.

Salvatierra, O., Vincenti, F., Amend, W. J. C., et al.: The role of blood transfusions in renal transplantation. Urol. Clin. North Am., 10 (2):243, 1983.

Salvatierra, O., Wolfson, M., Cochrum, K., et al.: End stage polycystic kidney disease: management by renal transplantation and selective use of preliminary nephrectomy. J. Urol., 115:5, 1976.

Sollinger, H., Cook, K., Sparks, E., et al.: Donor-specific transfusions in one haplotype mismatched high MLC donor recipient combinations and in vitro analysis. Paper presented at Ninth International Congress of The Transplantation Society. Transplant. Proc., *15*:935, 1983.

Southard, J. H., and Belzer, F. O.: The future of kidney preservation. Transplantation, *30*:161, 1980.

Starzl, T., Hakala, T., Rosenthal, J., et al.: The Colorado-Pittsburgh cadaveric renal transplantation study with cyclosporine. Transplant. Proc., *15*:2459, 1983.

Starzl, T., Klintmalm, G., Weil, R., III, et al.: Cyclosporin A and steroid therapy in sixty-six cadaver kidney recipients. Surg. Gynecol. Obstet., *153*:486, 1981.

Strom, T. B.: Immunosuppressive agents in renal transplantation. Kidney Int., *26*:353, 1984.

Thomas, F., Thomas, J., Flora, R., et al.: Effect of antilymphocyte globulin potency on survival of cadaver renal transplants. Prospective randomized double-blind trial. Lancet, *2*:671, 1977.

Tosato, G., Pike, S., Koski, I., et al.: Selective inhibition of immunoregulatory cell functions by cyclosporin A. J. Immunol., *128*:1986, 1982.

Vincenti, F., Amend, W. J. C., Feduska, N., et al.: Improved outcome following renal transplantation with reduction in immunosuppression therapy for rejection episodes. Am. J. Med., *69*:107, 1980.

Vincenti, F., Duca, R., Amend, W. J. C., et al.: Immunologic factors determining survival of cadaver kidney transplants. N. Engl. J. Med., *299*:793, 1978.

Wang, B., Heacock, E., Zheng, C., et al.: Restoration of allogeneic responsiveness of lymphocytes from cyclosporine A–treated animals with interleukin-2. Transplantation, *33*:454, 1982.

CHAPTER 67

Surgical Treatment of Renovascular Hypertension

JOSEPH J. KAUFMAN, M.D.

High blood pressure constitutes one of the major health problems in the United States, affecting between 30 and 50 million people. Fortunately, considerable progress has been made in drug therapy of this condition, but the morbidity and mortality resulting from hypertension still loom large and the medical profession cannot be complacent with regard to current methods of controlling this prevalent condition. Of particular concern to urologists, however, is the small but significant segment of the hypertensive population who have a remediable renal basis for their disease. This chapter will be devoted to a discussion of renovascular hypertension and the current state of its treatment.

PATHOGENESIS OF STENOSING LESIONS OF THE RENAL ARTERIES

The majority of stenosing renal arterial lesions in older patients are atherosclerotic, predominating in men and occurring more frequently on the left side than on the right. Lesions are bilateral in approximately one third of patients, but one side is nearly always more severely diseased than the other. They are frequently associated with atherosclerosis (AS) and hence their occurrence is generally assumed to be part of the aging process, but the renal, coronary, and carotid arteries appear particularly vulnerable and cause the major morbidity resulting from AS. Not infrequently, atheromatous narrowings of the renal arteries at their ostia appear disproportionate to AS of the aorta. It has been postulated that this may occur because of anatomic dispositions of these particular vessels (Fig. 67–1) (Rogers et al., 1971). In younger adults with precocious AS, a possible immune mechanism with intimal injury and subsequent deposition of cholesterol and salts has been suggested. Supporting this thesis is evidence that AS can be produced in mice and in human subjects by intravenous injection of viruses (Burch et al., 1973). Smoking and hypercholesterolemia appear to be other contributory factors. The cause and pathogenesis of fibrous stenoses of the renal arteries are more speculative subjects. In children, subintimal fibrosis affecting the proximal portion of the renal artery constitutes the most common disorder of this type, whereas in adults between the ages of 20 and 50 years, the pathologic change is more frequently found in the middle or distal segments of the renal arteries and has more varied patterns of fibrous dysplasia.

Medial fibroplasia is the most common variety of the disease and accounts for approximately 80 per cent of all cases. Women are affected more often than men by a ratio of 5:1 (Maxwell et al., 1972; Sheps et al., 1972; Stanley et al., 1975). The disease is frequently bilateral, but, as a rule, the right side is more severely affected than the left. In arteriographic appearance, the lesions are often long and multifocal with alternating stenotic and aneurysmal segments, producing the characteristic "string of beads" (Fig. 67–2). Bilateral involvement of the

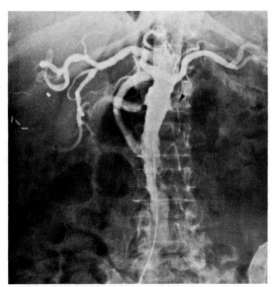

Figure 67–1. Bilateral atherosclerotic renal artery stenosis seen on aortogram. There is a high-grade ostial stenosis on the right side with poststenotic dilatation and a complete occlusion of the left renal artery by atherosclerosis.

renal arteries occurs in approximately 35 per cent of patients and branches are affected in approximately 45 per cent of these cases. On histologic examination, there is fibrous replacement of the media, disorientation of the smooth muscle fibers, and destruction and duplication of the internal elastic membrane (Mahoney and Waisman, 1975). It is generally believed that after the age of 35, progression is slow or

nonexistent, although we have witnessed patients with fibrous dysplasia of the renal arteries who subsequently developed atherosclerotic plaques. A major complication is mural dissection and aneurysm formation (Fig. 67–3) (Kincaid et al., 1968; Oxman et al., 1973).

Subadventitial fibroplasia composes 10 to 15 per cent of renal dysplasia. The disease occurs primarily in young or middle-aged women and usually affects the distal portion of the vessel. The stenoses tend to be tubular and affect shorter arterial segments than is the case with medial fibroplasia (Fig. 67–4). On histologic examination, dense collagen is present under the adventitia. The internal elastic membrane remains intact. The disease usually produces severe degrees of stenosis and is often rapidly progressive (Stewart et al., 1970; Sheps et al., 1972). Dissections are relatively uncommon.

Intimal fibroplasia is the least common of the three major forms of fibrous dysplasia and accounts for approximately 5 to 10 per cent of cases. The lesions appear as short or long tubular stenoses arteriographically (Fig. 67–5) and affect the right and left arteries of young men and women alike. On histologic examination,

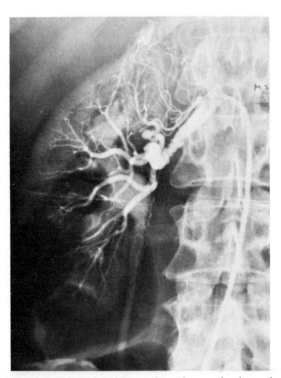

Figure 67–3. Selective right renal arteriogram showing multiple areas of stenosis and aneurysms at the terminal portion of the main renal artery. Note periureteral vascular collaterals.

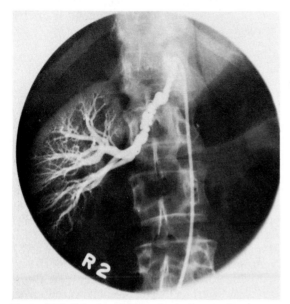

Figure 67–2. Selective right renal arteriogram showing medial fibroplasia of the renal artery.

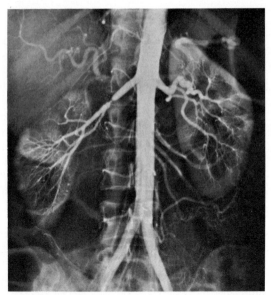

Figure 67–4. Subadventitial fibroplasia of the right renal artery seen on an aortogram. Note the short tubular stenosis of the midportion of the right renal artery.

collagenous tissue is seen inside the internal elastic membrane. Mural dissection is fairly frequent in this entity, and the disease progresses rather predictably (Stewart et al., 1970; Sheps et al., 1972). Since no single cause has yet been defined, and since the lesions are in many respects similar to the stenosing lesions of the main renal artery seen in some kidney transplant recipients (Doyle et al., 1975), an immune pathogenesis is an attractive explanation. The renal

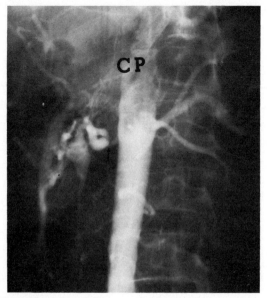

Figure 67–5. Aortogram showing a right renal artery stenosis typical of intimal fibroplasia.

arterial lesions resected from patients with post-transplant stenosis show subintimal fibrosis (Margules et al., 1973; Vidne et al., 1976), a histologic picture not unlike that seen in smaller vessels of the renal transplant being rejected. We have found positive immunofluorescence of these arteries by staining for IgG, IgM, and C_3 in the rejecting renal transplants (Kaufman et al., 1976).

The fibrous lesions of renal artery stenosis are often similar in histologic appearance, suggesting an initial insult in the form of a primary intimal injury. Derangement of the internal elastic membrane, combined with subintimal cellular proliferation and fibrosis, generally occurs. We have also demonstrated positive immunofluorescence in two such cases (IgG and fibrin). Both these immunoproteins are seen in response to arterial injury by immune complexes. Medial and subadventitial fibrosis may also occur as part of the healing process after arterial injury. Although the precise antigenic agent has yet to be identified, the natural history of the disease suggests that viral or bacterial infections can produce diffuse or focal arteritis. Months or years later the focal arterial lesion heals, with the formation of fibrous tissue in the subintima, media, or subadventitia. Hormonal factors may predispose the vessels to development of these lesions, as in cases of coronary artery and other vascular diseases of women who have been given estrogenic or progestational preparations (Almén et al., 1975). It is possible that pregnancy may likewise be a predisposing or contributing factor in the pathogenesis of the arteritis and subsequent arterial fibrosis.

ARTERITIS
(TAKAYASU'S DISEASE)

Takayasu's arteritis is an inflammation affecting the aorta and its primary branches. It is generally a disease that appears in two phases, the first consisting of fever, arthralgia, anorexia, headache, neck or chest pain, and cardiomyopathy. Some patients may have a subclinical onset with no symptoms recalled. The second phase of the disease is characterized by both stenoses and aneurysmal dilation of the aorta or major arteries (Butler, 1937; Ishikawa, 1978). Nonspecific autoimmune investigation (rheumatoid factor, antinuclear antibodies, LE [lupus erythematosus] factor) has not uncovered a clear mechanism. Our own series of cases of arteritis has failed to impugn tuberculosis as an etiologic agent. Rather, we submit that tuberculosis may be one of several antigenic factors leading to the development of arteritis.

Figure 67–6 is an example of the middle aortic syndrome with renal artery involvement. Although Takayasu's arteritis commonly implies involvement of the aorta with involvement of other arteries, we believe that a spectrum of arteritides is likely. We have witnessed a substantial number of cases of renal arteritis occurring with or without aortic involvement but sometimes with the disease affecting the splanchnic vessels. An appreciable cohort of such patients will have an inexorable progression of obliterative arterial disease causing global or segmental atrophy of the kidney (Fig. 67–7).

NEUROFIBROMATOSIS

Neurofibromatosis (von Recklinghausen's disease) (von Recklinghausen, 1882) is a hered-

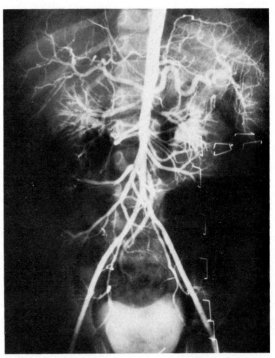

Figure 67–7. Arteriogram showing aortitis and arteritis, the latter affecting the first third of both renal arteries as well as branches of the superior mesenteric artery.

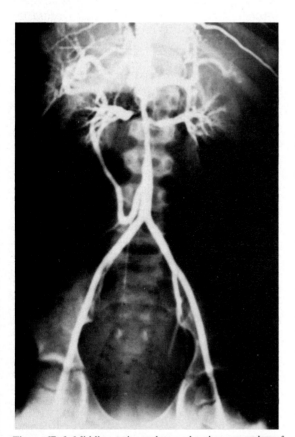

Figure 67–6. Middle aortic syndrome showing narrowing of the aorta and stenosis of both renal arteries in a young boy. Evidence of the coarctation is seen in the prominent subcostal arteries and the collateral course of inferior mesenteric artery.

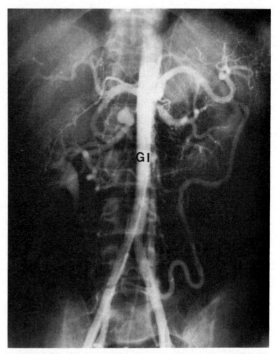

Figure 67–8. Neurofibromatosis with aneurysmal and stenotic lesions of the renal arteries and splanchnic vessels seen on an aortogram. Note the aneurysm of the right renal artery and the wandering inferior mesenteric artery, evidence of superior mesenteric artery stenosis.

itary disorder of ectodermal origin. It is characterized by café au lait spots, cutaneous fibromas, and neurofibromas. An association of pheochromocytoma with neurofibromatosis has been clearly established (Glushein et al., 1953). A variety of vascular lesions involving the renal arteries is associated with the disease. Our experience now includes 15 patients varying in age from 19 months to 45 years with a spectrum of vascular deformities, including aneurysms and stenoses (Fig. 67–8).

The vascular lesions of neurofibromatosis can be divided into three types: an intimal form consisting of endothelial proliferation in concentric layers; an intimal and aneurysmal form, which produces thickening of the intimal layer of the vessel, atrophy of the media, and disruption of the wall eventually leading to aneurysms; and a nodular form, which consists of cellular nodules located in the wall of the vessel. These vessels may show long areas of stenosis, and the aorta itself is frequently involved (Grad and Rance, 1972).

TREATMENT OF RENOVASCULAR HYPERTENSION

The choice of surgical versus medical treatment of renovascular hypertension is a subject receiving considerable attention. Many cases of renal and renovascular hypertension respond well to medical management, particularly since the introduction of better drugs, i.e., beta-blocking drugs used in conjunction with diuretics or converting enzyme inhibitors (CEI's) such as captopril. The major problems, then, involve drug acceptance, compliance, and tolerance by the patient, the true efficacy of medical treatment, and the natural history of the disease. For elderly patients who are poor risks for operation, serious consideration must be given to medical therapy. Likewise, for younger individuals with stable disease, i.e., without progression of the stenosis or renal function impairment, medical therapy should also be seriously considered.

Although effective antihypertensive drugs have become available, there are few hard data to aid in the decision as to whether operative or nonoperative therapy is preferable for a patient with renovascular hypertension. Of 214 patients with renovascular hypertension studied by Hunt and associates (1974) in a prospective study, 100 underwent operation and 114 were

treated medically. In a 7- to 14-year follow-up study, 16 per cent of surgically treated patients died, compared with 40 per cent of those treated medically. Furthermore, more than 90 per cent of the surgical survivors were cured or improved by the operation. Myocardial infarction, renal failure, and cerebrovascular accidents were more commonly encountered in the medical group than in the surgical cohort. Whether specific drugs such as CEI's (e.g., captopril) will change this picture is undetermined at present. A number of reports indicate that hypertension can be well controlled by CEI's (Gavras et al., 1974, 1978). However, there are significant side effects and occasional severe complications associated with this form of therapy.

Hall et al. (1977) showed that in chronic renin depletion produced by CEI's, the glomerular filtration rate (GFR) falls even though autoregulation of renal blood flow may be maintained. Curtis et al. (1983) and Hricik and associates (1983) have demonstrated that the renin-angiotensin system is central to the control of GFR at low renal perfusion pressure and warn that captopril and other CEI's cause deterioration of GFR in patients with bilateral renal artery stenosis or renal artery stenosis in the solitary kidney.

If partial or total nephrectomy is the treatment ultimately employed, reduction of renal reserve may, but will not necessarily, ensue, but in some cases will actually improve kidney function if the hypertension has been treated with multiple drugs, and particularly if captopril has been employed. The following case is illustrative of this feature of drug therapy in treating bilateral renal arterial disease.

Case 1
A 26-year-old man developed severe hypertension with progressive renal failure. Arteriograms disclosed severe bilateral disease with obliteration of the major branches supplying the upper two thirds of his right kidney and with dissection of a major branch to the lower half of the left kidney. Multiple drug therapy, including diuretics, beta-blockers, prazosin, and finally captopril, was employed but did not control his hypertension. Rather, the creatinine gradually rose from a pretreatment level of 2.5 to 6.3 when he was referred for treatment. Because the arterial disease was not amenable to revascularization by methods currently available, ablative surgery was employed and the upper two thirds of the right kidney was resected, leaving only the lower pole of the right kidney, which was adequately vascularized. Despite the loss of two thirds of the right kidney, the patient could be easily controlled with diuretics and beta-blocking agents alone, and on this regimen his creatinine fell to 2.2 despite the loss of a substantial amount of renal parenchyma (Fig. 67-9).

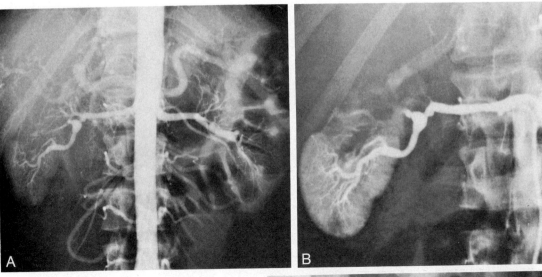

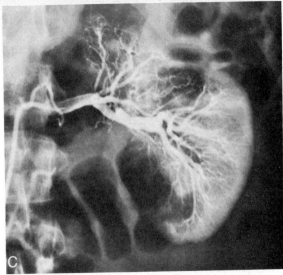

Figure 67–9. *A,* Diffuse obliterative vasculitis bilaterally with ischemia of the upper two thirds of the right kidney and a dissection of the lower branch of the left kidney. *B,* Selective right renal arteriogram showing absence of nephro-opacification of the upper two thirds of the right kidney secondary to obliterative arteritis. *C,* Selective left renal arteriogram showing poor vascularization of the upper portion of the left kidney and the medial aspect of the lower pole of the left kidney.

Obviously, ablative surgery of this type is rarely a satisfactory definitive treatment, since the primary vasculitis and obliterative arterial disease may progress and ultimately the patient may come to dialysis as a result of autonephrectomy or surgical nephrectomy.

Medical therapy aimed at the treatment of arteritis is unsatisfactory. We have employed agents such as azathioprine and prednisone in several cases and this has proved to be unsatisfactory, as illustrated in the following case.

Case 2

A 7-year-old boy had severe upper respiratory infection followed 1 month later by hypertension. When he was first seen he underwent hypertensive work-up, which disclosed a tubular stenosis of one of the major branches of his left kidney. On the assumption that he had an active arteritis in the wake

of a bacterial or viral disease, we employed azathioprine and prednisone over a period of 9 months. During this time his hypertension was controlled with medication, but an arteriogram revealed the progression of his obliterative arterial disease to the extent that he was left with an extreme atrophy of the kidney and the major arteries of the kidney. A nephrectomy was subsequently carried out with temporary improvement of the hypertension, but 1 year later he had a recurrence of hypertension and was found to have a tubular stenosis of a major right renal artery. Ultimately this required ex vivo repair with anastomosis of the two major vessels, one affected by stenosis and the other appearing to be normal. The patient ultimately did well in terms of renal function (Fig. 67–10), but his dénouement was further complicated by the appearance of an extra-adrenal pheochromocytoma discovered serendipitously on the anterior surface of the vena cava at the time of the autotransplantation of the right kidney,

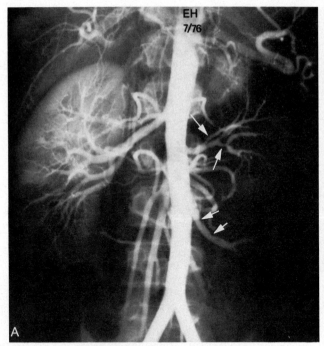

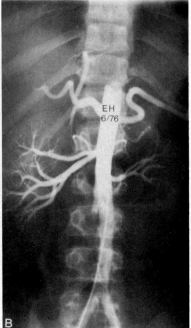

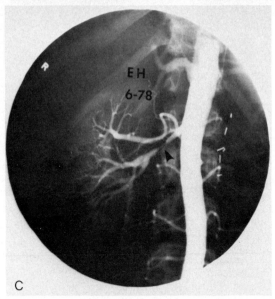

Figure 67–10. *A* and *B*, Aortograms showing stenosing lesions of the left renal arterial tree with poor nephro-opacification of the left kidney. *C*, Two and one-half years following the first appearance of hypertension, a stenosing lesion of the right renal artery, not present on the films of 7/76 *(A)*, appears.

and later by the appearance of a large left adrenal pheochromocytoma, which may have been present from the time of onset of his hypertension. Although in this case the coexistence of pheochromocytoma and progressive renal artery stenosis cannot be dissociated, we felt that the two processes were more likely independent or at least the corelationship of the progressive stenosing arterial lesions and pheochromocytoma was unclear.

With the advent of better drugs for immunosuppression, such as cyclosporin A, which has been suggested as treatment for rheumatoid and other collagen disorders, we may have better drugs with which to treat immune complex diseases such as arteritis.

Percutaneous Transluminal Dilation

Patients in satisfactory medical condition whose hypertension was correctable by reconstruction rather than nephrectomy have in the past been considered ideal candidates for operative angioplasty. However, with the development and wide use of percutaneous transluminal renal artery dilation (PTD), the indications for open surgery are considerably limited, and it is currently widespread practice to employ PTD prior to considering renal arterial reconstruction.

The development of the soft, flexible, double-lumen Gruntzig balloon catheter (Gruntzig et al., 1978) represents a remarkable advance over the bougie system of renal artery dilation originally described by Dotter and Judkins (1964). The technique of renal artery dilation is relatively simple and is currently used according to the method proposed by Katzen, Chang, and Knox (1979). Antihypertensive medications are discontinued 48 hours before dilation, if possible. If blood pressure control is a problem, nitroprusside may be used. Either the femoral artery or the axillary artery may be used. The Seldinger technique is used to introduce the catheter, and the renal artery is entered with a preshaped catheter. A small guidewire is advanced beyond the stenosis, a catheter exchange is made, and a Gruntzig catheter with appropriate balloon diameter is placed within the stenosis over the guidewire (Fig. 67–11). Heparin (5000 IU) is given through the catheter. When the catheter is properly positioned under fluoroscopic control, the balloon is inflated to between 5 atm and 8 atm of pressure (Fig. 67–12). The balloon is usually inflated and deflated two to three times.

Blood pressure response is somewhat variable, the lowest blood pressure usually occurring between 2 and 6 hours after dilation. When dilations have been successful as proved by the post-treatment angiographic appearance, between 85 and 90 per cent cure or improvement occurs for 6 months or longer in most series (Schwarten et al., 1980). Reports of the effectiveness of PTD in treating AS are variable. Sos and associates (1983) recently reported that following successful PTD, the blood pressure was reduced to normal or improved in 84 per cent of 17 patients with AS among 30 in whom successful dilation was accomplished. It is noteworthy, however, that partial success or failure to dilate atherosclerotic lesions occurred in 43 per cent of their patients. In bilateral renal artery stenosis, this group was successful in dilating both sides in only 4 of 21 cases (Sos et al., 1983). PTD has been used successfully in opening totally occluded arteries (Fig. 67–1).

The results of this group in treating patients with *fibromuscular dysplasia* (FMD) were better and comparable to those reported by other investigators. They were successful in dilating 24 of 28 patients with FMD and obtained cures and improvements in 93 per cent of their pa-

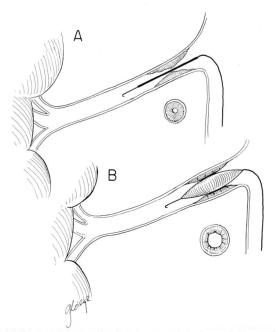

Figure 67–11. Artist's drawing showing the technique of percutaneous transluminal arterial dilation (PTD) using the wire *(A)* and balloon inflation to dilate an atherosclerotic plaque *(B)*.

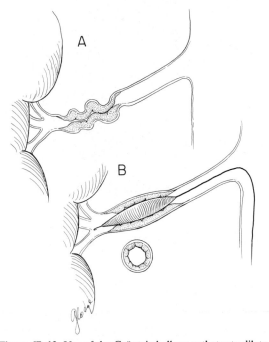

Figure 67–12. Use of the Grüntzig balloon catheter to dilate lesion of medial fibroplasia of the right renal artery by PTD.

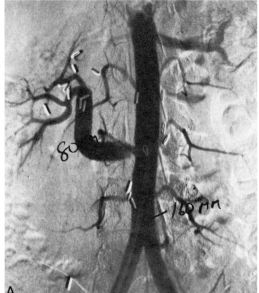

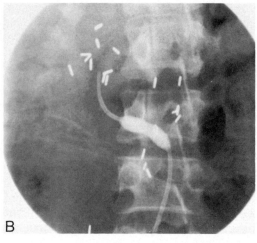

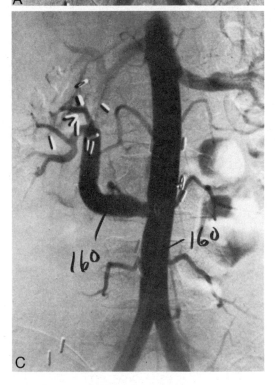

Figure 67–13. *A,* Subtraction aortogram showing stenosis of a Dacron graft at the take-off, with an 80-mm gradient measured at the time of arterial catheterization. *B,* Radiograph showing Grüntzig balloon catheter in area of narrowing of the graft take-off. *C,* Aortogram showing appearance of the Dacron graft following balloon dilation, with correction of the pressure gradient. (Courtesy of Dr. Barry Katzen.)

tients. The cures and improvements are notable. The patients were followed an average of 21.8 months. They caution, however, that in treating AS, the success rate is primarily among those patients who have unilateral nonostial atheroma. Our personal experience in treating 35 patients with renal artery stenosis indicates that the technique is more difficult, more hazardous, and less predictable in treating atherosclerotic disease than in treating fibrous dysplasia. How-

ever, in patients with fibrous dysplasia in whom successful passage of the guidewire and dilation of the stenosis was accomplished, the cure and improvement rate is 95 per cent and our mean follow-up in this group is 25.3 months. Transluminal dilation of arterial stenosis in renal transplant recipients has been quite successful. PTD has also been of value in dilating bypass grafts (Fig. 67–13*A*–*C*) (Katzen, 1982).

Complications of the technique should be

recognized. Massive hematoma formation in the inguinal or axillary regions, embolization to the toes that may even require amputation, perforation of the artery with dissections, or even retroperitoneal hemorrhage requiring operative intervention have all been reported. Figure 67–14*A* to *C* demonstrates a dissection produced during attempted PTD resulting in temporary occlusion of the artery. Fortunately, re-entry of the dissection preserved the kidney, which was subsequently revascularized by surgical bypass technique (Fig. 67–14*D*).

In terms of cost-effectiveness and patient discomfort alone, operative correction of stenosing lesions cannot effectively compete with PTD. However, surgical intervention will remain necessary for complicated cases with branch disease and for cases in which PTD has been unsuccessful in achieving or maintaining dilation of the renal artery.

Operative Procedures

Surgery for renal artery stenosis includes nephrectomy and partial nephrectomy; revascularization operations primarily of the bypass type; aneurysmectomy or aneurysmorrhaphy, with or without bypass surgery; and, in selected instances, autotransplantation with or without ex vivo repair.

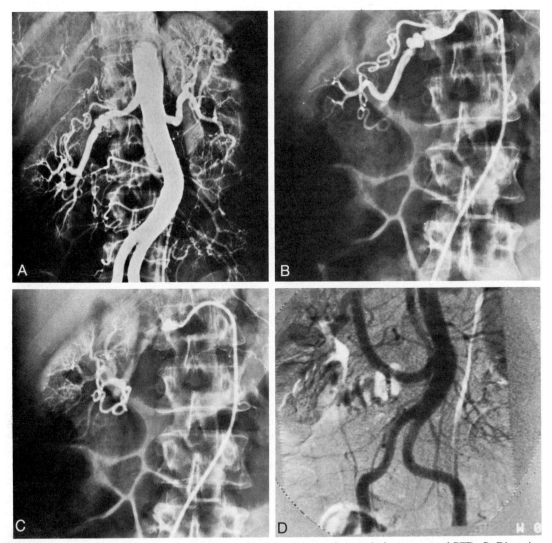

Figure 67–14. *A,* Aortogram showing medial fibroplasia of the right renal artery before attempted PTD. *B,* Dissection of the right renal artery caused by the angiographic wire preliminary to attempting PTD. *C,* Later phase of dissection of the right renal artery. *D,* Digital subtraction angiogram 4 days following a bypass using 6-mm knitted velour Dacron graft.

NEPHRECTOMY AND PARTIAL NEPHRECTOMY

In recent years, nephrectomy accounted for fewer than 20 per cent of primary operations performed for renovascular hypertension. It is indicated for unilateral renal infarction with nonfunction, for extremely poor-risk patients with a relatively healthy contralateral kidney, for kidneys that have multiple branch disease impossible to repair, for severe parenchymal disease with or without associated renal artery stenosis, and following unsuccessful previous arterial repair or partial nephrectomy.

Partial nephrectomy is performed when segmental renal disease makes this operation feasible, but, in our experience, fewer than 5 per cent of patients fall in this category. The cure and improvement rate following partial nephrectomy has been less than with either total nephrectomy or vascular repair; and with refined surgical techniques and magnification, it is now preferable to repair branch or segmental renal artery stenoses than to excise poorly defined ischemic renal segments. However, as described in Case 1, partial nephrectomy may be the only option in some instances. Angiographic infarction, either total or segmental and using embolization techniques with coils or other agents or ablation with absolute alcohol, may replace surgical ablative techniques. The principal problem with angioplastic infarction, however, may be the presence of collateral blood supply to the ischemic kidney through capsular, ureteral, or other parasitized vessels that may continue to keep portions of the kidney viable and capable of releasing renin to perpetuate the hypertension.

PREOPERATIVE PREPARATION OF THE SURGICAL PATIENT

An intravenous infusion is begun the night before to ensure that the patient is well hydrated. It is not necessary to discontinue antihypertensive drugs before operation. Potassium is repleted preoperatively, since many patients will have been on diuretic therapy and potassium depletion leads to myocardial irritability. Pulmonary wedge catheter is indicated in patients with questionable myocardial reserve. An arterial line for gas and blood pressure determinations is also a helpful adjunct during the operation. A catheter is usually placed in the bladder before operation. Intraoperatively, mannitol is given intravenously. We advise 25 gm of mannitol before renal artery clamping and another 25 gm following restoration of blood flow. Heparin is administered systemically

5 minutes before renal artery clamping (0.5 mg per kg). It has not been our practice to give heparin postoperatively because of the increased risk of secondary bleeding and the fact that other anticoagulation agents are equally effective. Dipyridamole and aspirin or ibuprofen have recently been shown to have platelet antiadhesive and aggregation effects that are equal to those of heparin, and are safer drugs to use.

Following renovascular surgery, vital signs and urine output are closely monitored. Exacerbation of hypertension is not uncommon following operation, even with a technically adequate repair, and sometimes requires management with intravenous nitroprusside or diazoxide. We do not customarily allow ambulation until 24 hours of bedrest. A renal scan or digital subtraction vascular imaging (DSA) or both are performed on the first or second postoperative day.

ACCESS FOR REVASCULARIZATION OPERATIONS

Revascularization operations are most commonly done through an anterior transperitoneal approach, using chevron, paramedian, or midline incisions.

Splenorenal Bypass

Splenorenal bypass is an operation that is still suited for left-sided lesions, particularly of the atherosclerotic type. Atherosclerosis predominates on the left side and not infrequently the aorta is in poor condition for the attachment of a free graft. Furthermore, the splenic artery is frequently spared severe atherosclerosis even when the renal arteries and infrarenal aorta are badly diseased. It is also extremely useful for proximal fibroplasias or dissections (Fig. 67–15). For this operation we prefer a thoracoabdominal extrapleural extracorporeal retroperitoneal approach, making an incision above the eleventh rib. The splenic flexure and left colon and duodenum are reflected medially and the plane between Gerota's fascia and the pancreas is developed. The pancreas and spleen are gently retracted cephalad to permit access to the splenic vessels. The splenic artery is usually palpated slightly posterior and superior to the splenic vein.

For right-sided lesions, it is best to mobilize the ascending colon and hepatic flexure along with the second portion of the duodenum and retract them to the left upper quadrant. In obese patients it may be necessary to incise along the root of the mesentery to the ligament of Treitz and to exteriorize the small bowel in a plastic

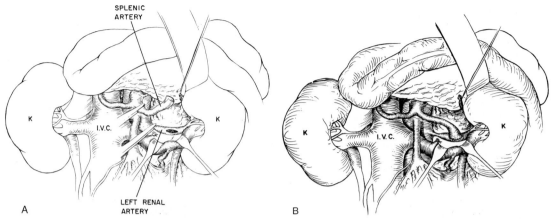

Figure 67–15. *A,* Artist's drawing showing technique of end-to-side splenorenal bypass. The duodenum and pancreas are lifted to gain access to the splenic artery. *B,* Artist's drawing showing completed end-to-side anastomosis of splenorenal bypass.

bag in order to provide optimal exposure of the right kidney, the aorta, and the root of the right renal artery. Dividing the right gonadal vein will allow full exposure of the vena cava, and the right renal vein and renal artery. The right renal artery is best secured by placing a tape about it just to the left of the vena cava. For repair of lesions in the distal portion of the right renal artery, it may not be necessary to secure the right renal artery medial to the vena cava. For most in situ operations on the renal vessels, it is not necessary to mobilize the kidney.

Left-sided lesions are best handled by reflecting the small bowel upward onto the chest or into the right upper quadrant and incising along the root of the mesentery much like the approach for transperitoneal retroperitoneal lymphadenectomy. The inferior mesenteric vein should be divided below where it enters the splenic vein. The left colon and splenic flexure can usually be left intact. If inadequate exposure is obtained, however, reflection of the splenic flexure and descending colon to the right will permit greater access. When autotransplantation is being done, with or without ex vivo branch repair, we use either a transperitoneal approach or an extraperitoneal incision with the patient in the torque position, making the incision from above the eleventh rib to the lateral border of the rectus above the symphysis. If it is necessary to reimplant the ureter into the bladder, we may divide the rectus muscle above the pubis.

SURGICAL ANGIOPLASTY TECHNIQUES

Endarterectomy was the first reconstructive procedure performed on the renal artery. The technique is applicable when patients have localized atheromatous stenosis of the renal artery. The approach to the atheroma is by renal, aortic, or aortorenal arteriotomy. Care must be taken to remove the plaque as completely as possible because residual roughened surfaces may invite subsequent dissection or thrombosis. In addition, caution must be exercised to prevent escape of particles of atheromatous material, which may cause atheroembolism and segmental renal infarction. Transaortic renal endarterectomy was proposed and popularized by Wylie (1975). In this approach the aorta is cross-clamped above and below the renal artery, a longitudinal aortotomy is made, and the plaques are removed from the aorta and the renal arterial ostia (Fig. 67–16). This method is useful for bilateral atherosclerotic renal arterial lesions, particularly those in which the atheroma is primarily aortic and "pours" into the renal ostia. It obviates the need to incise the renal arteries, which may require patch plasties to prevent narrowing.

The results of endarterectomy are not as favorable as with other types of revascularization. Long-term follow-up indicates that atrophy of endarterectomized vessels may occur. Therefore, it is rarely used as the operation of choice for repair of atherosclerotic narrowing.

The procedures that have gained greatest current popularity are *bypass operations* and *autotransplantation*. Although the choice of material for aortorenal bypass is still moot, the majority of vascular surgeons prefer autologous saphenous vein grafts because of the following advantages: (1) appropriate caliber and ample length; (2) ease of suturing; (3) lack of antigenicity; (4) their general success as bypasses for revascularization of the extremities and coro-

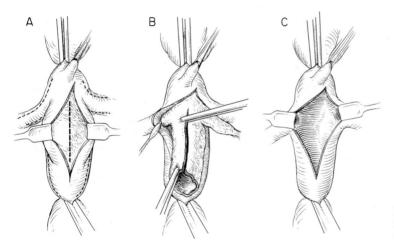

Figure 67–16. Artist's drawing showing technique of transaortic endarterectomy.

nary vessels; and (5) a relatively low incidence of early and late problems (Ernst et al., 1972; Foster and Dean, 1974). These advantages notwithstanding, stenoses, aneurysmal dilations, and thrombosis do occur in 10 to 20 per cent of cases where the saphenous vein is employed.

Saphenous Vein Bypass

The most upper portion of the greater saphenous vein is used for this procedure. A 10- to 15-cm segment is harvested and gently dilated with a diluted heparin solution. The aorta is exposed below the renal vessels and a tape or two is placed around the aorta for control in case of occlusion clamp slipping. On the anterolateral aspect of the aorta between the renal and inferior mesenteric arteries, an incision is made with an exclusion clamp or between aortic occlusion clamps. For the atherosclerotic aorta, isolation of the segment to be used is best achieved with two cross-clamps. The incision in the aorta is made with a sharp-pointed blade, then the aortic punch is used to remove as clean a full-thickness divet from the aorta as possible. This opening can be enlarged to accommodate the spatulated proximal end of the vein graft. An end-to-end anastomosis is generally done between the vein graft and the renal artery. On the right side the graft is brought anterior to the vena cava in preparation for the distal anastomosis. For most arterial anastomoses we prefer the use of interrupted sutures, although many surgeons employ continuous suture technique. Polypropylene sutures (5–0) are used for the anastomosis of the vein graft to the aorta, and 5–0 or 6–0 (interrupted) sutures are used for the vein-to–renal artery union. Generally the graft is placed on the aorta first to limit the time of renal artery clamping.

Two arterial trunks may be revascularized using bifurcated vein grafts or end-to-side and end-to-end anastomosis as shown in Fig. 67–17.

Long-term follow-up studies indicate that patency following vein grafts is fairly well maintained. Approximately 20 per cent of saphenous vein grafts, however, fail during the first year because of thrombosis, stenosis, or aneurysmal dilation (Ernst et al., 1972).

Arterial Autografts

Arterial autografts have the theoretical advantage over veins of having the same general caliber and viscoelastic characteristics as the renal artery. The hypogastric artery can be sacrificed with impunity and is not difficult to expose and resect. On occasion, it can be taken with several branches suitable for placement onto the branches of the renal artery. If more than two branches require anastomosis, we prefer ex vivo surgery in order to provide better cooling of the kidney and to optimize the anastomoses of the small branches to small renal vessels.

The disadvantages of the hypogastric artery are that it may be involved by atherosclerosis in patients over the age of 40 and that it may be too short. Our current choice for bypass grafts in young patients is the hypogastric artery autograft, which we have used in 87 reconstructions over the past 12 years (Kaufman, 1975; Wylie, 1975).

Aortorenal grafts are attached to the side of the abdominal aorta, as described for placement of saphenous vein grafts, and aortic occlusion is carried out in a similar fashion, except that long elliptical anastomoses are not considered mandatory, as they are for vein grafts. After the graft is placed on the aorta, the aortic

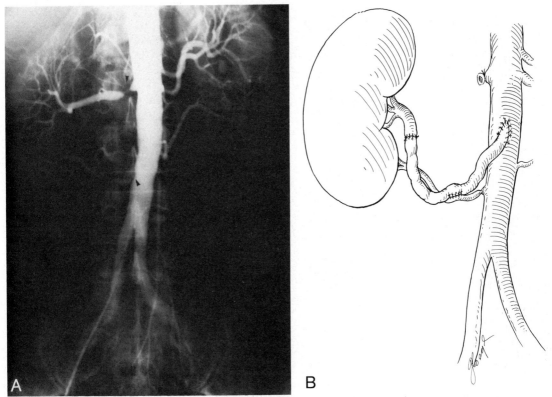

Figure 67–17. *A,* Aortogram showing duplex renal arterial supply to right kidney with stenoses of the take-off of both right renal arteries. *B,* Artist's drawing showing use of saphenous vein graft to revascularize the lower renal artery by side-to-side anastomosis and upper renal artery by end-to-end anastomosis.

blood flow is restored, and a clamp is customarily placed across the arterial graft. The renal artery is then divided, and an end-to-end anastomosis is made with interrupted fine sutures. Figure 67–18 shows the use of the hypogastric as a free autologous graft, and Figure 67–19 shows the postoperative arteriogram of a patient treated with a hypogastric artery graft using two branches.

In our series, 80 of 87 patients were cured of hypertension; two were improved, and five failed. One patient with a graft placed into a renal artery branch developed postoperative thrombotic occlusion, and another showed evidence of postoperative stenosis at the site of the hypogastric–renal artery anastomosis, the latter presumably occurring because the hypogastric artery was anastomosed to a diseased segment of renal artery. Forty-three patients observed for 9 to 12 years have demonstrated patency on arteriography and splendid functional results. Among these, eight had a solitary kidney.

Lye et al. (1975) reported the experience of Wylie's group and presented their long-term results with 45 patients undergoing aortorenal arterial autografts. In a comparison of their results with our series of 87 cases followed 1 to

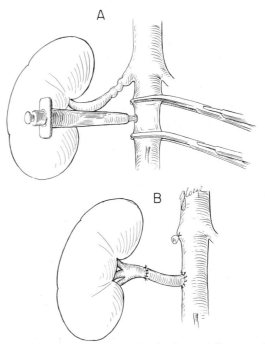

Figure 67–18. *A,* Artist's drawing showing use of hypogastric artery as interposition free graft. An aortic punch is used to remove a full thickness of aortic wall onto which the hypogastric artery is placed. *B,* Completed anastomosis using interrupted 5-0 prolene sutures.

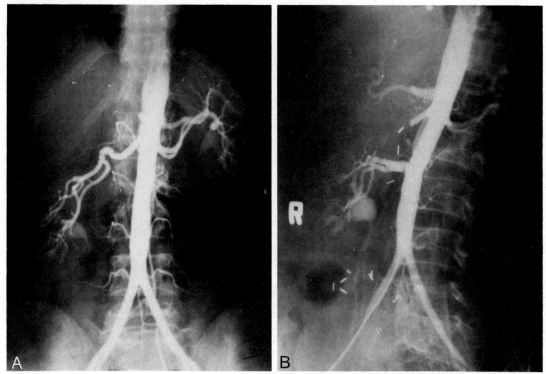

Figure 67–19. *A,* Aortogram showing fibromuscular dysplasia affecting the distal third of the right renal artery and its two major branches. *B,* Postoperative aortogram showing free hypogastric artery graft coursing from the aorta to two branches of the right renal artery beyond the area of disease.

12 years, the technique and results are roughly similar.

Synthetic Tubes

Synthetic tubes are less popular owing to the higher incidence of graft closure, particularly in cases where run-off is poor. Newer types of synthetic grafts with external or internal velour provide a more rapid formation of a smooth-lined neointima (Kaufman, 1974). The expanded polytetrafluoroethylene graft (Gore-Tex) appears to have application because the material is soft, somewhat elastic, and easy to suture. It also allows inner fibrous healing with minimal tissue reactivity. Although the material is reported to maintain patency over long periods of time, even in low-flow situations, this has yet to be established in large clinical series. The advantages of synthetics are that they are relatively easy to handle, they are readily available in a variety of sizes, and they entail no risk of subsequent involvement by the pathologic process (e.g., fibrosis, atheroma) for which they are inserted. Figure 67–20 shows our technique of aortorenal end-to-side Dacron bypass graft. Grafts should take origin from the anterolateral aspect of the mid-abdominal aorta. In the early postoperative period (i.e., first or second day), digital subtraction angiography is extremely useful to determine patency of any graft. It is also an excellent method of follow-up for graft patency (Fig. 67–14D). Long-term follow-up studies in patients undergoing Dacron aortorenal bypass grafts have recently been reported (Lawrie et al., 1980). These authors found an overall patency of 78.2 per cent on follow-up aortography in 201 patients at a mean interval of 31.5 months after operation. The patency rate was 76 per cent (113 of 149) for Dacron bypass grafts, 89.7 per cent (35 of 39) for saphenous vein bypass grafts, and 82 per cent (23 of 28) for arteries treated by endarterectomy or patch graft angioplasty.

AUTOTRANSPLANTATION OF THE KIDNEY

Autotransplantation of the kidney with and without ex vivo (bench) repair is a technique that has received increasing attention; its chief attraction is that it allows end-to-end anastomosis of the renal artery to the hypogastric artery or end-to-side anastomosis to the common or external iliac artery. The operation is done in the iliac fossa where the anatomic structures are more favorable for precise align-

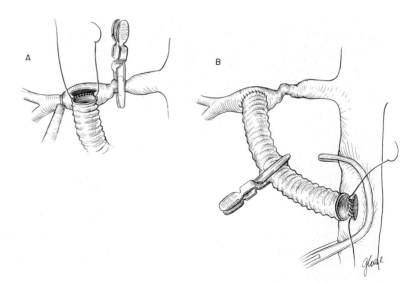

Figure 67–20. Technique of performing end-to-side anastomoses of a Dacron graft to the renal artery and to the aorta. The graft may be placed on the aorta initially and subsequently attached to the renal artery or attached to the renal artery first, as shown in the artist's drawing, allowing blood to flow to the kidney with the graft clamped until the graft-to-aorta anastomosis is accomplished. With larger-diameter grafts (6 mm), continuous suture technique is acceptable.

ment and suturing. Another indication for autotransplantation of the kidney may be middle aortic syndrome, in which the aorta is involved by inflammation, coarctations, or aneurysms. Often in this condition the iliac arteries are spared (Kaufman, 1973a). In the majority of such cases, the ureter need not be divided; the only additional surgical features, then, are mobilization of the kidney and anastomosis of the renal vein to the iliac vein. When there is a need to correct stenosis of branch vessels, removal of the kidney from the body is feasible with new cooling and preservation techniques that allow an ischemic period of at least 1½ to 2 hours for ex vivo macro- or microsurgical repair.

The technique of autotransplantation is not difficult. The torque position of the patient and the supracostal incision over the eleventh or twelfth rib allows good exposure of both the renal and the iliac vessels. The procedure is done entirely extraperitoneally, with reflection and retraction of the peritoneum and its contents medially. After the kidney is thoroughly mobilized and the renal vessels are isolated and freed of fat, the ureter is dissected down to the pelvic inlet. Bulldog clamps or an exclusion clamp is placed on the common iliac or external iliac vein, and polar sutures are prepared to receive the renal vein. The patient is heparinized, and both the renal artery and the renal vein are ligated and divided. The kidney is brought down to the iliac fossa without being rotated, and the venous anastomosis is then performed. Although the vein normally lies anterior to the artery, and the vessels must be transposed to some extent, there is no surgical

problem in anastomosing the hypogastric artery to the renal artery. After the venous anastomosis has been done with continuous or interrupted 6–0 sutures, the hypogastric artery is united to the normal post-stenotic renal artery end-to-end with interrupted 6–0 sutures. Sutures are customarily placed before tying is done so that maximal patency is ensured (Figs. 67–21 and 67–22). Figure 67–23 is an artist's drawings of techniques of managing branch anastomoses in the case of distal arterial disease. The ureter

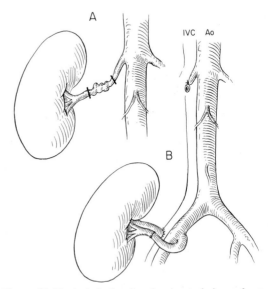

Figure 67–21. Artist's drawing showing technique of autotransplantation of the right kidney for fibrous dysplasia of the artery. End-to-end anastomosis is done to the hypogastric artery using interrupted sutures, and end-to-side anastomosis of the renal vein is made to the external or common iliac vein.

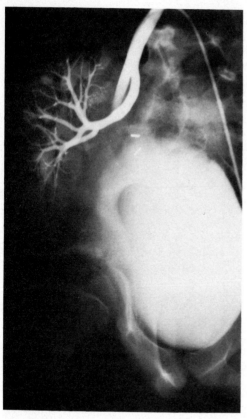

Figure 67–22. Postoperative angiogram showing smooth contour of the hypogastric–renal artery anastomosis after ipsilateral autotransplantation.

is allowed to take a serpiginous course to the bladder; this has not presented drainage problems in any of the 17 autotransplantations performed to date (Fig. 67–24).

A number of reports are appearing on the subject of autotransplantation of the kidney in cases of branch disease (Lim et al., 1972; Belzer et al., 1974; Orcutt et al., 1974). In such instances, renal preservation was accomplished with continuous pulsatile perfusion or initial perfusion with hypothermia (the preferred technique in our hands, inasmuch as the "bench" surgery can be done on the body surface without ureteral division). This technique allows 2 hours or even longer of operating time to perform branch surgery (Sacks et al., 1974; Barry et al., 1983). In some cases, segments of vein, artery, or Dacron have been used to bypass areas of stenosis involving the main renal artery and the first portions of its major branches. Vascular surgical techniques using 2× to 3.5× optical magnification aid in the performance of small vessel anastomoses, and on rare occasion microsurgical repair may be required.

The renal vein is easily handled, and generally a small divet of vena cava is taken if the renal vein is somewhat small. A Derra or Satinsky clamp is left on the vena cava while the kidney is moved to the iliac fossa, preferably without perfusion or cooling but with systemic mannitol and heparin administration. If simple

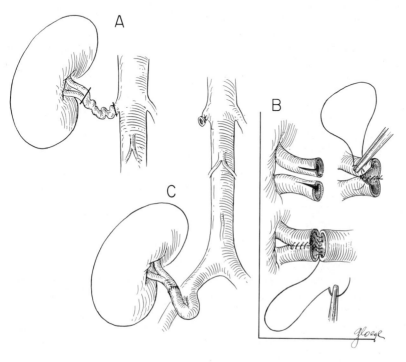

Figure 67–23. Artist's drawing showing method of performing conjoined anastomosis of renal artery branches to the hypogastric artery in renal autotransplantation.

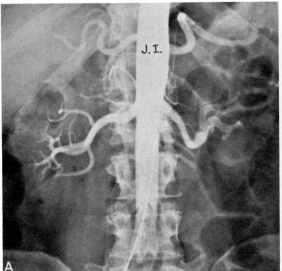

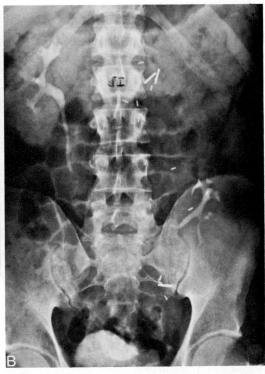

Figure 67–24. *A,* Aortogram showing dissection of left renal artery. Note decreased concentration of contrast beyond area of dissection. *B,* Postoperative intravenous urogram showing good function of the ipsilaterally autotransplanted kidney demonstrated in *A.*

autotransplantation is done, cooling should not be required. Double-armed sutures prevent separation of the intima from the media when passing the needle through the vessel wall from inside out on both sides of the anastomosis.

The use of segments of saphenous vein or hypogastric artery is practical for multiple vessel stenoses. The saphenous vein can be divided into three parts and segments, as illustrated in Figure 67–25 (Abeshouse, 1945). The segments must be oriented to maintain proper flow direction in keeping with the valves.

The headlamp, in addition to magnification, makes these anastomoses much easier. Furthermore, by threading a feeding tube or catheter through the open end of the free hypogastric artery graft and into each of the branches, the anastomoses can be performed over the "stenting" catheter. The base of the graft is then sewn with interrupted sutures to the end of the hypogastric artery or to the side of the external iliac artery (Fig. 67–26).

In addition to the advantages of the precise suturing for small vessel disease, ex vivo radiographic techniques are more easily performed with high resolution and magnification to demonstrate intrarenal arterial disease. Several pertinent references in the literature relative to ex

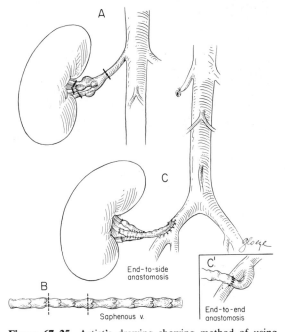

Figure 67–25. Artist's drawing showing method of using length of saphenous vein in several segments to design a branched vessel for ex-vivo repair of multiple aneurysms and stenoses of rami of the right renal artery. Take-off of the saphenous vein can be made from the external or common iliac artery or end-to-end with the hypogastric artery as shown in C′.

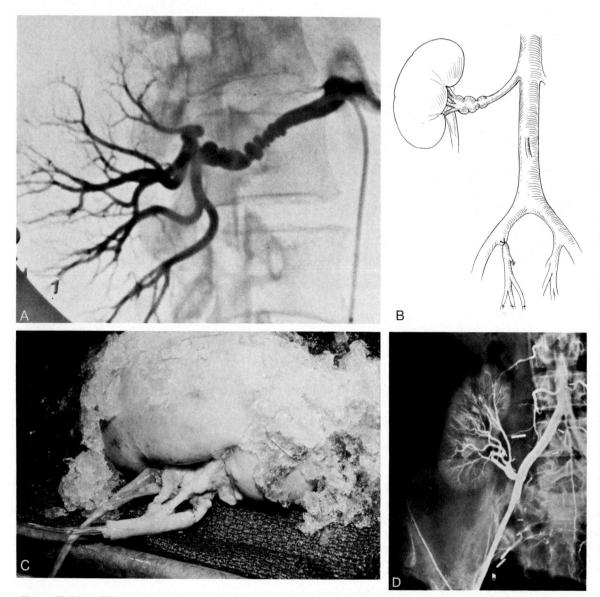

Figure 67–26. *A,* Right renal arteriogram subtraction study showing severe fibromuscular dysplasia of the middle and distal portions of the right renal artery. *B,* Artist's drawing showing the harvesting of the ipsilateral right hypogastric arterial trunk, which will be used to repair the branch lesions. *C,* Photograph showing ex vivo repair with a segment of hypogastric artery anastomosed to three branches of the renal artery. *D,* Postoperative aortogram of patient shown in *A* and *C,* with hypogastric artery transposed to the side of the common iliac artery and with anastomoses to the branches of the renal artery.

vivo surgery are cited (Ota et al., 1967; Kaufman et al., 1969; Lim et al., 1972; Kaufman, 1973a; Sacks, 1975; McLaughlin et al., 1976).

OTHER REVASCULARIZATION PROCEDURES

Resection and Reanastomosis

Resection of the diseased portion of the renal artery together with reanastomosis is ideal for selected cases in which the disease is well defined. The arteriogram, however, frequently fails to indicate the true extent of the disease and longer segments than may be apparent are often involved. In such cases, reanastomosis may be difficult and sometimes predisposes to stenosis at the area of the anastomosis. If resection of the diseased vessel requires an insertion graft, it is often easier to perform an aortorenal bypass, since the proximal anastomosis can be done at a lower level on the aorta, where exposure is better.

Patch Plasty

Patch plasty has been used successfully in a number of cases, but in general, it is not considered a first-choice operation except in unusual circumstances.

Renoaortic Reimplantation

Not only is renoaortic reimplantation more difficult than autotransplantation, but in addition the aorta may be involved by atherosclerosis, thus making satisfactory anastomosis difficult.

RENAL ARTERY STENOSIS AND RENAL FAILURE

In clinical practice, renal artery stenosis alone appears to be an extremely rare cause of end-stage renal disease (Kaufman, 1973b). Most patients with end-stage renal disease have intrinsic parenchymal disease, but this does not rule out the presence of renal artery stenosis, which may be a contributing factor. May and associates (1976) found eight patients with severe renal artery stenosis among a cohort with deteriorating renal function. Following renal revascularization, the average preoperative creatinine of 8 mg per dl declined to approximately 4 mg per dl when reassessed up to 36 months postoperatively. Other reports have appeared indicating that patients with rapidly progressive oliguric renal failure may benefit from vascular repair. Isolated reports indicate successful revascularization after long periods of nonfunction (Zinman and Libertino, 1977; Dean et al., 1979). The longest recorded nonfunction prior to surgical correction by atheromatous occlusion of the renal artery was 30 days (Besarab et al., 1976; Gulbrandson et al., 1977). It is logical, therefore, that renal arteriography should be considered more often in patients with renal failure, particularly when hypertension is an accompanying feature.

SUMMARY

Table 67–1 summarizes the results of surgical treatment in several series of cases of renovascular hypertension. As mentioned previously, the results have been better among younger individuals and among those with fibrous dysplasias than in the arteriosclerotic group. Predictably, morbidity and mortality rates are lower in younger than in older groups. One-stage bilateral procedures should be performed only after careful deliberation, owing to the increased morbidity and mortality, especially among older patients.

The medical treatment of renovascular hypertension is, in our view, a poor substitute for revascularization of the ischemic kidney and is usually associated with poor control of the hypertension or deterioration of renal function. Poor patient compliance, drug ineffectiveness, and unacceptable side effects are the principal reasons for failure to control the high blood pressure adequately and for the unacceptable high mortality.

On the other hand, percutaneous transluminal dilation of selected cases of stenosing renal lesions has proved to be a boon to the patients suffering from stenoses of the renal arteries, with cure and improvement rates comparable to those achieved in the past by surgical angioplasties. Furthermore, the reduced morbidity and mortality and the cost-effectiveness of PTD cannot be disputed. However, patients with atheromatous disease, particularly aortorenal ostial lesions, and patients with aneurysms or main and branch disease that is not amenable to PTD still have the prospect of kidney salvage and cure of hypertension by the surgical techniques that have evolved and been perfected over the last three decades.

TABLE 67–1. SURGICAL TREATMENT OF RENOVASCULAR HYPERTENSION
Combined Results

Author	Year	Patients	Cure	Improvement	Failure	Death
Kaufman	1979	568	364	133	71	—
Novick	1979	235	121	78	36	—
Starr	1980	216	161	22	33	3
Foster	1975	120	72	37	11	8
Hunt	1974	84	51	27	6	—
Morin	1980	44	22	19	3	1
Total		1267	791	316	160	12
%			62.4	24.9	12.6	

From Hillman, B. J. (Ed.): Imaging and Hypertension. Philadelphia, W.B. Saunders Co., 1983, p. 100.

References

Abeshouse, B. S.: Thrombosis and thrombophlebitis of the renal veins. Urol. Cutan. Rev., *49*:661, 1945.

Almén, T., Härtel, M., Nylander, G., and Olivecrona, H.: The effect of estrogen on the vascular endothelium and its possible relation to thrombosis. Surg. Gynecol. Obstet., *140*:938, 1975.

Barry, J. M., Fisher, S., Larson, B., Fearey, J. A., Lieberman, C., and Fuchs, E. F.: Comparison of imported with locally retrieved kidneys preserved by intracellular electrolyte flushing followed by cold storage. J. Urol., *129*:471, 1983.

Belzer, F. O., Salvatierra, O., Perloff, D., and Grausz, H.: Surgical correction of advanced fibromuscular dysplasia of the renal arteries. Surgery, *75*:31, 1974.

Besarab, A., Brown, R. S., Rubin, N. T., et al.: Reversible renal failure following bilateral renal artery occlusive disease: Clinical features, pathology and the role of surgical revascularization. JAMA, *235*:2838, 1976.

Burch, G. E., Harb, J. M., Hiramoto, Y., and Shewey, L.: Viral infection of the aorta of man associated with early atherosclerotic changes. Am. Heart J., *86*:523, 1973.

Butler, A. M.: Chronic pyelonephritis and arterial hypertension. J. Clin. Invest., *16*:889, 1937.

Cummings, K. C., Lecky, J. W., and Kaufman, J. J.: Renal artery aneurysms and hypertension. J. Urol., *109*:144, 1973.

Curtis, J. J., Luke, R. G., Whelchel, J. D., Diethelm, A. G., Jones, P., and Dustan, H. P.: Inhibition of angiotensin-converting enzyme in renal-transplant recipients with hypertension. N. Engl. J. Med., *308*:377, 1983.

Dean, R. H., Lawson, J. D., Hollifield, J. W., et al.: Revascularization of the poorly functioning kidney. Surgery, *85*:44, 1979.

Dotter, C. T., and Judkins, M. P.: Transluminal treatment of arteriosclerotic obstruction. Circulation, *30*:654, 1964.

Doyle, T. J., McGregor, W. R., Fox, P. S., Maddison, F. E., Rodgers, R. E., and Kauffman, H. M.: Homotransplant renal artery stenosis. Surgery, *77*:53, 1975.

Ehrlich, R. M.: Renal arteriovenous fistula treated by endofistulorhaphy. Arch. Surg., *110*:1195, 1975.

Ernst, C. B., Stanley, J. C., Marshall, F. F., and Fry, W. J.: Autogenous saphenous vein aortorenal grafts: A ten-year experience. Arch. Surg., *105*:855, 1972.

Foster, J. H., and Dean, R. H.: Changing concepts in renovascular hypertension. Symposium on Vascular Surgery. Surg. Clin. North Am., *54*:257, 1974.

Gavras, H., Brunner, H. R., Laragh, J. E., et al.: An angiotensin converting enzyme inhibitor to identify and treat vasoconstrictor and volume factors in hypertensive patients. N. Engl. J. Med., *291*:817, 1974.

Gavras, H., Brunner, H. R., and Turini, G. A.: Antihypertensive effect of the oral angiotensin converting–enzyme inhibitor SQ 14225 in man. N. Engl. J. Med., *298*:991, 1978.

Glushein, A. S., Mansuy, M. M., and Littman, D. S.: Pheochromocytoma: Its relationship to the neurocutaneous syndromes. Am. J. Med., *14*:318, 1953.

Grad, E., and Rance, C. P.: Bilateral renal artery stenosis in association with neurofibromatosis (Recklinghausen's disease): Report of two cases. J. Pediatr., *80*:804, 1972.

Gruntzig, A., Kuhlmann, U., Vetter, W., et al.: Treatment of renovascular hypertension with percutaneous transluminal dilation of a renal-artery stenosis. Lancet, *1*:801, 1978.

Gulbrandson, R. N., Al-Bermani, J., and Gaspard, D. J.: Successful renal revascularization after prolonged nonfunction. JAMA, *238*:2522, 1977.

Hall, J. E., Guyton, A. C., Jackson, T. E., Coleman, T. G., Lohmeier, T. E., and Trippodo, N. C.: Control of glomerular filtration rate by renin-angiotensin system. Am. J. Physiol., *233*:F366, 1977.

Hricik, D. E., Browning, P. J., Kopelman, R., Goorno, W. E., Madias, N. E., and Dzau, V. J.: Captopril-induced functional renal insufficiency in patients with bilateral renal-artery stenosis or renal-artery stenosis in a solitary kidney. N. Engl. J. Med., *308*:373, 1983.

Hunt, J. C., Sheps, S. G., Harrison, E. G., et al.: Renal and renovascular hypertension: A reasoned approach to diagnosis and management. Arch. Intern. Med., *133*:988, 1974.

Ishikawa, K.: Natural history and classification of occlusive thromboaortopathy (Takayasu's disease). Circulation, *57*:27, 1978.

Katzen, B. T., Chang, J., and Knox, W. G.: Percutaneous transluminal angioplasty with the Gruntzig balloon catheter. Arch. Surg., *114*:1389, 1979.

Katzen, B. T.: Personal communication, 1982.

Kaufman, J. J.: The middle aortic syndrome: Report of a case treated by renal autotransplantation. J. Urol., *109*:711, 1973a.

Kaufman, J. J.: Renal artery stenosis and azotemia. Surg. Gynecol. Obstet., *137*:949, 1973b.

Kaufman, J. J.: Long-term results of aortorenal Dacron grafts in the treatment of renal artery stenosis. J. Urol., *111*:298, 1974.

Kaufman, J. J.: Dacron grafts and splenorenal bypass in the surgical treatment of stenosing lesions of the renal artery. Urol. Clin. North Am., *2*:365, 1975.

Kaufman, J. J., Alferez, C., and Vela-Navarrete, R.: Autotransplantation of a solitary functioning kidney for renovascular hypertension. J. Urol., *102*:146, 1969.

Kaufman, J. J., Ehrlich, R. M., and Dornfeld, L.: Immunologic considerations in renovascular hypertension. J. Urol., *116*:142, 1976.

Kincaid, O. W., Davis, G. D., Hallerman, F. J., et al.: Fibromuscular dysplasia of the renal arteries: Arteriographic features, classification and observations on natural history of the disease. Am. J. Roentgenol. Radium Ther. Nucl. Med., *104*:271, 1968.

Lawrie, G. M., Morris, G. C., Jr., Sousson, I. D., et al.: Late results of reconstructive surgery for renovascular disease. Ann. Surg., *191*:528, 1980.

Lim, R. C., Jr., Eastman, A. B., and Blaisdell, F. W.: Renal autotransplantation. Adjunct to repair of renal vascular lesions. Arch. Surg., *105*:847, 1972.

Lye, C. R., String, S. T., Wylie, E. J., and Stoney, R. J.: Aortorenal arterial autografts. Late observations. Arch. Surg., *110*:1321, 1975.

Mahoney, A. D., and Waisman, J.: Lesions of the extrarenal segment of the renal artery and hypertension. Urol. Clin. North Am., *2*:259, 1975.

Margules, R. M., Belzer, F. O., and Kountz, S. L.: Surgical correction of renovascular hypertension following renal allotransplantation. Arch. Surg., *106*:13, 1973.

Maxwell, M. H., Bleifer, K. H., Franklin, S. S., et al.: Cooperative study of renovascular hypertension: Demographic analysis of the study. JAMA, *220*:1195, 1972.

May, J., Sheil, A. G. R., Horvath, J., et al.: Reversal of renal failure and control of hypertension in patients with occlusion of the renal artery. Surg. Gynecol. Obstet., *143*:411, 1976.

McLaughlin, M. G., Williams, G. M., and Stonesifer, G. L., Jr.: Ex-vivo surgical dissection. Autotransplantation in renal disease. JAMA, *235*:1705, 1976.

Orcutt, T. W., Foster, J. H., Richie, R. E., Wilson, J. P., and Warner, H. E.: Bilateral ex-vivo renal artery reconstruction with autotransplantation. JAMA, 228:493, 1974.

Ota, K., Mori, S., Awane, Y., et al.: Ex-situ repair of renal artery for renovascular hypertension. Arch. Surg., 94:370, 1967.

Oxman, H. A., Sheps, S. G., Bernattz, P. E., et al.: An unusual cause of renal arteriovenous fistula—fibromuscular dysplasia of the renal arteries. Mayo Clin. Proc., 48:207, 1973.

Rogers, W. H., Rukskiel, A., Camishion, R. L., and Padula, R. T.: In-vivo cinephotographic analysis of aortic and major arterial flow patterns. Arch. Surg., 103:93, 1971.

Sacks, S. A.: Renal autotransplantation and ex-vivo renal surgery: Surgical treatment of renovascular hypertension. Urol. Clin. North Am., 2:381, 1975.

Sacks, S. A., Petritsch, P. H., Linder, R., and Kaufman, J. J.: Renal autotransplantation: Further use of a new perfusate. Am. J. Surg., 128:402, 1974.

Schwarten, D. E., Yune, H. Y., Klatte, E. C., et al.: Clinical experience with percutaneous transluminal angioplasty (PTA) of stenotic renal arteries. Radiology, 135:601, 1980.

Sheps, S. G., Kincaid, O. W., and Hunt, J. C.: Serial renal function and angiographic observations in idiopathic fibrous and fibromuscular stenoses of the renal arteries. Am. J. Cardiol., 30:55, 1972.

Sos, T. A., Saddekni, S., Sniderman, K. W., Weiner, M., Beinart, C., Pickering, T. G., Case, D. B., Vaughan, E. D., Jr., and Larah, J. H.: Renal artery angioplasty: Techniques and early results. Urol. Radiol., 3:223, 1982.

Sos, T. A., Pickering, T. G., Sniderman, K., Saddekni, S., Case, D. B., Silane, M. F., Vaughan, E. D., Jr., and Larah, J. H.: Percutaneous transluminal renal angioplasty in renovascular hypertension due to atheroma or fibromuscular dysplasia. N. Engl. J. Med., 309:274, 1983.

Stanley, J. C., and Fry, W. J.: Renovascular hypertension secondary to arterial fibrodysplasia in adults: Criteria for operation and results of surgical therapy. Arch. Surg., 110:922, 1975.

Stanley, J. C., Rhodes, E. L., Gewertz, B. L., et al.: Renal artery aneurysms. Significance of macroaneurysms exclusive of dissections and fibrodysplastic mural dilations. Arch. Surg., 110:1327, 1975.

Stewart, B. H., Dustan, H. P., Kiser, W. S., et al.: Correlation of angiography and natural history in evaluation of patients with renovascular hypertension. J. Urol., 104:231, 1970.

Vidne, B. A., Leapman, S. B., Butt, K. M., and Kountz, S. L.: Vascular complications in human renal transplantation. Surgery, 79:77, 1976.

Von Recklinghausen, F.: Über die multiplen der Haut und ihre Beziehungen zu den multiplen Neurinomen. Berlin, Festshrift für Rudolf Virchow, 1882.

Wylie, E. J.: Endarterectomy and autogenous arterial grafts in the surgical treatment of stenosing lesions of the renal artery. Urol. Clin. North Am., 2:351, 1975.

Zinman, L., and Libertino, J. A.: Revascularization of the chronic totally occluded renal artery with restoration of renal function. J. Urol., 118:517, 1977.

CHAPTER 68

Surgery of the Ureter

WARREN W. KOONTZ, JR., M.D.
FREDERICK A. KLEIN, M.D.
M. J. VERNON SMITH, M.D., Ph.D.

The ureter is a muscular tube that transports urine from the ureteropelvic junction of the kidney to the bladder. It lies entirely in the retroperitoneal space and runs throughout most of the length of the abdomen and pelvis. It lies loosely in the retroperitoneum in its upper portion, but after crossing the iliac vessels, it becomes attached to the underside of the parietal peritoneum. It is more fixed in its course through the pelvis toward the bladder. The average ureteral length is approximately 20 to 30 cm, depending on the size of the patient and the distance from the kidney to the bladder.

In its proximal one third, the ureter courses up and over (anterior) to the psoas muscle and lateral to the transverse processes. The middle third of the ureter passes posterior to the gonadal vessels (spermatic or ovarian). More distally, the ureter crosses the iliac vessels and lies anterior to the sacroiliac joint. The ureter courses posteriorly and laterally, following the course of the hypogastric vessels, in close proximity to the wall of the pelvis. The ureter then turns medially toward the bladder, lying anterior to the hypogastric artery and medial to the obturator nerve and vessels.

In the male, the ureter crosses the vas deferens ventrally, penetrating the bladder wall posteriorly and above the prostate and seminal vesicles. In the female, the ureter crosses behind the uterine artery and vein and passes within 1 to 2 cm of the uterine cervix before entering the base of the bladder. The ureters enter the bladder obliquely, passing through a submucosal tunnel so that, when the bladder is filling, the tunnel will prevent vesicoureteral reflux.

There are three anatomic points of narrowing of the ureter. These are the ureteropelvic junction, the area where the ureter passes over the iliac vessels, and the ureterovesical junction.

The ureter develops its arterial blood supply from branches of the renal artery, which supplies the upper third of the ureter and the renal pelvis. Branches from the aorta and from the gonadal, iliac, hypogastric, and superior vesical arteries supply the middle third of the ureter. Branches of the uterine, vesical, and middle hemorrhoidal arteries supply the lower third of the ureter. There is a network of vessels in the adventitial tissue of the ureter, which allows interruption of the arterial supply in one area but will not ordinarily affect the vascular integrity of the ureter. The venous drainage of the ureter arises from the submucosal and muscular layers and courses through the adventitial tissue to drain into veins parallel to the arterial blood supply. A knowledge of ureteral blood supply is essential before undertaking ureteral surgery. If the surgeon follows anatomic and physiologic guidelines and uses gentle and accurate surgical techniques, the integrity of the urinary tract can be maintained even when threatened by a variety of pathologic conditions.

The ureter is composed of three anatomic layers: an outer adventitial sheath through which courses its blood supply; a medial layer of smooth muscle arranged in a spiral, circular, or longitudinal fashion; and, finally, an inner layer of transitional cells.

Ureteral contractions or peristaltic waves propel a bolus of urine from the kidney to the bladder. These contractions normally occur at a frequency of two to six times per minute. For efficient propulsion of the bolus, the contraction wave must completely coapt the ureteral wall and the urine must pass into the bladder. Any alteration that interferes with the function of this urinary transport mechanism may lead to renal deterioration and eventually to loss of that kidney unit.

The foundations for ureteral surgery were laid in the nineteenth century; with progress, ingenuity, and the diligence of many investigators, a variety of innovative approaches to the management of ureteral disorders have evolved (Persky et al., 1979).

If ureteral neoplasms are excluded, few diseases require ureterectomy; in most cases, the disease process affecting the ureter can be corrected and urinary continuity restored.

This chapter will include discussions on the disease states affecting the ureter, surgical approaches to the ureter, and general techniques of ureteral surgery. Other chapters will deal with the use of the intestine in ureteral surgery, ureteral reimplantation, and the use of endourologic procedures for the management of ureteral disorders.

Even though endourologic procedures will decrease the need for open surgical procedures, these newer techniques will not be applicable to all patients. The urologic surgeon must know and understand all aspects of the surgical management of the ureter. The indications for different surgical procedures on the ureter will also be discussed.

URETERAL DISORDERS THAT REQUIRE SURGERY

Congenital ureteral abnormalities may lead to minimal disturbances in ureteral function but may have significant manifestations owing to obstructive changes in the renal segment. Abnormalities of insertion or anastomosis at either end of the ureter or abnormalities in the midportion (such as megaureter, diverticula, or stricture) may lead to impairment of renal function. Congenital anomalies of the ureter are presented fully in Chapter 38.

Metabolic diseases, such as abnormalities in calcium, uric acid, and cystine metabolism, are well known to lead to calculi, which require surgical therapy. These diseases themselves do not generally cause a ureteral disorder. Gastrointestinal diseases that produce chronic diarrhea or malabsorption may lead to modification of oxalate metabolism, which will also result in formation of urinary calculi (Gregory et al., 1975; Hofman et al., 1970). Amyloidosis, both primary and secondary, is known to affect the

ureter (Andrews and Oosting, 1958; Johnson and Ankerman, 1964).

Inflammatory disease of bacterial or mycotic origin may affect the ureter. High concentrations of *Escherichia coli* and staphylococcal endotoxins inhibit contractions of in vitro guinea pig ureteral segments. Bacterial *E. coli* endotoxin can inhibit ureteral activity in monkeys and in man (Boyarsky et al., 1978). Irregular contractions with an often decreased amplitude have been recorded with infections. Ureteral dilatation has been reported to result from retroperitoneal inflammatory processes secondary to appendicitis, regional ileitis, ulcerative colitis, and peritonitis (Makker et al., 1972). An inflammatory process, such as ureteritis secondary to chronic urinary tract infection, would be expected to respond to the appropriate medication. If healing leads to scarring, obstructing strictures may require surgical intervention.

Tuberculous involvement of the upper urinary tract may cause ureteral scarring and stricture even after appropriate antituberculous therapy. Such stricture formation may require an open surgical procedure if more conservative ureteral dilation and stenting are not adequate. Intense scar tissue may accompany healing after prolonged drainage of uninfected as well as infected urine through the ureteral wall of a perinephric or intra-abdominal abscess; the fibrosis caused by idiopathic retroperitoneal fibrosis (the cause of which is disputed and unclear) frequently presents with ureteral involvement requiring operative intervention.

Primary neoplasms of the ureter are uncommon and may be either malignant or benign. All will require some form of surgical therapy. Benign tumors may be adequately managed with limited conservative procedures, such as local excision of the lesion with a reanastomosis of the ureter. A variety of benign lesions that have been described in the ureter are lipoma, leiomyoma, fibroma, neuroma, and endometrioma. In contrast, the appropriate surgical management of a malignant ureteral carcinoma may be the resection of the kidney and ureter in continuity. A more complete discussion of ureteral neoplasia and its surgical management is found in Chapter 29.

One of the more frequent indications for ureteral surgery is the repair of ureteral trauma. These injuries usually result from penetrating injury, such as a knife wound or gunshot wound, but a large number occur in the operating room. The pelvic ureter is most commonly injured by general surgical, gynecologic, and urologic procedures (Persky and Hoch, 1974). Only rarely does blunt trauma cause ureteral injury, and then this is usually an avulsion injury of the upper ureter. The reader is referred to Chapter 26 on renal and ureteral injury.

Fistulous tracts between the ureter and adjacent organs commonly occur in female patients following pelvic surgery. The ureter may be injured at any point along its course within the pelvis, but anatomically it is closely related to the vascular bundle and ligament of the uterus and ovaries. It is frequently injured during clamping or ligating of the uterine artery, the cardinal ligaments, or the infundibulopelvic ligament and ovarian vessels. During control of the pelvic blood vessels, the ureter may be kinked, crushed, sutured, excised, divided, or devascularized. If a urinary leak occurs, the urine may find the easiest way out, usually through the vaginal cuff. Inflammatory retroperitoneal processes may involve the ureter to such an extent that a fistulous tract will occur.

PRINCIPLES OF URETERAL SURGERY

Healing and Regeneration of the Ureter

A number of factors affect ureteral healing. At the time of the surgical procedure the delicate and gentle manipulation of ureteral tissue that results in minimal tissue trauma is most important. The use of noncrushing forceps and traction sutures will reduce crush injuries and maximize blood supply to the operated area. The ureter should never be intentionally grasped with a hemostat or other crushing instrument. The least amount of ureteral mobilization required to accomplish the operation lessens the possibility of vascular compromise. It is the ureteral adventitia that carries the blood supply to the ureter that is to be repaired. Several factors affect epithelialization of the ureteral defect. These include no tension on the area to be repaired, no urinary leakage, and a mucosa-to-mucosa approximation of the defect. A circumferential scar of the ureter may contract, causing a stricture, hydroureter, hydronephrosis, and possible renal damage.

Ureteral repair is enhanced since a longitudinal strip of ureter will allow bridging of a defect, around which new epithelium can spread to develop a new ureteral lumen. The ureter can close its own defect by regenerating all of its components. The defect is first bridged by transitional cell epithelium. A linear incision

with no intervening obstruction will allow the mucosa to span the defect in 8 to 10 days. A transverse ureteral incision will be rapidly closed by the urothelium. Prolonged and profuse urinary drainage may lead to abnormal epithelialization. Urinary flow across a repair may promote a lumen and stimulate transitional cell and muscle growth. However, newly formed epithelium may also be distracted and urinary extravasation may lead to a reactive fibrosis with subsequent stenosis and obstruction. After bridging of a defect by transitional cell epithelium, fibrous tissue will develop and then contract, pulling already present smooth muscle into the gap. This stimulates the growth of new smooth muscle to complete the repair.

The tissue surrounding the ureter is important in repair. Rigid tissue, such as fascia, produces a disorderly repair, whereas less rigid tissue, such as fat, allows the ureteral walls to renew with peristaltic activity. If a repaired ureter is to lie on fascia or bony tissue, the wrapping of the ureter with fatty tissues, such as omentum, may allow improved healing and more rapid return of normal peristaltic activity. For successful ureteral healing with regeneration of smooth muscle, minimal fibrosis is important for the re-establishment of peristaltic activity. Butcher and Sleator (1956) have shown that a period of 28 days is required for the resumption of the passage of electrical activity across an anastomotic ureteral site, and cineradiographic study after ureteral anastomosis in man was in accord with this observation (Caine and Hermann, 1970). This may account for the occasionally observed delayed pelvic emptying occurring after a dismembered pyeloplasty or ureteroureterostomy. Normally, electrical activity propagates from cell to cell as peristaltic activity is associated with the transport of urine. It is postulated that in the period immediately after anastomosis the electrical event propagates to the anastomotic site and then stops. There is some stasis of urine proximal to the anastomosis, with no urine passing the point of anastomosis until proximal ureteral pressure increases to a critical level and some urine passes beyond the anastomosis. This bolus then stretches the ureteral muscle just distal to the anastomotic site and serves to initiate peristaltic activity distal to the anastomosis (Weiss, 1979).

STENTING

A ureteral defect may exhibit improved healing with the use of a stenting agent. Davis (1943) popularized the use of stents and stimulated the investigation and controversy that continues to this day. Proponents of ureteral stenting believe that the stent will (1) immobilize the ureter until healing has occured; (2) inhibit the growth of granulation tissue and allow the orderly regrowth of an intact epithelial layer, followed by its muscular covering; (3) prevent the leakage of urine at the anastomotic site; (4) help to maintain an adequate lumen of the ureter during the healing phase; and (5) minimize any tendency to angulation of the ureter (Persky and Hoch, 1974). A well-fitting stent provides a mold around which the appropriate healing processes occur (Davis, 1958). The correct size is probably the one that fits comfortably without placing tension on the ureteral wall. Weaver (1957) noted fibrosis and stricture formation with large stents, which was not present with stents that were considerably smaller. Davis (1958) advocated larger stents but not to the point at which blanching of the ureteral wall occurred. Experimental evidence suggests that too large a stent places undue stress on the ureter and particularly on the area of the repair (Persky, 1967). Some investigators believe that complications may follow the use of stenting catheters, thus outweighing the possible merits of their use. One of the problems associated with the stent is an inflammatory stricture and calcification at the site of the repair. If the stent slips, angulation, distortion, and poor healing may result. The stent may develop deposits of amorphous phosphate material, causing obstruction with hydroureter and hydronephrosis.

Silastic tubing seems to be the material of choice. At body temperatures, it becomes quite soft and pliable. Care must be taken with these tubes to prevent them from becoming dislodged, obstructed, kinked, or encrusted. Stents may be held in place by suture materials, holding catheters such as nephrostomy tubes, or bladder Foley catheters. More popular today are the single- or double-ended pigtail catheters that prevent migration up or down the ureter.

In summary, there remains significant controversy over the use of the stent. The surgeon must weigh the advantages of the stent versus the disadvantages of this foreign body and the possible complications related to its use.

URINARY DIVERSION AND DRAINAGE

During the healing phase, a ureteral defect may be watertight within 24 to 48 hours. Large defects may take 4 to 6 weeks for complete epithelialization and regeneration of fibrotic tissue and smooth muscle without functional obstruction. Urine flow through an anastomosis does not seem to interfere with the organization

of repair; however, with continued urine flow the process requires a longer time. A longitudinal ureterotomy creates an adequate decompression, and after healing occurs, peristalsis will normalize throughout the ureter (Hamm and Weinberg, 1957). It would seem in such a case that proximal urinary diversion is not necessary for satisfactory ureteral regeneration. If there is a large defect, complete transection of the ureter, or a great deal of inflammatory reaction around the ureter, urinary drainage and diversion are applicable. Pooling of extravasated urine leads to disorganization of the healing process. Marked fibrous reaction and scarring may result, with poor muscular organization leading to stricture formation and obstruction.

The type of drain used is not as important as the efficiency of the drain. The Penrose drain has been the mainstay for years and can be left indwelling down to the site of any potential extravasation of urine or hemorrhage. It should be left as long as there is a possibility of urinary leakage and should be removed in steps over several days. A self-contained drainage system, such as a sump type (Jackson-Pratt or Hemovac), may also be utilized and can keep the wound cleaner and drier and the patient happier and more comfortable.

Urinary diversion may be of benefit to prevent the site of repair from being bathed in urine. This can be accomplished effectively by means of an indwelling stent. Effective diversion can also be accomplished by a nephrostomy (percutaneous or conventional) using a straight catheter, Foley catheter, mushroom catheter, or "U" tube. Another form of diversion may be a proximal ureterotomy or pyelotomy. The urologic surgeon should be adept at all techniques; the choice of diversion is left to the surgeon's preference, the patient's diagnosis and condition, the type of lesion, and the type of repair.

Of more importance is whether or not to divert. There continues to be controversy, and the guidelines to divert are variable. A patient who is considered a poor risk, such as one with a serious infection, widespread contaminated wound, impaired renal function, or other serious abnormality, will dictate whether diversion is necessary. A well-performed ureteral repair that is watertight in virgin tissue may not require a urinary diversion.

URETERAL SUTURING

There are several rules of thumb relating to the suturing of ureteral defects. The suture material should be fine (4-0 or smaller). It should be atraumatic and produce minimal tissue reaction. The suture should approximate and not strangulate the ureteral wall, and there should be no tension on the suture line. Lastly, the suture material should be absorbable. The use of silk, prolene, or other nonabsorbable materials may lead to fistula formation, encrustation, and calculi (Silbur and Thornburg, 1973). Fine, absorbable suture, such as 4-0 or 5-0 chromic catgut or Dexon, is preferable.

Approaches to Surgery of the Ureter

The ureter varies in length from 20 to 30 cm, depending on the size of the individual. The incision and surgical approach to the ureter depend on the segment to be operated upon. Surgical approaches to the upper third of the ureter are, in general, the same as those used for the kidney. These are covered in detail in Chapter 62. The subcostal flank incision approaches the upper third of the ureter. Rarely would this approach require the incision to go through the bed of the twelfth rib or above. A posterior lumbotomy incision may be of help, but, as pointed out elsewhere, the limitations of this incision are a problem if one is looking for an upper-third ureteral stone which then moves to an area that is very difficult to get to through the posterior lumbotomy approach (Figure 68–1C).

For calculi in the middle third of the ureter, an approach through a muscle-splitting incision at the appropriate level, sometimes called a high Gibson incision, provides easy access to the ureter with the possibility of extension of the incision if that is deemed necessary. The fascia and muscle bundles of the external oblique, internal oblique, and transverse abdominis are separated bluntly parallel to their fibers for a distance of 4 to 5 cm. The underlying peritoneum is mobilized and reflected medially, and as the fat is pulled aside anteriorly, the ureter is located (Fig. 68–1B).

The lower third of the ureter can be approached through a muscle-splitting, lower quadrant, modified Gibson incision. If necessary, the lower quadrant incision can be extended medially in order to retract the rectus muscle, or the rectus muscle can be divided for greater access to the lower ureter just before entry into the bladder.

Depending on the surgical procedure to be performed on the lower ureter, it may be ad-

vantageous to have as much exposure as possible in the area. This may mean that a transverse, Pfannenstiel, lower midline, or paramedian extraperitoneal approach would be better than a Gibson-type incision.

If special problems arise with scarring around the ureter, a low anterior midline incision, either extraperitoneal or transperitoneal, may be required. A transperitoneal approach to the ureter may provide access to the ureter from its insertion in the bladder to its origin at the ureteropelvic junction. An extraperitoneal approach is preferable because of the possibility of urine leakage postoperatively. However, in the appropriately chosen patient, the transperitoneal approach may be ideal when combined with adequate drainage, stenting, and a urinary diversion (Fig. 68–1A).

URETEROLYSIS

Ureterolysis as a primary procedure is indicated whenever there is ureteral entrapment with resultant obstruction and renal functional compromise. Ureteral entrapment or periureteral fibrosis may occur secondary to a number of pathologic processes, including intraperitoneal inflammatory disease, abscess formation from granulomatous bowel disease, pelvic inflammatory disease, endometriosis, neoplasm, previous radiation therapy, or drugs (methysergide maleate), or it may be idiopathic (Ormond's disease) (Ormond, 1948).

Although there may be some reversibility of fibrosis and obstruction by withdrawing methy-

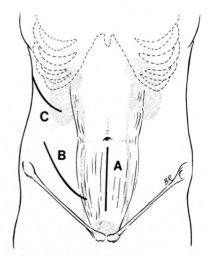

Figure 68–1. Incisions for surgical approaches to the ureter.

sergide maleate or with the use of steroids for idiopathic retroperitoneal fibrosis (Kearney et al., 1976), the majority of cases require surgical intervention, not only to relieve the obstruction but also to make a definitive diagnosis. Initial management and timing of surgical intervention are dicated by the extent of disease and renal compromise.

The primary objective of therapy is relief of obstruction, and this frequently can be accomplished by the passage of an indwelling catheter or stent. If the ureters cannot be catheterized and renal insufficiency or failure is present, temporary upper tract diversion by means of a percutaneous nephrostomy tube is mandatory to stabilize renal function before surgical exploration and definitive ureterolysis are undertaken.

Retroperitoneal fibrosis, whatever the etiology, may manifest itself initially as unilateral disease; however, even with what appears to be a totally normal opposite system, the opposite ureter will most likely be involved with the process and require "prophylactic therapy." For this reason a midline transabdominal incision is the preferable approach.

TECHNIQUE

A generous midline incision gives exposure from the renal pedicles to the level of the ureterovesical junction. Initially, routine abdominal exploration is performed. Ureteral exposure may be achieved in one of two ways: either through a single incision in the posterior peritoneum in the midline, between the duodenum and the inferior mesenteric vein, or on each side, by reflecting the colon along the white line of Toldt from the iliac bifurcation to the splenic and hepatic flexure. Tissue for biopsy and frozen-section examination should be obtained to rule out the presence of malignancy. The ureter is identified either at the level of the iliac vessel or at the ureteropelvic junction above the fibrotic process. Ureterolysis is accomplished from the ureteropelvic junction to below the iliac vessels. The fibrotic process can usually be stripped from the ureter rather easily with blunt dissection, using a right angle clamp. If the correct plane is entered, the fibrotic process usually comes off in a peel. If it does not strip off easily, malignancy should be considered. Since the fibrotic process is diffuse and covers the major vessels, injury is rare. After complete lysis, the ureter should promptly fill with urine. If it does not, significant fibrotic material may remain behind or the ureteral wall itself may be involved.

Ureterolysis alone is inadequate treatment to prevent reinvolvement by the fibrotic process. At this point, the ureters may be handled in one of two ways: (1) They may be transplanted to an intraperitoneal position; or (2) they may be transposed laterally and anteriorly, with retroperitoneal fat placed between the ureters and the fibrosis. With the former method, the parietal peritoneum is sutured with 2-0 chromic catgut posterior to the ureter, from the level of the ureteropelvic junction to the iliac vessels, leaving generous entrance and exit windows to prevent subsequent stenosis and obstruction (Fig. 68–2).

When fibrosis is especially extensive or when there is intraperitoneal involvement, lateral displacement and fixation offer better results. For this procedure, interrupted 2-0 chromic catgut sutures are placed between the parietal peritoneum and psoas or quadratus lumborum muscle, fixing it medial to the ureter. The peritoneal defect is then closed (Fig. 68–2). To further improve results, Tresidder and associates (1972) recommended wrapping the ureters in omentum; however, this addition is generally not necessary.

If stents can be placed preoperatively, they should remain in place for at least 3 to 4 days postoperatively to be sure that ureteral obstruction does not recur and to help the ureters remain in the position where they were operatively placed. The use of postoperative steroids is controversial but may be beneficial in helping to resolve fibrosis and in preventing recurrent fibrosis. Serum renal function studies should be performed at monthly intervals for several

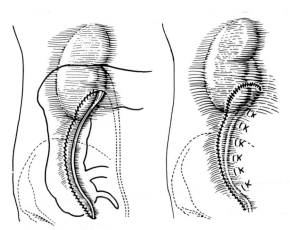

Figure 68–2. *Left,* The right ureter displaced laterally and intraperitonealized from the renal pelvis to the peritoneal reflection. *Right,* Lateral displacement of the right ureter with chromic sutures fixing the parietal peritoneum to the psoas or quadratus lumborum muscle.

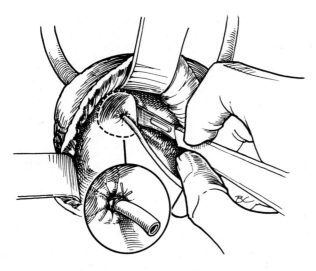

Figure 68–3. Excision of the ureterovesical junction by taking a 1-cm cuff of bladder mucosa and bladder wall with a ureteral catheter in place.

months, with a repeat intravenous pyelogram at approximately 3 months to assure that there has been no recurrence or progression of disease.

URETERECTOMY

Primary ureterectomy is most frequently done in combination with nephrectomy for the treatment of renal pelvic or ureteral urothelial neoplasms. Other indications for ureterectomy, with or without nephrectomy, include tuberculosis, severe hydronephrosis secondary to reflux, pyoureter, hydroureter, stricture, and complete duplication.

When ureterectomy is performed at the time of nephrectomy, either portion of the procedure may be done first. The most important consideration, if tumor is present, is to remove all of the tissue en bloc. If tumor is suspected but not proven, the ureteral exploration should be done first. Whether to do a nephroureterectomy through one flank incision or with two separate incisions primarily depends upon the patient's body habitus and whether a ureteral cuff excision (for carcinoma) is required.

Most commonly, the patient is placed in the 45 degree oblique position with the table flexed. A standard flank incision is made, and all renal attachments except the ureter are divided. If the distal ureterectomy with bladder cuff can be performed with adequate exposure, the incision is extended as a Gibson incision and the ureter freed by blunt dissection to the intramural portion. The distal ureterectomy may then be performed in one of two ways: either (1) by making a separate anterior incision in the bladder and circumscribing the ureteral orifice

with a 1-cm margin (Fig. 68–3) or (2) by staying completely extravesical and placing two right angle clamps across the ureterovesical junction, dividing the bladder between the clamps, and oversewing the distal clamp with a 2-0 chromic gut suture (Fig. 68–4). If the bladder was opened, the ureteral hiatus as well as the vesicotomy is closed in two layers with 0 or 2-0 chromic catgut. A Foley catheter for drainage should be left for 5 to 7 days. The major disadvantage for bladder cuff excision without vesicotomy is the inability to identify and prevent an occasional injury to the opposite ureteral orifice. If the distal ureterectomy is performed first for tumor, a sterile glove can be tied over the end of the ureter to prevent any tumor spillage and then tucked into the retroperitoneum. The remainder of the procedure can be accomplished through the flank, if necessary. If the ureterectomy is being done for benign disease, it is seldom necessary to remove a bladder cuff.

Secondary Ureterectomy—Excision of Ureteral Stump

Ureteral excision may be done at the time of nephrectomy or may be delayed. Depending upon the reason for excision, resection of an adjacent cuff of bladder may be necessary. The indications for secondary ureterectomy include reflux of the ureteral stump, pyoureter, tuberculous ureteritis, tumor, a ureter with a stricture and calculus above the stricture preventing adequate drainage, and ectopic ureters of dysplastic duplicated kidneys.

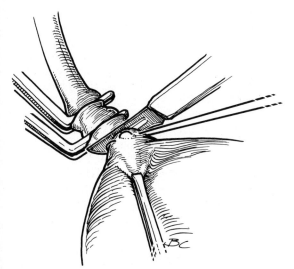

Figure 68–4. Division of the ureter across the ureterovesical junction. A figure-of-eight or purse-string suture is placed distal to the second clamp, and the ureter is excised.

Ureterectomy after nephrectomy may be performed through a midline infrapubic incision, a Gibson incision, or a Pfannenstiel incision. Even though dense adhesions may be present from previous surgery, an extraperitoneal approach is usually possible without too much difficulty. Blunt and sharp dissection is used to free the ureter from its attachments, with care taken not to injure the iliac vessels or overlying intraperitoneal structures. The ureter is freed to the ureterovesical junction and may be excised, as shown in Figure 68–4, by placing a right angle clamp as close as possible to the ureterovesical junction, excising the ureter, and oversewing the bladder wall distal to the clamp with a 2-0 chromic suture. If complete excision with a bladder cuff is required, a cystotomy is done, the ureteral orifice circumscribed and the stump removed, as shown in Figure 68–3. The ureteral hiatus and cystotomy are then closed in a standard two-layer fashion with 2-0 chromic sutures. Postoperatively, a Penrose drain should be left in the ureteral bed if the bladder was opened.

URETEROLITHOTOMY

With the advent of newer technologies and experience with shock-wave lithotripsy, ureteroscopy, and ureteroscopic ultrasonic lithotripsy, indications for ureterolithotomy will be changing. The limiting factors to the above-mentioned technologies are availability of the instruments and surgical expertise with transurethral stone dissolution. It is realistic to believe, however, that fewer open ureterolithotomies will be performed in the future.

The decision for operative intervention, or ureterolithotomy, depends on a number of factors. Alternatives to open surgery include expectant observation to see if the calculus will pass spontaneously, transurethral manipulation by means of basket extraction, or ureteroscopic ultrasonic lithotripsy or, possibly, shock-wave dissolution. As outlined by Persky and associates (1979), indications for open intervention can be divided into absolute indications and relative indications. Absolute indications include (1) the presence of a calculus with a transverse diameter greater than the width of the ureter. Although some calculi as large as 2 cm have passed, most calculi over 1 cm will hang up and not traverse the iliac vessels or ureterovesical junction; (2) a jagged or spurred calculus that will impale itself on the ureteral wall; (3) unresolving proximal hydroureteronephrosis or complete obstruction with no advance of the calculus; (4) sepsis from infection above the calculus; (5) severe symptoms that require intravenous narcotics for pain control; and (6) compromise or deterioration in renal function. Relative indications include (1) prolonged delay in progression of the calculus down the ureter; and (2) socioeconomic reasons when pain or symptoms interfere with the patient's livelihood.

As discussed earlier, the most appropriate incision for ureterolithotomy depends on the level of the calculus. For upper-third calculi, the extraperitoneal flank approach is preferred. For middle-third calculi, the approach may be extraperitoneal through a subcostal incision or a modified Gibson incision. For lower-third calculi, a midline Pfannenstiel or Gibson incision may be used. A transvaginal incision may be used for a calculus near the ureterovesical junction.

Upper Ureter

For an upper-third calculus a conventional subcostal flank incision is made. The skin, subcutaneous tissue, and external oblique, internal oblique, and transversalis muscles are incised sharply. The retroperitoneal space is entered carefully, so as not to open the peritoneum inadvertently. The ureter is gently exposed with blunt and sharp dissection, with care taken not to dislodge the calculus. After the calculus is located, a Babcock clamp is placed proximally to prevent dislodging the calculus upward. The ureter is then mobilized only enough to allow a ureterotomy directly over the calculus. The ureterotomy is made with a hook-blade knife. Fine chromic traction sutures may be placed before the ureterotomy, if desired. Whether a longitudinal or a transverse incision is used is left to the preference of the surgeon. As described by Cohen and Persky (1983), however, the chance of disrupting ureteral blood supply is less likely with a longitudinal incision than with a transverse incision, as the blood supply travels in the periureteral tissue. They also believe that the muscular sheath that composes the middle layer of the ureter tends to heal better after a longitudinal incision than it does after a transverse incision. The proponents of transverse ureterolithotomy, on the other hand, believe that there is less postoperative urinary extravasation with that incision than with the longitudinal incision.

The calculus is teased out of the ureter using the end of the knife blade or small forceps. After the calculus is removed, ureteral patency and urine flow should be established by passing an 8 F urethral catheter into the bladder and into the renal pelvis, irrigating continuously while withdrawing it. The ureterotomy may be just left open and the area drained, or, under most circumstances, several 4-0 or 5-0 chromic gut sutures may be placed to close the defect. A Penrose drain is brought out either through a stab wound or through the posterior portion of the incision. The wound is closed in appropriate layers with material of the surgeon's preference.

Calculi located around the transverse process of L3 or L4 may be removed either through a muscle-splitting incision as described by Foley (1935) or through a posterior lumbotomy approach or Gil-Vernet (1983) incision. Both these approaches offer the patient the advantages of reduced morbidity, hospital stay, and disability.

For the Foley muscle-splitting incision, the external oblique, internal oblique, and latissimus dorsi muscles are mobilized but not incised. The oblique muscles are retracted forward and the latissimus dorsi backward, exposing the lumbar fascia. The fascia is opened, the edges retracted, and the retroperitoneal space entered. The posterior layer of Gerota's fascia is separated from the posterior abdominal wall, and the ureter is located. The calculus is then extracted as described previously.

The Gil-Vernet incision is used with the patient either in the lateral position, without lumbar support, with the legs flexed to the point of maximal suppression of physiologic lordosis,

or in the prone position. A vertical incision is made 2 cm medial to the muscle mass of the lumbosacral muscles, from the twelfth rib to the posterosuperior iliac crest. The incision is carried through the posterior layer of the lumbodorsal fascia around the sacral spinalis and quadratus lumborum muscles, which are retracted medially to enter the perinephric space. A self-retaining retractor may then be placed in the wound. Gerota's fascia is entered by incising the thin layer of dorsal fascia that is the posterior extension of the transversalis fascia. With careful blunt dissection, the upper ureter is exposed and the calculus removed as previously described.

Middle Third

Calculi at L5 or in the middle ureter are approached through an appropriate level muscle-splitting incision (Gibson). The skin and subcutaneous tissues are divided and the fascia and muscles separated bluntly, parallel to the line of their fibers. The peritoneum is mobilized and retracted medially. The ureter should be easily identified clinging to the posterior peritoneum at the level of the iliac vessels. The calculus is located and isolated, and a Babcock clamp is placed above the calculus as previously described. A ureterotomy is done, the calculus extracted, and the ureteral incision closed with several 4-0 or 5-0 chromic gut sutures. After draining the wound with a Penrose drain, the wound is closed in standard fashion.

Lower Ureter

Although a lower-third ureteral calculus may be removed through a Gibson incision as described earlier, we prefer a midline approach through either a vertical incision or a Pfannenstiel incision. After incision of the rectus abdominis fascia, the peritoneum is mobilized medially and upward. The ureter is identified at the pelvic brim where it crosses the iliac vessels and is traced to the level of the calculus. A ureterotomy is made, and the calculus is extracted as already described. The ureterotomy is closed and drainage effected with a Penrose drain. The drains are left 5 to 7 days or until all drainage ceases. If calculi are present on the opposite side, the midline incision offers the advantage of simultaneous surgical correction without another incision.

For the special instance in which the calculus is impacted in or near the intramural ureter, a transvesical approach is most efficacious. The bladder is opened in the midline, a meatotomy done, and the calculus extracted either by forceps or by being milked out by means of extravesical palpation. Only under rare circumstances when a calculus might be impacted should ureteroneocystostomy be necessary. If a calculus is dislodged at any time and not easily seen or retrieved, a basket extractor or Fogarty catheter may be passed up the ureter and, with the use of intraoperative fluoroscopy, the calculus located and retrieved.

COMPLICATIONS

The most common complication following a ureterolithotomy is persistent urinary leakage. In general, if drainage persists for longer than 5 to 7 days, a retrograde study should be performed to rule out distal obstruction and an indwelling ureteral catheter passed for a period of 24 to 48 hours. Rarely will leakage continue longer; however, as is the case with intubated ureterotomies, stents and drains may be left in for a period of 6 weeks, the patient discharged, and removal done on an outpatient basis in an office setting.

Sepsis and infection may occur in any type of urologic surgery. If a specific organism has been cultured from the urine or blood preoperatively, appropriate antibiotic coverage should be employed. The judicious and appropriate use of prophylactic antibiotics, under most circumstances, will usually prevent any significant complications in this regard. Although the exact incidence of ureteral stricture and urinoma following ureterolithotomy is unknown, these complications are uncommon.

TRANSVAGINAL APPROACH TO THE URETER

One way to approach distal ureterolithotomy in the female is transvaginally. Before attempting this procedure, the calculus must be palpable. The advantages of the transvaginal approach are the following: (1) it is rapid and involves a minimum of tissue dissection and trauma; (2) it eliminates the complications of transabdominal surgery; and (3) the periods of hospitalization and recuperation are short. The disadvantages of this approach include minimal total ureteral exposure and control of the proximal ureter and the risk of a postoperative ureterovaginal fistula. If the calculus is dislodged and migrates proximally, retrieval can be diffi-

cult. Attempts at recovery can be made with a stone basket or Fogarty catheter assisted by intraoperative fluoroscopy. Since there is little tissue between the ureter and vagina, the suture lines may be in proximity. If any sort of infection, hematoma, distal obstruction, vascular compromise, or prolonged drainage occurs, the risk of a fistula is high. The use of an internal double J stent placed after the ureterotomy may help to prevent fistula formation.

TECHNIQUE

The basic technique is shown in Figure 68–5 (Persky et al., 1979). With the patient in the lithotomy position, a weighted vaginal speculum is placed deep in the vagina. The cervix is grasped with a tenaculum forceps and retracted down into the side opposite the calculus. The calculus is palpated, and an incision is made in the vaginal mucosa overlying the calculus with a No. 15 blade. The ureter is mobilized above and below the calculus with blunt and sharp dissection to allow placement of a Babcock clamp proximal to the calculus. A ureterotomy is made, the calculus is extracted, and a No. 8 red rubber catheter is passed in both directions to be sure there are no retained calculi. The incision is closed with interrupted 5-0 chromic sutures, the vagina is closed with a running 4-0 chromic catgut suture, and the area is drained. If an indwelling ureteral stent can be left, the incidence of postoperative ureterovaginal fistula can be reduced. If the stone cannot be palpated, Walsh (1984) suggests that the patient be placed

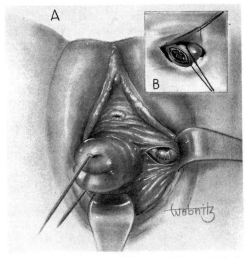

Figure 68–5. Vaginal ureterolithotomy. The cervix is drawn forward and laterally toward the opposite side. In inset *B* the ureter has been incised over the calculus after placement of a holding suture immediately above the obstruction.

in the exaggerated lithotomy position as for a radical perineal prostatectomy and the bladder filled to push the lower ureteral segment and stone down to where the stone is more easily found.

URETEROURETEROSTOMY

Ureteroureterostomy is defined as the end-to-end anastomosis of any two ureteral segments, including ipsilateral duplicated ureters. Ureteroureterostomy may be performed following resection of short fibrotic strictures due to operative injury or infection; ureteral disruption secondary to intraoperative injury; blunt or penetrating trauma; short segments of periureteral inflammation; short segments of radiation injury; obstruction or reflux in an ectopic or duplicated ureter; congenital stricture; vascular obstruction from a retrocaval ureter; or segmental resection for a localized carcinoma. The primary contraindication for ureteroureterostomy is inadequate length to assure a tension-free anastomosis. Other relative contraindications include the presence of abscess, hematoma, or urinoma; vascular compromise of the ureter from dissection or mobilization; previous ureteral injury; and previous therapeutic doses of radiation.

TECHNIQUE

To rationally discuss surgical approach, the ureter should be divided into upper-, middle-, and lower-third segments and the reason for repair divided into primary elective repair or repair at the time of exploration for another problem (operative ureteral injury). In the latter instance, repair can usually be made through the incision at hand. In the case of upper-third injury, the best approach is via the flank or twelfth rib. For middle-third exposure, a Gibson incision is appropriate, as it can be extended upward to the twelfth rib for better kidney exposure or across the midline for better exposure of the distal ureter, if necessary. The lower-third approach is best made through a midline infraumbilical incision.

The upper-third ureter or middle-third ureter should be easily located through the aforementioned incisions by dissecting posteriorly along the psoas muscle and reflecting the peritoneum medially. The ureter will come into view anteriorly attached to the peritoneum. The area of pathology is isolated, the ureter dissected free to obtain length, and the edges prepared for anastomosis. For lower-third exposure, the

midline approach is preferred. The rectus muscles are separated and the retropubic space entered by careful blunt dissection. This dissection is continued around the bladder on the side of the diseased area, exposing the ureter at the level of the iliac vessels. Exposure may be expedited by dividing the obliterated umbilical artery. Although injuries in this area are best handled by ureteroneocystostomy, often requiring a psoas hitch or Boari flap, ureteroureterostomy may be indicated in injuries more than 5 cm from the bladder. If the ureteral injury is discovered at the time of an intra-abdominal or retroperitoneal procedure, access to the ureter may be sufficient by the exposure at hand. If not, additional exposure may be obtained in one of two ways: either by reflecting the colon along its lateral gutter or by incising the posterior peritoneum medial to the inferior mesenteric artery from the ligament of Treitz to the sacral promontory.

As stated by Young (1983), once the ureteral segment is identified and exposed, various factors are evaluated to determine if ureteroureterostomy is appropriate. These include the length of the defect, previous irradiation, no previous injury, no previous surgical mobilization, no involvement by inflammation, no duplication, and the presence of an adequate blood supply. Once it is determined that there is enough length for a tension-free anastomosis, ureteral mobilization should be wide, including all periureteral tissue and the gonadal vessels. Once dissection has been performed and anastomosis deemed possible, a number of anastomotic techniques are available.

Stents can be a valuable aid to ureteroureterostomy if there is any question of viability or tension of the anastomosis. The size should be the largest caliber that loosely fits in the ureter, and the length should extend from the renal pelvis to well inside the bladder. Modern, flexible, silicone type double J catheters are ideal. Although T-tubes have been used in the past, there is little place for them today. Advantages of the T-tube are ready access for contrast studies and drainage, a decreased need for venting nephrostomy, and removal without the necessity for cystoscopy. Disadvantages are ureteral angulation when pulling the tube and prolonged drainage after removal.

Different techniques of anastomosis are shown in Figure 68–6. The ends may be spatulated and sutured obliquely as a fishmouth, with running or interrupted suture, or by Z-plasty and interrupted suture. The most commonly used anastomotic technique is spatulation with

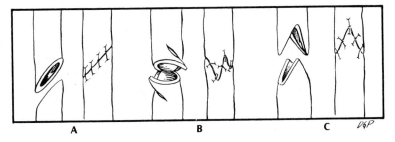

Figure 68–6. Ureteroureterostomy: techniques of anastomosis. *A*, Oblique. *B*, Z-plasty. *C*, Fishmouth. (From Young, J. D., Jr.: *In* Glenn, J. F. (Ed.): Urologic Surgery. 3rd ed. Philadelphia, J. B. Lippincott Co., 1983. Used by permission.)

sutures of 5-0 chromic placed at the right angle of each cut end into the angle of the spatulating incision on the opposing ureteral cut end. After the first suture is tied, the second and third sutures are placed 1 to 2 mm apart and tied. If a stent is used, it should be placed at this point. The remainder of the sutures are then placed and tied. Spatulation is necessary only if the ureter is less than 1 cm in diameter, to prevent narrowing or stenosis.

The goal in ureteroureterostomy is a watertight suture line with good vascular supply and no luminal compromise. Some sort of drainage is necessary. A Penrose drain, red rubber catheter, or suction catheter may be brought out through a separate stab incision or through the incision itself. As much as possible, the repair should be retroperitonealized. Drains are removed, usually, by the fifth to seventh postoperative day or when there is no evidence of any further leakage. Stents should be left in place for at least 4 weeks and removed only after appropriate postoperative healing is demonstrated on intravenous pyelography.

Ureteroureterostomy of duplicated ureters on the same side may be performed for reflux or ectopia or whenever there is one abnormal or damaged ureter and one normal ureter. This anastomosis is usually performed end-to-side with care being taken not to damage the recipient ureter (Fig. 68–7). Likewise, to assure a successful anastomosis, as little dissection as possible should be done of the recipient ureter to maintain the best possible blood supply. The incision in the recipient ureter should be parallel to its long axis and the exact length of the obliquely cut end of the donor ureter. The end-to-side anastomosis is performed with 5-0 chromic interrupted sutures, 1 to 2 mm apart. Whether or not to stent this anastomosis and use a diverting nephrostomy remains controversial. If there is a large discrepancy in size, stenting and diversion may be indicated. Of course, extraureteral drains should be placed in the same manner described earlier. The results of properly performed ureteroureterostomies

can be quite good, as reported by Carlton et al (1969, 1971). In 1969, they reported excellent results in 83 per cent in conjunction with ureteral injuries. In 1971, they reported 92 per cent satisfactory results when this technique was used in 25 patients with a watertight anastomosis.

TRANSURETERO-URETEROSTOMY

The operation transureteroureterostomy was first reported as an experimental technique by Sharpe in 1906. The first successful clinical application was by Higgins in 1934. Initial reluctance to use the procedure was based on the anastomosis of a diseased nephroureteral unit to a clinically normal unit. Since 1934, clinical experience with this technique has been considerable and results now show that there is little risk to the recipient ureter if patients are selected properly and there is strict adherence to surgical technique.

Clinically, transureteroureterostomy may be applied when it is necessary to reconstruct a lower-third or, occasionally, a middle-third defect. For the operation to succeed, there must

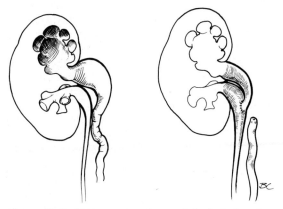

Figure 68–7. Ureteroureterostomy of duplicated ureters. The refluxing upper pole segment is sutured end-to-side to the normal lower pole segment.

be sufficient length for the ureter to cross the midline for a tension-free anastomosis to its mate on the opposite side. A gentle sweeping path without kinking is desired. The more proximal the end of the donor ureter, the more acute the sweep and the greater the possibility of mechanical obstruction. The optimal place for crossing the midline is at the level of the bifurcation of the aorta, where the ureters lie closest to one another. Contraindications to transureteroureterostomy include inadequate length to permit a tension-free anastomosis, previous dissection or ureteral mobilization, a previously injured ureter, a ureter previously exposed to therapeutic doses of radiation, ureteral or renal tuberculosis, stones in either or both kidneys, the presence of uroepithelial tumors, retroperitoneal fibrosis, chronic pyelonephritis in either kidney, or reflux of the recipient ureterovesical unit.

TECHNIQUE

Transureteroureterostomy is best performed through an anterior midline transperitoneal incision. If previous cystoscopy and passage of ureteral catheters were possible, localization and dissection of the ureter may be facilitated; in most situations, however, they are not needed. The area where the two ureters are closest together is above the bifurcation of the aorta; therefore, the diseased area should be well enough away from the pelvic brim to allow the donor ureter to cross the spine without tension.

The intestines are reflected upward and packed out of the way. Each ureter is identified and the overlying posterior peritoneum incised for a length of several centimeters. The donor ureter is freed from its area of involvement proximally and transected, and the distal end is ligated with a 0 or 2-0 chromic catgut ligature. The proximal end of the ureter may then be tagged with a fine chromic suture to facilitate later manipulation and traction when the ureter is drawn to the opposite side. The area of the recipient ureter for anastomosis is isolated with minimal mobilization in an attempt to preserve as much blood supply as possible.

After the donor ureter is sufficiently free proximally to allow a gentle sweep across the retroperitoneal space, a tunnel beneath the sigmoid and preferably above the inferior mesenteric artery is created bluntly. If the inferior mesenteric artery is a barrier to mobilization, it may be divided provided that the remainder of the left colon vascular supply is intact. The suture on the donor ureter is grasped, and using gentle tension, the ureter is drawn through the

tunnel to the opposite side, with care taken to avoid any inadvertent rotation.

The donor ureter is spatulated to a length of about 1.5 cm. An incision, just as long, is made on the anteromedial surface of the recipient ureter. The anastomosis is performed with interrupted 4-0 or 5-0 chromic catgut sutures placed approximately 2 mm apart. The first suture is placed from the apex of the spatulated ureter to the proximal apex of the ureterostomy in the recipient ureter, with the knot tied extraluminally. The remaining sutures are then placed in the posterior and anterior walls in a stepwise fashion (Fig. 68–8). Continuous sutures can be used on the posterior and anterior walls without any untoward problems. The area should be drained extraperitoneally through a stab wound, preferably with a Penrose drain. The posterior peritoneal incision is then reapproximated with 3-0 chromic catgut sutures and the incision closed according to the surgeon's preference.

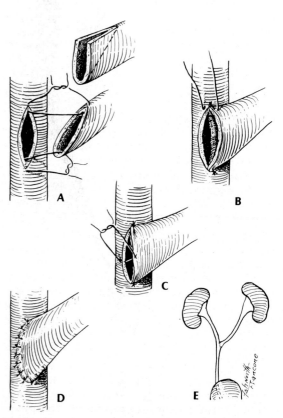

Figure 68–8. Transureteroureterostomy. The ureteroureteral anastomosis is done end-to-side using a running layer of 4-0 chromic catgut suture for the posterior layer. The anterior layer is approximated with interrupted sutures of the same material. (From Young, J. D., Jr.: *In* Glenn, J. F. (Ed.): Urologic Surgery. Philadelphia, J. B. Lippincott Co., 1983. Used by permission.)

Stenting the anastomosis is optional but should not be required in a technically well-performed anastomosis in which the ureters are well vascularized. If stenting is desired, 5 F or 6 F Silastic tubing, pediatric feeding tubes, or soft double J catheters may be employed. One end of the stent should lie in the donor renal pelvis and traverse the recipient ureter into the bladder. If the recipient ureter is large enough, a second stent may be passed from the recipient renal pelvis into the bladder. If necessary, the catheters could be brought out through a stab wound in the normal proximal recipient ureter; however, this would seldom be necessary. Drains should remain until all leakage has stopped. Stents can remain for an indeterminate time if they are indwelling and not obstructed. After a pyelogram shows no leakage or obstruction, the stents may be removed cystoscopically.

RESULTS

In general, reports by authors using transureteroureterostomy have been favorable, with mention of few complications (Van Arsdalen and Hackler, 1983; Hendren and Hensler, 1980; Udall et al., 1973; Schmitt et al., 1972; Hodges et al., 1980; Brannan, 1975). Ehrlich and Skinner (1975), on the other hand, reported six cases of severe complications. Four patients had damage to the recipient unit, necessitating ileal substitution in two; one had persistent mild ureteral stricture, and one required an extensive vesicopsoas hitch. Three donor kidneys required subsequent nephrectomy. Sandoz and associates (1977) reported on 4 patients out of 23 who had injuries to the recipient ureter. Of these, three eventually had good results after reoperation, and one died secondary to operative complications.

On the other hand, good results from transureteroureterostomy have been reported in over 400 cases (Hodges et al., 1980). Udall et al. (1973) reported good results in 61 of 67 patients. Of the six patients who had unsatisfactory results, three required cutaneous diversion secondary to reflux, one developed stenosis of the diseased donor ureter at the anastomosis site, one developed tumor obstruction of both ureters at the anastomosis site, and one had progression of pre-existing pyelonephritis leading to donor nephrectomy. Brannan (1975) reported on 17 patients with no complications or renal deterioration. Hendren and Hensle (1980) reported on 112 patients, mostly children, who underwent transureteroureterostomy for reflux or undiversion. There were no deaths, leaks, or nephrectomies in their series; however, three patients did require reoperation for technical mistakes.

Hodges and associates (1980) also have reported on 25 years' experience with 100 transureteroureterostomies done primarily for ureteral stricture, injury, or lower ureteral tumors. There were two deaths secondary to myocardial infarction, and one patient died of mycotic sepsis. A total of 23 complications were reported. Three of these involved the recipient ureter and were secondary to the development of tumor and subsequent obstruction at the anastomotic site. The investigators believed that these could have been prevented by the use of frozen sections at the time of surgery. There was one anastomotic leak subsequently leading to nephrectomy, two nephrectomies secondary to persistent pyelonephritis, and two patients who required reoperation for the inferior mesenteric artery syndrome. Hodges and Coworkers did report 97 per cent success with no damage to the recipient ureter, and 92 per cent of the patients had excellent results of both renal units.

In summary, transureteroureterostomy is a successful procedure with a low complication rate if strict attention is paid to technique and proper patient selection. Every urologic surgeon should be familiar with this procedure and be able to use it when the situation dictates.

INTUBATED URETEROTOMY

The Davis intubated ureterotomy arose from the classic work of Davis, reported in 1943. Since then, ureteral physiology, the process of ureteral healing, ureteral regeneration, and ureteral reconstruction have been the subjects of numerous reports (Boyarsky and Duque, 1955; Hinman, 1957; Lapides and Caffrey, 1955; Persky and Carlton; 1972; Weinberg, 1967; Weinberg et al., 1960). Basically, uroepithelial outgrowth to cover a ureteral defect occurs in 4 to 7 days. This is followed by slower ingrowth of muscular tissue into the granulation tissue covering the defect. For this type of regeneration or healing to occur, there must be normal uroepithelial mucosa present without abnormal folds, pockets, or diverticula. The lumen must be patent and distensible and offer a low resistance such that the flow of urine is unimpeded from the renal pelvis to the bladder. Likewise, the surrounding muscularis must show normal amounts of smooth muscle bundles with appropriate vascular and nerve supply. The surrounding adventitia should also be free of inflammation, foreign bodies, necrotic debris, and periureteral adhesions. If not, the healing process may be incomplete and normal ureteral

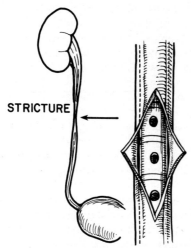

Figure 68–9. For the intubated ureterotomy, the ureteral defect is left to close spontaneously around a catheter.

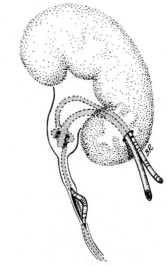

Figure 68–10. Pyelotomy for placement of nephrostomy tube and splint.

architecture may not be formed. Under these circumstances, false passages, diverticula, and stricture formation can occur. With the addition of periureteral fatty coverage, adherence to surrounding muscle may be prevented as well as fixation, angulation, traction, and dense encapsulation.

TECHNIQUE

The primary indications for intubated ureterotomy are a long, strictured ureteral segment or long ureteral gap that is not amenable to conventional repair. This technique is readily applicable to strictures of the ureter as long as 10 to 12 cm. After the ureter is exposed and the involved segment isolated, a longitudinal ureterotomy is performed through the desired area, with care being taken not to spiral the incision (Fig. 68–9). A posterior incision has been advocated by some authors (Persky, 1967; Persky et al., 1979; Smart, 1961) as the better approach. After the ureterotomy has been performed, the stent is chosen and placed. The stent catheter may be a multi-eyed Silastic or a polyethelene double J, running from the renal pelvis to the bladder; or polyethelene tubing, which bridges the defect and is brought out with a nephrostomy tube (Fig. 68–10). All intubated ureterotomies should have proximal urinary diversion by means of a nephrostomy. To assure optimal healing, the stent and ureter should be in close proximity. This can be achieved by wrapping the ureter with fat or omentum. Drainage of the periureteral and renal bed area is accomplished by Penrose drains.

Postoperatively, the drains are left until drainage subsides and the stent should be left for a minimum of 6 to 8 weeks. To assure healing, a nephrostogram is performed before the stent is removed. When healing is deemed satisfactory, the nephrostomy may be removed. Long-term follow-up should include repeated urinalysis and pyelograms at appropriate intervals.

RENAL DECENSUS

The addition of renal decensus to the techniques of ureteral surgery was originally made by Popescui in 1964 for the management of the pelvic ureter in postsurgical ureterovaginal fistula. This maneuver, however, can be applied whenever extra ureteral length is needed to bridge a gap or to relieve tension on a ureteral anastomosis.

TECHNIQUE

Through a transperitoneal approach, the colon on the affected side is reflected medially from the colonic flexure to the level of the diseased ureteral area in the pelvis. Gerota's fascia is incised anteriorly and, using blunt and sharp dissection, the kidney is completely mobilized. After the kidney is completely free, the vessels and the proximal ureter are displaced downward and inward by pressure exerted on the upper pole to define the suture placement. With constant pressure holding the kidney in this position, the lower pole is fixed to the iliac fossa with three or four 2-0 chromic catgut sutures (Fig. 68–11). The redundant ureter is

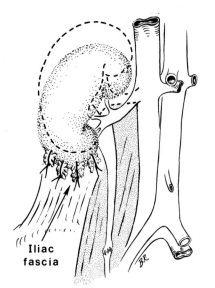

Figure 68–11. Suture placement in renal descensus.

freed from the peritoneum with care to preserve as much periureteral tissue as possible in order to decrease the possibility of postoperative vascular injury. After primary ureteral repair, the peritoneum is reapproximated and the retroperitoneum drained. As much as an 8-cm section of ureter may be replaced with this technique.

PSOAS HITCH

Trauma to the distal 3 to 5 cm of ureter is not uncommon. Even when the injury is discovered immediately, the technical problems of repairing a ureter deep in the pelvis have prompted most urologists to employ some form of ureteral reimplantation procedure. The anastomosis should be as near the trigone as possible. It is well understood that an essential part of a successful operation to prevent reflux is fixation of the ureter to the trigone with adequate ureteral backing. Paquin, in 1959, mentioned the use of the bladder hitch procedure to reduce anastomotic tension. This procedure was popularized in the United States by Harrow (1968) and in Europe by Turner-Warwick and Worth (1969), who gave it its name. The technique itself is simple and is based on the fact that distortion of the bladder does not usually interfere with function and will gain the surgeon between 3 and 5 cm of additional length. The relative contraindications for this procedure are a contracted scarred bladder or previous pelvic surgery in which the blood supply to the bladder was compromised.

It is essential, prior to attempting this adjunctive technique, to ensure that there is sufficient mobility of the bladder. This can be assessed by means of a preoperative cystogram. If this luxury is not available to the surgeon, passage of a Van Buren sound intraoperatively and "tenting" of the appropriate wing will facilitate the decision as to whether a hitch is possible. This becomes particularly important if the surgeon intends a concomitant flap procedure, because the base of the flap and its blood supply should not be compromised by the immobilizing sutures. Additional mobility of the bladder can be obtained (at the discretion of the surgeon) by mobilizing the contralateral bladder pedicle after division of all the umbilical ligaments.

TECHNIQUE

The lateral walls of the bladder are mobilized and the peritoneum stripped from the dome and the posterior wall. Through a small and appropriately placed vesicotomy the index finger is inserted, directing a bladder horn toward the proximal ureter. Some surgeons anchor the bladder at this point, while others create the submucosal tunnel and then anchor the bladder. Ideally, the bladder is sutured to the tendon of the psoas minor muscle with several 2-0 chromic catgut sutures (Fig. 68–12). Frequently, this tendon is absent, and in this case it is important to ensure that large bites of

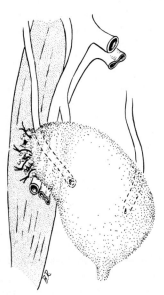

Figure 68–12. Suture placement in psoas bladder hitch.

the muscle are taken with the suture, being careful to avoid the genitofemoral nerve. Once the bladder has been fixed to the psoas muscle above the iliac vessels, the ureter can be reimplanted, either by an antireflux anastomosis with a submucosal tunnel or by direct anastomosis if adequate length is not present. The anterior vesicostomy should be closed in two layers, utilizing a submucosal layer and a burying muscular closure. Ureteral stents may be left at the discretion of the surgeon. Prout and Koontz (1970) pointed out that occasionally it is possible to fix the bladder to the lateral pelvic wall. They also observed that a hitch will often produce enough trigonal movement to allow reimplantation directly. It is very important to be sure that no kinking of the ureter is occasioned by this hitch maneuver. This procedure is quite satisfactory for short defects, and it has gained popularity by allowing tension-free anastomoses in the operation of ureteroneocystostomy (Middleton, 1980).

RESULTS

The technique is excellent in many surgeons' hands, and indeed the psoas hitch has generally replaced the Boari bladder flap procedure for bridging gaps in the lower one third of the ureter.

BLADDER FLAP PROCEDURE

The use of a bladder tube to bridge large ureteral defects in dogs was successfully demonstrated in 1894 by Boari (Spies et al., 1933). It was not until 1947, when Ockerblad reported his 10-year follow-up of the bladder flap technique to bridge defects of 10 to 15 cm on a single patient, that this technique assumed its present popularity (Ockerblad and Carlson, 1939; Ockerblad, 1947). This standard urologic procedure has been modified in many ways, yet the underlying principle of creating a pedicle tube graft from the bladder to bridge the defect has stood the test of time. Thompson and his colleagues have reported excellent results in the long-term follow-up of patients who have undergone this surgery and thus reinforced the confidence of most surgeons in this maneuver (Thompson and Ross, 1974). This technique has come under question recently because of the introduction of tailoring techniques of the bowel with direct reimplantation to the bladder. It is essential for a surgeon to understand that attention to the minute details of the operation are important and that a tension-free anastomosis

is absolutely essential. Major controversy exists as to the use of stents, and certain authors feel urinary diversion should be done prior to the construction of the tube. It is important to remember that a successful result also depends upon adequate vascular supply to the vesical pedicle and the ureter. Principles of plastic surgery usually require graft length-to-width ratio of 3:2; however, the surgeon should carefully identify the superior vesical artery or one of its major branches and base the pedicle upon this. Many surgeons also forget that the tubularized flap is, in essence, an artificially created diverticulum of the bladder and has no functional activity as a tube, so that the opening must always be wide-mouthed to drain satisfactorily.

TECHNIQUE

The bladder flap operation can be performed through a variety of incisions, using whichever is appropriate to approach and resect the distal and damaged ureter. Once this diseased ureter has been resected back to normal tissue, implantation can be undertaken. The bladder should be fully mobilized, particularly on its lateral and medial-posterior aspects. This always involves dividing all of the umbilical ligaments so that bladder mobility is maximal. It is helpful to distend the bladder with normal saline, following which the previously placed Foley catheter is clamped. A bladder flap is created from the posterior wall with a base of at least 4 cm and an apex of approximately 3 cm. This trapezoid-shaped pedicle should be marked and supported with sutures and then based upon the superior vesical artery or one of its major branches. Under most circumstances, up to 12 cm of bladder tube can be created in this manner. If increased length is required, a spiral flap placed across the anterior surface of the bladder may be helpful (Fig. 68–13). The flap should be handled mainly by means of supporting stay sutures and not with instruments. Minimal trauma should occur, since edema of the bladder mucosa may lead to partial obstruction during the postoperative period. The vesical flap should be closed with interrupted sutures of 0 or 2-0 chromic catgut. The ureter may then be sutured to the end of the flap or tunneled submucosally as an antirefluxing anastomosis (Scott, 1962). This antireflux anastomosis should not be established at the sacrifice of a tension-free suture line. Stents are probably best avoided. However, if there is fear of inadequate primary healing, particularly with (1) infection, (2) tension at the anastomosis, (3) ureteral fibrosis, (4) ischemia, or (5) poor func-

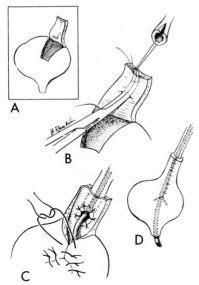

Figure 68–13. Bladder flap procedure for ureteral replacement.

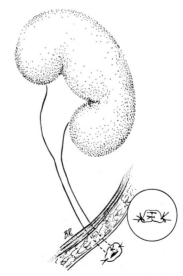

Figure 68–14. Cutaneous ureterostomy with a single stoma.

tion (dilation) of the proximal ureter, it might be wise to leave stents for at least 12 to 14 days. Adequate drainage of the anastomosis and closure site must be maintained for at least 5 days postoperatively. Use of a suprapubic catheter is left to the surgeon's discretion.

RESULTS

As mentioned earlier, Thompson and Ross (1974) followed a series of 23 patients for up to 14 years after completion of a bladder flap procedure. All patients were documented to have reflux postoperatively. Twenty of these patients had sterile urine. There was no deterioration of renal function specifically referable to the bladder flap procedure.

CUTANEOUS URETEROSTOMY

Cutaneous ureterostomy was the common form of urinary diversion until the 1950's, when the Bricker conduit was introduced. The main advantages of this procedure are that it is simple and speedy and there are no complex intestinal anastomoses to worry about. If both ureters have to be brought to the skin, they ideally should come to a single stoma (Fig. 68–14).

The various forms of temporary ureterostomies, most frequently used in children, are discussed elsewhere. There are three major disadvantages to cutaneous ureterostomy, and these should always be in the mind of the surgeon who undertakes such a procedure.

1. *The problem of two stomas.* Many techniques have been advanced to try to surmount this problem. Swenson and Smyth (1959) described a double-barreled stoma placed in an infraumbilical position over which a single appliance could be worn. Straffon and his colleagues (1969) described several methods whereby both ureters could be joined on their medial borders and combined with a Z-plasty technique. The skin is interposed to prevent stenosis of the stoma. The technique of transureteroureterostomy and end-cutaneous ureterostomy has been advocated by Young and Aledia (1966). These investigators also made the very useful suggestion that the ureter and the ovarian (or spermatic) vessel be mobilized as a single unit. These modified procedures may solve the problem in selected patients but, unfortunately, are not applicable to all.

2. *The problem of stricture formation.* The very poor ureteral blood supply frequently leads to a distal ureteral slough, recession of the stoma, or stomal stricture. These events are primarily responsible for the major complications seen with this diversionary procedure. The very large number of technical modifications designed to enhance ureteral blood supply speak to the importance of these complications. Some examples of these are internal and external splinting, pedicle grafts, and omental wraps; none, however, has gained wide acceptance. Some authors have had remarkable success with skin flaps, and others find that they only make the problem worse. Stomal stricture remains a significant risk of cutaneous ureterostomy, especially when the ureters are essentially normal

at the time of the operation. It is advisable in this situation to seek other methods of diversion.

3. *Problems of urinary collection.* The advent of the enterostomal therapist certainly has made handling of the collection device and patient educational support simple matters. It is very important, however, that the surgeon and the therapist pay particular attention to the placement of the stoma. The site of the stoma should be assessed in the sitting, standing, and lying positions. The body habitus of the patient and the avoidance of skin creases play a significant role in planning the site of the stoma. It is also important to make sure that the muscular backing of the stoma is able to support the filled collection device. Thus, the ideal site is at or on the lateral border of the rectus muscle, about one third of the way down a line from the umbilicus to the anterior superior iliac spine.

TECHNIQUE

The ureters may be approached through the peritoneum or extraperitoneally, depending upon the circumstances of the cutaneous diversion. In the transperitoneal technique, the posterior parietal peritoneum overlying the right ureter is opened, usually at the level of the iliac vessels. The ureter is then mobilized very carefully down, as far as is feasible, toward the bladder. During the mobilization, it is essential that the periureteral tissue be preserved and that no cautery be used. Prior to transection of the ureter, a stay suture should be placed on the ureter so as to facilitate mobilization and allow handling of the ureter; it also serves to identify anterior and posterior relationships, thus preventing twisting of the ureter when it is brought out through the abdominal tissues. The ureter should be mobilized in a cranial direction as far as is necessary to make sure that there is a smooth, gentle curve of the ureter to reach the skin with a protrusion of at least 2 cm without tension.

Transperitoneal mobilization of the left ureter is always best accomplished by mobilization lateral to the sigmoid colon. In the obese individual, ureteral length may become a particular problem, such that certain authors have suggested that the ureter be brought transperitoneally. Clinical experience with transperitoneal cutaneous ureterostomy is very small, and it is difficult to provide an assessment of its ultimate role. Ideally, the site for the emergence of the ureteral stoma has been selected and marked by an intradermal injection of methylene blue by the stoma therapist prior to surgery; however, if this has not been done, the site should be selected so that the patient will be

able to easily see and manage the stoma in a position below the belt line.

Once the stomal site has been selected and an incision made, a very liberal opening must be made in the muscle and fascial layers, using a cruciate incision with excision of the fascial components. Very careful attention must be paid to preventing angulation or rotation of the ureter, because the shuttering effect of various muscle layers can compromise the ureteral blood supply. It must be stressed that the opening in the abdominal wall should be generous, i.e. wide enough to admit at least the finger of the operating surgeon. The distal 1 cm of ureter is then spatulated and a "U" flap of skin sewn into the spatulated area, using four to six interrupted sutures of 4-0 chromic catgut (or equivalent Dexon). Some authors suggest that the ureter should also be fixed to the internal oblique. It is our feeling that this is unwise and may result in compromise of the blood supply.

Temporary catheter drainage of the cutaneous ureterostomy is a matter of individual preference. We prefer to use a small indwelling catheter that in no way occludes the ureter. It probably should be left indwelling for the first 7 to 10 days postoperatively. An excessively large catheter will lead to large abrasion or necrosis of the ureteral wall and must be avoided. This preference for catheter drainage is based upon the unpredictable ultimate success of the ureterocutaneous anastomosis and the potential difficulties and hazards that may attend catheterization that is delayed until frank evidence of terminal ureteral slough, extravasation, or obstruction appears. In this regard, all catheters have the distal end punched out so that a guide wire may be passed through, if and when a new catheter has to be placed (particularly if satisfactory union between the skin and the ureter does not occur). This splinting catheter should probably be left in place for 3 to 6 weeks. Whenever satisfactory primary union between the skin and the ureter does not occur, it is almost a foregone conclusion that a stricture will develop. It is important to allow these to mature, after which attempts for surgical revision may be made. This is usually accomplished by an elliptical incision in the skin around the area, with dissection of the fibrous tract down to its junction with viable ureter, and interposition of a skin tube. Not infrequently, the Gibbons catheter has proved highly useful as a permanent catheter in the management of cutaneous ureterostomy. Certainly, it is better than the Foley balloon. The single-ended J stent probably also would be suitable, but we have only limited experience with this

RESULTS

Feminella and Lattimer (1971) reported long-term follow-up of cutaneous ureterostomies with a stomal stricture rate of 64 per cent in 70 patients. They related this stricture formation to three factors: (1) Ureters with radiographic diameters of greater than 8 mm had a lower stricture rate than normal-caliber ureters; (2) an everted stoma had a stricture rate of 56 per cent, whereas a flush stoma had a stricture rate of 92 per cent; and (3) preoperative irradiated ureters and skin predisposed to stomal stenosis. Holden and Whitmore (1981) reported on experience with 135 patients with elective bilateral cutaneous ureterostomies and found that almost two thirds of the patients developed unilateral or bilateral ureteral strictures. In those patients with strictures, the use of indwelling catheters was mandatory and was invariably associated with infection and stone formation. These investigators also reported that about one third of the patients manifested hyperchloremic acidosis, which began 6 months or more following the operation. Other investigators have not reported this finding. Despite the low operative mortality of the cutaneous ureterostomy in the patient with good renal function, the problems associated with sloughing and stricture have been sufficiently serious to lead many to abandon this procedure. It is predictable, however, that it will become more common again now that chemotherapy, which requires good renal function, is an integral part of the management of carcinoma.

References

Andrews, B. F., and Oosting, M.: Primary amyloidosis of the ureter. J. Urol., 79:929, 1958.

Boyarsky, S., and Duque, O.: Ureteral regeneration in dogs. An experimental study bearing on the Davis intubted ureterotomy. J. Urol., 73:53, 1955.

Boyarsky, S., Labay, P., and Teague, N.: Aperistaltic ureter in upper urinary tract infection—cause or effect? Urology, 12:134, 1978.

Brannan, W.: Useful applications of transureteroureterostomy in adults and children. J. Urol., 113:460, 1975.

Butcher, H. P., and Sleator, W., Jr.: The effect of ureteral anastomosis upon the conduction of peristaltic waves: An electroureterographic study. J. Urol., 75:650, 1956.

Caine, M., and Hermann, G.: The return of peristalsis in the anastomosed ureter: a cine-radiographic study. Br. J. Urol., 42:164, 1970.

Carlton, C. E., Jr., Guthrie, A. G., and Scott, R., Jr.: Surgical correction of ureteral injury. J. Trauma, 9:457, 1969.

Carlton, C. E., Jr., Scott, R., Jr., and Guthrie, A. G.: The initial management of ureteral injuries: A report of 78 cases. J. Urol., 105:335, 1971.

Cohen, J. D., and Persky, L.: Ureteral stones. Urol. Clin. North Am., 10:699, 1983.

Davis, D. M.: Intubated ureterotomy: A new operation for ureteral and ureteropelvic stricture. Surg. Gynecol. Obstet., 76:513, 1943.

Davis, D. M.: The process of ureteral repair: A recapitulation of the splinting question. J. Urol., 79:215, 1958.

Davis, R. M.: Intubated ureterotomy. J. Urol., 66:77, 1951.

Ehrlich, R. M., and Skinner, D. G.: Complications of transureteroureterostomy. J. Urol., 113:467, 1975.

Feminella, J. G., and Lattimer, J. K.: A retrospective analysis of 70 cases of cutaneous ureterostomy. J. Urol., 106:538, 1971.

Foley, F. E. B.: Management of ureteral stone. JAMA, 104:13, 1935.

Gil-Vernet, J. M.: Pyelolithotomy. In Glenn, J. F. (Ed.): Urologic Surgery. Philadelphia, J. B. Lippincott Co., 1983, pp. 159–162.

Gregory, J. G., Starkloff, E. B., Miyai, K., and Schoeubing, H. W.: Urologic complication of iliac bypass operation for morbid obesity. J. Urol., 113:521, 1975.

Hamm, F. C., and Weinberg, S. R.: Management of the severed ureter. J. Urol., 77:407, 1957.

Harrow, B. R.: A neglected maneuver for ureterovesical reimplantation following injury at gynecologic operations. J. Urol., 100:280, 1968.

Hendren, W. H., and Hensle, T. W.: Transureteroureterostomy experience with 75 cases. J. Urol., 123:826, 1980.

Higgins, C. C.: Transuretero-ureteral anastomosis: report of a case. Trans. Am. Assoc. Genitourin. Surg., 27:279, 1934.

Hinman, F., Jr.: Ureteral repair and the splint. J. Urol., 78:376, 1957.

Hodges, C. B., Barry, J. M., Fuchs, E. F., Pearse, H. D., and Tank, E. S.: Transureteroureterostomy: twenty-five year experience with 100 patients. J. Urol., 123:834, 1980.

Hofman, A. F., Thomas, P. J., Smith, L. H., and McCall, J. T.: Pathogenesis of secondary hyperoxalemia in patients with ileal resection and diarrhea. Gastroenterology, 58:960, 1970.

Holden, S., and Whitmore, W. F., Jr.: Ureteral diversion. In Bergman, H. (Ed.): The Ureter. 2nd. ed., New York, Springer-Verlag, 1981, p. 722.

Johnson, H. W., and Ankerman, G. J.: Bilateral ureteral primary amyloidosis. J. Urol., 92:275, 1964.

Kearney, G. P., Mahoney, E. M., Sciammas, F. D., et al.: Venacavography, corticosteroids and surgery in the management of idiopathic retroperitoneal fibrosis. J. Urol., 115:32, 1976.

Lapides, J., and Caffrey, E. L.: Observation on the healing of ureteral muscle: relationship to intubated ureterotomy. J. Urol., 73:47, 1955.

Makker, S. P., Tucker, A. S., Izont, R. J., Jr., and Heymann, W.: Nonobstructive hydronephrosis and hydroureter associated with peritonitis. N. Engl. J. Med., 287:535, 1972.

Middleton, R. G.: Routine use of the psoas hitch in ureteral reimplantation. J. Urol., 123:352, 1980.

Ockerblad, N. F.: Reimplantation of the ureter into the bladder by a flap method. J. Urol., 57:845, 1947.

Ockerblad, N. F., and Carlson, H. E.: Surgical treatment of ureterovaginal fistula. J. Urol., 42:263, 1939.

Ormond, J. K.: Bilateral ureteral obstruction due to envelopment and compression by an inflammatory retroperitoneal process. J. Urol., 59:1072, 1948.

Paquin, A. J., Jr.: Ureterovesical anastomosis: the description and evaluation of a technique. J. Urol., 82:573, 1959.

Persky, L.: Splinting vs. nonsplinting in ureteral surgery. In Bergman, H. (Ed.): The Ureter. New York, Harper & Row, 1967.

Persky, L., and Carlton, C. E., Jr.: Urinary diversion in ureteral repair. *In* Scott, R. (Ed.): Current Controversies in Urologic Management. Philadelphia, W. B. Saunders Co., 1972, pp. 169–173.

Persky, L., and Hoch, W. H.: Iatrogenic ureteral and vesical injuries. *In* Kerafin, L., and Kendall, A. R. (Eds.): Lewis Practice of Surgery. New York, Harper & Row, 1974.

Persky, L., Hoch, W. H., and Kursh, E. D.: Surgical management of the ureter. *In* Harrison, H. J., Gittes, R. F., Pearlmutter, A. D., Stamey, T. A., and Walsh, P. C. (Eds.): Campbell's Urology. Philadelphia, W. B. Saunders Co., 1979.

Popescui, C.: The surgical management of postoperative ureteral fistulas. Surg. Gynecol. Obstet. *119*:1079, 1964.

Prout, G. R., Jr., and Koontz, W. W., Jr.: Partial vesical immobilization: an important adjunct to ureteroneocystostomy. J. Urol., *103*:147, 1970.

Sandoz, I. L., Paull, D. P., and MacFarlane, C. A.: Complications with transureteroureterostomy. J. Urol., *117*:39, 1977.

Schmitt, J. D., Flocks, R. H., and Arduino, L.: Transureteroureterostomy in the management of distal ureteral disease. J. Urol., *108*:240, 1972.

Scott, F. B.: Submucosal flap ureteroplasty: experimental study. J. Urol., *88*:42, 1962.

Sharpe, N. W.: Transuretero-ureteral anastomosis. Ann. Surg., *44*:687, 1906.

Silber, S. J., and Thornburg, J.: The fate of non-absorbable intraureteral suture. J. Urol., *110*:40, 1973.

Smart, W. R.: An evaluation of intubated ureterotomy with a description of surgical technique. J. Urol., *85*:512, 1961.

Spies, J. W., Johnson, C. E., and Wilson, C. S.: Reconstruction of the ureter by means of bladder flaps. Proc. Soc. Exp. Biol. Med., *230*:425, 1933.

Straffon, R. A., Kyle, K., and Corvalan, J.: Techniques of cutaneous ureterostomy and results in 51 patients. Trans. Am. Assoc. Genitourin. Surg., *61*:130, 1969.

Swenson, O., and Smyth, B. T.: Aperistaltic megalureter: treatment by bilateral cutaneous ureterostomy using a new technique. Preliminary communication. J. Urol., *82*:62, 1959.

Thompson, I. M., and Ross, G., Jr.: Long-term results of bladder-flap repair of ureteral injuries. J. Urol., *3*:483, 1974.

Tresidder, G. C., Blandy, J. P., and Singh, M.: Omental sleeve to prevent retroperitoneal fibrosis under the ureter. Urol. Int., *27*:144, 1972.

Turner-Warwick, R., and Worth, P. H. L.: The psoas bladder-hitch procedure for the replacement of the lower third of the ureter. Br. J. Urol., *41*:701, 1969.

Udall, D. A., Hodges, C. V., Harper, H. M., and Burns, A. B.: Transureteroureterostomy: a neglected procedure. J. Urol., *109*:817, 1973.

Van Arsdalen, K. N., and Hackler, R. H.: Transureteroureterostomy in spinal cord injury patients for persistent vesicoureteral reflux: six to fourteen year followup. J. Urol., *129*:1117, 1983.

Walsh, P. C.: Personal communication, 1984.

Weaver, R. G.: Ureteral regeneration: experimental and clinical: Part II. J. Urol., *77*:164, 1957.

Weinberg, S. R.: Injuries of the ureter. *In* Bergman, H. (Ed.): The Ureter. New York, Harper & Row, 1967, p. 355.

Weinberg, S. R., Harmon, F. C., and Berman, B.: The management and repair of lesions of the ureter and fistula. Surg. Gynecol. Obstet., *110*:575, 1960.

Weiss, R. M.: Clinical implications of ureteral physiology. A review article. J. Urol., *121*:403, 1979.

Young, J. D., Jr.: Ureteroureterostomy and transureteroureterostomy. *In* Glenn, J. F. (Ed.): Urologic Surgery. Philadelphia, J. B. Lippincott Company, 1983, pp. 427–432.

Young, J. D., and Aledia, F. T.: Further observations on flank ureterostomy and cutaneous transureteroureterostomy. J. Urol., *95*:327, 1966.

CHAPTER 69

Ureterointestinal Diversion

JEROME P. RICHIE, M.D.
DONALD G. SKINNER, M.D.

The need for a satisfactory form of urinary diversion has taxed the imagination of many urologists from the late 1800's to the present. Numerous types of supravesical urinary diversion have been described, but no one variety has received universal acceptance, and each has limitations that require the urologic surgeon to be familiar with several techniques. In this chapter, operative techniques of the more popular types of ureterointestinal diversions will be considered along with the complications and possible advantages of each.

URETEROSIGMOIDOSTOMY

Simon (1852) was probably the first to describe urinary diversion to the bowel, but the modern era of ureterointestinal diversion really began in 1911 with Coffey's description of a "tunneled" technique for implantation of the ureters into the intact colon (Coffey, 1911). Ureterosigmoidostomy remained the most popular form of urinary diversion until 1950, when Bricker (1950) described the ureteroileal cutaneous operation, and when the long-term hazards of urinary diversion into the intact colon were becoming increasingly apparent. Most of the problems of ureterosigmoidostomy relate to the ureterocolonic anastomosis, and the early techniques described by Coffey (1911) and Nesbit (1949) either allowed free reflux of fecal contents to the kidney or were associated with a high incidence of stenosis and obstruction. Leadbetter's description of a combined technique that created a submucosal tunnel with a direct mucosa-to-mucosa ureterocolonic anastomosis (Leadbetter, 1950) was reported at the

same time that Ferris and Odel (1950) described the serious problem of electrolyte imbalance affecting many of these patients. Other authors were also reporting serious long-term complications with the older techniques of ureterosigmoidostomy (Harvard and Thompson, 1951; Whisenand and Moore, 1951; Zincke and Segura, 1975). Most surgeons, weary of the problems of ureterosigmoidostomy, abandoned the procedure in favor of Bricker's operation. Subsequently, Goodwin and associates (1953) described a transcolonic technique similar to Politano and Leadbetter's operation (1958) for preventing reflux with ureteroneocystostomy. A comparison of Leadbetter's combined technique with Goodwin's technique reveals similar success in reducing the incidence of pyelonephritis. Both are based on the principle of creating a long submucosal tunnel (Ridlon, 1963). It would appear that one of these techniques should be used whenever ureterosigmoidostomy is contemplated (Woodruff et al., 1952; Wear and Barquin, 1973; Zincke and Segura, 1975).

Combined Technique

Bowel preparation is employed as described later in this chapter under Ileal Conduit Diversion, except that neomycin retention enemas are given the night before surgery and again early on the morning of surgery (200 ml of 1 per cent neomycin solution). Cystectomy is done first when performed in conjunction with ureterosigmoidostomy. During cystectomy, it is helpful to place a large hemoclip on the end of the proximal ureter. This allows the ureter to dilate, facilitating ureterocolonic anastomosis.

Some surgeons prefer to pass ureteral catheters, but we have seen considerable ureteral spasm from this and believe there is real advantage to hydrostatic ureteral dilatation as well as to minimal manipulation of the ureters by catheters.

The operative technique has been described in detail (Leadbetter, 1950; Woodruff et al., 1952; Leadbetter and Clarke, 1954) and is illustrated in Figure 69–1. The important parts of the operation involve creating the submucosal tunnel, bringing the left ureter through the sigmoid mesentery without angulation or tension, and making certain that obstruction does not occur as a result of closing the proximal end of the tunnel too tightly over the ureter.

The procedure usually begins on the left side. If cystectomy has not been performed, the retroperitoneum is incised lateral to the sigmoid colon at the pelvic rim. The left ureter is exposed, mobilized, and divided between large hemoclips. It is freed proximally to a point behind the sigmoid mesentery, where a small transverse incision is made. The end of the ureter is pulled through the mesentery, and one should make certain that it is not twisted and that angulation from adhesive retroperitoneal bands does not occur. Leadbetter stressed that it was better to bring the left ureter through the sigmoid mesentery and to implant it in the anterior tenia rather than to implant it laterally in the posterior tenia (Leadbetter and Clarke, 1954).

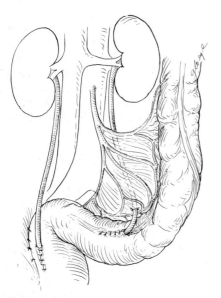

Figure 69–1. Leadbetter's combined technique of ureterosigmoidostomy. Note that the left ureter is brought through the sigmoid mesentery and implanted on the anterior tenia. The rectosigmoid is fixed to the lateral pelvic wall or psoas muscle in the region of the right ureterocolonic anastomosis.

The ureter is then allowed to lie, without tension, along the anterior tenia to allow the surgeon to determine the location for creation of the submucosal tunnel. Marking sutures of 4–0 silk are then placed in the tenia, approximately 4 cm apart, to determine the length of the desired tunnel. (A technique of creating the submucosal tunnel in the tenia is described later in this chapter under Sigmoid Conduit Diversion and is illustrated in Fig. 69–11.) One then prepares the end of the ureter by incising it obliquely, spatulating the medial margin with fine scissors, and placing a marking suture through the most distal lateral margin of the ureter (illustrated in Fig. 69–7). A small circular opening in the colonic mucosa is made approximately 0.5 cm proximal to the distal extent of the tunnel. One can best perform this by picking up the mucosa and snipping out a small circular piece with fine curved scissors (see Fig. 69–11).

A careful, precise mucosa-to-mucosa anastomosis is then performed with interrupted 4–0 Dexon sutures beginning at the proximal apex of the ureteral spatulation. Meticulous care is taken not to handle the ureter with forceps nor to strip the adventitia of the ureter. The authors do not use a stent in this ureterocolonic anastomosis.

The muscularis is then closed over the ureter, beginning approximately 1 cm distal to the beginning or proximal portion of the incision in the tenia. Interrupted 4–0 silk sutures are used, and care is taken not to incorporate any of the ureter with the sutures. After the muscularis has been closed, it is important to make certain that the ureter is not obstructed proximally. A right-angle clamp should pass easily along the ureter; if it does not, the first suture should be removed (see Fig. 69–12). It is unnecessary to anchor the ureter to the bowel, inasmuch as this may result in a ureteral fistula.

The right ureter is implanted by the same technique, except that it remains lateral to the colon and does not have to be brought through to the sigmoid mesentery. The site for anastomosis is chosen where the sigmoid lies adjacent to the proximal end of the divided right ureter. It is important to fix the colon to the retroperitoneum of the pelvic wall or psoas muscle at this point before anastomosis to prevent angulation of or tension on the ureterocolic anastomosis.

After the right ureterocolonic anastomosis is completed, the sigmoid is fixed to the retroperitoneum between the two anastomotic sites to immobilize the sigmoid and prevent small bowel herniation behind the bowel or its mesentery.

Two large rectal tubes with numerous perforations are passed through the anus at the conclusion of the procedure and sutured to the perineum. These remain in place approximately 7 days. A routine intravenous pyelogram is obtained prior to discharge for use as a baseline in later studies.

Transcolonic Technique

In this procedure, the lower rectosigmoid is opened through a 6- to 8-cm vertical incision in its antimesenteric border. A 0.5-cm transverse incision is made in the mucosa of the posterior bowel wall at the site determined for ureteral anastomosis. A 2.5- to 3.0-cm submucosal tunnel is then created with the curved scissors or a hemostat in a superior lateral direction. Once the desired length of tunnel has been created, the instrument is pushed down through the muscularis, with care taken to avoid injuring mesenteric blood vessels. The ipsilateral ureter is then brought through the tunnel, and the procedure is repeated on the contralateral side (Fig. 69–2). It is easier to bring both ureters into the bowel before beginning the mucosal anastomosis; care must be taken not to twist the ureter and to make sure that it is not angulated where it enters the bowel muscularis.

Goodwin (1976) prefers to suture the medial border of the ureters together and then anastomose the mucosa of the bowel to the joined ureters circumferentially, using interrupted fine chromic catgut. There must be no tension on the ureter, and a small stenting catheter should pass easily up both ureters without obstruction. The stents are carefully positioned, irrigated, and secured to the mucosa of the bowel with a fine chromic suture. They are then passed out the anus, and two rectal tubes with multiple perforations are placed and are secured to the perineum.

The bowel is then closed with a running chromic suture to the mucosa and with a second layer of interrupted 4–0 silk muscular inverting sutures. Drains are not used.

It is important that submucosal tunnels of adequate length are created. The principles and technique of the operation are very similar to those described by Politano and Leadbetter for ureteroneocystostomy. A film illustrating Goodwin's technique is available from the American College of Surgeons Film Library and the Eaton Laboratories Medical Film Library (1975).

The ureteral stents usually fall out by the seventh day, and the rectal tubes are removed on the eighth postoperative day. If the stents do not drain well, they are best removed, but the rectal tubes should remain at least 7 to 8 days.

Complications of Ureterosigmoidostomy

EARLY

The most feared early complication of ureterosigmoidostomy is anuria, usually secondary

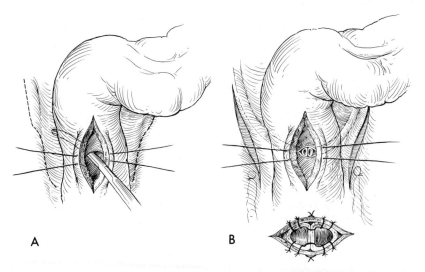

A   B

Figure 69–2. Goodwin's transcolonic technique of ureterosigmoidostomy. Note that both ureters are brought through individual submucosal tunnels in the posterior rectal wall *(A)*. The ureters are then sewn together medially before they are secured to the colonic mucosa circumferentially *(B)*. (Redrawn with permission from Goodwin, W. E.: Surg. Gynecol. Obstet., 97:296, 1953.)

to edema or obstruction of the rectal tubes by fecal matter or mucous plugs. The use of two rectal tubes with multiple perforations will generally eliminate this problem, and patency of the tubes can be assured by irrigation with 20 to 30 ml of saline. Anuria secondary to obstruction of the stents can be alleviated by removal of the stents. If anuria continues after these measures, intravenous pyelography should be performed to search for a urinary leak.

The most distressing complication is leakage of urine from the ureterocolonic anastomosis or from the colotomy suture line. Abdominal distention with ileus, increasing blood urea nitrogen out of proportion to the serum creatinine, and poor urinary output signify such a complication. Small leaks will usually seal without intervention; however, evidence of a major leak calls for immediate reoperation, drainage, reanastomosis, or possibly cutaneous diversion or nephrectomy.

Pelvic abscess may be heralded by unexplained spiking fevers. Ultrasonography, or computed tomography, is valuable in diagnosing and localizing a pelvic abscess. Once the diagnosis has been confirmed, drainage should be performed through the lower abdominal incision or through a perineal stab wound. Occasionally, in the male patient, passage of a urethral catheter into the space formerly occupied by the bladder will allow adequate drainage.

LATE

Even with the use of the combined technique (Leadbetter, 1950) or the transcolonic technique (Goodwin et al., 1953), pyelonephritis continues to be a significant problem. Wear and Barquin (1973) reported an 81 per cent incidence of acute pyelonephritis in patients with ureterosigmoidostomy using the older refluxing techniques of Coffey or Nesbit as compared with a 57 per cent incidence using the combined technique of Leadbetter. All patients should receive antibacterial medications for the first 3 months after surgery, and many patients should be advised to remain on antibiotics permanently.

Ureteral obstruction at the ureterocolonic anastomotic site may occur as a late complication in 32 to 62 per cent of patients (Wear and Barquin, 1973). This condition can be minimized by use of a careful mucosa-to-mucosa anastomosis combined with minimal manipulation of the ureter at surgery.

Renal calculi may occur as a late complication and are usually associated with stasis and recurrent pyelonephritis. The incidence increases with the length of follow-up and is of the same magnitude as that observed after ileal conduit cutaneous diversion.

In 1950, Ferris and Odel described an unusual electrolyte disturbance characterized by hypokalemia, hyperchloremia, acidosis, and absorption of ammonia from the rectal bladder. About half of all patients undergoing ureterosigmoidostomy will demonstrate some degree of electrolyte abnormality, and those with poor renal function may have recurring serious difficulties. This complication results from an extended contact between urine and the colonic mucosa and can be minimized by instructing the patient to evacuate his rectum at frequent intervals during the day and at least twice at night. All patients should be placed on a low-chloride diet supplemented by sodium potassium citrate. One such supplement, Scholl's solution, is composed of 5 gm of sodium citrate and 5 gm of potassium citrate per 100 ml of water (10 per cent solution of sodium potassium citrate). The patient is instructed to take one tablespoon by mouth two to three times per day for the rest of his life.

Depletion of serum magnesium may also occur in connection with ureterosigmoidostomy and may result in strange behavior and serious changes in the patient's mental status (Goodwin, 1976).

Colonic Neoplasia

A growing awareness in recent years has been the increased incidence of colon cancer at the site of ureterosigmoidostomy, adding apprehension to patients with long-standing ureterosigmoidostomy diversion. Hammer first reported the association of ureterosigmoidostomy with tumor in 1929. In the ensuing 50 years, 45 documented cases of tumor at the site of ureterosigmoidostomy have been reported (Leadbetter et al., 1979). The majority of these have been adenocarcinoma of the colon, although four cases of transitional cell carcinoma have been reported. The average size of the lesions is 5 cm, and the earliest time of appearance has been 2 years. The mean lag period is 8.7 years in patients older than 40 and 21.4 years in patients under 40. It has been estimated that a patient with ureterosigmoidostomy has about a 5 per cent risk of developing cancer of the colon at the implant site within 6 to 50 years (Preissig et al., 1974). Experimental studies postulate that the mixing of fecal and urinary streams is associated with higher risk (Crissey et al., 1979). Follow-up should include periodic occult tests for blood in the stool and yearly colonoscopy in order to detect changes at an early time. If tumors are found, treatment should be resection of the involved segment and conversion to cutaneous diversion.

In summary, there are numerous major complications that can occur following ureterosigmoidostomy, and it would appear that only about one third of patients will be spared at least one of these at some time following this type of diversion. Because of these side effects, many urologists no longer consider doing this form of diversion, even though many patients prefer diversion without an external collecting device. Recent reports by Spence and associates (1975), Wear and Barquin (1973), and Goodwin and his colleagues (1975) appeal for greater utilization of this type of diversion and record good long-term results for the properly selected patient operated upon by a surgeon with experience in the technique.

Strict attention to patient selection is essential. It should be emphasized that the relative contraindications to this procedure include previous radiation to the pelvis, dilated upper tracts with evidence of pyelonephritis on radiographic examination, poor renal function, poor rectal sphincter tone, and less than average intelligence in the patient. If none of these contraindications is present, ureterosigmoidostomy might be considered as an alternative long-term form of urinary diversion.

URETEROENTEROCUTANEOUS DIVERSION

Although cutaneous ureteroileostomy was described as early as 1911 by Zaayer, Bricker was the first to popularize this form of cutaneous diversion (Bricker, 1950; Murphy, 1972). His report in 1950 provided a welcome alternative for the urologic surgeon weary of the complications of ureterosigmoidostomy. Thus, the "era of ureterosigmoidostomy" ended, and urologists were quick to adopt the ileal conduit form of diversion, which they thought would eliminate most problems previously encountered with diversion into the intact colon.

Unfortunately, the long-term results of ileal conduit diversion are now appearing in the literature (Schwarz and Jeffs, 1975; Sullivan et al., 1980), and it is obvious that the ideal form of supravesical diversion has not yet been developed.

In 1967, Mogg redirected attention to the colon and recommended its use as an isolated conduit, suggesting certain advantages over the ileal segment of intestine. Subsequent laboratory data tend to support his contention and are briefly discussed later in this chapter under Sigmoid Conduit Diversion. Others have reported experience with the use of jejunal conduits (Golimbu and Morales, 1973, 1975; Morales and Whitehead, 1973), the transverse colon (Schmidt et al., 1975), and the ileocecal segment (Zinman and Libertino, 1975) for diversion. Each of these is briefly discussed.

Ileal Conduit Diversion

Since 1950, the ileal conduit has been by far the most common type of supravesical urinary diversion, and there have been only a few surgical modifications of Bricker's original description, related to ureteral implantation into the ileal segment. Figure 69–3 illustrates the traditional method described by Bricker. Barzilay (1960, 1968) and Wallace have described methods of joining the two ureters and either implanting them into the side of the ileal segment (Barzilay) or sewing them to the open end of the proximal conduit (Wallace). Leadbetter felt that it was important to anchor the base of the conduit to the sacral promontory or retroperitoneum and then implant the ureters end-to-side just above the closed end of the segment (Fig. 69–4) (Parkhurst and Leadbetter, 1960). A review of Leadbetter's experience with more than 500 patients and of the authors' personal experience with more than 250 indicates that this technique works effectively and is virtually free of early technical failures.

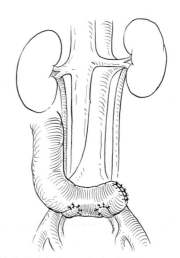

Figure 69–3. Bricker's method of ureteral placement for ileal loop cutaneous diversion.

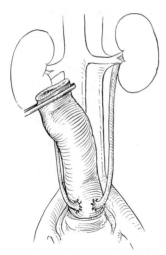

Figure 69–4. Leadbetter's technique of ileal loop diversion. Note that the base of the ileal loop is sutured to the sacral promontory or to the fibrous tissue at the aortic bifurcation. The ureters are anastomosed end-to-side, either at the same level or staggered, according to the individual's anatomic characteristics.

PATIENT PREPARATION

Unless the patient is undergoing diversion for a neurogenic bladder, a brief but efficient bowel preparation is utilized. The patient is admitted 2 days prior to surgery and started on a low-roughage diet. This is continued through breakfast the day before surgery, after which a clear liquid diet is initiated. A castor oil preparation (Neoloid, 120 ml, or castor oil, 60 ml) is given for mechanical cleansing immediately after breakfast, 24 hours before surgery, and oral neomycin (1 gm every hour for four doses, followed by 1 gm every 4 hours until midnight) and erythromycin base (1 gm every 4 hours for three doses) are administered beginning at 10 o'clock the morning before operation. Erythromycin is added to neomycin to inhibit more effectively the growth of colonic anaerobia, particularly *Bacteroides fragilis*. Neomycin retention enemas (200 ml of a 1 per cent solution) are used the night before, as well as the morning of, surgery if a colonic segment is to be incorporated or if ureterosigmoidostomy has been chosen for diversion.

Patients with neurogenic bladder and rectal sphincter spasticity are started on a low-roughage diet, oral Sulfathalidine (phthalylsulfathiazole) (2 gm four times per day), and laxatives (citrate of magnesia, 45 ml four times per day) 4 days before admission.

Adequate preoperative hydration is imperative, and intravenous volume expanders are

begun the night before operation. When diversion is to be an adjunct to radical cystectomy, a central venous catheter is placed and checked for position, and the patient is further hydrated with lactated Ringer's solution to achieve a central venous pressure between 6 and 10 cm of water. In addition, slow preoperative digitalization (1 mg digoxin) over the course of 48 hours is utilized routinely.

Preparation is not complete until a responsible physician, preferably with the aid of an enterostomal therapist, has examined the patient in the supine, sitting, and standing positions to determine the proper location for the stoma. In order to accommodate a collecting appliance, the stomal site should not impinge on any adjacent bony structures, such as the anterosuperior iliac spine or the costal margin, and should not be near any abdominal deformity such as the umbilicus, a previous surgical scar, or a crease (Fig. 69–5). The ideal site is usually just below the center of a line connecting the umbilicus with the anterosuperior iliac spine. In an obese patient or in one whose status is questionable, fitting with an appliance for several days preoperatively will ensure the best placement. An additional consideration in obese individuals is placement of the stoma at a slightly higher level than usual, because visualization is an important aspect in the proper positioning of the appliance. A preoperative scratch mark or tattoo made at the site selected for the stoma will prevent accidental erasure of ink marking during the preoperative shaving for operation.

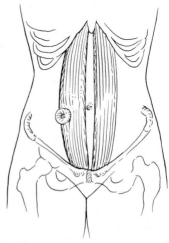

Figure 69–5. Correct placement of the stoma. The loop should be brought through the rectus muscle and the optimal placement determined before surgery with the patient placed in the supine, standing, and sitting positions. Care must be taken not to place the stoma too close to the umbilicus or bony protuberances, or in a skin fold.

OPERATIVE TECHNIQUE

A paramedian incision (above the umbilicus) converted to a lower midline incision is employed, depending on the proposed location of the stoma. The ascending colon and the terminal ileum are mobilized up to the second portion of the duodenum, thus freeing the base of the small bowel mesentery from its peritoneal attachment to the sacral promontory. The descending and sigmoid colon is then mobilized to the same level. Obstructing bands between the base of the sigmoid mesentery and the sacral promontory must be divided to allow free passage of the left ureter without obstruction. The ureters identified during the colonic mobilization are divided at a convenient level, usually several centimeters distal to the iliac vessels. Ligation of the distal end of the proximal ureteral segment with a large hemoclip allows the ureter to dilate, facilitating subsequent ureteroileal anastomosis.

In patients with carcinoma of the bladder, obtainment of frozen sections of the ureter is essential to ascertain lack of epithelial or periureteral involvement with tumor prior to implantation into the bowel segment. In patients undergoing radical cystectomy in addition to ileal loop diversion, it is usual to finish the cystectomy part of the operation first. Occasionally, it may be advantageous to isolate the ileal segment, close its proximal end, and anastomose the ureters to the ileum immediately after completing the proximal pelvic node dissection, before proceeding with the cystectomy portion of the operation. In this way, the operative team is fresh, and more careful attention can be paid to the important details of the ureteroileal anastomosis. One disadvantage of this, however, is potential harm to the conduit from overzealous retraction during subsequent cystectomy. The authors' preference is to finish the node dissection and the cystectomy and then perform the urinary diversion.

A suitable segment of distal ileum is identified and isolated, as illustrated in Figure 69–6. Traction on the terminal ileum identifies the broad pedicle containing the ileocolic artery or a suitable branch of the terminal superior mesenteric artery. Digital palpation confirms the presence of this vessel, and the avascular space between the ileocolic artery and the right colic artery is readily apparent. A similar avascular space exists between the terminal branch of the superior mesenteric artery and the ileocolic vessel. It is seldom necessary to change the operating lights to identify a satisfactory segment. The most important principle in isolation of the

segment is to make the distal mesenteric division as long as possible, extending into the base of the mesentery, and to make the proximal diversion as short as possible, thus providing a broad vascular pedicle to the segment (Fig. 69–6). The length and mobility of the segment that is to reach the skin are dependent only on the distal mesenteric division. The bowel is then divided, and the proximal end of the conduit is closed immediately with a running inverting Parker-Kerr suture of 3–0 chromic catgut in two layers. A third layer of interrupted 4–0 silk inverting serosal sutures is used for reinforcement.

A standard bowel anastomosis is then performed above the conduit; we use a two-layer interrupted 4–0 silk technique. The trap in the mesentery is then closed, and great care must be taken not to injure any of the mesenteric vessels, potentially causing a serious hematoma or even infarction of the segment.

The base of the conduit is then secured, either to the sacral promontory, to the retroperitoneal fibrous tissue in the region of the aortic bifurcation, or, in the case of a solitary kidney, to the ipsilateral muscle. An end-to-side ureteroileal anastomosis is then performed approximately 2 to 3 cm above the closed end of the loop (Fig. 69–7). The ureter should be freshly incised and spatulated medially (Fig. 69–7). A stay suture is placed to avoid trauma to the ureter by forceps, and it may be necessary to place a small hemoclip on the periadventitial blood vessel, usually present along the medial side of the ureter. It is important to make certain that the ureter has not been twisted and that the left ureter passes under the base of the sigmoid mesentery without angulation or tension. A meticulous mucosa-to-mucosa anastomosis of interrupted 4–0 Dexon sutures is performed after a small full-thickness ellipse of ileum has been excised. The anastomosis starts proximally at the apex of the spatulation along the ureter, and all knots are tied on the outside.

An important feature is the placement of the suture in the ileum. This suture should include the very edge of the mucosa but should also incorporate a large bite of muscularis and serosa (Fig. 69–7). This tends to telescope the anastomosis into the ileum and takes the tension off the mucosal portion of the anastomosis. The last three or four sutures are placed before the knots are tied, and a probe is gently passed to assure patency of the anastomosis. Stents are not used, and the anastomosis is not drained. Because radical cystectomy is performed concomitantly in many of these cases, it is usually impossible for the ureteroileal anastomosis to become retroperitoneal, and we have not seen

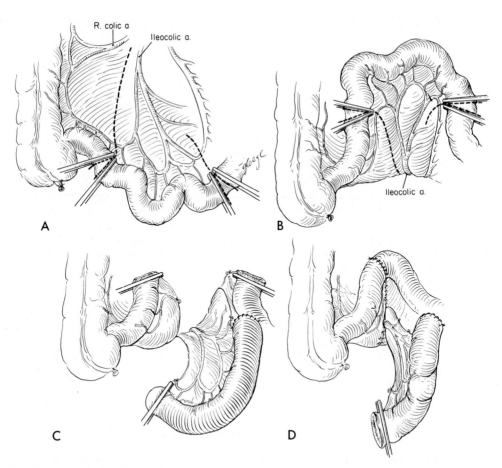

Figure 69–6. Selection of a suitable segment of ileum. Note that the distal mesenteric division should extend to the base of the mesentery, almost to the origin of the right colic artery *(A, B)*. This provides maximal mobility and sufficient length to reach the skin without being under tension. The proximal mesenteric division should be quite short to assure an adequate blood supply to the segment. The proximal end of the ileal loop is usually closed immediately following division of the bowel *(C)*; a standard bowel anastomosis is performed above the segment, and the mesenteric trap is closed *(D)*.

any problems related to this area. We do suture the base of the sigmoid mesentery above and distal to the left ureteroileal anastomosis on the ileal conduit to prevent ureteral angulation where the ureter passes under the mesentery.

There is usually a small trap left between the sigmoid mesentery, the base of the small bowel mesentery, and the base of the ileal loop. This should be closed carefully with several 4–0 interrupted silk sutures to prevent late small bowel herniation and obstruction.

PREPARATION OF THE STOMA

All layers of the abdominal wall are grasped with heavy clamps or towel clips to avoid the shifting of muscle layers during wound closure. A button of skin and subcutaneous tissue ap-

proximately the size of a quarter is excised at the predetermined location. Care must be taken not to undermine the skin edges and to make sure that the diameter of excised subcutaneous tissue is less than the diameter of excised skin. Excision of excessive subcutaneous tissue may cause recession of the stoma. A longitudinal incision is then made in the anterior rectus fascia; the rectus muscle is split; and a longitudinal incision is made in the posterior fascia and peritoneum sufficiently large to permit two fingers to be inserted in it. The segment is then brought through the opening and should protrude at least 2 inches above the skin. If this cannot be accomplished without undue tension on the conduit mesentery, a loop stoma should be created according to the method of Turnbull

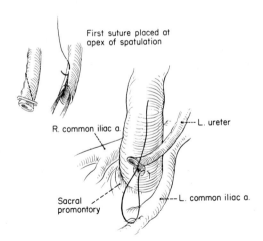

First suture placed at
apex of spatulation

R. common iliac a.

L. ureter

Sacral
promontory

L. common iliac a.

Figure 69–7. Left ureteroileal anastomosis. Note medial spatulation of the ureter with placement of the first suture at the apex of the spatulation. A traction suture should be placed through the distal lateral margin of the ureter for traction, and care must be taken not to injure the ureter by mechanical manipulation of forceps. Correct placement of the sutures in the ileum should include the lateral edge of mucosa with a generous portion of the muscularis and serosa. This essentially telescopes the ureteroileal anastomosis into the ileum and takes tension off the direct mucosa-to-mucosa anastomosis.

(1975) (Fig. 69–8). If the segment has sufficient mobility to protrude 2 inches above the skin, it should be sutured to the anterior and posterior fascia in four quadrants, with care taken not to injure the mesentery. If a loop stoma is created, Turnbull (1975) claims it is necessary to fix the loop only to the subcutaneous fascia (Scarpa's fascia). We feel, however, that if possible, the loop of ileum should be sewn to the anterior fascia with four to six interrupted sutures of 3–0 chromic catgut. This obviates the need for the use of a glass rod, as described by Turnbull—a feature that makes appliance placement difficult during the immediate postoperative period. The ileum is sutured to the skin with interrupted 3–0 Dexon sutures. These are placed through the subcuticular tissue at the cutaneous skin edge, through the seromuscular layer of the ileum at the level of the skin, and through the full thickness of the bowel at its distal edge. This will create a nipple or bud of approximately 1 inch in length (Fig. 69–9). Patients do much better if they have a protruding nipple at least 1 inch long; the results obtained by Turnbull (1975) in more than 500 stomas lend great support to the use of his loop technique, a method we have found highly successful.

Other methods of ureteroileal anastomosis

have been advocated, perhaps the most popular of which is Bricker's original technique (see Fig. 69–3). Wallace's method of joining the ureters and then anastomosing them end-to-end with the ileum may save some time, and it is particularly suitable for thick-walled dilated ureters resulting from long-term ureteral obstruction (Esho et al., 1974). This technique is least suitable for normal-sized ureters and for patients in whom diversion is done for malignancy. Severe epithelial atypia in one ureter occurs in nearly 20 per cent of the patients undergoing cystectomy for bladder cancer, and up to a third of these patients may develop subsequent malignancy in that ureter or renal pelvis. It would seem that the Wallace technique might jeopardize the contralateral collecting system in those cases in which the two ureters are sutured together.

A gastrostomy tube may be placed in patients undergoing cystectomy in addition to urinary diversion, as well as in those with neurogenic bladder (particularly paraplegic or quadriplegic patients in whom prolonged ileus is expected). Drains are not placed routinely; if a significant ooze of blood within the pelvis occurs and drainage seems desirable, large hemovacs are placed and should be removed in 48 hours. The abdominal incision is closed, and anterior retention sutures of heavy nylon are utilized in all cases in which extirpative surgery for cancer has also been performed.

Stents may be used at the discretion of the operating surgeon. In our review of 141 patients undergoing radical cystectomy, the incidence of complications was not reduced by the use of stents (Richie et al., 1975). Stents may be a source of obstruction, in which case they should be removed promptly. We have found that with a meticulous ureteroileal anastomosis, stents are not necessary, and we do not routinely utilize them for urinary diversion.

For patients who have received greater than 6500 rads of radiation therapy, it is often desirable to stage cystectomy and ileal conduit diversion. In these cases, the urinary diversion is performed through an upper transverse incision. Precise judgment must be exercised in the selection of a suitable segment of small bowel. Pale color and thickened serosa indicate significant radiation damage, and the portion of bowel with these findings should be avoided. Proximal ileum, jejunum, or even transverse colon may be preferable; the urologic surgeon should be familiar with all techniques of diversion for these patients.

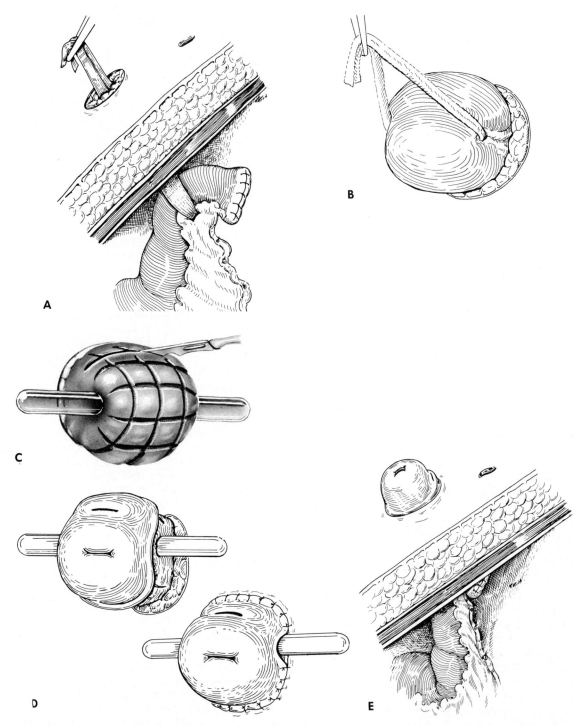

Figure 69–8. Turnbull's method of loop ileocutaneous stoma. The distal end of the segment is closed, and the most mobile portion of the ileum is brought through the rectus musle and foramen in the abdominal wall *(A)*. The loop should extend at least 2 inches in length above the level of the skin *(B)* and should be secured to the anterior rectus fascia or to Scarpa's subcutaneous fascia. Longitudinal and transverse myotomies are made with either a knife or a scissors *(C)*, and the loop is opened four fifths of the way across the nonfuntional segment at the level of the skin. The stoma is matured to the subcuticular tissue *(D)*, as illustrated in Figure 69–9. This method produces a dependent, protruding, prominent, functioning stoma and a recessive nonfunctioning loop *(E)*. (Turnbull recommends use of a glass rod for 7 days, but we feel that this inconvenience can be avoided if the loop is sutured to the anterior fascia.) (Reproduced from Dr. R. Turnbull, *In* Stewart, B. [Ed.]: Operative Urology. The Kidney, Adrenal Glands and Retroperitoneum. Baltimore, The Williams & Wilkins Co., 1975. © (1975) The Williams & Wilkins Co., Baltimore.)

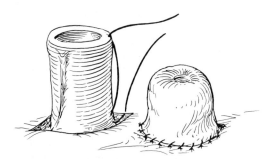

Figure 69-9. Method of stomal maturation to create a protruding "nipple" stoma. The suture should incorporate the subcuticular portion of the skin and the serosa of the loop at the level of the skin with the muscularis and mucosa of the distal end of the segment.

Ureterojejunal Cutaneous Diversion

The surgical technique of jejunal loop urinary diversion varies minimally from that described in the section on ileal conduit diversion; it should be considered for patients with severe radiation damage to the ileum (Morales and Whitehead, 1973; Golimbu and Morales, 1975). It was originally thought that the jejunum might be superior to the ileum for urinary diversion, inasmuch as early experiments suggested that jejunal segments might absorb less than ileal segments (Rangel et al., 1969). Recent studies by Clark (1974) and Golimbu and Morales (1973, 1975), however, reveal an unusual electrolyte disturbance that develops in some patients with jejunal conduits, characterized by hypochloremic acidosis, hyponatremia, hyperkalemia, and azotemia. This abnormality was seen in 11 of 25 patients and was most serious in those with poorest renal function.

Experimental data based on jejunal conduits in dogs and perfusion through isolated intestinal segments have helped explain the pathophysiology of the jejunal conduit syndrome. A two-way movement of electrolytes exists between extracellular fluid and the jejunal lumen. If the urine entering the jejunal conduit is lower in sodium chloride than the plasma, sodium and chloride will move across the intestinal mucosa into the jejunal urine to restore isotonicity. A low urinary sodium results in an outpouring of sodium chloride from the extracellular fluid and hence a low serum sodium and chloride. This diminishes the intravascular volume, reducing renal blood flow and the glomerular filtration rate. This activates the renin-angiotensin-aldosterone system to cause increased reabsorption of sodium and chloride and increased excretion of potassium in the kidney. This results in a lower urinary sodium and chloride and a higher urinary potassium to the jejunal conduit, leading to a vicious circle of increased salt loss and potassium absorption. It is essential that patients with jejunal diversion add salt to their diet (Morales and Whitehead, 1973; Golimbu and Morales, 1975). Evidence currently suggests that jejunal segments are not as good as ileal segments and that they should be reserved for use in those patients with heavily irradiated ileum.

Sigmoid Conduit Diversion

In 1967, Mogg reported on 65 patients who underwent diversion by means of an isolated ureterosigmoid cutaneous conduit, claiming good results without operative mortality. Mogg used the nipple technique described by Mathisen (1953) to prevent reflux, but either the Leadbetter combined technique or Goodwin's transcolonic technique appears to be more effective and reliable in preventing this (Richie and Skinner, 1975). Recent reports suggest that the main advantage of use of the colon rather than small bowel conduits is the ability to prevent reflux and to provide a more trouble-free stoma (Kelalis, 1974; Altwein and Hohenfellner, 1975; Hendren, 1975; Morales and Golimbu, 1975; Richie and Skinner, 1975; Scardino et al., 1975; Skinner et al., 1974, 1975).

PREPARATION

Bowel preparation is the same as that described earlier in this chapter under Ileal Conduit Diversion, except that neomycin retention enemas (200 ml of 1 per cent solution) are given the night before and the morning of surgery.

The sigmoid stoma works best on the left side, although placement on the right side is possible if previous surgery or deformities preclude satisfactory placement on the left. Barium enemas are usually obtained in advance to rule out significant bowel disease. Diverticulosis is not a contraindication to sigmoid loop diversion unless it is severe, but diversion by means of a sigmoid conduit should not be done if there is a history or evidence on radiographic examination of active inflammatory disease.

At the present time, sigmoid conduit diversion is indicated for (1) those patients with neurogenic bladder requiring cutaneous diversion whose upper tracts are normal, (2) those undergoing total pelvic exenteration for malignancy, and (3) those requiring temporary cutaneous diversion while major reversible bladder disease is being corrected. Until recently, dilated ureters were considered a contraindication to either ureterosigmoidostomy or sigmoid conduit diversion. Nevertheless, Hendren (1975, 1976) has demonstrated that dilated ureters can be tapered and implanted according to Leadbetter's combined technique. Patients with atonic ureters, however, are best managed by pyeloileocutaneous diversion or ileocecal cutaneous diversion (King and Scott, 1964; Holland et al., 1968; Markland and Kelly, 1968; Perlmutter and Tank, 1969).

OPERATIVE TECHNIQUE

A right paramedian or midline skin incision is used, and the descending and sigmoid colons are extensively mobilized from the retroperitoneum. It is important that the base of the sigmoid mesentery be freed from the sacral promontory and distal aorta up to the origin of the inferior mesenteric artery. There is usually sufficient redundancy of the sigmoid to obviate the need for mobilization of the splenic flexure.

A suitable length of sigmoid is then selected; it should be made longer than is anticipated to be necessary because it tends to contract once it is divided (Fig. 69–10). A segment 6 to 8 inches long is usually sufficient. The distal mesenteric division extends all the way to the sacrum to provide maximum mobility. This divides the superior hemorrhoidal artery and assures an excellent blood supply to the segment from the inferior mesenteric artery. Blood supply to the rectal segment is derived from the middle and inferior hemorrhoidal arteries arising from the internal pudendal branch of the hypogastric artery. Sigmoid diversion may be hazardous if performed concomitly with radical cystectomy, because ligation of the hypogastric blood vessels compromises the blood supply to the distal rectal segment. The proximal mesenteric division should be very short, and meticulous care must be taken to assure adequate venous return.

The segment is then placed laterally, and a careful end-to-end sigmoid bowel anastomosis is performed; we use interrupted 4–0 silk sutures in two layers (Fig. 69–10B).

The proximal end of the sigmoid is then closed with a two-layer Parker-Kerr suture of 3–0 chromic catgut as well as a third layer of interrupted 4–0 silk inverting serosal sutures. The mobility of the segment allows it to be brought out of the incision for the creation of the submucosal tunnels under direct vision (Fig. 69–11).

Two 4–0 silk marking sutures are then placed in each tenia, approximately 4 cm apart (Fig. 69–11). The incisions in the tenia are staggered; the incision for the right ureter begins distal to the bowel closure, and the one for the left tenia begins 2 to 3 cm distally (Fig. 69–11).

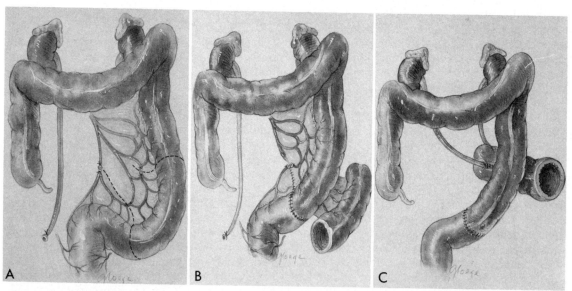

Figure 69–10. Isolation of a suitable sigmoid segment for sigmoid loop urinary diversion. Note that the distal sigmoid mesentery is divided all the way to the sacral promontory, including division of the superior hemorrhoidal artery (A). This provides maximal mobility of the loop and allows it to function in an isoperistaltic manner. Division of the proximal mesentery should be quite short, and care should be taken to avoid injury to the venous drainage from the segment. The proximal end of the isolated segment is closed, and a standard bowel anastomosis is performed medial to the isolated segment (B). The right ureter is brought under the sigmoid mesentery (C).

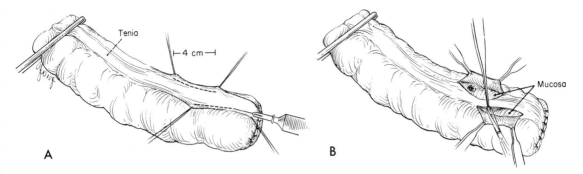

Figure 69–11. Creation of the submucosal tunnels in preparation for ureterosigmoid anastomosis. Marking sutures are placed in the tenia approximately 4 cm apart. Note that the incisions in the tenia are slightly staggered to prevent devascularization of the muscularis between the two tunnels and that the right ureter is implanted closer to the base of the segment than is the left ureter *(A)*. A solution containing 1:100,000 parts epinephrine to saline is injected beneath the muscularis to facilitate dissection. An incision is made in the tenia, and the muscularis is dissected off the mucosa. This dissection should be directed toward the mesentery and should be adequate to avoid ureteral obstruction *(B)*. A small opening in the mucosa is made approximately 1 cm proximal to the distal limits of the tunnel.

It is helpful to inject several milliliters of a 1:100,000 solution of epinephrine and saline beneath the muscularis. This reduces bleeding and facilitates development of the submucosal plane. A longitudinal incision is made in the tenia and carried down through the circular muscle fibers until the mucosa can be visualized. Blunt and sharp dissection with fine scissors, with traction placed on the muscularis by forceps, allows the submucosal plane to be developed. Dissection should be directed toward the mesenteric side to prevent devascularization of the bowel between the two tenia (Fig. 69–11). Creation of these tunnels is similar to the technique described by Leadbetter (1950) for ureterosigmoidostomy, and the entire procedure has been depicted on film by Skinner and Richie (1973), available from the American College of Surgeons Film Library and the Eaton Laboratories Medical Film Library.

If the mucosa is inadvertently entered during creation of the tunnel, closure should be done with fine Dexon sutures. These tunnels should be at least 4 cm long and should be developed sufficiently to provide ample room for the ureter, with good muscular backing.

Once the tunnels have been completed, the base of the conduit is secured to the left psoas by one suture of 4–0 silk. The right ureter is brought beneath the sigmoid mesentery without being twisted and is spatulated in the same manner described earlier in the section on Ileal Conduit Diversion.

A small elliptical section of bowel mucosa is then excised with fine forceps and scissors, immediately proximal to the distal extent of the tunnel in the right tenia (Fig. 69–11). A careful mucosa-to-mucosa anastomosis between the ureter and the bowel mucosa is then performed with interrupted 4–0 Dexon sutures.

The muscularis of the tenia is thereafter reapproximated over the ureter with interrupted 4–0 silk sutures. This closure should start approximately 1 cm distal to the proximal incision in the tenia and should not in any way obstruct the ureter (Fig. 69–12). Care must be taken not to catch the ureter during the placement of any of these sutures. Once the tenia has been reapproximated, a right-angle clamp should pass easily along the ureter where it enters the tunnel. If this passage is tight, the first suture should be replaced; otherwise, ureteral obstruction may occur.

Leadbetter and Hendren (1975) prefer to position the conduit medial to the reconstituted bowel, anchor it on the sacral promontory, and bring it out on the right side. It is our opinion that this might increase the possibility of small bowel obstruction, and that the most natural position for the conduit is on the left side. If a total pelvic exenteration is performed, however, then the conduit needs to be anchored at the sacral promontory and brought out on the right, inasmuch as permanent sigmoid colostomy is performed on the left.

CREATION OF THE STOMA

The foramen through the abdominal wall is made in the same manner as that described earlier in the section on Ileal Conduit Diversion. It is important that the opening in the skin be no more than 1.5 inches in diameter, inasmuch as colonic stomas have a tendency to be larger than ileal stomas. The colon is brought through

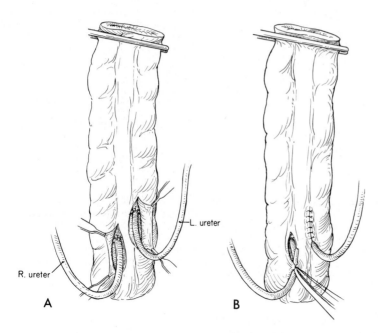

R. ureter

L. ureter

A   B

Figure 69–12. Ureterocolonic anastomosis. The base of the sigmoid loop is secured to the retroperitoneum at a location where the ureters will lie without tension and form a gentle curve into the submucosal tunnel (A). The tenia is closed over the ureter starting approximately 1 cm distal to the beginning of the proximal incision (B). Care must be taken not to obstruct the ureter with this suture. A right-angle clamp should pass easily along the ureter; if not, the suture must be replaced.

the foramen and secured to the anterior and posterior fascia with interrupted 3–0 chromic sutures. An everting nipple stoma is created with interrupted 3–0 Dexon sutures joining the cutaneous edge of the skin to the serosa of the colon at that level and to the full thickness of the distal bowel. The technique is similar to that described in the section on Ileal Conduits (see Fig. 69–9). Myotomies or loop stomas are not necessary because long-term complications from colonic stomas are unusual. It is important, however, to create protruding stomas.

Gastrostomies are performed routinely in those patients with neurogenic bladders and spastic rectal sphincters.

Ileocecal Cutaneous Diversion

Zinman and Libertino (1975) reported on 15 patients who underwent ileocecal cutaneous diversion (Fig. 69–13). Further details of surgical technique are discussed in Chapter 70. This method has certain appeal because it combines the advantage of colonic stomas with an antireflux mechanism (ileocecal valve) (Fig. 69–14) and is particularly suited to augmentation cystoplasty by the cecal segment if urinary tract reconstruction should subsequently be desirable. The authors believe, however, that the primary application of this type of diversion is in patients with dilated upper tracts, and particularly in those for whom secondary urinary tract reconstruction may be possible (Skinner, 1974). Sigmoid conduits would seem preferable to the

ileocecal segment for diversion of normal upper collecting systems because a more reliable and effective antireflux valve can be created (Hendren, 1975; Richie and Skinner, 1975; Skinner et al., 1974, 1975). Sullivan and his associates (1973) advocate employing the reversed ileocecal segment as a substitute bladder, using the cecum as a reservoir, and creating an ileal stoma (Fig. 69–15); they instruct their patients to catheterize the ileocecal segment intermittently every 4 or 6 hours during the day and once at night. An antireflux ureterocecal anastomosis is created by means of the Leadbetter combined technique. The authors report complete continence in 37 of 40 patients (94 per cent) and have 6 long-term survivors doing well 13 to 20 years following diversion (Sullivan et al., 1973).

Transverse Colon Cutaneous Diversion

Use of the transverse colon for diversion should be considered for patients who have undergone heavy pelvic radiation and who have dilated upper tracts requiring high cutaneous diversion. Schmidt and coauthors (1975) have described the technique, which has the advantage of using nonirradiated bowel, and which is best performed through a high transverse incision. A pyelocolonic anastomosis is preferable, and the authors claim no problems with stasis in the antiperistaltic segment (Schmidt et al., 1975). Only short follow-up is available. Most patients considered candidates for this proce-

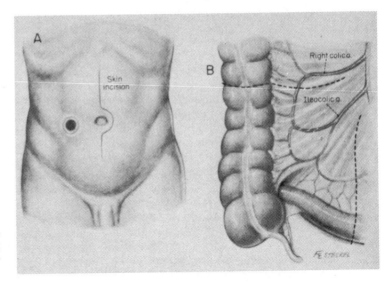

Figure 69–13. Ileocecal cutaneous diversion. (Courtesy of Dr. L. Zinman; by permission of the Journal of Urology.)

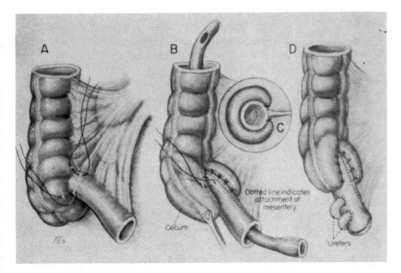

Figure 69–14. Preferred method of enhancing competency of ileocecal valve to prevent reflux *(B and C)*. *D,* Plication-intussusception of the ileocecal valve. (Courtesy of Dr. L. Zinman; by permission of the Journal of Urology.)

Figure 69–15. Placement of stoma after completed ureteroileocecal cutaneous diversion. (Courtesy of Dr. L. Zinman; by permission of the Journal of Urology.)

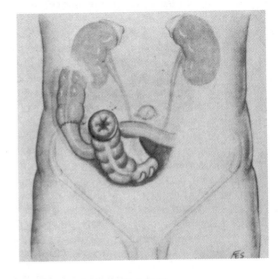

dure will have been treated for advanced pelvic malignancy.

Continent Cutaneous Diversion

Many attempts have been made in the past to develop a continent form of urinary diversion. Complex procedures such as the rectal bladder or reconstruction to the urethra have failed because of the complexity of procedures involved and the inability to control infection. Medical advances, especially the use of intermittent self-catheterization, have changed the premise for construction of continent supravesical diversion and renewed interest in continent diversion procedures. Encouraging results with a continent ileal reservoir after proctocolectomy have led to the adaptation of a continent ileal reservoir for urinary diversion (Kock et al., 1982). The technique involves isolation of a 60- to 70-cm segment of bowel, creation of a U-shaped reservoir, and intussusception of afferent and efferent segments with fixation of nipple valves by stapling instruments. Although results are preliminary, this type of technique does offer some promise for a continent type of urinary diversion that includes an antireflux technique.

Complications of Ureteroileal Cutaneous Diversion

Early complications are, fortunately, rare, but include obstruction, urinary leakage, vascular infarction of the conduit, and problems relating to the bowel anastomosis. Detailed discussions about the management of early as well as late complications of ureterointestinal diversion have been published; therefore, only a few remarks are made here.

Anuria, which may result from edema at the ureterointestinal anastomosis, usually resolves in 12 to 18 hours. A straight No. 20 Robinson catheter with extra perforations should be passed into the conduit proximal to the fascia in these cases to make certain that anuria is not due to obstruction of the loop where it passes through the fascia. A fluid challenge or placement of a central venous line might reveal hypovolemia as the main cause of poor urine output.

As in ureterosigmoidostomy, urine leak either from the ureteroileal anastomosis or from the base of the conduit is the most distressing early complication. Abdominal distention with prolonged ileus, an elevated serum creatinine level, or poor urine output despite adequate hydration may indicate such a complication, which can be confirmed by gravity radiographic examination of the loop performed under fluoroscopic control. Most small leaks will seal if adequately drained, but formal revision by means of re-exploration may be necessary and should be considered early in treatment. Percutaneous techniques have been particularly helpful in these situations.

Infarction of the conduit can result from tension on the mesentery or as a complication of closure of the mesenteric traps at surgery. Arterial insufficiency is usually obvious at surgery, and the intestinal segment involved must be replaced. Late infarction may result from venous insufficiency or from tension on the mesentery due to abdominal distention. A dusky stoma is seen initially, followed by obvious nonviability. Infarction may occur early or may not be obvious for 5 to 7 days. Panendoscopy of the conduit will reveal the extent of infarction and will indicate a possible need to replace the entire segment or simply to revise the stoma.

Late complications include stomal stenosis, ureterointestinal stenosis, pyelonephritis, and calculi. The incidence of these complications is smaller than in ureterosigmoidostomy, but it clearly increases with increased length of follow-up (Richie, 1974; Orr et al., 1981). Most long-term experience reported has been with the ileal conduit diversion, and only limited, short follow-up is available for other types of cutaneous diversion.

Stomal stenosis is seen in up to 38 per cent of children followed longer than 5 years and is probably related to disproportionate growth (Ellis et al., 1971; Malek et al., 1971; Cass and Geist, 1972; Richie, 1974). Early revision is mandatory to prevent elongation of the conduit and obstruction of the upper tracts. Effective stomal care to prevent encrustations is helpful (Esho and Cass, 1972), and the review of the subject by Jeter et al. (1971, 1974) is recommended.

Ureteroileal stenosis occurs in about 10 per cent of patients, usually on the left side where the ureter is brought beneath the sigmoid mesentery (Ellis et al., 1971; Harbach et al., 1971; Richie, 1974). Antegrade pyelography is helpful in the determination of the level of obstruction and also provides urine for cytologic examination. Extrinsic ureteral obstruction due to recurrent cancer vis-à-vis benign fibrosis can usually be determined only at surgery. It is important to follow cytologic studies of urine from the loops in patients who underwent diversion for bladder cancer, inasmuch as malignant cells found on cytologic examination may herald the presence of a transitional cell carcinoma of the upper collecting system (Soloway et al., 1972).

Clinical chronic pyelonephritis occurs in 10 to 33 per cent of patients followed less than 5 years, and its incidence would appear to increase as the length of follow-up increases (Cordonnier and Nicolai, 1960; Delgado and Muecke, 1973; Bergman and Nilson, 1974; Richie, 1974; Goodwin et al., 1975). Recently, reports of ileal conduit urinary diversion in children followed more than 10 years indicate that in up to 40 per cent of normal kidneys, prediversion will have deteriorated by the tenth year (Murphy and Schoenberg, 1967; Retik et al., 1967; Arnarson and Straffon, 1969; McCoy and Rhamy, 1970; Delgado and Muecke, 1973; Schmidt et al., 1973; Gregory et al., 1974; Richie, 1974; Koziol and Hackler, 1975; Rabinowitz and Price, 1975; Schwarz and Jeffs, 1975). Many are silent and occur after 5 years, indicating that close, continued long-term follow-up is mandatory. We routinely give patients antibacterial medication for 3 months following diversion, and thereafter treat specific infection only if there is clinical evidence of pyelonephritis or if catheter specimens of urine from the proximal loop indicate more than 100,000 colonies of *Proteus mirabilis* per milliliter of urine. The meaning of positive cultures obtained from ileal loops is uncertain and depends largely on the method of collection (Needham et al., 1970; Bishop et al., 1971; Spence et al., 1972; Schmidt et al., 1973; Steward et al., 1974). Experimental data, however, demonstrate that freely refluxing ileal conduits cause histologic evidence of pyelonephritis and suggest that an antirefluxing type of ureterointestinal cutaneous diversion may prevent the late complications of pyelonephritis (Kelalis, 1974; King et al., 1974; Hendren, 1975). Renal calculi may develop in 4 to 30 per cent of patients with ileal conduits, usually associated with *Proteus mirabilis* urinary infection, and almost always occur in kidneys damaged prior to urinary diversion (Cordonnier and Nicolai, 1960; Bowler and Tall, 1967; Engel, 1969; Malek et al., 1971; Delgado and Muecke, 1973; Schwarz and Jeffs, 1975). Dretler (1973) has postulated that poor renal function and urinary stasis with reflux of infected, alkaline urine predispose to calculus formation. He further notes that many of these patients have a relative metabolic acidosis resulting in calcium mobilization, which further enhances stone development. Treatment of such patients with acidifying agents such as ascorbic acid is contraindicated. Management should consist of elimination of stasis and long-term antibacterial therapy.

COMMENT

Since 1950, the ileal conduit has been by far the most popular type of cutaneous diversion, and it remains a tested, reliable form of diversion. Like ureterosigmoidostomy, however, it has taken almost 25 years for long-term results in a significant number of patients to have been reported. Also, like ureterosigmoidostomy, long-term results reveal that it is not a panacea and that late complications, many similar to those seen in ureterosigmoidostomy, occur in a significant number of patients (Creevy, 1960; Madsen, 1964; Richie, 1974; Schwarz and Jeffs, 1975). A significant incidence of long-term complications following ileal conduit diversion has now become apparent, and the ileal loop has not proved to be the ideal form of diversion hoped for by Bricker in 1950. It remains, however, a tested, effective means of diversion and is our preference when combined with cystectomy for the treatment of bladder cancer. Use of Turnbull's technique for creation of the stoma would seem to offer a real advantage.

The best method of diversion for benign disease remains controversial. There is increasing evidence that ileoureteral reflux is detrimental to the normal upper collecting system (King et al., 1974) and that long-term survival of patients (mainly children) undergoing diversion for benign disease is dependent on the preservation of renal function (Richie, 1974).

The use of the sigmoid colon for cutaneous diversion has recently become popular for patients with benign disease, but it needs further evaluation (Mogg, 1967; Kelalis, 1974; Altwein and Hohenfellner, 1975; Hendren, 1975, 1976; Morales and Golimbu, 1975; Richie and Skinner, 1975; Skinner et al., 1974, 1975). Its main advantage over the ileum is the thicker musculature, which allows creation of effective antirefluxing ureterocolonic anastomoses (Kelalis, 1974; Hendren, 1975; Richie and Skinner, 1975). One long-term (13-year) study, of Mogg's original patients, found that 73 per cent of patients without reflux maintained normal kidneys as opposed to 21 per cent of patients with reflux (Elder et al., 1979). We believe that the isolated sigmoid conduit is preferable for diversion in children or adults with benign disease and normal upper collecting systems (Skinner et al., 1974; Richie and Skinner, 1975; Skinner et al., 1975).

Use of the ileocecal segment for cutaneous diversion has appeal, particularly in those patients with dilated ureters, but long-term experience is lacking, and the lasting effectiveness of the ileocecal valve in the prevention of reflux is not known.

References

Altwein, J. E., and Hohenfellner, R.: Use of the colon as a conduit for urinary diversion. Surg. Gynecol. Obstet., *140*:33, 1975.

Arnarson, O., and Straffon, R. A.: Clinical experience with the ileal conduit in children. J. Urol., *102*:768, 1969.

Barzilay, B.: Experimental study of the technique of uretero-ileal anastomosis. J. Urol., *83*:612, 1960.

Barzilay, B., and Goodwin, W. E.: Clinical application of an experimental study of uretero-ileal anastomosis. J. Urol., *99*:35, 1968.

Bergman, B., and Nilson, A. E. V.: Intussusception of the ileal loop: An operative method for preventing urinary backflow in ileal conduits. J. Urol., *112*:735, 1974.

Bishop, R. F., Smith, E. D., and Gracey, M.: Bacterial flora of urine from ileal conduit. J. Urol., *105*:452, 1971.

Bowler, W. T., and Tall, B. A.: Urinary diversion in children. J. Urol., *98*:597, 1967.

Bricker, E. M.: Bladder substitution after pelvic evisceration. Surg. Gynecol. Obstet., *30*:1511, 1950.

Cass, A. S., and Geist, R. W.: Results of conservative and surgical management of the neurogenic bladder in 160 children. J. Urol., *107*:865, 1972.

Clark, S. S.: Electrolyte disturbance associated with jejunal conduit. J. Urol., *112*:42, 1974.

Coffey, R. C.: Physiologic implantation of the severed ureter or common bile duct into the intestine. JAMA, *56*:397, 1911.

Cordonnier, J. J., and Nicolai, C. H.: An evaluation of the use of an isolated segment of ileum as a means of urinary diversion. J. Urol., *83*:834, 1960.

Creevy, C. D.: Renal complications after iliac diversion of the urine for non-neoplastic disorders. J. Urol., *83*:394, 1960.

Crissey, M. M., Steele, G. D., Jr., and Gittes, R. F.: Carcinoma in colonic urinary diversion in rats. Surg. Forum, *30*:554, 1979.

Delgado, G. E., and Muecke, E. C.: Evaluation of 80 cases of ileal conduits in children: Indication, complication and results. J. Urol., *109*:311, 1973.

Dretler, S. P.: The pathogenesis of urinary tract calculi occurring after ileal conduit diversion: I. Clinical study. II. Conduit study. III. Prevention. J. Urol., *109*:204, 1973.

Elder, D. D., Moisey, C. U., and Rees, R. W. M.: A long term follow-up of the colonic conduit operation in children. Br. J. Urol., *51*:462, 1979.

Ellis, L. R., Udall, D. A., and Hodges, C. U.: Further clinical experience with intestinal segments for urinary diversion. J. Urol., *105*:345, 1971.

Engel, R. M.: Complications of bilateral uretero-ileocutaneous urinary diversion: A review of 208 cases. J. Urol., *101*:508, 1969.

Esho, J. O., and Cass, A. S.: Management of stomal encrustation in children. J. Urol., *108*:797, 1972.

Esho, J. O., Vitko, R. J., Freland, G. W., and Cass, A. S.: Compression of Bricker and Wallace methods of ureteroileal anastomosis in urinary diversion. J. Urol., *111*:600, 1974.

Ferris, D. O., and Odel, H. M.: Electrolyte pattern of the blood after bilateral ureterosigmoidostomy. JAMA, *142*:634, 1950.

Golimbu, M., and Morales, P.: Electrolyte disturbances in jejunal urinary diversion. Urology, *1*:432, 1973.

Golimbu, M., and Morales, P.: Jejunal conduits: Technique and complications. J. Urol., *113*:787, 1975.

Goodwin, W. E.: Personal communication, 1976.

Goodwin, W. E., Harris, A. P., Kaufman, J. J., and Beal, J. M.: Open, transcolonic ureterointestinal anastomosis; new approach. Surg. Gynecol. Obstet., *97*:295, 1953.

Goodwin, W. E., Kaufman, J. J., and Dale, G.: Uretero-sigmoidostomy and closure of exstrophy of the urinary bladder. Film; produced 1975. Available from the American College of Surgeons Film Library and the Eaton Laboratories Medical Film Library.

Gregory, J. G., Gursahani, M., and Schoenberg, H. W.: Five-year radiographic review of ileal conduit. J. Urol., *112*:326, 1974.

Hammer, E.: Cancer du colon sigmoide dix ans apres implantation des ureteres d'une vessie exstrophiee. J. Urol. Nephrol., *28*:260, 1929.

Harbach, L. B., Hall, R. L., Cockett, A. T. K., Kaufman, J. J., Martin, D. C., Mims, M. M., and Goodwin, W. E.: Ileal loop cutaneous urinary diversion: A review. J. Urol., *105*:511, 1971.

Harvard, R. M., and Thompson, G. J.: Congenital exstrophy of the bladder: Late results of treatment by the Coffey-Mizo method of ureterointestinal anastomosis. J. Urol., *65*:223, 1951.

Hendren, W. H.: Nonrefluxing colon conduit for temporary or permanent urinary diversion in children. J. Pediatr. Surg., *10*:381, 1975.

Hendren, W. H.: Reconstruction ('undiversion') of the diverted urinary tract. Hosp. Pract., *11*:70, 1976.

Holland, J. M., Schirmes, H. K. A., King, L. R., Gibbons, R. P., and Scott, W. W.: Pyeloileal urinary conduit: An 8-year experience in 37 patients. J. Urol., *99*:427, 1968.

Jeter, K. F., and Bloom, S.: Management of stomal complications following ileal or colonic conduit operation in children. J. Urol., *106*:425, 1971.

Jeter, K. F., and Lattimer, J. K.: Common stomal problems following ileal conduit urinary diversion. Urology, *3*:399, 1974.

Kelalis, P. P.: Urinary diversion in children by the sigmoid conduit: Its advantages and limitations. J. Urol., *112*:666, 1974.

King, L. R., and Scott, W. W.: Pyeloileocutaneous anastomosis. Surg. Gynecol. Obstet., *119*:281, 1964.

King, L. R., Kazmi, S. O., and Belman, A. B.: Natural history of vesicoureteral reflux. Outcome of a trial of non-operative therapy. Urol. Clin. North Am., *1*:441, 1974.

Kock, N. G., Nilson, A. E., Nilsson, L. O., Norden, L. J., and Philipson, B. M.: Urinary diversion via a continent ileal reservoir: Clinical results in 12 patients. J. Urol., *128*:469, 1982.

Koziol, I., and Hackler, R. H.: Cutaneous ureteroileostomy in the spinal cord injured patient: A 15-year experience. J. Urol., *114*:709, 1975.

Leadbetter, G. W., Jr., Zickerman, P., and Pierce, E.: Ureterosigmoidostomy and carcinoma of the colon. J. Urol., *121*:732, 1979.

Leadbetter, W. F.: Consideration of problems incident to

performance of uretero-enterostomy: Report of a technique. Trans. Am. Assoc. Genitourin. Surg., *42*:39, 1950.

Leadbetter, W. F., and Clarke, B. G.: Five years' experience with uretero-enterostomy by the "combined" technique. J. Urol., *73*:67, 1954.

Madsen, L. O.: The etiology of hyperchloremic acidosis following urointestinal anastomosis: An experimental study. J. Urol., *92*:448, 1964.

Malek, R. S., Burke, E. C., and De Weerd, J. H.: Ileal conduit diversion in children. J. Urol., *915*:892, 1971.

Markland, C., and Flocks, R. H.: The ileal conduit stoma. J. Urol., *95*:344, 1966.

Markland, C., and Kelly, W. D.: Experiences with the severely damaged urinary tract. J. Urol., *99*:327, 1968.

Mathisen, W.: New method for uretero-intestinal anastomosis. Surg. Gynecol. Obstet., *96*:255, 1953.

McCoy, R. M., and Rhamy, R. K.: Ileal conduits in children. J. Urol., *103*:491, 1970.

Mogg, R. A.: The treatment of urinary incontinence using the colonic conduit. J. Urol., *97*:684, 1967.

Morales, P. A., and Golimbu, M.: Colonic urinary diversion: Ten years of experience. J. Urol., *113*:302, 1975.

Morales, P. A., and Whitehead, E. D.: High jejunal conduit for supravesical urinary diversion: Report of 25 cases. Urology, *1*:426, 1973.

Murphy, J. J., and Schoenberg, H. W.: Survey of long-term results of total urinary diversion. Br. J. Urol., *39*:700, 1967.

Murphy, L.: The History of Urology. Springfield, Illinois, Charles C. Thomas, Publishers, 1972.

Needham, R. N., Smith, M. M., and Matsen, J. M.: Differences in the bacteriology of intestinal loop urinary diversions. J. Urol., *104*:831, 1970.

Nesbit, R. M.: Ureterosigmoid anastomosis by direct elliptical connection: A preliminary report. J. Urol., *61*:728, 1949.

Orr, J. D., Shand, J. E. G., Watters, D. A. K., and Kirkland, I. S.: Ileal conduit urinary diversion in children. An assessment of the long-term results. Br. J. Urol., *53*:424, 1981.

Parkhurst, E. C., and Leadbetter, W. F.: A report on 93 ileal loop urinary diversions. J. Urol., *83*:398, 1960.

Perlmutter, A. O., and Tank, E. S.: Ileal conduit stasis in children: Recognition and treatment. J. Urol., *101*:688, 1969.

Politano, V. A., and Leadbetter, W. F.: Operative technique for correction of vesicoureteral reflux. J. Urol., *79*:932, 1958.

Preissig, R. S., Barry, W. F., Jr., and Lester, R. G.: The increased incidence of carcinoma of the colon following ureterosigmoidostomy. Am. J. Roentgenol., *121*:806, 1974.

Rabinowitz, R., and Price, S. E., Jr.: Ileal conduit urinary diversion in children. J. Urol., *114*:444, 1975.

Rangel, D. M., Yakeishi, Y., Stevens, G. H., and Fonkalsrud, E. W.: Absorption of urinary contents from isolated segments of jejunum and ileum. Surg. Gynecol. Obstet., *129*:1189, 1969.

Retik, A. B., Perlmutter, A. D., and Gross, R. E.: Cutaneous ureteroileostomy in children. N. Engl. J. Med., *277*:217, 1967.

Richie, J. P.: Intestinal loop urinary diversion in children. J. Urol., *111*:687, 1974.

Richie, J. P., and Skinner, D. G.: Urinary diversion: The physiological rationale for non-refluxing colonic conduits. Br. J. Urol., *47*:269, 1975.

Richie, J. P., Skinner, D. G., and Kaufman, J. J.: Radical cystectomy for carcinoma of the bladder: 16 years of experience. J. Urol., *113*:186, 1975.

Ridlon, H. C.: Ureterosigmoidostomy: A comparison of two techniques. J. Urol., *89*:167, 1963.

Scardino, P. T., Bagley, D. F., Javadpour, N., and Ketcham, A. S.: Sigmoid conduit urinary diversion. Urology, *6*:107, 1975.

Schmidt, J. D., Hawtrey, C. E., and Buchsbaum, H. J.: Transverse colon conduit: A preferred method of urinary diversion for radiation-treated pelvic malignancies. J. Urol., *113*:308, 1975.

Schmidt, J. D., Hawtrey, C. E., Flocks, R. H., and Culp, D. A.: Complications, results and problems of ileal conduit diversions. J. Urol., *109*:210, 1973.

Schwarz, G. R., and Jeffs, R. D.: Illeal conduit urinary diversion in children: Computer analysis of follow-up from 2 to 16 years. J. Urol., *114*:285, 1975.

Simon, J.: Ectopic vesical (absence of the anterior walls of the bladder and pubic abdominal parietes); operation for diverting the orifices of ureters into the rectum: temporary success: subsequent death: autopsy. Lancet, *2*:568, 1852.

Skinner, D. G.: Secondary urinary reconstruction: Use of the ileocecal segment. J. Urol., *112*:48, 1974.

Skinner, D. G., and Richie, J. P.: Urinary diversion: The isolated sigmoid conduit. Film; produced 1973. Available from the American College of Surgeons Film Library and the Eaton Laboratories Medical Film Library.

Skinner, D. G., Gottesman, J. E., and Richie, J. P.: The isolated sigmoid segment: Its value in temporary urinary diversion and reconstruction. J. Urol., *113*:614, 1975.

Skinner, D. G., Richie, J. P., and Gottesman, J. E.: Experience with sigmoid conduits in urinary diversion. Surg. Forum, *25*:556, 1974.

Soloway, M. S., Myers, G. H., Jr., Burdick, J. F., and Malmgren, R. A.: Ileal conduit exfoliative cytology in the diagnosis of recurrent cancer. J. Urol., *107*:835, 1972.

Spence, B., Steward, W., and Case, A.: Use of a double lumen catheter to determine bacteruria in intestinal loop diversion in children. J. Urol., *108*:800, 1972.

Spence, H. M., Hoffman, W. M., and Pate, V. A.: Exstrophy of the bladder: Long-term results in a series of 37 cases treated by ureterosigmoidostomy. J. Urol., *114*:133, 1975.

Steward, W., Cass, A. S., and Matsen, J. M.: Variation in bacteriuria with intestinal loop urinary diversions. J. Urol., *111*:117, 1974.

Sullivan, H., Gilchrist, R. K., and Merricks, J. W.: Ileocecal substitute bladder: Long-term follow-up. J. Urol., *109*:43, 1973.

Sullivan, J. W., Grabstald, H., and Whitmore, W. F., Jr.: Complications of ureteroileal conduit with radical cystectomy: Review of 336 cases. J. Urol., *124*:797, 1980.

Turnbull, R. B., Jr., and Fazio, V.: Advances in the surgical technique and ulcerative colitis surgery. In Nyhus, L. (Ed.): Surgery Annual. New York, Appleton-Century-crofts, 1975, p. 315.

Wear, J. B., Jr., and Barquin, O. P.: Ureterosigmoidostomy: Long-term results. Urology, *1*:192, 1973.

Whisenand, J. M., and Moore, V.: Hydrodynamics of upper urinary tract after mucosal ureterosigmoidostomy: Case report. J. Urol., *65*:564, 1951.

Woodruff, L. M., Coyua, J. F., and Leadbetter, W. F.: Uretero-enterostomy: Experimental studies. J. Urol., *76*:873, 1952.

Zincke, H., and Segura, J. W.: Ureterosigmoidostomy: Critical review of 173 cases. J. Urol., *113*:324, 1975.

Zinman, L., and Libertino, J. A.: Ileocecal conduit for temporary and permanent urinary diversion. J. Urol., *113*:317, 1975.

CHAPTER 70

Use of Intestinal Segments in the Urinary Tract

GARY LIESKOVSKY, M.D.
DONALD G. SKINNER, M.D.

The use of intestinal segments in the urinary tract has evolved from cutaneous diversion to the most sophisticated methods of urinary tract reconstruction. For many years, isolated segments of bowel have been used successfully to augment the contracted bladders of patients afflicted with tuberculosis or interstitial cystitis, and for those undergoing cystectomy for non-urothelial pelvic malignancy while perserving the continence-providing mechanism (Charqhi et al., 1967; Goodwin and Winter, 1959; Kerr et al., 1969; Kuss, 1959; Kuss et al., 1970; Maged, 1968; Orr et al., 1958; Shanket and Muhsen, 1967, Skinner, 1982). Goodwin pioneered the use of the ileum for ureteral replacement, and candidates for this procedure now include selected patients with nephrocalcinosis or recurrent staghorn calculi (Goodwin and Crockett, 1961; Goodwin et al., 1959; Skinner and Goodwin, 1975). Gil-Vernet popularized the use of the ileocecal segment for bladder augmentation as well as for ureteral replacement (Gil-Vernet, Jr., 1965), and since then Skinner (1974), Gittes (1976), Skinner (1982), Whitmore and Gittes (1983) and Zinman and Libertino (1975) have demonstrated its value in urinary reconstruction. Sigmoid segments have also proved useful for urinary tract reconstruction in patients undergoing cutaneous diversion for benign or malignant disease, for those undergoing staged cutaneous diversion while major bladder disease is corrected, for reconstruction of the urinary tract by means of a sigmoid cystoplasty (Althausen et al., 1978; Hendren, 1975; Skinner et al., 1975). Hendren has popularized the concept of urinary tract "undiversion," often using various intestinal segments. He has demonstrated that urinary tract reconstruction is usually possible in children with severely abnormal urinary tracts if bladder innervation is present and if the surgeon is able to use imagination together with experienced surgical judgment and skill (Dretler et al., 1973; Hendren, 1976; Hendren, 1974; Hendren, 1972; Hendren and Skinner, 1981; Hendren, 1983a; Hendren, 1983b).

It is thus apparent that the use of intestinal segments in the intact urinary tract is no longer a curiosity or reserved for simple bladder augmentation but should be considered a part of the urologic surgeon's armamentarium in solving major urologic problems. One point should be stressed, however; major reconstructive surgery of the urinary tract is complex and difficult under the best of circumstances and should be undertaken only by those who are thoroughly familiar with the various operative procedures and are able to select the best alternative for the particular case. Sound judgment and operative skill are equally important; for this reason it is probably best to refer complicated cases to surgeons who have made this work their particular interest, and who therefore see a number of patients that is sufficient to provide continuing experience and to help them gain and maintain expertise.

AUGMENTATION CYSTOPLASTY

Bladder augmentation by intestinal segments has proved extremely effective in the rehabilitation of the contracted bladder of small capacity caused by tuberculosis or interstitial cystitis refractory to more conservative methods of management. Ileal, cecal, or sigmoid segments have been reported to be effective, and each has proponents claiming certain advantages (Goodwin et al., 1958; Kerr et al., 1969; Kuss et al., 1970; Maged, 1968; Winter and Goodwin, 1958). In the properly selected patient, there would appear to be little difference; selection depends more on the anatomic particulars of the case and on the experience or preference of the surgeon (Kerr et al., 1969). Bowel preparation for all types of augmentation cystoplasties is the same as that described in Chapter 69, under the heading Ileal Cutaneous Diversion.

Ileal Cystoplasty

Numerous types of ileal augmentation cystoplasty have been described since von Mikulicz made the first attempt to enlarge the bladder by using an isolated segment of bowel, in 1898 (Fig. 70–1) (Orr et al., 1958). Goodwin's technique of "cup-patch" ileal cystoplasty, however, seems preferable (Goodwin et al., 1958). In this procedure, a suitable segment of distal ileum is chosen, which is usually 20 to 25 cm in length and is located in the same general area as that selected for ileal conduit diversion. A segment is isolated, with particular care taken not to injure its blood supply. The isolated segment is irrigated with a triple antibiotic solution and is then opened along its antimesenteric border. After the ileum has been opened, it is molded into a U shape, and adjacent edges are sewn together with a continuous 3-0 chromic catgut suture (Fig. 70–2). Once the "cup patch" has been formed, the peritoneum is stripped from the dome and the posterior wall of the bladder. A portion of the dome and the posterior wall is usually excised, taking care not to injure the ureters. If the bladder is very small, a cruciate incision may be made to provide as wide an anastomosis as possible between the ileum and the bladder.

Gil-Vernet (1965) and Kerr and associates (1969) state that it is important to remove all of the bladder except the trigone and the bladder neck. We have not found this to be necessary in most cases. The ileovesical anastomosis can be either continuous, with 2-0 and 3-0 chromic catgut sutures or interrupted, with 3-0 chromic sutures (Fig. 70–2C). A urethral catheter is positioned, and a cystotomy tube is placed through a stab incision in the anterior bladder wall. This tube should not be placed through the ileum or through the suture line to avoid prolonged drainage when the tube is removed, the peritoneum should be loosely closed around the vascular pedicle to the ileal segment, and at least one large Penrose drain should be placed. The suprapubic tube is removed on the seventh postoperative day, and the drain is removed on the eighth day. The urethral catheter is then removed 24 hours later.

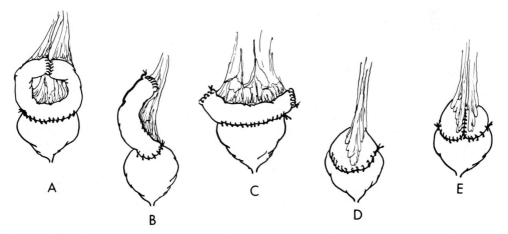

Figure 70–1. Various types of augmentation ileocystoplasty. *A*, "Ring plastic"; *B*, "rat-tail"; *C*, "U-shaped tube"; *D*, "flap" or "patch"; *E*, "cup patch." (From Goodwin, W. E.: Surg. Gyne. Obstet., *108*:370, 1958. By permission of Surgery, Gynecology and Obstetrics.)

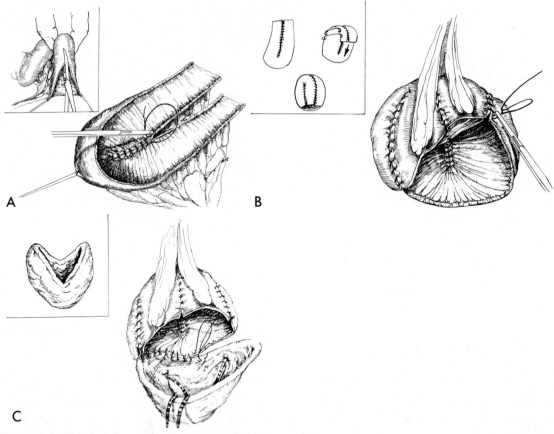

Figure 70–2. Technique for creating "cup patch" ileocystoplasty. *A,* The isolated loop is incised along its antimesenteric border *(inset)* and is then sewn into a U with a continuous 3-0 chromic catgut suture. *B,* After the U-shaped patch has been formed, it is again sewn on itself to form the "cup patch" structure shaped like the dome of the bladder. *C,* The "cup patch" is then sewn to the bladder, beginning posteriorly in the midline and working laterally toward each side with a continuous 3-0 chromic catgut suture. (From Goodwin, W. E.: Surg. Gynecol. Obstet., *108:*370, 1958. By permission of Surgery, Gynecology and Obstetrics.)

Sigmoid Cystoplasty

Use of the sigmoid for augmentation cystoplasty has certain advantages because of its anatomic proximity, thicker muscularis, and enhanced ability to accommodate to increasing volume without significant increases in pressure (Goodwin and Winter, 1959). Goldschmidt and Dayton (1919) also pointed out that the colon absorbs less than the ileum. The anastomosis can be accomplished without major mobilization or relocation of the intra-abdominal viscera.

The rectosigmoid is separated from the retroperitoneum, and a redundant segment conveniently close to the bladder is selected. A 10- to 15-cm segment is isolated, making certain that the bowel can be reapproximated without tension. It is not necessary to divide deeply into the mesentery as for sigmoid conduit diversion. A standard bowel anastomosis is performed below the segment; we use interrupted 4-0 silk sutures in two layers. The colonic segment is then opened along the tenia to form a flat patch. The patch of sigmoid is anastomosed to the prepared bladder, making certain that the anastomosis is as wide as possible (Fig. 70–3) (Goodwin and Winter, 1959). Catheters and drains are placed as just described under Ileal Cystoplasty.

Cecal Cystoplasty and Ileocecal Cystoplasty for Reconstruction

The ileocecal segment is the author's preference for either augmentation cystoplasty or lower urinary tract reconstruction if augmentation is necessary and ureteral substitution is required. Although it was originally described by Couvilier in 1950 (Gittes, 1976), Gil-Vernet in 1956 was the first to popularize the use of the

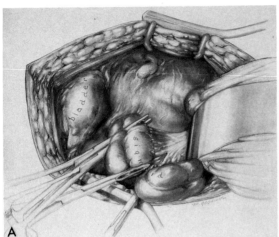

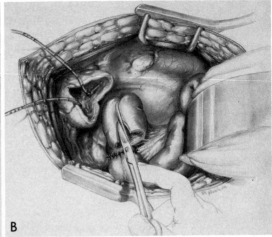

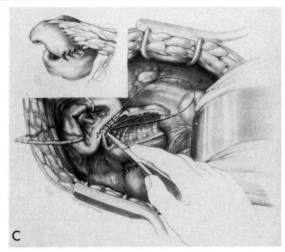

Figure 70–3. Technique of sigmoid cystoplasty. *A,* A 10- to 15-cm segment of redundant sigmoid is isolated conveniently close to the bladder. *B,* The bowel anastomosis is completed posteriorly, and the sigmoid segment is opened along its tenia. *C,* The isolated sigmoid patch is sutured to the opened bladder. (From Goodwin, W. E.: Surg. Gynecol. Obstet., *108*:370, 1958. By permission of Surgery, Gynecology and Obstetrics.)

ileocecal segment for enlargement of a small bladder and for the provision of a suitable substitute for the distal ureter. In 1965, he described its successful use in 26 patients with probable interstitial cystitis, stenosing ureteritis, and small bladders with reflux (Gil-Vernet, Jr., 1965). The ileocecal segment is a surgical unit based on an excellent vascular pedicle, the ileocecal artery. The cecum is ideally suited for bladder augmentation because of its shape, its ability to accommodate without the high peristaltic pressure activity noted in the ileum, and the thick muscularis of the colon. When ureteral substitution is also required, the advantage of the ileocecal segment over an ileal segment is its ability to prevent reflux either by relying on the ileocecal valve itself or, preferably, by intussuscepting a 6 to 8 cm segment of terminal ileum into the cecal segment as described by Hendren (Fig. 70–4).

Preventing slippage of the intussuscepted segment should be attempted by circumferential plication of the base of the segment to the seromuscular wall of the cecum with interrupted 4-0 silk sutures as described by Gittes (Gittes, 1976; Skinner et al., 1975) or by stapling the nipple and anchoring the outside base to a collar of Marlex mesh analogous to that described in the section on the Ileal Reservoir.

The surgical techniques of ileocecal cystoplasty and simple cecal cystoplasty are similar. In the latter, the terminal ileum is excised with the ileum closed and is turned in at the ileocecal junction. In either procedure, the ascending colon is mobilized from the right gutter, and the peritoneal attachments between the terminal ileum and the sacral promontory are divided, thus mobilizing the ascending colon and the terminal ileum up to the point at which the retroperitoneal portion of the duodenum crosses the midline. The ileocecal artery is identified, and the avascular region of the mesentery between this vessel and the right colic artery is noted. The length and mobility of the segment

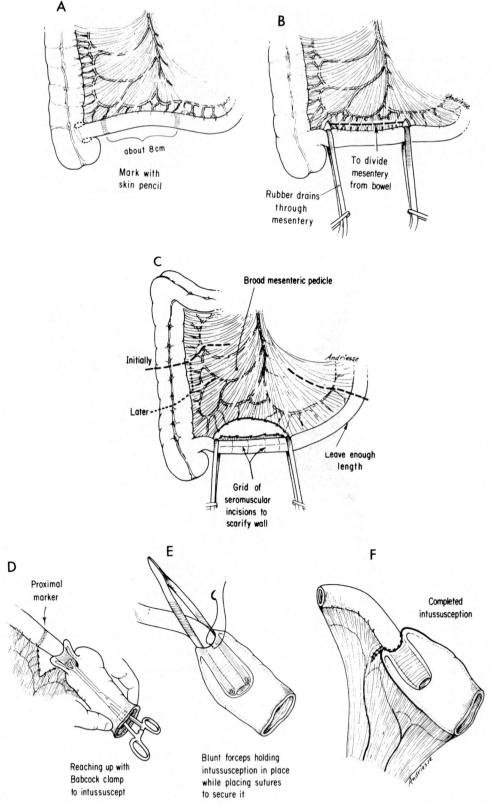

Figure 70–4. Hendren's technique of intussusception of a 6- to 8-cm segment of terminal ileum to create antirefluxing ileocecal segment for lower urinary reconstruction. (From Hendren, W. H.: J. Pediatr. Surg., *15*:770, 1980. Used with permission.)

depend on an adequate incision in the mesentery between these vessels, almost to the origin of the right colic artery. The surgeon may keep as much terminal ileum as required and then divide the ileal mesentery on the other side of the ileocolic artery (Fig. 70–5). A standard end-to-end ileal ascending colonic bowel anastomosis is done above the isolated segment; we use interrupted 4-0 silk sutures in two layers (Fig. 70–6). At this point, a small window is made in the posterior peritoneum, and the segment is passed out of the peritoneal cavity to the right gutter. The mesenteric trap is closed, and the peritoneum is then closed around the vascular pedicle to the segment. Finally, the remainder of the peritoneum is completely closed, thus making the segment entirely retroperitoneal. Thereafter, the segment is rotated 180 degrees so that it will function in an isoperistaltic manner (Figs. 70–6 and 70–7).

If a simple augmentation cystoplasty is to be performed, the terminal ileum is discarded, and the ileum at the ileocecal junction is closed with a running Parker-Kerr suture of 3-0 chromic in two layers. A third layer of interrupted 4-0 silk serosal sutures is added, and an appendectomy is performed.

Anastomosis of the opened distal cecum to the bladder is accomplished after a generous amount of bladder dome has been excised. The cecum should be incised along one of the tenia so that a wide isoperistaltic anastomosis can be accomplished. The anastomosis is done in two layers of 3-0 chromic catgut—an inner mucosal layer and an interrupted outer muscular serosal

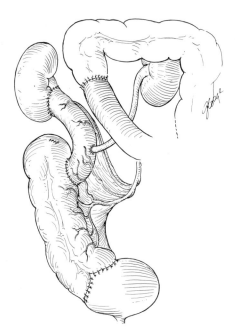

Figure 70–6. Method of urinary reconstruction by use of the ileocecal segment. Note plication and intussusception of the ileocecal valve to prevent reflux, and the use of the terminal ileum for ureteral replacement. (From Goodwin, W. E.: J. Urol., *81*:406, 1959. © The Williams & Wilkins Co., Baltimore.)

layer. Catheters and drains are used as discussed in the section entitled Ileocystoplasty.

If ureteral substitution is required, a segment of terminal ileum as long as necessary is used (see Figure 70–7). This may extend all the way to the renal pelvis or may be closed with a ureteroileal anastomosis similar to that described in Chapter 69, in the section entitled Ileal Conduit Diversion.

Comments on Augmentation Cystoplasty

In properly selected patients, results of augmentation cystoplasty with respect to frequency of micturition, control, and presence or absence of residual urine are about the same for all three segments (Goodwin et al., 1958; Kerr et al., 1969; Kuss et al., 1970; Maged, 1968; Winter and Goodwin, 1958; Chan et al., 1980; Dounis et al., 1980; DeKlerk et al., 1979). We have observed, however, that the ileocystoplasty as created by Goodwin et al. (1958) or utilization of the ileum as a hemi-Kock method to augment the bladder as well as to prevent reflux serves as a better reservoir and accommodates to increasing volumes without intermittant pressure spikes, whereas the cecum

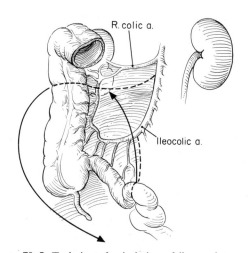

Figure 70–5. Technique for isolation of ileocecal segment based on the ileocolic vasculature pedicle. Note that the segment must be rotated 180 degrees to function in an isoperistaltic direction. (From Goodwin, W. E.: J. Urol., *81*:406, 1959. © The Williams & Wilkins Co., Baltimore.)

Types of Ileal Ureters

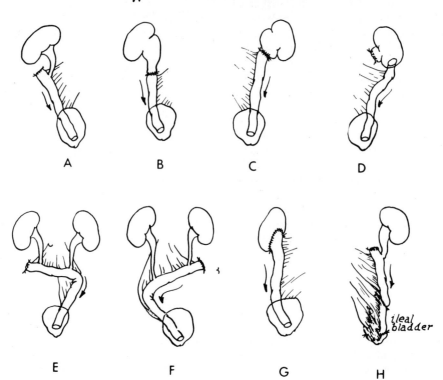

Figure 70–7. Various anatomic arrangements of successful ureteral replacement with an isolated ileal segment. (From Goodwin, W. E.: *In* Modern Trends in Urology, 172, 1960. Used by permission.)

when distended develops mass contractions, causing occasional nocturnal incontinence. Nocturnal incontinence is particularly a problem when the majority of the bladder is excised. Late complications from the procedure include intestinal obstruction, build-up of residual urine, chronic infection, and the development of calculi.

Kerr and associates (1969) and Gil-Vernet (1965) claim that all of the bladder except the trigone and the bladder neck must be excised before enterocystoplasty, otherwise frequency will not be relieved. Our experience does not confirm this, and the results have been uniformly good provided that a wide anastomosis is created between the bowel segment and the bladder, which is a view supported by Dounis and associates (1980). It should also be noted that the incidence of nocturnal incontinence is directly related to the extent of bladder resected (Kuss et al., 1970).

Goodwin routinely performs a Y-V plasty to the bladder neck whenever bowel is used in the intact urinary tract, and Chan and associates (1980) emphasize the need for this in patients undergoing cecocystoplasty. We have not done

so, and have had excellent results in those patients who empty completely and who have an entirely normal urethra and bladder neck. Preoperative evaluation with urethral pressure profiles is very important to make certain that there is no pelvic floor spasticity; cystoscopy with possible biopsy should rule out extension of interstitial cystitis into the urethra. In these cases, a generous Y-V plasty might provide a good result, but failure is not uncommon (Smith, 1975).

Close long-term follow-up is essential to detect bladder calculus formation and the silent but progressive build-up of residual urine (Charqhi et al., 1967; Kerr et al., 1969; Kuss et al., 1970). Next to infection, renal calculi constitute the major cause of renal deterioration; they should be treated by administration of long-term antibacterial medication and elimination of residual urine. Many of these patients have pre-existing reflux, which persists in about 80 per cent following augmentation cystoplasty (Kuss et al., 1970). Our current practice in patients with reflux who are considered candidates for bladder augmentation is to utilize Kock's principles to create a hemi-Kock pouch with implantation of the ureters into the afferent limb of ileum of the pouch with creation of an intussuscepted nipple valve to prevent reflux (See section on continent urinary diversion).

Mucous secretion may initially be a problem but usually subsides as the mucoid secretory cells of the intestinal segment atrophy (Roblejo and Malamenet, 1973; Watson and Crockett, 1973).

Intestinal augmentation cystoplasty has thus proved to be therapeutically valuable for patients with small bladders that have contracted owing to tuberculosis, interstitial cystitis, or chemical injury. Its use in the management of neurogenic bladder remains questionable, however, and would seem contraindicated in those patients with spasticity of the pelvic floor and external sphincter (Kuss et al., 1959; Smith, 1975).

ILEOURETERAL SUBSTITUTION

Use of the small intestine to replace a segment of damaged ureter was probably first performed by Shoemaker in 1906 (Goodwin, 1960), but the procedure was not popularized until the mid-1950's, when Goodwin and associates (Winter and Turner, 1959), Annis (1953), Britker (1954), Moore and his colleagues (1956), Wells (1956), Baum (1954), and Goldstein with his associates (1956) reported early experience in the clinical replacement of the ureter by ileum. Since then, the ileal ureter operation has become established as a useful and safe method of replacing damaged segments of ureter that are not amenable to repair with more conservative techniques, such as a vesicopsoas hitch, a Boari flap, or a transureteroureterostomy. In a recent review of 92 patients undergoing the ileal ureter operation approximately one third were performed for ureteral stricture or fistula (Boxer et al., 1979). In 1959, Goodwin and associates used the ileal ureter operation in a patient with bilateral staghorn calculi and severe infection to eliminate obstruction and provide maximum drainage of the renal pelvis and lower calyces (Goodwin and Crockett, 1961). Further experience in more than 47 patients with multiple recurrent renal calculi refractory to traditional forms of therapy has indicated that the ileal ureter technique should be considered early in the management of some patients with multiple renal calculi and a history of having passed stones from both kidneys. It should also be considered in patients with a solitary kidney and multiple calculi as well as in those with staghorn

calculi and evidence on radiographic examination of nephrocalcinosis (Skinner and Goodwin, 1975; Boxer et al., 1979). In such cases, the principle of the procedure is to provide maximum drainage of the renal pelvis and the lower calyces in order to prevent recurrence or to allow free passage of stones if they do recur.

The procedure should not be done in those patients who have poor renal function (creatinine greater than 2 mg per dl) or in those with neurogenic bladders and spasticity of the pelvic floor or external sphincter.

OPERATIVE TECHNIQUE

It is important to evaluate the bladder neck mechanism preoperatively to identify those individuals who fail to empty their bladder completely, since those patients are at greater risk for bladder outlet obstruction from mucous production when an ileal segment is incorporated in the intact urinary tract. In such patients, particularly females, a bladder neck revision such as a Y-V plasty seems indicated, whereas when mucous retention is less or in males, this condition can usually be dealt with postoperatively by TUR of the bladder neck. Of 90 patients reported by Boxer et al., 24 (25 per cent) were felt to have impending outlet obstruction and underwent some form of bladder neck revision, 19 of whom (79 per cent) had a successful outcome. However, no mention was made regarding the outcome of the remaining five patients.

The various anatomic arrangements of the isolated ileal ureters are depicted in Figure 70–7. It should be noted that when the procedure is being done for calculi, the proximal segment should be anastomosed to the renal pelvis, with extension into the lower pole infundibulum. This may be a very difficult and time-consuming procedure because of previous surgery and inflammation. Therefore, maximum exposure is essential, and in such cases only one side should be done at a time. Exposure for this procedure is best provided by a thoracoabdominal approach, with the patient placed in the torqued position (Fig. 70–8). Depending on the location of the kidney, the incision usually starts over the 11th or 12th rib, extends into the epigastrium just lateral to the midline, and then proceeds caudally as a paramedian incision. It is the authors' preference to perform an extrapleural resection of the 11th or 12th rib, transect the rectus muscle, and reflect it laterally to prevent denervation of the rectus muscle. The peritoneum is then mobilized from the entire gutter over to the great vessels. Dissection in the area

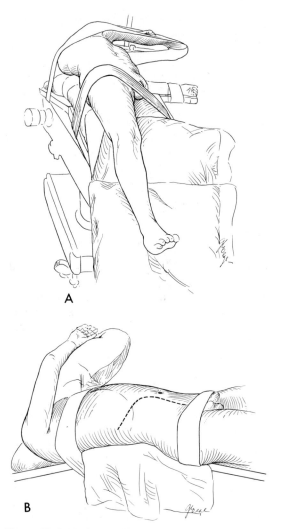

A

B

Figure 70–8. Patient position *(A)* and outline of incision *(B)* for the ileal ureter operation.

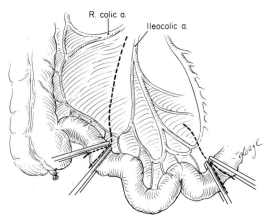

Figure 70–9. Isolation of a suitable segment of distal ileum for ureteral replacement. Note long division of distal mesentery.

of the kidney is not done until the ileal segment has been prepared, inasmuch as that is the most difficult and bloodiest part of the operation.

Once the peritoneum has been completely mobilized, it is entered. The ascending colon and the peritoneal reflection attaching the mesentery of the terminal ileum to the sacral promontory are then incised, thus mobilizing the ascending colon and the terminal ileum up to the region of the duodenum.

The most dependent portion of the ileum is chosen, usually based on the ileocolic artery or on the terminal ileal artery off the superior mesenteric. It is important to divide the distal mesentery as far as possible, inasmuch as length and mobility are dependent on that division (Fig. 70–9). Although the required incision in the proximal mesentery is shorter, the authors

routinely remove a small triangular wedge of mesentery and bowel, which eliminates tension on the short proximal vascular arcades and allows maximum mobility of the mesentery to the proximal limb of the intestinal segment. This should allow the proximal portion to reach the kidney easily. The distal end of the segment should be marked with a silk suture for later identification to assure that it is used in an isoperistaltic manner. A standard bowel anastomosis is performed above the isolated segment (we use interrupted 4-0 silk sutures in two layers), and the trap in the mesentery is then closed.

The next step is to make a small opening or a window in the peritoneum behind the cecum on the right or through the descending colonic mesentery on the left. The segment is passed through this opening and is rotated 180 degrees to lie in an isoperistaltic direction (Fig. 70–10). The defect in the mesentery or peritoneum is then closed, with great care taken not to injure the vascular pedicle. The peritoneum is then completely closed. The isolated segments should be thoroughly irrigated with saline and an antibiotic solution.

If the proximal ureter is still present, the proximal end of the segment is closed with a running 3-0 chromic catgut Parker-Kerr suture in two layers, and the ureter is spatulated and anastomosed end to side with interrupted 4-0 Dexon sutures (Fig. 70–11).

If the operation is being done for stone disease, or if there is no satisfactory proximal ureter, the lower pole of the kidney is separated from the Gerota fascia. This is often very difficult and bloody because of previous surgery. Identification of the renal pelvis may be facili-

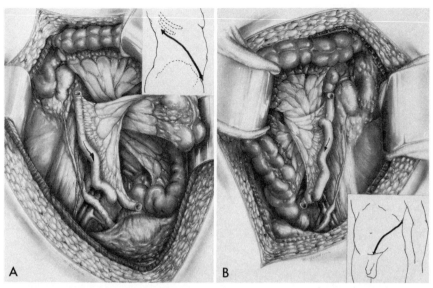

Figure 70–10. Isolated ileal segment has been passed through an opening in the colonic mesentery and rotated 180 degrees to lie on the iliopsoas muscle in an isoperistaltic direction. *A,* Right side; *B,* left side. (From Goodwin, W. E.: *In* Riches, E. (Ed.): Modern Trends in Urology [second series]. London, Butterworth and Co., Ltd., 1960, p. 172.)

tated in those patients with a pre-existing nephrostomy tube by passing a stone-searching forceps along the nephrostomy tract and cutting down over the end of the forceps, located in the renal pelvis (Fig. 70–12).

It is important that the renal pelvis be opened widely, with the incision extending into the lower pole infundibulum or, for stone disease, into the lower pole calyx. Usually it is possible to identify the proximal ureter just below the ureteropelvic junction. The ureter can then be opened with a lateral incision extended into the renal pelvis and lower pole infundibulum. All calculi should be removed; if a nephrostomy tube is not already present, it should be positioned through a convenient calyx at this time.

The anastomosis between the proximal ileum and the renal pelvis begins at the mesenteric border of the ileum and the medial portion of the renal pelvis or at the apex of the incision along the ureter. Sufficient length of ileum to extend to the lower pole calyx can be obtained by longitudinal incision of the antimesenteric

Figure 70–11. Use of the ileal ureter with the proximal ureter still patent. Note medial spatulation of the ureter with an end-to-side ureteroileal anastomosis. (From Goodwin, W. E.: *In* Riches, E. (Ed.): Modern Trends in Urology [second series]. London, Butterworth and Co., Ltd., 1960, p. 172.)

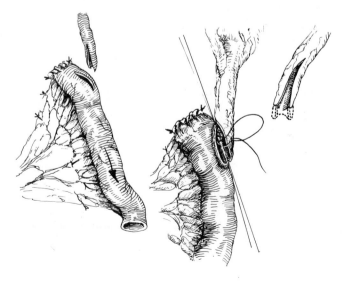

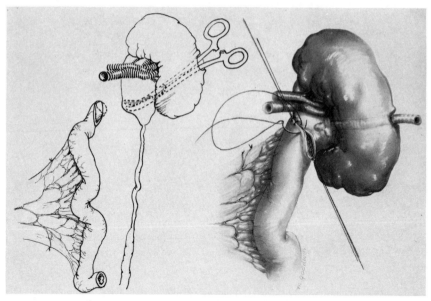

Figure 70–12. Use of stone-searching forceps inserted through a pre-existing nephrostomy site to facilitate dissection of renal pelvis. (From Goodwin, W. E.: *In* Riches, E. (Ed.): Modern Trends in Urology [second series]. London, Butterworth and Co., Ltd., 1960, p. 172.)

border of the ileum. The authors prefer an interrupted anastomosis of 3-0 chromic catgut, though a running suture can also be used. It is important that this anastomosis be as wide as possible and free of tension (Fig. 70–13). When used for stone disease, the ureter is left in situ, because it may be desirable to pass a catheter at a later date for retrograde pyelography or for irrigation. Irrigation of the nephrostomy tube will demonstrate that the anastomosis is watertight and patent.

A Foley catheter is purposely not placed at the beginning of the procedure so that the bladder can fill and distend during the opera-

tion, making it easy to identify rising out of the pelvis. A small cystotomy is made. The posterior wall of the bladder can be attached to the psoas above the iliac vessels with three or four sutures of 2-0 chromic catgut. A small divot of muscularis is excised just above its attachment to the psoas, which is the point at which the ileovesical anastomosis will be located (Fig. 70–14). Redundant distal ileum is then excised, with the surgeon being careful not to interrupt the main blood supply to the segment. The ileovesical anastomosis is completed with interrupted 3-0 chromic catgut suture. If the procedure is not done for stone disease, an antirefluxing nipple

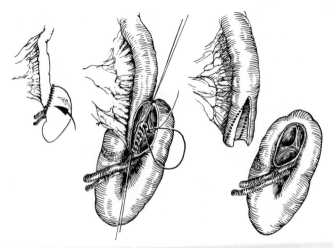

Figure 70–13. Correct placement of a proximal ileal segment with renal pelvis, lower pole infundibulum, and lower pole calyx. Although missing from the diagram, the ureter is generally left in situ and is incorporated in the anastomosis. (From Goodwin, W. E.: *In* Riches, E. (Ed.): Modern Trends in Urology [second series]. London, Butterworth and Co., Ltd., 1960, p. 172.)

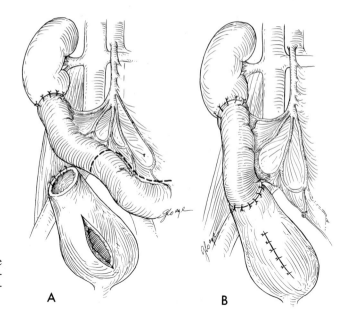

Figure 70–14. Use of vesicopsoas hitch with the ileal ureter operation. Redundant ileum is dissected *(A)*, and an ileovesical anastomosis is performed *(B)* with interrupted 3-0 catgut sutures.

A

B

can be created (Reiner and Jeffs, 1979; Hendren, 1980) or the distal segment can be tapered and implanted into the bladder with a long submucosal tunnel as described by Hendren (1976). However, Goodwin feels that an antirefluxing procedure is unnecessary and may in fact contribute to iatrogenic stricture of the intestinal ureter (Hendren, 1983*b*). For stone disease, however, we feel that reflux is desirable and make no effort to prevent it. Goodwin likes to implant the segment into the posterior bladder wall just above the trigone, and he routinely performs a Y-V plasty to the bladder neck (Goodwin, 1960). The authors prefer to use a vesicopsoas hitch, which elongates the trigone and fixes the posterior bladder wall. Angulation or obstruction of the segment does not occur when this is done, and the technique shortens the length of small bowel within the intact urinary tract, which is important in those with impaired renal function. Use of the vesicopsoas hitch also reduces operating time and minimizes blood loss when dissection in the deep pelvis can be avoided. The segment should not be implanted in the dome or mobile part of the bladder, inasmuch as obstruction may occur owing to angulation when the bladder fills.

A cystotomy tube is usually placed, and both anastomoses are drained with soft Penrose drains.

Nephrotomography and cystography are performed on the eighth to tenth postoperative days prior to the removal of the drains, provided that no leak is demonstrated. The drains are removed 24 hours later. Administration of antibacterial medication is continued for at least 6

weeks, and a follow-up intravenous pyelogram is obtained after 3 months. A film demonstrating this procedure is available from the A.U.A. Film Library or the Eaton Laboratories Medical Film Library (Skinner and Goodwin, 1976).

Comments on the Ileal Ureter Operation

Since the original report by Moore and his associates in 1956 concerning four patients in whom isolated segments of ileum were used for repair of ureteral injuries (Moore et al., 1956), considerable clinical and experimental data have accumulated indicating that it is a safe and useful procedure for the properly selected patient. Recently, Tveter and Goodwin (1982) and Boxer et al. (1979) updated the experience of Fritzche and her associates (1975) in patients undergoing the ileal ureter operation. Overall, the operation was judged successful in 81 per cent of the cases and 92 per cent for the 36 patients followed more than 5 years. Significant alteration of serum electrolytes or creatinine was uncommon in those patients whose preoperative creatinine was less than 2 mg per dl. In contrast, 5 of 11 (45 per cent) patients developed progressive renal impairment when the preoperative creatinine exceeded 2 mg per dl. Reflux into the interposed intestinal segment was not associated with deterioration of renal function or adverse pyelographic changes. Radiographic assessment of the upper tracts revealed no change or improvement in approximately 90 per cent of the patients studied. Symptomatic urinary tract infections were uncommon despite finding significant bacterial colonization in most patients. Tanagho, however, has reported six patients who needed to be converted to cutaneous diversion or who underwent reconstruction because of obstructed, malfunctioning segments (Tanagho, 1975). It must be emphasized that proper patient selection is essential; the operation is difficult and complex, and it should be performed only when other, more conservative procedures using normal tissues of the urinary tract are not possible.

CONTINENT URINARY DIVERSION

The development of a continent cutaneous form of urinary diversion dates to 1950 when both Gilchrist et al. (1950) and Bricker and Eiseman (1950) simultaneously described a technique of ureterocecocutaneous ileostomy. Reflux was prevented by implanting the ureters in a cecal submucosal tunnel, and continence was provided mainly by the action of the ileocecal valve and a tight cutaneous stoma. In 1973, Sullivan et al. (1973) reported their long-term results in 40 patients undergoing the Gilchrist procedure. Complete continence was achieved in 94 per cent of the patients, whereas 3 patients (7 per cent) developed ureteral reflux or ileocecal calculi. No patient demonstrated significant electrolyte disturbances. Since these initial reports, others (Ashken, 1974, 1978; Tanagho, 1975; Winter and Turner, 1959) have modified the technique and incorporated an intussuscepted segment of ileum into the cecal segment to provide additional continence. However, despite these encouraging results, this technique failed to gain widespread acceptance. Bricker, for example, noted that the ileocecal valve usually failed to provide acceptable continence and that leakage got worse with time. He soon abandoned the procedure in favor of the more accepted ileal conduit (Bricker) procedure, in which a good modern appliance prevented leakage (Bricker, 1984).

More recently Kock et al. (1982) have repopularized the concept of a continent form of urinary diversion and have described a technique for construction of an internal ileal reservoir similar to that developed for patients undergoing proctocolectomy (Kerr et al., 1969). In 10 of 12 patients currently alive, all are continent without ureteral reflux or dilatation of the upper tracts, with volumes of the reservoir averaging more than 500 ml. Symptomatic urinary tract infections or electrolyte disturbances have not been encountered. However, it should be noted that 12 reoperations in 8 patients were necessary because of malfunction of the continence valve mechanism or to prevent reflux. We have modified Kock's original description to avoid slippage of the intussuscepted nipple valves, and we describe our technique of creating a continent ileal reservoir in the following segment of this chapter (Skinner et al., 1984).

TECHNIQUE OF CREATING A CONTINENT ILEAL RESERVOIR (KOCK POUCH)

The ascending colon and peritoneal attachments to the small bowel mesentery are divided up to a point at which the retroperitoneal portion of the duodenum crosses the midline. The descending colon is likewise mobilized by incising the avascular line of Toldt, and a window is developed underneath the colonic mesentery to allow either the left or right ureter to be brought under the mesentery without tension or angulation. The distal avascular region of the mesentery between the ileocolic artery and the terminal branches of the superior mesenteric artery is identified and incised (Fig. 70–15). The small bowel is then transected between well-positioned Welch-Allyn bowel clamps at a point approximately 15 cm from the ileocecal junction. Proximal to the transected small bowel, approximately 80 cm of ileum, which will eventually form the completed ileal reservoir, is measured. The proximal small bowel is then divided between Welch-Allyn bowel clamps after first removing a small, short triangular wedge of mesentery and bowel, which eliminates tension on the short proximal vascular arcades and allows maximum mobility of the mesentery supplying the proximal limb of the intestine. The proximal end of the isolated intestinal segment is then closed with our standard 3-0 chromic Parker-Kerr suture and is reinforced by an interrupted seromuscular layer of 4-0 silk. The continuity of the small bowel is then reestablished and the trap in the mesentery is closed.

This isolated portion of small intestine is, in turn, divided into four segments: one 17-cm efferent limb that is destined to form the continence-providing intussuscepted nipple, two 22-cm segments to form the reservoir of the pouch itself, and another 17-cm afferent limb that will eventually form a reflux-preventing intussuscepted nipple (Fig. 70–15). The medial two

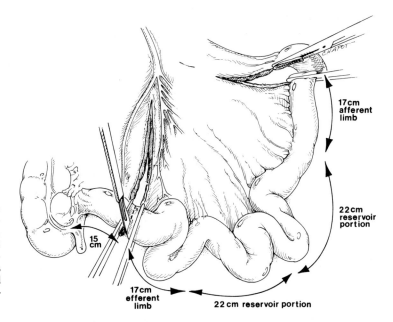

Figure 70–15. Isolated small bowel segment measuring 78 cm used for contruction of a continent ileal reservoir. Note the longer distal incision into the avascular mesentery between the ileocolic artery and the terminal branches of the superior mesenteric artery and the shorter proximal mesenteric division.

limbs, each measuring 22 cm, are then brought together to form a U with the bottom of the U jdirected in a caudal direction toward the side of the predetermined stoma site. This is important in order to allow proper alignment of the pouch and efferent and afferent limbs when performing the ureteroileal anastomosis and constructing the cutaneous stoma.

The antimesenteric borders of the two medial ends are attached to one another using a continuous suture of 3-0 PGA, and the bowel is opened by making close parallel incisions on either side of the suture line using diathermy (Fig. 70–16). This incision is extended an addi-

tional 2 to 3 cm into the efferent limb to stagger the final position of the intussuscepted nipples and to prevent their direct contact within the completed pouch. Additional reinforcement of the inner layer of the approximated U is provided by a transmural continuous 3-0 PGA suture, which is run forward and back (Fig. 70–17). In an attempt to prevent extussusception of the nipples resulting in either reflux or leakage from the stoma, we have implemented a technique popularized by Hendren (1983) of dividing the mesentery of the afferent and efferent limbs close to the bowel wall for a distance of approximately 8 cm to facilitate intus-

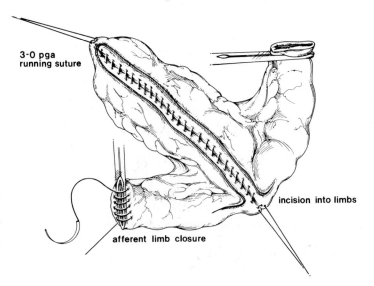

Figure 70–16. Incision alongside the approximated medial two limbs opens the reservoir portion of the pouch. The afferent limb is closed using a Parker-Kerr 3-0 chromic and interrupted silk sutures.

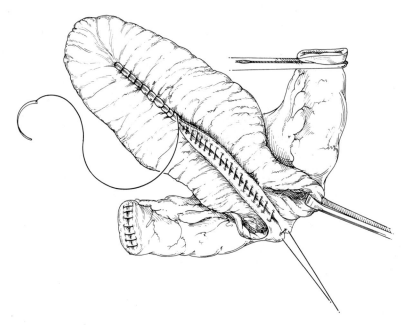

Figure 70–17. Inner layer of reservoir portion reinforced with a two-layer running suture of 3-0 PGA.

susception of the bowel and creation of the nipples.

Two additional openings in the mesentery are made through the windows of Deaver approximately 1 cm from the future base of either nipple to allow the passage of a 2-cm-wide strip of Marlex mesh, which will eventually form a collar around the base of each nipple (Fig. 70–18).

Two Allis clamps are passed through the open ends of the afferent and efferent limbs, grasping the intraluminal bowel wall at a point approximately 5 cm from the proximal end of the divided mesentery. Gentle traction on the Allis clamps results in formation of two 5-cm

intussuscepted nipples (Fig. 70–19). In a further attempt to prevent extussusception of these nipples, three vertical rows of staples are placed along the entire length of each nipple using a TA-55, 4.8-mm autosuture stapling device. Since staples at the end of the nipple do not contribute to the maintenance of the intussusception, remain exposed, and may form a nidus for subsequent stone formation, we routinely remove the proximal five staples from the apparatus before stapling (Fig. 70–20).

An index finger is then passed into one nipple at a time, and the ends of each previously placed Marlex strip are approximated with interrupted 2-0 nylon to form an outside collar

Figure 70–18. Diagram showing 8-cm openings in the mesentery of both afferent and efferent limbs and positioning of a Marlex strip around the future site of the intussuscepted nipple base.

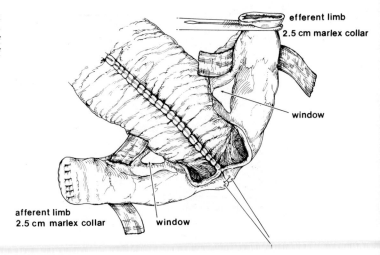

efferent limb

2.5 cm marlex collar

window

afferent limb
2.5 cm marlex collar

window

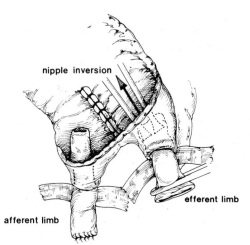

Figure 70–19. Formation of the continent-providing and reflux-preventing nipples by grasping the mucosa of the efferent and afferent limb, approximately halfway to the Marlex strip and intussuscepting the ileum into the pouch.

around the base of each nipple. The positioning of the finger is critical to prevent making the collar too tight, which, in turn, may lead to obstruction or erosion of the cuff through the intestinal wall. Additional interrupted sutures of 3-0 nylon are placed circumferentially in the

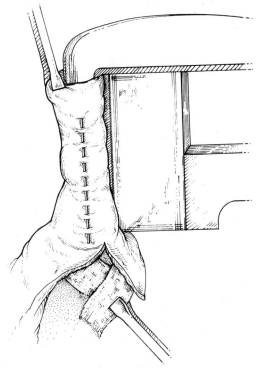

Figure 70–20. Placement of four well-positioned longitudinal rows of staples into both afferent and efferent intussuscepted nipples using a TA-55 4.8-mm automatic stapling device. Note the absence of staples at the end of the nipple.

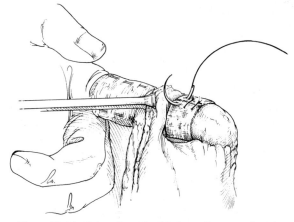

Figure 70–21. Formation of a Marlex collar around each nipple base and attachment of each edge to the adjacent seromuscular layer using interrupted 2-0 nylon sutures.

seromuscular layer and then to each edge of the Marlex strip to provide additional protection against slippage of the intussuscepted nipples (Fig. 70–21).

The midpoint at the bottom of the opened intestinal plate is then sutured to the apex joining the afferent and efferent limbs using 3-0 PGA. Each half of the reservoir is then approximated with a double continuous layer of 3-0 PGA suture, completing closure of the ileal reservoir (Fig. 70–22).

The afferent limb is then anchored to the promontory of the sacrum with interrupted 4-0 silk, and a standard 4-0 PGA interrupted mucosal-to-mucosal Leadbetter-type ureteroileal anastomosis is performed. The ureters are stented with fenestrated polyethylene No. 8

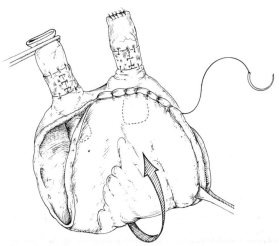

Figure 70–22. Completing closure of the ileal reservoir portion of the pouch with a double running layer of 3-0 PGA provides a meticulous watertight closure.

French catheters that are left indwelling within the pouch.

After completion of the ileal reservoir and ureterointestinal anastomosis, a small flush stoma is constructed at a predetermined site, usually in the right lower quadrant below the normal stomal position employed for intestinal conduits. A circular plug of skin without the underlying subcutaneous fat is removed using the butt end of a 20-cc syringe as a template. The underlying subcutaneous tissue is incised vertically and retracted using narrow Richardson retractors, exposing the anterior rectus fascia. A longitudinal incision is then made in the anterior rectus fascia, and the belly of the rectus muscle is bluntly separated, exposing the underlying posterior rectus fascia and peritoneum. This, in turn, is vertically incised to easily admit two fingers through the abdominal wall opening. Two horizontal mattress sutures of No. 1 nylon are then positioned on either side of the split in the anterior rectus fascia and are secured to both medial and lateral aspects of the Marlex cuff (Fig. 70–23). This allows the Marlex collar

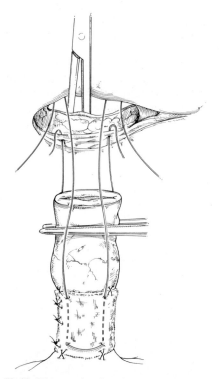

Figure 70–23. Diagram showing placement of two horizontal mattress sutures of No. 1 nylon from the anterior rectus fascia to the medial and lateral aspects of the efferent Marlex collar. This secures the Marlex to the posterior rectus fascia and allows for a short segment from the Marlex to the skin.

of the efferent limb to be accurately positioned at the level of the posterior rectus fascia. The mattress sutures are then tied, and any excessive efferent limb is removed. The stoma is completed by suturing circumferentially the mucosal edge to the subcuticular tissue using 3-0 PGA suture on a CE-6 needle. A well-positioned No. 32 French Medena tube is placed into the base of the reservoir and is well secured to the abdominal wall with heavy nylon suture material. A 1-inch Penrose drain placed through a separate stab wound is positioned beneath the intra-abdominal reservoir and is secured to the psoas muscle with a 3-0 chromic catgut suture to prevent the possible migration of the drain into the reservoir itself. This drain should remain in place at least 48 hours after the Medena tube is removed. In patients with existing ileal conduits, we anastomose the pre-existing ileal conduit end to end with the afferent limb of the Kock pouch, provided that there is no ureteroileal obstruction. Redundant ileum from the conduit is discarded, and the length of the afferent limb used for the pouch is reduced to 13 to 15 cm.

Postoperatively, the Medena tube is irrigated at least every 4 hours to remove excessive mucus and prevent obstruction of the tube. Three weeks following surgery, patients are readmitted for 1 day for Kockoscopy and retrieval of the ureteral stents, a Kockogram of the ileal reservoir, and an intravenous pyelogram. In the absence of significant extravasation from the pouch, the patient is instructed on the technique of clean self-catheterization of the reservoir. It is recommended that catheterization be performed every 2 hours at first and then the interval between catheterization be increased by 1 hour per week up to a maximum of 6 hours or until the patient experiences a feeling of fullness or distention of the pouch. Patients are followed every four months, at which time a Kockogram, an intravenous pyelogram, determination of serum electrolytes, and a urine culture from the pouch are obtained.

References

Althausen, A. F. et al.: Non-refluxing colon conduit: Experience with 70 cases. J. Urol., *120*:35, 1978.
Annis, D.: Replacement of the ureter by small intestine: An experimental study. Br. J. Urol., 25:69, 1953.
Ashken, W. H.: An appliance-free ileocecal urinary diversion: Preliminary communication. Br. J. Urol. 46:631, 1974.
Ashken, W. H.: Continent ileocecal urinary reservoir. J. Roy. Soc. Med., *71*:357, 1978.

Baum, W. C.: The clinical use of terminal ileum as a substitute ureter. J. Urol., 72:16, 1954.

Boxer, R. J., Fritzcshe, P., Skinner, D. G., Kaufman, J. J., Belt, E., Smith, R. B., and Goodwin, W. E.: Replacement of the ureter by small intestine: Clinical application and results of the ileal ureter in 89 patients. J. Urol., 121:728, 1979.

Bricker, E., and Eiseman, B.: Bladder reconstruction from cecum and ascending colon following resection of pelvic viscera. Ann. Surg., 132:77, 1950.

Bricker, E.: Personal communication, 1984.

Bricker, E.: Bladder substitution after pelvic evisceration. Surg. Clin. North Am., 30:1511, 1950.

Britker, M. P.: Les uretero-ileo-plasties. J. Urol. Med. Chir., 60:474, 1954.

Chan, S. L., Ankenman, G. J., Wright, J. E., and McLoughlin, M. G.: Cecocystoplasty in the surgical management of the small contracted bladder. J. Urol., 124:338, 1980.

Charqhi, A., Charbonneau, J., and Gauthier, G. E.: Colocystoplasty for bladder enlargement and bladder substitution: A study of late results in 31 cases. J. Urol., 97:849, 1967.

DeKlerk, J. N., Lambrechts, W., and Viljoen, I.: The bowel as substitute for the bladder. J. Urol., 121:22, 1979.

Dounis, A., Abel, B. J., and Gow, J. G.: Cecocystoplasty for bladder augmentation. J. Urol., 123:164, 1980.

Dretler, S. P., Hendren, W. H., and Leadbetter, W. F.: Urinary tract reconstruction following ileal conduit diversion. J. Urol., 109:217, 1973.

Fritzsche, P., Skinner, D. G., Goodwin, W. E., Craven, J. D., and Cahill, P.: Long-term radiographic changes of the kidney following the ileal ureter operation. J. Urol., 114:843, 1975.

Gilchrist, R. K., Merricks, J. W., Hamlin, M. H., and Rieger, I. T.: Construction of substitute bladder and urethra. Surg. Gynecol. Obstet., 90:752, 1950.

Gil-Vernet, J. M., Jr.: The ileocolic segment in urologic surgery. J. Urol., 94:418, 1965.

Gittes, R. F.: Augmentation cystoplasty. In Libertino, J. (Ed.): Reconstructive Surgery in Urology. Philadelphia, W. B. Saunders Co., 1976.

Goldschmidt, S., and Dayton, A.: Studies in the mechanism of absorption from the intestine. Am. J. Physiol., 48:419, 1919.

Goldstein, A. E., Abeshouse, B. S., Yildiran, C., and Siberstein, H.: Experimental studies of ileo-ureteral substitutes in dogs. J. Urol., 76:371, 1956.

Goodwin, W. E.: Replacement of the ureter by small intestine—the ileal ureter. In Riches, E. (Ed.): Modern Trends in Urology (second series). London, Butterworth and Co., Ltd., 1960, p. 172.

Goodwin, W. E., and Crockett, A. T. K.: Surgical treatment of multiple, recurrent, branched, renal (staghorn) calculi by pyelo-nephro-ileovesical anastomosis. J. Urol., 85:214, 1961.

Goodwin, W. E., and Winter, C. C.: Technique of sigmoidocystoplasty. Surg. Gynecol. Obstet., 108:370, 1959.

Goodwin, W. E., Turner, R. D., and Winter, C. C.: Results of ileocystoplasty. J. Urol., 80:461, 1958.

Goodwin, W. E., Winter, C. C., and Turner, R. D.: Replacement of the ureter by small intestine: Clinical application and results of the "ileal ureter." J. Urol., 81:406, 1959.

Hendren, W. H.: Restoration of function in the severely decompensated ureter. In Johnston, J. H., and Scholt-meijer, R. J. (Eds.): Problems in Pediatric Urology. Amsterdam, Excerpta Medica, 1972, p. 1.

Hendren, W. H.: Urinary tract refunctionalization after prior diversion in children. Ann. Surg., 180:494, 1974.

Hendren, W. H.: Nonrefluxing colon conduit for temporary or permanent urinary diversion in children. J. Pediatr. Surg., 10:381, 1975.

Hendren, W. H.: Reconstruction ("undiversion") of the diverted urinary tract. Hosp. Prac., 11:70, 1976.

Hendren, W. H.: Reoperative ureteral reimplantation: management of the difficult case. J. Pediatr. Surg., 15:770, 1980.

Hendren, W. H.: Urinary undiversion. In Glenn, J. F. (Ed.): Urologic Surgery. Philadelphia, J. B. Lippincott Co., 1983a.

Hendren, W. H.: Ureterocolic diversion of urine: Management of some difficult problems. J. Urol., 129:719, 1983b.

Hendren, W. H., and Skinner, D. G.: Visits in urology—Urinary undiversion: a movie. Presented at Annual Meeting of American Urological Association, Boston, Mass., May 10 to 14, 1981. Film available from Eaton Laboratories Film Library, Eaton Laboratories, Norwich, N. Y.

Kerr, W. K., Gale, G. L., and Peterson, K. S. S.: Reconstructive surgery for genitourinary tuberculosis. J. Urol., 101:254, 1969.

Kock, N. G., Nilson, A. E., Nilsson, L. D., Norlen, L. J., and Philipson, B. M.: Urinary diverson via a continent ileal reservoir: Clinical results in 12 patients. J. Urol., 128:469, 1982.

Kuss, R.: Colocystoplasty rather than ileocystoplasty. J. Urol., 82:587, 1959.

Kuss, R., Bitker, M., Camey, M., Chatelain, C., and Lassau, J. P.: Indications and early and late results of intestino-cystoplasty: A review of 185 cases. J. Urol., 103:53, 1970.

Maged, A.: Evaluation of different techniques of ileocystoplasty: An analysis of complications in 32 cases. J. Urol., 99:267, 1968.

Moore, E. V., Weber, R., Woodward, E. R., Moore, J. G., and Goodwin, W. E.: Isolated ileal loops for ureteral repair. Surg. Gynecol. Obstet., 102:87, 1956.

Orr, L. M., Thomley, M. W., and Campbell, J. L.: Ileocystoplasty for bladder enlargement. J. Urol., 79:250, 1958.

Reiner, W. G., and Jeffs, R. D.: Ileal intussusception as an antireflux mechanism in urinary diversion for myelomeningocele. J. Urol., 121:212, 1979.

Roblejo, P. G., and Malamenet, M.: Late results of an ileocystoplasty: A 12-year follow-up. J. Urol., 109:38, 1973.

Shanket, T. N., and Muhsen, J.: Treatment of Bilharzial contracted bladder by ileocystoplasty or colocystoplasty. J. Urol., 97:285, 1967.

Skinner, D. G.: Secondary urinary reconstruction: Use of the ileocecal segment. J. Urol., 112:48, 1974.

Skinner, D. G.: Further experience with the ileocecal segment in urinary reconstruction. J. Urol., 128:252, 1982.

Skinner, D. G., and Goodwin, W. E.: Indications for the use of intestinal segments in management of nephrocalcinosis. J. Urol., 113:436, 1975.

Skinner, D. G., and Goodwin, W. E.: The use of the ileal ureter for recurrent renal calculi. Film, produced 1976. Available from the A.U.A. Film Library or the Eaton Laboratories Medical Film Library.

Skinner, D. G., Gottesman, J., and Richie, J.: The isolated sigmoid segment: Its value in temporary urinary diversion and reconstruction. J. Urol., 113:614, 1975.

Skinner, D. G., Lieskovsky, G., and Boyd, S. D.: Technique of creaton of a continent internal ileal reservoir (Kock pouch) for urinary diversion. Urol. Clin. North Am., *11*:741, 1984.

Smith, R. B.: Use of ileocystoplasty in the hypertonic neurogenic bladder. J. Urol., *113*:125, 1975.

Sullivan, H., Gilchrist, R. K., and Merricks, J. W.: Ileocecal substitute bladder: Long-term followup. J. Urol., *109*:43, 1973.

Tanagho, E. A.: A case against incorporation of bowel segments into the closed urinary system. J. Urol., *113*:796, 1975.

Turnbull, R. B., Jr., and Higgins, C. C.: Ileal valve pouch for urinary tract diversion. Cleve. Clin. Q., *24*:187, 1957.

Tveter, K. J., and Goodwin, W. E.: The use of ileum as substitute for the ureter. Cur. Trend. Urol., *1*:1, 1982.

Watson, D. W., and Crockett, A. T. K.: Intestinal mucosa of dogs with ileocystoplasties: Long-term histologic and histochemical changes. Urology, *2*:385, 1973.

Wells, C. A.: The use of the intestine in urology, omitting ureterocolic anastomosis. Br. J. Urol., *28*:335, 1956.

Whitmore, W. F., and Gittes, R. F.: Reconstruction of the urinary tract by cecal and ileocecal cystoplasty: Review of a 15-year experience. J. Urol., *129*:494, 1983.

Winter, C. C., and Goodwin, W. E.: Results of sigmoido-cystoplasty. J. Urol., *80*:467, 1958.

Winter, C. C., and Turner, R. D.: Replacement of the ureter by small intestine: Clinical application and results of the ileal ureter. J. Urol., *81*:406, 1959.

Zingg, E., and Tscholl, R.: Continent cecoileal conduit: preliminary report. J. Urol., *118*:724, 1977.

Zinman, L., and Libertino, J.: Ileocecal conduit for temporary and permanent urinary diversion. J. Urol., *113*:317, 1975.

CHAPTER 71

Open Bladder Surgery

MICHAEL M. LIEBER, M.D.
DAVID C. UTZ, M.D.

Open bladder surgery is one of the most usual and ancient of urologic endeavors. All urologic surgeons must be familiar with the safe and effective performance of a variety of surgical procedures affecting the urinary bladder. The most common open bladder operations are described in this chapter. Other surgical techniques requiring open bladder surgery are described in related chapters: Repair of vesicovaginal fistulae is described in Chapter 74, augmentation cystoplasty is described in Chapter 70, the Boari bladder flap and psoas hitch operations are described in Chapter 68, and ureteroneocystostomy is described in Chapter 66.

Sterilization or suppression of urinary tract infection, even if this requires prior hospitalization to administer aminoglycoside antibiotics parenterally, should be carried out before open bladder surgery is performed; this markedly reduces the possibility of postoperative wound sepsis.

SURGICAL APPROACH TO THE BLADDER

For open operations, the urinary bladder is usually approached through incisions in the lower abdomen. A lower midline abdominal incision is most commonly used to expose the anterior bladder wall (Fig. 71–1). The transverse Pfannenstiel and the Cherney incisions are also useful for bladder surgery, particularly in the obese patient. A transverse incision, beneath the bulk of the abdominal wall fat, often provides a more facile approach to the bladder than a midline abdominal incision in the obese individual. We commonly make the Pfannenstiel incision two fingerbreadths above the pubic symphysis (Fig. 71–1). With the lower midline or with a Pfannenstiel incision, the anterior fascia is divided in the midline and the rectus muscles are separated and retracted laterally. With the Cherney approach, after the fascia has been divided in the midline, the rectus abdominis tendon is dissected from the pubis.

For most operations on the urinary bladder, there is no reason to enter the peritoneal cavity. The prevesical-retropubic space can be developed readily by inserting two index fingers behind the pubic symphysis and then opening the potential space; this procedure provides access to the anterior surface of the bladder wall. Distending the bladder with urine or saline (via a urethral catheter) often facilitates location of the anterior bladder wall.

Incisions in the bladder wall are usually closed in two layers by using absorbable suture material. The mucosal layer is usually run with 3-0 or 4-0 catgut. The muscular and serosal layers are closed as a single layer by using interrupted simple, interrupted figure of eight, or running, heavier sutures, such as 2-0 chromic catgut or one of the new synthetic absorbable sutures. Distending the bladder with saline through a urethral catheter or suprapubic tube after the cystotomy has been closed is a prudent way to check for leaks in the bladder closure. Drains are usually left near any closed incision through the bladder wall because cystotomy sites may leak urine. Most commonly, we use a Hemovac-type suction catheter in the prevesical space. These drains appear to work more efficiently than the Penrose-type drain used formerly and require a smaller incision in the abdominal wall to assure good drainage. If possible, vesical drains should be brought out through a separate stab incision rather than being passed through the main abdominal incision; this reduces the risk of wound sepsis, which is significantly increased when a drainage catheter or other foreign body is led through the wound.

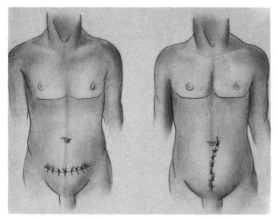

Figure 71–1. Abdominal incisions for open bladder surgery. Open operations on the bladder are normally performed through a lower midline abdominal incision or a transverse Pfannenstiel incision as illustrated here.

In closing lower abdominal incisions, we loosely reapproximate the rectus muscles with interrupted, heavy absorbable sutures. The anterior fascia is then approximated by using interrupted, heavy absorbable sutures, such as 1-0 Dexon or Vicryl. We avoid the use of nonabsorbable sutures at any stage of open bladder surgery. The subcutaneous tissues are reapproximated with running 3-0 chromic; a small Hemovac suction catheter is often left in the subcutaneous space in obese patients. The skin edges are then approximated with the use of a buried subcuticular absorbable suture, such as Dexon or Vicryl, or by skin staples.

SUPRAPUBIC CYSTOSTOMY

Punch Cystostomy

Indications

When drainage of the bladder is indicated and it is impossible, unsafe, or unwise to use an indwelling urethral catheter, percutaneous placement of a suprapubic tube is necessary. The availability of a number of commercially marketed, suprapubic catheterization kits expressly designed for this purpose makes the procedure much easier now than in the past. Cystocaths and their relatives are an elegant and simple means to drain the bladder. They are not useful, however, in the presence of hematuria or clot retention because of their small caliber (8 to 14 F).

Technique

Safe performance of percutaneous cystostomy is greatly facilitated by a markedly distended bladder. The procedure may be per-

formed under local anesthesia. The suprapubic area is shaved and prepared in sterile fashion, the midline skin 2 to 3 cm above the pubic symphysis is infiltrated with a local anesthetic, and a stab incision is made in the skin with a scalpel blade. The trocar and cannula are then pushed posteriorly until urine returns ("aim for the anus"). Prospecting for urine beforehand with a long spinal needle may help to locate the bladder in obese patients or in those who have had prior surgery. The specially prepared and designed cystostomy tube is then passed through the cannula into the bladder. The cystostomy catheter is anchored to the skin with several nonabsorbable sutures, and a sterile dressing is applied.

Open Suprapubic Cystostomy

Indications

This technique is usually used to place a large-caliber drainage tube into the bladder. Often, long-term drainage of the bladder is the goal and the use of a long-term indwelling urethral catheter is being avoided. Tube suprapubic cystostomy, however, should rarely be used as a permanent method of urinary diversion because of the common occurrence of urinary tract infection, reflux, and calculus formation in the bladder and about the catheter.

Technique

Placement of a suprapubic cystostomy is facilitated by a full bladder. A short incision (6 to 8 cm) is made in the lower midline just above the symphysis pubis (Fig. 71–2). The anterior fascia is divided and the rectus muscles are separated. The retropubic space is defined by digital dissection and the anterior wall of the bladder is identified. In patients who have undergone previous bladder or pelvic surgery, even "simple" placement of a suprapubic tube can be challenging, and prospecting for the bladder lumen by using an aspirating syringe with a 22-gauge spinal needle can be helpful. When the bladder is identified, the bladder wall near the fundus is grasped with Allis forceps or several heavy traction sutures, and a 1.5 cm stab wound is made between the clamps using cautery. A 24 to 26 F Malecot or Pezzer catheter is inserted into the bladder lumen, and the cystostomy is closed tightly around the catheter with several 0 absorbable sutures. The cystotomy site in the bladder wall can be fixed to the anterior abdominal fascia with several absorbable sutures to facilitate replacement of the cath-

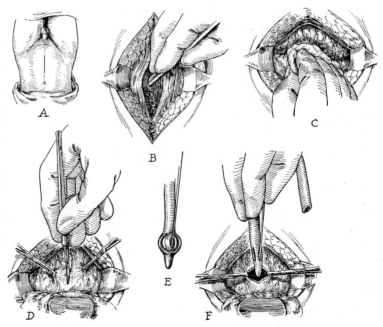

Figure 71–2. Suprapubic cystotomy. *A,* Incision. *B,* Separation of the rectus muscles in the midline. *C,* The prevesical fascia has been divided transversely behind the pubis and the peritoneum is stripped upward on the bladder. *D,* By grasping the bladder with two Allis clamps, a stab wound is made in the bladder into which the winged or balloon-type catheter tube is introduced. The introduction of a four-wing Malecot catheter *(E)* is shown, and it or the balloon type is preferred to the mushroom variety because, by extension with a grooved director, the wing catheter can be made into a straight tube that can be *(F)* changed, inserted, or withdrawn practically without pain. (From Campbell, M. F., and Harrison, J. H. (Eds.): Urology, Vol. 3, 3rd ed. Philadelphia, W. B. Saunders Co., 1970.)

eter if it should fall out before a tract is well established. The anterior fascia is closed with heavy absorbable sutures after a Hemovac drain is placed in the prevesical space. Ideally, the suprapubic tube is brought out through a separate stab incision on either side of the midline or Pfannenstiel abdominal incision and is fixed to the skin with several nonabsorbable sutures.

Cystolithotomy

Indications

Open removal of bladder calculi is indicated when the calculi cannot be totally removed transurethrally. Although the surgical removal of very large or very hard stones was formerly a common occurrence, the availability of endoscopically guided visual lithotrites as well as the newer ultrasonic and electrohydraulic lithotriptors should make cystolithotomy, performed solely to remove vesical calculi, an unusual procedure.

Technique

Cystolithotomy is usually performed through a small open suprapubic cystotomy as described earlier. Calculi are removed with a forceps and fragments are aspirated. Because most bladder stones in adults form in the presence of bladder outlet or urethral obstruction, this blockage should be corrected concurrently with or prior to removal of vesical stones.

Cystotomy with Tumor Excision and Fulguration

Indications

Transurethral excision of superficial papillary transitional cell carcinomas (T_0, T_1) is always the procedure of choice within reasonable limits of tumor extent; open cystotomy for tumor resection should be avoided, if possible. Seeding of tumor cells onto wound surfaces is always a possibility when the bladder is opened. Nevertheless, there are often patients with tumors that cannot be totally resected transurethrally because of their position, size, and multiplicity. Occasionally, the presence of a single, large-sized tumor makes excision and fulguration through a cystostomy preferable. This should not be done without prior biopsy and staging of the tumor.

Technique

Preoperative external beam irradiation for 1 to 5 days before surgery may be used to suppress the seeding of malignant cells (van der Werf–Messing, 1969). The bladder is preirrigated with distilled water or a chemotherapeutic agent such as thiotepa as additional means to suppress proliferation and seeding of malignant cells. The bladder wall is opened with an anterior cystotomy that is well removed from the area where tumors have been identified in the bladder lumen. The wound is carefully packed to contain malignant cells that may be shed.

With the use of the loop electrode and then the ball electrode attached to the electric cautery, papillary bladder tumors are excised and their bases are fulgurated. Random biopsies of bladder mucosa that appears nearly normal also can be made with the cold-cup biopsy instrument while the bladder is open. The bladder wall is then closed in several layers with absorbable sutures, and a urethral catheter is used for vesical drainage. Placement of a suprapubic tube in patients with an open cystotomy for tumor excision is best avoided to prevent possible wound contamination by tumor cells. A hemovac drain in the retropubic space is put in place and is brought out through a separate stab incision.

Postoperative intravesical chemotherapy with agents such as thiotepa or mitomycin C is strongly recommended to reduce the risk of tumor recurrence for patients with large, recurrent, or multiple T_0 or T_1 papillary bladder tumors (Gavrell et al., 1978).

Y-V PLASTY OF THE BLADDER NECK

Indications

Y-V plasty of the bladder neck is usually required to treat a recalcitrant fibrous bladder neck contracture following open or transurethral prostatectomy. Initially, bladder neck contractures should be treated by endoscopic incision, preferably with a cold-knife urethrotome instrument. If one or more attempts at endoscopic incision fail, an open Y-V plasty of the bladder neck is necessary.

Technique

The anterior surface of the bladder and prostate is exposed by a standard lower abdominal incision. A curved transverse, semicircular incision is made in the lower anterior bladder wall (Fig. 71–3). The scarred bladder neck can then be visualized directly from within the bladder interior as it is incised longitudinally with cautery, the stem of the Y incision extending caudad into the midprostatic urethra. After bleeding points in the bladder and prostatic incisions are controlled with cautery, the apex of the bladder flap is approximated to the apex of the incision in the prostatic urethra by using a 0 absorbable suture. The mucosal edges are then approximated with running, fine chromic catgut sutures, and the bladder muscle–prostate capsule incision is closed with interrupted 2-0

absorbable sutures. The retropubic space is drained with a Hemovac. An indwelling urethral catheter is left in place to drain the bladder for about 1 week; cystography is performed to assess incisional healing before the urethral catheter is removed.

PARTIAL RESECTION OF THE BLADDER

Reduction Cystoplasty

At present, partial cystectomy to reduce the size of an atonic bladder that empties poorly is rarely performed. Most patients, both male and female, with large atonic bladders achieve good results through chronic intermittent self-catheterization. Repeated attempts to open the bladder outlet by surgical and pharmacologic techniques in both male and female patients are also indicated. Surgical removal of the anterior bladder wall, sparing the bladder neck, trigone, and posterolateral bladder, can be carried out technically; however, the long-term results from such a procedure in an atonic bladder generally have not been favorable, and the patient is often left with an atonic and poorly emptying bladder remnant that continues to require intermittent catheterization.

Vesical Diverticulectomy

Indications

Most diverticula of the bladder develop in patients who also have bladder outlet obstruction. Treatment of the cause of the outlet obstruction, usually an obstructing prostate gland, should precede or accompany vesical diverticulectomy. Most small vesical diverticula do not require treatment; merely relieving the obstructive process with a transurethral resection will suffice. Large vesical diverticula with resultant significant residual urine, however, may cause chronic urinary infection and an unsatisfactory voiding pattern; these do require excision. Diverticula that contain superficial bladder tumors that cannot be resected safely or fulgurated transurethrally should also be resected, but full-thickness partial cystectomy is usually the procedure of choice.

Technique

The tactical goal in treating a vesical diverticulum is to excise the mucosal lining carefully. Excision of the fibrous sac surrounding the

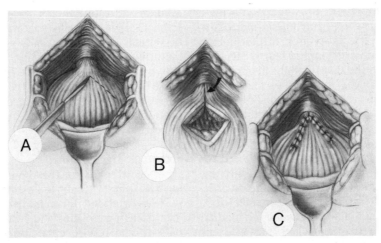

Figure 71–3. Y-V plasty of the bladder neck. The anterior surfaces of the bladder and capsule of the prostate are exposed (a). A curved or wide-angled transverse, full-thickness incision is made in the anterior wall of the bladder with its apex toward the prostate. Use of the cautery limits bleeding from the bladder mucosa and muscle wall. With the bladder lumen open, the contracture of the bladder neck can be visualized from within the bladder (b). A longitudinal incision of the anterior prostate capsule extending into the prostatic urethra then can be carried out under direct vision, again using the cautery for hemostasis. The apex of the bladder wall incision is then sewn to the apex of the incision in the prostatic urethra to complete the Y-V plasty (c). A urethral catheter is left indwelling for 1 week.

mucosal hernia is not necessary. Rather, the mucosa of the diverticulum should be considered as a peritoneal hernia sac; it should be excised and the neck of the diverticulum should be closed securely with suture. Relatively small diverticula, particularly those arising laterally on the bladder, can be excised by an intravesical approach alone. This technique is illustrated in Figure 71–4. The bladder wall is opened with an anterior cystotomy. The vesical mucosa surrounding the neck of the diverticulum is incised circumferentially, and the plane between the mucosa, the bladder, and the diverticular fibrous sac is carefully developed. The mucosa is stripped from within the diverticular sac and the bladder muscle wall of the neck of the diverticulum is closed securely with interrupted, heavy absorbable sutures. The mucosa is then closed with fine, running chromic catgut. The cystotomy is closed in two layers and a Hemovac drain is retained in the retropubic space.

For larger diverticula, which generally arise posterolaterally, a combined intravesical and extravesical approach is usually necessary to avoid injury to surrounding structures. The bladder wall is opened in the anterior midline. The diverticular orifice is identified and circumscribed as described. The ureteral orifice on the

Figure 71–4. Intravesical diverticulectomy. *A,* Circular incision about the neck of the diverticulum. *B,* Transvesical resection of the sac. *C,* Transvesical inversion of the sac by grasping its fundus with a clamp; this is the usual procedure. *D,* Incision of the inverted sac through the open bladder. *E,* Closure of the site of sac resection. (From Campbell, M. F.: *In* Campbell, M. F., and Harrison, J. H. (Eds.): Urology, Vol. 3, 3rd ed. Philadelphia, W. B. Saunders Co., 1970.)

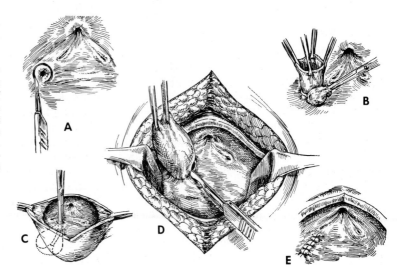

side of the diverticulum is cannulated with a ureteral catheter to aid in avoiding and identifying ureteral injury. Dissection of the mucosa from within the diverticulum is begun intravesically. A finger in the diverticulum then permits safe dissection of the anterior surface of the diverticular fibrous capsule from the lateral pelvic sidewall. Quite often, division of the ipsilateral superior vesical artery and its associated vascular pedicle structures is necessary so that the bladder wall can be rolled medially and the diverticulum can be dissected safely. Once the anterolateral extravesical surface of the diverticulum is clearly identified, an extravesical incision is made at the junction between the bladder wall and the diverticular neck to permit facile dissection of the bladder mucosa from within the large diverticular sac. Again, it is important to emphasize that resection of the fibrous capsule around the mucosal diverticulum is not necessary. This capsule is best left in place so as to avoid unnecessary bleeding and damage to adjacent structures, such as the rectum and the ureter. After the diverticular mucosa is excised, the bladder muscle wall and bladder mucosa are carefully closed from within. A Hemovac drain is left in the diverticular sac extravesically for external drainage. A suprapubic tube or urethral catheter is retained in the bladder for 7 to 10 days. Cystography is performed 1 week after surgery to evaluate the repair of the diverticular neck. If the cause of the bladder outlet obstruction has been satisfactorily rectified, permanent healing of the bladder mucosal hernia will generally follow uneventfully.

Segmental Cystectomy for Tumor

Indications

The indications for partial cystectomy in patients with bladder carcinoma remain controversial. One or two decades ago, this procedure was commonly performed for invasive transitional cell carcinoma (stages T_2 [B_1] or T_3 [B_2 and C] bladder tumors). Numerous series of patients who had undergone segmental resection for invasive transitional cell carcinoma yielded results suggesting that the survival expectation for these patients, corrected for stage and grade, is not greatly different from that seen for similar patients treated by total cystectomy (Utz and DeWeerd, 1978; Kiker and Crawford, 1982). Problems arise, however, because of the often diffuse "field change" nature of the urinary

bladder transitional cell carcinoma diathesis. Even though a specific solitary, invasive transitional cell carcinoma tumor mass can be satisfactorily excised technically, recurrence elsewhere in the bladder occurs in 50 per cent or more of patients if they are followed over a long enough time. Therefore, many patients who formerly would have been treated by partial cystectomy now undergo radical cystectomy when an apparent solitary invasive bladder carcinoma is first identified.

Nevertheless, in the presence of a suitably located solitary tumor in an elderly or otherwise poor-risk patient, for palliative tumor resection in a patient with metastatic disease, or for the patient who refuses cystectomy and urinary diversion, segmental resection of the bladder for transitional cell carcinoma still has a place. Solitary tumors located on the posterior wall of the bladder or on the dome well away from the bladder neck and trigone are ideally suited for partial cystectomy. Tumors occurring in a vesical diverticulum or elsewhere in the bladder where adequate transurethral resection cannot be performed also are appropriate for partial cystectomy. In the setting of high-grade, muscle-invasive transitional cell carcinoma, extensive cystoscopic examination and random mucosal biopsies are indicated to rule out the presence of carcinoma in situ elsewhere in the bladder prior to partial cystectomy. Partial cystectomy is also a useful procedure when the bladder wall is invaded by tumors from other primary sites, such as cervical, colonic, or endometrial carcinomas. In all instances, the tumor must be of limited size so that the bladder capacity after segmental resection is adequate for voiding comfort.

Surgical Procedure

With the patient under anesthesia, a preliminary cystoscopic examination is carried out immediately before the partial cystectomy. The bladder tumor to be excised is encircled with the coagulating electrode approximately 2 cm from the base of the tumor; this is the planned line of bladder resection. Sterile water is used as the irrigant because of its cytocidal effect and a urethral catheter is left indwelling. Short-course, low-dose (500 to 2000 R) external beam radiation therapy should be used preoperatively in this situation to reduce the incidence of tumor cell implantation in the pelvis and abdominal wall (van der Werf–Messing, 1969).

The patient is placed in a supine position and the lower abdomen is sterilely prepared with the penis or female urethra included in the operative field. A lower midline abdominal incision is made. If the tumor is located on the bladder dome, the peritoneal cavity is opened in the midline and the intestine is packed cephalad. Careful palpation of the bladder and pelvic sidewalls is performed to check for evidence of local tumor extension and nodal metastases. Unilateral or bilateral pelvic lymphadenectomy may be indicated, depending on the clinical circumstances as well as the location of the tumor and its preoperative stage and grade. This procedure is described further on.

The operative field is carefully packed off in an attempt to prevent tumor cell seeding. The dome of the bladder is grasped with Allis clamps and the bladder is incised using diathermy well away from the location of the tumor. The edges of the bladder incision are grasped with Allis clamps or fixed with suture ligatures so that the tumor to be resected can

be exposed clearly (Fig. 71–5). The tumor and its surrounding cuff of presumed normal bladder wall are excised en bloc by using cautery. This technique facilitates hemostasis. A full-thickness segment of the bladder wall is removed with its underlying perivesical fat. If the tumor is located in the dome of the bladder, excision of the overlying fat and peritoneum is required. If the tumor is located close to the trigone, full mobilization of the bladder on the side of the tumor with ligation and division of the ipsilateral vascular pedicle and excision of the intramucosal ureter is often required to obtain adequate resection margins. An indwelling ureteral stent may help to prevent ureteral injury.

Frozen-section histologic examination of the tumor and the resection margins is performed. If the specimen resection margins are free of tumor, the bladder wall is then closed in two layers. Reimplantation of the ureter may

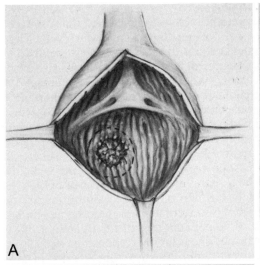

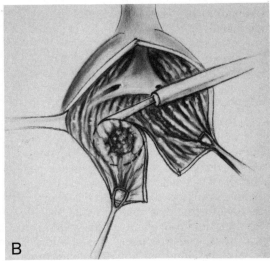

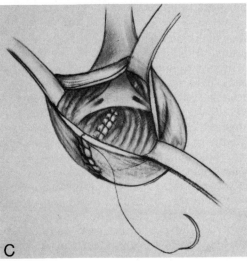

Figure 71–5. Partial cystectomy for bladder tumor. *A,* The bladder is opened anteriorly well away from the known location of the bladder neoplasm. The tumor is visualized within the coagulating marks placed transurethrally to outline the proposed margins of resection. *B,* The bladder tumor and its surrounding cuff of normal-appearing mucosa are excised with a full-thickness segment of bladder wall. Use of the electric cautery reduces blood loss at this time. Care must be taken to not injure the distal ureter. *C,* The defect in the bladder wall is then closed in two layers. The seromuscular layer is closed with interrupted or running 2-0 absorbable sutures; the mucosa is closed with running 3-0 chromic catgut.

be required. The mucosa and submucosa are closed as a single layer with running, 3-0 chromic catgut, and the seromuscular layer is closed with running or interrupted 2-0 chromic catgut or a synthetic absorbable suture. Bladder drainage is provided by a urethral catheter. Suprapubic catheter drainage after a partial cystectomy for transitional cell carcinoma is contraindicated because of the risk of tumor recurrence in the cystostomy tract or incision. After the bladder is closed, a large Hemovac drain is positioned in the retropubic space and brought out through a separate stab incision. The peritoneum is closed with running, heavy chromic catgut and the incision is closed by the usual techniques. A cystogram should be obtained after about 7 to 10 days to check for vesical healing before removal of the drainage catheter. Prolonged drainage may be necessary for healing to occur in a bladder that has been heavily irradiated. Routine and frequent postoperative cystoscopic examinations should be performed because the rate of tumor recurrence after partial cystectomy is quite high.

RADICAL CYSTECTOMY

Definitions

This procedure in the male patient denotes removal of the urinary bladder, prostate, and seminal vesicles with a wide margin of surrounding adipose tissue and the overlying pelvic peritoneum. In the female patient, radical cystectomy implies surgical excision of the bladder, urethra, and surrounding adipose tissue, usually with en bloc removal of the uterus, fallopian tubes, ovaries, and a segment of the anterior vaginal wall. Bilateral pelvic lymphadenectomy is commonly performed at the time of radical cystectomy. Simple cystectomy describes removal of the bladder alone, usually performed by excision close to the bladder wall, for benign conditions such as pyocystis or interstitial cystitis. In these procedures, the prostate and seminal vesicles or both are usually preserved. Simple cystectomy is contraindicated in the presence of malignant disease.

Indications

Radical cystectomy is indicated most often in the presence of biopsy-proven, muscle-invasive primary carcinoma of the urinary bladder (Stages T_2 or greater). Usually, radical cystectomy is performed with curative intent in patients who have been carefully staged by radiologic imaging methods and who appear free of metastatic disease. Radical cystectomy may also be necessary for patients with bladder cancer treated with primary radiotherapy who have failed to respond or who have recurrent tumor growth. Occasionally, radical cystectomy may be necessary in the setting of known metastatic bladder carcinoma, to be used as a palliative procedure to alleviate severe local symptoms, such as bleeding. Radical cystectomy is often indicated as well for diffuse, high-grade transitional cell carcinoma in situ of the bladder and prostate epithelium (Stage T_{is}) or for other multifocal, high-grade superficial transitional cell carcinomas (Stage T_1).

Preoperative Irradiation

The results of the excellent studies by Bloom, Wallace, and colleagues in England (Wallace and Bloom, 1976; Bloom et al., 1982) and by other clinical investigators (reviewed by Droller, 1983), as well as our own personal experience, have convinced us that primary external beam radiotherapy *alone* (with curative intent) is not the most generally useful method of treatment for patients with invasive bladder cancer. We do continue to recommend this treatment method for late octagenerians and nonagenerians with invasive bladder cancer and for certain younger patients with severe medical problems or those who categorically refuse extirpative bladder surgery. Although there is no question that approximately 20 per cent of patients with invasive bladder cancer will have their bladder tumor successfully sterilized by high-dose external beam radiotherapy alone, at least 50 per cent of patients treated in this way will not show tumor response or will have recurrent tumor growth within a period of several years. We and other surgeons have found so-called salvage cystectomy, carried out after previous high-dose external beam radiotherapy for curative intent, to be more technically difficult than per primum radical cystectomy, and have found it to be associated with a much higher incidence of complications (Crawford and Skinner, 1980). Other surgeons have had a more sanguine experience with salvage cystectomy (Blandy et al., 1980; Hope-Stone et al., 1981).

The combination of preoperative external-beam radiation therapy and subsequent radical cystectomy has been a popular treatment method over the last 20 years for managing invasive bladder cancer. The exact role, if any, for preoperative external-beam radiotherapy in patients with invasive bladder cancer is now a topic of intense debate among urologic oncologists and radiotherapists (Radwin, 1980; Droller, 1983). During the 1960's and early 1970's, most patients at the Mayo Clinic and other urologic oncology centers were treated with 4000 to 5000 R of whole-pelvis external beam radiotherapy preoperatively followed by radical cystectomy approximately 1 month later. There is little debate that those patients treated with this technique, whose bladder specimens after cystectomy showed no evidence of residual cancer, have had a relatively good prognosis (Prout et al., 1970). In addition, the 2- to 3-month preoperative period required for patients to receive this type of external-beam radiotherapy allowed micrometastases in certain patients to be declared clinically, thus avoiding unnecessary radical cystectomy. For example, in a number of patients, the results of bone scans became positive or new pulmonary nodules were evident on chest radiography during the several months between documentation of their invasive bladder cancer and the planned time of radical cystectomy, during the time interval allotted for preoperative radiation therapy. Since the middle 1970's, beginning with the successful results from 2000 R short-course treatment reported by Whitmore and colleagues at Memorial Sloan-Kettering Cancer Center (Whitmore et al., 1977), other urologic oncologists have moved to lower doses and shorter courses of preoperative radiotherapy (Reid et al., 1976; Skinner et al., 1982). The use of 1600 to 2000 R, delivered in four to five fractions the week before radical cystectomy, has been a common treatment plan. It has been suggested that this treatment may be as effective for sterilizing micrometastatic disease remaining in the pelvis as higher dose radiotherapy given over a longer time.

Many urologists now believe that systematic radical cystectomy in conjunction with definitive bilateral pelvic lymphadenectomy is adequate local treatment for invasive bladder carcinoma, and that prolonged high-dose preoperative radiotherapy adds little to local control. Many urologists have continued to use high-dose, short-course radiotherapy simply to reduce the risk of pelvic recurrence of tumor should the bladder be opened inadvertently and tumor cells spilled at the time of total cystectomy. At our own institution at the present time, most patients receive short-course radiotherapy prior to radical cystectomy for muscle-invasive transitional cell carcinoma. Treatment regimens have ranged from 500 R in 1 day to 2000 R in 5 days. Such treatment regimens may serve to reduce the incidence of seeding. The short course causes relatively little inconvenience to the patient, in marked contrast to the 3- to 4-month schedule disruption found with the previously standard treatment of 4500 to 5000 R.

Whether preoperative radiation therapy, in fact, does contribute to the somewhat increased survival rates seen recently after radical cystectomy for patients with invasive transitional cell carcinoma remains controversial (Radwin, 1980; Droller, 1983). Many urologic oncologists believe the improved survival figures seen now (in comparison to historical controls) simply result from improved preoperative staging tests (e.g., radionuclide bone scans, CT scanning of the abdomen and chest, magnetic resonance imaging, periaortic lymphadenectomy) from those used in series of patients who had surgery 20 to 30 years ago. There is a continuing need for carefully controlled prospective studies that investigate the value of preoperative radiotherapy for apparently localized, invasive bladder cancer treated by radical cystectomy. Clearly, the trend is away from the use of prolonged high-dose (4000 to 5000 R) preoperative radiation treatment; indeed, many urologic oncologists in current clinical pilot studies have not employed preoperative radiotherapy at all. Some investigators have changed to the use of preoperative systemic cytotoxic chemotherapy.

At present, most patients who have high-grade, deeply invasive (stage P_3 or greater) bladder cancer will eventually die from metastatic transitional cell carcinoma. In general, local control of the tumor is not the problem. It is believed that most patients die from the progressive growth of systemic micrometastases already seeded before the time of radical cystectomy. The abiding hope of all urologic oncologists is that highly active systemic therapy for transitional cell carcinoma will be identified and will permit the development of effective chemotherapy protocols that can be given pre- or postoperatively for patients with deeply invasive or nodal metastatic transitional cell carcinoma. Such adjuvant chemotherapy protocols are under continuous investigation but have not yet been proven efficacious.

Until the demonstration that such pre- or postoperative adjuvant chemotherapy protocols are useful for patients with invasive transitional cell carcinoma, we continue to recommend short-course pelvic radiotherapy prior to cystectomy.

Preoperative Preparation

Combined radical cystectomy and bilateral pelvic lymphadenectomy plus a urinary diversion is one of the most extensive operative procedures performed by urologic surgeons. Many elderly patients or younger patients with major medical problems are not good candidates for this procedure; some alternative form of treatment for their bladder cancer, such as segmental resection or definitive external-beam radiotherapy, should be selected. For patients who do appear to have adequate physiologic reserve to undergo radical cystectomy, it is imperative for them to be in optimal condition prior to surgery. Thus, preoperative preparation for radical cystectomy requires "fine-tuning" of the patient's other medical problems, particularly cardiovascular disease, pulmonary problems, and obesity. The urinary tract should be sterilized preoperatively. Our patients are usually hospitalized 2 days before anticipated surgery, and a combined mechanical and antibiotic (erythromycin-neomycin) bowel preparation is performed to clean and decompress the intestine and to reduce the risk of sepsis should rectal injury occur during pelvic dissection. This measure is particularly important for patients who have had previous pelvic surgery or high-dose pelvic irradiation. A vigorous pulmonary toilet is carried out preoperatively for patients with chronic bronchitis. All patients receive intravenous hydration for 12 hours before surgery to neutralize the fluid and electrolyte loss generated by the bowel preparation and the restriction of oral intake. Finally, the surgeon and an enterostomal therapist locate and mark the best skin site for the stoma of the ileal conduit. Several units of blood for possible transfusion should also be available.

Surgical Technique

After anesthesia is induced, male patients are positioned supine on the operating table. Female patients are placed in a modified lithotomy position or "frog-legged" so that the perineum and vaginal introitus can be visualized. Male patients who require concurrent en bloc urethrectomy are also initially placed in a modified lithotomy position. If a difficult pelvic dissection with increased risk of rectal injury is anticipated because of the patient's history or physical examination (previous pelvic surgery, high-dose pelvic irradiation, extremely large tumor), a large-bore rectal tube is placed at this time to aid identification of rectal injury. The abdomen is prepared from the nipples to the thighs, and the perineum and external genitalia are included in this sterile operative field. An indwelling urethral catheter is placed in the bladder.

A midline abdominal incision is made, extending from the pubis to the epigastrium. The skin incision is brought lateral to the midline on the side away from the anticipated conduit stoma site to facilitate placement of the urine collection device (Fig. 71–6). The midline urachal remnant is identified near the umbilicus and divided, and the peritoneum is incised along the lateral umbilical ligaments toward the bladder. Careful abdominal exploration is then performed. The liver is palpated for metastases and the gallbladder is carefully inspected; if stones have formed, cholecystectomy should be considered. The retroperitoneal lymph node chains are palpated; any suspicious nodes are excised for biopsy. We do not ordinarily perform routine para-aortic lymph node dissection in the absence of palpable nodal enlargement. But some surgeons do sample such nodes, finding that normal-sized nodes are occasionally involved and thus aborting the radical procedure. The pelvic organs are then carefully inspected, particularly the obturator fossa and the iliac lymph node chains bilaterally, in search of macroscopic metastases that might preclude the performance of radical cystectomy. The pelvic visceral structures are also palpated to assess the extent of extravesical tumor extension. If exploration suggests that the patient is still a candidate for radical extirpation of the bladder, the intestine is mobilized. The peritoneal attachments of the sigmoid colon laterally are incised from the pelvis up to the level of the lower pole of the left kidney. The posterior

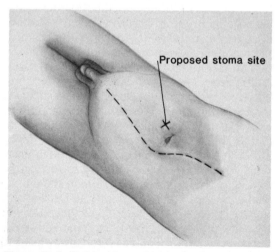

Proposed stoma site

Figure 71–6. Incision for radical cystectomy. A midline incision is made extending from the pubis to the epigastrium. The incision is swung to the contralateral side from the previously marked proposed stomal site on the skin in order to leave more virgin territory to attach the urinary collection device.

peritoneal attachments of the right colon, cecum, and small bowel mesentery are also incised, and the right colon and small bowel are packed superiorly in the abdomen so that unencumbered dissection of the pelvis can be carried out (Skinner, 1982a).

Pelvic Lymphadenectomy

Patients who have received prior (more than 8 weeks before surgery) high-dose (more than 5000 R) external-beam radiotherapy to the pelvis often have a fibrotic, even woody, texture to the fat and connective tissue in the pelvis, which makes all pelvic surgery difficult, particularly the performance of a technically satisfactory pelvic lymphadenectomy. We usually do not perform a systematic bilateral pelvic lymphadenectomy for patients who have received prior high-dose radiotherapy when such scarred pelvic tissues are found. However, in most other patients with transitional cell carcinoma of the urinary bladder who are candidates for radical

cystectomy, a bilateral pelvic lymphadenectomy is performed concurrently to detect and remove nodal metastases.

Patients who have extensive macroscopic nodal metastases in the pelvic lymph nodes (or retroperitoneal nodes) generally have a grim prognosis. At present, such patients are not usually treated by radical cystectomy and urinary diversion but receive postexploration systemic cytotoxic chemotherapy. Occasionally, patients will have a small number of microscopic nodal metastases. (Such nodal metastases are even found occasionally in patients with pathologically proven diffuse transitional cell carcinoma in situ, which would suggest undetected microinvasion in the bladder. We believe that patients who receive radical cystectomy for the indication of diffuse carcinoma in situ therefore also should undergo pelvic lymphadenectomy.) Some patients with a few nodal metastases apparently can be cured by radical cystectomy that includes a systematic bilateral lymphadenec-

Figure 71–7. Technique of pelvic lymphadenectomy. *A,* First, the posterior peritoneum overlying the presumed course of the ureters as they cross into the pelvis is incised on each side. *B,* The ureter is identified where it crosses the common iliac artery and is dissected free from the retroperitoneal structures. A narrow Penrose drain is placed around it to retract the ureter out of the way during subsequent pelvic lymphadenectomy. The anterior surfaces of the common, external, and internal iliac arteries are dissected free from the overlying peritoneum. *C* and *D,* The fibrofatty and nodal tissue surrounding the distal common iliac artery and vein, the internal iliac artery, and the external iliac artery and vein is then systematically stripped from around these vessels. Numerous hemoclips are used to control the afferent and efferent lymph vessels. Total removal of the fatty connective tissue surrounding the vessels from the mid–common iliac artery to the inguinal ligament is performed. *E,* The connective tissue contents of the obturator fossa are completely removed, with care taken to protect the obturator nerve.

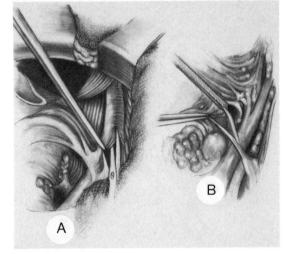

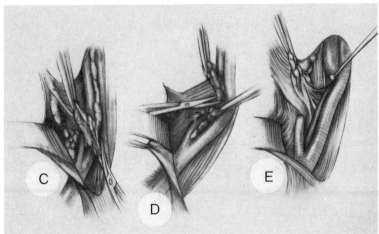

tomy (Dretler et al., 1973; Skinner, 1982b). Most patients with nodal metastases of any extent, however, will subsequently show metastatic recurrences, just as is commonly true for patients with pelvic nodal metastases from prostate adenocarcinoma (Barzell et al., 1977). Because of the few patients with limited nodal metastatic disease who can be salvaged by this technique, we believe that most patients with transitional cell carcinoma of the bladder should be offered pelvic lymphadenectomy at the time of radical cystectomy. It is to be hoped that, in the near future, patients with "positive nodes" will be treated routinely with active adjuvant systemic chemotherapy and will come to enjoy a more favorable prognosis than is observed now in its absence. When this time comes, formal staging pelvic lymphadenectomy will become a nearly mandatory procedure for determining subsequent therapy.

Technique. The posterior peritoneum is incised bilaterally, and the ureters are identified as they cross the common iliac vessels (Fig. 71–7). They are dissected free from the retroperitoneum, and Penrose drains are placed around the ureters to retract them out of the operative field during the lymphadenectomy. To initiate this procedure, the pelvic peritoneum overlying the common and external iliac arteries is sharply incised. The incision in the peritoneum is extended anteriorly to the level of the previous anterior peritoneal incision. Ligation and division of the vasa deferens or the round ligaments are then carried out.

The tactical goal of pelvic lymphadenectomy is to remove all the pelvic lymph nodes constituting the first echelon of lymph drainage from the bladder (Fig. 71–8) (Lieber, 1982). Consequently, the lymph nodes and adjacent tissues surrounding the internal and external iliac vessels and the distal common iliac arteries must be systematically resected. The fibrofatty areolar and nodal tissue surrounding these vessels and the fatty tissue in the obturator fossae

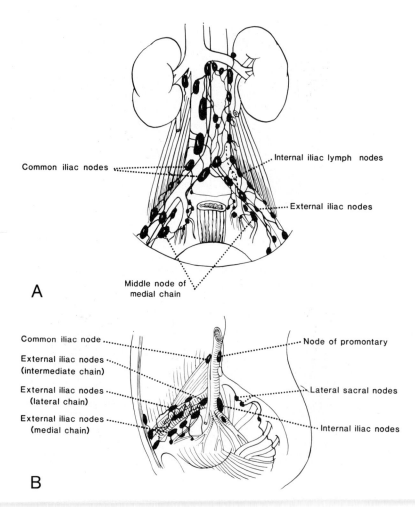

A

Common iliac nodes

Internal iliac lymph nodes

External iliac nodes

Middle node of medial chain

B

Common iliac node

External iliac nodes (intermediate chain)

External iliac nodes (lateral chain)

External iliac nodes (medial chain)

Node of promontary

Lateral sacral nodes

Internal iliac nodes

Figure 71–8. *A* and *B,* Lymph node anatomy of the pelvis. The strategic goal of pelvic lymphadenectomy is to remove the first echelon of lymph node drainage from the bladder and prostate. Numerous anatomic studies have demonstrated that the nodes that constitute this first echelon of drainage lie along the common, external, and internal iliac vessels in the pelvis. There are the nodes to be removed by meticulous pelvic lymphadenectomy. The so-called obturator lymph node, which is so commonly involved in metastatic bladder and prostate cancer, in fact is the middle node of the medial external iliac lymph node chain.

on each side must be cleanly excised. Pelvic lymph node dissection on the side of the pelvis in which the bladder tumor is located is usually performed first because metastatic nodal deposits are most likely found on the ipsilateral side of the pelvis. The margins of lymph node dissection are the inguinal ligament distally, the mid common iliac artery proximally, the genitofemoral nerves laterally, and the endopelvic fascia and contents of the obturator fossae medially.

Node dissection is begun by incising the fibroareolar tissue from the anterior surface of the common and external iliac arteries (Fig. 71–7). A rake retractor is used to elevate the abdominal wall in the region of the inguinal ligament. The lymph vessels coursing cephalad along the external iliac artery and vein are ligated with hemoclips. The fibronodal tissue overlying Cooper's ligament is totally removed with care to avoid injuring an accessory obturator vein, if present. Fibrofatty nodal tissues around the external artery and vein are then systematically stripped cephalad. Small hemoclips are used to control the few small branch vessels. Large hemoclips are used to control the proximal limit of the pelvic node dissection at the level of the mid–common iliac artery. The nodal tissue at the bifurcation of the common iliac artery and along the internal iliac or hypogastric artery is also excised. The pelvic fascia along the genitofemoral nerve is incised and the fatty nodal tissue is passed behind the external iliac vein into the obturator fossa (Fig. 71–9). The obturator nerve is identified and carefully preserved as the contents of the obturator fossa down to the endopelvic fascia, in particular the medial external iliac lymph node chain, are carefully removed.

The pelvic lymph node tissue is sent for frozen-section pathologic examination. If extensive metastatic involvement of the pelvic lymph nodes with transitional cell carcinoma indicates that radical cystectomy will not be potentially curative, the surgeon must re-evaluate the situation. The presence of even one microscopic nodal metastasis is a bad prognostic sign. Nevertheless, a few patients with limited nodal metastases can still be cured by an aggressive surgical approach, including meticulous bilateral pelvic lymphadenectomy and radical cystectomy (Skinner, 1982*b*). Taking the patient's age and overall medical condition into account, radical cystectomy for *palliation* may still be advisable to alleviate the potential for symptoms such as vesical bleeding and pelvic pain.

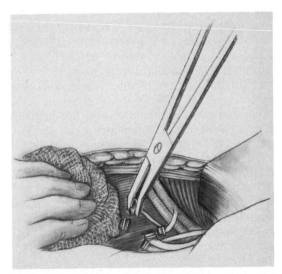

Figure 71–9. Radical cystectomy. Radical cystectomy is begun by dividing the vascular pedicles coming into the bladder posterolaterally from the anterior branches of the internal iliac artery and vein. These structures are usually well identified after a preceding pelvic lymphadenectomy. The technique illustrated by Skinner (1982a) and others, of formally separating the bladder pedicles into a lateral and a posterior group by using one's fingers, can be most helpful in an obese patient or one without extensive previous pelvic irradiation. We generally use large metal hemoclips to control the vascular pedicles, dividing between the clips. Care must be taken subsequently to avoid wiping the clips off the vascular stumps. The usual routine is to divide the lateral pedicles down to the area of the endopelvic fascia on each side prior to incising the peritoneum in the cul-de-sac.

Technique of Radical Cystectomy

To proceed with radical cystectomy, the ureters are ligated and divided deep in the pelvis, and biopsy specimens of the terminal ureters are sent for frozen-section analysis. The presence of carcinoma in situ or atypia in the distal ureters mandates resection of the ureters at a higher level. Large hemoclips are usually used to ligate the distal ureteral stumps deep in the pelvis. If the patient has received high-dose radiation to the pelvis, the pelvic ureters are sacrificed and a more proximal level on the ureters is used for the ureteroileal anastomosis.

Next, the hypogastric (internal iliac) arteries are ligated just distal to the posterior superior gluteal artery branch on each side. A heavy silk suture, or umbilical tape, is usually used for this purpose. Ligation of the hypogastric arteries at this time can markedly reduce subsequent blood loss during radical cystectomy. Occasionally, in patients who previously have had extensive pelvic radiation therapy or pelvic surgery, the hypogastric arteries are ligated at their origins. These patients may experience claudication in their buttocks postoperatively if they are physically active, so it is advisable to preserve blood flow to the posterior superior gluteal arteries if this is technically possible.

The dome of the bladder is retracted anteriorly by using a heavy traction suture or a tenaculum. An assistant retracts the rectosigmoid superiorly. The upper part of the so-called lateral bladder pedicle, consisting of the umbilical artery, the superior vesical artery, and the associated structures, is usually quite prominent (after pelvic lymph node dissection), and it is ligated with large hemoclips and then divided (Fig. 71–9). Alternatively, the vascular pedicles to the bladder can be controlled with standard heavy sutures of 0 chromic catgut. The routine use of large metal hemoclips, however, accelerates the pelvic dissection and avoids the necessity for a series of large clamps on the bladder pedicles, which somewhat clutter the operative field. After the superior portion of the lateral bladder pedicle is ligated and divided on each side, the peritoneum in the cul-de-sac is sharply incised with a scissors so that the dissection plane between the posterior bladder wall, seminal vesicles, and prostate anteriorly and the rectum posteriorly can be developed (Fig. 71–10).

Developing this plane is one of the critical events of radical cystectomy and must be skill-fully carried out to avoid injury to the rectum. The most common error at this point, however, is to establish this dissection plane too far anterior out of fear of injuring the rectum. This leads the novice into the plane between the posterior bladder wall and the seminal vesicles. We believe the surgeon should aim for a plane directly anterior to the rectum, behind or between Denonvilliers' fascia, which in the non-irradiated pelvis readily leads down the anterior surface of the rectum behind the prostate and the membranous urethra. As this plane is gently developed, careful blind digital dissection is used to separate the rectum from the posterior vascular pedicles coming anteriorly from the region of the middle hemorrhoidal arteries and going from along the rectum toward the bladder. If at this point a satisfactory plane cannot be easily created between the posterior prostate and the rectum, it is often advisable to beat a retreat and use another tactic to establish this plane, incising the endopelvic fascia along the lateral aspect of the prostate and then developing the plane between the posterior prostate and the rectum, such as one would commonly perform during a radical retropubic prostatectomy. This alternative tactic is more desirable than continuing to dissect digitally from above in a forceful way behind the bladder, with risk of injuring the anterior rectal wall or of breaking into the tumor-filled bladder.

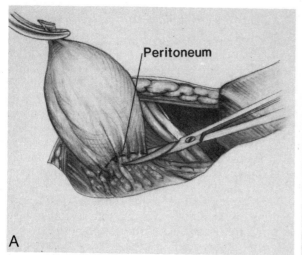
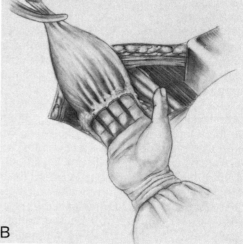

Figure 71–10. Radical cystectomy. *A,* After the lateral vascular pedicles to the bladder have been divided, the peritoneum in the cul-de-sac between the posterior bladder wall and the rectum is sharply divided with a scissors. *B,* The potential plane between the anterior rectal wall and the posterior bladder, seminal vesicles, and prostate is then developed blindly, using one's fingers. The goal is to push the rectum posteriorly away from the bladder, seminal vesicles, and prostate and to delineate the so-called posterior pedicles coming to the bladder from alongside the rectum. Staying close to the rectum usually leads into this plane most easily. The vas deferens can often be visualized in thin individuals and can be used to identify the correct latitude for dissection as well. A common error is to stay too far anteriorly. In seeking to avoid a rectal injury, one enters the plane between the back of the bladder and the seminal vesicles, which is a temporary dead end.

Once the plane between the posterior bladder, seminal vesicles, prostate, and rectum has been fully developed, the bladder is again retracted anteriorly and the remaining vascular pedicles attaching the bladder to the posterior and posterolateral pelvis are ligated and divided. Digital separation of these pedicles into lateral and posterior groups facilitates control and ligation (Skinner, 1982a). Once again, large metal hemoclips or standard heavy-caliber sutures may be used to ligate the pedicles. After the lateral and posterior pedicles have been ligated on each side, the bladder and prostate are left attached anteriorly to the endopelvic fascia, the puboprostatic ligaments, and the urethra. At this juncture, some surgeons instill a small volume of 10 per cent formalin into the bladder via the Foley catheter, to prevent seeding if any urine leaks out in subsequent steps. The endopelvic fascia is incised on each side of the prostate, and the plane between the distal prostate and rectum is further extended. The puboprostatic ligaments are then ligated with hemoclips and divided (Fig. 71–11). The tissue at the prostatic apex and around the membranous urethra is incised. Bleeding from the periprostatic veins may be profuse at this point. Nevertheless, careful attentive dissection must be performed at this stage to dissect and telescope as much membranous urethra as possible proximally, and to place a heavy clamp around the urethra, well past the prostatic apex, before the urethra is sharply divided, with one finger behind to protect the rectum. The bladder specimen is then free and can be removed from the operative field. A fresh urethral catheter is then passed retrograde, inflated with 50 ml of water in the

balloon, and placed on traction to tamponade venous bleeding from the urogenital diaphragm. A pack is placed in the true pelvis. Attention is then turned to fashioning the ileal conduit urinary diversion. After an hour or so, the urogenital diaphragm is again inspected for bleeding. Suture ligatures will usually control any residual arterial or extensive venous bleeding from the urogenital diaphragm; we often leave the indwelling urethral catheter with the balloon inflated on gentle traction for 24 hours to tamponade slow bleeding. The rectum is again carefully inspected for any injury.

Potency-Preserving Radical Cystectomy Technique. A technique for avoiding the paraprostatic nerves coursing down to the corpora cavernosa has been developed for radical retropubic prostatectomy by Walsh. His modification of the radical cystectomy technique to achieve the same goal is appended to Chapter 76.

Radical Cystectomy in the Female Patient

This procedure is usually an anterior exenteration with removal of the bladder, urethra, anterior vaginal wall, uterus, fallopian tubes, and ovaries (Nelson, 1977). The vascular pedicles to the ovaries, the infundibulopelvic ligaments, are ligated and divided early in the operation. The vascular pedicles to the bladder and uterus and the plane between the posterior vagina and the rectum can be developed in a fashion similar to the operative approach used in the male. For large bladder tumors, particularly those close to the bladder neck or involving the proximal urethra, which require excision of an extensive amount of neighboring vaginal

Figure 71–11. Radical cystectomy. After the lateral and posterior pedicles to the bladder have been divided, the specimen is attached only at the prostate apex and by the membranous urethra. The endopelvic fascia is incised along the prostate laterally. Hemoclips are placed across the puboprostatic ligaments, which are sharply divided. The urethra is dissected carefully from within the mass of tissue at the prostatic apex. By pulling cephalad and dissecting sharply, 4 to 5 cm of urethra can be telescoped from within the urogenital diaphragm and perineum, making subsequent urethrectomy much easier. A heavy clamp is placed across the urethra and the catheter to prevent spillage of tumor cells into the wound, and the urethra and catheter are divided with a heavy scissors.

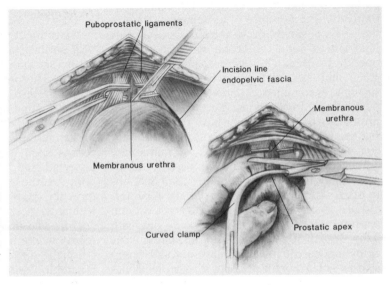

Puboprostatic ligaments

Incision line
endopelvic fascia

Membranous
urethra

Membranous urethra

Curved clamp

Prostatic apex

tissue, we often remove the entire vagina to the introitus with this approach. Generally, however, only the anterior one third of the vaginal wall is removed with the bladder, including the entire urethra. With the surgeon's fingers in the vagina, the cutting cautery is used to incise the vagina laterally beginning at the posterior fornix, while the lateral vascular pedicles to the uterus and bladder are controlled with hemoclips or sutures. The usual technique of leaving the posterior vaginal wall on the anterior surface of the rectum avoids risk of rectal injury and can be particularly useful in the presence of previous pelvic irradiation or surgery. If an adequate amount of the vagina remains, i.e., the posterolateral two thirds, a vaginal cuff can be reconstructed; we close the vagina with a heavy absorbable suture. Alternatively, a smaller posterior vaginal flap can be left on the anterior rectal wall; the introitus is then closed. In any event, female patients must be apprised of the possible or probable loss of a functional vagina prior to the time of radical cystectomy.

Postoperative Care

Radical cystectomy with bilateral pelvic lymphadenectomy and ilial conduit urinary diversion is an extensive procedure that often requires an operating time of 4 to 6 hours (or more in patients who are massively obese or who have had previous surgery or irradiation). Vigorous replacement of blood and fluid losses must proceed intraoperatively and postoperatively, sometimes assisted by a central venous catheter. A heating blanket may be useful to prevent profound intraoperative hypothermia in difficult cases. The loss of plasma from the large raw spaces created ("third spacing") can be particularly large and should be replaced quantitatively. The presence of a Hemovac drain in the pelvis postoperatively helps to measure this fluid loss as well as to detect evidence of postoperative bleeding. Vigorous pulmonary hygiene and early activity and ambulation are strongly encouraged to prevent postoperative pulmonary complications. Certain experienced urologic-oncologic surgeons have recommended the use of intraoperative or postoperative anticoagulation to reduce the risk of pulmonary embolism in the postoperative period; this is one of the most common major complications to occur after extensive pelvic surgery (Skinner, 1982a). A common regimen is to start sodium warfarin on the second postoperative day with a low dose of 10 to 15 mg either intramuscularly or by nasogastric tube. We have not had extensive experience with perioperative anticoagulation for radical cystectomy at our institution.

URETHRECTOMY

Indications

In general, we usually do not perform concurrent or en bloc urethrectomy at the time of radical cystectomy in male patients. Total urethrectomy is, of course, performed at the time of standard radical cystectomy in women. It is only male patients with transitional cell carcinoma in their anterior or prostatic urethras for whom we consider it imperative to perform an en bloc urethrectomy. These patients constitute only a small minority of patients coming to radical cystectomy. En bloc urethrectomy adds significantly to the operating time of an already extensive procedure, usually 45 to 60 minutes in our experience. Moreover, the moderate lithotomy position in which the patient is placed at the time of concurrent cystectomy is less ideal for urethrectomy in the male patient than is the exaggerated lithotomy position, which may be employed at the time of a secondary urethrectomy. Therefore, for patients with transitional cell carcinoma at the bladder neck or multifocal high-grade carcinoma in situ in the bladder, we do recommend urethrectomy, but only 3 to 6 months after the patient has recovered from radical cystectomy. The progress of other patients with bladder cancer treated by radical cystectomy is followed by cytologic evaluation of urethral washings, and urethrectomy is recommended if neoplastic or atypical cells become evident. For patients who have penile prostheses inserted to restore potency after radical cystectomy, a perineal approach affords a good opportunity to perform a urethrectomy at the same time.

Technique

Urethrectomy is performed through a vertical perineal incision extending from the base of the scrotum to a point near the anus (Fig. 71–12). The presence of a sound or a catheter in the urethra greatly facilitates efforts to stay in the midline and to come right down on the dorsal surface of the urethra. The bulbocavernosus muscle is divided in the midline and the corpus spongiosum containing the urethra is dissected free from its attachments to the corpora cavernosa. We dissect and invert the urethra and penis into the perineum, using the technique described by Whitmore and Mount (1970). The urethra is dissected distally to the region where it enters the glans penis and then is usually ligated at this point. Because of unfavorable cosmetic results, we have not been particularly satisfied with any of the procedures

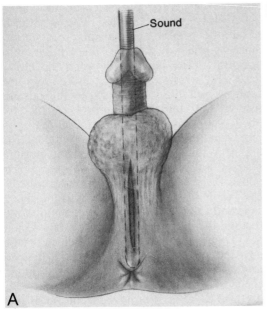 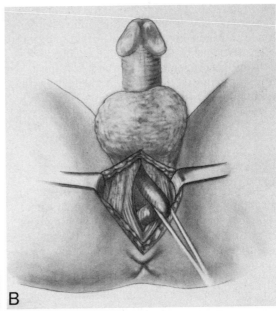

Figure 71–12. Urethrectomy. Urethrectomy is greatly facilitated by having the patient placed in the exaggerated lithotomy position. *A,* A midline incision in the perineum is made over a sound or relatively rigid catheter present in the urethra. Keeping the incision strictly in the midline over the urethra reduces bleeding. *B,* After the bulbocavernosus muscle is divided, the corpus spongiosum is separated from the corpus cavernosum by sharp dissection. A Penrose drain is placed around the bulbous urethra and the urethra and penis are inverted into the perineum using the technique of Whitmore and Mount (1970). Sharp dissection is required to separate the corpus spongiosum and urethra from the corpus cavernosum as the inversion operation proceeds. Cautery is required to control numerous small bleeding points. Blood loss can be reduced if careful dissection is used to avoid entering the substance of the corpus spongiosum or corpus cavernosum. Two assistants holding retractors in the perineum are often required to allow visualization of the proximal urethral dissection up to the urogenital diaphragm. Extensive use of the cautery and suction is needed to allow anatomic dissection and to prevent unnecessary blood loss during the proximal dissection of the urethrectomy.

recommended to remove the terminal 2 cm of urethra from within the glans penis. Therefore, we have generally avoided removing the very distal glandular urethra unless tumor is present within it. After the distal urethra is ligated and divided, we dissect proximally toward the urogenital diaphragm. If possible, the small arteries to the bulb are identified visually at the 4 and 8 o'clock positions and are ligated with fine sutures. Care is taken to separate the proximal urethra from the central tendon of the perineum and to carefully mobilize the urethra dorsally to avoid any potential rectal injury.

The urethral dissection proximally requires good visualization, and care must be taken to have adequate local exposure and to cauterize the small blood vessels encountered as one moves cephalad. Otherwise, one may dissect a small, blood-filled hole. With generous use of diathermy and suction, and two or three carefully placed perineal retractors, the proximal corpus spongiosum is dissected up to the urogenital diaphragm and is severed at this point. Cautery is again used to obtain complete hemostasis from the generally oozing urogenital

diaphragm. A small Hemovac drain is left against the urogenital diaphragm and is brought out into the urethral bed distally. The end of the Hemovac drain is brought out through a separate stab wound lateral to the perineal incision. The subcutaneous fascia in the perineum is approximated with a running absorbable suture and the skin incision is similarly closed with a buried absorbable suture.

For patients with known tumors of the prostatic, membranous, or penile urethras who do require en bloc urethrectomy, the same general technique is utilized. The urethra is mobilized in the perineum *after* it has been determined by intra-abdominal surgery that radical cystectomy is indicated and technically can be performed. The urethral portion of the operation should not be performed if the bladder is not to be removed. Subsequently, after the bladder is fully mobilized and dissected free, the urethrectomy portion of the procedure is performed through the perineum. This is one instance in which availability of a second surgical team to perform the perineal portion of the operation while another team proceeds with the ileoconduit urinary diversion can save time. If en bloc or concurrent urethrectomy is performed, an indwelling urethral catheter cannot be left in the pelvis to tamponade venous bleeding from the urogenital diaphragm; suture ligatures are required to close the defect in the pelvic floor and to control bleeding.

SIMPLE CYSTECTOMY

Indications

Simple cystectomy is and should be an uncommon operation. Occasionally, however, it may be required in the presence of nonmalignant disease affecting the bladder. Typical instances would be a chronically infected neurogenic bladder (pyocystis) in a patient who had already received a supravesical urinary diversion or in a patient with chronic interstitial cystitis who is not a candidate for augmentation cystoplasty and who remains symptomatic (pelvic pain) after urinary diversion. In such male patients, removal of the prostate and seminal vesicles is not necessary and potency often can be preserved by simply removing the supraprostatic bladder wall itself. In female patients, removal of the bladder and urethra can be performed without removing a significant amount of anterior vaginal wall, and the uterus and female genital organs in the pelvis need not be removed at the time of bladder excision.

Technique

Patients who require simple cystectomy often have undergone previous supravesical urinary diversion. In such patients, the pelvic surgery can be performed satisfactorily through a small, lower midline or transverse abdominal incision. Entering the peritoneal cavity may not be necessary. The pelvic peritoneum is stripped off the dome of the bladder with care to maintain adequate hemostasis. Dissection is carried out along the serosal surface of the bladder wall. In the female patient, careful dissection continues along the bladder wall circumferentially, with the arteries and veins entering the bladder muscle controlled by cautery, hemoclips, or suture ligatures. Dissection of the bladder wall away from the lower uterus and anterior vaginal wall is carefully performed, hemostasis is assured, and the defect in the vagina resulting from removal of the bladder neck and urethra is closed with heavy absorbable sutures.

In the male patient, simple cystectomy can be readily performed as an extraperitoneal pro-

cedure. The peritoneum overlying the dome of the bladder is dissected free. The junction between the prostate and bladder is identified, much as one would in forming a radical prostatectomy. The junction between the bladder neck and prostate is then divided by using cautery, and the plane between the posterior bladder wall and the seminal vesicles is developed just as is done for a radical retropubic prostatectomy with the modified Campbell technique. With the plane between the posterior bladder wall and the seminal vesicles and ampullae of the vasa well established, it is relatively easy to hug the bladder wall posteriorly and superiorly and to develop the plane between the rectum, the overlying peritoneum, and the bladder. The posterolateral vascular pedicles coming into the bladder are then divided serially by using hemoclips, working retrograde, beginning at the bladder neck and coming superiorly. The urethral catheter is removed from the prostatic urethra, which is closed with several absorbable sutures. A large Hemovac drain is retained in the bed of the bladder and is brought out through a separate stab incision to drain the former vesical space.

CONCLUSION

The urinary bladder is a wonderful and forgiving organ. Its extensive blood supply permits ready healing and extensive plastic surgery. Conversely, the anatomic location of the bladder deep in the true pelvis, its close relation to the rectum, and its immense blood supply can lead to formidable challenges for the urologic surgeon. In general, we have found that open bladder surgery can be a safe and straightforward surgical pursuit if concentrated attention is directed toward the relevant anatomy. Moreover, much consideration also must be given to controlling blood vessels and hemorrhage during vesical surgery. The use of cautery to control bleeding at the time of cystotomy is one such method. Systematic control of the vascular pedicles to the bladder along the pelvic sidewalls at the time of cystectomy can be accomplished by careful anatomic dissection and visual ligation of the feeding arteries and veins, and is also desirable to prevent unnecessary blood loss. Bladder surgery, particularly radical cystectomy or an extensive vesical diverticulectomy, simply need not be carried out in a pool of blood. Attention to basic surgical techniques, particularly anatomy and thorough hemostasis, will almost inevitably lead to highly successful bladder surgery and the absence of injuries to adjacent structures.

References

Barzell, W., Bean, M. A., Hilaris, B. S., and Whitmore, W. F., Jr.: Prostatic adenocarcinoma: relationship of grade and local extent to the pattern of metastases. J. Urol., *118*:278, 1977.

Blandy, J. P., England, H. R., Evans, S. J., Hope-Stone, H. F., Mair, G. M., Mantell, B. S., Oliver, R. T., Paris, A. M., and Resdon, R. A.: T3 bladder cancer—the case for salvage cystectomy. Br. J. Urol., *52*:506, 1980.

Bloom, H. J. G., Hendry, W. F., Wallace, D. M., and Skeet, R. G.: Treatment of T3 bladder cancer: controlled trial of pre-operative radiotherapy and radical cystectomy versus radical radiotherapy. Second report and review (for the Clinical Trials Group, Institute of Urology). Br. J. Urol., *54*:136, 1982.

Crawford, E. D., and Skinner, D. G.: Salvage cystectomy after irradiation failure. J. Urol., *123*:32, 1980.

DeWeerd, J. H., Colby, M. Y., Jr., Segura, J. W., Utz, D. C., and Cupps, R. E.: Invasive bladder carcinoma managed by irradiation and surgery. Urology, *20*:471, 1982.

Dretler, S. P., Ragsdale, B. D., and Leadbetter, W. F.: The value of pelvic lymphadenectomy in the surgical treatment of bladder cancer. J. Urol., *109*:414, 1973.

Droller, M. J.: The controversial role of radiation therapy as adjunctive treatment of bladder cancer. J. Urol., *129*:897, 1983.

Gavrell, G. J., Lewis, R. W., Meehan, W. L., and Leblanc, G. A.: Intravesical thio-tepa in the immediate postoperative period in patients with recurrent transitional cell carcinoma of the bladder. J. Urol., *120*:410, 1978.

Hope-Stone, H. F., Blandy, J. P., Oliver, R. T. D., and England, H.: Radical radiotherapy and salvage cystectomy in the treatment of invasive carcinoma of the bladder. *In* Oliver, R. T. D., Hendry, W. F., and Bloom, H. J. G. (Eds.): Bladder Cancer: Principles of Combination Therapy. London, Butterworths, 1981, p. 127.

Kiker, J. D., and Crawford, E. D.: Partial cystectomy. *In* Crawford, E. D., and Borden, T. A. (Eds.): Genitourinary Cancer Surgery. Philadelphia, Lea & Febiger, 1982, p. 217.

Lieber, M. M.: Pelvic lymphadenectomy. *In* Crawford, E. D., and Borden, T. A. (Eds.): Genitourinary Cancer Surgery. Lea & Febiger, 1982, p. 142.

Nelson, J. H., Jr.: Atlas of Radical Pelvic Surgery. 2nd ed. New York, Appleton-Century-Crofts, 1977.

Prout, G. R., Jr., Slack, N. H., and Bross, I. D. J.: Irradiation and 5-fluorouracil as adjuvants in the management of invasive bladder carcinoma. A cooperative group report after 4 years. J. Urol., *104*:116, 1970.

Radwin, H. M.: Radiotherapy and bladder cancer: a critical review. J. Urol., *124*:43, 1980.

Reid, E. C., Oliver, J. A., and Fishman, I. J.: Preoperative irradiation and cystectomy in 135 cases of bladder cancer. Urology, *8*:247, 1976.

Skinner, D. G.: Radical cystectomy. *In* Crawford, E. D., and Borden, T. A. (Eds.): Genitourinary Cancer Surgery. Philadelphia, Lea & Febiger, 1982*a*, p. 207.

Skinner, D. G.: Management of invasive bladder cancer: meticulous pelvic node dissection can make difference. J. Urol., *128*:34, 1982*b*.

Skinner, D. G., Tift, J. P., and Kaufman, J. J.: High dose, short course preoperative radiation therapy and immediate single stage radical cystectomy with pelvic node dissection in management of bladder cancer. J. Urol., *127*:671, 1982.

Utz, D. C., and DeWeerd, J. H.: The management of low grade, low stage carcinoma of the bladder. *In* Skinner, D. G., and deKernion, J. B. (Eds.): Genitourinary Cancer. Philadelphia, W. B. Saunders Co., 1978.

van der Werf–Messing, B.: Carcinoma of the bladder treated by suprapubic radium implants. The value of additional external irradiation. Eur. J. Cancer Clin. Oncol., *5*:277, 1969.

Wallace, D. M., and Bloom, H. J. G.: The management of deeply infiltrating (T3) bladder carcinoma: controlled trial of radical radiotherapy versus preoperative radiotherapy and radical cystectomy (first report). Br. J. Urol., *48*:587, 1976.

Whitmore, W. F., Jr., Batata, M. A., Ghoneim, M. A., Grabstald, H., and Unal, A.: Radical cystectomy with or without prior irradiation in the treatment of bladder cancer. J. Urol., *118*:184, 1977.

Whitmore, W. F., Jr., Batata, M. A., Hilaris, B. S., Reddy, G. N., Unal, A., Ghoneim, M. A., Grabstald, H., and Chu, F.: A comparative study of 2 preoperative radiation regimens with cystectomy for bladder cancer. Cancer, *40*:1077, 1977.

Whitmore, W. F., Jr., and Mount, B. M.: A technique of urethrectomy in the male. Surg. Gynecol. Obstet., *131*:303, 1970.

CHAPTER 72

The Treatment of Male Urinary Incontinence

H. ROGER HADLEY, M.D.
PHILIPPE E. ZIMMERN, M.D.
SHLOMO RAZ, M.D.

Although incontinence is not a life-threatening disease, the embarrassment, humiliation, and inconvenience it causes make it a "social cancer." Since pediatric incontinence will be discussed in detail elsewhere, we will focus primarily on the prevalence, anatomy, physiology, etiology, evaluation, and treatment of adult male urinary incontinence.

PREVALENCE

In the community, the prevalence of unrecognized incontinence (those men between the ages of 15 and 64 years not actively seeking medical attention for their wetness) was determined by use of a postal survey to be 1 to 2 per cent. Recognized incontinence (those men seeking medical attention) in the same age group, however, was approximately 0.1 per cent (Thomas et al., 1980; Feneley et al., 1979). For those over the age of 65 years and residing in the community, 7 to 17 per cent were incontinent (Vetter et al., 1969; Brocklehurst, 1978). Among elderly patients residing in long-term care institutions, 18 to 55 per cent were incontinent (Brocklehurst, 1978; U.S. DHEW Study, 1975).

Prostatectomy is one of the major causes of urinary incontinence in the nonelderly population. In 1978, approximately 300,000 prostatectomies were recorded in the United States (DHEW Statistics, 1980). The number of prostatectomies performed increases each year in disproportion to the population growth. This difference may be explained by safer operations, better patient acceptance, better health insurance, longer life expectancy, and greater numbers of urologists (Birkhoff, 1983). If 0.1 to 1.0 per cent of these procedures are complicated by incontinence, then one may extrapolate that 300 to 3000 men become incontinent each year.

ANATOMY OF CONTINENCE

Detrusor

Most anatomists agree that the detrusor muscle coat consists of numerous interlacing, intricately connecting smooth muscle bundles that are similar histologically and histochemically. This arrangement is ideally suited to cause reduction in all dimensions of the bladder during contraction of the intramural muscle coat.

The trigone of the bladder is composed of two layers: The deep layer is a continuation of the detrusor, and the superficial layer is very thin, extends posteriorly to the level of the verumontanum, and consists of small muscle bundles (Gosling, 1979). The contribution of the superficial layer to continence is probably minimal. It may, however, assist in opening of the bladder neck and closure of the ureterovesical junction during micturition.

Urethra

In the male anatomy, there appear to be two functional urethral sphincters: (1) the proximal urethral sphincter, and (2) the distal urethral sphincter (Fig. 72–1).

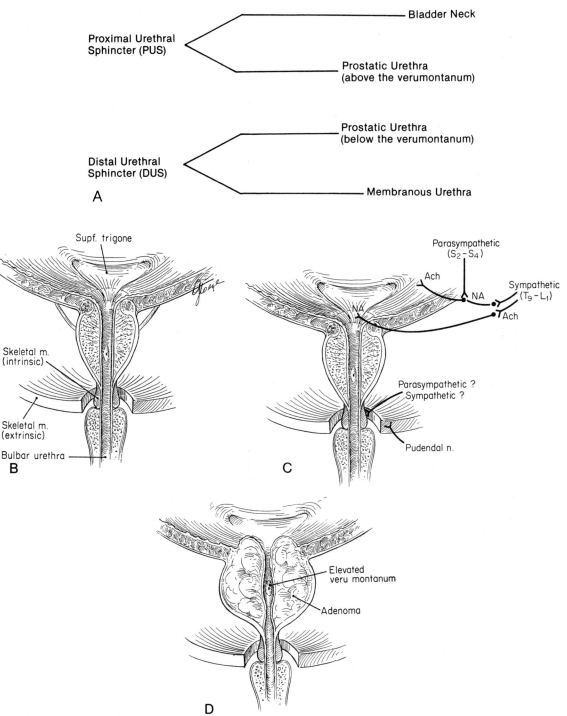

Figure 72–1. *A* and *B*, Normal anatomy of male continence. We have empirically divided the continence mechanism into the proximal urethral sphincter (PUS) and the distal urethral sphincter (DUS). The PUS includes the bladder neck and the prostatic urethra down to the verumontanum. The DUS extends from the verumontanum to the bulbar urethra and consists of (1) smooth muscle that is continuous from the prostatic apex; (2) intrinsic skeletal muscle; and (3) extrinsic skeletal muscle. The latter is attached to the urethra only on its posterior aspect. The bulbar urethra does not contribute to continence. *C,* Innervation of the lower urinary tract. Parasympathetic fibers stimulate contraction of the detrusor. Sympathetic fibers stimulate the bladder neck and inhibit bladder contraction by a blocking effect on the parasympathetic ganglia. The nerve supply to the intrinsic portion of the distal urethra may be autonomic in origin. The pudendal somatic efferents innervate the extrinsic portion of the distal urethral sphincter. *D,* Growth of a prostatic adenoma tends to elevate the verumontanum. This commonly leaves a significant amount of resectable tissue between the verumontanum and the apex of the prostate.

Illustration continued on following page

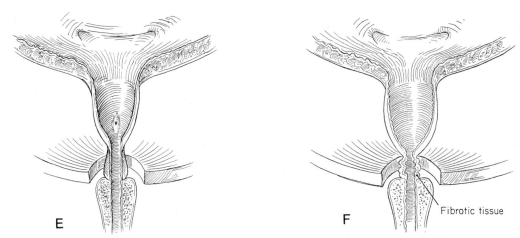

Figure 72–1 *Continued. E,* Continence in a patient after a simple prostatectomy. The infolding of the epithelium, the vascular supply, the smooth musculature, and the "slow-twitch" intrinsic skeletal muscle provide passive continence. Active continence and support of the distal urethra during stress is supplied by the "fast-twitch" pudendal innervated extrinsic muscles. *F,* Scarring of the distal urethral sphincter in a postprostatectomy incontinent patient. Damage is usually to the structures that are responsible for passive continence in the DUS. Rarely is the extrinsic skeletal muscle of the DUS involved.

PROXIMAL URETHRAL SPHINCTER (PUS)

In this discussion, PUS will refer to the bladder neck and prostatic urethra above the verumontanum. It is made up of smooth muscle that is different histologically and histochemically from the detrusor. It is believed that the bladder neck is arranged as a complete circular collar that surrounds the preprostatic portion of the urethra. Distally, this muscle merges with, and is indistinguishable from, the musculature of the prostatic capsule (Gosling, 1979). This fact is in contradiction to the belief that the detrusor extends through the bladder neck and is continuous with the smooth muscle of the urethra (Tanagho and Smith, 1968; Hutch, 1966). In the male urinary tract, the smooth muscle of the bladder neck is richly innervated by noradrenergic (sympathetic) nerve terminals (Gosling et al., 1977). Most investigators agree that this smooth muscle plays an important role in the prevention of retrograde ejaculation. Controversy exists, however, on the exact role of this muscle in the maintenance of passive urinary continence (see further on).

DISTAL URETHRAL SPHINCTER (DUS)

In this discussion, DUS will refer to all the anatomic structures of the urethra extending from the verumontanum, through its membranous portion, and to, but not including, the bulbar urethra (Fig. 72–1*B*). It consists of:

1. An inner layer of epithelial folds that have an abundant vascular supply to make the urethra supple. This adaptability allows sufficient urethral coaptation to result from a minimal amount of circular pressure. This "washer effect" is an important factor in the maintenance of passive continence.

2. A middle layer composed of elastic tissue and smooth muscle.

3. An outer layer of intrinsic and extrinsic skeletal muscles. The intrinsic skeletal muscle is intimately attached to the underlying urethra and is composed of "slow-twitch" fibers that are probably innervated by the autonomic system (Gosling, 1979; Gosling et al., 1981). Because its fibers can maintain tonus for prolonged periods without fatigue, this muscle is ideal for passive continence. The outer or extrinsic layer of skeletal muscle is similar to the surrounding pelvic floor muscles. It is attached to the urethra only on its posterior aspect and acts mainly as a sling. The "fast-twitch" fibers of this muscle are innervated by the pudendal nerve, fatigue more quickly, and contract on voluntary command (Gosling, 1979). This muscle contributes minimally to passive continence, although voluntary contraction of the extrinsic layer permits the interruption of the urinary stream and reinforces the DUS during coughing and straining (Gosling, 1979).

The relative ratio of smooth muscle to skeletal muscle decreases from the proximal to the distal portion of the DUS. A cross-sectional histologic analysis of the proximal portion of the DUS would show primarily smooth muscle, whereas distally, skeletal muscle would predominate.

The innervation of the lower urinary tract is by the sympathetic and parasympathetic divisions of the autonomic system and somatic portions of the pudendal nerves. These regulate the voluntary control of coordinated micturition, continence, penile erection, and ejaculation. The parasympathetic efferents control bladder contraction and are involved in the maintenance of a sustained penile erection. The sympathetic afferents transmit bladder sensations. The sympathetic efferents inhibit detrusor contraction and promote seminal emission (peristalsis of the vas deferens and contraction of the seminal vesicles), psychogenic erection, and bladder neck contraction during ejaculation. The pudendal (somatic) afferents transmit proprioception and exteroception from the urethra, penis, and pelvic floor. The pudendal efferents control jet-type ejaculation and pelvic floor muscle activity, including the extrinsic portion of the DUS (Fig. 72–1C).

The smooth muscle of the bladder is rich in beta receptors that initiate relaxation when stimulated by norepinephrine. This is in contrast to the bladder neck and urethra, which possess mainly alpha receptors that, when stimulated by norepinephrine, respond by contraction.

The nerve supply of the DUS is not well known. The fact that continence is preserved in a postprostatectomy patient whose pudendal nerve has been blocked demonstrates that the extrinsic muscles of the DUS are not needed for passive continence. There may be separate innervation from the pelvic nerve for the intrinsic "slow-twitch" skeletal and smooth muscle of the DUS (Gosling, 1979). Whether this innervation is mediated via the sympathetic, parasympathetic, or both divisions is not well delineated (Elbadawi, 1982). Histochemically, there is evidence that there are alpha receptors in this region (Elbadawi, 1982). Clinically, the administration of an alpha antagonist and agonist will decrease and increase, respectively, the urethral closing pressure in the DUS (Nordling, 1978; Koyanagi, 1980). Some believe that this noradrenergic effect is on the surrounding urethral blood vessels, rather than directly on the intrinsic muscle (Nordling, 1983).

PHYSIOLOGY AND PATHOPHYSIOLOGY OF CONTINENCE

Continence is dependent on the ability of the detrusor to accommodate filling without a significant increase in intravesical pressure, and on passive maintenance of sufficient urethral resistance to prevent leakage of urine. These two factors depend on the neural, muscular, and mechanical properties of the lower urinary tract.

It is accepted that the PUS can maintain passive urinary continence. The role and significance of the sympathetic influence in the maintenance of this continence are subjects of considerable controversy (Nordling, 1983). It seems unlikely that the mechanism of continence of the PUS is dependent exclusively on neural innervation because adrenergic receptors in the PUS are found only in the male anatomy (Gosling et al., 1977), and patients who have had neurologic trauma that obliterates the sympathetic supply to the lower urinary tract do not consistently have an open PUS when studied radiographically (Nordling, 1983). Operative sympathectomy, in general, does not produce any measurable change in lower urinary tract function. This observation may indicate that continuous sympathetic influence is not required to keep the PUS closed. Instead, continence is probably due to the spontaneous activity of the smooth muscle and the arrangement of the muscle fibers around the bladder neck.

Longitudinally, there are three zones of continence in the DUS: (1) verumontanum to the apex of the prostate, (2) apex of the prostate, and (3) apex to the bulbar urethra. These zones play an important part in the understanding of continence and incontinence after prostatectomy (Nordling, 1978) (Fig. 72–2).

Because the PUS is removed during prostatectomy, postoperative continence is dependent on the DUS. This fact is demonstrated by a urethral pressure profile that shows no increase in pressure at the level of the bladder neck (prostatic fossa) but a sufficient elevation of pressure in the region of the DUS (Fig. 72–3). Removal of the proximal one third of the DUS (i.e., verumontanum to apex) during simple prostatectomy (TURP [transurethral resection of the prostate] or open prostatectomy) is not followed by incontinence (Fig. 72–D and E). A radical prostatectomy removes the proximal two thirds (i.e., verumontanum to and including the apex) of the DUS and leaves only the distal one third to maintain continence. Therefore, avoidance of damage to the latter (apex to the bulbar urethral) is of paramount importance for maintenance of passive continence after either type of prostatectomy (Turner-Warwick, 1983).

During a radical retropubic prostatectomy, the extrinsic skeletal portion of the DUS is rarely damaged. This is demonstrated by the

Proximal 1/3	Verumontanum to Apex of the Prostate	Prostatic smooth muscle
Middle 1/3	Apex of the Prostate	Smooth Muscle and Skeletal Muscle, Intrinsic
Distal 1/3	Apex of the Prostate to Bulbar Urethra	Smooth Muscle, Skeletal Muscle — Intrinsic / Extrinsic

Figure 72–2. Distal urethral sphincter (DUS) functional anatomy.

fact that active (voluntary) continence is maintained in most patients with postprostatectomy incontinence (Tanagho, 1981). This sphincter is unavoidably damaged, however, during a radical perineal prostatectomy, with continence being reliant on the intrinsic skeletal layer. Because of the preservation of the mechanism of passive continence (intrinsic smooth and skeletal portions of the DUS), a pudendal block will not render a continent postprostatectomy patient incontinent. On the other hand, incontinent postprostatectomy patients are worse after such a block (Raz, 1978).

During TURP, limitation of the resection to the level of the verumontanum is the most reliable way to assure future continence. When damage occurs to the DUS, it is most frequently located anteriorly between the 10 and 2 o'clock positions (Turner-Warwick, 1983). This damage may be prevented by the use of a 0 degree lens and a nonbeaked resectoscope that allows vision of the verumontanum during the delicate anterior phase of the procedure. Coagulation must be avoided in the vicinity of the verumontanum to prevent fibrosis, which leads to a lack of

compliance of the sphincter zone as well as to narrowing of the urethra (Fig. 72–1F).

After simple retropubic prostatectomy, opening the prostatic urethra on the anterior surface of the adenoma is recommended to visualize precisely the position of the verumontanum and apex prior to incising the apical portion. During radical retropubic prostatectomy, continence is best preserved by avoidance of (1) excessive coagulation and dissection of the membranous urethra, (2) tension on the urethra during its transection and (3) anastomotic leaks that may lead to fibrosis.

ETIOLOGY OF MALE URINARY INCONTINENCE

Urinary incontinence results when the bladder has (1) an inability to store, or (2) a combination of an inability to store and empty (overflow) (Fig. 72–4). The inability to store may be due to urethral insufficiency or bladder instability. Urethral insufficiency occurs only when both the PUS and the DUS have been

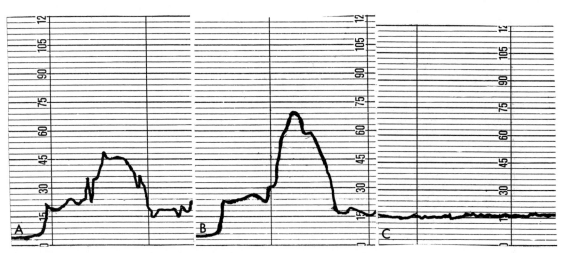

Figure 72–3. Urethral pressure profile studies in a patient with postprostatectomy incontinence. A, Maximal closing pressure of 45 cm of water. B, Closing pressure of 70 cm of water upon active contraction of pelvic floor. C, A flat curve after spinal anesthesia.

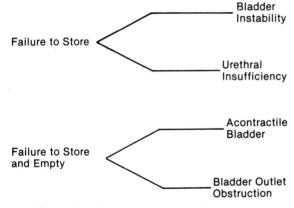

Figure 72–4. Clinical classification of incontinence.

compromised. Either sphincter, by itself, is capable of maintaining continence. The inability to empty may be due to an acontractile bladder, an unsustained bladder contraction (seen in spinal cord injury), or a bladder outlet obstruc-

tion secondary to benign prostatic hyperplasia (BPH), urethral stricture, detrusor-sphincter dyssynergia, and the like.

After discussing urethral insufficiency and detrusor instability, we will comment briefly on the unique aspects of postprostatectomy incontinence as well as incontinence in the elderly.

Urethral Insufficiency

An etiologic classification is delineated in Figure 72–5. Urethral insufficiency after prostatectomy is the most common cause of urinary incontinence (Turner-Warwick, 1983). Less than 1 per cent of simple prostatectomy (including TURP) (Bergman et al., 1955; Chilton et al., 1978) and 5 to 10 per cent of radical prostatectomy patients suffer from postprostatectomy incontinence (Lindner et al., 1983). Resection of posterior valves with a concurrent decompensated bladder neck may also result in

Figure 72–5. Etiology of urethral insufficiency.

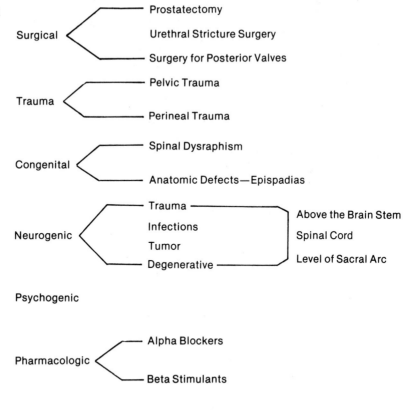

incontinence. Another cause is traumatic posterior urethral disruption, commonly associated with severe pelvic trauma. This disruption usually occurs at the prostatomembranous urethral junction (region of the DUS) with continence preserved because of the intact PUS. If there is an associated PUS deficiency either before or at the time of injury, the patient may be incontinent. A third cause is congenital anatomic abnormalities, such as epispadias or duplicated urethra. Congenital or acquired neurogenic abnormalities may result in incontinence. The former includes spinal dysraphia (myelomeningocele), sacral agenesis, or tethered cord syndrome. Acquired neurologic lesions may be traumatic, operative, neoplastic, metabolic, infectious, or inflammatory. The urinary symptoms that are manifested depend upon the location of the lesion (above the brain stem, below the brain stem, at the level of the sacral arc or peripheral nerve roots). There are also psychogenic causes. These incontinent patients have intact innervation of an anatomically normal bladder. Alpha-adrenergic blockers may render a patient with an already compromised urethra incontinent. Radiotherapy to the pelvis may impair the coaptation of the urethra, and may also decrease bladder compliance. And finally, carcinoma of the prostate may bring about urinary incontinence. Neoplastic invasion of the sphincter may result in poor elasticity and inadequate coaptation of the urethra.

Detrusor Instability

Detrusor instability may be motor or sensory in nature. During a filling cystometrogram, sensory instability is demonstrated by an early sensation of fullness and urge to void, without motor instability (increase in detrusor pressure).

Motor instability is reflected by poor bladder compliance or bladder hyperreflexia. Its origin may be neurogenic, vesicogenic, idiopathic, psychogenic (Fig. 72–6). Neurogenic motor instability may result from (1) lesions above the brain stem (e.g., CVA, trauma), which may cause a coordinated but uninhibited bladder; (2) lesions below the brain stem, such as a cord lesion (e.g., trauma, surgery, tumor), which results in detrusor-sphincter dyssynergia; or (3) lesions at the level of the sacral arc (e.g., dysraphism, arachnoiditis) (see appropriate chapter for further details).

Vesicogenic motor instability is due to an intrinsic disease of the bladder or urethra. Chronic infection, chronic retention, or radiation may cause poor compliance. Fifty-six per cent of patients complaining of "prostatism" demonstrate detrusor instability during cystometrography (CMG). Three fourths of these patients have outlet obstruction, and one fourth have no obstruction (Abrams and Feneley, 1978; Abrams et al., 1976). After correction of their obstruction, many of these patients continue to have instability because of permanent

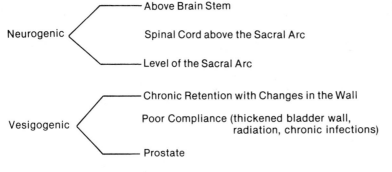

Figure 72–6. Detrusor instability.

changes in their bladder wall. Idiopathic motor instability occurs normally in approximately 10 per cent of the population.

Postprostatectomy Incontinence (PPI)

The main cause of PPI is weakness of the DUS (anatomic structures between the apex of the prostate and the bulbar urethra). This inefficient sphincteric mechanism may be due to iatrogenic or pre-existing conditions. It is important to recognize the latter by careful evaluation prior to prostatectomy. Patients at high risk for PPI may have a history of radical pelvic surgery (abdominoperineal resection), previous inlay urethroplasty, neuropathy (diabetes, alcohol), fractured pelvis (with prostatomembranous urethral disruption), cancer of the prostate, or pelvic irradiation.

Patients after abdominoperineal resection or inlay urethroplasty may have an inadequate intrinsic portion of the DUS as a result of injury to the pelvic nerves and impairment of the blood supply to the inner layer, respectively. Patients with root lesions or peripheral neuropathy may have damage of the pelvic nerves. This problem may occur in the presence of autonomic neuropathy, herpes zoster, cauda equina tumors, protruded lumbar disc, and so forth.

Cancer of the prostate also demands careful attention. Incontinence may result from malignant invasion of the sphincters, a TURP of the PUS with tumor invasion in the DUS, or unclear landmarks from the tumor. Previous radiotherapy for the carcinoma may in itself damage sphincteric function, placing the patient at high risk for a TURP.

The second cause of PPI that must always be ruled out is detrusor instability. After prostatectomy, 60 per cent of patients who suffered from detrusor instability associated with obstructive symptoms were cured (Abrams, 1978). A persistent unstable bladder may be explained by (1) permanent residual damage of the bladder wall (compensatory hypertrophy of the detrusor (Borg and Comarr, 1971); (2) normal decline in cortical inhibitory stimuli in an otherwise neurologically intact elderly population (Isaacs and Walkey, 1964; Milne et al., 1972); or (3) underlying subclinical neurologic disorders, such as parkinsonism or multiple sclerosis, which must be demonstrated by electrophysiologic testing.

The third principal cause of PPI is a combination of urethral insufficiency and failure to empty the bladder ("overflow incontinence"). This condition may result from an outlet obstruction (urethral stricture or bladder neck stenosis); a chronic and acontractile distended bladder, due either to the sequela of BPH or to a pre-existing neuropathy (e.g., diabetes, ethanol); or a residual obstruction. (Some authors contend that residual apical tissue may "hold open" the DUS and lead to incontinence [Yalla et al., 1982]. In any case, a complete urodynamic evaluation must establish this fact clearly before any new TURP is performed.)

In many patients, incontinence is caused by more than one factor. The most common combination is sphincter weakness and detrusor instability (Fitzpatrick et al., 1979; Mayo and Ansell, 1979). The possibility of such a combination is why a complete evaluation with urodynamic studies is indispensable when attempting to demonstrate the mechanism responsible for PPI.

Advanced Age

As mentioned at the beginning of this chapter, the incontinence rate in elderly men may be as high as 55 per cent. The causes are listed in Table 72–1. There are several types of incontinence:

1. *Detrusor instability.* This is the most common source and results from damage to the cortical center that controls micturition.

2. *A combination of a failure to store and an inability to empty.* This occurs less frequently and is related to anatomic obstruction (e.g., prostate, urethral stricture) and atonic bladder (e.g., diabetes, syphilis, and spinal cord diseases).

3. *Stress incontinence.* This is relatively rare and essentially is caused by sphincter damage.

4. *Total incontinence.* This may be seen in severe cases of dementia and sphincter or nerve damage.

EVALUATION OF MALE URINARY INCONTINENCE

The evaluation of the incontinent male patient may include the history, physical examination, cystourethroscopy, radiographs of the bladder and urethra, and urodynamic studies. This information assists in determining the type of incontinence and the specific diagnosis (Fig. 72–4). The factors that determine the most appropriate treatment are the type and severity

TABLE 72–1. CAUSES OF URINARY INCONTINENCE IN THE ELDERLY

Causes of Transient Incontinence
Urinary tract infection
Acute illness—especially when accompanied by
    Fatigue
    Immobilization
    Hospital admission and environmental barriers
    Confusion
Other acute confusional disorders
Retention with overflow incontinence
    Fecal impaction
    Anticholinergic drugs
    Spinal cord compression
Drugs
    With effects on the autonomic nervous system
    Sedatives and tranquilizers
Psychologic
    Depression with regression and dependency
    Hostility
Causes of Established Incontinence
Previous surgical procedure
    With damage to sphincters or pelvic innervation
Diseases of the cerebral cortex
    Stroke
    Dementia
    Parkinson's disease
Diseases of the spinal cord
    Compression by tumor, spondylosis, herniated disc
    Trauma
    Demyelination
Retention with overflow
    Atonic bladder due to diabetes, alcoholism
    Prostatic obstruction
    Urethral stricture
Diseases of the bladder
    Chronic cystitis
    Carcinoma
    Calculi
Uninhibited bladder
Stress incontinence

From Ouslander, J. G.: Urinary incontinence in the elderly. West. J. Med., *135*:482, 1981.

of the incontinence, the presence of strictures, the bladder capacity, and any associated conditions.

History

The history should determine if the patient is wet all the time or if the incontinence is associated with urgency, frequency, nocturia, stress, position (standing or supine), or sensation of fullness. The urologist should inquire if the patient has ever been capable of generating a urinary stream; if so, it should be determined how much is voided and how soon afterward the patient becomes incontinent. Other important information is the need for protective pads, penile clamps, and external catheters. The physician must be cognizant of previous lower uri-

nary tract surgery or trauma and resultant complications (e.g., blood loss, duration of surgery, length of catheter drainage); previous neurologic surgery or trauma, the presence or absence of diabetes; urinary tract infections; muscular disorders; or neurologic diseases. The review of systems should include erectile and ejaculatory potency, bowel habits, and symptoms of neurologic disorders, specifically multiple sclerosis. The urologist must realize that associated impotence may be secondary to the same underlying organic disease or may be psychologic in origin as a result of incontinence. The sexual function of the latter patient should return to normal after the incontinence is cured.

Physical Examination

The emphasis of the physical examination is placed on the following areas:

1. *Abdomen*—check for an enlarged bladder in retention, the integrity of the abdominal muscles, and the presence of any masses.

2. *Back*—evaluation for spinal column deformities, dimples indicative of dysraphism, and evidence of an operation or trauma.

3. *Neurologic*—a complete neurologic examination, including perianal and perineal sensations and bulbocavernosus reflex.

4. *Rectum*—assessment of anal tone, voluntary activity of the anal sphincter, and evaluation for neoplasm. It is helpful to assess the quality and quantity of the patient's voiding stream and to note his ability to stop micturition voluntarily.

Urinalysis

Evaluation or treatment of the patient should not be done until the patient is free of infection. Incontinent patients are more likely to have a urinary tract infection because of the loss of the natural barrier between the bladder and the outside environment, the need for an indwelling urethral catheter, and the use of external collection devices.

Cystourethroscopy

During this procedure, the urologist searches for (1) false passages that may result from traumatic or vigorous urethral dilatation; (2) obstruction that may contribute to overflow incontinence, including BPH, carcinoma of the prostate, and urethral strictures; (3) damage to the DUS that occurs most commonly at the 12 o'clock (anterior) position; (4) voluntary activity of the DUS; (5) presence or absence of the verumontanum; (6) postprostatectomy residual apical tissue or rigidity of the distal urethra that does not allow proper coaptation of the distal intrinsic urethra (further resection of residual tissue will rarely, if ever, improve continence); and (7) concomitant pathologic states of the bladder, such as poor bladder capacity (best assessed with the patient under anesthesia), trabeculation, neoplasm, diverticula, and so forth.

Radiologic Evaluation of the Lower Urinary Tract

Radiologic studies of the lower urinary tract may include both a retrograde urethrogram and a voiding cystourethrogram, preferably performed under fluoroscopic control. Findings on the scout film may include congenital or acquired spinal deformities, a large amount of residual urine, calculous disease, or evidence of previous surgery. The retrograde study will delineate false passages (Fig. 72–7), strictures, urethral sinuses, and diverticula. With the patient standing, it is possible to identify the level of continence (PUS or DUS) (Fig. 72–8), the adequacy of a previous prostatic resection, the presence or absence of stress incontinence, blad-

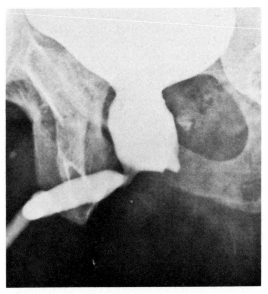

Figure 72–8. A cystogram in a patient who suffers from postprostatectomy incontinence. The region of the distal urethral sphincter is scarred and nonfunctional.

der diverticula, trabeculation, ureterovesical reflux, or fistula. The voiding phase permits identification of a bladder neck stricture, detrusor-sphincter dyssynergia, and occult vesicoureteral reflux. The quantity of residual urine is estimated on the postvoid radiographs.

Urodynamic Studies

The four main types of urodynamic diagnostic studies in the incontinent male are noninvasive urinary flow, filling CMG, combined pressure-flow EMG studies, and urethral pressure profile (UPP). Urinary flow factors that are useful include volume voided, peak flow, voiding time, and average flow. Coughing or straining before the initiation of urinary flow will objectively demonstrate stress incontinence. Information from the filling CMG includes capacity, compliance, and sensory or motor instability. If leakage occurs around the filling catheter, it may be necessary to place traction on a Foley catheter to assess bladder stability properly. The combined pressure-flow EMG records detrusor pressures generated during micturition, a concomitant flow rate, and pelvic floor EMG (with either needle or surface electrodes). This aids in the evaluation of detrusor-sphincter dyssynergia (an increase of sphincteric activity simultaneous with a detrusor contraction) and outflow obstruction (low flow and high detrusor pressure). Because of transurethrally placed trans-

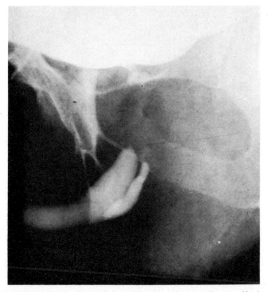

Figure 72–7. Retrograde urethrogram in a patient suffering from urinary incontinence after TURP. A fistula can be seen in the area of the bulbar urethra and the prostatic fossa. The area of the distal urethral sphincter, endoscopically as well as functionally, was intact.

ducer catheters, the pressure-flow study must be interpreted with caution. Therefore, the non-invasive urinary flow rate when compared with the pressure-flow study is helpful in diagnosing bladder outlet obstruction. If there is no significant change in intravesical pressure during the flow phase, the patient should be instructed to stop his stream abruptly ("hold maneuver"). A sudden increase of detrusor pressure indicates the presence of bladder contractility. The UPP, the value of which is questionable, yields the functional urethral length, the closing pressure, and the level of continence (the last is possible only with the aid of concomitant radiography). The UPP in the normal individual usually reveals a functional length of 5 to 6 cm and a maximal urethral pressure in the region of the DUS. In the continent postprostatectomy patient, the functional length is 1.5 to 2.0 cm, with

a maximal urethral pressure that is decreased but is still greater than 50 per cent of normal levels. In the patient with PPI, the functional urethral length is also 1.5 to 2.0 cm, but the maximal urethral pressure is usually less than 50 cm of water (Mayo and Ansell, 1979).

An algorithm (Fig. 72–9) is supplied for the evaluation and treatment of PPI. If a patient complains of incontinence 6 to 8 weeks after prostatectomy, we believe that evaluation according to this algorithm is indicated.

TREATMENT

When treating male incontinence, certain priorities must be kept in mind:

1. *Maintenance of renal function.* At no time is continence more important than renal function.

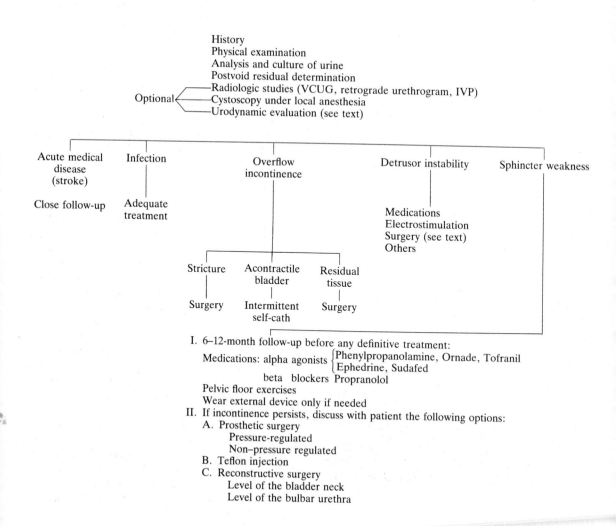

Figure 72–9. Assessment of postprostatectomy incontinence.

2. *Patient's dryness.* Patients who are free of wetness and external collection devices are forever grateful. Even the patient who is in retention and on intermittent catheterization is thankful to be rid of the social embarrassment of a constant uriniferous odor.

3. *Normal voiding pattern.* This is the ideal end result of treatment, although one must never forget that the first two priorities are more important.

Treatment of urinary incontinence is in essence dependent on its type and severity. Urethral insufficiency, detrusor instability, and obstruction may all be treated by pharmacologic agents, electrical stimulation, or surgery.

Pharmacologic Agents

Since the pharmacology of the lower urinary tract is discussed in detail elsewhere, only a brief summary is presented. Because most incontinent patients suffer from an inability to store urine, the physician must either improve functional bladder capacity or increase urethral resistance. Drugs that improve detrusor stability (and thus bladder capacity) include those that block the cholinergic transmission (atropine derivatives) and those that have a direct inhibitory effect on the bladder wall. Examples of anticholinergics are belladonna, propantheline bromide (Pro-Banthine), and methantheline bromide (Banthine). Among the drugs acting directly on the smooth muscle are oxybutynin (Ditropan), flavoxate hydrochloride (Urispas), and imipramine hydrochloride (Tofranil).

Urethral resistance may be improved by an alpha agonist. Examples include phenylpropanolamine, ephedrine, and imipramine. Incontinent patients with a combination of the inability to store and the inability to empty, e.g., sphincter-detrusor dyssynergia, may benefit from the alpha blocker phenoxybenzamine hydrochloride (Dibenzyline) to facilitate bladder emptying. Parasympathomimetics (Urecholine) have been used with limited success in improving detrusor function. Most clinicians find, however, that significant improvement in bladder contractility requires such high doses of Urecholine that the side effects (gastrointestinal disturbance) become prohibitive (Raz, 1978).

Nerve Stimulation

Intermittent electrical stimulation of the pelvic muscles may produce relaxation of the detrusor or contraction of the urethral sphincter, or both. Three different techniques have been used: (1) implantable, which requires an operative procedure to place the electrodes directly on the pelvic floor muscles; (2) nonimplantable, in which a rectal plug is used on the surface, thereby obviating an operation, and (3) acute maximal functional electrical stimulation (AMFES), which is done periodically on an outpatient basis. The amplitude and frequency of stimulation are just below the patient's threshold of tolerance. The first two methods involve chronic stimulation with lower amplitudes in contrast to AMFES. Recently, the emphasis has been on the less invasive, superficial methods (numbers 2 and 3) because the results are essentially the same as the implantable method without the obvious increase in morbidity.

In general, those patients suffering primarily from myogenic incontinence are best treated by chronic, nonimplantable functional electrical stimulation, whereas those suffering from mild to moderate detrusor instability respond best to periodic AMFES.

Depending on the selection of patients, the rate of those improved or cured is in the range of 40 to 66 per cent. Some patients are cured after only a short course of treatment, while others depend on chronic stimulation or repeated AMFES (Godec and Cass, 1978; Plevnik and Janez, 1979; Suhel and Kralj, 1983).

Operative Approach

The history of the treatment of male urinary incontinence is characterized by trial, error, early rejoicing, and late frustration (Kaufman, 1978). Table 72–2 is a classification and summary of a wide range of treatments that have been reported since the turn of the century.

RECONSTRUCTIVE SURGERY

Region of the Bladder Neck. The use of bladder wall to construct a neourethra (neosphincter) has been applied to patients with a nonfunctioning urethra as a result of surgery, trauma, or congenital anomalies such as epispadias. The anterior tube reconstruction of Tanagho is based on his observation that the anterior detrusor muscle is similar histologically to the bladder neck. He describes the technique as follows: After the bladder is transected from the urethra, a tube is constructed over a urethral catheter by using an anterior bladder flap. After prostatic fossa reduction (narrowing of the prostatic urethral), the neourethra is reanastomosed to the urethra. He reports that the operation

TABLE 72–2. CLASSIFICATION OF TREATMENTS OF
URINARY INCONTINENCE

I. Nonsurgical
  A. Expectant, 9 months to 1 year
  B. Training
  C. Pharmacologic
    1. Alpha-adrenergic simulators
    2. Cholinolytic agents
  D. Electrical stimulation (Plevnik and Janez, 1979)
  E. Injection
    1. Sclerosing fluids (Sachse, 1963)
    2. Paraffin (Quackels, 1955)
    3. Supportive material—Teflon (Politano, 1982)
II. Surgical
  A. "Surrogate sphincter" formation
    1. Abdominal muscle and fascial slings
      a. Pyramidalis and/or rectus fascia and muscle
        (Goebell, 1910; Stoeckel, 1917; Frangenheim,
        1914; Cooney and Horton, 1951)
    2. Gracilis muscle slings
      a. Gracilis muscle (Deming, 1926; Player, 1927)
    3. Fascia lata strips (Boer and Ivanovici, 1973)
    4. Perineal muscles
      a. Ischiocavernosus (Lowsley, 1936)
      b. Levator ani (Squier, 1911)
      c. External sphincter ani (Verges-Flaque, 1951;
        Mathisen, 1970)
    5. Bladder flaps
      a. Tube (Tanagho et al., 1969)
      b. Spinal (Flocks and Boldus, 1973)
    6. Muscle transplant (Gierup and Hakelius, 1983)
    7. Prosthetic devices
      a. External (Foley, 1947)
      b. Implanted (Scott, 1973; Scott, personal com-
        munication; Rosen, 1978)
  B. Vesicourethral suspension and angulation (Kelly,
    1928; Marshall et al., 1949)
  C. Posterior urethral lengthening (Young, 1919;
    Thompson, 1961; Leadbetter and Fraley, 1967)
  D. Urethral plication and twists (Young, 1908; Bene-
    venti, 1966; Petersen, 1967; Firlit, 1977)
  E. Urethral compression—passive
    1. Acrylic, Silastic (Berry, 1961)
    2. Collagen (Girgis and Veenema, 1965)
    3. Autologous rib (Hinman et al., 1970)
    4. Fascia lata
    5. Kaufman
      a. Crural cross (1970)
      b. Crural approximation (1972)
      c. Silicone gel prosthesis, SGP (1973)
    6. Crural approximation (Puigvert, 1971)
    7. Marlex (Salcedo, 1972)
    8. SGP and Marlex (Yarbrough, 1975)
    9. Intercavernous embedding (Lenzi et al., 1983)
  F. Electrical stimulation (with electronic implants)
    (Caldwell, 1963; Merrill, 1971)
  G. Urinary diversion
    1. Ileal conduit
    2. Colon conduit
    3. Cutaneous ureterostomy
    4. Vesicostomy and bladder neck closure
    5. Nephrostomy
  H. Continent urinary diversion
    1. Ureterosigmoidostomy
    2. Ileocecal
    3. Ileal reservoir (Kock and Philipson, 1982)
    4. Continent vesicostomy

has been used for PPI and traumatic incontinence, epispadias, and other causes of incontinence. The success rate (those patients who
were cured or markedly improved) was approximately 70 per cent. Those patients treated for
incontinence after TURP did better than those
treated for either post–open prostatectomy incontinence or traumatic urethral injuries (Tanagho, 1981). A modification of the anterior
bladder flap technique, which may improve urethral resistance, is to advance the tubularized
flap through the prostatic fossa and membranous
urethra (Neto, 1978).

In addition to anterior bladder neck reconstruction, patients with epispadias may be
treated by (1) posterior urethral lengthening by
tubularization of the trigone, with concomitant
ureteral reimplantation, as described by Leadbetter and Fraley (1967); or (2) by the Young-
Dees operation (Young, 1919). Epispadic patients treated with either of these procedures
should be expected to achieve close to a 70 per

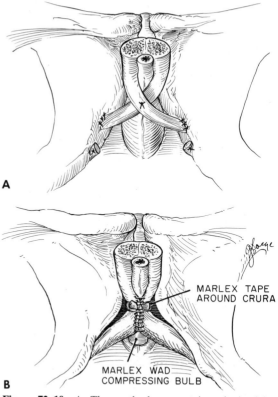

Figure 72–10. *A,* The urethral compression obtained by
crossing the crura of the corpora cavernosa (Kaufman I).
B, The urethral compression operation by approximation
of the crura of the corpora. Further modification entailed
the addition of a Marlex wad to provide better compression
of the bulbous urethra.

cent cure rate after puberty (Kramer and Kelalis, 1982).

Free autogenous muscle transplantation has been used to increase urethral resistance. In children, Hakelius from Sweden uses a segment of skeletal muscle (usually extensor digitorum brevis of the foot) that has been denervated 2 to 3 weeks before surgery. This muscle is then transplanted to the posterior urethra, close to the normally innervated muscles of continence; the latter act as a reinnervating source for the transplanted muscle. During the following 6 months, the patient gradually gains continence. The overall results have been considered good (i.e., increased functional bladder capacity and no need for protective pads during the day) in 10 of 16 patients (Gierup and Hakelius, 1983). Other researchers have not had such successful results (Medgyese et al., 1979).

Region of the Bulbar Urethra. Continence may be achieved by passive compression of the bulbar urethra. The Kaufman I (crural cross) and its modification, the Kaufman II (crural approximation), were introduced in the early 1970's (Kaufman, 1970) (Fig. 72–10). Fifty per cent of patients were markedly improved or cured with a minimum of 6 months' follow-up (Kaufman, 1972). In an attempt to obtain a longer length of urethral compression, other investigators have mobilized the entire bulbar urethra and buried it beneath the two corpora that have been approximated in the midline (Lenzi et al., 1983). Another concept in urethral compression is that of telescoping a transected bulbar urethra into and through the prostato-membranous urethra. This retrograde urethral advancement may increase the resistance sufficiently to maintain continence 55 per cent of the time (Guzman, 1983). It also provides a relatively easy means for urethral reconstruction in the patient with a seemingly irreparable posterior urethra (Fig. 72–11).

PROSTHETIC SURGERY

Non–pressure regulated. With the advent of relatively inert plastics came prostheses used for urinary continence. The silicone gel prosthesis (Kaufman) maintains passive continence via bulbar urethral compression. Its position is secured by four straps. Two straps are placed around the crura of the penis; the other two are placed around staples previously inserted into the rami of the pelvis (Fig. 72–12). Postoperatively, urethral compression may be increased by percutaneous injection of saline into the prosthesis (Fig. 72–13). Of 184 cases reported, 61 per cent had an excellent or good result. There were 20 (11 per cent) major complications, including 12 instances of urethral or perineal skin erosions. Eight subjects had infections that required surgical removal of the prosthesis (Kaufman and Raz, 1979). In other reports, the success rate ranged from 30 to 82 per cent (Graham et al., 1982; Confer and Beall, 1981).

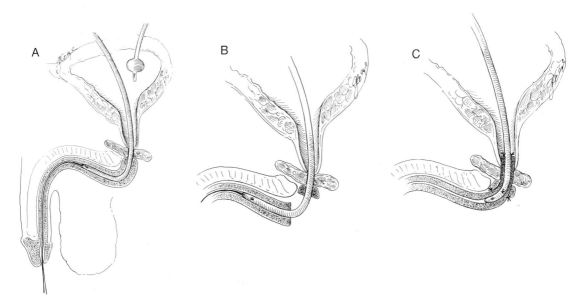

Figure 72–11. Urethral advancement technique. *A,* A suprapubic catheter is passed antegrade into the bulbar urethra. *B,* The bulbar urethra is transected close to the membranous urethra through a perineal incision. *C,* The catheter is secured to the urethra with absorbable sutures. After dilation of the membranous urethra, the bulbar urethra is advanced (telescoped) into the membranous urethra by pulling on the attached suprapubic catheter.

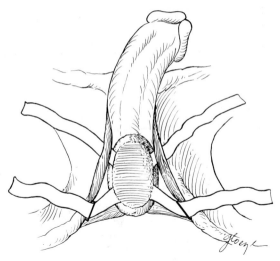

Figure 72–12. Preferred method of anchoring the silicone-gel prosthesis. Bone staples are inserted in the pubis above the insertion of the crura of the corpora. Better compression of the bulb is obtained by deeper fixation of the prosthesis.

In reviewing the results and complications of the silicone gel prosthesis, the following conclusions may be drawn. (1) The silicone gel prosthesis should not be used in patients with previous pelvic radiotherapy (Confer and Beall, 1981). (2) Concomitant penile prostheses significantly increase the risk of implantation. (3)

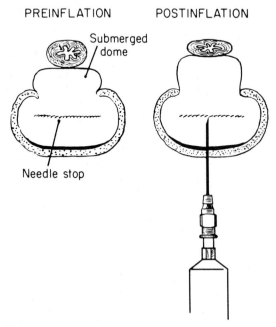

PREINFLATION   POSTINFLATION

Submerged dome

Needle stop

Figure 72–13. The effect of injecting the prosthesis to elevate the submerged dome and to compress the urethra. A needle stop in the chamber prevents puncture of the thin dome.

Success is likely only if preoperative manual perineal compression will significantly increase urethral closing pressure (Kaufman, 1978). (4) Intravesical pressure while standing, coughing, or straining should not exceed 90 cm of water.

The Rosen prosthesis consists of an inflatable urethral occluding device and a scrotally placed pump-reservoir. The amount of urethral resistance is dependent on how much fluid the patient pumps into the occluder. Because the reservoir is not in the abdomen, there is no compensatory increase in urethral pressure at the time of abdominal straining. The cure rate of incontinence ranges from 23 to 77 per cent, with follow-up to 34 months. Complications include aneurysmal dilatation of the occluder pillow, kinking of the tubing, erosion, and infection (Rosen, 1978; Small, 1980; Augsberger, 1981; Giesy et al., 1981).

Periurethral and Transurethral Teflon Injections. Teflon (polytetrafluoroethylene) can be injected periurethrally, creating adequate urethral coaptation and improving resistance. Injection may be done transperineally while observing the effects cystoscopically, or transurethrally via a cystoscopic needle (Fig. 72–14). Politano reported a 6-month to 16-year follow-up of 103 male patients who had undergone transperineal Teflon injection between the years 1964 and 1980. Seventy-five per cent had a good to excellent result. Each patient had an average of 1.8 injections (Politano, 1982). Results from transurethral Teflon injection after TURP and open simple prostatectomy have been successful in 85 and 75 per cent, respectively, of incontinent patients. In incontinent patients with a neurogenic bladder, 40 to 50 per cent had an excellent result from transurethral injection, whereas only 25 per cent of patients with prostate surgery and radiotherapy were cured (Politano, 1983). The obvious advantages of this procedure are (1) a brief hospital stay (only 1 to 2 days); (2) few and only minor complications (occasional urethritis, temporary retention, and one case of abscess formation); and (3) the opportunity for repeated injections.

Pressure-Regulated Sphincters. In 1973, the first artificial inflatable urinary sphincter was introduced (Scott, 1973). In men, the cuffs of these devices are placed around the bulbar urethra or, less commonly, the bladder neck. Over the ensuing 10 years, these devices have evolved into a more simplified and more effective means to treat incontinence; approximately 5500 have been implanted. Still inherent in the device, however, are the inevitable problems associated with implantation of a foreign body,

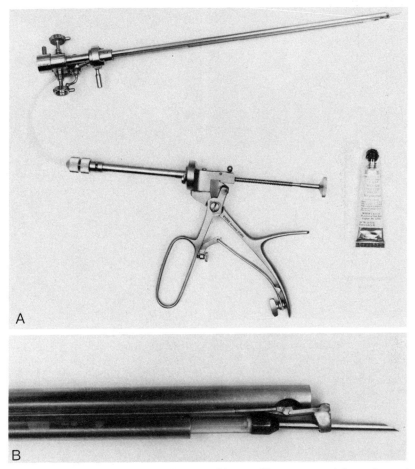

Figure 72–14. *A,* Teflon is supplied in 7-ml tubes. Because of its pastelike nature, an injector is required to instill the Teflon transurethrally. *B,* Close-up of the transurethral needle.

persistent urethral pressure, and fluid hydraulics and moving parts.

The two devices marketed most recently by American Medical Systems are the AS/791/792 and the AS/800 (Fig. 72–15). Both have an abdominally placed, pressure-regulated reservoir that maintains a constant predetermined pressure on the periurethral cuff. Because of the connection between the reservoir and the cuff, any increase in intra-abdominal pressure will transmit more fluid into the urethral cuff. This mechanism allows for a compensatory increase in urethral resistance during straining or coughing. When squeezed, a scrotally placed pump temporarily shifts fluid out of the cuff into the reservoir; this decreases the urethral pressure to allow bladder emptying, and fluid then automatically returns to the cuff via a resistor. This resistor, which allows a slow (60 to 120 seconds) re-equalization of pressure, is a separate device in the AS/791/792, whereas it is incorporated within the pump in the AS/800. A

locking button, which traps the fluid in the reservoir, is equipped in the pump of the AS/800. This button leaves the physician the option to deactivate (decompress for a prolonged period of time) and reactivate the urethral cuff (Fig. 72–16).

Indications for placement of the artificial sphincter in addition to incontinence are:

1. Incontinence of 9 to 12 months' duration after surgery or trauma.

2. No response to conservative measures.

3. Unobstructed urinary flow.

4. Sterile urine.

5. Adequate functional bladder capacity and compliance.

6. Absence of bladder hyperreflexia or good response to pharmacologic therapy.

7. Absence of ureterovesical reflux.

8. Adequate patient motivation.

9. Adequate manual dexterity.

10. Absence of residual urine (Furlow, 1981).

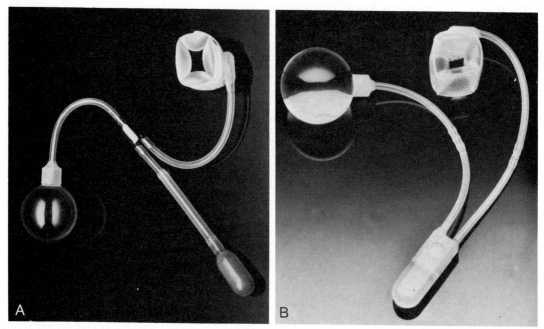

Figure 72–15. *A*, AS/791. The device includes a periurethral cuff, a pump that is placed in the scrotum, a control assembly, and an abdominally placed reservoir. Squeezing of the pump transfers fluid from the cuff to the reservoir. A resistor in the control assembly allows the slow return (1–3 minutes) of fluid to the cuff. This delay in fluid return provides sufficient time for bladder emptying. *B*, AS/800. Similar to the AS/791 except that the control assembly is incorporated into the pump. It is also equipped with an activating and deactivating button on the upper aspect of the pump. (Courtesy of American Medical Systems, Minnetonka, Minn.)

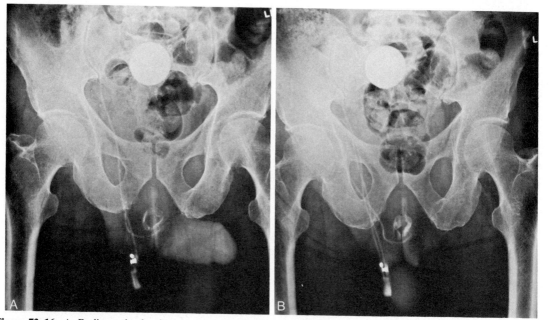

Figure 72–16. *A*, Radiograph of a deactivated AS/800. Note the relative paucity of contrast material in the periurethral cuff. *B*, Radiograph of an activated AS/800, showing the periurethral cuff filled with contrast. Both views demonstrate the abdominally placed reservoir and the pump in the right hemiscrotum.

The successful use of these artificial sphincters depends on two important factors: selection of the appropriate cuff size, and use of a low-range balloon pressure reservoir. An oversized cuff will not give adequate or well-distributed urethral pressure. An undersized cuff or a cuff with a pressure balloon greater than 90 cm will produce pressure necrosis and subsequent erosion. Other high-risk factors for cuff erosion are (1) penile blood pressure less than 50 to 60 mm Hg, (2) accidental injury to the urethra during placement, (3) marked fibrosis from previous surgery or trauma, (4) previous irradiation to the urethra, and (5) pedicle flap reconstruction of the urethra done at the time of cuff placement (Furlow, 1981).

To obviate erosion in the high-risk patient, it is suggested that the cuff remain deactivated from 2 to 6 weeks to allow healing of the surrounding tissues (Scott, 1981). Activation requires only a push of a button in the newer AS/800 model, whereas a second surgical procedure is required with the AS/791/792.

After a preoperative evaluation indicates the individual is a candidate for the artificial sphincter, instruction is given as to its use and proper care. Parenteral antibiotics are administered perioperatively. With the patient in a modified lithotomy position (one leg is lowered to allow access to the lower abdomen), inguinal and perineal incisions are made. The bulbar urethra is circumferentially mobilized. Care must be taken to avoid perforating the urethra—especially in the thin portion on its back (anterosuperior) side. A transverse incision is made just above the inguinal ligament and lateral to the pubic tubercle. The reservoir is placed in the prevesical space (Fig. 72–17A). If the cuff is to be placed around the bladder neck, the patient is put in the supine position and exposure of the bladder neck is made through a lower abdominal incision. This latter approach is preferred when the patient is young or if the bulbar urethra is severely scarred (Fig. 72–17B). The pump is introduced through the abdominal incision and is transferred to the scrotum through a subcutaneous tunnel. The right-handed patient should have the pump placed in his right scrotum (vice versa for the left-handers). The reservoir, cuff, and pump are filled to the appropriate volume with 12.5 per cent Hypaque. The system can then be checked by pumping the device. The cuff should deflate easily, remain flat (like a crushed jelly bean) for 60 to 120 seconds, and then refill completely.

Intraoperative perfusion sphincterometry may be then done with the use of a Foley catheter placed just inside the meatus. The

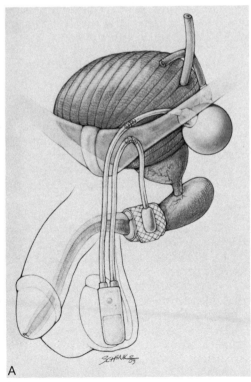

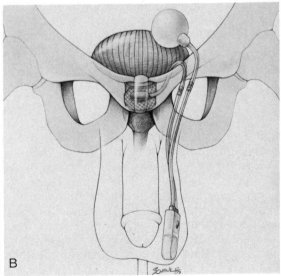

Figure 72–17. *A,* In situ AS/800 placed around the bulbar urethra. *B,* In situ AS/800 placed around the bladder neck. (Courtesy of American Medical Systems, Minnetonka, Minn.)

pressure when flow commences should be greater than the cuff pressure. After compression of the pump, flow should occur at a much reduced pressure (Leach and Raz, 1983). For the first 24 hours after surgery, ice packs are placed over the scrotum and perineum to diminish postoperative swelling. For those patients whose artificial sphincter is left activated, a urethral catheter is not usually placed. Instead, the nurses and the patient are instructed to deflate the cuff every 2 hours for the first 72 hours and then every 4 hours for the next 2 weeks.

Reported results of the more recent models involve only limited follow-up time intervals. In a series of 348 patients who received an AS/791/792, Scott (1983) reported an overall success rate of 80 per cent, with follow-up from 1 month to more than 3 years. Failures were due to erosion (6 per cent), infection (5 per cent), and device malfunction (9 per cent). Device malfunction was usually the fault of the cuff. In a follow-up study of 6 to 30 months, the treatment of 43 of 47 (91 per cent) patients at the Mayo Clinic was considered successful. Complications included erosions (5 to 10 per cent) and infection (5 per cent) (Furlow, 1981).

Erosions of the cuff without clinical or operative evidence of a gross purulent infection may be treated by removal of only the cuff, leaving in place the pump, reservoir, and tubing. If gross pus is encountered in any part of the device, it is recommended that the entire apparatus be removed. A new cuff or an entire new device may be replaced 6 to 12 weeks later if a cystoscopic examination shows adequate healing of the urethra and the patient is free of any residual infection.

URINARY DIVERSION

In those patients whose bladder or urethra is incapable of storing or transporting urine despite all treatment measures, the most appropriate option may be urinary diversion. Diversion may be either incontinent or continent. Incontinent diversions include ileal conduit, colon conduit, cutaneous ureterostomy, vesicostomy with bladder neck closure, and nephrostomy. (A complete review is found elsewhere in this book.)

The ileum, ileocecum, and sigmoid colon have all been used to create continent pouches. Kock, who obtained encouraging results from a continent ileostomy in proctocolectomy patients, applied his technique to create a urinary reservoir. This reservoir, which has two intussuscepted limbs, is designed to maintain conti-

nence and prevent ureterovesical reflux. Self-intermittent catheterization of the pouch is required three or four times each day. Because the stoma is flush with the skin, only a small dressing is required for coverage. The total amount of ileum required is approximately 75 cm. Kock has reported excellent results in 16 patients (Kock et al., 1982; Kock and Philipson, 1983).

Some patients may best be treated by closure of the bladder neck and placement of a continent vesicostomy. Simple ligation around the bladder neck rarely cures urethral incontinence; rather, the bladder neck must be well mobilized, denuded from the inside, and then closed with opposing concentric sutures. Only with good drainage and healing of the denuded tissues will the bladder neck remain closed. Reid formed a continent vesicostomy in 24 patients with neurogenic bladder. In this procedure, a tubularized bladder flap is brought through the lower abdominal wall. Through this stoma, intermittent catheterization is performed (Reid et al., 1978; Schneider et al., 1974).

The continent reservoir described by Zingg intussuscepts the terminal ileum into the cecum, which has been removed from the fecal stream. The proximal portion of this ileal segment is brought to the skin as a stoma, which is intubated intermittently. Antirefluxing ureterocecostomies are placed on the antimesenteric border. Two of four patients were dry without reflux 5 to 14 months after surgery (Zingg and Tscholl, 1977; Benchekroun, 1982).

SURGICAL TREATMENT OF DETRUSOR INSTABILITY

If detrusor instability is the cause of, or is a major factor in, urinary incontinence, and if the patient's symptoms are not improved after conservative or pharmacologic therapy, the urologist may then consider an operative alternative.

Bladder distention has been used for treatment of patients with detrusor instability. After epidural anesthesia, the bladder is distended to a pressure equal to the systolic blood pressure of the patient for four 30-minute periods. Of 51 patients, 40 (80 per cent) were either cured of symptoms or were greatly improved; 13 (26 per cent) patients had a relapse and received a second bladder distention. Eight of these 13 patients eventually were cured or improved (follow-up of 13 months). Complications consisted of transient urinary retention in three cases and extraperitoneal bladder rupture treated by catheter drainage in two cases. Follow-up histologic evaluation revealed axonal degeneration but no increase in collagen deposition (Ramsden et al., 1976; Wolk and Bishop, 1981).

Central or peripheral denervation has also been done for the treatment of detrusor instability. A subarachnoid block with alcohol or a rhizotomy have been used for central denervation (Torrens and Hald, 1979). Discussion of these procedures is found elsewhere in this book. Peripheral denervation may be done at the nerve plexus or perivesically. Perivesical operations include detrusor myotomy, detrusor transection, and cystolysis. Decreasing instability by disrupting the innervation of the detrusor is the principle of these procedures.

Bladder transection with and without myotomies involves detaching and then reattaching the bladder and its trigone. Satisfactory improvement of urge incontinence ranges from 53 to 81 per cent (Hindmarsh et al., 1977; Parsons et al., 1977; Mundy, 1982).

Cystolysis is the mobilization of the supratrigonal bladder from its surrounding attachments. The results have been encouraging in women with interstitial cystitis and detrusor hyperreflexia (Worth and Turner-Warwick, 1973; Worth, 1980; Freiha and Stamey, 1980). In men, however, the procedure is done rarely because of the possibility of resultant impotence.

Bladder augmentation by cecocystoplasty, ileocystoplasty, or sigmoidocystoplasty has generally been employed for the patient with detrusor instability and a limited bladder capacity (less than 150 ml when studied with the patient under spinal anesthesia). The procedure can be performed alone, with the intent of increasing the intravesical volume, thereby decreasing intravesical pressure at the time of an uninhibited detrusor contraction. Alternatively, bladder augmentation may be performed in combination with a perivesical denervation procedure, with the goal of simultaneously ablating the detrusor instability and providing an adequate "holding capacity" to minimize urinary incontinence. When bladder emptying is impaired after the combined procedure, clean, intermittent self-catheterization is performed.

The results of bladder augmentation alone are generally good (Smith et al., 1977; Linder et al., 1983; Bramble, 1982). Linder et al. reported an excellent result in 14 of 17 patients (82 per cent) with follow-up ranging from 12 to 120 months. Bramble reported satisfactory results in 13 of 15 patients (86 per cent) with urge incontinence, with follow-up ranging from 6 months to 5 years.

References

Abrams, P.H.: The urodynamic changes following prostatectomy. Urol. Int., *33*:181, 1978.

Abrams, P.H., and Feneley, R.C.L.: The significance of the symptoms associated with bladder outflow obstruction. Urol. Int., *33*:171, 1978.

Abrams, P.H., Roylance, J., and Feneley, R.C.L.: Excretion urography in the investigation of prostatism. Br. J.Urol., *48*:681, 1976.

Andersen, J.T.: Detrusor hyperreflexia in benign intravesical obstruction: a cystometric study. J. Urol., *115*:532, 1976.

Augspurger, R.R.: Pitfalls of the Rosen anti-incontinence prosthesis. J. Urol., *125*:201, 1981.

Benchekroun, A.: Continent caecal bladder. Br. J. Urol., *54*:505, 1982.

Beneventi, F.A.: A new operation for the correction of postoperative urinary incontinence in the male patient. J. Urol., *96*:740, 1966.

Bergman, R.T., Turner, R., Barnes, R.W. and Hadley, H.L: Comparative analysis of 1000 consecutive cases of transurethral prostatic resection. J. Urol., *74*:533, 1955.

Berry, J.L.: A new procedure for correction of urinary incontinence. Preliminary report. J. Urol., *85*:771, 1961.

Birkhoff, J.D.: Natural history of benign prostatic hypertrophy. *In* Hinman, F. (Ed.): Benign Prostatic Hypertrophy. New York, Springer-Verlag, 1983, p. 7.

Boer, P.W., and Ivanovici, F.C.: The fascia lata strip method for postoperative urinary incontinence correction. Transactions XVI Congres de la Societé Internationale D'Urologie, Amsterdam, 1973. Paris, Diffusion Doin Editeurs, 1974, pp. 471–473.

Bors, E.H., and Comarr, A.E.: Neurological Urology: Physiology of Micturition. Its Neurological Disorders and Sequelae. Baltimore, University Park Press, 1971.

Bramble, F.J.: The treatment of adult enuresis and urge incontinence by enterocystoplasty. Br. J. Urol., *54*:693, 1982.

Brocklehurst, J..C.: The genitourinary system. *In* Brocklehurst, J.C. (Ed.): Textbook of Geriatric Medicine and Gerontology. New York, Churchill Livingstone, 1978.

Caldwell, K.P.S.: The electronic control of sphincter incompetence. Lancet, *2*:174, 1963.

Chilton, C.P., Morgan, R.J., England, H.R., Paris, A.M.I., and Blandy, J.P.: A critical evaluation of the results of transurethral resection of the prostate. Br. J. Urol., *50*:542, 1978.

Confer, D.J., and Beall, ME.: Evolved improvements in placement of the silicone gel prosthesis for post-prostatectomy incontinence. J. Urol., *126*:605, 1981.

Cooney, C. J., and Horton, G. R.: An operation for the cure of urinary incontinence in the male. J. Urol., *66*:586, 1951.

Deming, C.L.: Transplantation of the gracilis muscle for incontinence of urine. JAMA, *86*:822, 1926.

Elbadawi, A.: Neuromorphologic basis of vesicourethral function. Neurourol. Urodyn. *1*:3, 1982.

Feneley, R.C.L., Shepherd, P.H., Powell, P.H., and Blannin, J.: Urinary incontinence: prevalence and needs. Br. J. Urol., *51*:493, 1979.

Firlit, C.F.: Management of total urinary incontinence in boys by urethral plication. Surg. Gynecol. Obstet., *144*:239, 1977.

Fitzpatrick, J.M., Gardiner, R.A., and Worth, P.H.L.: The evaluation of 68 patients with postprostatectomy incontinence. Br. J. Urol., *51*:552, 1979.

Flocks, R.H., and Boldus, R.: The surgical treatment and prevention of urinary incontinence associated with disturbance of the internal urethral sphincter mechanism. J. Urol., 109:279, 1973.

Foley, F.E.B.: An artificial sphincter: a new device and operation for control of enuresis and urinary incontinence: general considerations. J. Urol., 58:250, 1947.

Frangenheim, P.: Zur operativen behandlung der inkontinenz der mannlichen harnohre. Verh. Dtsch. Ges. Chir., 43:149, 1914.

Freiha, F.S., and Stamey, T.A.: Cystolysis: a procedure for the selective denervation of the bladder. J. Urol., 123:360, 1980.

Furlow, W.L.: Implantation of a new semiautomatic artificial genitourinary sphincter: experience with primary activation and deactivation in 47 patients. J. Urol., 126:741, 1981.

Gierup, H.J.W., and Hakelius, L.: Further experience of free muscle transplantation in children with urinary incontinence. Br. J. Urol., 55:211, 1983.

Giesy, J.D., Barry, J.M., Fuchs, E.F., and Griffith, L.D.: Initial experience with the Rosen incontinence device. J. Urol., 125:794, 1981.

Girgis, A.S., and Veenema, R.J.: Perineal urethroplasty. A new operation for correction of incontinence in the male patient. J. Urol., 93:703, 1965.

Godec, C., and Cass, A.: Acute electrical stimulation for urinary incontinence. Urology, 12:340, 1978.

Goebell, R.: Zur operativen beseitigung der angeborenen incontinentia vesicae. Z. Gynakol. Urol., 2:187, 1910.

Gosling, J.: Symposium on clinical urodynamics. Urol. Clin. North Am., 6:31, 1979.

Gosling, J.A., Dixon, J.S., Critchley, H.O.D., and Thompson, S.A.: Comparative study of the urinary external sphincter and periurethral levator muscle. Br. J. Urol., 53:35, 1981.

Gosling, J.A., Dixon, J.S., and Lendon, R.G.: The anatomic innervation of the human male and female bladder neck and proximal urethra. J. Urol., 118:302, 1977.

Graham, S.D., Culley, C.C., and Anderson, E.E.: Long-term results with the Kaufman prosthesis. J. Urol., 128:328, 1982.

Guzman, J.M.: Personal communication, 1983.

Hindmarsh, J.R., Essenhigh, D.M., and Yeates, W.K.: Bladder transection for adult enuresis. Br. J. Urol., 49:515, 1977.

Hinman, F., Schmaelzle, J.F., and Cass, A.S.: Autogenous perineal bone graft for post-prostatectomy incontinence. J. Urol., 104:888, 1970.

Hutch, J.A.: A new theory of the anatomy of the internal urinary sphincter and the physiology of micturition. 2. The base plate. J. Urol., 96:182, 1966.

Isaacs, B., and Walkey, F.A.: A survey of incontinence in the elderly. Geront. Clin., 6:367, 1964.

Kaufman, J.J.: A new operation for male incontinence. Surg. Gynecol. Obstet., 131:295, 1970.

Kaufman, J.J.: Surgical treatment of post-prostatectomy incontinence. Use of the penile crura to compress the bulbous urethra. J. Urol., 107:293, 1972.

Kaufman, J.J.: Symposium on male incontinence. Urol. Clin. North Am., 5:265, 1978.

Kaufman, J.J.: The silicone-gel prosthesis for the treatment of male urinary incontinence. Symposium on male incontinence. Urol. Clin. North Am., 5:393, 1978.

Kaufman, J.J., and Raz, S.: Urethral compression procedure for the treatment of male urinary incontinence. J. Urol., 121:605, 1979.

Kelly, H.A. (Ed.): Gynecology. New York, D. Appleton and Co., 1928, 821–823.

Kock, N.G., Nilson, A.E., Nilsson, L.W., Norlen, L.J., and Philipson, B.M.: Urinary diversion via a continent ileal reservoir: clinical results in 12 patients. J. Urol., 128:469, 1982.

Kock, N.G., and Philipson, A.E.: Urinary diversion via a continent reservoir. Proceedings II of the International Continence Society in Aachen, Federal Republic of Germany, 1983, p. 503.

Koyanagi, T.: Studies on the sphincteric system located distally in the urethra: the external urethral sphincter revisited. J. Urol., 122:655, 1980.

Kramer, S.A., and Kelalis, P.: Assessment of urinary continence in epispadia: review of 94 patients. J. Urol., 128:290, 1982.

Leach, G.E., and Raz, S.: Perfusion sphincterometry. Urology, 21:312, 1983.

Leadbetter, G.W., and Fraley, F.E.: Surgical correction of total urinary incontinence. Five years after. J. Urol., 97:869, 1967.

Lenzi, R., Barbagli, G., Stomaci, N., and Selli, C.: Surgical treatment of male urinary incontinence. J. Urol., 130:463, 1983.

Linder, A., Leach, G.E., and Raz, S.: Augmentation cystoplasty in the treatment of neurogenic bladder dysfunction. J. Urol., 129:491, 1983.

Linder, A., DeKernion, J.B., Smith, R.B., and Katske, F.A.: Risk of urinary incontinence following radical prostatectomy. J. Urol., 129:1007, 1983.

Lowsley, O.S.: New operations for the relief of incontinence in both male and female. J. Urol., 36:400, 1936.

Marshall, V.F., Marchetti, A.A., and Krantz, K.E.: The correction of stress incontinence by simple vesicourethral suspension. Surg. Gynecol. Obstet., 88:509, 1949.

Mathisen, W.: A new operation for urinary incontinence. Surg. Gynecol. Obstet., 130:606, 1970.

Mayo, M.E., and Ansell, J.S.: Urodynamic assessment of incontinence after prostatectomy. J. Urol., 122:60, 1979.

Medgyese, S., Mortensen, S., and Nerstrom, B.: The failure of free muscle transplants in the treatment of urinary incontinence. Br. J. Plast. Surg., 32:336, 1979.

Merrill, D.C., Glover, E., and Conway, C.: Recent advances in electronic bladder control. Med. Elec. Data, 2:72, 1971.

Milne, J.S., Williamson, J., Maule, M.M., et al.: Urinary symptoms in older people. Mod. Geriatr., 2:198, 1972.

Mundy, A.R.: The surgical treatment of urge incontinence of urine. J. Urol., 128:481, 1982.

Neto, M.: Pull-through intraurethral bladder flap. J. Urol., 119:699, 1978.

Nordling, J.: Alpha blockers and urethral pressure in neurological patients. Urol. Int., 33:304, 1978.

Nordling, J.: Influence of the sympathetic nervous system on the lower urinary tract in man. Neurourol. Urodyn., 2:3, 1983.

Ouslander, J.G.: Urinary incontinence in the elderly. West. J. Med., 135:482, 1981.

Parsons, K.F., O'Boyle, P.J., and Gibbon, N.O.K.: A further assessment of bladder transection in the management of adult enuresis and allied conditions. Br. J. Urol., 49:509, 1977.

Petersen, R.A.: Plastic repair of the external urethral sphincter. A new technique for correction of postoperative incontinence in man. J. Urol., 97:1050, 1967.

Player, L.P., and Callander, C.L.: A method for the cure of urinary incontinence in the male: preliminary report. JAMA, 88:989, 1927.

Plevnik, S., and Janez, J.: Maximal electrical stimulation for urinary incontinence. Urology, 14:638, 1979.

Politano, V.A.: Periurethral polytetrafluoroethylene injection for urinary incontinence. J. Urol., *127*:439, 1982.

Politano, V.A.: Personal communication, 1983.

Puigvert, A.: Surgical treatment of urinary incontinence in the male. Urol. Int., *26*:261, 1971.

Quackels, R.: Deux incontinences après adeńomectomie guefies par injection de paraffine dans le périnee. Acta Urol. Belg., *23*:259, 1955.

Ramsden, P.D., Smith, J.C., Dunn, M., and Andran, G.M.: Distention therapy for the unstable bladder; later results including an assessment of repeat distentions. Br. J. Urol., *48*:623, 1976.

Raz, S.: Symposium on male incontinence. Urol. Clin. North Am., *5*:298, 323, 1978.

Reid, R., Schneider, K., and Fruchtman, B.: Closure of the bladder neck in patients undergoing continent vesicostomy for urinary incontinence. J. Urol., *120*:40, 1978.

Rosen, M.: The Rosen inflatable incontinence prosthesis. Symposium on male incontinence. Urol. Clin. North Am., *5*:405, 1978.

Sachse, K.: Sclerosing therapy in urinary incontinence—indications-results-complications. Urol. Int., *15*:225, 1963.

Salcedo, H.: Surgical correction of post-prostatectomy urinary incontinence using Marlex mesh—preliminary report. J. Urol., *107*:440, 1972.

Schneider, K.M., Ewing, R.S., and Signer, R.D.: Continent vesicostomy. Urology, *3*:654, 1974.

Scott, F.B: Editorial comment on Furlow, W.L. (1981). J. Urol., *126*:141, 1981.

Scott, F.B.: Personal communication, 1983.

Scott, F.B.: Treatment of urinary incontinence by implantable prosthetic sphincter. Urology, *1*:252, 1973.

Small, M.P.: The Rosen incontinence procedure: a new artificial urinary sphincter for the management of urinary incontinence. J. Urol., *123*:507, 1980.

Smith, R.B., Van Cangh, P., Skinner, D.G., Kaufman, J.J., and Goodwin, W.E.: Augmentation enterocystoplasty: a critical review. J. Urol., *118*:35, 1977.

Squier, JB.: Post-operative urinary incontinence: urethroplastic operation. Med. Rec., *79*:868, 1911.

Stoeckel, W.: Uber die verwendung der muscli pyramidales bei der operativen behandlung der incontinentia urinae. Z. Gynakol., *41*:11, 1917.

Suhel, P., and Kralj, B.: The treatment of urinary incontinence using functional electrical stimulation. In Raz, S. (Ed.): Female Urology. Philadelphia, W.B. Saunders Co., 1983.

Tanagho, E.A.: Bladder neck reconstruction for total urinary incontinence: 10 years of experience. J. Urol., *125*:321, 1981.

Tanagho, E.A.: Post-prostatectomy incontinence. I. Physiology and pathophysiology of micturition. In Weber, D., and Jonas, D. (Eds.): Postoperative Urinary Incontinence. Stuttgart, Georg Thieme Verlag, 1981, pp. 1–17.

Tanagho, E.A., and Smith, D.R.: Mechanisms of urinary incontinence. 1. Embryologic, anatomic and pathologic considerations. J. Urol., *100*:640, 1968.

Tanagho, E.A., Smith, D.R., Meyers, F.H., et al.: Mechanism of urinary continence. II. Technique for surgical correction of incontinence. J. Urol., *101*:305, 1969.

Thomas, T.M., Plymat, R.B., Blannin, J., and Meade, T.W.: Prevalence of urinary incontinence. Br. Med. J., *281*:1243, 1980.

Thompson, I.M.: Incontinence following prostatectomy. J. Urol., *86*:130, 1961.

Torrens, M., and Hald, T.: Symposium on clinical urodynamics. Urol. Clin. North Am., *6*:283, 1979.

Turner-Warwick, R.: Sphincter mechanism and prostatic enlargement. In Hinman, F. (Ed.): Benign Prostatic Hypertrophy. New York, Springer-Verlag, 1983, pp. 809–828.

U.S. DHEW: Longterm care facility improvement study. Washington, D.C.: U.S. Government Printing Office, 1975.

Verges-Flaque, A.: Flaque-Lowsley operation for urinary incontinence: preliminary report. J. Urol., *65*:427, 1951.

Vetter, N.J., Jones, D.A., and Victor, C.R.: Urinary incontinence in the aged. Gerontol. Clin. *11*:330, 1969.

Vital and Health Statistics—Utilization of Short Stay Hospitals. Series 13, No. 4G. Washington, D.C., DHEW publication No. (PHS)80-1797, 1980.

Wolk, F.N., and Bishop, M.C.: Effectiveness of prolonged hydrostatic dilatation of bladder. Urology, *18*:572, 1981.

Worth, P.H.L.: The treatment of interstitial cystitis by cystolysis with observations on cystoplasty. A review after 7 years. Br. J. Urol., *52*:232, 1980.

Worth, P.H.L., and Turner-Warwick, R.: The treatment of interstitial cystitis by cystolysis with observations on cystoplasty. Br. J. Urol., *45*:65, 1973.

Yalla, S.V., Karsh, L., Kearney, G., Frases, L., Finn, D., Defelippo, N., and Dyro, F.M.: Postprostatectomy urinary incontinence: urodynamic assessment. Neurourol. Urodyn. *1*:77, 1982.

Yarbrough, W.J., Semerdjian, H.S., and Miller, H.C.: George Washington University technique for surgical correction of post-prostatectomy incontinence. J. Urol., *113*:47, 1975.

Young, H.H.: An operation for the cure of incontinence of urine. Surg. Gynecol. Obstet., *28*:84, 1919.

Young, H.H.: Suture of the urethra and vesical sphincters for the cure of incontinence of urine, with report of a case. Trans. South. Surg. Gynecol. Assoc., *28*:84, 1908.

Zingg, E., and Tscholl, R.: Continent cecoileal conduit: preliminary report. J. Urol., *118*:724, 1977.

CHAPTER 73

Urinary Incontinence in the Female*
Stress Urinary Incontinence

LINDA M. DAIRIKI SHORTLIFFE, M.D.
THOMAS A. STAMEY, M.D.

Most of what we know about urinary continence in the normal female is from what we have learned about stress urinary incontinence (SUI). For this reason, plus the fact that SUI is very common, most of the emphasis in this chapter is on SUI, but the urologist should remember that much of the information is applicable to patients with total urinary incontinence from widely diverse causes such as pelvic fractures, radiation incontinence, and iatrogenic surgical incontinence. The various causes of urinary incontinence are best classified on an anatomic basis; the list in Table 73–1 is based upon our experience at Stanford.

The most common causes of urinary incontinence in the female are SUI and nonobstructive, detrusor instability (spontaneous, unsuppressible contractions of the detrusor muscle). We have had only one female patient with obstructive instability of the bladder; retention was a greater component of her condition than incontinence. Women can, of course, have urinary incontinence from more than one cause (Table 73–1) (for example, SUI and detrusor instability). There are some women in whom neither SUI nor detrusor abnormalities can be demonstrated, despite the most careful examinations. It is clear that patients with SUI and iatrogenic and pelvic trauma represent the vast

TABLE 73–1. CAUSES OF URINARY INCONTINENCE IN THE FEMALE

Urethral
  Stress urinary incontinence (SUI)*
  Iatrogenic trauma
    Transurethral resection
    Vesical neck Y-V plasty
    Urethral diverticulectomy
    Operations for SUI
    Radiation
  Pelvic trauma
  Congenital anomalies
    Ectopic ureterocele
    Congenitally defective "sphincter" (short urethra)
    Epispadias with or without exstrophy

Bladder (Detrusor)
  Involuntary contractions (instability)
    *Non-obstructive**
    Obstructive
  Acontractile detrusor (overflow)
  Vesicovaginal fistulae
  Functional (psychiatric)

Ureteral
  Uretero-vaginal fistulae
  Ectopic ureter

Unknown
  Women who have neither SUI nor detrusor instability*

*SUI, nonobstructive detrusor instability, and women who lose urine in whom neither detrusor instability nor SUI can be demonstrated account for 95 per cent or more of all incontinent women.

majority of surgically curable cases, and that surgical correction in these women requires restoration of the vesical neck from a dependent position in the pelvis to a new high behind the symphysis pubis.

*Some of the written material and a few figures in this chapter have been reproduced or adapted from Stamey, T. A.: Endoscopic suspension of the vesical neck for surgically curable urinary incontinence in the female. Monogr. Urol., 2:65, 1981.

DEFINITION, HISTORY, AND PHYSICAL EXAMINATION OF PATIENTS WITH SUI

Definition

SUI is the most common cause of involuntary loss of urine in women. Indeed, several investigators have shown, from careful interviews with normal women, that about 50 per cent of nulliparous women occasionally experience SUI; however, the occurrence is neither frequent enough nor in sufficient quantity to be socially embarrassing. Precisely because SUI is so common, it is best defined as the involuntary loss of urine through the intact urethra, which is caused by an increase in intra-abdominal pressure and is of sufficient quantity to be socially embarrassing. It is nearly always worse when the patient is in the erect position, it is aggravated by any action or disease that increases abdominal pressure, it is never caused by contraction of the detrusor muscle, and, most important, it can be diagnosed on physical examination.

History

The history is important. It should exclude at least overt neuromuscular disease, it should emphasize any associated cause if the onset of incontinence was abrupt (such as pelvic surgery), and it should include a careful analysis of the physical forces producing SUI. The classic patient will lose urine with sudden increases in abdominal pressure, but never in bed at night (Grade I). As the incontinence worsens, lesser degrees of physical stress—such as walking, standing erect from a sitting position, or sitting up in bed—will produce incontinence (Grade II). In the severest problems, especially after operative failures or severe pelvic fractures, total incontinence occurs, and urine is lost without any relation to physical activity or to position (Grade III). It is important to note the grade of incontinence and even to estimate the amount of urine loss (1 to 10 sanitary napkins per day), because many basically inadequate operations will cure Grade I incontinence but not Grade II or III.

The history obtained from the patient depends in substantial part on how severe the urinary incontinence is. Although the historic circumstances of urinary loss are important, in surgically curable incontinence these circumstances are helpful only in Grade I incontinence

and may be misleading in Grades II and III; for example, it is helpful to know if the patient is dry in the recumbent position, especially at night when movement is minimal, but patients with Grade II incontinence can be wet at night, whereas those with Grade III incontinence are wet all of the time. The distinction between loss of urine in small spurts from a sharp rise in abdominal pressure and the loss of urine in large amounts from a detrusor contraction that has emptied the bladder is obviously useful in suspecting a neuropathic bladder.

These introductory questions represent an attempt to characterize the degree and circumstances of urinary leakage and are listed in Table 73–2 as the first set of questions. The next set of questions represents an attempt to characterize urgency incontinence. It is clear that patients who present only with urgency incontinence, that is, loss of urine that occurs only after they sense a desire to urinate, cannot be cured by surgery. The difficulty, however, is that at least one third of patients with surgically curable incontinence also have urgency incontinence, and they can be cured of both problems by surgical elevation of the vesical neck. It is possible that the urgency component in patients with surgically curable incontinence is due to the well-recognized funneling and low pressure of the internal vesical neck; as detrusor pressure starts to rise, urine flows immediately into the proximal urethra, causing an uncontrollable desire to urinate. With restoration of the vesical neck from a dependent position in the pelvis to one high behind the symphysis pubis, urine presumably cannot enter the proximal urethra during the early rise in pressure just prior to voiding.

In our 1975 series of 44 patients with SUI, we carefully analyzed the preoperative and postoperative interrelationships of urgency incontinence (Stamey et al., 1975). Preoperatively, 27 of the 44 patients had some degree of urgency incontinence, and in 5 patients it was so marked that it accounted for most of their urinary loss. Postoperatively, 18 patients had some urgency incontinence, a group that included some who had no preoperative urgency, but the problem disappeared within 6 months in all except for two patients, one of whom lost her sensation of urgency at 18 months and another whose condition was controlled with anticholinergic drugs at 10 months after surgery.

It is interesting that in half of the 27 patients, there was a diminution or complete disappearance of preoperative urgency incontinence in the postoperative period, whereas

TABLE 73–2. STANFORD INCONTINENCE QUESTIONNAIRE

History

CHARACTERIZATION OF URINARY LEAKAGE

Do you lose urine with any of the following?	Always	Sometimes	Never	Comments
Coughing or sneezing......................				
Laughing.................................				
Lifting..................................				
Active exercise (running, and so on)				
Minimal exercise (walking, light housework) ...				
Sleeping				
Nervousness or increased anxiety				
Leakage unrelated to any specific cause........				

Is your clothing damp_____, wet_____, or soaking wet_____?

Do you use sanitary napkins_____, tissue paper_____, or diapers_____ for protection?

How many protective pads to you change per day_____?

Are they damp_____, wet_____, or saturated_____ at each change?

	YES	NO
Do you leave puddles of urine on the floor?...		
Do you lose urine by continuous dribbling?...		
Do you lose urine in small spurts?...		
If yes, is the loss of urine related to physical activity?..		
Do you lose urine in sudden, large amounts as if your whole bladder has emptied uncontrollably? ...		

CHARACTERIZATION OF URGENCY INCONTINENCE

When you have the desire to urinate, do you lose urine before you can get to the bathroom or toilet seat?..........

If yes, please indicate which of the following most accurately describes how often you lose urine before you can get to the toilet: Every time I have a strong desire to pass urine_____; half of the time I pass urine_____; only occasionally when I pass urine_____.

Does this urgency leakage represent a small amount_____, a moderate amount_____, or most of the total urine you lose in a 24-hour period_____?

CHARACTERIZATION OF VOIDING HABITS

	YES	NO
Do you have pain over your bladder when it is full?..		

How often do you pass urine during the day? Every hour or less_____; 1 to 2 hours_____; 2 to 3 hours_____; 3 to 4 hours_____; greater than 4 hours_____.

How often do you pass urine after going to bed? Every hour or less_____; 1 to 2 hours_____; 2 to 3 hours_____; 3 to 4 hours_____; greater than 4 hours_____.

Is the volume of urine you usually pass large_____, average_____, small_____, or very small_____?

Do you empty your bladder frequently, before you experience the desire to pass urine just so you can stay dry? Yes_____, No_____.

MISCELLANEOUS

	YES	NO
Have you had your uterus removed (a hysterectomy)?..		
Have you had orthopedic or neurosurgical operations on your back or spinal cord?		

Have you had previous abdominal_____ or vaginal_____ operations to cure your urinary leakage?

several patients who had no preoperative urgency incontinence experienced some for a short period postoperatively. The second section of the questionnaire in Table 73–2 is designed to determine if urgency incontinence is present and, if so, how much of a problem it is to the patient; it also attempts to quantitate how much of the total urinary leakage is attributable to the urgency component. In general, our impression is that those patients with demonstrable stress incontinence on physical examination who also have a strong component of urgency incontinence often have some problems with a sensation of urgency for the first few months after surgery, even though they no longer have stress incontinence. This is particularly true of those patients older than 65 years of age. In our 1980 series of 203 patients, 69 patients had some component of urgency incontinence in the immediate postoperative period, but little remained after 6 months (Stamey, 1980a).

The third group of questions shown in Table 73–2 relates to characterization of voiding habits. An affirmative answer to the first question concerning suprapubic pain when the bladder is full may suggest interstitial cystitis; several patients in our series had surgically curable urinary incontinence and interstitial cystitis. The latter disease, of course, is not helped by preventing urinary incontinence.

These, then, are the questions we have found helpful in evaluating the history of patients who present with urinary incontinence. Many other questions are found in some questionnaires (e.g., queries relating to childhood history, sensations of losing urine, the sight or sound of running water causing urinary incontinence, and so on), but we have not found such questions useful. One of the advantages to the questionnaire presented in Table 73–2 is that the nurse or office assistant can easily fill it out before the patient sees the urologist.

Physical Examination

Determination of Maximum Voided Volume and Residual Urine. While the patient's history is being taken, she is asked to force fluids until her bladder is very full and she has a strong desire to urinate. Once the bladder is filled to capacity from oral hydration, she is asked first to empty her bladder in the privacy of a bathroom using a standard toilet with a measuring pan beneath the seat; this gives the surgeon an objective measurement of maximal functional volume. Immediately after the voided volume is measured, the patient is placed on an examining table, and the bladder is catheterized with a No. 14 French straight polyethylene catheter; the residual urine is recorded, and a specimen for urinalysis and urine culture is obtained from the catheter. Significant residual urine is often a sign of a neuropathic bladder. The absence of residual urine, however, does not exclude neurologic disease. Large residuals of several hundred milliliters are usually caused by acontractile bladders; if these patients also have surgically curable incontinence, they invariably require intermittent catheterization after their vesical neck is suspended behind the symphysis pubis because they will be unable to void.

Filling the Bladder. We attach the open barrel of a 50-ml syringe to the end of the catheter and fill the bladder by gravity flow to a comfortable volume, usually somewhat less than the amount the patient voided. Using the simple technique of holding the catheter vertically with the attached open syringe, the filling rate is about 60 to 100 ml per minute. When the syringe is filled to the 50-ml mark, the water height is about 40 cm above the urethra. This column of water in the syringe and catheter should fall steadily throughout bladder filling until the bladder is comfortably full. At this time the column of water in the catheter neither falls nor rises and should be less than 15 cm of water above the urethral meatus. Bladder instability is often defined as uninhibited spontaneous bladder contractions of 15 cm H_2O or greater; therefore, if the open syringe and catheter are carefully observed during filling, a spontaneous contraction of this magnitude is usually detected as a sudden rise in the column of the water, which had been falling during bladder filling.

The primary purpose of the catheter, however, is to determine the amount of the patient's residual urine and, even more importantly, to fill the bladder with a known amount of fluid at a volume comfortable to the patient. This needs to be emphasized because though these observations on the presence or absence of spontaneous detrusor contractions as well as the final filling pressure are interesting and represent "free" information without increasing the time or expense of the procedure, they are rarely helpful in patients with surgically curable incontinence and are only occasionally contributory in women with nonsurgically curable incontinence.

Demonstration of Surgically Curable Incontinence. With the bladder comfortably full, the catheter removed, and the patient in the lithotomy position, the urologist is ready for the only critical diagnostic step: demonstration of urinary incontinence directly related to coughing. So critical is this observation that we believe surgically curable urinary incontinence in females should be defined literally as the visual demonstration of a simultaneous loss of urine with the rise and fall of abdominal pressure during coughing. Without this simple demonstration, no patient should be operated on for urinary incontinence. With the exception of Grade III total urinary incontinence, the surgeon must be wary of any patient who loses urine unrelated to increased abdominal pressure. Four of the 19 failures in the 1980 series of 203 patients (Stamey, 1980a) were operated on because of a highly suggestive history, even though loss of urine could not be demonstrated on physical examination; not one of these patients was helped even partially. We should also emphasize how unreliable the patient's history of urinary incontinence can be, even when the highly focused and selected questionnaire presented in Table 73–2 is used. With this questionnaire, we have often entered the examining room convinced we would be dealing with uncomplicated, surgically curable urinary incontinence, only to find that incontinence could not be demonstrated with sudden elevations in abdominal pressure. However, it is also true that we have often expected nonsurgical incontinence based on the questionnaire findings only to discover gross leakage of urine with coughing. Our estimate is that the questionnaire is misleading at least 20 per cent of the time, which is why the surgeon must personally examine the patient with a full bladder.

If the patient does not lose urine when examined in the lithotomy position, she is then tilted to a 45 degree upright position on the cystoscopy table to increase the resting pressure of the bladder by adding the weight of some of the abdominal contents. In the 45 degree tilted position, the surgeon can still observe the urethral meatus by spreading the labia during coughing. About 80 per cent of patients with surgically curable incontinence lose urine in the lithotomy position with coughing, whereas another 10 per cent require tilting to the 45 degree position. The last 10 per cent demonstrate loss of urine directly related to coughing only when examined in the standing position. In the erect position, the full weight of the abdominal contents (about 35 cm H_2O) is exerted on the bladder and becomes additive to the pressure generated by the cough.

The urologist, however, must be very careful and patient when examining his subject in the erect position. For one thing, the urethral meatus can no longer be seen when the patient coughs. Because the labia cover the urethra somewhat like a dam, leakage of urine may appear a second or so after coughing and even continue to drip after the rise in pressure from coughing has returned to normal. Furthermore, the examiner must be careful also because 90 per cent of patients with surgically curable incontinence have already been eliminated by failure to observe leakage in the lithotomy or tilted position; thus, there is a greater chance that he is now dealing with nonsurgical urinary incontinence or even an overt neuropathic bladder.

Most of our patients with nonsurgical urinary incontinence simply fail to demonstrate urinary leakage with coughing in the standing position. There are a few, however, whose cough causes a spontaneous detrusor contraction, and 5 to 15 seconds after the cough they begin to pass a small volume of water. Because this loss of urine requires a detrusor contraction, it is clearly evident on physical examination that urinary leakage is not simultaneous with cough pressure. Moreover, the urinary loss is usually a stream of urine that slowly ceases after an ounce or two has been voided.

Hodgkinson (1965), who was the first to recognize these patients, called this condition "idiopathic detrusor dyssynergia." This is not common in the patients we examine with urinary incontinence, but the phenomenon is fascinating to observe and is astonishingly reproducible; most patients with nonsurgical incontinence simply fail to lose urine in any of the three positions in which we examine them.

The reader will note that those patients who lose urine exactly coincident with the rise and fall of abdominal pressure have been referred to here as having surgically curable urinary incontinence (Stamey, 1980a). We prefer this term to SUI simply because patients with total urinary incontinence (Grade III), and even some with Grade II incontinence, simply do not recognize the stress component of their incontinence. Surgically curable incontinence is also a better term than anatomic incontinence, or a number of other terms nicely reviewed by Hodgkinson (1965), because it emphasizes that these patients can be cured of their incontinence. Thus, we would propose that surgically curable urinary incontinence be defined on the basis of physical examination, and that the definition be confined to those patients in whom the surgeon has visually demonstrated loss of urine exactly coinciding with the rise in abdominal pressure. All other types of incontinence, except for that in a few selected patients with neuropathic bladders and severe spontaneous detrusor contraction in whom cystolysis (Freiha and Stamey, 1979) or vaginal resection of the inferior hypogastric plexus (Hodgkinson and Drukker, 1977) can successfully denervate the bladder, have surgically incurable incontinence, according to the present state of our knowledge.

Presence of Rectocele or Cystocele. Every patient who is a potential candidate for endoscopic suspension of the vesical neck should be examined for the presence of a rectocele or cystocele. Endoscopic suspension corrects mild and even moderate relaxation of the anterior vaginal wall, but of course does nothing for rectoceles. In the first 100 of our patients, 3 of them returned in the early postoperative course with symptomatic rectoceles protruding from the vaginal introitus; these had not been observed by the patient preoperatively. Presumably, counterpressure from the cystocele buttressed against the rectocele prevented prolapse of the rectocele from the introitus. Whatever the reason, we soon learned to recognize significant rectoceles and to repair them after suspending the bladder neck. If very large cystoceles that protrude from the introitus upon straining or standing are present, the anterior vaginal incision is simply extended to the vaginal vault or the cervix, and the cystocele is fixed before suspending the vesical neck. It is important to recognize, however, that mild to moderate cystoceles never require an extension of the routine incision and are readily corrected by the suspending bolster of Dacron at the urethrovesical junction (see the section on operative technique later in this chapter).

We much prefer a tongue blade to the vaginal speculum in assessing the degree of anterior or posterior vaginal wall relaxation. By lifting the cystocele or depressing the rectocele with the tongue blade in the midline, and then having the patient perform the Valsalva maneuver, we can determine the degree of anterior or posterior relaxation. The vaginal speculum is required, of course, to evaluate an enterocele or vaginal vault prolapse, both of which should be excluded during the physical examination.

The Role of Urethroscopy. In summary, the instruments needed to diagnose surgically curable urinary incontinence in the urologist's office include an inexpensive urethral catheter, a 50-ml syringe, and a bottle of water (Table 73–3). Observe that cystoscopes, urethroscopes, cystometry, urethral pressure profiles, electromyography recordings, cystograms, and videotape cystourethrography are not only unnecessary but also clearly add needless expense to the evaluation of these patients.

Preoperative urethroscopy, with or without gas cystometry to measure the opening pressure

TABLE 73–3. INSTRUMENTS USED TO DIAGNOSE STRESS URINARY INCONTINENCE

1. URETHRAL CATHETER
2. SYRINGE
3. BOTTLE OF WATER
NOTE: Unnecessary Measures
    URETHROSCOPE
    CYSTOMETROGRAM
    URETHRAL PRESSURE PROFILE
    EMG

of the urethra as advocated by an increasing number of gynecologists, is even more useless than cystometry and should not be tolerated in a health system already overburdened by skyrocketing costs. It is true that urethroscopy often shows an open, lax urethra in the proximal two thirds, but this observation contributes nothing to the diagnosis already made by simple physical examination. Some proponents of urethroscopy attempt to justify its use for observing "trigonitis," "urethritis," and urethral polyps. It should be clear to the most casual observer, however, that none of these conditions has anything to do with surgically curable urinary incontinence. Indeed, it is highly doubtful if any of these diagnoses has anything to do with any symptomatic diseases in the female. For example, "trigonitis" does not even exist; the cystoscopic findings of a "cobblestone" or "furry-appearing" trigone actually represent congenital inclusion of normal vaginal epithelium within the bladder, which occurs in all women, (Cifuentes 1947). True "urethritis" in the female cannot be documented bacteriologically (Stamey, 1980b) and has no endoscopic hallmarks, even in the presence of overt, proven bacterial cystitis; to be sure, urethral "polyps" are secondary to chronic bacteriuria, but they disappear with sterilization of the infection and long-term prophylaxis to prevent reinfection. It is also true that an incidental urethral diverticulum may be seen on urethroscopy, but it has no pathologic significance unless it presents as a symptomatic urethral mass. Thus, though it is almost impossible to justify urethroscopy in the female in terms of true urethral disease, the medical profession is faced with a surge of urethroscopic interest among gynecologists. This is based on the false premise that the female urethroscope offers important diagnostic information in SUI.

Marshall-Marchetti or Bonney Test. We routinely perform the Marshall-Marchetti or Bonney test of elevating the internal vesical neck while the patient coughs, thereby preventing loss of urine that would otherwise appear at the urethral meatus. It is important, however, to recognize that the test is not discriminatory in a diagnostic sense, because it is inappropriate and cannot be done in the case of urinary loss from a neuropathic bladder (i.e., there is no leakage to stop with coughing), and in surgically curable urinary incontinence the test is almost always positive. We have seen only one patient with surgically curable incontinence in whom urinary leakage with coughing could not be stopped by elevating the internal vesical neck;

this patient had a skin graft of the anterior vaginal wall that was so thick that we could not put pressure on the vesical neck. At surgery, however, the vesical neck was easily elevated to a position of continence once the anterior vaginal wall was dissected free. Thus, though the Marshall-Marchetti or Bonney test is nondiscriminating for diagnostic evaluation, it is psychologically comforting to the surgeon to see the urinary leakage cease with elevation of the vesical neck. Moreover, the ease of the surgical repair is usually proportional to the mobility and ease with which the tissues lateral to the vesical neck can be elevated behind the symphysis pubis. For this reason, even if the Marshall-Marchetti test is not done to prevent leakage of urine while coughing, the pliability of these tissues around the vesical neck should always be examined by the surgeon.

Before the patient is removed from the lithotomy position, a bimanual pelvic examination is performed to complete the physical examination, the rectum is examined for any masses, and the S_2, S_3, and S_4 dermatomes on the perineum are checked for sensory loss by using a sharp, broken cotton stick. Because the patient has been catheterized and may have been infected by the catheter, she is given 24 hours of an oral antimicrobial agent prophylactically, usually nitrofurantoin or trimethoprim-sulfamethoxazole.

Our practice is to record these few crucial observations from the physical examination on the form presented in Table 73–4; the last entry in this table is used to assign a grade to the degree of urinary incontinence.

The Role of Urinary Tract Infections in Incontinence. Although urinary tract infection is commonly mentioned in the literature as a cause of urinary incontinence, and patients with acute cystitis often have urgency incontinence, we have never helped a patient with stress incontinence by clearing their bacteriuria. In fact, urodynamic studies have amply shown that most patients with urinary tract infections have stable bladders.

TABLE 73–4. RECORD OF IMPORTANT OBSERVATIONS FROM PHYSICAL EXAMINATION

Volume of urine voided before examination:_____ml.
    Residual urine:_____ml.

Volume of water used to fill bladder by gravity (should be less than volume voided before examination):_____ml.
    Intravesical pressure at final bladder volume:_____cm H_2O.

How much leakage occurs when the patient coughs hard?
    None_____; Minimal (barely dribbles out the urethra)_____; Moderate (water spurts 2 or 3 inches beyond the urethral meatus)_____; Large (water spurts 6 inches or more beyond the urethral meatus)_____.

Was it necessary to tilt the patient to a partial upright position (30 to 45 degrees) to demonstrate loss of urine with coughing? Yes_____; No_____.

Did patient have to stand in the erect position to demonstrate stress incontinence with coughing? Yes_____; No_____.

Is sensation to pin prick at S_2, S_3, and S_4 dermatomes normal? Yes_____; No_____.
    If no, describe abnormality: _____

Is anal sphincter tone normal? Yes_____; No_____.

Rectocele: None_____; Slight_____; Moderate_____; Marked (protrudes through vaginal introitus)_____.

Cystocele: None_____; Slight_____; Moderate_____; Marked (protrudes through vaginal introitus)_____.

Enterocele: None_____; Slight_____; Moderate_____; Marked (protrudes through vaginal introitus)_____.

Uterine-vault descent: None_____; Slight_____; Moderate_____; Marked (protrudes through vaginal introitus)_____.

Grade the degree of incontinence:
    Grade   I: Leakage with severe stress only (coughing, sneezing, lifting). _____

    Grade II: Leakage with minimal stress only (walking, standing, shopping). _____

    Grade III: Leakage all the time regardless of activity or position. _____

Radiologic Studies to Determine the Anatomic Position of the Vesical Neck in Relation to the Symphysis Pubis

Every successful operation for SUI is dependent upon moving the vesical neck to a higher position behind the symphysis pubis; failure to move the vesical neck is tantamount to surgical failure. Thus, there is a practical reason—at least in surgically difficult cases—for knowing the position of the vesical neck in relation to the symphysis pubis, that is, if the patient remains incontinent after surgery, and the surgeon has not moved the vesical neck, he does not need to look elsewhere for the cause of failure.

Although we rarely perform radiologic studies today in our evaluation of SUI, they are of historic interest because pre- and postoperative radiologic studies on the anatomy of SUI have done more to add to our understanding of curable incontinence in the female than has any other investigative technique. The credit belongs to Jeffcoate and Roberts (1952), who introduced the lateral urethrocystogram and to Hodgkinson (1953), who introduced and popularized the metallic bead chain urethrocystogram. Whether a catheter (Jeffcoate and Roberts, 1952) or a chain is used to visualize the urethrovesical junction in relation to the symphysis pubis, the radiographs must be carefully done with the patient straining (but not voiding) in the erect position, and the radiograph must be taken in a true lateral view across both hips.

The relationship of the urethrovesical junc-tion to the symphysis pubis in the young, normal, nonparous female is shown in Figure 73–1 and is diagramatically represented in Figure 73–2. The "normal" anatomic position (Fig. 73–2A) is compared to two types of Valsalva urethrocystograms seen in women with SUI (Fig. 73–2B and C); in both of these incontinent configurations, the urethrovesical junction tends to be cone-shaped and is located at the lowest bladder level. Typical lateral urethrocystograms in an incontinent patient before and after endoscopic suspension of the vesical neck are shown in Figures 73–3 and 73–4. Note that the position of the urethrovesical junction has been moved from below the symphyseal-fifth sacral vertebral line to several centimeters above it. We reported on the pre- and postoperative lateral radiographs in 44 consecutive patients undergoing endoscopic suspension of the vesical neck (Stamey et al., 1975). In those patients operated on for the first time, the average preoperative position of the urethrovesical junction was almost 2 cm below the symphyseal-S_5 line compared to a postoperative position of 3.5 cm above the line, making the average movement of the urethrovesical junction nearly 5.5 cm (Figure 73–5). To appreciate this movement of the urethrovesical junction fully, the surgeon should remember that the maximal movement achieved by anterior colporrhaphy (Kelly plication) is only 1 cm (Low, 1967; Hodgkinson, 1970).

It is important to recognize that the configuration of these radiographs does not correspond with either the incidence or the severity of the urinary incontinence, an observation rec-

Figure 73–1. A normal, direct lateral urethrocystogram taken in the straining position from a continent female who was not operated upon. Note the high position of the urethrovesical junction behind the symphysis pubis, the flat and posteriorly directed baseplate, and the definite but slight posterior direction of the proximal urethra.

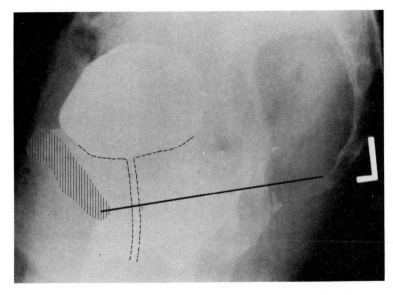

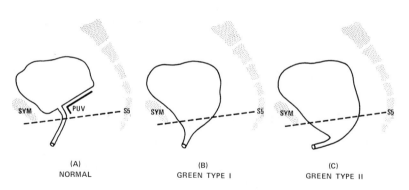

Figure 73–2. *A,* Relationship of the baseplate of the bladder (directed inferiorly and slightly posteriorly toward the sacrum) in the normal continent female who has not had surgery. Note the posterior urethrovesical angle (PUV) of 90 degrees, indicating a flat baseplate with the proximal urethra; the proximal urethra is directed somewhat posteriorly. *B,* Downward and backward displacement with funneling of the urethrovesical junction, characteristic of the Green Type I anatomic configuration in SUI. *C,* Further downward and backward displacement of the urethrovesical junction (Green Type II).

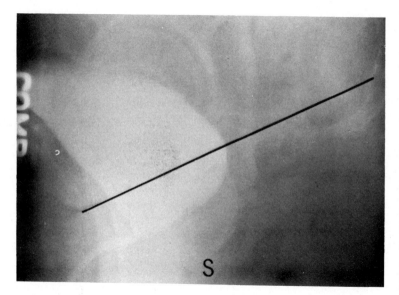

Figure 73–3. Typical preoperative lateral cystourethrogram with straining in a patient with stress urinary incontinence (Green Type II). Note complete loss of posterior urethrovesical angle (180°) and, more important, the fact that the urethrovesical junction is far below the inferior border of the symphysis, marked by the symphyseal-S5 line. (From Stamey, T. A., et al.: Surg. Gynecol. Obstet., *140*:355, 1975. Used by permission.)

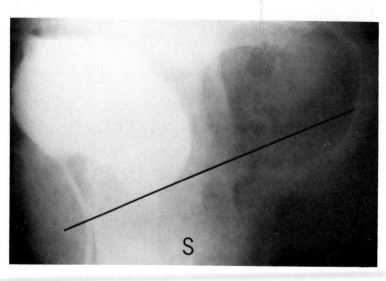

Figure 73–4. Postoperative studies in the same patient as Figure 73–3 but following endoscopic suspension with permanent cure of her urinary incontinence (15-year follow-up). Observe that the urethrovesical junction is now at the upper to middle third of the symphysis pubis and that the posterior baseplate forms an acute angle with the urethrovesical junction. (From Stamey, T. A., et al.: Surg. Gynecol. Obstet., *140*:355, 1975. Used by permission.)

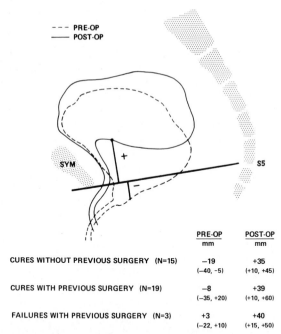

	PRE-OP mm	POST-OP mm
CURES WITHOUT PREVIOUS SURGERY (N=15)	−19 (−40, -5)	+35 (+10, +45)
CURES WITH PREVIOUS SURGERY (N=19)	−8 (−35, +20)	+39 (+10, +60)
FAILURES WITH PREVIOUS SURGERY (N=3)	+3 (−22, +10)	+40 (+15, +50)

Figure 73–5. The preoperative and postoperative position of the posterior baseplate of the bladder, 1 cm from the posterior urethrovesical junction during straining. The mean of the three patient groups, together with the minimal and maximal values observed, is presented for each category. The plus sign (+) indicates those positions above the symphyseal (SYM)–fifth sacral vertebral (S5) line, and the minus sign (−) those below the line. (From Stamey, T. A., et al.: Surg. Gynecol. Obstet., *140*:355, 1975. Use by permission.)

ognized by both Jeffcoate and Hodgkinson. Moreover, if one measures the various angles of these radiographs in relation to the urethrovesical junction—for example, the posterior urethrovesical angle (Fig. 73–2*A*)—there is a substantial overlap between continent and incontinent women (Ala-Ketola, 1973; Greenwald et al., 1967). Despite this radiographic overlap in bladder base configuration in continent and incontinent women, the unique place of the lateral urethrocystogram lies in evaluating the efficacy of the surgery designed to restore the urethrovesical junction to a position of continence behind the symphysis pubis. In addition to performing lateral urethrocystograms in the 44 consecutive patients we reported in 1975, we continued this routine for another 100 patients. Our observations, as well as those reported in the literature when these radiographs were consistently performed, are absolutely convincing that every successful operative procedure is always accompanied by a forward and upward displacement of the urethrovesical junction; unsuccessful operations are usually characterized by failure to move the urethrovesical junction.

Indeed, in those few patients in whom we continue to obtain preoperative lateral urethrocystograms to check for postoperative movement of the urethrovesical junction in case of failure, we do not measure any "angles" but rely instead on the position of the urethrovesical junction in relation to the symphysis pubis and its subsequent postoperative movement upward behind the symphysis pubis. Tanagho (1974) has also emphasized the relationship of the urethrovesical junction to the fixed bony structures of the pelvis. In this way, the surgeon can answer the crucial question in an operative failure: Did he successfully move the urethrovesical junction with the operation? If he did not achieve upward and forward displacement, he does not need to blame the failure on some hypothetic functional mechanism such as an "unstable bladder."

For these reasons, we reserve preoperative radiographs of the urethrovesical junction for those patients with very complicated cases, having had multiple previous surgeries or radiation fibrosis and in whom we expect substantial difficulty in elevating the internal vesical neck. In the last several years, at the suggestion of Dr. Kenneth Wishnow, who was one of our urologic residents at Stanford, we have placed several small surgical clips on one end of the Dacron buttress; this allows postoperative identification of the position of the urethrovesical junction with only a plain film lateral radiograph, thereby avoiding urethral catheterization and the use of contrast medium. To be sure, without preoperative assessment, one cannot be certain of the net change, but one of the reasons we ceased these radiologic measurements is that following endoscopic suspension, the urethrovesical junction was virtually always elevated to a position halfway up and behind the symphysis pubis (Figure 73–4); simple surgical clips placed on the end of the Dacron tube (see section on surgical procedure) positioned away from the urethra, allow the postoperative observation to be made with a single, uncomplicated x-ray study. At times this is surprisingly useful. For example, one of our colleagues recently was distressed to find that his patient was as incontinent in the immediate postoperative period as she was before surgery. SUI was easily demonstrable on physical examination. Since he had expected some difficulty because of several previous operations, he had obtained a preoperative lateral chain urethrocystogram. The operation seemed uneventful; excellent anatomic and functional closure of the vesical neck was observed by lifting the suspending sutures singularly and in unison (see operative description). The postoperative lateral chain cystogram not only showed no change in the position of the urethrovesical junction, but also, as can be observed in Figure 73–6, the metallic clips marking the Dacron buttresses (indicated by the two arrows) showed them to have pulled through all of the fasical levels and to be resting beneath the rectus muscle above the symphysis pubis! This was not appreciated by the surgeon when he tied the suspending sutures, and we have not seen this complication before; single buttresses on one side have pulled through in a few radiated patients, but this occurrence has always been recognized at the time of surgery. Perhaps this incident serves as a reminder that these suspending sutures must not be tied tightly and that the technique described later in this chapter should be carefully followed.

Preoperative radiographs that show normal bladder base configuration with a flat base plate and a good posterior urethrovesical angle in patients who have had previous retropubic procedures should not be disconcerting to the surgeon. We have observed and reported several patients with such normal-appearing anatomy who were cured by surgical movement of the urethrovesical junction farther upward behind the symphysis pubis, as illustrated in Figure 73–7.

From an investigative viewpoint, radiographic evaluation of the lateral urethrocystogram represents the only objective way to compare the efficacy of different operations proposed to restore the vesical neck to a higher position behind the symphysis pubis. As seen in Figure 73–5, the mean elevation of the posterior bladder base at a point 1 cm from the urethrovesical junction, achieved by endoscopic suspension of the vesical neck, is about 5 cm. A well-performed Marshall-Marchetti operation (Marshall et al., 1949), or colposuspension of the anterior vaginal wall to the iliopectineal ligament at the pelvic brim (Burch, 1961), probably gives this much elevation, but we are unaware of any substantial series in which consecutive patients have undergone pre- and postoperative radiography. It is clear that anterior colporrhaphy, even in the best of hands, achieves only about 1 cm of elevation. In a careful radiologic study of pre- and postoperative lateral urethrocystograms in all patients undergoing anterior colporrhaphy for SUI, Low (1967) noted a 1-cm "upward and forward elevation of the bladder neck" in 50 per cent of the patients who were cured by surgery.

Because of these generally poor results when all patients with surgically curable urinary incontinence are treated by anterior colporrhaphy, Green (1968) divided urinary incontinence into Type I and Type II, based on the lateral urethrocystogram. He believed that although Type I (Fig. 73–2*B*) could be successfully treated by the vaginal route, Type II (Fig. 73–2*C*) required retropubic urethropexy. One of the advantages to endoscopic suspension of the vesical neck is that it makes no difference whether Green's Type I or Type II bladder configuration is present.

It is clear that most anterior colporrhaphy surgery does little to restore the urethrovesical

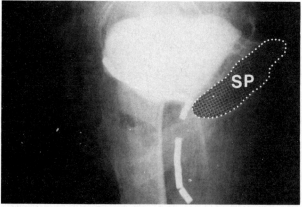

PRE OP

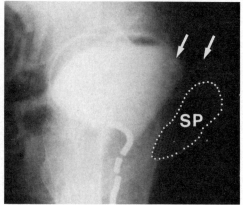

POST OP

Figure 73–6. Pre- and postoperative lateral chain cystourethrograms in a patient whose incontinence was not changed by uneventful endoscopic suspension of the vesical neck. Observe that the position of the urethrovesical junction in relation to the symphysis pubis is essentially unchanged, allowing for the slight difference in laterality of the radiograph. Also observe the metallic clips, placed on the end of the Dacron buttress at the time of surgery. These clips (arrows) are clearly in the space of Retzius beneath the symphysis pubis and had pulled through the pubocervical and endopelvic fasciae, unknown to the surgeon. (From Stamey, T. A.: Monogr. Urol., 2:65, 1981. Used by permission.)

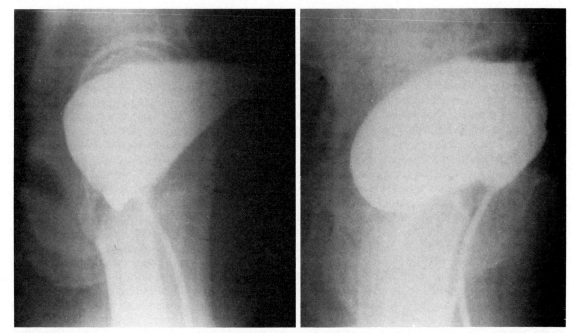

Figure 73–7. *Left,* Preoperative lateral cystourethrogram with straining in patient with total urinary incontinence (Grade III) who had previously undergone multiple suprapubic and vaginal operations. Note that the baseplate is not funneled in relation to the urethra; indeed, it is flat (90 degrees). Position of the urethrovesical junction is at the lower third of the symphysis pubis, which is not seen well in this radiograph. *Right,* Postoperative lateral cystourethrogram during straining. Following endoscopic suspension of the vesical neck, this patient was cured of her incontinence (12-year follow-up). Note that the urethrovesical junction has been moved farther upward and forward behind the symphysis pubis, despite previously normal position of the vesical neck. (From Stamey, T. A.: Monogr. Urol., *2*:65, 1981. Used by permission.)

junction and that the 1-cm elevation achieved by this surgery in the best of hands can help only the mildest form of urinary incontinence. To be sure, if the patient requires a vaginal hysterectomy for uterine prolapse and also has mild stress incontinence, attempted plication of the internal vesical neck is clearly worthwhile. The danger, however, of overcorrection of the accompanying cystocele is that urinary incontinence can be created or stress incontinence can be made worse; this distressing complication of cystocele repair, apparently caused by creating a funnel at the vesical neck by extensive elevation of the bladder base, is recognized by most gynecologists but was emphasized by Green (1968). These difficulties have often caused the well-informed gynecologist to perform vaginal hysterectomy and retropubic exploration to suspend the vesical neck. It should be apparent that vaginal hysterectomy combined with endoscopic suspension of the vesical neck through the same vaginal incision offers substantial advantages to the patient; the fear of postoperative incontinence from overcorrection of a cystocele would be removed completely.

There is, in our opinion, no place for micturition cystography—either single-shot static or cineradiographs—in the diagnosis and practical management of surgically curable urinary incontinence in the female.

THE ROLE OF INFLOW CYSTOMETRY, PRESSURE FLOW STUDIES OF VOIDING, AND URETHRAL PRESSURE MEASUREMENTS

If the surgeon follows these simple office evaluation procedures and demonstrates SUI on physical examination, there is usually no reason to perform routine cystometrograms with voiding and urethral pressure studies. We have recently performed cystometrograms with urethral pressure profiles in a number of consecutive, unselected patients in our university urodynamics laboratory: They do *not* add to the practical decision of whether or not to operate. Indeed, they have not predicted such aspects of the patient's postoperative course as how long postoperative residual urine may persist or whether urgency will continue, subside, or develop anew. In short, cystometry and urethral pressure studies, like cystoscopy, are procedures that do not add to the evaluation of women with straightforward SUI, and, therefore, most patients can be spared this medical expense. There are, however, women in whom these measurements may be useful. Rare patients (less than 1 per cent) with SUI and large postvoid residual urines preoperatively, who can be shown by pressure-flow studies during voiding to have an acontractile bladder, can still be treated with surgical evaluation of the vesical neck, but this must be combined with a permanent program of intermittent catheterization. The even rarer patient (we have seen 5 in some 500 cases) who leaks urine continuously when examined in the lithotomy position can be shown to have a "stovepipe" urethra with virtually no closure pressure on urethral pressure studies. Although endoscopic suspension and urethral plication cured all five, our series is too small to know whether the simple urethral plication we added to the endoscopic suspension of the vesical neck is necessary. The information gained in these rare bladder or urethral conditions—which may be predicted by a good physical examination—probably does not justify routine urodynamic evaluation of patients with demonstrable SUI.

Constantinou and Stamey (1985) have performed urodynamics on 151 consecutive unselected women seen in consultation for urinary incontinence. On physical examination, 84 demonstrated SUI (56 per cent) while 67 did not (44 per cent). Upon urodynamic evaluation, 62 per cent of the 84 patients with SUI had stable detrusors when examined in the upright (sitting) position; 30 per cent were unstable (8 per cent showed marginal instability but are not considered further). Of those patients without demonstrable SUI, 51 per cent were stable while 43 per cent were unstable (6 per cent were marginal). Excluding the marginal instability groups (11 patients), 140 consecutive patients were available for analysis—77 with SUI and 63 without (Table 73–5).

After their maximum urinary flow rate and voided volume were measured, a 10 F double-lumen urethral catheter was passed into the bladder and the residual volume was recorded. With the patients in the upright position, the bladder was filled with warm water at about 20 ml per minute. The bladder volume at first sensation and at urgency to void, the maximum detrusor pressure and urine flow rate during voiding, and the bladder capacity and residual volume after voiding were recorded. Simultaneous recordings of rectal and bladder pressures (accompanied by electronic subtraction), urine flow rates, and EMG tracings were made, as seen in a copy of the original tracing in Figure 73–8. Upon refilling the bladder, isometric pressures were measured in the sitting position by acutely obstructing the vesical neck with a Foley

TABLE 73–5. URODYNAMIC EVALUATION OF 140 CONSECUTIVE, UNSELECTED, INCONTINENT WOMEN WITH AND WITHOUT STRESS URINARY INCONTINENCE (SUI)

Detrusor Function	SUI (77)		Non-SUI (63)	
	STABLE	UNSTABLE	STABLE	UNSTABLE
N = Number of patients	52	25	34	29
Age	56 ± 13	60 ± 11	50 ± 16	43 ± 18
Catheter-free voiding				
Max. flow rate (ml/sec)	22 ± 13	21 ± 16	21 ± 15	21 ± 16
Vol. voided (ml)	260 ± 186	182 ± 117	289 ± 231	168 ± 122
Residual vol. (ml)	39 ± 71	30 ± 41	146 ± 163	84 ± 92
Cystometrograms				
Vol. at first sensation (ml)	211 ± 94	179 ± 95**	190 ± 165	144 ± 77**
Vol. at urgency (ml)	410 ± 145	337 ± 179	436 ± 211	214 ± 101
Max. detrusor pressure (cm H_2O)	20 ± 13†	26 ± 15*	28 ± 15†	56 ± 26*
Max. flow rate (ml/sec)	21 ± 11	28 ± 19††	19 ± 9	20 ± 17††
Capacity (ml)	531 ± 165	384 ± 201	534 ± 204	283 ± 177
Residual vol. (ml)	40 ± 71	30 ± 41	210 ± 191	195 ± 190
Isometric tests				
Max. isometric pressure	52 ± 65 (N=35)	52 ± 22 (N=17)	46 ± 22 (N=9)	46 ± 21 (N=4)
Vol. at Max. isometric pressure	430 ± 185	284 ± 205*	494 ± 152	407 ± 127*

   * = p < 0.001 between the two values indicated by *
   ** = p < 0.05 between the two values indicated by **
   † = p < 0.001 between the two values indicated by †
   †† = p < 0.01 between the two values indicated by ††
   Unstable = Involuntary unsuppressible, spontaneous or provoked, detrusor contraction(s) during bladder filling that leads to loss of urine.

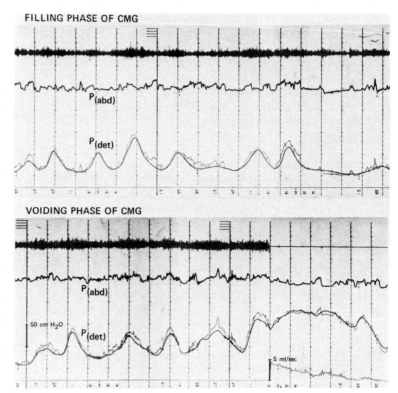

FILLING PHASE OF CMG

VOIDING PHASE OF CMG

Figure 73–8. A cystometrogram tracing from a healthy control volunteer woman, without urinary symptoms, representative of the five-channel recording used to obtain the data in Table 73–6 during filling and voiding phases. The top line represents EMG activity of the external sphincter; $P_{(abd)}$, the abdominal pressure recorded from a rectal balloon; and $P_{(det)}$, the detrusor pressure from an intravesical catheter. The solid line along the $P_{(det)}$ tracing is an electronic subtraction of $P_{(det)}$ minus $P_{(abd)}$ and therefore represents true intravesical pressure. The declining tracing in the right lower corner illustrates urine flow rate caused by the detrusor contraction shown just above it; note the sharp diminution in CMG activity during contraction of the detrusor muscle. The spontaneous detrusor contractions of 50 cm H_2O or more are readily apparent in this healthy volunteer control.

catheter balloon after the initiation of urine flow by a detrusor contraction (Constantinou et al., 1984).

Recognizing the substantial controversy over the definition of instability (Turner-Warwick, 1979), we defined unstable to mean an involuntary, unsuppressible detrusor contraction(s)—spontaneous or evoked—during bladder filling that leads to loss of urine. Marginal instability was defined as an unsuppressible detrusor contraction(s) with a pressure greater than 15 cm of water during bladder filling for which urine loss, if it occurs, cannot be determined to be voluntary or involuntary.

The data in Table 73–5 show that there is no single characteristic of the detrusor response that distinguishes an incontinent patient with SUI from one without SUI. We believe it is best to compare stable SUI with stable non-SUI and unstable SUI with unstable non-SUI. It is true that patients with non-SUI have a significantly higher maximum detrusor pressure during voiding (p < 0.001) and that the unstable non-SUI women void at slower flow rates than the unstable SUI group (p < 0.01). These characteristics, however, are compatible with the accepted observation that women with SUI have less urethral resistance and therefore demonstrate a smaller rise in maximum detrusor pres-

sure, often accompanied by a faster urine flow rate. The maximum isometric pressures (the maximum detrusor pressure in the presence of complete bladder outlet obstruction) are the same in SUI and non-SUI (Table 73–5), indicating that the detrusor of the SUI patient is capable of generating a normal pressure in the presence of increased urethral resistance. These cystometry data reflect accepted differences in urethral resistance between women with SUI and non-SUI—differences that are more easily recognized during the physical examination by directly observing the patient to lose urine through the urethra simultaneously with a cough-induced rise in abdominal pressure (SUI). It is also clear that even at a p-value difference of < 0.001 for maximum detrusor pressures during voiding, the standard deviations are such that these parameters do not differentiate between incontinent individuals with SUI or non-SUI. Lastly, the residual volumes in Table 73–5, measured both after the initial voiding before the urethral catheterization and after the later voiding around the catheter, are obviously larger in non-SUI women than those with SUI. Whether this reflects a component of even greater urethral resistance in women with non-SUI induced by the study conditions per se, we do not know;

these non-SUI patients did not show a significant residual when first seen in the outpatient setting, where they were examined in less stressful circumstances.

Because we knew that endoscopic suspension of the vesical neck consistently elevated the urethrovesical junction upward and forward behind the symphysis pubis (Stamey et al., 1975), and that such elevation was curative in 90 to 95 per cent of patients operated upon, we were interested in measuring urethral closure pressures after endoscopic suspension. These urethral pressure profiles were measured in the lithotomy position with a specially made 11 F catheter that contained two microtip transducers equally spaced 180 degrees apart at the tip. This allowed us to evaluate static urethral pressure profiles in the anterior and posterior urethra. As can be seen in Table 73–6, the maximum urethral closure pressures are very much lower in women with SUI than in healthy controls without incontinence, an observation well documented in the literature (Enhörning, 1961; Toews, 1967). Urethral closure pressure is known to decline dramatically with age, and the controls here are less than half the age of the patients, accentuating the difference in urethral closure pressures. Observe, however, that the anterior and posterior maximum closure pressures are approximately equal in the controls and in the non-SUI women, but that the SUI patients demonstrate significantly decreased pressures in the posterior urethra in comparison with pressures observed in the anterior urethra. Endoscopic suspension of the vesical neck does not change the pressure in the anterior urethra but doubles it in the posterior urethra, making it approach the pressure of the anterior quadrant. Thus, the maximum impact of endoscopic suspension on these resting urethral pressures appears to be in restoring the posterior urethral resistance to equal that of the anterior urethra.

Hilton and Stanton (1983) were among the first to point out that rotational variations in the urethral closure pressure profile may not be as artifactual as earlier observers thought.

The resting urethral pressure profiles do not afford a complete picture of urethral competence because they are static studies. Enhörning (1961) was the first to measure differential pressures between the bladder and urethra at rest and during cough-induced increases in abdominal pressure. He demonstrated that while cough-induced increases in abdominal pressure added to the pressure measured in the continent urethra, they were not as efficiently transferred to the incontinent urethra, thereby allowing leakage of urine with coughing because the bladder pressure exceeded the urethral pressure. Dynamic urethral pressure profiles performed at Stanford University (Constantinou et al., 1981; Constantinou and Govan, 1982) have shown that the cough-induced rise in urethral pressure measured in the distal urethra of control volunteers is significantly attenuated in patients with SUI. After endoscopic suspension of the vesical neck, transmission of pressure is enhanced in the distal, as well as in the proximal, urethra. More recently, Constantinou (personal communication, 1985), using a four-quadrant microtip transducer, found that these cough-induced increases in urethral pressure appear to localize to the anterior region of the urethra. This is contrary to the static studies, which clearly demonstrated a posterior urethral weakness that was corrected with endoscopic suspension. The explanation of these various urethral responses must await further research.

The gynecologic literature, and much of the European urologic literature as well, often warn against operating upon women with SUI who also have urgency incontinence (presumably unstable bladders). Indeed, urgency incontinence is the usual reason given for referral of patients

TABLE 73–6. ANTERIOR AND POSTERIOR MAXIMUM URETHRAL CLOSURE PRESSURES IN INCONTINENT WOMEN WITH AND WITHOUT SUI IN COMPARISON WITH VOLUNTEER CONTROLS

| | Volunteer Controls | | Women With SUI | | | | Women Without SUI | |
| | | | STABLE BLADDERS | | UNSTABLE BLADDERS | | | |
	STABLE	UNSTABLE	Pre-operative	Post-operative	Pre-operative	Post-operative	STABLE BLADDERS	UNSTABLE BLADDERS
Number of subjects	17	4	52	47	25	18	34	29
Age	24 ± 4	27 ± 6	56 ± 13	55 ± 15	60 ± 11	63 ± 10	50 ± 16	43 ± 18
Maximum anterior closure pressure (cm H_2O)	119 ± 25	116 ± 27	60 ± 33	45 ± 43	47 ± 38*	45 ± 43	51 ± 29	82 ± 29*
Maximum posterior closure pressure (cm H_2O)	113 ± 17	107 ± 23	44 ± 25**	58 ± 42	33 ± 20†	51 ± 34	60 ± 42**	82 ± 42†

* = $p < 0.01$ between the two values indicated by *
** = $p < 0.01$ between the two values indicated by **
† = $p < 0.001$ between the two values indicated by †

with SUI for urodynamic evaluation; we have repeatedly emphasized, however (see references), that the presence of urgency incontinence—as long as it is clearly and demonstrably accompanied by loss of urine through the urethra exactly coinciding with the cough-induced rise in abdominal pressure—is *not* a contraindication to surgery. Neither does it appear to have an adverse influence on the ultimate course of the patient's incontinence. In fact, about one third of our patients operated upon for SUI have some degree of urgency incontinence by history. Moreover, our consecutive unselected series of 151 incontinent patients increases insight into the role of urgency incontinence. Since 30 per cent of those with SUI showed unstable bladders at cystometry, and 51 per cent of patients with non-SUI (despite a history of urgency incontinence) failed to show detrusor instability, the presence of instability on cystometry clearly does not separate SUI from non-SUI patients. More important, the presence of preoperative instability in SUI patients is not predictive of a poor outcome following endoscopic suspension of the vesical neck. We recently contacted 38 patients who were operated on for SUI who also had urgency incontinence by history. Twenty-five patients (mean follow-up 11 ± 9 months) had stable preoperative cystometry; 68 per cent of them were cured of their urgency, 25 per cent were improved, and only one was worse. Of the 13 patients with SUI and instability on preoperative cystometry, 31 per cent were cured of their urgency, 54 per cent said they were better, 15 per cent were the same, and none was worse (mean follow-up 12 ± 6 months). While the numbers of patients are small, they support a strong clinical impression that the presence of urgency incontinence—in a patient with demonstrable SUI regardless of whether instability is present on preoperative cystometry—is not a contraindication to endoscopic suspension of the vesical neck. It should be clear, however, that surgical evaluation of the vesical neck for pure urgency incontinence will not benefit the patient and may make her worse. The surgeon should recognize that to suspend the vesical neck of a patient who claims to lose urine only when she has the urge to urinate and in whom only a drop or two of urine (if any) can be demonstrated with severe coughing in the standing position is a mistake.

It should be apparent that while these research data are interesting from the physiologic view of characterizing continence and incontinence, they are of little practical importance in determining who will benefit from surgery.

Why, then, have urodynamic investigations become so popular in recent years as a part of the evaluation of patients with urinary incontinence, especially stress urinary incontinence?

One reason is the failure of the surgeon to identify loss of urine with coughing on physical examination. Many physicians fail to take the time and trouble to make this important observation while knowing how much water is in the bladder and while looking directly at the urethra when the patient coughs. It is interesting that four major authors in a recent text on this subject did not even mention this aspect of the physical examination in the preoperative evaluation of their patients with urinary incontinence (Stanton and Tangho, 1980). Other authors have gone so far as to *define* stress incontinence on the basis of cystometrographic criteria, even dismissing the validity of directly observing the physical loss of urine on coughing (Drutz et al., 1978); it is not surprising that in such studies there was a poor correlation between all parameters that were measured. If the surgeon does not examine the patient for urinary loss directly related to coughing, then referral to a urodynamic unit with videocystourethrographic capability will probably make the diagnosis, but this is an expensive way to determine that a patient leaks urine simultaneously with coughing.

Another reason for excessive usage of urodynamic studies in patients with urinary incontinence may relate to surgical techniques that inconsistently elevate the urethrovesical junction to a permanent position of urinary continence. If the surgeon does not recognize the anatomic reason for his operative failure, he may look for a physiologic explanation. It is the use of an operation that consistently and reliably elevates the vesical neck (in this case, endoscopic suspension) that has allowed us to simplify the evaluation of women with SUI at Stanford.

TREATMENT OF STRESS URINARY INCONTINENCE

Pharmacologic Treatment

The sympathetic nervous system exercises important control over the bladder and urethra. Since the bladder neck and proximal urethra contain mainly α-adrenergic receptors (Awad et al., 1974), α-adrenergic stimulation of the smooth muscle in these areas increases urethral resistance. For this reason, sympathomimetic agents that stimulate α-adrenergic receptors are sometimes useful in females with mild SUI.

SYMPATHOMIMETIC AGENTS

Ephedrine. Ephedrine is a natural sympathomimetic agent that stimulates both α- and β-receptors and causes peripheral release of norepinephrine. In human studies this drug has increased the urethral pressure throughout its length (Diokno and Taub, 1975). In 27 of 38 patients with mild incontinence, 25 mg three times daily improved urinary continence (Diokno and Taub, 1975). The side effects, however, were substantial. Patients suffered increased irritability, cardiac palpitations, and anxiety, and some became refractory to its effect. Furthermore, ephedrine is contraindicated in patients with hypertension, cardiovascular disease (especially angina), and hyperthyroidism.

Pseudoephedrine Hydrochloride. This drug is a stereoisomer of ephedrine and acts similarly. Thirty to 60 mg four times daily gives an effect similar to that seen with ephedrine (Wein, 1979).

Phenylpropanolamine Hydrochloride. This is another sympathomimetic agent with activity similar to ephedrine, but it has fewer central side effects. This agent has been used in 25- and 50-mg doses with effectiveness; it is present in a sustained-release form combined with chlorpheniramine maleate as Ornade,* which needs to be taken only once or twice daily. While taking Ornade, 11 of 12 patients with moderate SUI increased their maximal urethral pressures by greater than 20 per cent (Montague and Stewart, 1979). The only important side effect was occasional drowsiness.

Estrogen. Estrogens may act synergistically with the sympathomimetic agents. In a study confirming the increase in the urethral pressure profile generated by α-adrenergic agents, addition of oral estrogen to the α-adrenergic drugs increased even further the urethral pressures (Schreiter et al., 1976). The mechanism of this change is unclear.

Although these agents may be useful in patients with mild SUI, surgical correction is often preferable to chronic medication with its associated side effects. Moreover, none of these drugs cure severe stress incontinence.

ANTICHOLINERGIC AGENTS

The anticholinergic agents are usually not helpful for treating pure SUI. They may, however, be helpful in patients with reflex detrusor contractions and stress incontinence. In these people, anticholinergic drugs suppress symptoms of urgency and urgency incontinence.

Propantheline Bromide. Propantheline is a synthetic quarternary ammonium compound that competitively inhibits cholinergic transmission in the pelvic and detrusor ganglia. Although its exact site and mode of action are unknown, it suppresses reflex detrusor contractions (Hald and Bradley, 1982). Propantheline is similar to methantheline, but is more potent (Innes and Nickerson, 1970; Wein, 1979). The dose is 15 to 30 mg four times daily. Side-effects are those of any of the anticholinergic drugs—dry mouth, visual blurring, and decreased gastrointestinal motility with resulting constipation. It is contraindicated in patients with glaucoma, ulcerative colitis, cardiovascular disease, and cardiac arrhythmias.

Oxybutynin Chloride. Oxybutynin is a tertiary amine that suppresses reflex detrusor contractions. Its mechanism of action is unknown (Hald and Bradley, 1982). The adult dosage is 5 mg two to four times daily, and the side effects and contraindications are the same as for propantheline.

Imipramine. This agent is often referred to as one of the "tricyclic antidepressants," because it is used most frequently as an antidepressant. It is a dibenzazepine derivative that has some anticholinergic activity and is useful for treating childhood enuresis. Although the drug's mechanism of stopping enuresis is unknown, it is thought to suppress abnormal detrusor reflex contractions and potentiate urethral α-adrenergic activity (Hald and Bradley, 1982). Since this drug increases urethral resting pressure (Mahony et al., 1973), it might be useful in managing stress incontinence. One and a half to 2 mg per kg is recommended in childhood enuresis. The drug is contraindicated in patients with cardiovascular disease, arrhythmias, glaucoma, hyperthyroidism, and seizure disorders.

Although other drugs, such as emepronium bromide, are reported to be useful for treating incontinence, these drugs are not easily available in the United States (Hald and Bradley, 1982; Ulmsten and Andersson, 1977).

---

*Smith Kline & French Laboratories, Philadelphia, PA 19101.

Kegel Exercises

Although Kegel exercises with extensive practice periods of contraction and relaxation of the levator ani muscles (especially the pubococcygeal muscle, through which the urethra passes) can undoubtedly cure patients with mild SUI (Jones, 1963), these exercises require extraordinary devotion and persistence on the part of the patient. In view of the minimal elevation of the urethrovesical junction that accompanies Kelly plications that cure SUI in its milder form, it is possible that exercise of the levator muscles achieves some elevation of the urethrovesical junction. It is unfortunate that those who advocate these exercises have not sought objective evidence of anatomic changes before and after cure of SUI by this method. Nevertheless, many women with minimal SUI and a strong pubococcygeus muscle contraction on vaginal examination should try these exercises. The urologist should read the paper by Jones (1963) before instructing the patient. A positive attitude and frequent encouragement are required of the physician. The patient must contract the levator muscles 10 times every 30 minutes, holding the contraction about 3 seconds before relaxing. The secret of success is clearly a highly motivated patient with a strong pubococcygeus muscle.

Operative Treatment

Surgical procedures designed to correct female SUI elevate the bladder neck to a position behind the symphysis pubis. The techniques used to accomplish this goal are multiple and have varying success. Proper evaluation of incontinence and careful selection of the appropriate surgical procedure increase the likelihood of success and avoid a haphazard approach to incontinence. As others have clearly stated: "There is no doubt that the prime operation for (stress urinary incontinence) is the initial one and that for every subsequent operation, the 'cure' rate declines more or less proportional to the number of subsequent operations. . . . (It) is no longer necessary to follow the once popular gynaecological adage 'do a vaginal plastic first and, if this fails, go above.'" (Hodgkinson and Stanton, 1980).

Operations can be classified by incision: (1) transvaginal, (2) retropubic, and (3) a combination of transvaginal and retropubic (Table 73–7). Artificial sphincters (Bruskewitz et al., 1981) and endoscopic periurethral Teflon injec-

TABLE 73–7. OPERATIONS FOR THE CORRECTION OF STRESS URINARY INCONTINENCE (SUI)

Transvaginal Procedures
  Anterior colporrhaphy (Kelly plication)
Retropubic Procedures
  Suprapubic vesicourethral suspension (Marshall-Marchetti-Krantz)
  Ileopectineal ligament urethrovesical suspension (Burch procedure)
Combination Transvaginal and Retropubic Incisions
  Sling procedures
  Combined urethrovesical suspension and vaginourethroplasty (Pereyra and Raz procedures)
  Endoscopic suspension of the vesical neck (Stamey procedure)
Other Procedures
  Periurethral Teflon injection
  Artificial sphincter

tion (Lewis et al., 1984) have been used in complicated stress incontinence refractory to other surgical procedures or incontinence related to neurologic dysfunction. These procedures differ in principle from the other operations designed to correct SUI; continence in these two latter methods is maintained by mechanical obstruction of the urethra. Although these modalities might be considered for the intractable case of SUI, to date neither has been widely used for routine stress incontinence.

ANTERIOR COLPORRHAPHY, KELLY PLICATION

Currently, the anterior colporrhaphy is performed with only a few modifications (Drukker, 1978; Green, 1980) from its original description by Kelly in 1911 (Kelly and Dumm, 1914). With the patient in the dorsolithotomy position, and a posterior retractor in place, a 14 F urethral catheter is placed in the bladder, and the balloon is inflated to mark the urethrovesical junction. A midline anterior vaginal incision is made below the urethra, and the vaginal mucosa is dissected off the urethra proximally toward the bladder neck and laterally to expose the periurethral tissues. Once the urethra, the surrounding tissues, and the urethrovesical area are exposed, two or three mattress sutures of 2–0 or 0 chromic catgut or polyglycolic acid are placed at the bladder neck by taking bites of the periurethral tissues on both sides of the bladder neck (Fig. 73–9); some surgeons place two or three additional sutures slightly distal to these initial ones along the proximal urethra (Drukker, 1978). Excess vaginal mucosa is excised, and the vagina is reapproximated with a running 0 or 1–0 chromic catgut suture. In the surgically successful case, this imbrication of the periurethral fascia at the vesical neck produces a

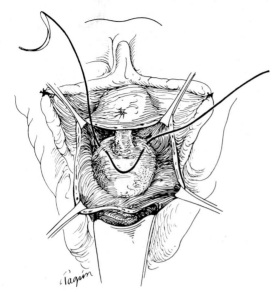

Figure 73–9. After the vaginal mucosa is dissected off the proximal urethra and bladder neck, several sutures are placed into the periurethral tissues on both sides of the neck in the anterior colporrhaphy. (From Green, T. H., Jr.: *In* Stanton, S. L., and Tanagho, E. A. (Eds.): Surgery of Female Incontinence. New York, Springer-Verlag, 1980. Used by permission.)

0.9- to 1.1-cm elevation of the urethrovesical junction behind the symphysis pubis (Low, 1967).

Although this operation can be performed quickly and with minimal morbidity, long-term evaluation shows that only 40 to 50 per cent of patients are permanently cured (Green, 1968). In select patients (68 from a total of 341) with SUI, anterior colporrhaphy had a 95 per cent primary success rate, but this group represented only 20 per cent of the patients with stress incontinence, and the remaining 80 per cent of patients needed other operations (Green, 1978). As a result, this procedure is not applicable to all females with SUI. It is most appropriate in women who have minimal stress incontinence and need a vaginal hysterectomy for organic disease as well.

SUPRAPUBIC VESICOURETHRAL SUSPENSION, MARSHALL-MARCHETTI-KRANTZ PROCEDURE

Suprapubic vesicourethral suspension is performed through a suprapubic incision with the patient in the dorsolithotomy position. A urethral catheter is placed in the bladder, and the balloon is inflated to define the urethrovesical junction. The surgeon uses blunt dissection to expose the bladder neck. Two or three interrupted 2–0 chromic sutures are placed in the paraurethral tissues from the proximal urethra to the urethrovesical junction and are fixed to the subpubic periosteum. If nonabsorbable suture material is used, only two sutures, one on each side of the urethrovesical junction, are needed. These sutures elevate the proximal urethra and urethrovesical junction toward the symphysis pubis. This important operation is described in detail in the second part of this chapter.

When this operation was first described in 1949, it represented a turning point in the surgical correction of SUI. This procedure had cure rates of 75 to 85 per cent (Marchetti, 1956; Marchetti et al., 1957), rates that were far superior to those for any other procedure of its time. More recently, a 96 per cent success rate has been reported (Krantz, 1980). In Green's critical evaluation of 230 patients undergoing the Marshall-Marchetti-Krantz operation, he emphasized that 97 per cent (144 of 149) of patients who had the procedure concomitantly with abdominal hysterectomy were cured and 90 per cent (37 of 41) who had the procedure and had had previous hysterectomy were cured, but only 82 per cent who had the procedure with intact uteri were cured (Green, 1980). On the basis of these data, he recommended that unless a contraindication exists, a hysterectomy should be performed with the Marshall-Marchetti-Krantz operation.

ILEOPECTINEAL LIGAMENT URETHROVESICAL SUSPENSION, BURCH PROCEDURE

The Burch operation elevates the urethrovesical angle by attaching the vaginal fascia near the urethra to the ileopectineal ligament (Cooper's ligament). The patient is draped in the dorsolithotomy position, and a sterile plastic bag or large glove is inserted into the vagina and is sutured to the surrounding skin and drapes. Alternatively, the patient is draped with access to the vagina, and the surgeon's gloves are changed after vaginal palpation. An indwelling urethral catheter with the balloon inflated at the vesical neck is placed. A paramedian, low midline, or Pfannenstiel incision is used to gain access to the retropubic space. Using sharp and blunt dissection, the surgeon separates the bladder from the symphysis and exposes the retropubic space and the superior and lateral pubis, which is covered by the ileopectineal ligament. The surgeon's or the assistant's second and third fingers are placed in the vagina to elevate the urethrovesical junction, which is identified by palpation of the urethral catheter balloon (Fig. 73–10). The bladder and urethra are displaced medial to the area of vaginal finger pressure by blunt dissection. A suture of 2–0 chromic catgut (Burch, 1968), 2–0 nonabsorbable plastic or nylon, or No. 1 polyglycolic suture (Hodgkinson and Stanton, 1980) is placed through the paravaginal tissues and the vaginal wall through all layers except the vaginal mucosa. Usually one to three similar sutures are placed near the urethrovesical junction with the ends tagged. Similar sutures are placed on the opposite side of the urethra. Once this is accomplished, the sutures are passed through the ipsilateral ileopectineal ligament, at the point where apposition of the anterior vaginal wall and the ligament causes the least tension. While the fingers elevate the vaginal wall toward the ileopectineal ligaments to decrease tension, the sutures are tied (Fig. 73–11). Enteroceles may become more apparent, and indeed, may be caused by the Burch urethropexy. If the uterus is absent and preoperative descent of the vaginal vault is detected, the rectovesical pouch (pouch of Douglas) should be obliterated by placing successive purse-string sutures in the pelvic peritoneum. Routine abdominal closure is performed. Postoperatively an indwelling urethral catheter or percutaneous

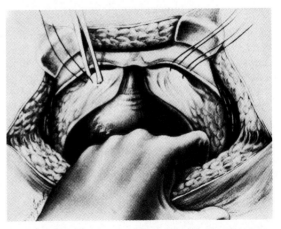

Figure 73–11. Placement of the periurethral sutures near the vesicourethral junction is shown. These sutures are placed through all layers of tissue except the vaginal mucosa. They are then attached to the iliopectineal (Cooper's) ligament. (From Hodgkinson, C. P., and Stanton, S. L.: *In* Stanton, S. L., and Tanagho, E. A. (Eds.): Surgery of Female Incontinence. New York, Springer-Verlag, 1980. Used by permission.)

suprapubic catheter drains the bladder. These catheters are described in detail in the section on postoperative management of endoscopic suspension of the vesical neck.

Ileopectineal ligament urethrovesical suspension was described by Burch (1961). In 1968 he reported satisfactory results in 93 per cent of patients. More recently, in an evaluation of 180 patients (43 of whom were reviewed at 2 years or longer), the overall cure rate was 87 per cent at 1 year and 86 per cent at 2 years (Stanton and Cardozo, 1979). When ileopectineal urethropexy was performed as the primary surgical procedure, the cure rate was 96 per cent at 1 year, but for those with previous procedures it was 76.5 per cent at 1 year. This procedure offers two advantages over the suprapubic vesicourethral suspension (Marshall-Marchetti-Krantz procedure): (1) use of the ileopectineal ligament often provides a sturdier anchorage point than does the pubic periosteum and (2) use of the ligament rather than the periosteum avoids osteitis pubis. It is emphasized by Hodgkinson (Burch, 1968), however, that ileopectineal fixation may be difficult or impossible in patients who have had multiple previous incontinence procedures or those who have other causes, such as radiation and infection, for scarring and rigidity of the anterior vaginal wall and paraurethral tissues. Moreover, placement of the suspending sutures too lateral can actually pull the vesical neck open and cause total incontinence.

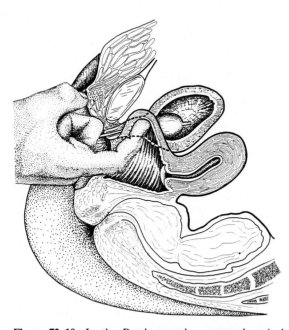

Figure 73–10. In the Burch procedure, upward vaginal pressure by the operator's or assistant's finger aids dissection and suture placement performed through the suprapubic incision (From Hodgkinson, C. P., and Stanton, S. L.: *In* Stanton, S. L., and Tanagho, E. A. (Eds.): Surgery of Female Incontinence. New York, Springer-Verlag, 1980. Used by permission.)

SLING PROCEDURES

Since the 1900's, suburethral slings of tissue, and more recently synthetic materials, have been used to elevate the bladder neck in the surgical treatment of SUI. Gracilis muscle, pyramidalis muscle and rectus fascia, round ligament, levator ani, fascia lata, external oblique fascia, lyophilized dura, and synthetic substances such as nylon, Mersilene, and inert polypropylene mesh have all been used as suburethral slings. Whether the sling is of attached fascia, free fascial graft, or synthetic material, the operative principles are similar, so only the fascia lata sling procedure will be described here.

The fascia lata to be used as the sling is harvested through an incision 3- to 4-cm long overlying the iliotibial tract just above the patella. A piece of fascia aproximately 1.5 cm in width is pulled through the fascial stripper until a length of 17 cm or more is obtained. The proximal end is then cut. This free fascial strip is then placed in Ringer lactate solution until it is needed. The leg wound is sutured closed, and circumferential pressure bandages are applied. The patient is then repositioned, reprepped, and redraped in the dorsolithotomy position. An in-dwelling urethral catheter is placed to define the urethrovesical junction. An 8- to 10-cm transverse suprapubic incision 3 to 4 cm above the pubic tubercle is made and is extended down the anterior rectus sheath. If the patient has had no previous retropubic surgery, only two 2-cm stab wounds on both sides of the midline are made in the anterior rectus sheath. Previous retropubic operations will necessitate entry into the retropubic space and dissection of the bladder from the symphysis. A midline (Lee, 1978) or V-shaped (Beck, 1978) vaginal suburethral incision is made. The vaginal mucosa is dissected from the urethra and away from the region of the urethrovesical junction. A curved, blunt-tipped clamp is passed into one of the fascial incisions, into the retropubic space, and alongside the urethrovesical junction to exit from the vaginal incision. One end of the prepared fascial strip is placed in the clamp and is withdrawn suprapubically. This end is fixed to the anterior rectus fascia using No. 1 chromic catgut (Beck, 1978) or several nonabsorbable sutures. On the opposite side of the urethra similarly, the other end of the fascial strip is passed from the vagina into the suprapubic incision and is then sutured to the anterior rectus fascia (Fig. 73–12). Since it is difficult to determine the proper tension with which to fix the sling, different tests have been devised (Beck,

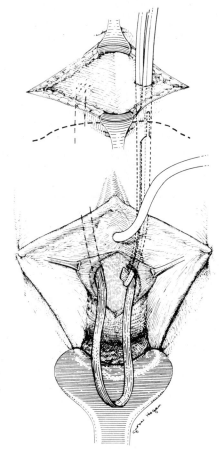

Figure 73–12. In the fascia lata sling procedure, the fascial strip is passed from the vaginal incision to the suprapubic incision by using a curved clamp. The strip is anchored to the rectus fascia on the patient's right side. When both ends of the strip are anchored to the fascia, a sling is formed below the urethra. (From Ridley, J. H.: Gynecologic Surgery. Baltimore, The Williams & Wilkins Co., 1974. Used by permission.)

1978), but most often tension is determined empirically. The fascial strip may be attached to the urethrovesical junction vaginally by placing several 2–0 chromic catgut sutures into the strip and the periurethral tissues at the bladder neck; this is often difficult, however, because the bladder neck may have elevated away from easy access. Routine closure of the suprapubic and vaginal incisions is performed, and the retropubic space is usually drained.

Before endoscopic suspension of the vesical neck (Stamey, 1973) and other newer operations were devised, the sling procedures were reserved for patients with severe SUI that was refractory to previous surgical correction, because these procedures were long operations with frequent postoperative complications. Typical patients who had the sling operations had already failed multiple attempts to correct incontinence surgically and had unusually severe stress from asthma or bronchitis. Postoperative complications were common. The average time before the patient started voiding was 24 days, and as many as one third of the women were unable to completely empty their bladders for as long as 2 years after the operation (Beck, 1978). Furthermore, occasional slings, especially when synthetic material was used, eroded into or sloughed the urethra. In 50 patients who had had one to five other unsuccessful incontinence procedures, the fascia lata sling cured 80 per cent, but half of these patients had been followed for less than 1 year (Beck, 1978). At this time, however, more recent operations make the sling procedures virtually obsolete.

COMBINED URETHROVESICAL SUSPENSION AND VAGINOURETHROPLASTY, PEREYRA PROCEDURE

Since Pereyra described his "simplified surgical procedure for the correction of stress incontinence in women" in 1959 (Pereyra, 1959) and results in 1967 (Pereyra and Lebherz, 1967), the procedure has had considerable modification (Pereyra and Lebherz, 1978). The revised procedure elevates the region of the vesical neck by placing helical sutures into the paraurethral tissues and tying them to the anterior rectus fascia. For this procedure the patient is placed in the dorsolithotomy position; the anterior vagina is incised from 1 cm from the urethral meatus to the bladder base. The vaginal epithelium is dissected away from and lateral to the

urethra to expose the paraurethral tissues. An indwelling urethral catheter empties the bladder and identifies the urethrovesical junction; a superficial suture is placed to mark this junction. Through the vaginal incision, the anterolateral attachments of the paraurethral tissues and endopelvic fascia are freed from the pubic ramus bilaterally by blunt and sharp dissection. This exposes the retropubic space to the vagina. With an Allis clamp, the released paraurethral tissue from one side of the urethra is pulled down and over the surgeon's index finger, which rests against the bladder. A No. 3 half-circle tapered Mayo needle on a 0 polypropylene monofilament suture is placed through the released paraurethral tissue half an inch distal to the urethrovesical junction. This needle is reinserted repeatedly into this tissue at quarter inch spacings three or four more times until a "helical" suture is created (Fig. 73–13). The same suture is placed on the other side of the urethra. The surgeon now directs his attention to the suprapubic area. A 1-inch skin incision is made just above the pubic symphysis to expose the rectus fascia. The Pereyra ligature carrier instrument is used to puncture the rectus fascia an inch to the right of midline while the index finger of the opposite hand guides the needle into the retropubic space and through the vaginal incision. Both ends of the "helical" suture are threaded onto the needle, and the instrument is pulled through the suprapubic incision (Fig. 73–14). Since both suture ends exit the suprapubic incision through the same hole, one of the ends

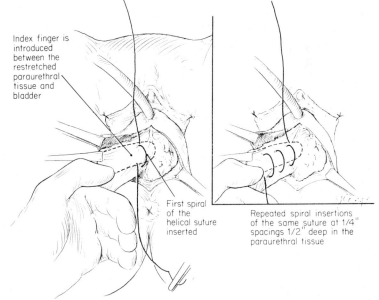

Figure 73–13. In the Pereyra procedure, after the anterolateral attachments of the paraurethral and endopelvic tissues are freed from the pubic ramus, these tissues are pulled laterally over the index finger. A needle is then placed into the paraurethral tissues slightly distal to the urethrovesical junction. This same needle is reinserted repeatedly into these tissues, forming a "helical" suture as illustrated in the inset. (From Pereyra, A. J., and Lebherz, T. B.: *In* Buchsbaum, H. J., and Schmidt, J. D. (Eds.): Gynecologic and Obstetric Urology. Philadelphia, W. B. Saunders Co., 1978. Used by permission.)

Index finger is introduced between the restretched paraurethral tissue and bladder

First spiral of the helical suture inserted

Repeated spiral insertions of the same suture at 1/4" spacings 1/2" deep in the paraurethral tissue

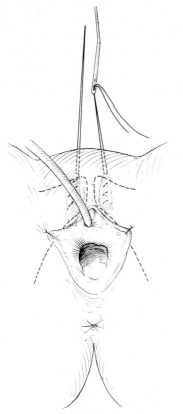

Figure 73–14. In the Pereyra procedure, the two "helical" sutures containing the paraurethral tissues are passed to the suprapubic incision using the Pereyra needles. Each suture is tied independently over rectus fascia lateral to the midline. (From Pereyra, A. J., and Lebherz, T. B.: *In* Buchsbaum, H. J., and Schmidt, J. D. (Eds.): Gynecologic and Obstetric Urology. Philadelphia, W. B. Saunders Co., 1978. Used by permission.)

is passed under the fascia parallel to the midline for half an inch. This creates a fascial bridge over which the suspending suture can be tied. The procedure is repeated on the other side of the urethra. One of the right polypropylene suture ends is then passed under the fascia for half an inch parallel to the midline so that a fascial bridge over which the suspending suture will be tied is formed. The same procedure is performed on the left. While an assistant views the urethrovesical junction with the cystoscope, the surgeon ties the two suspending sutures at the tension at which the lower bladder neck appears to flatten. The suprapubic and vaginal incisions are then closed.

The 1978 version of the Pereyra procedure (Pereyra and Lebherz, 1978) is very different from the original version described in 1959 (Pereyra, 1959). The sutures were changed from wire to polypropylene, the needle from double- to single-headed, and the helical sutures and

cystoscopic examination were added. This procedure is similar to that described by Raz (Raz, 1981), except that Raz ties the right and left suspending sutures together across the rectus fascia, he incises the anterior vagina in a "U," and he attempts to dissect the paraurethral tissues more laterally.

ENDOSCOPIC SUSPENSION OF THE VESICAL NECK, STAMEY PROCEDURE

Endoscopic suspension of the vesical neck was first described in 1973 (Stamey, 1973). It has advantages over open retropubic urethrovesical suspensions such as the Marshall-Marchetti-Krantz or Burch procedures; the incision is superficial, the bladder and bladder neck are not dissected, and the parauraethral tissues that suspend the vesical neck are buttressed vaginally with knitted Dacron. Furthermore, this is the first incontinence operation to use the cystoscope to place the sutures exactly at the vesical neck. The operation is still performed as originally described. Because of the distinct advantages and relative simplicity of this operation, this technique will be discussed in detail.

Preoperative Management. The evening before the operation the patient undergoes routine preparations including soap suds enemas, povidone-iodine douche, and perineal and suprapubic shaving and scrubbing. Urinalysis and urine culture are obtained. Blood is not usually cross-matched for this procedure. Although any known urinary infection should be treated before the patient enters the hospital, the night before the operation a parenteral aminoglycoside (tobramycin or gentamicin 80 mg) is given to sterilize the patient's urine in case a urinary infection is present. A second antibiotic injection is given an hour before the operation is started; this dose produces a tissue level of antimicrobial agent during the operation, which reduces the risk of postoperative pelvic infection.

Anesthesia. The operation can usually be performed under a spinal block with a sensory level of anesthesia to at least T_{10}; however, the patient should be given the form of anesthetic that is best suited to her general health. At least 90 to 120 minutes of anesthetic time should be planned.

The Operation. The surgeon performs the operation while standing or sitting, with the patient in the modified lithotomy position. The patient's legs are extended laterally and the knees are bent slightly to ensure a flat lower abdomen. The patient's buttocks should be placed well below the edge of the table in order to use the weighted posterior vaginal retractor.

After careful shaving and scrubbing of the entire perineum, vagina, and suprapubic area, a half towel covered by a sticky plastic drape is sutured across the perineum to exclude the rectum from the surgical field. Both labia minora are sutured laterally to expose the vaginal introitus. The legs and abdomen are draped, but the pubis and 4 to 5 cm of the suprapubic area and perineum are kept within the operative field. The cystoscope fiberoptic cord and water tubing are draped over one leg and the suction tubing and electrocautery are draped over the other leg.

Two symmetric transverse 2- to 3-cm skin incisions are made to the left and right of midline at the upper border of the symphysis pubis. A Mayo clamp is used to bluntly spread the subcutaneous tissue down to the anterior rectus fascia (Fig. 73–15). A dry 4 × 4 gauze sponge is packed into each incision while the vaginal portion of the operation is continued.

The urethral length is measured by inserting a urethral catheter into the bladder and inflating the balloon with air; the catheter balloon is placed at the internal vesical neck without traction while the urethral meatus is marked on the catheter with a hemostat. When the catheter is

withdrawn, the balloon is reinflated so that the urethral length, from balloon to hemostat, can be measured. The catheter is reinserted into the bladder, and the balloon is inflated with 10 ml of air. The weighted posterior vaginal retractor is placed. The anterior vaginal mucosa is incised in the shape of a "T." If the urethra is short (2.5 cm or less), the transverse part of the "T" incision (Fig. 73–16A) is started near the urethral meatus. If the urethra is longer, this incision is made deeper in the vagina. This transverse incision is started with the scalpel and should be 2 to 2.5 cm. The anterior vaginal tissue is separated from the urethra by gently spreading the blunt, curved scissors in the plane between these tissues. The scissors must be kept parallel to the floor with the tips pointed down to prevent inadvertent entry into the bladder or urethra. The vertical tissues alongside the vesical neck and urethra should be left undisturbed, because dissection in this area would weaken the pubocervical fascia that forms part of the suspending tissue. The vertical portion of the "T" incision (Fig. 73–16B) is made after the mucosa is separated from the urethra. When the vaginal incision permits the tip of the index finger to rest against the bladder neck on each side of the catheter, it is complete.

The long, blunt, steel Stamey needles are

Figure 73–15. A urethral catheter is in place to aid palpation of the urethrovesical junction. Two small skin incisions are made just lateral to midline at the upper border of the pubic symphysis (inset). A Mayo clamp is used to bluntly spread the subcutaneous tissue down to the anterior rectus fascia in each incision. (From Shortliffe, L. M. D., and Stamey, T. A.: *In* McDougal, W. S. (Ed.): Operative Urology. Kent, England, Butterworth, 1985.)

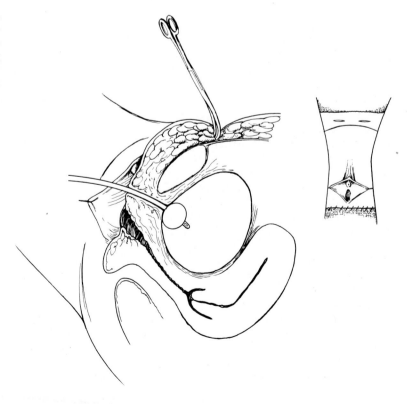

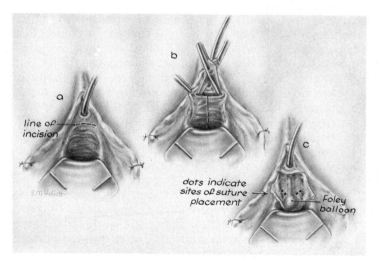

Figure 73–16. *A,* The vaginal mucosal incision is made in the shape of a T. The transverse portion of the T is started near the urethral meatus if the urethra is short (2.5 cm or less); if it is longer, this incision is made deeper in the vagina. *B,* The anterior vaginal tissue is separated from the overlying urethra before the vertical portion of the incision is made. *C,* Once the mucosal incision is complete, dissection is continued until the incision permits the tip of the index finger to rest against the bladder neck on each side of the catheter. (From Stamey, T. A.: Surg. Gynecol. Obstet., *136*:547, 1973. Used by permission.)

specially designed for this procedure.* The straight needle is used in 90 per cent of cases. The needles with the tips angled 15 or 30 degrees are useful when the patient has had earlier open retropubic surgery for urinary incontinence and the bladder is easily punctured by the straight needle.

After the weighted retractor is removed, both the surgeon's hands are used to insert the Stamey needle into the medial edge of one of the suprapubic incisions and through the rectus fascia just above the symphysis pubis (Fig. 73–17). The superior edge of the symphysis is probed with the tip of the needle to find the undersurface of the symphysis, and the needle is now passed about 1 to 2 cm parallel to the posterior surface of the symphysis pubis. The left (nondominant) index finger is now placed in the vaginal incision at the ipsilateral bladder neck while the right (dominant) hand moves the needle onto the tip of this finger. Sometimes bouncing the needle vertically in the retropubic space without advancing it helps to locate the point of the needle by the left index finger. The needle is then guided alongside the vesical neck, through the endopelvic and pubocervical fascia, and into the periurethral tissues adjacent to the bladder neck while controlled by the surgeon's left (nondominant) index finger, which is still on the needle point. During this maneuver, the urethral catheter is held without tension in the left hand palm so that the catheter balloon can be felt at the bladder neck (Fig. 73–18). The urethral catheter must not be tugged on because this would telescope the urethra and cause the surgeon to misjudge the natural position of the vesical neck.

The right-angle (70 or 110 degree lens) cystoscope is now passed into the bladder and is withdrawn to the urethrovesical junction (half in the urethra and half in the bladder) to make sure that the needle is exactly at the urethrovesical junction. If the needle is in the correct position it will indent the ipsilateral vesical neck when the suprapubic end is moved slowly from right to left (Fig. 73–19). The dome and ipsilateral bladder wall are also examined to ensure that the needle did not pass into the bladder. The course of the needle outside the bladder is seen by pushing the entire needle medially, which indents the side of the bladder. If the needle is intramural rather than outside the bladder muscle, the same bladder indentation or fold is seen without pushing the needle medially; in such cases, especially when the fold is seen at volumes less than 250 ml, the needle should be removed and passed again more laterally. If the needle passes into the bladder or if its position is incorrect, it is removed and repassed. It should be emphasized that the posterior weighted retractor must be removed when the needles are passed so that the tissues are not distorted by posterior pressure.

Once the surgeon is satisfied with the needle placement, the posterior vaginal speculum is replaced, a No. 2 monofilament nylon suture is threaded through the eye of the needle, and the needle is pulled suprapubically. Hemostats are placed on both the suprapubic and vaginal ends of the nylon suture.

The urethral catheter empties the bladder, the vaginal speculum is removed, and the needle is passed a second time 1 cm lateral to the first time, as described previously. While this pass is made, the nylon suture is put on tension by placing two additional Mayo clamps on the dangling vaginal suture. This weighted suture is

---

*These needles are available from the Pilling Company, Delaware Drive, Fort Washington, Pa. 19034.

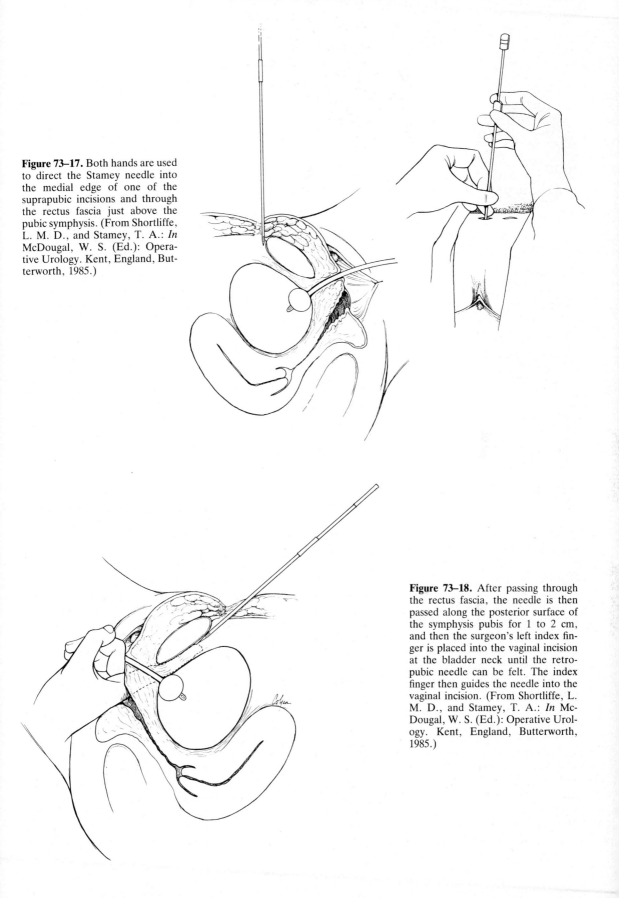

Figure 73–17. Both hands are used to direct the Stamey needle into the medial edge of one of the suprapubic incisions and through the rectus fascia just above the pubic symphysis. (From Shortliffe, L. M. D., and Stamey, T. A.: *In* McDougal, W. S. (Ed.): Operative Urology. Kent, England, Butterworth, 1985.)

Figure 73–18. After passing through the rectus fascia, the needle is then passed along the posterior surface of the symphysis pubis for 1 to 2 cm, and then the surgeon's left index finger is placed into the vaginal incision at the bladder neck until the retropubic needle can be felt. The index finger then guides the needle into the vaginal incision. (From Shortliffe, L. M. D., and Stamey, T. A.: *In* McDougal, W. S. (Ed.): Operative Urology. Kent, England, Butterworth, 1985.)

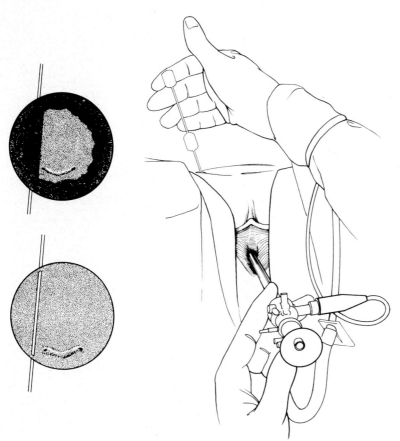

Figure 73–19. Once the needle is in place, the right angle cystoscope is passed into the bladder and withdrawn to the urethrovesical junction to make sure that the needle is placed exactly at the urethrovesical junction. If the needle is in the correct position it will indent the ipsilateral vesical neck when moved medially by the surgeon, as shown in the upper inset. Should the needle penetrate the bladder, as shown in the lower inset, the needle must be removed and repassed. (From Shortliffe, L. M. D., and Stamey, T. A.: *In* McDougal, W. S. (Ed.): Operative Urology. Kent, England, Butterworth, 1985.)

used to guide the needle 1 cm laterally. Once passed, the needle position is checked cystoscopically as before. After the vaginal speculum is replaced, the vaginal end of the nylon suture is passed through a 1-cm tube of 5-mm knitted Dacron arterial graft, to buttress the vaginal tissues, and then through the eye of the needle. If the Dacron tube is grasped lengthwise with an Allis clamp while the needle is pulled suprapubically, the two ends of the nylon suture can be balanced in the suprapubic incision, and the Dacron tube can be visually guided into the area of the urethrovesical junction. The periurethral tissues on one side of the urethra are now suspended at the vesical neck. The same steps are repeated on the other side of the bladder neck (Fig. 73–20).

Now for the first time the foroblique (30 or 150 degree) lens is put in the distal urethra to evaluate closure of the bladder neck when either one or both of the suspending nylon sutures is lifted (Fig. 73–21). Functional closure of the vesical neck is tested by filling the bladder with 300 to 500 ml of irrigating solution and removing the cystoscope while gently pushing down to remove the suspending tension of the Dacron tubes. A stream of fluid will immediately leak from the urethral meatus, but will stop promptly and easily with gentle elevation of either or both suspending nylon sutures. In an occasional person with severe periurethral scarring, unusual suture positions can cause the vesical neck to close when an individual suture is suspended, but open paradoxically when both periurethral sutures are suspended; in such instances, the suspending sutures are replaced to avoid paradoxical opening of the vesical neck, or one suture is removed and the operation is concluded with only one suspending suture at the vesical neck. When placement of both sutures is satisfactory, the vaginal incision is irrigated with an aminoglycoside solution (usually 80 mg of tobramycin or gentamicin in 200 to 300 ml sterile water) and is closed with a continuous 3–0 chromic stitch. Both pieces of Dacron graft should be buried well beneath this suture line. The vaginal incision should be closed before tying the suprapubic nylon sutures, because the elevation of the bladder neck and periurethral tissues that accompanies suspension makes the

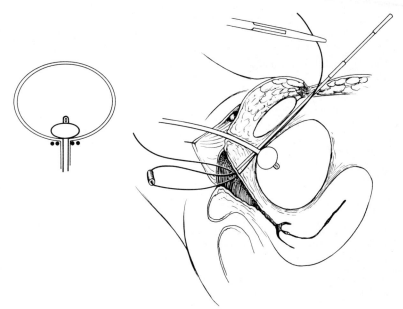

Figure 73–20. When the needle is passed the second time, 1 cm lateral to the first pass, the vaginal end of the nylon suture is passed through a 1-cm tube of 5-mm Dacron arterial graft before it is pulled suprapubically. This buttresses the periurethral tissue, which holds up the suspending suture. (From Shortliffe, L. M. D., and Stamey, T. A.: *In* McDougal, W. S. (Ed.): Operative Urology. Kent, England, Butterworth, 1985.)

incision difficult or impossible to reach afterward. A dry vaginal pack is left in the vagina overnight.

While the bladder is still full, a percutaneous polyethylene 14 F suprapubic Malecot (Stamey suprapubic catheter) or other percutaneous catheter may be placed. Position of the bladder is confirmed by aspirating bladder fluid with a 21-gauge spinal needle. A 3- to 4-mm

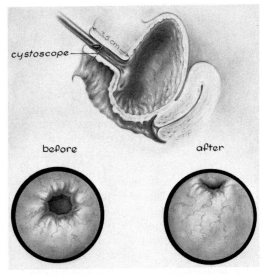

Figure 73–21. When sutures have been placed on both sides of the bladder neck, the panendoscope is put into the distal urethra to evaluate closure of the bladder neck when either or both suspending sutures are lifted. The cystoscopic views of the bladder neck before and after elevation of the sutures are shown in the insets. (From Stamey, T. A.: Surg. Gynecol. Obstet., *136*:1547, 1973. Used by permission.)

incision is made 3 to 4 cm above the suprapubic incision. The polyethylene catheter with its obturator locked in position is then passed into the bladder with the needle entering the skin at a 30 degree angle above the vertical position. The obturator is removed and the catheter is taped into position when the operation is finished. The final position of the catheter in the bladder can be examined with the cystoscope. If the patient has had previous low abdominal surgery and there is concern that low-lying bowel may be punctured, if the catheter drains poorly, or if the patient is so obese that her pannus interferes with the suprapubic tube, a 16 F urethral catheter can be used to drain the bladder.

Before the two suprapubic suspending sutures are tied, the incisions are irrigated with an aminoglycoside solution, and the weighted vaginal retractor is removed. The bladder is emptied with the cystoscope sheath. The two suprapubic suspending sutures are gently lifted until the loops are taut. Occasionally it is necessary to press a finger onto the rectus fascia to remove extra slack. The tension is now released and both sutures are tied without tension so that the knot lies flat on the rectus fascia with at least five to six additional throws placed on the knot (Fig. 73–22). As the surgeon can see with the panendoscope and the physiologic tests to stop bladder leakage, only minimal lifting of the suspending loops closes the neck and prevents incontinence; therefore, no tension is needed. Skin and subcutaneous tissue are closed in one layer with several interrupted vertical mattress

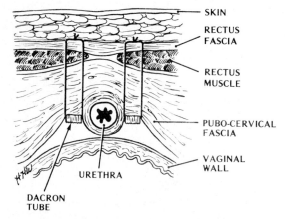

SKIN
RECTUS FASCIA
RECTUS MUSCLE
PUBO-CERVICAL FASCIA
VAGINAL WALL
URETHRA
DACRON TUBE

Figure 73–22. The two suprapubic suspending sutures should be tied on the rectus fascia without tension, so that the knot lies flat. Silicone bolsters (buttons cut by the surgeon from flat silicone sheets are adequate) can be threaded onto the suture above the rectus fascia if the fascia is weak. These bolsters should then lie flat on the rectus fascia just below the knot. (From Stamey, T. A.: Surg., *192*:465, 1980. Used by permission.)

stitches of 3–0 nylon. If the rectus fascia is shredded and weak from previous surgery or lax musculature, two flat silicone bolsters may be made and placed on the sutures so that the knot is tied over them.

The suprapubic tube is taped onto the abdomen using waterproof adhesive tape with benzoin placed on the catheter and skin before adhesion. A mesentary on the tape extending from the catheter to the abdomen will help prevent the catheter from being dislodged. In addition, the taping should start from the point at which the tube exits from the abdomen. No gauze needs to be placed around the base of the catheter. A dry gauze dressing may be placed over the two suprapubic incisions.

Postoperative Management. Each patient receives only two or three additional doses of gentamicin at 8-hour intervals after surgery; then all antimicrobial therapy is stopped until the suprapubic tube is removed. The patient can be discharged on the second or third postoperative day if necessary, though because of the older age of these patients, we tend to keep them hospitalized for 4 or 5 days after surgery. On the second or third postoperative day, the patient is taught the following regimen: on awakening in the morning, the stopcock on the percutaneous Malecot tube is turned at right angles to the tubing to stop dependent drainage in order to fill the bladder, and fluids are forced throughout the day. When the patient has a strong urge to urinate and thinks her bladder is

very full, she attempts voiding in the privacy of a bathroom; a plastic disposable catch pan is placed below the toilet rim to measure the voided volume. It should be emphasized that the patient must wait for a strong desire or urgency to urinate before attempting to void; the Valsalva maneuver will not help her to urinate so she must rely on detrusor contraction. Once the urgency occurs, however, if the patient is unsuccessful in voiding (usually the case at first), she need not prolong her suprapubic discomfort for more than a full minute while attempting to initiate urination; she simply turns the stopcock on line or parallel to the drainage tubing in order to empty her bladder. The tube has a very fast flow rate (200 ml per minute) and less than 5 minutes' time serves to empty the bladder regardless of the volume of residual urine. One of the values of the suprabic percutaneous catheter is that the patient herself has complete control over her discomfort. She is taught to measure and record the amount she voids and the amount of residual urine. If the patient is uncomfortable with the tube, she can be taught intermittent, self-catheterization.

Unlike retropubic operations for incontinence, very few of these patients can void by the second or third postoperative day. They should be told that every patient ultimately voids satisfactorily without residual urine. The percutaneous suprapubic Malecot catheter is removed postoperatively or self-catheterization is terminated when the patient is able to consistently void about 75 per cent of her total bladder volume. The time required for patients to achieve this degree of bladder emptying varies between 1 and 120 days; in half of the 203 patients in the 1980 series (Stamey, 1980a), the tube was removed by the seventh postsurgical day. In 14 of the 203 patients, more than 30 days were required to establish satisfactory voiding. It is very important not to remove the catheter when voided volumes are accompanied by equal residual urines, for example, 200 ml voided and 200 ml residual. Such premature removal of the catheter is accompanied by so much frequency and urgency that it usually has to be reinserted. Oral antibiotics are started only when the catheter is removed or when intermittent self-catheterization is terminated. If the patient has been discharged with her catheter attached to a leg bag, as is our practice, the closed drainage system used in the hospital has obviously been broken, and *Pseudomonas* is not an uncommon pathogen in the urine. Because of this possibility, inexpensive tetracycline hydrochloride at 250 mg four times a day is our first choice for an antimicrobial agent, because the urinary levels of tetracycline are bactericidal to 80 per cent of all strains of *Pseudomonas aeruginosa* (Stamey, 1980*b*). The important culture, as always with any urinary tract infection, is that done 2 weeks after stopping all antimicrobial therapy in order to be sure that the patient is returned to society with a sterile urine. This can be determined along with the residual urine at one of the postoperative visits, but catheterization should be followed by 24 hours of oral antimicrobial prophylaxis to prevent reinfection of the bladder.

Postoperative Complications. Few complications have been incurred (Stamey, 1981). While the procedure was being developed silk and braided nylon were used for the suspending sutures, and several suprapubic wound infections occurred with both these materials. Since monofilament nylon has been used, only one patient has developed a suprapubic wound infection that forced removal of both the sutures. This occurred in a diabetic women in whom a small periurethral abscess was discovered intraoperatively; she developed suprapubic and vaginal *Staphylococcus aureus* wound infections postoperatively. Another complication from the suture occurred in a patient 7 years after her surgery, when the suture and bolster eroded into her bladder. This complication was discovered when the patient developed irritative bladder symptoms without an infection and was cystoscoped. The intravesical suture and bolster were excised flush with the mucosa endoscopically; the patient is asymptomatic and continent with only one intact suture. In fact, in about 10 of 400 patients who have had this procedure, one suprapubic suture has been removed under local anesthesia for either infection or pain; the stress incontinence in these patients is cured with only one suture. Osteitis pubis has not been and should not be a complication with this operation.

The vaginal Dacron bolsters became a routine part of the operation after three or four of the initial patients had the nylon suture pull through the pubocervical and endopelvic fascia. Since the bolsters have been used, only the patient just mentioned has had the suture erode into the bladder. In three patients the anterior vaginal incision failed to heal completely, resulting in an exposed Dacron tube. In each case the exposed tube and suture were removed, and the patient remained continent with the single remaining suture.

One death from a cardiopulmonary event occurred on the fourth postoperative day; the operation had been uneventful.

Surgical Results. The results of this procedure have been reported before (Stamey, 1973; Stamey et al., 1975; Stamey, 1980*a*). This method of elevating the bladder neck has cured 91 per cent of 203 consecutive patients. All have had at least 6 months of follow-up and 47 have had longer than 4 years; cure was defined by absence of urinary incontinence 6 months after surgery. Nearly all of the failures occurred early in the postoperative period, and there was only one failure after 1 year. Of these 203 patients, 188 had had previous surgical attempts to correct their SUI, so few of these patients had simple Grade I stress incontinence (Stamey, 1980*a*). In fact 20 per cent (41 of these patients) had total urinary incontinence, that is, they could hold no more than 30 ml in their bladder when standing, and 32 of these women were cured by this operation (Stamey, 1980*a*). These figures reveal that even women with total urinary incontinence should undergo an endoscopic suspension of the vesical neck prior to more complicated procedures or attempts at implantation of artificial sphincters.

The presence or absence of a uterus has not affected the success of this operation. Of the 203 patients evaluated in 1980, 65 had not had a hysterectomy, and the surgical result was independent of this (Stamey, 1980*a*). Indeed, in the absence of uterine prolapse, a hysterectomy for urinary incontinence alone is difficult to justify.

Conclusion. This method of elevating the urethrovesical neck with two permanent heavy nylon sutures is a successful means of correcting female SUI and even total urinary incontinence. The cystoscope guides placement of the nylon sutures at the vesical neck, and the Dacron buttress strengthens the suspending tissues in a way that is not accomplished in other open retropubic urethropexies. This technique is less invasive and causes less blood loss and postoperative discomfort than many other operations; as a result, blood transfusion may be avoided and hospitalization shortened. It may be used in women who have undergone other procedures unsuccessfully and may be combined with other abdominal or vaginal procedures with good results. Furthermore, the operation is no more difficult in obese women than in thin women. Endoscopic suspension of the vesical neck is the ideal operation for the patient who has already had multiple pelvic operations, previous trauma with pelvic fractures, or prior pelvic irradiation for carcinoma. Since it has been so successful in these surgically difficult cases, it is an excellent surgical choice for the routine case.

References

Ala-Ketola, L.: Roentgen diagnosis of female stress urinary incontinence: roentgenological and clinical study. Acta Obstet. Gynecol. Scand. (Suppl.) 23:1, 1973.

Awad, S., Bruce, A. W., Carro-Ciampi, G. et al.: Distribution of alpha and beta-adrenoceptors in human urinary bladder. Br. J. Pharmacol., 50:525, 1974.

Beck, E. P.: The sling operation. In Buchsbaum, H. J., and Schmidt, J. D. (Eds.): Gynecologic and Obstetric Urology. Philadelphia, W. B. Saunders Co., 1978.

Brown, M., and Wickham, J. E. A.: The urethral pressure profile. Br. J. Urol., 4:211, 1969.

Bruskewitz, R., Raz, S., and Kaufman, J. J.: Treatment of urinary incontinence with the artificial sphincter. J. Urol., 126:469, 1981.

Burch, J. C.: Urethrovaginal fixation to Cooper's ligament for correction of stress incontinence, cystocele, and prolapse. Am. J. Obstet. Gynecol., 81:281, 1961.

Burch, J. C.: Cooper's ligament urethrovesical suspension for stress incontinence. Am. J. Obstet. Gynecol., 100:764, 1968.

Cifuentes, L.: Epithelium of vaginal type in the female trigone: the clinical problem of trigonitis. J. Urol., 57:1028, 1947.

Constantinou, C. E.: Personal communication, 1985.

Constantinou, C. E., and Govan, D. E.: Spatial distribution and timing of transmitted and reflexly generated urethral pressures in healthy women. J. Urol., 127:964, 1982.

Constantinou, C. E., Djurhuus, J. C., Silverman, D. E., et al.: Isometric detrusor pressure during bladder filling and its dependence on bladder volume and interruption to flow in control subjects. J. Urol., 131:87, 1984.

Constantinou, C. E., Faysal, M. H., Rother, L. et al.: The impact of bladder neck suspension on the mode of distribution of abdominal pressure along the female urethra. In Zinner, N. R., and Sterling, A. M. (Eds.): Female Incontinence. New York, Alan R. Liss, 1981, p. 121.

Constantinou, C. E., and Stamey, T. A.: The relative value of the physical exam, history, and urodynamics in predicting the cure rate of endoscopic suspension of the bladder neck. Submitted for publication.

Diokno, A. C., and Taub, M.: Ephedrine in treatment of urinary incontinence. Urology, 5:624, 1975.

Drukker, B. H.: Anterior colporrhaphy. In Buchsbaum, H. J., and Schmidt, J. D. (Eds.): Gynecologic and Obstetric Urology. Philadelphia, W. B. Saunders Co., 1978.

Drutz, H. P., et al.: Do static cystourethrograms have a role in the investigation of female incontinence? Am. J. Obstet. Gynecol., 130:516, 1978.

Enhörning, G.: Simultaneous recording of intravesical and intra-urethral pressure. Acta Chir. Scand., 276:3, 1961.

Freiha, F. S., and Stamey, T. A.: Cystolysis: a procedure for the selective denervation of the bladder. Trans. Am. Assoc. Genitourin. Surg., 71:50, 1979.

Green, T. H., Jr.: The problem of urinary stress incontinence in the female: an appraisal of its current status. Obstet. Gynecol. Surv., 23:603, 1968.

Green, T. H., Jr.: Urinary stress incontinence: pathophysiology, diagnosis, and classification. In Buchsbaum, H. J., and Schmidt, J. D. (Eds.): Gynecologic and Obstetric Urology. Philadelphia, W. B. Saunders Co., 1978.

Green, T. H., Jr.: Vaginal repair. In Stanton, S. L., and Tanagho, E. A. (Eds.): Surgery of Female Incontinence. New York, Springer-Verlag, 1980.

Greenwald, S. W., Thornbury, J. R., and Dunn, L. J.: Cystourethrography as a diagnostic aid in stress incontinence. An evaluation. Obstet. Gynecol., 29:324, 1967.

Hald, T., and Bradley, W. E.: The Urinary Bladder, Neurology and Dynamics. Baltimore, The Williams & Wilkins Co., 1982.

Hilton, P., Stanton, S. L.: Urethral pressure measurements by microtransducer: the results in symptom-free women and in those with genuine stress incontinence. Br. J. Obstet. Gynaecol., 90:919, 1983.

Hodgkinson, C. P.: Relationships of the female urethra and bladder in urinary stress incontinence. Am. J. Obstet. Gynecol., 65:560, 1953.

Hodgkinson, C. P.: Stress urinary incontinence in the female. Surg. Gynecol. Obstet., 120:595, 1965.

Hodgkinson, C. P.: Stress urinary incontinence—1970. Am. J. Obstet. Gyencol., 108:1141, 1970.

Hodgkinson, C. P., and Drukker, B. H.: Infravesical nerve resection for detrusor dyssynergia. The Ingelman-Sandberg operation. Acta Obstet. Gynecol. Scand., 56:401, 1977.

Hodgkinson, C. P., and Stanton, S. L.: Retropubic urethropexy or colposuspension. In Stanton, S. L., and Tanagho, E. A. (Eds.): Surgery of Female Incontinence. New York, Springer-Verlag, 1980.

Innes, I. R., and Nickerson, M.: Drugs inhibiting the action of acetylcholine on structures innervated by postganglionic parasympathetic nerves (antimuscarinic or atropinic drugs). In Goodman, L. S., and Gilman, A. (Eds.): The Pharmacological Basis of Therapeutics. New York, The Macmillan Co., 1970.

Jeffcoate, T. N. A., and Roberts, H.: Stress incontinence of urine. J. Obstet. Gynecol. Br. Commonw., 59:685, 1952.

Jones, E. G.: Nonoperative treatment of stress incontinence. Clin. Obstet. Gynecol., 6:220, 1963.

Kelly, H. A., and Dumm, W. M.: Urinary incontinence in women, without manifest injury to the bladder. Surg. Gynecol. Obstet., 18:444, 1914.

Krantz, K. E.: The Marshall-Marchetti-Krantz Procedure. In Stanton, S. L., and Tanagho, E. A. (Eds.): Surgery of Female Incontinence. New York, Springer-Verlag, 1980.

Lee, R. A.: Surgical incontinence procedures for recurrent stress incontinence. In Buchsbaum, H. J., and Schmidt, J. D. (Eds.): Gynecologic and Obstetric Urology. Philadelphia, W. B. Saunders Co., 1978.

Lewis, R. I., Lockhart, J. L., and Politano, V. A.: Periurethral polytetrafluoroethylene injections in incontinent female subjects with neurogenic bladder disease. J. Urol., 131:459, 1984.

Low, J. A.: Management of anatomic urinary incontinence by vaginal repair. Am. J. Obstet. Gynecol., 97:308, 1967.

Mahoney, D. T., Laferte, R. O., and Mahoney, J. E.: Studies of enuresis. Part VI. Observations on sphincter-augmenting effect of imipramine in children with urinary incontinence. Urology, 1:317, 1973.

Marchetti, A. A.: Urinary incontinence. JAMA, 162:1366, 1956.

Marchetti, A. A., Marshall, V. F., and Shultis, L. D.:

Simple vesicourethral suspension for stress incontinence of urine. Am. J. Obstet. Gynecol., *74*:57, 1957.

Marshall, V. F., Marchetti, A. A., and Krantz, K. E.: The correction of stress incontinence by simple vesicourethral suspension. Surg. Gynecol. Obstet., *88*:590, 1949.

Montague, D. K., and Stewart, B. H.: Urethral pressure profiles before and after Ornade administration in patients with stress urinary incontinence. J. Urol., *122*:198, 1979.

Pereyra, A. J.: A simplified surgical procedure for the correction of stress incontinence in women. West. J. Surg., *65*:223, 1959.

Pereyra, A. J., and Lebherz, T. B.: Combined urethrovesical suspension and vaginourethroplasty for correction of urinary stress incontinence. Obstet. Gynecol., *30*:537, 1967.

Pereyra, A. J., and Lebherz, T. B.: The revised Pereyra procedure. *In* Buchsbaum, H. J., and Schmidt, J. D. (Eds.): Gynecologic and Obstetric Urology. Philadelphia, W. B. Saunders Co., 1978.

Raz, S.: Modified bladder neck suspension for female stress incontinence. Urology, *17*:82, 1981.

Ridley, J. H.: Gynecologic Surgery: Errors, Safeguards, and Salvage. Baltimore, The Williams & Wilkins Co., p. 114, 1974.

Rud, T.: Urethral pressure profile in incontinent women from childhood to old age. Acta Obstet. Gynecol. Scand., *59*:331, 1980.

Schreiter, F., Fuchs, P., and Stockamp, K.: Estrogenic sensitivity of alpha-receptors in the urethra musculature. Urol. Int., *31*:13, 1976.

Shortliffe, L. M. D., and Stamey, T. A.: Endoscopic suspension of the vesical neck for the correction of urinary stress incontinence in the female. *In* McDougal, W. S. (Ed.): Operative Urology, London, Butterworth, 1985.

Stamey, T. A.: Endoscopic suspension of the vesical neck for urinary incontinence. Surg. Gynecol. Obstet., *136*:547, 1973.

Stamey, T. A.: Urinary incontinence in the female: stress urinary incontinence. *In* Harrison, J. H., Gittes, R. F., Perlmutter, A. D. et al. (Eds.): Campbell's Urology. Vol. 3. Philadelphia, W. B. Saunders Co., p. 2282, 1979.

Stamey, T. A.: Endoscopic suspension of the vesical neck for urinary incontinence in females: Report of 203 consecutive patients. Ann. Surg., *192*:465, 1980*a*.

Stamey, T. A.: Pathogenesis and Treatment of Urinary Tract Infections. Baltimore, The Williams & Wilkins Co., 1980*b*.

Stamey, T. A.: Endoscopic suspension of the vesical neck for surgically curable urinary incontinence in the female. Monogr. Urol., *2*:65, 1981.

Stamey, T. A., Schaeffer, A. J., and Condy, M.: Clinical and roentgenographic evaluation of endoscopic suspension of the vesical neck for urinary incontinence. Surg. Gynecol. Obstet., *140*:355, 1975.

Stanton, S. L., and Cardozo, L.: Results of colposuspension operation for incontinence and prolapse. Br. J. Obstet. Gynecol., *86*:693, 1979.

Stanton, S. L., and Tanagho, E. A. (Eds.): Surgery of Female Incontinence. Chaps. 3, 5, 6, and 8. New York, Springer-Verlag, 1980.

Tanagho, E. A.: Simplified cystography in stress urinary incontinence. Br. J. Urol., *46*:295, 1974.

Toews, H. A.: Intraurethral and intravesical pressures in normal and stress-incontinent women. J. Obstet. Gynecol., *29*:613, 1967.

Turner-Warwick, R.: Observations on the function and dysfunction of the sphincter and detrusor mechanisms. Urol. Clin. North Am., *6*:(1)13, 1979.

Ulmsten, U., and Andersson, K. E.: The effects of emeprone of intravesical and intra-urethral pressures in women with urgency incontinence. Scand. J. Nephrol., *11*:103, 1977.

Wein, A. J.: Pharmacologic approaches to the management of neurogenic bladder dysfunction. J. Cont. Ed. Urol., *18*:17, 1979.

Suprapubic Vesicourethral Suspension (Marshall-Marchetti-Krantz) for Stress Incontinence

VICTOR F. MARSHALL, M.D.
E. DARRACOTT VAUGHAN, JR., M.D.
JEROME P. PARNELL, M.D.

THE STRESS TEST

A principal objective indication for the correction of stress incontinence is the stress test, which can also predict the degree of success. At least one such test has evolved as a standard (Marshall et al., 1946; 1949; Bonney, 1964; Marchetti, 1956). The bladder is filled to 250 ml with bland solution via catheterization, the catheter is then removed, and the patient coughs in the lithotomy position. If the patient leaks on such sudden strain (characteristically by spurt), she* has stress incontinence. She may have additional disorders, but she certainly has stress incontinence. Supporting the vesical base via the vagina with one or two fingers approximately under the trigone should eliminate the spurt or leak (Fig. 73–23). Care must be taken not to compress the urethra for a falsely favorable result. An Allis clamp can seize the vaginal wall without anesthesia at the same site and provide support without the danger of inadvertently occluding the urethra. Downward traction on the Allis clamp usually exaggerates leakage.

Probably the best prognostic approach is to insert in the vagina three or four 4 inch × 4

*For purposes of this section, the patient will be considered female, though stress incontinence occurs also in males.

inch flat gauze sponges in a tight roll, like a large vaginal menstrual tampon; have the patient observe the effect on her urinary control for 15 to 20 hours; and then remove the tampon. This modification of the Marshall test provides vesical support for some hours while the patient continues a good fluid intake. A favorable test is one in which leakage stops while the tampon is in place, yet the patient can void regularly (not unlike the effect of the old-fashioned pessary). This simple test should retract the sphincteric mechanism away from the introitus toward the umbilicus, and *any* technique that consistently duplicates that effect should cure stress incontinence. This is not to say that all urinary complaints will go away but only that the stress incontinence itself will cease. Which of the many

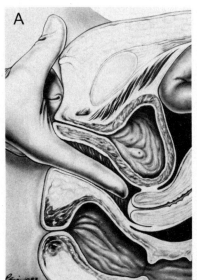
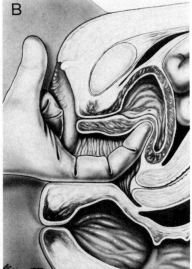
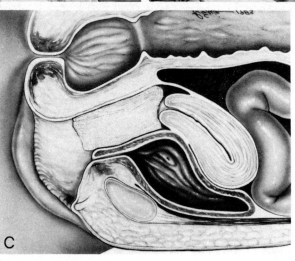

Figure 73–23. *A*, The stress test, which temporarily supports the sphincteric mechanism away from the introitus toward the umbilicus. *B*, Notice curved finger not compressing urethra. *C*, The extended Marshall stress test, using a gauze vaginal tampon for several hours.

types of operations will do this most consistently and permanently at the least risk remains to be seen in a comparative study of large numbers operated upon by competitive methods.

STATISTICS

We reviewed 140 cases under our complete responsibility on our urologic service at The New York Hospital–Cornell Medical Center when the patient's first operative procedure for incontinence was our suprapubic vesicourethral suspension, the Marshall-Marchetti-Krantz operation (Marshall et al., 1982). Ninety per cent of these individuals were completely cured of the incontinence, and an additional 7 per cent had objectively and greatly improved control during an average follow-up of 46 months. During the same period, 99 women who had failures following previous vaginal repairs or through suprapubic approaches were also treated (Marshall et al., 1983). Nearly all these women were considered to have favorable stress tests. Eighty per cent of them who had had one or more previous failures had excellent results, and an additional 10 per cent had major objective improvement during a similar follow-up.

A third group under our responsibility comprised miscellaneous patients who desperately desired even a modest improvement. Most of these women had unfavorable or equivocal stress tests. In general, the results were dismal but did clearly indicate the value of our test: For instance, only three had excellent results in spite of "fond hopes" and a willingness to have another operation. Another 12 could be labeled "improved." Included were eight men who experienced leakage with damage to the sphincters on endoscopic examination following prostatic surgery: Only two of them were merely "improved" during 30 months' follow-up. Not included in this group are some even earlier cases in which a perineal hernia following an abdominoperineal resection of the rectum restored control in men by means of our suprapubic approach (Marshall et al., 1946). Performing the Pereyra-Lebherz-Stamey (Pereyra and Lebherz, 1967; Stamey, 1979) type of operation on men would seem hazardous to the rectum.

STRESS VERSUS URGENCY

A balancing of the amount of stress incontinence versus mere urgency frequency has been important in selecting candidates. Characteristically, the patient with stress incontinence has no warning that she may leak (except as past experience may have taught her) until she actually becomes wet, whereas the patient with urgency frequency, mainly with the urethral syndrome (as well as any vesical infection), nearly always has a preliminary desire to void, albeit momentarily, before she actually leaks. A 2-week trial of therapy aimed against the irritation that is present can indicate the nature of this syndrome, as opposed to the purely mechanical inadequacies of stress. The therapy consists of hot sitz baths twice a day for 10 minutes by the clock and urinary antiseptics, such as nitrofurantoin 100 mg three times per day or sulfisoxazole 1 gm three times per day. For those women past menopause, diethylstilbestrol 1 mg three times per day is often added for the 2-week trial. Careful examination of the vagina for infection was part of the preliminary study (Marchetti, 1956), as was a search for intrinsic vesical neck damage from previous surgery, tuberculosis, interstitial cystitis, neurogenic bladder, foreign bodies, and fistula. Cystoscopy was done routinely at the time of stress testing but probably was not necessary in the easily defined typical case of stress incontinence.

THE OPERATION

Suprapubic vesicourethral suspension, the Marshall-Marchetti-Krantz operation (Marshall et al., 1949), has been modified many times, but not by us. Our only routine change has been to place the paraurethral sutures clearly into the vagina and to avoid suturing into the urethra proper. Our plan always was to insert the suspending sutures into the cartilage of the symphysis, since the cartilage provides a strong anchorage. Whether a transverse or a vertical incision is made depends on the demands of exposure. We have usually favored a vertical incision, since exposure of the distal vagina and urethra has seemed better. After the muscles were retracted, a sponge on ring forceps was applied down on the vesical neck, the urethra, and the top of the vagina. About 1 pound of force sufficed to open widely the space of Retzius in virgin subjects (indeed, this lack of support was fundamental in causation of the stress incontinence). Following previous operations for stress incontinence, however, a scalpel was commonly necessary to separate the back of the symphysis from the vagina-urethra. Any remains of pubourethral ligaments were routinely divided. We have ignored the endopelvic fascia, incising it regularly to move the sphincteric mechanism away from the introitus toward the umbilicus.

Cleaning out the fat on top of the urethra and vagina would seem to provide future better adherence to the posterior aspect of the symphysis. The fat was removed by gently skeletonizing the veins (just boldly wiping out the fat tears many vessels). Since the bleeding was venous, packing for a few minutes nearly always allowed the operator to continue to proceed directly, and the eventual closure approximating these structures to the back of the symphysis did control further venous bleeding. The upper surface of the urethra, vagina, and vesical neck were thus freed down within 1 cm of the external urethral meatus, permitting the tips of three fingers of the operator to be inserted under the lower symphyseal edge as if to lift the patient with a satchel handle. The lack of such extensive freeing was the apparent cause of failure in a number of reported cases. Three 2-0 chromic catgut sutures were inserted equidistantly on

either side near the urethra into the vaginal wall (Fig. 73–24). A double insertion provided a firmer hold and later applied more tissue to the back of the symphysis for adherence there. A Mayo needle reduced the chance of breakage. Next, on either side of the vesical neck the same sutures were inserted—probably the most important pair (Fig. 73–25). The vesical neck was defined by a 5-ml Foley balloon catheter placed preoperatively. These sutures were tagged with different clamps identifying the various echelons.

Then, the ends of these sutures were passed into the cartilage and periosteum at points estimated to retract the freed vesical neck, urethra, and top of the vagina away from the introitus and toward the umbilicus (Fig. 73–26). An assistant's fingers in the vagina aided in the selection of sites of insertions on the posterior aspect of the symphysis. Tying these sutures was facilitated by having the assistant periodically press up to close the space of Retzius. Rarely, these upper two sutures were put into the lowermost attachments of the recti muscles if such a measure seemed indicated. The space of Retzius was additionally closed by suturing the vagina upward at points that might seem to sag unduly. If the vagina was unusually large, we have occasionally used the Burch (Burch, 1961) modification of suturing to the lacunar (Cooper's) ligaments further laterally in the pelvis on both sides. Only in the rarest instances have we used combined suprapubic and vaginal approaches, mostly in cases in which the structures have been stuck down, as for example in extreme fibrosis that might occur following old lymphogranuloma venereum (Marshall et al., 1983; Ball, 1952). Any ordinary cystourethrocele has been routinely cured without a vaginal approach! If cystocele is still present, our operation has probably been performed inadequately (Stanton, 1982). A transurethral catheter fastened to a leg with adhesive was maintained for 3 to 5 days (Fig. 73–27); and a small suprapubic drain was removed at about the same time as the catheter. No vaginal packing was employed in any case.

Since a degree of retention following the removal can be anticipated, our habit was to test for residuum some 6 to 8 hours later, even if the patient appeared to progress smoothly. If there was major residuum of more than 100 ml, intermittent catheterization was employed until it was reduced to about 50 ml. The administration of bethanechol chloride, mild urinary antiseptics, and hot sitz baths seemed to help in these retentive cases. We had one patient who

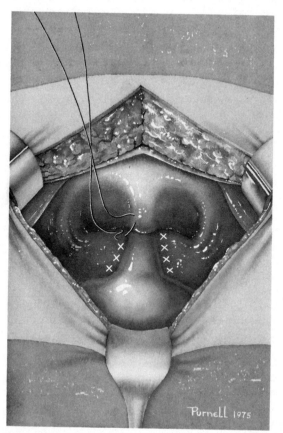

Figure 73–24. Downward view in the space of Retzius showing the sites of placement of the catgut sutures.

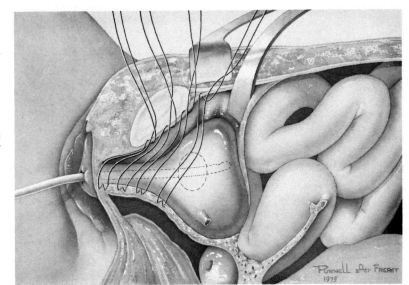

Figure 73–25. Sagittal view before sutures have been tied. (After Freret.)

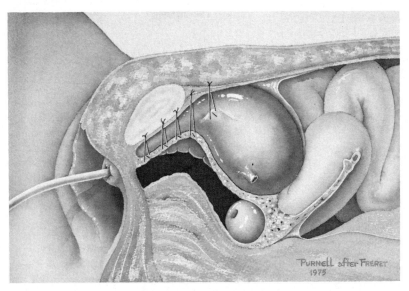

Figure 73–26. After sutures have been tied, showing retraction of the urethra from the introitus toward the umbilicus. Actually, the space of Retzius is snugly closed and not strung across as for illustrative purposes here.

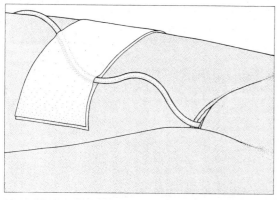

Figure 73–27. The transurethral catheter has been attached to adhesive on the thigh postoperatively to forestall undue traction counter to the purposes of the operation.

had significant retention for 2 months, but such retention nearly all resolved in less than 2 weeks, even in seemingly obstinate cases. Nearly all our patients have been mobilized out of bed within 12 hours after the operation. We guess that 2 per cent of the early successes will come down in the next 5 years, but the operation can, of course, be repeated.

Complications

This suprapubic vesicourethropexy has been widely popularized. As with other often repeated operations we have discovered complications. Table 73–8 lists those accompanying

TABLE 73–8. TWO HUNDRED THIRTY-NINE PATIENTS HAVING MARSHALL-MARCHETTI-KRANTZ OPERATIONS FOR ORDINARY STRESS INCONTINENCE, INCLUDING FAILURES OF EARLIER PROCEDURES FOR STRESS INCONTINENCE

	No.	Percentage
Urinary infection, more than 10^5 organisms (Marshall et al., 1982)	2	0.8
Wound infection	7	3
Hernia	2	0.8
Dehiscence	1	0.4
Osteitis pubis	14	6
Osteomyelitis pubis	1	0.4
Immediate urinary retention, requiring recatheterization	38	16
Prolonged urinary retention	15	6
Urinary fistula 3 weeks or more	0	0
Frequency, urgency	6	3
Pulmonary embolus	6	3
Myocardial infarct	2	0.8
Failure to improve urinary control at all	2	0.8
Worse urinary control	0	0
Deaths	0	0

the aforementioned first two groups (virginal and straightforward recurrent cases), comprising 239 patients. In the group having secondary operations for recurrences, the incidence of openings made into the urinary tract was significant, but all closed spontaneously within 3 weeks or less. We usually left a cystostomy for about a week in such cases and formally closed the opening into the urinary tract. The results seem to be essentially unchanged even in this group of previous operated upon patients—and there were no permanent fistulae or secondary closures.

Each complication has been counted so that if a patient had two or more complications, it would be counted two or more times. Conversely, this review indicates that 50 per cent of the whole group (130) had completely smooth postoperative courses without any complications, and if minor urinary retentions were omitted as being considered to be expected transiently, 195 or 82 per cent (195 of 239) had no complications (Marshall et al., 1982, 1983).

On our service with these and similar cases, we have never ligated a urethra or a ureter, nor have we produced a vesicovaginal fistula even temporarily. All suprapubic fistulae closed spontaneously before discharge within 3 weeks. Several pregnant patients have had vaginal deliveries without recurrences of stress incontinence (we have suggested keeping the bladder empty during delivery). We have not indulged in elaborate cystourethrographic preliminaries, such as chain cystograms (Hodginson, 1965; Green, 1968) or pressure profiles, yet our results seem to compare favorably.

THE MECHANISM

What is the mechanism of correction? All sharply functioning sphincters have points of peripheral fixation. Observe the drastic difference between the pupil of the eye, which has complete fixation all around, and the ileocecal valve, a notoriously poor sphincter, which is almost floating. If proper fixation is restored to an intrinsically intact sphincter—not one internally damaged or neurologically deficient—the surgeon should have greater than a 90 per cent rate in restorations. In such cases, displacement away from the introitus and toward the umbilicus seems essential, as favorably shown by the preliminary Marshall test. As emphasized at the beginning of this chapter, any procedure that does this routinely will eliminate stress incontinence. How permanent is restoration? We have tried to provide a bit more information than immediate results here and hope that comparisons can still be made with significant numbers of cases operated upon differently. When suprapubic vesicourethral suspension was first devised in 1949, practically all earlier patients had had vaginal repairs for stress incontinence. In fact, the first concept seems to have been to tighten by plicating the vesical neck: the Kelly procedure with the Kelly stitch (Green, 1968). After a while it was realized that these vaginal operations produce a floor of fibrous tissue (scar) under the bladder. Attention was then centered on the downward herniation (cystourethrocele), and elaborate operations were devised on this basis. There were even a few suprapubic approaches in which slings were employed to suspend the herniation from above (Aldridge, 1942). Indeed, some approaches were combined suprapubic and vaginal ones (Ball, 1952). Included in these approaches would be the recently repopularized Pereyra-Lebherz (Pereyra and Lebherz, 1967) and its modification known as the Stamey procedure, in which endoscopy and special instruments are essential (Stamey, 1979).

The Marshall-Marchetti-Krantz procedure was devised not by studying women exclusively but by observing mainly men who had had abdominal perineal excision of the rectum (Marshall et al., 1946). This then new operation in 1949 (Marshall et al., 1949) opened a vista and a fresh concept: If the sphincteric mechanism were intrinsically intact (as demonstrated by the Marshall stress test), restoration of mechanical advantage could be achieved *suprapubically* by displacing that mechanism away from the introitus toward the umbilicus. Indeed, the operation opened the management of stress incontinence, hitherto limited to gynecologists, to urologists and general surgeons. Others had stumbled upon similar preoperative tests, but they failed to emphasize or exploit them (Bonney, 1964) (after all, it has been known for more than half a century that fitting, supporting pessaries could often alleviate stress incontinence). Finally, the Marshall-Marchetti-Krantz operation does not require esoteric tools, and so it can be performed by any good surgeon on proper indication.

References

Aldridge, A. H.: Transplantation of fascia for relief of urinary stress incontinence. Am. J. Obstet. Gynecol., 44:398, 1942.

Ball, T. L.: Combined vaginal and abdominal plication and cystopexy urinary stress incontinence. Am. J. Obstet. Gynecol., 63:1245, 1952.

Burch, J. E.: Urethrovaginal fixation to Cooper's ligament for the correction of stress incontinence. Am. J. Obstet. Gynecol., 81:281, 1961.

Green, T. H., Jr.: The problem of urinary stress incontinence in the female: An appraisal of its current status. Obstet. Gynecol. Surv., 23:603, 1968.

Hodginson, C. P.: Stress incontinence in the female. Surg. Gynecol. Obstet., 102:595, 1965.

Kelly, H. A., and Dumm, W. M.: Urine incontinence in women without manifest injury to the bladder. Surg. Obstet. Gynecol., 18:444, 1914.

Macleod, D., and Hawkins, J. (Eds.): Bonney's Gynecological Surgery. 7th ed. London: Cassell, 1964.

Marchetti, A. A.: Urinary incontinence. JAMA, 162:1366, 1956.

Marshall, V. F., Marchetti, A. A., and Krantz, K. E.: Correction of stress incontinence by simple vesicourethral suspension. Surg. Gynecol. Obstet., 88:509, 1949.

Marshall, V. F., and Nelson, J.: Visits in urology, suprapubic vesicouretheral urethral suspension of stress incontinence in females. 1977. Produced by and obtainable from Norwich Eaton Pharmaceuticals, Inc., 17 Eaton Ave., Norwich, N.J. 13815.

Marshall, V. P., Pollock, R. S., and Miller, C.: Observations on urinary dysfunction after excision of the rectum. J. Urol., 55:409, 1946.

Parnell, J. P. II, Marshall, V. F., and Vaughan, E. D., Jr.: Primary management of urinary stress incontinence by The Marshall-Marchetti-Krantz vesicourethropexy. J. Urol., 127:679, 1982.

Parnell, J. P. II, Marshall, V. F., and Vaughan, E. D., Jr.: Management of recurrent stress incontinence by Marshall-Marchetti-Krantz vesicourethropexy. J. Urol., 132:912, 1984.

Pereyra, A. J., and Lebherz, T. B.: Combined vesicourethral suspension and vaginourethroplasty for correction of urinary stress incontinence. Obstet. Gynecol., 30:537, 1967.

Stamey, T. A.: Urinary incontinence in the female. Stress urinary incontinence. In Harrison, J. H., et al. (Eds.): Campbell's Urology. 4th ed. Philadelphia, W. B. Saunders Co., 1979, p. 2272.

Stanton, S. L.: The choice of surgery for incontinence. Br. J. Urol., 54:74, 1982.

CHAPTER 74

Urinary Fistulae in the Female

RICHARD TURNER-WARWICK, B.Sc., D.M. (Oxon.), M.Ch., F.R.C.P., F.R.C.S., F.A.C.S., F.R.A.C.S.

It is almost always possible to close a urinary tract fistula; meticulous surgical technique is essential, but success with the more complicated problems is equally dependent upon both the selection of a procedure that is suited to the particular clinical situation and the ability of the surgeon to vary it appropriately during the course of the operation, according to the findings and his personal experience.

Simple traumatic vesicovesical fistulae can often be resolved reliably by simple closure in layers from either a vaginal or an abdominal approach; however, failure with either reflects upon the surgical judgment or the technique, because the possibility of a failure should have been anticipated. Even recurrent fistulae and those associated with severely impaired healing or local tissue loss can be most reliably repaired by the addition of an omental interposition graft procedure.

VESICOVAGINAL FISTULAE

ETIOLOGY

Simple vesicovaginal fistulae are usually the result of local trauma. The commonest cause of these, worldwide, is tissue necrosis resulting from pressure between the head of the child and the pubis during an unduly prolonged labor. The incidence of this has been largely eradicated with improvements in the overall obstetric care in many countries.

In communities with sophisticated medical care, the commonest residual cause of a simple vesicovaginal fistula is gynecologic surgery. This risk is inherent in paravesical surgery and it can never be entirely eradicated; even the most experienced gynecologists are confronted with this complication, often quite unexpectedly, after an apparently easy hysterectomy; the chance of it is considerably increased when the procedure is technically difficult or when the local tissue healing is impaired by fibrosis, infection, tumor, irradiation, or generalized debilitating conditions such as diabetes.

SYMPTOMS

Incontinence is the primary symptom; it is usually total but occasionally, when a fistula is small, it may be remarkably intermittent, so that the leakage is less obviously fistulous in origin. It may become apparent immediately postoperatively or it may develop after a delay of several days.

DIAGNOSIS

Both the suspicion and the confirmation of the diagnosis are usually all too obvious. A large vesicovaginal fistula is easy to feel on vaginal examination; the smaller the fistula, the more difficult the diagnosis is likely to be. Occasionally, when there is very little surrounding telltale inflammation, it can be very difficult to detect a long-standing pinhole fistula endoscopically.

Intravenous Urography. Intravenous urography is essential to the diagnostic evaluation of a vesicovaginal fistula; in the uncomplicated case, both upper urinary tracts drain normally. Obstruction or hold-up of the drainage of ureteral contrast medium indicates either a coincident ureteral abnormality or involvement of the ureter in the fistula; such a finding requires further evaluation and often determines the need for an abdominal approach to the repair of the fistula.

Cystography. Cystographic examination may be helpful in the evaluation of small fistulae but it contributes little or nothing to that of the larger ones. The detection of minute vesicovaginal fistulae may be particularly difficult because urine that is passed normally through the urethra quite frequently refluxes into the vagina and may confuse the picture; occasionally, it is helpful to insert a loose vaginal pack of absorbent gauze before cystographic examination of a doubtful case, so that a relatively small fistulous leakage of contrast into the vault will be located separately from any urethral leakage that may reflux into the vagina.

Examination Under Anesthesia. Detailed examination with the patient under anesthesia is essential to the evaluation of a fistula and the choice of approach is often dependent upon it. In complicated cases, it may be undertaken as a separate preoperative procedure, but in a relatively simple case, it is usually an immediate preliminary to the operative procedure.

Endoscopy. When a vesicovaginal fistula is large, the escape of irrigating fluid from the bladder or from the vagina must be prevented so that the bladder can be adequately distended for proper examination. If the fistula itself is too large to be occluded by a finger in the vagina, the introitus can usually be closed sufficiently with the overdistended balloon of a Foley catheter or even by lateral compression of the labia.

It is very important to exclude the existence of additional, less obvious, collateral fistulae, especially if a vaginal repair is contemplated, because it is easy to miss these in the course of a limited dissection from this approach (Fig. 74–1).

If the fistula is close to a ureteral orifice, it may be advisable to elect the better exposure provided by an abdominal approach in case ureteral reimplantation becomes necessary, even if the preoperative urographic evaluation showed the ureteral drainage to be unimpaired. It is also important to assess the relationship of the fistula to the functional area of the bladder neck because local scarring may compromise its sphincteric function and thus require an extension of the reconstructive procedure.

Local tissue biopsy is obviously indicated if there is any possibility of a specific underlying pathologic condition so that this may be taken into account. However, a positive biopsy after radiation of a tumor is not necessarily a contraindication to an omental graft fistula repair; not only is this usually a simpler surgical procedure than a surface diversion, but it is remarkably reliable and provides patients with a better quality of life for their remaining days.

While the confirmation of a good bladder capacity is encouraging at this stage, it is often impossible to obtain immediate distention of bladders that have been leaking continuously for considerable periods, even if the escape of irrigating fluid is effectively occluded; this does not necessarily imply, however, that it is permanently "contracted" and incapable of gradual distention once the fistula is closed.

Simple defunctionalization of the bladder, with or without a fistula, even over a period of years, does not in itself lead to a permanently contracted bladder or to dysfunction; in general, this occurs only as a result of a recognizable local pathologic condition such as interstitial cystitis, tuberculosis, tumor, or irradiation. Occasionally, the bladder may become incarcerated by perivesical fibrosis resulting from a pelvic hematoma, infection, or scarring; function in such cases can sometimes be restored by a decortication similar to the technique used for "frozen lung," especially if reformation of the scar tissue is prevented by a pliable omental wrap (Turner-Warwick, 1976).

A "systolic" bladder with uninhibited detrusor contractions may appear to have a small capacity, but this can easily be shown to be due to muscular activity, rather than fibrosis, because it readily distends under effective general or spinal anesthesia that relaxes the detrusor activity.

Additional Maneuvers. Small vesicovaginal fistulae can be best identified, with the patient under anesthesia, by distending the bladder and observing the site of leakage into the vagina with the aid of a suitable vaginal speculum; good illumination provided by a special fiberlight suction tube is often particularly helpful. A spectacular but less useful alternative is to distend the vagina with air and to observe endoscopically the stream of bubbles escaping into the bladder through a small fistulous tract. In practice, it is rare that the site of a small fistula is so "clean" that it cannot be identified by inflammatory changes around its margin.

Dye Test. The dye test is occasionally helpful in determining whether a urinary leakage arises from a ureterovaginal fistula, a vesicovaginal fistula, or urethral incontinence. A light gauze pack is placed in the vagina, and a suitable dye such as methylene blue is introduced into the bladder with a urethral catheter. If, over a

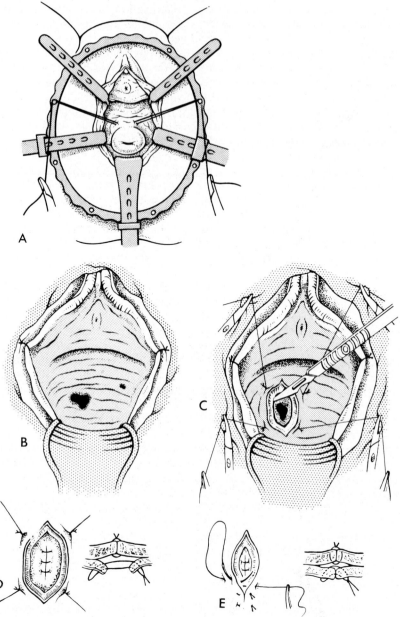

Figure 74–1. Vaginal repair of vesicovaginal fistulae.

A, The exposure of the fistula facilitated by lateral labial stay-sutures, and a wide-blade weighted posterior vaginal or a perineal ring retractor with stay-suture guide-knobs (Turner-Warwick 1977). A careful check to exclude additional fistulae is made.

B, Development of the tissue plane between the vagina and bladder around the fistula.

C, Closure of the bladder wall with 3–0 absorbable sutures; knots tied on the lumen.

D, Closure of the vaginal layer with everting 3–0 PGA aPG sutures or removable 3–0 nylon sutures.

period of several hours, the pack remains dry and only the outer end becomes colored, the origin of the leakage is obviously urethral; if the proximal end becomes colored, it is probably the result of a fistulous vesicovaginal leak. If the proximal part of the pack becomes wet with unstained urine, its source must be ureteral, but occasionally dyed urine can escape from a ure-terovaginal fistula if there is free vesicoureteral reflux.

Principles of Surgical Repair

The successful closure of a fistula is essentially dependent upon the healing of the surrounding tissues; if the surgical procedure is not in sympathy with this, even the most painstaking repair may fail.

Failure to close a fistula should be a rare occurrence and should always stimulate a surgeon to reflect upon the reasons; although it may be the result of a hematoma, an infection, or some other relatively unpredictable circumstance, it is the selection of a procedure appropriate to the local circumstances and to the surgeon's technique that is really the most important factor in successful closure.

TISSUE HANDLING

It is always distressing to a reconstructive surgeon to see tissue margins roughly handled with so-called tissue forceps; many of these are sufficiently crushing to create an area of necrosis, even in normal tissues. A simple guide is to avoid the use of any instrument that causes discomfort when applied to a fold of one's finger skin. In general, stay sutures are tissue-preserving, and when they are used as retractors over the margin of a ring retractor, either perineal or abdominal (Fig. 74–4), they are much more helpful than supernumerary assistants, however willing.

LAYER CLOSURE

The development of tissue planes for layer closure requires careful judgment. In general, when the tissue margins around the fistula are relatively normal, it is helpful to develop the planes and to close them separately; if, however, they are densely scarred or the healing reaction is impaired as a result of infection, irradiation, and so forth, separation of the tissue layers can be a self-defeating exercise, since their survival may be interdependent. Thus, any attempt to develop an intervening plane, instead of providing the basis for better healing, may well result in spontaneous marginal necrosis.

SUTURES AND SUTURE LINES

The selection of sutures and the technique of their use may well be critical to the result of a difficult fistula repair.

All absorbable suture materials create some degree of tissue reaction, so the gauge selected should be as small as possible, compatible with the necessary strength; in general, this is more commonly overestimated than underestimated. Polyglycolic acid (PGA) sutures cause much less tissue reaction than catgut, and the tensile strength of finer sizes is particularly good and reliable. The choice of suture material is a matter of individual surgical preference, but currently this author has a strong preference for Dexon or Vicryl sutures for reconstructive surgery in general and for fistula repair in particular; however, special care is necessary to achieve secure locking of the knot when using these materials. Since knot-tying must be a habitual procedure, many surgeons prefer to use either catgut or synthetic sutures, rather than both.

The extent to which the tissue bite is tightened can be more important to the tissue reaction that a suture causes than is the material from which it is made; great care must be taken to avoid strangulating the tissue enclosed within the suture bite by overtightening it, and allowance must be made for the natural swelling of the healing reaction of different tissues.

The knot of a suture represents the point of maximal tissue reaction; every "throw" adds twice its thickness, so that its placement may be important. It has become a generally accepted surgical habit to bury the knot in the tissue, but this is not necessarily the best place for it; when healing is critical, there seems to be an advantage in placing the knots of the inner layer of lower urinary tract sutures in the lumen, so that they fall off and are voided as soon as the suture releases.

INFECTION AND TISSUE HEALING

Local infection can prove a serious complication of any delicate reconstructive procedure, particularly when tissue healing is somewhat impaired for any reason. If antibiotic treatment of this is delayed until infection becomes clinically obvious, it is likely to be too late to save the suture line; therefore, many surgeons use prophylactic broad-spectrum antibiotics routinely to cover the more critical reconstructive procedures.

POSTOPERATIVE URINARY DRAINAGE

It is, of course, technically impossible to keep a urinary tract suture line "dry" postoperatively, and indeed the endeavor is quite unnecessary, because the urinary tract tissues are naturally adapted to healing in a wet environment. High intravesical pressures and overdistention during the early stages of the healing of a critical bladder suture line, however, risk urinary extravasation, which impairs healing; it may be wise to use two catheters to drain the bladder.

There are considerable advantages in suprapubic catheter drainage as a routine postoperative procedure after all but the simplest fistula closures; it is efficient, reliable, and considerably less uncomfortable than a urethral catheter and it probably reduces infection. Furthermore, at the conclusion of the drainage period, it is easy to restore voiding and to verify its efficiency by clamping a suprapubic catheter and releasing it to verify the postvoiding residual volume before deciding to remove it; this compares favorably with the emotionally charged situation that occasionally arises when a urethral catheter has to be repeatedly inserted—the "yo-yo" catheter state. A urethral catheter can be used in addition, but if the fistula lies close to the internal meatus, it is advisable to retain the catheter with a sling suture anchored by a button on the abdominal wall; the presence of a catheter balloon in contact with a bladder base suture line probably does little harm, but inadvertent traction upon it can be disastrously disruptive.

Few reconstructive urologists now advocate the vaginal cystotomy route for catheter drainage, and nearly all of us have long since abandoned the old-fashioned mushroom de Pezzer catheter, with its grotesque and irreducible end.

TIMING OF SURGICAL INTERVENTION

It is impossible to generalize usefully about the timing of a fistula repair; this is determined by clinical estimation of the state of the local tissues of a particular case in relation to the proposed procedure.

If a repair is to be entirely dependent upon a layered closure, it is obviously of great importance that the local tissue be in the best possible condition. It is often possible to resolve the problem of simple traumatic and postoperative fistulae by early exploration—within a day or two—before a compromising degree of tissue reaction has developed; however, once this is established, it is usually better to wait several months, until the local inflammatory response has stabilized as much as possible.

The main disadvantage of delaying a closure is the discomfort it causes the unfortunate patient, for she is likely to be intractably wet until the fistula is closed; nevertheless, if this course of action is decided upon, it must be carried through with determination, for disasters can result from impatience and premature intervention.

A reasonably efficient interim collection of urine can sometimes be achieved by Foley catheter drainage of the vagina, retained by overdistending the balloon within the introitus.

Although it is obviously important to ensure that any acute inflammatory element has resolved, the timing of a fistula repair is relatively less critical when the success of the procedure is largely dependent upon an interposed omental pedicle graft; just as this procedure has enabled us to repair fistulae resulting from permanent severe tissue damage due to such causes as irradiation, which were way beyond the potential of a layer closure technique, so it also makes us somewhat less time-dependent as far as the local tissue healing of a relatively simple fistula is concerned.

Thus, the timing of a repair must be considered carefully in relation to each individual fistula. It would certainly be unjustifiable to use a relatively major abdominoperineal procedure involving a full-length median incision if the same fistula could be simply repaired using a vaginal approach layer closure merely by waiting a few months. There are occasions, however, when it is quite clear that the ultimate repair is going to be difficult anyway, and provided that the element of acute infection has been reduced to a minimum, there may be little point in waiting for maximal resolution of the local inflammation.

The Repair of Simple Vaginal Fistulae

The emphasis on practical details in this chapter leaves little room for the historical aspects of fistula repair, but nothing that could have been included would have substituted for the excellent monograph of John Chassar Moir (1967); this and the review of Russell (1962), Everett and William's chapter in the previous edition of this work, and the chapters of Carlton (1975) and O'Connor (1976) provide many references; however, so many have contributed so much to the subject for so long that it is often difficult and even invidious to identify individual originators.

The majority of simple traumatic vesicovaginal fistulae can be repaired by simple layer closure techniques. The decision whether to use the vaginal or the abdominal route is sometimes dictated by the nature and extent of the fistula, but for those that are not critically close to the ureteral orifices, it is often largely a matter of the individual surgeon's training and preference. Surgeons who have a gynecologic training naturally elect a vaginal approach for simple fistulae, and this certainly has the advantage of causing less postoperative discomfort to the patient; careful selection should, however, ensure that this procedure is almost always successful; otherwise, one would suspect that the approach was being overused. An abdominal or a synchronous abdominoperineal approach is more reliable for the repair of difficult cases, especially since these can be further extended, when necessary, to the almost invariably successful interposition of an omental pedicle graft.

POSITIONING OF THE PATIENT

Although it is possible to repair many simple vesicovaginal fistulae by the vaginal route, it is important to be aware of the limitations imposed by this relatively restricted access; it is inappropriate for extensive fistulae and for those lying close to the ureteral orifices.

In the case of a simple fistula, if after preliminary examination under anesthesia the surgeon is quite certain that a simple vaginal repair will be sufficient, it may be reasonable to place the patient in the standard hip-flexed lithotomy position, suited only for this; otherwise, if there is any doubt about the procedure that might be required, the patient should be positioned so that the procedure can be extended without interruption to a combined abdominoperineal approach (flat, head slightly down, with legs widely abducted in minimal hip flexion). This modified position can be arranged to provide very good exposure for vaginal surgery, particularly if a self-retaining retractor such as a perineal ring with stay suture guides is used, so that the number of perineal assistants can be reduced to one, at most.

If an abdominal approach is elected, there is an advantage to using the same flat, legs-apart position and including the perineum in the operation field: not only does an orientating finger in the vagina greatly facilitate the layer dissection around the fistula, but it also provides space for a synchronous surgical approach from the perineum if the situation proves unexpectedly complicated. When no perineal surgery is required, it is convenient to position the instrument table and the scrub nurse between the legs of the patient.

VAGINAL REPAIR OF SIMPLE VESICOVAGINAL FISTULAE

Most gynecologic surgeons prefer to operate with the patient in the standard dorsal, hip-flexed lithotomy position; the alternative prone knee-chest position has been particularly advocated by Lawson (1967) as a routine approach for obstetric fistulae. Once the surgeon is used to having the patient in the prone position, it may have some advantages, especially in obese patients, because the abdominopelvic contents tend to fall away from the operative site and retropubic visualization may be improved; how-

ever, it is important to remember that the bladder is dependent in this position, so that any clots that have accumulated in it during the operation must be carefully removed before the bladder is closed. Neither the flexed lithotomy position nor the prone position offers the immediate facility of extension to a synchronous abdominal exploration, if this becomes advisable.

Proper exposure and retraction is one of the keys to success. The inner labial fold can be simply retracted with temporary lateral skin sutures, and if the vaginal introitus is less than adequate, it can be enlarged by simple midline or posterolateral Schuchardt incisions to enable a wide-blade self-retaining retractor to be inserted (in the standard lithotomy position). The steps of the procedure are illustrated in Figure 74–1.

Since this is primarily a layer closure technique, meticulous attention to detail is essential; if there is any reason to doubt the success of the procedure, either the closure should be reinforced by the addition of a Martius (1928) interposition rotation graft of labial tissue (Fig. 74–2), or it should be extended so that a more extensive synchronous abdominoperineal repair with omental interposition can be achieved.

TRANSABDOMINAL REPAIR OF SIMPLE VESICOVAGINAL FISTULAE

The abdominal approach can be used for the repair of any vesicovaginal fistula. The patient is positioned as previously described so that the sterile area permits a synchronous approach to be made from below; even though a formal vaginal approach may not be initially intended, it is often very helpful to the separation of the layers around the fistula if the surgeon can orient the dissection with a finger in the vaginal vault.

A suprapubic V incision provides an access to the pelvis and the lower abdomen that is superior to that obtainable with either a Pfannenstiel incision or a midline incision (Turner-Warwick et al., 1974); however, if there is any possibility that a formal omental interposition graft may be needed, it is important to use a median incision that can be extended to the xiphisternum to provide access to the gastrosplenic area if formal mobilization of the omental pedicle proves necessary.

A simple transvesical approach to the repair of a vesicovaginal fistula provides a relatively restricted access, so this time-honored procedure has been largely abandoned (Fig. 74–3).

The supravesical approach has many advan-

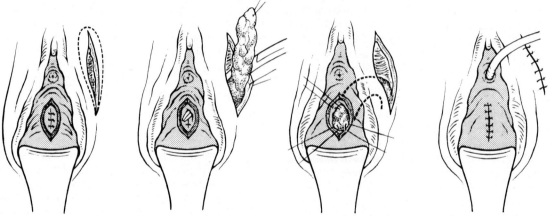

Figure 74–2. Optional reinforcement of the vaginal layer closure by interposition of a posteriorly based pedicle graft of labial tissue (the Martius procedure).

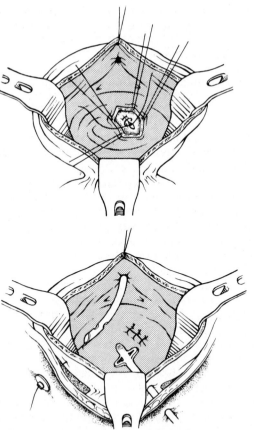

Figure 74–3. The classic transvesical layer-closure of a simple vesicovaginal fistula. This approach has been generally abandoned in favor of the alternative supravesical approach.

tages (Fig. 74–4). It provides wide exposure of the fistulous area and direct extravesical access to the terminal ureter, so that it is relatively easy to reimplant this into the bladder, if necessary. The transperitoneal supravesical approach to a fistula is also basic to the creation of the abdominoperineal tunnel required for an interposition graft closure of a complex fistula; thus it is simple to proceed to a reinforced repair when necessary.

COMPLEX URINARY FISTULAE

If the healing potential of the tissue margins of the fistula is compromised by scarring due to infection, previous attempts at repair, or irradiation, the success rate of a simple layer closure technique falls abruptly, and some form of viable tissue interposition is advisable. A sizable flap of parapelvic peritoneum sometimes provides sufficient extra support for a layer closure; however, in complicated situations, the use of local tissues is generally contraindicated, since they are likely to be involved in the same scar reaction resulting from infection and especially from irradiation.

Pedicle grafts of skeletal muscle are available in the region of the pelvis, but this tissue is not ideal for the purpose because (1) although its blood supply has excellent potential, it is available only in response to exercise; furthermore, without exercise, muscle undergoes fi-

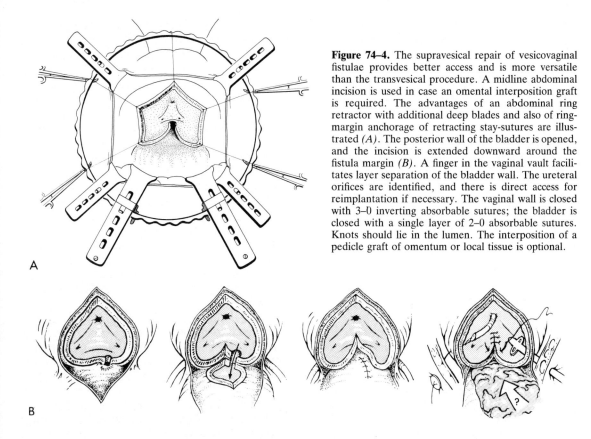

Figure 74–4. The supravesical repair of vesicovaginal fistulae provides better access and is more versatile than the transvesical procedure. A midline abdominal incision is used in case an omental interposition graft is required. The advantages of an abdominal ring retractor with additional deep blades and also of ring-margin anchorage of retracting stay-sutures are illustrated *(A)*. The posterior wall of the bladder is opened, and the incision is extended downward around the fistula margin *(B)*. A finger in the vaginal vault facilitates layer separation of the bladder wall. The ureteral orifices are identified, and there is direct access for reimplantation if necessary. The vaginal wall is closed with 3–0 inverting absorbable sutures; the bladder is closed with a single layer of 2–0 absorbable sutures. Knots should lie in the lumen. The interposition of a pedicle graft of omentum or local tissue is optional.

brotic atrophy; and (2) muscle is ill adapted to resist the infection that is commonly associated with complex fistulae resulting from impaired tissue healing and irradiation. The mobilized gracilis and other muscles have, however, been used successfully for fistula repair (Ingleman-Sundberg, 1960; Hamlin and Nicholson, 1969).

INTERPOSITION OF OMENTAL PEDICLE GRAFT REPAIR

The omentum is unique in that it is the only body tissue that is specifically developed for the resolution of local inflammatory processes. In its normal resting state the omentum has superficial resemblance to extraperitoneal fat, but here the similarity ends because its healing potential is greatly superior, deriving from a combination of its blood supply and its abundant lymphatic drainage. Every inflammatory response creates cell debris and macromolecular protein exudates into the tissue spaces; these cannot be reabsorbed directly into the blood stream, and unless they are removed efficiently by lymphatic drainage, they accumulate to form pus.

Inasmuch as the omentum has several special qualities that are not shared by the natural surroundings of the urinary tract, its use as a graft is of great value to the urologist.

It can provide:

1. Healing tissue support for complicated urinary tract reconstructions.

2. A vascular graft to local tissue when its healing is impaired by infection, irradiation, diabetes, and so forth.

3. Replacement of tissue loss in the pelvis and the perineum.

4. A supple surrounding tissue allowing urodynamic mobility, because unlike extraperitoneal fat, once its inflammatory response is complete it regains its normal suppleness and never forms dense fibrosis.

5. An easily separable tissue plane, which facilitates any subsequent re-exploration.

Thus, the use of the omentum is well established for the more complex reconstructions of the urinary tract in general (Turner-Warwick et al., 1967; Turner-Warwick, 1976). Bastiaanse (1954, 1960) and Kiricuta and Goldstein (1956, 1972) pioneered the omental repair of vesical fistulae in particular, but of course the use of omental pedicle flaps has been such a long-established routine in abdominal surgery for the repair of lesions in the gastrointestinal tract that it is quite impossible to identify the actual surgeon who first used it for a pelvic fistula.

The omental apron is often long enough to reach the pelvic floor without tension; in such cases, it can be used as an interposition graft without mobilization of its vascular pedicle. It is usually advisable, however, to separate it from the transverse colon and its mesocolon by development of the intervening avascular plane to reduce the chance that postoperative bowel distention may dislocate it.

When the omental apron is short it must be mobilized so that it will reach the pelvis; this is not particularly difficult, but it does require great attention to detail. A patient has only one omentum; properly handled, it will almost always ensure the closure of a complicated fistula in the pelvis. It is a disaster for such a patient to lose the omentum as a result of careless mobilization, and this must be constantly borne in mind during the somewhat time-consuming and tedious procedure. It is of course entirely naive to suppose that the magic of the omentum can be transposed by a free graft in the manner of a postage stamp.

The blood supply of the omentum derives from the gastroepiploic arch on the greater curvature of the stomach. The right element of this arises from the gastroduodenal vessels below the pylorus and is almost always larger than the left, which arises somewhat higher in the abdomen, from the splenic flexure. The gastroepiploic arterial arch is sometimes incomplete, and in such cases the interruption of continuity is almost invariably located toward its left extremity. The omental branches of the gastroepiploic arch descend from it vertically, with few major collateral anastomoses.

Consequently, when omental mobilization is indicated, the vascular anatomy almost always favors its basement on the larger right gastroepiploic vessels (Turner-Warwick et al., 1967) rather than the left, as advocated by Bastiaanse (1954, 1960) and by Kiricuta and Goldstein (1956, 1972); furthermore, since the right pedicle arises lower than the left, even the shortest omental apron will reach the pelvis, provided the full length of the gastroepiploic arch is mobilized. Thus, it is almost always possible to avoid horizontal elongating incisions into the apron, which inevitably divide some of the main vertical omental vessels.

While the transposition of a viable omental flap based on the left gastroepiploic vessels may be sufficient to close most pelvic fistulae, the author believes that the provision of a graft that is visibly pulsating down to the pelvic floor may occasionally be critical to the success of the procedure in the most difficult of the problems for which the use of the omentum is indicated.

A subumbilical incision provides sufficient access to enable a conveniently long omental apron to be used to support a pelvic procedure; however, one cannot assume or prejudge its length, so if there is any possibility that the omentum will be required for the repair of a particular fistula, it is important to start with a median incision, because this can be extended to the xiphisternum to provide access to the splenic pedicle in the event that the omentum proves to be short and requires formal mobilization.

The fundamental principles of mobilization of the gastroepiploic omental pedicle are the following:

1. Adequate access for division of the splenic origin of the left gastroepiploic vessels must be obtained; if this does not provide sufficient length, a formal mobilization of the gastroepiploic vascular pedicle is required (Fig. 74–5).

2. The 20 to 30 short gastric branches must be individually ligated with absorbable suture material without damaging the main gastroepiploic vessels. Ligation of a bunch of branches shortens the pedicle and adds the risk that one might escape and bleed.

3. Nonabsorbable sutures should never be used on the omental graft; any one could come to lie exposed within the fistulous area and cause stone formation as a result of urinary encrustation.

4. It is important to pay particular attention to the technique of ligation of the short gastric branches; the escape of the proximal end of any of these is a potential disaster because this rapidly creates an interstitial hematoma, and great care is then necessary to retrieve the end for secure religation if damage to the main vessels is to be avoided. It is generally safer to ligate the proximal end of these vessels in continuity before dividing them; however, hemostat ligation of the gastric end is quite appropriate, because this is easy to retrieve if it inadvertently escapes in the process of tying off (Fig. 74–5).

5. Once started, the mobilization of the gastroepiploic arch should usually be completed to its gastroduodenal origin; otherwise, there is a risk that traction on the pedicle might tear the last undivided branch (Fig. 74–6).

6. The omental pedicle should lie in an extraperitoneal position as far as possible; this

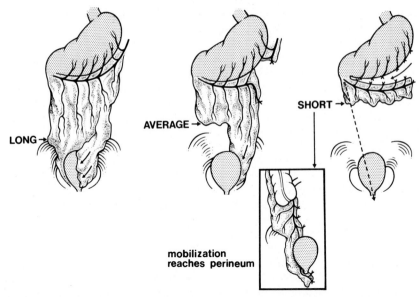

Figure 74–5. Mobilization of the omentum. The omental apron is quite often long enough to reach the perineum without formal mobilization of its pedicle. If it is of only average length, mobilization of the gastroepiploic vessels is necessary. Even a short apron, commonly found in children, will reach the perineum if the full length of the gastroepiploic vessels is mobilized, because the length of the greater curvature of the stomach is approximately equal to the distance between the duodenum and the perineum.

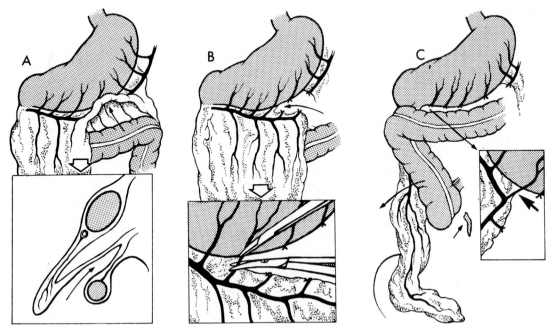

Figure 74–6. Mobilization of the vascular pedicle of the omentum *(A)*. A long omental apron will reach the pelvis without mobilization; a short one requires definitive mobilization of the gastroepiploic vessels from the full length of the greater curvature of the stomach, based on the right gastroepiploic pedicle.

Individual ligation of each gastric branch separately with 2–0 absorbable sutures *(B)*. Proximal ligation in continuity before division of each short gastric vessel is advisable. Complete mobilization of the gastroepiploic arch to its origin from the gastroduodenal pedicle avoids traction on the last undivided gastric branch. The omental pedicle is positioned behind the ascending colon *(C)*; prophylactic appendectomy is optional.

is easy to achieve in the abdomen by placing it behind the mobilized ascending colon. It is not usually necessary to extend this extraperitoneal approach into the pelvic area except in females with a childbearing potential that could be compromised by occlusion of the fallopian tubes.

7. The pedicle of a mobilized omental graft lies immediately adjacent to the appendix; routine appendectomy is advisable to avoid the possibility that appendicitis might compromise the immediately adjacent pedicle, either by inflammatory response or by inadvertent ligation during an emergency appendectomy.

8. Gastric suction for a mild ileus is often required for 2 or 3 days after a full-length mobilization of a gastroepiploic vascular pedicle; a gastrostomy tube is a humane alternative to a nasogastric tube and quite simple to insert because the stomach is well exposed. However, technique and management of this is important to avoid complications of leakage when it is removed. A No. 18 Foley catheter is pulled through the abdominal wall to the left of the upper extremity of the midline incision and inserted into the antrum with a pursestring suture. The anterior wall of the stomach is then invaginated with a running suture to form a tunnel about 5 cm long, and at the proximal end of this the stomach is fixed to the anterior abdominal wall around the tube with a few interrupted sutures. As an added precaution, the gastrostomy can be spigoted when gastric suction is no longer required and left in situ for 5 or 6 days to ensure a complete track is formed before it is removed.

The mobilization of the omentum may be compromised if a preliminary transverse colostomy has been established in a case with rectal involvement; this does not prevent mobilization, but it adds considerably to the time involved. The probable need for the use of the omentum in the definitive repair of such cases should be borne in mind during the initial management, and a defunctionalizing sigmoid colostomy should be positioned in the left iliac fossa.

TECHNIQUE OF OMENTAL INTERPOSITION

The success of an interposition omental pedicle graft is also fundamentally dependent upon the creation of a large abdominoperineal tunnel between the fistulous cavities; this should readily accept four fingers in the adult and should extend the full width of the pelvis to ensure that there is a good overlap of the tissues and that there are no residual lateral fistulous tracts.

If the local tissue-healing situation is particularly precarious, the success of the procedure may be more dependent upon the omentum than upon the suture line closure of the bladder and the vagina (or the rectum). If the bladder suture line breaks down, the omental graft is exposed to its lumen; however, provided the omental bulk overlaps the margin of the fistula sufficiently, it usually heals without significant urinary leakage, and the omentum exposed to the lumen of the bladder is rapidly covered by regenerating urothelium. If a fistula should persist after an omental interposition, its reexploration is facilitated by the omental tissue plane, once the tissue reaction has settled several months later. The omentum never becomes densely fibrotic so that, provided the original mobilization achieved a good bulk of well-vascularized omental tissue in the pelvis, it can be redeployed in relation to a reclosure.

COMPLEX FISTULAE

A synchronous abdominoperineal approach is usually advisable for the repair of complex urinary vaginal fistulae; the tissue plane used to create the abdominoperineal tunnel for the omental interposition graft is dictated by the type of fistula.

Complex Vesicovaginal Fistulae

In these cases, the abdominoperineal interposition tunnel is developed between the anterior vaginal wall and the urethra; it is important that this should lie as close to the vagina as possible to avoid injury to the residual urethral mechanism. The fistulous opening into the bladder is freshened and is closed with a single layer of 2–0 absorbable sutures, with the knots tied so that they lie in the lumen as far as possible. The anterior vaginal wall is often extensively scarred from previous surgery in such cases, but it is helpful to reconstruct it as far as possible to keep the omental graft in position; it is of no consequence if its reapproximation is incomplete in places.

Complex Vesicovaginorectal Fistulae

Such fistulae occasionally result from the treatment of uterine and cervical tumors by a combination of hysterectomy and irradiation; the vault of the residual vagina is usually stenosed and surrounded by dense scar tissue. The abdominoperineal tunnel is created through the vagina by circumcising its wall at the upper limit of reasonably healthy tissue and developing a plane between the bladder and the rectum by synchronous abdominoperineal dissection. It is usually impossible to identify the individual tissue layers around the stenotic vaginal vault, but the excess of scar tissue should be excised and the tunnel fully developed laterally so that it will admit four fingers; particular care must be taken to avoid leaving islands of vaginal epithelium in this area, since they could predispose to the persistence of a fistulous tract. The steps of the procedure are outlined in Figure 74–7.

VAGINOPLASTY FISTULAE

A vaginal reconstruction for atresia naturally lies in close proximity to the urinary tract so that, occasionally, an otherwise satisfactory split-skin vaginoplasty may develop a fistula into the bladder (or indeed into the rectum). This situation presents a special problem because a reconstructed vagina has no wall thickness, and an additional grafting procedure is essential to recreate a septal bulk if the fistula is to be closed without sacrificing the otherwise satisfactory inlay.

It is usually possible to resolve this situation quite simply by incising the vaginal inlay longitudinally on the side of the fistula and developing an abdominoperineal tunnel in such a way that the skin graft opens to form a flat strip of epithelium lying opposite to the fistula. The fistulous tract is then loosely closed, and an omental pedicle graft, folded so as to present a smooth surface to the inlay, is interposed and sutured into position; its bare area epithelializes to complete the circumference of the vagina. Provided that the lateral margins of the vaginal skin strip are anchored laterally with sutures so that it presents its full width to the omental graft, the ultimate diameter of the reconstructed vagina will be considerably increased; this is important because the primary cause of such fistulae is often an insufficiently capacious vaginal reconstruction (Figs. 74–8 and 74–9). In practice, there are advantages in using the cecum rather than a skin graft to augment or replace a vagina (Turner-Warwick and Handley Ashken, 1967).

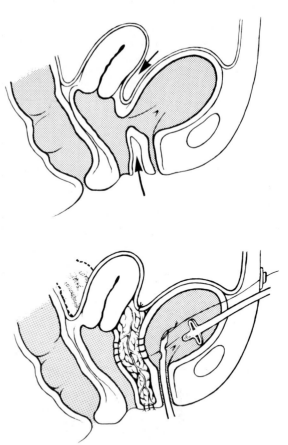

Figure 74–7. Omental repair of vesicovaginal fistulae. The interposition tunnel created by a synchronous abdominoperineal approach between the bladder and vagina should be as close as possible to the vagina to avoid injury to the urethral sphincter mechanism. The tunnel should be extended laterally to admit 3 or 4 fingers. The bladder and the vagina are closed with 2–0 absorbable sutures, with knots on the lumen where possible. The appropriately mobilized omentum fills the capacious abdominoperineal tunnel with good lateral overlap of the fistula closure; its distal margin is included in the perineal suture line. Free drainage of the pelvis occurs around the omentum; no additional drains are necessary, but two-catheter bladder drainage is advisable, by suprapubic and suture-slung urethral catheters.

URETHROVAGINAL FISTULAE AND THE SPHINCTER MECHANISMS

Failure to close a urinary vaginal fistula should be a rare indication for urinary diversion; this is more often required for urinary incontinence when the sphincter mechanisms subsequently prove to have been irreparably damaged. It is most important that this situation not be prejudged, even if the fistula extends into

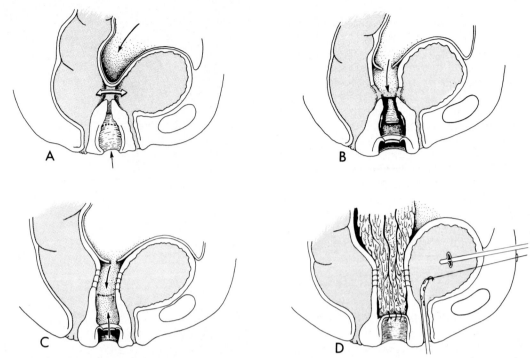

Figure 74–8. The omental repair of vesicovaginorectal fistulae. Preliminary left iliac colostomy. The abdominoperineal tunnel is developed through the vault of the vagina *(A)*. The vaginal wall is circumcised at the upper limit of its normality, and the stenosed vault above this is carefully denuded of vaginal epithelium *(B)*. The tunnel is fully developed laterally to accept 3 or 4 fingers, and the excess scar tissue around the fistulous orifices of the bladder and the rectum are trimmed away before they are closed with 2–0 absorbable sutures *(C)*. The lower border of the appropriately mobilized omental interposition graft is included in the loosely tied closure sutures of the vaginal cuff. This allows free pelvic drainage without additional drains *(D)*. Two-catheter urinary drainage, by suprapubic and stitch-slung urethral catheters, is used. The defunctioning colostomy is maintained 2 months.

the sphincter mechanism, because continent function may sometimes be restored by an effective reconstructive urethral repair.

A basic understanding of the sphincter mechanism is therefore essential to the repair of urethrovaginal fistulae, and indeed much of our knowledge of the function of isolated mechanisms derives from the urodynamic study of patients such as those with partial sphincter damage (Turner-Warwick and Whiteside, 1979).

It is well recognized that the bladder neck mechanism can maintain continence on its own; an efficient bladder neck mechanism is particularly important in females because their urethral mechanism is relatively inefficient. Spence's method of treating a urethral diverticulum is based upon the creation of an intentional urethrovaginal fistula by marsupializing the diverticulum into the vagina (Spence and Duckett, 1970); provided that the bladder neck mechanism is functioning normally, the patient will be continent. Distal urethrovaginal fistulae most commonly result from complications following anterior colporrhaphy; if the original colporrha-

phy was undertaken for stress incontinence, this is quite likely to persist after fistula repair, because the bladder neck is essentially incompetent in stress incontinence.

It is most important to appreciate that the assessment of bladder neck function requires careful urodynamic evaluation; it cannot be "guessed at" on the basis of simple endoscopic appearances or static anatomic radiologic concepts such as the "posterior angle." Furthermore, even if the bladder neck is proven to be truly normal, its competence is also dependent upon the stability of the detrusor function; it seems that the neck mechanism is inevitably opened in association with any abnormal uninhibitable detrusor contractions (Turner-Warwick, 1974).

It follows that a bladder neck mechanism should not be divided or encroached upon unnecessarily in the course of the repair of a vesical or urethral fistula; furthermore, unless or until follow-up urodynamic studies indicate that it is incompetent, it is probably inadvisable to proceed directly to any variety of Flocks-Young-

OMENTO-VAGINOPLASTY

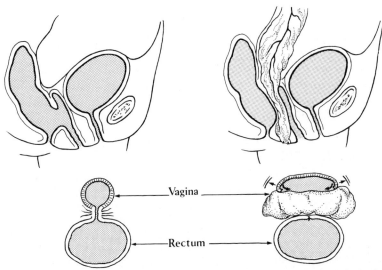

Figure 74–9. The omental repair of vaginoplasty fistulae. The split-skin vaginal inlay graft is incised throughout its length on the side of the fistula. The abdominoperineal tunnel is developed laterally so that the circumference of the vaginal graft lies flat on the side opposite the fistula; its lateral margins are sutured laterally to prevent its rolling up. The fistula is closed with interrupted 2–0 absorbable sutures. The appropriately mobilized omental graft is folded so as to present a flat surface to the vaginal strip, and its margins are sutured to the margins of the bare area of the tunnel. A light vaginal pack is inserted to keep the omental graft in apposition with the bare area of the tunnel. Two-catheter bladder drainage is maintained for 2 to 3 weeks for a vesicovaginal fistula; the defunctioning colostomy for a vesicourectal fistula is maintained 2 months.

Dees-Tanagho bladder tube reconstructions, because the intrinsic sphincteric functions of these seem generally less reliable than a definitive reconstruction of the actual bladder neck mechanism by a reduction sphincteroplasty.

URETHRAL MECHANISM

The intrinsic urethral mechanism of the female is both weaker and less reliable than that of the male, so that when the bladder neck is dysfunctional (whether due to intrinsic weakness or unstable detrusor contractions) the risk of stress incontinence is much greater. The closing pressure of the urethral sphincter derives from its various components, including smooth muscle, striated muscle, and elastic tissue; this pressure normally extends the whole length of the female urethra, but it is maximal at about the middle third. An important point, so far as urethral reconstruction and fistula repair are concerned, is that the voluntary striated muscle, such as it is, is eccentric and concentrated in the anterior urethral wall, becoming almost aponeurotic posteriorly; consequently, it is generally advisable to approach the female urethra from behind, and it is sometimes possible to improve

the competence of a urethral sphincter with a posterior tightening closure. In practice, it seems advisable from the functional point of view to reduce the lumen so that it is relatively snug around a No. 12 or 14 F sound (if a stenting catheter is left in the urethra, it should be relatively small to avoid suture line tension—about 10 F). Once effective urethral closure is obtained, the lumen can usually be recalibrated to a larger size, if necessary, with simple dilatation.

PELVIC FLOOR

The relationship of the pelvic floor to urethral function is indirect. The normal intra-abdominal position of the vesicourethral mechanism is generally related to its natural functions of voiding and control; this becomes increasingly critical if the efficiency of the detrusor or the urethral mechanism is impaired. In general, therefore, although the pelvic floor and the uterocervicovaginal structures are helpful in maintaining the normal intra-abdominal anatomic position of the bladder base and urethra, the striated muscle element of the pelvic floor lies remote from the urethra, so that it cannot effect a significant direct compression, comparable to that of the male. Since a considerable proportion of urethrovaginal fistulae result from operations that were primarily designed to improve urinary continence, it is important that reconstructive surgery be directed not only toward the closure of the fistula and the reapproximation of the sphincteric defect, but also toward the elevation of the bladder base into the high normal intra-abdominal anatomic position that seems to improve the efficiency of substandard urethral mechanisms.

URETEROVAGINAL FISTULAE

Vaginal ectopia of the ureteral orifice is not particularly uncommon as one of the varieties of congenital urinary tract malformations, only very rarely does such a situation complicate the diagnosis of an acquired fistula.

A ureterovaginal fistula quite frequently occurs in association with a vesicovaginal fistula; technically, it exists whenever the ureter opens into the fistulous tract rather than onto the bladder mucosa.

True ureterovaginal fistulae can be created by penetrating or lacerating injuries, but the commonest cause by far is pelvic surgery. Fistulae may present immediately or after a few "dry" postoperative days.

SYMPTOMS

The natural consequences of an established isolated ureterovaginal fistula are continuous urinary leakage from the vagina and intermittent bladder voiding, but this pattern is not entirely diagnostic, since it may occasionally result from small vesicovaginal fistulae. When the fistulous upper tract is grossly infected and partially obstructed, it may give rise to a continuous purulent vaginal discharge that can be diagnostically confusing.

DIAGNOSIS

The cause of a ureterovaginal fistula is usually self-evident, but its detection occasionally presents a diagnostic problem in relation to a vesicovaginal fistula. One important feature is that it is rare for a ureterovaginal fistula to exist without some degree of radiologically identifiable obstruction of the upper urinary tract, so in most cases it can be excluded on the basis of the finding of a normal upper tract on intravenous urography. Conversely, ureteral involvement should always be suspected whenever an upper tract proves to be partially obstructed in association with a vesical fistula. Once suspected, it is usually quite easy to demonstrate

or exclude a ureteral fistula by retrograde bulb-catheter ureterography. The bladder dye test, using a vaginal pack, may indicate a ureteral as opposed to a vesical origin of a vaginal urinary leak, but the expenditure of time and effort on such an empirical maneuver in the investigation of a suspected ureteral fistula would generally be wasted, because definitive radiographic studies are simple and accurate.

Treatment of Ureteral Fistulae

If a traumatic ureteral fistula is associated with an incomplete circumferential defect, and if a retrograde ureteral catheter can be introduced past it into the upper tract, there is a fair chance that the leakage will heal spontaneously if the catheter is left in situ on continuous drainage.

FENESTRATED URETERAL STENT DRAINAGE

To obtain efficient drainage of urine from the ureter, the catheter should be provided with multiple drainage holes throughout its length. A standard ureteral catheter with two or three holes in the region of the tip may provide effective drainage of the pelvicalyceal system, but the peristaltic activity of the ureter results in the propulsion of urine into the space around the catheter, so that unless holes are specifically provided for its re-entry into the catheter, there is a natural tendency for urine to be extravasated at peristaltic pressure through any fistula or suture line. This is especially true since the resistance to the passage of urine beyond this point may be increased by the presence of an unfenestrated catheter that is supposedly improving ureteral drainage. It is probable that this simple mechanical point is one of the factors contributing to some of the unexpected complications after anastomotic repair of the ureter (Turner-Warwick, 1972, 1976).

REPAIR OF FISTULAE OF THE LOWER URETER

The majority of lower ureteral fistulae originate at or very close to the termination of the ureter, so that continuity can be restored by a simple reflux-preventing reimplantation into the bladder; one of the particular advantages of a supravesical approach to the repair of a vesicovaginal fistula is immediate access for ureteral reimplantation.

Occasionally, there is a sufficient length of normal ureter distal to a ureterovaginal fistula to enable ureteral continuity to be restored by a spatulated reanastomosis to the mobilized proximal ureter, optionally supported by an omental wrap and by ureteral drainage with a fenestrated catheter.

THE PSOAS BLADDER HITCH PROCEDURE

A simple technique for the resolution of the more complicated ureterovaginal or ureterovesicovaginal fistulae is to reimplant the ureter into the bladder fixed in a suprailiac position; the mobilization of the bladder involved in this helps to separate the fistulous tract closures (Zimmerman et al., 1960). The psoas hitch procedure has distinct advantages over the standard Boari technique (Turner-Warwick and Worth, 1969); not only is it easier to perform, but it also facilitates a reflux-preventing reimplantation of the ureter (Fig. 74–10).

An important point of technical detail is the primary incision in the bladder, which should be horizontal and at least hemi-circumferential; the upward extension of the bladder is much increased, often enabling it to reach the middle third of the ureter without tension, by closing this vertically.

FISTULAE INVOLVING THE MIDDLE THIRD OF THE URETER

Restoration of ureteral continuity may present a particular problem when a fistula involves the middle third of the ureter; ideally, restoration can be achieved by a simple spatulated overlap anastomosis of the mobilized ends of the proximal and distal ureter, but the length of the ureteral defect or the extent of the periureteral inflammation often prevents this.

The closure of any fistula is fundamentally dependent upon the healing potential of the surrounding tissue; that of the periureteral tissue is notoriously poor, and any inflammation of it tends to result in dense fibrosis and adhesions, so it is not surprising that the results of simple intubated ureterotomy left much to be desired, although they were considerably improved by omental wrapping.

Omentoureteroplasty

Omental support can be used to advantage for the support of any ureteral overlap reanas-

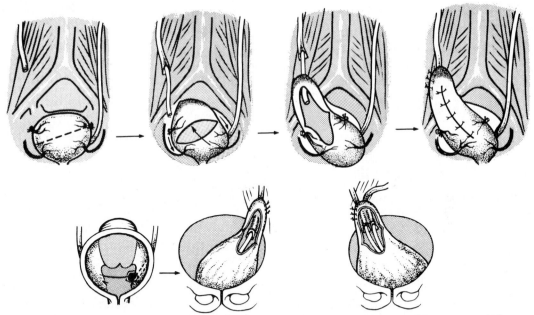

Figure 74–10. The psoas hitch repair of ureterovesicovaginal fistulae. The fistula is exposed by a supravesical approach through a suprapubic V incision. The anterior wall of the bladder is opened with a horizontal incision, which is subsequently closed vertically to increase bladder elevation. The bladder is effectively mobilized by circumcision of its peritonealized area and division of the supravesical vessels; the plane of mobilization is extended to the base, if necessary, preserving the ascending branches of the inferior vesical vessels on the bladder wall where possible. The fistulous tract is divided, and the bladder and the vagina are closed with 2-0 absorbable sutures. The elevation of the bladder usually separates the fistula closure lines quite widely—otherwise, an interposition graft may be advisable. The ureter is mobilized and its abnormal lower segment excised; it is reimplanted into the psoas-hitched bladder, above the iliac vessels, by a reflux-preventing procedure, usually a simple submucosal tunnel. The psoas-hitched position of the bladder is maintained with several strong absorbable sutures (1-0), anchoring the peritonealized area of the bladder (which provides good suture anchorage) to the psoas (including the psoas minor tendon, when present, but carefully avoiding the genitofemoral nerve and the lumbosacral trunk). The psoas hitch of the bladder should not be under tension when the detrusor is at rest; however, the deep anchor sutures must be inserted with care to prevent distraction as a result of detrusor contraction (although we have not yet encountered this complication in our series over a 10-year period) (Turner-Warwick and Worth, 1972). Two-catheter drainage is maintained for 2 to 3 weeks. The psoas-hitched position of a bladder does not impair its voiding efficiency.

tomosis, since its healing potential is incomparably superior to that of the periureteral tissue, to which it bears only a superficial resemblance. The principles of omentoureteroplasty are detailed elsewhere (Turner-Warwick et al., 1967; Turner-Warwick, 1976). In practice, the omentum will usually reach an upper urinary tract reconstruction without formal mobilization of its vascular pedicle; all that is necessary is to make a midline incision in the apron between the vertical vessels and to separate the omentum from the transverse colon on that side.

Omental support is particularly helpful for the prevention and treatment of renal transplant ureteric fistulae.

SKIN-PATCH OMENTOURETEROPLASTY

If, after appropriate mobilization, it is impossible to restore urethral continuity by an overlap anastomosis, it may be possible to obtain a simple end-to-end anastomosis of the spatulated ends and to complete the urethral circumference by a full-thickness graft of foreskin supported by an omentoplasty (Figs. 74–11 and 74–12).

Appendix Ureteroplasty

Occasionally, the appendix provides an appropriate substitution for a segment of the middle part of the right ureter.

Ureteroureterostomy or Autotransplantation?

When it is impossible to restore direct ureteral continuity after appropriate mobilization of the proximal and distal ends of the ureter, the options lie between a renal autotransplant and a ureteroureterostomy.

URETEROURETEROSTOMY

Ureteroureterostomy is a valuable operative procedure when the proximal end of the ureter is long enough to reach across; however, the potential complications of it must be carefully weighed. It is a urologic disaster to compromise a normal contralateral urinary tract and kidney, which is more than sufficient in itself, by an attempt to preserve the other, unless the circumstances are really appropriate and do not increase the risk of potential complications; the sequelae of suture line urinary extravasation, periurethral fibrosis, and the development of stricture-obstruction can be reduced by the use

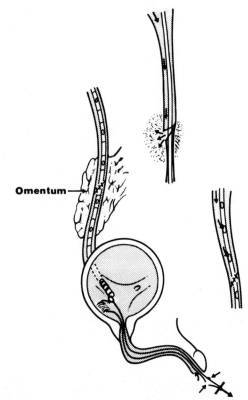

Figure 74–11. Repair of ureteral defect/fistula by spatulated overlap reanastomosis with an omental pedicle wrap. A fenestrated stent reduces the risk of suture line extravasation of peristalted urine due to distal ureteral obstruction by an unfenestrated stent. In this illustration, one limb of a transurethral nylon loop stitch is used to retain an internal stent; when this limb is cut externally, the other limb withdraws both stent and stitch (Turner-Warwick, 1980).

of appropriately fenestrated ureteric stents and omental pedicle graft wrapping.

AUTOTRANSPLANTATION

The advantage of renal autotransplantation to the pelvis is that the risk is confined to the affected kidney and, in experienced hands, the results are excellent, especially if the potential complications are also reduced by omental pedicle graft wrapping.

VESICOENTERIC FISTULAE

Although fistulization between the bowel and the bladder may be caused by penetrating injuries or by the synchronous spontaneous drainage of a pelvic abscess, it most commonly results from a specific gastrointestinal tract disease such as diverticulitis, neoplasm of the large bowel, or Crohn's disease.

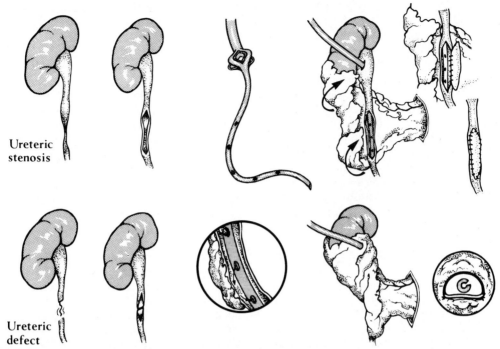

Ureteric
stenosis

Ureteric
defect

Figure 74–12. Omentoureteroplasty. When there is sufficient length of ureter for an overlap anastomosis the spatulated ends of the mobilized proximal and distal ureter are approximated by an oblique suture line and the ureteric circumference completed with a full-thickness graft of foreskin. A proximal pyelostomy drain is preferred, and it is most important to ensure that the stenting ureteric catheter is fenstrated to allow the re-enry of peristalted urine into it and thus avoid extravasation; the Cummings tube illustrated combines both features and is self-retaining. Continuous drainage is maintained until fenestrated cathetergram studies show no radiographic evidence of contrast extravasation.

DIAGNOSIS

The characteristic symptoms of a bowel fistula are pneumaturia and urinary infection; when the fistula is sizable, the patient may also recognize the passage of bowel content through the urethra. The diagnosis is usually self-evident once a fistula is established; cystoscopy reveals a generalized cystitis with gross focal inflammatory change, often bullous, in the region of the fistula. Contrast medium escaping from the bladder shows a bowel pattern on cystography. Barium studies from above or below are required to identify the underlying bowel disease.

TREATMENT

In most cases, the urinary tract is only secondarily and incidentally involved, so that from the urologic point of view, the resolution of a fistula is a relatively simple mechanical problem involving separation and closure. When a fistula results from primary bowel disease, the priority is almost always the expert surgical management of the intestinal disease; the urologic element is incidental to this and is usually a simple matter to resolve.

CONCLUDING DATA

The patients that a referral center receives are naturally heavily loaded with complex problems, and many have undergone previous attempts at closure; nevertheless, a simple review of 100 consecutive cases of vesical fistulae may appropriately highlight a few concluding points.

Only 8 of these 100 patients were treated with simple vaginal repair; this grossly underestimates the relative value of this procedure for the routine resolution of simple vesicovaginal fistulae. In 3 further cases, it was considered advisable to reinforce the vaginal repair with a Martius interposition labial rotation flap.

All 11 vaginal repairs closed the fistula. This is as it should be, because although the occasional failure is inevitable after any reconstructive procedure, a significant failure rate would have indicated that the simple approach had been overexercised; at the first hint of doubt or difficulty during the operation, it should be extended to a supravesical abdominal approach, and again, if the result of this appears in any way doubtful, then an additional omental interposition support should be used.

In practice, when a transperitoneal supravesical repair is used, it is the author's routine to use the omentum in the interposition between the closure lines whenever it will reach without formal mobilization; this adds greatly to the security and takes only a few minutes. Therefore, only 13 fistulae in this series were repaired with an unsupported multilayer supravesical procedure, but this number would probably have been more than doubled had the omentum not been readily available, because the relatively extensive procedure of formal omental mobilization would not have been undertaken without fair indication. None of the 13 simple supravesical closures failed; had they done so, one would certainly have regretted not mobilizing the omentum.

There were no simple transvesical repairs in this series.

The repair of vesicovaginal fistulae with an omental interposition graft is a reliable and reasonably simple procedure; closure on our first attempt was achieved in 70 out of the 73 cases in which it was used. It must be stressed again that the disproportionately high incidence of the use of the omentum in this series was partly the result of the complexity of the referred cases, and partly due to its free use in the course of a transperitoneal supravesical repair whenever it was easily available without mobilization being necessary.

The omentum required formal mobilization in 28 of the 73 cases; the need for its use was clearly felt in all these cases, and it was probably considered equally important to the repair in about half the cases in which its formal mobilization proved unnecessary.

One of these patients with multiple pelvic fistulae died postoperatively as a result of septicemia.

One of the two patients in whom the initial closure failed had a tumor that proved to be extending more rapidly than anticipated. We do not consider the presence of a tumor to be a definitive contraindication to an attempt at the omental closure of a relatively simple fistula if this procedure seems to offer a simple alternative to palliative diversion, although presence of a tumor would almost certainly contraindicate a simple layer closure.

In the other case in which the fistula persisted, it was quite easily closed on the second attempt 3 months later with re-exploration and redeployment of the omentum; the original problem had been a particularly extensive vesicourethrovaginal fistula. Re-exposure of the fistulous area is greatly facilitated by the use of the omental tissue plane, which remains supple and separates remarkably easily.

Four patients were referred who had had an omental repair fail elsewhere. In one of these, the fault clearly lay in an inappropriate attempt at mobilization of a relatively short omentum with a random incision (this was one of the 28 closed with formal omental mobilization). The 3 remaining fistulae in this group were closed by re-exploration and redeployment of the graft; it seemed that the width of the original abdominoperineal tunnel in these patients had been insufficiently developed laterally to provide a good tissue overlap.

Five patients whose fistulae were successfully closed with omentum subsequently required urinary diversion because of intractable urinary incontinence due to sphincter damage.

The only late complication directly relating to omental interposition repair that we have seen is the development of an omental bulge of the anterior vaginal wall. This has the appearance of a cystocele and can easily be mistaken for one, but it is simple to differentiate by combining vaginal examination with cystoscopy. On two occasions, we have had to treat this by incising the vaginal wall and simply reclosing it after resecting the excess omental tissue.

INSTRUMENTATION

A surgeon's armamentarium is even more personal than his selection of procedure; this author, for instance, would find it almost impossible to do any operation without his insulated diathermy scissors and insulated short-handled scalpel with No. 15 blade.

There are, however, a small number of instruments, both old and new, that are particularly useful for the repair of vesical fistulae (Fig. 74–13).

1. A fiberlight suction tube. An important combination of "suck and see" for dark narrow places; it can also be used for retracting small view-obstructing tissue folds. Some surgeons find a headlamp useful.

2. Perineal and abdominal ring retractors with self-retaining abdominal wall blades and a selection of deep retraction blades (Figs. 74–1 and 74–4).

3. A delicate, angled needle holder, which keeps the hand out of the line of vision when suturing at the bottom of a deep narrow access.

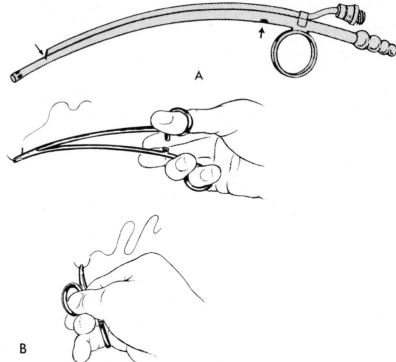

Figure 74–13. *A,* The fiberlight suction tube. *B,* The delicate angled needle holder, which keeps the hand out of the line of vision when suturing.

ACKNOWLEDGEMENT

Special appreciation—as ever—of Miss Freda Wadsworth, M. B. E., Medical Artist to the London University Institute of Urology, for her illustrations.

INSTRUMENTS

The instruments described are available from V. Mueller, Chicago, and The Genito-Urinary Company, London and Leibinger, West Germany.

References

Bastiaanse, M. A.: The repair of vesicovaginal fistulae, including so-called radium fistulae. Proc. R. Soc. Med., 47:610, 1954.

Bastiaanse, M. A.: The omental repair of vesicovaginal fistulae. *In* Youssef, A. H. (Ed.): Gynaecologic Urology. Springfield, Ill., Charles C. Thomas, 1960, pp. 280–296.

Carlton, E.: Vesicovaginal fistulae. *In* Glenn, J. F. (Ed.): Urologic Surgery. 2nd ed. New York, Harper & Row, 1975.

Chassar Moir, J.: Vesicovaginal fistula. Paris, Ballière, Tindall, and Cannell, 1967.

Everett, H. S., and Williams, T. J.: Vesical fistulae. *In* Campbell, M. F., and Harrison, J. H. (Eds.): Urology. 3rd ed. Philadelphia, W. B. Saunders Co., 1970.

Hamlin, R. H. J., and Nicholson, E. C.: Reconstruction of the urethra totally destroyed in labour. Br. Med. J., 2:147, 1969.

Ingleman-Sundberg, A.: The pathogenesis and treatment of urinary fistulae in irradiated tissue. *In* Youssef, A. H. (Ed.): Gynaecologic Urology. Springfield, Ill., Charles C Thomas, 1960, pp. 263–279.

Kiricuta, I., and Goldstein, A. M. B.: Epiplooplastia vezicala metoda da tratament curativ al fistulelor vezico vaginale. Obstet. Gynaecol. Bucuresti, *1*:163, 1956.

Kiricuta, I., and Goldstein, A. M. B.: The repair of extensive vesicovaginal fistulas with pedicle omentum. J. Urol., *108*:724, 1972.

Lawson, J. B., and Stewart, D. B.: Obstetrics and Gynaecology in the Tropics and Developing Countries. London, Edward Arnold, 1967.

Martius, H.: The repair of vesicovaginal fistulae with interposition pedicle graft of labial tissue. Zentralbl. Gynaecol., *52*:480, 1928.

O'Connor, V. J.: Vesicovaginal fistulas. *In* Smith, R. B., and Skinner, D. G. (Eds.): Complications of Urologic Surgery: Prevention and Management. Philadelphia, W. B. Saunders Co., 1976.

Russell, C. S.: Vesicovaginal fistulae and related matters. Springfield, Ill., Charles C Thomas, 1962.

Spence, H. M., and Duckett, J. W.: Diverticulum of the female urethra—Clinical aspects and presentation of simple operative technique for cure. J. Urol., *104*:432, 1970.

Turner-Warwick, R. T.: A urodynamic view of isolated sphincter mechanisms. First Int. Symp. Urodynamics. Aachen. Berlin, Springer Verlag, 1970b.

Turner-Warwick, R. T.: The use of pedicle grafts in the repair of urinary tract fistulae. Br. J. Urol., *44*:644, 1972.

Turner-Warwick, R. T.: Some clinical aspects of detrusor dysfunction. J. Urol., *66*:61, 1974.

Turner-Warwick, R. T.: The use of the omentum in urinary tract reconstruction. J. Urol., *116*:341, 1976.

Turner-Warwick, R. T.: Vesicovaginal fistula. *In* Williams, D. I.: Urology. Reading, Mass., Butterworths, 1977.

Turner-Warwick, R. T., and Handley Ashken, M.: The functional results of caecocystoplasty. Br. J. Urol., *39*:3, 1967.

Turner-Warwick, R. T., and Whiteside, C. G.: Clinical urodynamics. Urol. Clin. North Am., *6*:1, 1979.

Turner-Warwick, R. T., and Worth, P. H. L.: Psoas bladder hitch procedure for the repair of the lower third of the ureter. Br. J. Urol., *41*:701, 1969.

Turner-Warwick, R. T., Wynne, E. J. C., and Handley Ashken, M.: The use of the omental pedicle graft in the repair and reconstruction of the urinary tract. Br. J. Surg., *54*:849, 1967.

Turner-Warwick, R. T., Worth, P. H. L., Milroy, E. G. J., and Duckett, J.: Suprapubic V incision. Br. J. Urol., *36*:39, 1974.

Zimmerman, I. J., Precourt, W. E., and Thompson, C. C.: Direct uretero-cysto-neostomy with a short ureter in the cure of the uretero-vaginal fistula. J. Urol., *83*:113, 1960.

CHAPTER 75

Suprapubic and Retropubic Prostatectomy

JOHN E. NANNINGA, M.D.
VINCENT J. O'CONOR, JR., M.D.

SUPRAPUBIC PROSTATECTOMY

Suprapubic prostatectomy designates the procedure by which the enlarged and obstructing prostate gland is removed through the cavity of the bladder after extraperitoneal incision of its superior wall. This procedure may be termed transvesical prostatectomy to distinguish it from the transcapsular operation, which is usually spoken of as retropubic prostatectomy.

History

The first suprapubic *cystotomy* was performed over 400 years ago by Pierre Franco of Lausanne, who in 1561 deliberately opened the urinary bladder through an incision above the pubes for the removal of a vesical calculus. In 1827, Amussat of France performed the first partial suprapubic prostatectomy, removing a tumor the size of a large hazelnut that protruded from the neck of the bladder in a patient upon whom he was operating for a bladder calculus. The patient survived, but considering that anesthesia was not in vogue until some 30 years later, it is not surprising that this operation did not gain widespread approval. In the latter part of the 19th century more aggressive surgeons performed cystotomy for stones, and it was only natural that a bold surgeon would attempt complete removal of obstructing prostatic tissue. This indeed was done by von Dittel in 1885. The patient was a physician with bladder neck obstruction; he died of diffuse infection and urinary extravasation 6 days following the operation. In 1886, William T. Belfield of Chicago (without knowledge of von Dittel's experience) performed what must have been at least the second deliberately planned suprapubic prostatic enucleation. Eight months after Belfield's initial report, McGill of Leeds reported a series of three patients subjected to suprapubic prostatectomy. McGill was apparently unaware of Belfield's earlier report; however, his contribution stimulated enthusiasm for this operation in the surgical world of Europe. From notes of personal conversations with Dr. Belfield, it is apparent that he believed that, on an historical basis, priority for this operation should be accorded to von Dittel, himself, and McGill, in that order. In 1890, Belfield presented a series of 80 patients subjected to this operation and analyzed the reasons for the rather high mortality and frequent poor result. Subsequent observations suggest that much of this early difficulty resulted from incomplete removal of the obstructing tissue. The necessity for complete enucleation was later stressed by Eugene Fuller of New York in 1895, when he reported six successive and successful cases wherein the obstructing tissue had been completely enucleated.

Fascinating controversy developed in the early 1900's following the report of Sir Peter Freyer of London, who performed this operation in 1900, and who was credited throughout Europe and Great Britain with having originated suprapubic prostatectomy. Fuller pointed out that Freyer's description of the procedure followed Freyer's having heard a paper by Guiteras of New York, which was read at a meeting of the International Congress in Paris in 1900.

This priority is rather well established and well documented in Fuller's subsequent publication of 1905. Although it appears that Freyer was surely undeserving of priority as the originator of suprapubic enucleation of the prostate, he must be given credit for popularizing the operation previously described by Fuller, and for enlarging our knowledge of the pathologic aspects of prostatic enlargement.

Subsequent improvements in the technique have centered on the method of drainage and means of hemostasis. Fuller utilized perineal drainage, whereas Freyer and most subsequent surgeons have utilized both urethral and suprapubic tubes, obviating a second incision. Hemostasis in the early years was often effected by either packing the prostatic fossa with gauze or flushing the fossa with extremely hot solutions. Rubber bag compression of the prostatic fossa with or without traction on the bag was popularized by Hagner and Pilcher. More recently, direct methods of achieving hemostasis by ligature have refined this operation. A more detailed historical summary of suprapubic prostatectomy may be found in *Perspectives in Urology,* published under the sponsorship of the American Urological Association.

Indications

Each surgeon interested in prostatic surgery will have his own indications for the type of procedure he feels will best apply to the individual patient with significant prostatic obstruction. Every properly qualified urologic surgeon should have the skill and experience to permit him to utilize any of the four standard approaches for relief of this condition.

In the experience from the Northwestern Memorial Hospital during the past 25 years, the great majority of patients with benign prostatic hyperplasia have been relieved of their urinary obstruction and residual urine by either transurethral resection or suprapubic enucleation. Consecutive reviews by Bulkley and Kearns (1952), by O'Conor and colleagues (1963), and by O'Conor and Nanninga (1972) indicate that transurethral resection was utilized in approximately 80 per cent of cases. Currently, only about 10 per cent of such patients have open prostatectomy, whereas 90 per cent undergo transurethral resection. The perineal approach is used infrequently; this is advised primarily for the exposure of a prostatic abscess, or occasionally in an obese poor-risk patient with a large intraurethral gland.

In general, when the obstructing tissue is estimated to weigh more than 60 gm, the patient is subjected to open (suprapubic or retropubic) prostatectomy. Smaller glands are subjected to transurethral resection. When a patient is returning to a foreign country, or to a location where adequate urologic care is not available, we favor open prostatectomy over transurethral resection. The reason for this attitude on our part is that severe late hemorrhage from the prostatic bed rarely occurs after enucleation but is not uncommon months or even years after transurethral resection (Ignatoff and O'Conor, 1977).

Patients with sizable diverticula of the bladder and significant bladder neck obstruction should undergo excision of the diverticulum as well as removal of the obstructing prostatic tissue. All too frequently in past years these patients have been submitted to transurethral resection without removal of the diverticulum. In this situation the diverticulum frequently empties incompletely, and persistent infection results. On several occasions a fragment of prostatic tissue from transurethral resection has lodged in a diverticulum, producing persistent urinary infection. Occasionally the orifice of the diverticulum can be enlarged by transurethral resection when an associated small gland is being resected, and the diverticulum will empty completely postoperatively. These patients seem to be the exception rather than the rule.

Vesical calculi not easily fragmented transurethrally must be removed through the open bladder and often serve as a primary indication for the open operation. Bladder calculi have been associated with prostatic enlargement in 13 per cent of those patients subjected to suprapubic prostatectomy. Additional indications for an open operation are severe strictures of the posterior urethra that cannot be bypassed by perineal urethrotomy; marked limitation of bladder capacity, which precludes satisfactory transurethral resection; and ankylosis of the hips, preventing proper positioning for transurethral resection. Patients who have marked intravesical enlargement, as evident in Figure 75–1, are technically difficult to subject to either retropubic or perineal procedures. The selection of which procedure to perform is arrived at only after complete evaluation, including excretory urography and cystoscopic examination. Cystoscopic examination aids greatly in determining the size of the prostate as well as identifying other possible lesions of the bladder. Prostatic ultrasound is also of value in determining the size of the prostate. We have found this of

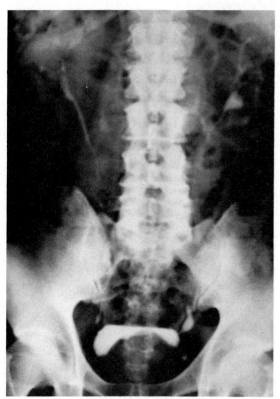

Figure 75–1. The excretory urogram demonstrates a large intravesical projection of an enlarged prostate. The gland was found to weigh 120 gm following suprapubic prostatectomy.

particular value in the prostate estimated to weigh 40 to 60 gm.

Preoperative Evaluation

Over the past 10 years, the average age of patients undergoing suprapubic prostatectomy on our service has been about 70 years. About a third of these patients have heart disease as evidenced by ECG abnormalities, history of heart failure, angina, or demonstrated coronary artery narrowing. Of these patients, 12 per cent have a history of a myocardial infarct. In patients who have experienced a recent myocardial infarct, elective prostatectomy is usually delayed for 3 to 6 months (von Knorring, 1981).

Marked pulmonary obstructive disease was present in 5 per cent of patients. Such patients should be seen preoperatively by the pulmonary and anesthesia services in order to provide optimal care pre- and postoperatively.

Other medical diseases present preoperatively included diabetes, which was present in 12 per cent of patients. Cerebrovascular disease

including stroke was present in 5 per cent of patients.

The preoperative evaluation of potential bleeding problems includes a history of bleeding during dental procedures, previous surgery, or relatively minor injury. Anticoagulation medication will have to be stopped prior to prostatectomy. It has been our recent policy to obtain a prothrombin time, partial thromboplastin time, and bleeding time prior to surgery. A platelet estimate is done routinely with the preoperative blood count. The yield from these studies may be small, but they do occasionally detect an abnormality in clotting that could be troublesome during a surgical procedure. We have been surprised on more than one occasion by patients taking aspirin who fail to reveal this prior to elective surgery.

Urinary retention now occurs in about 40 per cent of patients undergoing open prostatectomy on our service. A persistent azotemia is present in only 3 per cent of these patients. A serum sodium is monitored in these patients for several days when the urinary retention is relieved so that a diuresis and possible hyponatremia can be identified. Also, age in itself will impair renal sodium conservation (Epstein and Hollenberg, 1976).

Bladder calculi associated with benign prostatic enlargement were present in 13 per cent of patients. These are usually removed at the time of prostatectomy.

Urinary tract infection was present in 10 per cent of patients either prior to surgery or at the time of admission for prostatectomy.

Bladder function was evaluated by cystometrogram in patients with residual urine above 150 ml and in those patients where the frequency of urination seemed out of proportion to the residual or where the flow was near normal. Diabetic patients usually have a cystometrogram performed. If patients have spasticity of the lower extremities, a sphincter electromyogram is performed to evaluate the degree to which the striated sphincter contributes to obstruction.

Finally, it should be mentioned that patients with cardiac valvular abnormalities and patients with implanted prosthetic devices are treated with prophylactic antibiotics, usually ampicillin and an aminoglycoside.

Anesthesia

Spinal anesthesia is the procedure of choice. If a patient is particularly anxious or requests general anesthesia, the spinal is gen-

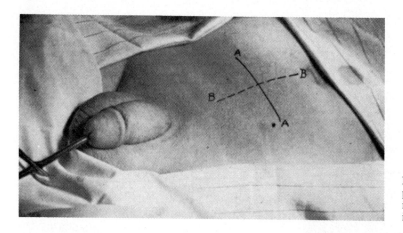

Figure 75–2. Incisions for suprapubic prostatectomy. A-A, transverse (horizontal) skin incision; B-B, vertical incision.

erally supplemented by intravenous pentobarbital. Only in rare instances, usually when a spinal puncture is unsuccessful owing to technical difficulties, is general inhalation anesthesia utilized. We have had no reason to regret the almost routine use of spinal anesthesia, which affords complete and comfortable relaxation of the patient.

Operative Procedure

The procedure to be described is a modification of low suprapubic prostatectomy, as originally suggested by Dr. B. Marvin Harvard (Harvard and White, 1960). The basic principle involves a low transverse incision in the bladder, through which the bladder neck and the prostatic fossa are exposed, facilitating hemostasis under direct vision.

The patient is placed in a recumbent position, with shoulder braces in place to allow any degree of Trendelenburg position that may be necessary. The heels and legs are positioned so that no interruption of venous return results. Pulmonary embolism accounted for 30 per cent of deaths in the original reported series of suprapubic prostatectomies from our institution, and careful attention to proper positioning of the patient during surgery seems to have been an important preventive measure in the last 30 years' experience.

The entire abdomen, scrotum, penis, perineum, and upper thighs are thoroughly cleansed with antiseptic detergent and painted with a skin antiseptic of choice. If a catheter is not in place, a 16 to 18 F Foley catheter is introduced, 200 to 300 ml of sterile saline instilled into the bladder, and the catheter clamped. Removal of this catheter later in the operation is easily performed by an assistant, who will reach under the drapes without contaminating the operative field. Distention of the bladder facilitates extraperitoneal mobilization of the anterior wall and dome and is employed in all suprapubic cystotomies on our service.

Drapes are applied as shown in Figure 75–2, with a half-folded towel often placed across the symphysis as well. Incision of the skin is generally made transversely at a point approximately 4 cm above the symphysis pubis. A vertical incision may be used when an additional procedure such as excision of a diverticulum is planned. After incision of the skin and subcutaneous tissue, we have found the small Gilpi vaginal retractors to be of great value in effecting adequate exposure. The rectus sheath is then incised transversely, and as shown in Figure 75–3, the underlying rectus muscle bellies are separated from the sheath by blunt and sharp dissection. The tendinous portions of the rectus muscles are exposed, but we have not found it necessary to *incise* these to gain adequate exposure. The rectus muscle bellies are retracted laterally and held in position by either a Balfour or self-retaining Farr retractor. The prevesical space is then developed to effect exposure of the bladder neck and anterior prostatic capsule. The bladder wall is then grasped with Allis clamps; the clamp on the catheter is released, allowing the sterile solution to run out of the bladder; and, by elevation of the Allis clamps, the bladder is opened transversely about 2 cm above the bladder neck. At this point the bladder contents are aspirated, the Foley catheter is removed from beneath the drapes by an assistant, and two stay sutures of 0 chromic catgut are placed at the margins and held with clamps. These stay sutures enable the easy reintroduction of the operating finger later in the procedure (Fig. 75–4).

After the bladder incision has been ex-

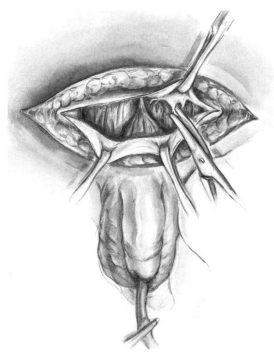

Figure 75–3. Suprapubic prostatectomy. Transverse incision in anterior rectus sheath separating underlying rectus muscle bellies.

tended laterally, bleeding points are either spot coagulated or transfixed with suture ligatures, and the interior of the bladder is inspected. This is aided by either a self-retaining Judd retractor or, if assistance is available, several Deaver retractors of variable sizes used to expose the bladder neck. Three loose sponges placed on

the floor of the bladder beneath a broad Deaver retractor often give the best exposure. Under direct vision the mucosa overlying the enlarged prostate is circumcised with a long-handled knife, or preferably with the cutting electrode, using partial coagulation (Fig. 75–5). This maneuver allows a clean break of the mucosa, and some of the troublesome bleeding from the bladder neck area is eliminated. If the circumference of this incision is too small, difficulty may be encountered later during removal of the adenomatous tissue; the incision must therefore be adequate to remove the tissue and yet must stay well away from the ureteral orifices.

Retractors are removed from the bladder, and enucleation of the gland is carried out with the index finger (Fig. 75–6). If necessary, two fingers are inserted in the rectum and the prostate is elevated to aid definition of the proper cleavage plane. The urethral mucosa is broken at the apex of the prostate in the midline, and the finger is pushed forcibly through against the symphysis and then swept either right or left around the lateral lobes to the opposite side. If possible, the mucosal attachment at the apex should be broken through early in the enucleation, for later traction on the gland may injure or tear the external sphincter. However, when the mucosa is not easily broken through at the apex, then the enucleation should start at the bladder neck, where the mucosa overlying the adenoma was incised. If the gland as a whole does not shell out easily, it is often advisable to enucleate each enlarged lobe separately, particularly when the aggregate weight of the enlarged

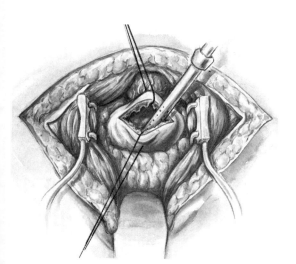

Figure 75–4. Suprapubic prostatectomy. Aspiration of bladder contents. Stay sutures in place.

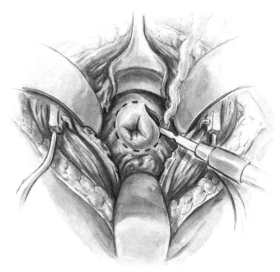

Figure 75–5. Suprapubic prostatectomy. Circumcision of mucosa over adenoma with electrocautery.

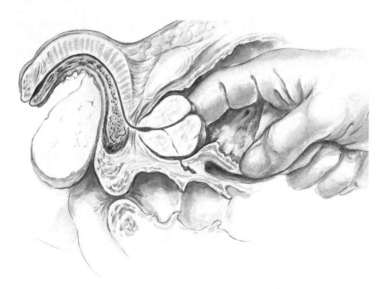

Figure 75–6. Suprapubic prostatectomy. Digital enucleation of adenoma.

lobes is over 200 gm. If the gland is excessively adherent, it may be grasped with lobe forceps and freed by scissors dissection under direct vision.

Immediately after removal of the gland it is our custom to pack the prostatic fossa tightly with 3-inch gauze of the head-roll type, and maintain steady pressure for approximately 5 minutes (Figs. 75–7 and 75–8). If rectal direction has been used, the surgeon then changes gown and gloves. The retractors are then reintroduced, and as the 3-inch gauze is slowly removed anteriorly, the posterior lip of the bladder neck

is visualized and grasped with Kocher clamps in the regions of 4 o'clock and 8 o'clock. Deep mattress sutures of 0 chromic catgut are placed in these regions, leaving the remaining prostatic fossa packed (Figs. 75–9 and 75–10). These sutures are used to exert moderate traction for progressively deeper inspection of the prostatic cavity. Several maneuvers are valuable at this stage. The anterior edges of the prostatic fossa may also be grasped with traction sutures or Kocher clamps and elevated, revealing the occasional bleeders at 11 o'clock or 1 o'clock. Stick sponges may be inserted into the fossa and

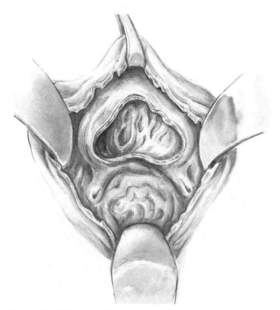

Figure 75–7. Suprapubic prostatectomy. Prostatic fossa after enucleation; 12 o'clock position is at the top of the drawing.

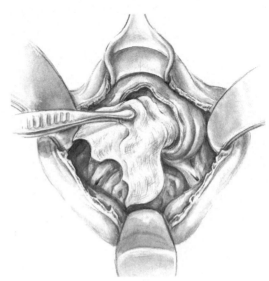

Figure 75–8. Suprapubic prostatectomy. Packing fossa with 3-inch roller gauze.

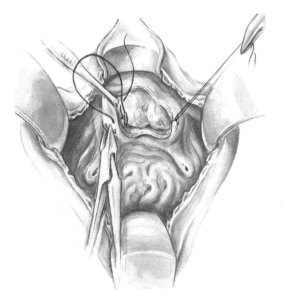

Figure 75–9. Suprapubic prostatectomy. Sutures placed at 4 o'clock and 8 o'clock to control major arterial bleeders.

pulled laterally, inspecting first one side and then the other, utilizing either spot coagulation for small vessels or suture ligatures for the larger arteries. A boomerang needle may be used, although our preference is for an atraumatic catgut suture on a ⅝ curved needle, which is readily available. As the bladder neck area is elevated circumferentially, the deep packing is removed and the deeper recesses of the prostatic

fossa are examined for bleeders. It is a mistake to believe that there are no significant arteries near the apex of the fossa, and complete inspection of the entire fossa *must* be effected *under direct vision* (Fig. 75–11). When the major arterial bleeding is under control, one or more loose sponges are placed in the deep recesses of the prostatic fossa, and attention is turned to the bladder neck area. Ragged or redundant mucosa is trimmed away, and if significant bladder neck contracture is present, a deep V incision is made in the midline. When this is done we frequently approximate the mucosa of the bladder neck to the posterior prostatic urethra or capsule with one or more sutures of plain catgut and occasionally run a continuous suture from 4 o'clock to 8 o'clock, bringing the mucosa down into the posterior capsule. These maneuvers are variations of what Harris (1929) described as the "retrigonalization" suture. In our experience, with these maneuvers, it is rarely necessary to incise the bladder neck and anterior prostatic capsule longitudinally to obtain hemostasis. Occasionally, there is persistent oozing from an area on the prostatic capsule. If so, one or more plicating sutures can be placed transversely in the region from which the bleeding appears to be coming (Fig. 75–12) (O'Conor, 1982).

When bleeding is under control, a 24 F Foley catheter is inserted per urethram, and the 30-ml bag is inflated so that the balloon will lie

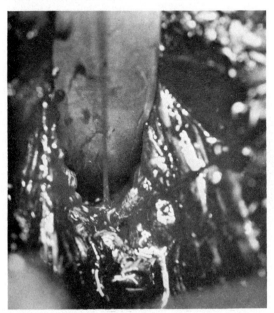

Figure 75–10. Here a retractor is being used to hold the packing so that a suture ligature can be placed in the posterior bladder neck as shown.

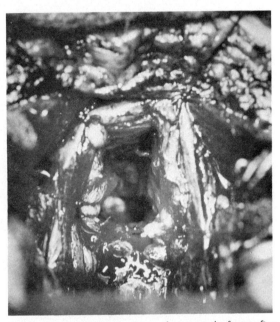

Figure 75–11. This view shows the prostatic fossa after removal of a 76 gm adenoma. Under direct vision the walls can be inspected for bleeding points or residual tissue.

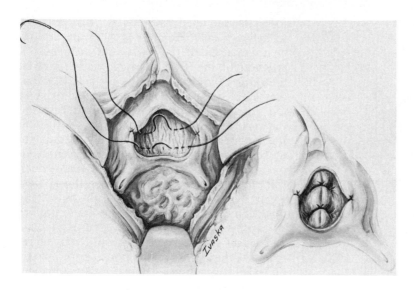

Figure 75–12. Transverse sutures have been placed in the posterior capsule to stop venous bleeding.

in the bladder and with gentle traction compress the bladder neck but not enter it (Fig. 75–13). A 30-ml bag will easily hold up to 100 ml, and this inflation prevents the bag from slipping into the prostatic fossa. The bag *should not* be drawn into the prostatic fossa because this prevents the normal contraction of these tissues, which aids hemostasis, and, moreover, the presence of the bag in the prostatic fossa produces severe postoperative discomfort and may contribute to postoperative incontinence. If venous oozing remains troublesome, we place a small piece of Surgicel deep in the fossa, pulling the Foley bag down snugly on the bladder neck. The other hemostatic substances, such as Oxycel and Gel-foam, have the disadvantage of being relatively nonabsorbable, and often it is necessary to remove unabsorbed pieces of these materials by cystoscopic manipulation. Delayed calculus formation on a piece of Oxycel or Gelfoam has occasionally been noted, and if these agents are used, one method of ensuring dissolution of the substances is the irrigation of the bladder with an alkaline solution such as sodium bicarbonate prior to the removal of the last catheter.

At this point a decision must be made about the use of primary closure of the bladder with urethral drainage only or the addition of suprapubic drainage. If the bladder is closed primarily, conditions must be such that close observa-

Figure 75–13. Suprapubic prostatectomy. Foley catheter snug against bladder neck. Prevesical drain and Pezzar suprapubic catheter.

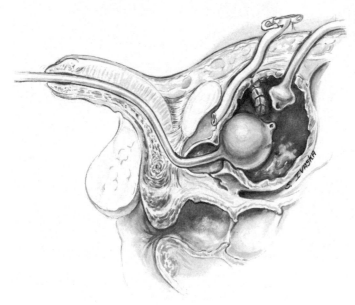

tion of the patient and irrigation by a skilled assistant are available whenever necessary. As Brown (1933) so aptly stated the problem with primary closure of the bladder, "Under favorable conditions the results have been highly satisfactory, but at other times have been such that my desire to continue with surgery, and urology in particular, has almost ceased." The problems arising from clot retention and reactivation of bleeding in the early postoperative period have led us more or less routinely to use a suprapubic catheter, regardless of how dry the operative site appears. A No. 32 right angle Pezzer catheter is brought through a stab wound at the dome of the bladder and the bladder is closed in two layers with 0 or 2–0 chromic catgut. The first layer is generally a continuous suture reinforced by a second layer of interrupted sutures. Irrigation of the bladder is carried out at this time, and if a small leak is present, this is reinforced with additional sutures. A split-rubber drain is led out through the incision from the prevesical space, and when the transverse incision is used, the suprapubic tube is brought up through a stab wound superior to the incision (Fig. 75–13). The high exit of the cystotomy tube prevents the peritoneum from obliterating the prevesical space and allows rapid closure of this sinus when the tube is subsequently removed. The rectus muscle bellies are approximated in the midline, the anterior rectus sheath is closed with interrupted chromic sutures, and the subcutaneous tissue and skin are closed in the usual manner. The

suprapubic tube is generally fixed to the skin with a heavy silk stitch and a dressing applied with either Montgomery or Senn straps to facilitate frequent changing during the first few postoperative days when drainage may be considerable.

Invariably, newer modifications of prostatectomy have been proposed. Malament (1965) has described a pursestring suture around the bladder neck for hemostatic control. The suture is tied tightly over the catheter and the ends of the suture are brought out through the abdominal incision (Fig. 75–14). Nicoll et al. (1978), using an absorbable pursestring suture, have reported a transfusion rate of only 8 per cent in a series of 300 patients.

Combined methods of prostatectomy using a vesicocapsular incision have been described by Bourque (1954) and Leadbetter et al. (1959). The latter included a Y–V plasty enlargement of the bladder neck after enucleation of the adenoma. We have not found that the vesicocapsular incision offers any greater advantage in hemostasis over that afforded by either the low suprapubic or standard retropubic approach.

Postoperative Care

General aspects of postoperative care are covered in detail in other texts (Beal, 1982). Blood is given only when the blood loss has been sufficient to justify its administration, and

Figure 75–14. A pursestring suture has been placed around the bladder neck. This is then brought out below the incision and tied down over a button, gauze, or other material. After 24 to 48 hours, the suture is loosened and shortly after that is pulled out.

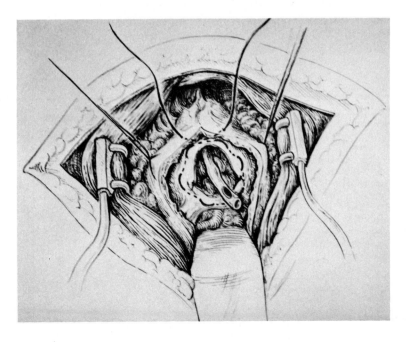

in the past 10 years less than 15 per cent of patients undergoing suprapubic prostatectomy have received whole blood or packed red blood cells. In general, those patients who required blood transfusions had larger adenomas than those not requiring blood (86 gm vs. 67 gm, p <0.05). Intravenous fluid administration is determined by individual requirements; however, the average patient receives approximately 1000 ml per 8-hour period during the first 24 hours following operation. After the first 12 hours postoperatively and when the effects of the anesthesia have worn off and there is no nausea or abdominal distention, oral fluids may be started. The diet is then advanced as tolerated over the next 24 to 48 hours. Deep breathing, coughing, and leg exercises are encouraged from the recovery room onward—measures that undeniably reduce the risk of pneumonia, phlebothrombosis, and subsequent pulmonary embolism. The patient is generally allowed to sit up in bed the night of the operation and progresses rapidly to walking in the first few postoperative days. Antibiotics are given for a specific infection usually just prior to catheter removal. However, as mentioned earlier, patients with prosthetic devices or cardiac valvular disease are given antibiotics prior to the procedure and postoperatively.

The postoperative management of the urethral and suprapubic catheters varies widely among urologic surgeons and, indeed, has varied considerably in our own experience. *In the past,* our practice was to remove the suprapubic catheter on the second or third postoperative day, and when the wound was sufficiently dry the urethral catheter was removed, usually on the fifth to seventh postoperative day. In the past 15 years we have removed the urethral catheter first, usually on the second or third postoperative day. If bladder spasm is significant on the first postoperative day, the amount of fluid exceeding 30 ml in the Foley bag is removed, with attendant relief in many cases. Removal of the urethral catheter seems to significantly reduce discomfort and bladder spasm and certainly decreases the incidence of persistent urethritis and development of subsequent urethral stricture. The suprapubic catheter is removed on about the fifth postoperative day, and as a rule patients void spontaneously at this time, with minimal leakage from the suprapubic site. If suprapubic leakage persists for 24 hours, a small urethral catheter is inserted for an additional 48 hours, after which most patients void freely without leakage. Over the past 10 years, about 12 to 14 per cent of patients have required the urethral catheter because of this suprapubic leakage.

Complications

The difference in complications, as analyzed over the past 40 years, shows marked improvement since utilization of the low suprapubic approach (Table 75–1).

The surgical mortality rate for open prostatectomy has decreased to less than 1 per cent in recent years (Nicoll et al., 1978). On our service, fatalities from myocardial infarction, pneumonia, and pulmonary embolism have accounted for about three fourths of postoperative deaths. For patients with known heart or lung disease, placement in a surgical intensive care unit will aid in identifying early postoperative complications and speed therapy (Beal, 1982). Cardiac monitoring will detect arrhythmias and

TABLE 75–1. SUPRAPUBIC PROSTATECTOMY MORBIDITY AND MORTALITY

	1942–1950	1953–1961	1961–1965	1965–1970	1971–1982
Hemorrhage*	5 (2)	1	—	1	—
Postoperative bleeding†	not recorded	1	5	5	5
Pyelonephritis	4 (2)	1	—	—	—
Myocardial infarct	2 (1)	1 (1)	1 (1)	—	1
Congestive heart failure	3 (3)	—	—	2	1
Pneumonia	4	1 (1)	1 (1)	4 (1)	—
Pulmonary embolus	5 (4)	—	—	1 (1)	2
Gastrointestinal hemorrhage	—	—	1 (1)	—	—
Incontinence (partial)	2	—	—	3	3
Wound infection	not recorded	1	1	4	6
Staphylococcal enterocolitis	—	1 (1)	—	—	—
Epididymitis	3	7	5	4	4
mortality	8.5%	2.1%	2.1%	1.4%	0%

( ) = expired.
*4 units of blood.
†Required catheterization or cystoscopy.

ischemic changes. Patients with impaired lung function are able to have diagnostic studies performed quickly, which will guide respiratory therapy. Deep vein thrombosis has been reported as occurring in 47.6 per cent of patients after open prostatectomy (Nicolaides et al., 1972). However, the clinical incidence seems much less. We have not used prophylactic anticoagulation with heparin. However, some patients with a history of thrombophlebitis have been started on Coumadin within the first week after prostatectomy. Measures that seem to reduce the incidence of deep vein thrombosis in the lower extremities include early ambulation, elastic stockings, and leg movement in bed.

Wound infection has occurred in 6 patients (4 per cent) over the past 10 years. This is a slight increase and may be due to more diligent reporting of suspicious incisions by the surgeon, house staff, or infectious disease clinicians. Of interest is the fact that none of the patients who had a urinary infection before surgery had a wound infection.

Incontinence of urine is less common following suprapubic enucleation than after perineal or even transurethral resection. In the last 700 patients there was no instance of permanent incontinence following this operation. An occasional patient complains of some stress incontinence in the first week or two following removal of the catheter, and most patients experience some urgency, as is expected following any prostatic operation.

Impotence has been studied and found to be relatively uncommon following this operation or transurethral resection. Retrograde ejaculation is a frequent occurrence and is easily understood if explained beforehand to the patient.

Urethral stricture is rarely encountered following suprapubic prostatectomy. This is in significant contrast to a greater number of patients who have had transurethral resection, in which this is a significant postoperative annoyance. All patients have the urethra calibrated at some time during the first few postoperative months, and it is rare to find a significant stricture.

RETROPUBIC PROSTATECTOMY

The first report of retropubic prostatectomy was from van Stockum, who performed this procedure in 1908 and reported two cases in 1909. Sporadic reports appeared after this, but the operation did not gain general popularity.

In 1933, Jacobs and Casper from San Francisco reported the first two operations done in this country. Unaware of van Stockum's work, they referred to the operation as "the Casper technique." The largest series in these early years was reported by Hybbinette from Sweden (1935); he described excellent results in 15 patients. Credit for reintroducing and popularizing retropubic prostatectomy among urologic surgeons must go to Terence Millin, who reported on 20 such procedures in 1945. Coming to this country and demonstrating his technique, this genial Irishman effectively convinced urologic surgeons of the virtues of this approach. The operation is not difficult to perform, the exposure allows good visualization of the bladder neck, and direct hemostasis can be effected more easily than by the *blind* suprapubic technique in use at that time. Early concern regarding the complication of osteitis pubis was unfounded, since the incidence of this over the years has been low. The major advantage afforded by improved hemostasis is the ability to eliminate a suprapubic catheter, allowing speedy recuperation and earlier discharge from the hospital.

Indications

In our practice over 80 per cent of the patients requiring prostatic surgery undergo transurethral resection; the estimated weight of the gland is the deciding factor, and glands over 60 gm are enucleated by either the suprapubic or retropubic approach. These procedures are done with about equal frequency in our hospital, depending primarily on the surgeon's preference and the patient's individual physical characteristics.

Operative Technique

Following the usual low spinal anesthetic, the skin is widely prepared and the patient placed in a modified Trendelenburg position. Although we frequently flex the table gently, the extreme Walcher position is not used. Extreme positioning as used in some clinics results in long-standing back discomfort and is generally unnecessary. In contrast to the preparation for the suprapubic operation, the bladder is not distended and, indeed, some surgeons prefer emptying the bladder prior to surgery.

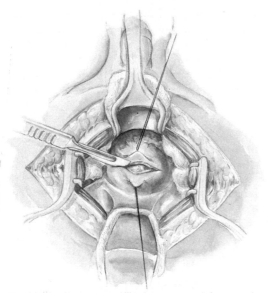

Figure 75–15. Retropubic prostatectomy. Transverse incision of capsule after placement of stay sutures.

A transverse incision similar to that used in the suprapubic procedure (Fig. 75–3) exposes the rectus sheath, which is opened transversely. After freeing of the rectus muscles in the midline, the preperitoneal fat is swept upward. At this point two moist sponges are placed over the rectus muscle bellies and a standard Balfour retractor is placed. A wet laparotomy pad is placed on the bladder, which is then depressed with a broad Deaver retractor. A single self-retaining Millin or Beneventi retractor will accomplish the same effect, which depresses the bladder and seemingly elevates the prostate into view. The loose areolar and fatty tissue is then gently dissected away with a Küttner dissector, and any large veins are coagulated and transected. The basic maneuver consists of pushing the tissue from the midline laterally until the prostatic capsule is well defined. A single loose moist sponge is placed in each lateral fossa to aid both exposure and hemostasis. Two traction or stay sutures are then placed, the distal one about 2 cm beyond the bladder neck. Atraumatic 0 chromic catgut suture on a ⅝ curved needle is used to take a deep bite through the capsule. The proximal suture is placed just at the junction of the bladder and prostate. These sutures are tied doubly and tagged with different length hemostats to afford easy later recognition.

The proposed capsular incision is lightly traced with the electrocautery blade to aid coagulation of small vessels, and the incision is made sharply with a scalpel. The incision should be as short as possible, avoiding potential wide lateral extension, which makes closure more difficult (Fig. 75–15).

Bleeding is brisk at this point; however, only major arteries are tied off. Blood loss is less if one proceeds quickly with enucleation. The plane between adenoma and capsule is now readily apparent, and the Richter or Metzenbaum scissors are used to extend this cleavage laterally (Fig. 75–16).

Our preference is to free the apex early and transect the apical prostatic urethra by pinching it between thumb and index finger or, if necessary, carefully sectioning the urethra with the scissors, avoiding injury to the external sphincter. The lateral lobes are then enucleated and delivered through the prostatotomy incision. At this point the only attachment is at the bladder neck. (Fig. 75–17). With one hand holding the lateral lobes, the other index finger frees the attachment to the bladder neck and trigone, and if adherent, this is transected with the scissors under direct vision.

The prostatic fossa is then packed with long roller gauze and pressure applied for approximately 5 minutes. Some surgeons take this opportunity to perform bilateral vasectomy. The exposure of the fossa is then effected by means of either small Deaver retractors or empty ring forceps. These are used to visualize the bladder neck area first, where the major arterial sources at 5 o'clock and 7 o'clock are controlled with mattress sutures. A search is made for the occasional arterial bleeder at 11 o'clock or 2

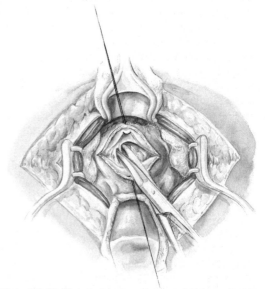

Figure 75–16. Retropubic prostatectomy. Scissor dissection of adenoma from capsule.

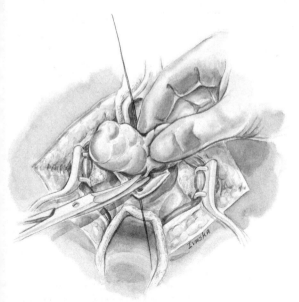

Figure 75–17. Retropubic prostatectomy. Section of adherence to bladder neck.

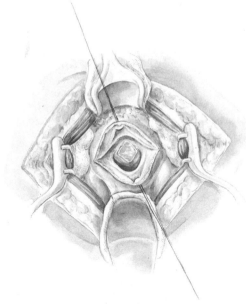

Figure 75–19. Retropubic prostatectomy. Wedge excised.

o'clock, and these are either sutured or coagulated. The remainder of the fossa is visualized, and hemostasis is carried out by electrocoagulation. At this point a sponge is placed in the fossa and attention turned toward the bladder neck area. The trigone and ureteral orifices are identified, and usually a generous wedge is removed from the posterior lip (Fig. 75–18). This excision is made well into the muscle, and the mucosa is then approximated with a running suture of 3–0 plain catgut (Figs. 75–19 and 75–20).

The pack in the fossa is then removed, and

most venous oozing will have ceased. If there is persistent bleeding from the apical area, we do not hesitate to place a small piece of Surgicel deep into this area. A 24 F Foley catheter is inserted, the 30-ml bag inflated, and capsular closure performed with a continuous 0 chromic suture, again utilizing the atraumatic ⅝ curved needle (Fig. 75–21). Irrigation may reveal a small leak, usually at the lateral margins of closure, and single reinforcing sutures are used to make this watertight. Split-rubber drains are led out from the lateral fossas, and abdominal closure is carried out as previously described.

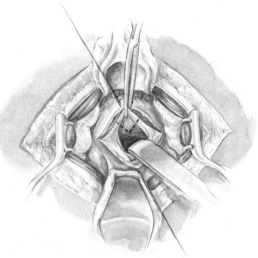

Figure 75–18. Retropubic prostatectomy. Dotted line shows wedge to be excised at bladder neck.

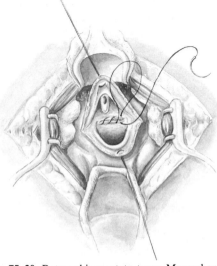

Figure 75–20. Retropubic prostatectomy. Mucosal approximation with 3–0 plain catgut.

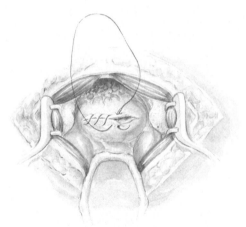

Figure 75–21. Retropubic prostatectomy. Closure of capsule with continuous 0 chromic catgut.

Postoperative Care

The Foley catheter is attached to closed drainage, and irrigation is *not* carried out routinely. If the catheter becomes plugged, or the patient complains of discomfort, gentle irrigation is done by the physician or nurse trained in postoperative urologic surgery care. The Foley catheter is removed when the urine clears, and this is generally in 2 to 5 days. Patients are usually ambulatory, and unless experiencing complications, are discharged by the seventh postoperative day.

Complications

In our experience at Northwestern University Medical Center, the complications of prostatic enucleation are similar for both the suprapubic and retropubic approaches, the exception being in the rare patient who develops osteitis pubis. This problem occurred more commonly in early experience, and the decrease of its appearance in both retropubic prostatectomy and retropubic vesicourethropexy is not explainable. This rare complication generally responds to bed rest and corticosteroids.

SUMMARY

Prostatic enucleation done by either the low suprapubic or retropubic approach is the operation of choice in approximately 10 per cent of patients with significant bladder neck obstruction. The operative mortality with these procedures approaches that of transurethral resection. The overall morbidity of these procedures has been significantly lowered, so that results are more permanent and definitely more satisfactory from a functional point of view.

References

Amussat: Leçons sur les Rétentions d'Urine Saucees par les Rétrécissements du Canal de l'Urètre et sur les Maladies de la Prostate. Paris, Ballière, 1832.

Beal, J. (Ed.): Critical Care for Surgical Patients. New York, MacMillan, 1982.

Belfield, W. T.: Prostatic myoma—a so-called "middle lobe" of the hypertrophied prostate—removed by suprapubic prostatectomy. JAMA, 8:303, 1887.

Belfield, W. T.: Operations on the enlarged prostate, with a tabulated summary of cases. Am. J. Med. Sci., 100:439, 1890.

Bourque, J. P.: Transvesicocapsular prostatic adenectomy (transcommissural): preliminary report on 80 cases. J. Urol., 72:918, 1954.

Brown. R. K. L.: Primary closure in prostatectomy. Aust. N.Z. J. Surg., 2:344, 1933.

Bulkley, G. J., and Kearns, J. W.: Analysis of results of prostatic surgery in 866 cases. J. Urol., 68:724, 1952.

Epstein, M., and Hollenberg, N.: Age as a determinant of renal sodium conservation. J. Lab. Clin. Med., 87:411, 1976.

Franco, P.: Traité des Hernies Contenant, une Example. Déclaration de toutes Leurs Effeces et autres Excellentes Pertics de la Chirurgie, affoir de la Pierre, etc. Ed. I. Lyon, Payan, 1561, p. 140.

Freyer, P. J.: A new method of performing prostatectomy. Lancet, 1:774, 1900.

Fuller, E.: Six successful and successive cases of prostatectomy. J. Cutan. Genitourin. Dis., 13:229, 1895.

Fuller, E.: The question of priority in the adoption of the method of total enucleation, suprapubically, of the hypertrophied prostate. Am. Surg., 41:520, 1905.

Harris, S. H.: Suprapubic prostatectomy with closure. Br. J. Urol., 1:285, 1929.

Harvard, B. M., and White, R. R.: A technic for transvesical prostatectomy. Conn. Med., 24:286, 1960.

Hybbinette, S.: Suprapubische transurethrale Prostatectomie. Arch. Klin. Chir., 183:145, 1935.

Ignatoff, J., and O'Conor, V. J., Jr.: Transurethral resection: A review. Int. Urol. Nephrol., 9:33, 1977.

Jacobs, L. C., and Casper, E. J.: Prevesical prostatectomy. Urol. Cutan. Rev., 37:729, 1933.

Leadbetter, G. W., Jr., Duxberry, J. H., and Leadbetter, W. F.: Can prostatectomy be improved? J. Urol., 82:600, 1959.

Malament, M.: Maximal hemostasis in suprapubic prostatectomy. Surg. Gynecol. Obstet., 120:1307, 1965.

McGill, A. F.: Suprapubic prostatectomy. Br. Med. J., 2:1104, 1887.

Millin, T.: Retropubic prostatectomy: New extravesical technique. Report on 20 cases. Lancet, 2:693, 1945.

Nanninga, J. B., and O'Conor, V. J., Jr.: Suprapubic prostatectomy: A 28 year review, 1942–1970. Int. Urol. Nephrol., 4:377, 1972.

Nicolaides, A., Field, E., Kakkar, V., Yeats-Bell, A., Taylor, S., and Clarke, M.: Prostatectomy and deep-vein thrombosis. Br. J. Surg., 59:487, 1972.

Nicoll, G. A., Riffle, G., and Andersen, F.: Suprapubic prostatectomy. The removable purse: a continuing comparable analysis of 300 consecutive cases. J. Urol., *120*:702, 1978.

O'Conor, V. J.: Observations on the blood pressure in cases of prostatic obstruction. Arch. Surg., *1*:359, 1920.

O'Conor, V. J., Jr.: Suprapubic prostatectomy. *In* Landes, R., Bush, R., and Zorgniotti, A. (Eds.): Perspectives in Urology. Nutley, N.J., American Urological Association and Roche Laboratories, 1976.

O'Conor, V. J., Jr.: An aid for hemostasis in open prostatectomy: capsular plication. J. Urol., *127*:448, 1982.

O'Conor, V. J., Jr., and Nanninga, J. B.: Low suprapubic prostatectomy: A continuing report. J. Urol., *108*:453, 1972.

O'Conor, V. J., Jr., Bulkley, G. J., and Sokol, J. K.: Low suprapubic prostatectomy: Comparison of results with the standard operation in two comparable groups of 142 patients. J. Urol., *90*:301, 1963.

van Stockum, W. J.: Prostatectomia suprapubica extravesicales. Zentralbl. Chir., *36*:41, 1909.

von Dittel: Blasenpunction und nachtragliche Resection des mittleren Lappens wegen hochgradiger Hypertrophie der Prostata. Wien. Med. Bl., *8*:270, 1885.

von Knorring, J.: Postoperative myocardial infarction: A prospective study on a risk group of surgical patients. Surgery, *90*:55, 1981.

CHAPTER 76

Radical Retropubic Prostatectomy

PATRICK C. WALSH, M.D.

Radical prostatectomy is the most effective form of treatment for the patient with localized prostatic cancer (Walsh and Jewett, 1980; Walsh 1980; Paulson et al., 1982). Yet radical prostatectomy has never gained widespread popularity because critics claim that the morbidity associated with the procedure does not justify its therapeutic advantages. In addition, many urologists are not familiar with perineal exposure of the prostate, which for many years was the preferred approach to radical prostatectomy.

Millin (1945) pioneered the retropubic approach to the prostate. Subsequently Millin (1947) and Memmelaar (1949) and Lich et al. (1949) described total prostatovesiculectomy using the retropubic approach. The technique was then adopted by others (Chute, 1954) and modified (Ansell, 1959; Campbell, 1959). These advances offered an approach to radical prostatectomy that has proved over the years to have many advantages. The retropubic anatomy is not only less complicated than the perineal approach but is also more familiar to the surgeon experienced in radical pelvic surgery. The retropubic approach leads to fewer rectal injuries than does the perineal approach, and because the urogenital diaphragm is left intact, urinary incontinence is a rare complication. More recently the anatomy of Santorini's plexus has been clarified (Reiner and Walsh, 1979) and the anatomic relationships between the branches of the pelvic plexus that innervate the corpora cavernosa and the structures surrounding the prostate have been delineated (Walsh and Donker, 1982). These observations have further reduced the morbidity of the procedure by making it possible to lessen blood loss and reduce the incidence of impotence (Walsh et al., 1983).

This chapter describes an anatomic approach to radical retropubic prostatectomy. The retropubic technique reduces the morbidity of the procedure to a minimum without altering its therapeutic efficacy. It is hoped that these advances may lead to widespread acceptance of radical prostatectomy as the most effective form of treatment for the management of localized prostatic cancer. When performed correctly, the side effects of this procedure should be equal to or even less than those associated with radiation therapy (see Chapter 32). A film depicting the surgical technique is available (Walsh, 1984).

SURGICAL ANATOMY

The prostate is confined to a small recess in the pelvis, at which point it is surrounded by the levator ani musculature and pubis, as well as other more vulnerable structures, such as the rectum, the urogenital diaphragm with the external sphincter, Santorini's plexus, and the autonomic branches of the pelvic plexus to the corpora cavernosa. Consequently, if one hopes to minimize the morbidity of radical prostatectomy, it is necessary to understand fully the following anatomic concepts and relationships.

Pelvic Fascia

The prostate is covered with two distinct and separate fascial layers: Denonvilliers' fascia and the lateral pelvic fascia. The urologist is well acquainted with the concept of Denonvilliers' fascia, which is a filmy delicate layer of connective tissue located between the anterior wall of the rectum and the prostate. This fascial layer extends cranially to cover the posterior surface of the seminal vesicles and lies snugly against the posterior prostatic capsule (Fig. 76–1A). The fascia is most prominent and dense near the base of the prostate and seminal vesicles; it thins dramatically as it extends caudally to its termination at the rectourethralis musculature. Microscopically it is impossible to discern a "posterior" and "anterior" layer to this fascia (Jewett et al., 1972). One must therefore excise this fascia completely to obtain an adequate surgical margin. In addition to Denonvilliers' fascia, the prostate is also invested with a second important layer of fascia—the lateral pelvic fascia, which covers the levator ani musculature (Fig. 76–1A). This fascia has also been called the prostatic fascia or the parietal layer of the endopelvic fascia. Anteriorly and anterolaterally this fascia is in direct continuity with the true capsule of the prostate. The major tributaries of the dorsal vein of the penis and Santorini's plexus travel within this fascia (Fig. 76–1A). Posteriorly the lateral pelvic fascia separates from the prostate to travel immediately adjacent to the levator ani musculature surrounding the rectum. The prostate receives its blood supply and autonomic innervation through the leaves of this fascia. In performing radical perineal prostatectomy, the lateral pelvic fascia is reflected off the prostate in an effort to avoid the dorsal vein of the penis and Santorini's plexus (Fig. 76–1B). Avoiding these veins accounts for the reduced blood loss associated with radical perineal prostatectomy. As described by Young and Davis (1927), once the posterior surface of

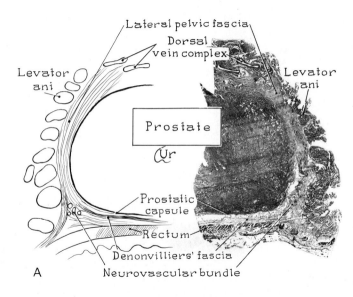

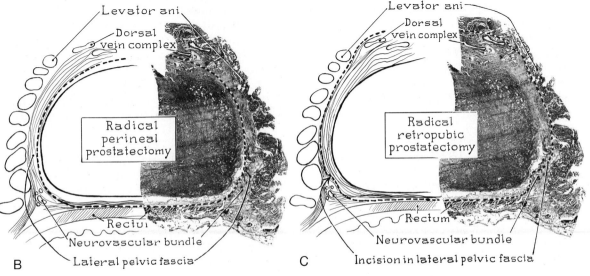

Figure 76–1. *A,* Cross section through an adult prostate demonstrating the anatomic relationships between the lateral pelvic fascia, Denonvilliers' fascia, and the neurovascular bundle. *B,* and *C,* Schematic diagrams of surgical planes (dashed line) employed in radical perineal prostatectomy *(B)* and in radical retropubic prostatectomy *(C)*. Note the site for incision in the lateral fascia, which avoids injury to the neurovascular bundle. (From Walsh, P. C., Lepor, H., and Eggleston, J. C.: Prostate, *4*:473, 1983. Used by permission.)

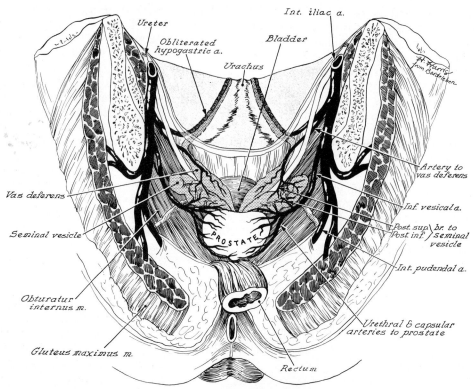

Figure 76–2. Posterior view of the arterial supply to the prostate. The rectum has been removed to expose the posterior surface of the prostate and pelvis. (From Weyrauch, H. M.: Surgery of the Prostate. Philadelphia, W. B. Saunders Co., 1959. Used by Permission.)

the prostate has been exposed, "the next procedure is to search for the point along the lateral surface of the prostate where the fascia coming from the lateral wall of the pelvis divides to encircle the prostate. By making an incision through the posterior layer close to the prostate one can then by blunt dissection easily separate the anterior layer from the prostate on each side until the membranous urethra is reached." In performing radical retropubic prostatectomy, the prostate is approached from outside the lateral fascia (Fig. 76–1C); for this reason the dorsal vein complex must be ligated, and the lateral pelvic fascia must be divided.

Arterial Supply and Venous Drainage

The prostate receives its arterial blood supply from the inferior vesical artery, which has also been termed the "prostatovesicular artery." According to Flocks (1937), after the inferior vesical artery provides small branches to the inferior, posterior extent of the seminal vesicle

and the base of the bladder and prostate, the artery terminates in two large groups of prostatic vessels: the urethral and capsular groups (Fig. 76–2). The urethral vessels enter the prostate at the posterolateral vesicoprostatic junction; these vessels provide arterial supply to the vesical neck and periurethral portion of the gland. The capsular branches run along the pelvic side wall in the lateral pelvic fascia posterolateral to the prostate, providing branches that course ventrally and dorsally to supply the outer portion of the prostate. The capsular vessels terminate as a small cluster of vessels that supply the pelvic floor. Histologically, the capsular group of vessels is surrounded by an extensive network of nerves (Fig. 76–1) (Walsh et al., 1983). The capsular vessels—both arteries and veins —provide the macroscopic landmark that aids in the identification of the microscopic branches of the pelvic plexus innervating the corpora cavernosa.

The prostatic veins drain into the plexus of Santorini. One must be completely familiar with the anatomy of these veins in order to avoid excessive bleeding and to ensure a bloodless field when exposing the membranous urethra and apex of the prostate. The deep dorsal vein leaves the penis under Buck's fascia between the corpora cavernosa and penetrates the urogenital diaphragm, dividing into three major branches: the superficial branch and the right and left lateral venous plexuses (Fig. 76–3) (Reiner and Walsh, 1979). The superficial branch, which travels between the puboprostatic ligaments, is the centrally located vein overlying the bladder neck and the prostate (Fig. 73–3B). This vein, which is easily visualized early in retropubic operations, has communicating branches over the bladder itself and into the endopelvic fascia. The superficial branch lies outside the pelvic fascia; the common trunk and lateral venous plexuses are covered and concealed by this fascia. The lateral venous plexuses traverse posterolaterally (Fig. 72–3B) and communicate freely with the pudendal, obturator, and vesical plexuses. These plexuses interconnect with other venous systems to form the inferior vesical vein, which then empties into the internal iliac vein. With the complex of veins and plexuses anastomosing freely, any laceration of these rather friable structures can lead to considerable blood loss.

Pelvic Plexus

The autonomic innervation of the pelvic organs and external genitalia arises from the pelvic plexus, which is formed by parasympathetic visceral efferent preganglionic fibers—nervi erigentes—that arise from the sacral center (S2 to S4) and sympathetic fibers from the thoracolumbar center (T11 to L2) (Fig. 76–4A) (Walsh and Donker, 1982). In men, the pelvic plexus is located retroperitoneally beside the rectum and forms a fenestrated rectangular plate situated in the sagittal plane. The branches of the inferior vesical artery and vein that supply the bladder and prostate perforate the pelvic plexus. For this reason, ligation of the so-called lateral pedicle in its midportion not only interrupts the vessels but also transects the nerve supply to the prostate, urethra, and corpora cavernosa. The pelvic plexus provides visceral branches that innervate the bladder, ureter, seminal vesicles, prostate, rectum, membranous urethra, and corpora cavernosa. In addition, branches that contain somatic motor axons travel through the pelvic plexus to supply the levator ani, coccygeus, and striated urethral

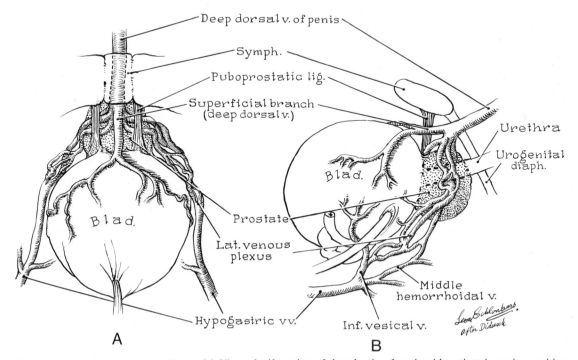

Figure 76–3. Santorini's venous plexus. (a) View of trifurcation of dorsal vein of penis with patient in supine position; relationship of venous branches to puboprostatic ligaments is depicted. (b) Lateral view shows anatomic relationships at trifurcation. In this schematic illustration, the lateral pelvic fascia has been removed. In reality, these structures are never visualized in this skeletonized manner because they are encased by the lateral pelvic fascia. (From Reiner, W. G., and Walsh, P. C.: J. Urol., *121*:198, 1979. Used by permission.)

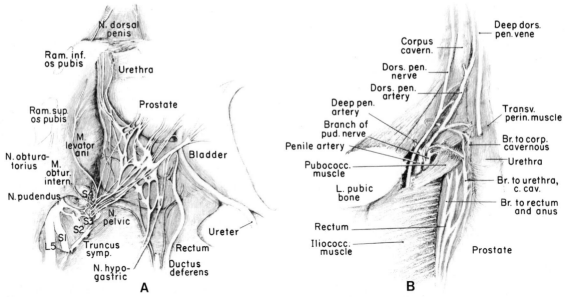

Figure 76–4. *A,* Dissection of left pelvic plexus in male newborn with peritoneum, pelvic vessels, pelvic fascia, and pubic symphysis removed. *B,* Close-up view of the dissection demonstrating the anatomic location of the branches of the pelvic plexus that innervate the corpora cavernosa. (From Walsh, P. C., and Donker, P. J.: J. Urol., *128*:492, 1982. Used by permission.)

musculature. The nerves innervating the prostate travel outside the capsule of the prostate and Denonvilliers' fascia until they perforate the capsule, at which point they enter the prostate. The branches to the membranous urethra and corpora cavernosa also travel outside the prostatic capsule in the lateral pelvic fascia. Recently, Walsh and Donker (1982) demonstrated the exact anatomic course of these branches. The found that the branches innervating the corpora cavernosa are located dorsolaterally in the lateral pelvic fascia, between the prostate and rectum. Near the apex of the prostate they course slightly anteriorly to travel on the lateral surface of the membranous urethra at the 3 and 9 o'clock positions. After piercing the urogenital diaphragm, they pass behind the dorsal penile artery and dorsal penile nerve before entering the corpora cavernosa (Fig. 76–4*B*). Although these nerves are microscopic, their anatomic location can be estimated intraoperatively by using the capsular vessels as a landmark. For this reason, throughout the remainder of the chapter, I will refer to this structure as the neurovascular bundle (see Fig. 76–1).

SURGICAL TECHNIQUE

Indications for Surgery

In Chapter 32, the diagnosis and staging of prostatic cancer and the indications for radical prostatectomy have been outlined extensively.

The ideal candidate for radical prostatectomy is a patient who is under the age of 70 years, is in good health, and has a tumor confined solely to the prostate. These requirements limit the candidates for surgery to those patients with stages A2, B1, or low-grade B2 disease. The preoperative evaluation of surgical candidates consists of a careful rectal examination which is performed to exclude palpable evidence of extraprostatic extension; a serum acid phosphatase determination; a chest x-ray and intravenous pyelogram (IVP); and bone scan with selective radiographs of any suspicious areas. In addition, the histologic slides from the needle biopsy are carefully reviewed to exclude the presence of high-grade disease. One of the major advantages of the retropubic approach is that a staging pelvic lymphadenectomy can be performed at the time of surgery. We have found this to be useful in avoiding unnecessary surgery in patients with more advanced disease than was clinically suspected.

Preoperative Preparation

Surgery is deferred for 6 to 8 weeks following the needle biopsy of the prostate. This delay enables any inflammatory adhesions or hematoma resulting from the needle biopsy to resolve, and thus allows the anatomic relationship between the prostate and the surrounding structures to return to a more normal state prior to surgery. Such healing is especially important if one hopes to preserve the neurovascular bundles intraoperatively and to avoid rectal injury. If the patient either has undergone a needle aspiration of the prostate as a diagnostic procedure or can be operated on within a week after the needle biopsy before inflammatory complications occur, there is no reason for delay.

Since 1 or 2 units of transfusions are frequently required in the perioperative period, patients may donate blood for autotransfusion during the 6 to 8 week waiting period. Use of the patient's own blood is certainly the safest way to avoid complications from transfusion. Patients are admitted to the hospital the day before surgery, and they undergo standard preoperative evaluation. The night before surgery they are given a Fleet enema.

Special Instruments

Unlike radical perineal prostatectomy, radical retropubic prostatectomy requires very few special instruments. A fiberoptic headlight is most useful, because much of the procedure is performed beneath the pubis in an area in which visualization can be difficult. A standard Balfour retractor with a malleable center blade is useful during the lymph node dissection and subsequently during the radical prostatectomy to provide cranial and posterior retraction on the peritoneum and bladder, respectively. Coagulating forceps, vessel loops, and long bulldog clamps are the only other special instruments that should be available.

Anesthesia, Incision, and Lymphadenectomy

A spinal or epidural anesthetic is preferable for this procedure. They are safer and their use seems to be associated with less blood loss. The patient is placed in the supine position, with the table broken in the midline to extend the distance between the pubis and the umbilicus slightly. The table is then tilted to 20 degrees in the Trendelenburg position. The skin is prepared and draped in the usual way. A No. 22 catheter with a 30-cc balloon is passed into the bladder, and the catheter is connected to sterile, closed-continuous drainage. A right-handed surgeon always stands on the left side of the patient. A midline extraperitoneal lower abdominal incision is made extending from the

pubis to the umbilicus. The rectus muscles are separated in the midline, and the transversalis fascia is opened sharply to expose the space of Retzius. Care is taken to incise the anterior fascia down to the pubis and to incise the posterior fascia above the semicircular line to the umbilicus. Laterally the peritoneum is dissected off the external iliac vessels to the point of bifurcation of the common iliac artery. Isolating, dividing, and ligating the vas deferens bilaterally facilitates this maneuver. At this point, a self-retaining Balfour retractor is placed, and the staging pelvic lymphadenectomy on the right side is commenced. Exposure is facilitated by using the malleable blade attached to the Balfour retractor to retract the peritoneum superiorly.

The lymphadenectomy is considered a staging, not a therapeutic, procedure. Its value is in identifying those patients with occult metastases to pelvic lymph nodes in whom a radical prostatectomy would be of little benefit. For this reason we use the modified technique of Whitmore and associates (Fisher et al., 1981). The dissection begins along the external iliac vein. The lymphatics overlying the external iliac artery are preserved. The dissection proceeds inferiorly to the femoral canal, at which point care is taken to ligate the lymphatic channels at the node of Cloquet. Next, the obturator lymph nodes are removed, carefully avoiding injury to the obturator nerve. The obturator artery and vein are usually left undisturbed and are not ligated unless excessive bleeding occurs. The dissection then proceeds superiorly to the bifurcation of the common iliac artery, at which point the lymph nodes in the angle between the external iliac and hypogastric arteries are removed. At the completion of the dissection, the vasculature in the hypogastric and obturator fossae should be neatly skeletonized (Fig. 76–5). These lymph nodes are sent for frozen section, and a similar procedure is carried out on the left side. The pathologist is requested to section all lymph nodes and perform frozen sections only on those lymph nodes that look suspicious. Using this procedure we have encountered only three false-negative frozen section evaluations in more than 100 cases. The three falsely classified lymph nodes were only 4 mm in diameter. For this reason, we feel that frozen section analysis of lymph nodes has great value. To reduce blood loss during the remainder of the procedure, the hypogastric arteries are encircled with vessel loops and bulldog clamps are placed proximal to the origin of the obliterated umbilical artery.

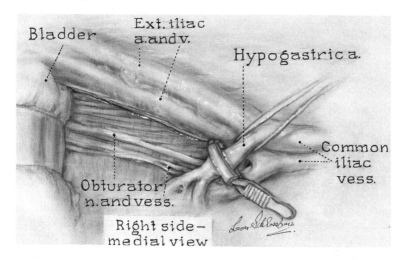

Bladder
Ext. iliac a. and v.
Hypogastric a.
Common iliac vess.
Obturator n. and vess.
Right side — medial view

Figure 76–5. View of the right pelvis following completion of the staging lymph node dissection. Note that the fibrofatty tissue overlying the external iliac artery and vein has not been disturbed and that a bulldog clamp has been placed on the hypogastric artery.

Incision in Endopelvic Fascia

At this point, the malleable blade is repositioned to retract the bladder. If the Foley balloon in the bladder is placed beneath the blade, maximal cranial and posterior displacement of the bladder will be achieved, providing excellent exposure of the anterior surface of the prostate. The endopelvic fascia is entered at the point at which it reflects over the pelvic side wall, well away from its attachments to the bladder and prostate (Fig. 76–6). The lateral venous plexuses, along with the branches of the inferior vesical artery and pelvic plexus, traverse adjacent to the prostate and the lower portion of the bladder. Therefore an incision in the endopelvic fascia adjacent to the bladder or the prostate risks laceration of these important structures and potentially severe blood loss. At the point of incision, the fascia is usually quite transparent, revealing the underlying levator ani musculature. After the fascia has been opened, one can usually see the bulging lateral venous plexus of Santorini, which is located medially. Beneath this venous complex lies the prostatovesicular artery and the branches of the pelvic plexus that course together toward the prostate, urethra, and corpora cavernosa. The incision in the endopelvic fascia is then carefully extended in an anteromedial direction toward the puboprostatic ligaments, thus enabling the surgeon to palpate the lateral surface of the prostate.

Division of the Puboprostatic Ligaments

The fibrous, fatty tissue covering the superficial branch of the dorsal vein and puboprostatic ligaments is gently teased away to prepare for division of the ligaments without inadvertent injury to the superficial branch of the dorsal vein. This maneuver enables the surgeon to incise the puboprostatic ligaments sharply at their attachment to the pubis. According to a microscopic study by Albers and associates (1973), the puboprostatic ligaments consist mostly of collagen; variable amounts of smooth muscle tend to cause retraction when the ligaments are severed. Albers and his colleagues found no vessels of significance on microscopic section. Thus, there is no need to ligate the ligaments. With the puboprostatic ligaments transected, the superficial branch of the dorsal vein is readily apparent over the bladder neck in the midline. This vein should be dissected carefully from the undersurface of the pubis, thereby exposing the trifurcation of the dorsal vein over the region of the prostatourethral junction (Fig. 76–7).

Ligation of Dorsal Vein Complex

The lateral wall of the urethra is identified by palpating the in-dwelling catheter. Using a right-angle clamp, the surgeon perforates the lateral pelvic fascia and passes the clamp through the avascular plane between the anterior surface of the urethra and the posterior surface of the dorsal vein complex (Fig. 76–7B). At this level, the complex with its associated fascia is 1 to 2 cm thick. A 0 silk ligature is then passed around the dorsal vein and tied (Fig. 76–7A). The dorsal vein complex, together with its investment of fascia, is then transected on the bladder side of the ligature with a No. 15 blade on a long handle (Fig. 76–7A). Generally,

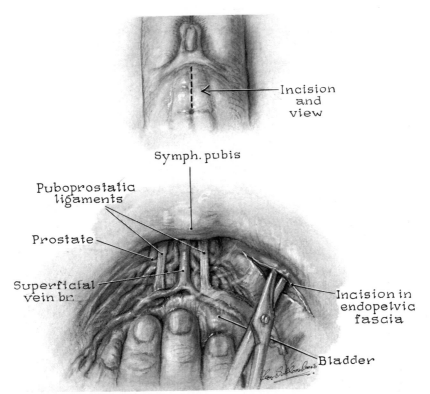

Figure 76–6. The incision in the endopelvic fascia is made at the junction with the pelvic side wall well away from the prostate and bladder.

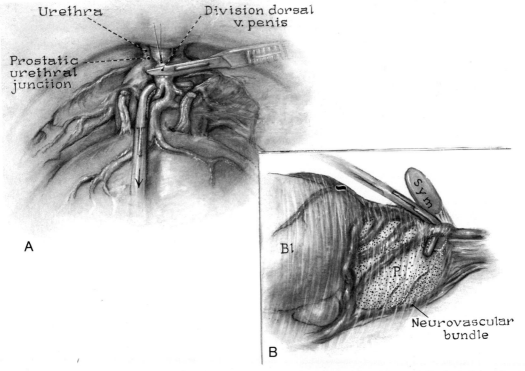

Figure 76–7. Division of the dorsal vein complex. *A,* A right angle clamp is positioned beneath the ligated dorsal vein at the time of division. *B,* Separation of the lateral pelvic fascia between the dorsal vein complex and urethra.

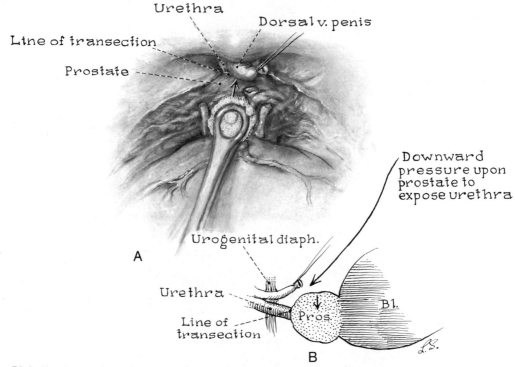

Figure 76–8. The dorsal vein has been transected, and a sponge stick is used to displace the prostate posteriorly to expose the prostatourethral junction.

little or no back flow from the untied lateral plexus occurs at this point, presumably because of the valves in the venous system. This is especially true in patients under epidural or spinal anesthesia; in patients under general anesthesia, there may be more back bleeding as a result of the increased venous pressure associated with increased intrathoracic pressure. If back bleeding is a problem, the venous channels over the anterior surface of the prostate can be oversewn with a 00 chromic catgut suture.

Division of Urethra

At this point, it is often useful to use a sponge stick to displace the prostate downward in order to see the prostatourethral junction (Fig. 76–8). During this stage of the procedure, venous bleeding from the dorsal vein complex must be controlled so that visualization can be achieved in a bloodless field. If the ligature has fallen off the dorsal vein or if there is significant oozing, a 00 chromic catgut suture on a large needle (T-12) can be used to oversew the fascial edges of the ligated distal vein to perfect hemostasis. Posterior sponge stick displacement of the prostate should result in a good view of the

prostatovesicular junction. Intact bands of lateral fascia are present on either side of the urethra (Fig. 76–9). These fascial bands must not be disturbed, since they contain the branches of the pelvic plexus that innervate the corpora cavernosa. In the past, these fascial bands were routinely divided in an effort to

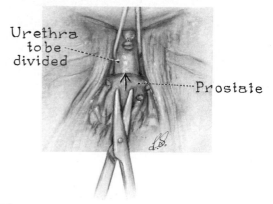

Figure 76–9. Exposure of the prostatourethral junction prior to transection of the urethra at site indicated by the arrow. Note that the intact lateral pelvic fascia on either side of the urethra has not been disturbed. The autonomic branches to the corpora cavernosa travel in this fascia posterior to the urethra.

skeletonize the urethra and mobilize the apex of the prostate. As a result, most patients were impotent after the operation.

Sharp dissection then develops the plane between the urethra and the lateral fascia, and an umbilical tape is passed around the urethra with care not to injure the adjacent fascia (Fig. 76–9). The anterior wall of the urethra is then incised at its junction with the apex of the prostate. The Foley catheter can then be brought through this incision, clamped, and divided. Next, the posterior wall of the urethra is divided (Fig. 76–10). At this point in the procedure, some authors advocate placing sutures in the distal urethra for use later during anastomosis. These sutures, however, are often pulled out during the subsequent maneuvers, and their accurate placement later in the procedure is not especially difficult.

Division of the Rectourethralis Muscle and Lateral Fascia

Using upward traction on the divided catheter, the rectourethralis muscle is incised in the midline, thus freeing the apex of the prostate from the underlying rectum (Fig. 76–10). With traction on the catheter, one can visualize bands of skeletal muscle and fibrous tissue that tether

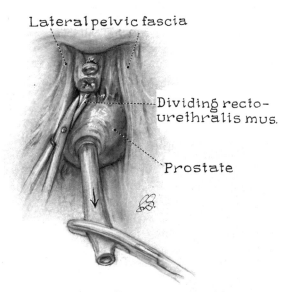

Figure 76–10. The urethra has been transected, and the divided catheter, which has been clamped, is used to retract the apex of the prostate superiorly, exposing the rectourethralis muscle. The muscle is divided to open the plane posteriorly between the anterior rectal wall and Denonvilliers' fascia, which covers the posterior prostatic surface.

the apex of the prostate to the pelvic floor musculature (Fig. 76–11A). When viewed laterally, these bands travel outside the lateral pelvic fascia, anteriorly. Consequently, they can be divided without fear of injury to the neurovascular bundles that are inside the lateral pelvic fascia (Fig. 76–11B). Once this has been accomplished, division of the rectourethralis muscle can be completed under direct vision, with care taken not to injure the neurovascular bundles that are located at the edges of this muscle bilaterally (Fig. 76–11B). Using finger dissection, the plane between the anterior wall of the rectum and the prostate with its investment of Denonvilliers' fascia is developed (see Fig. 76–11C). After this plane has been established, a right-angle clamp separates the lateral pelvic fascia from the lateral surface of the prostate at the apex (Fig. 76–12). At this point, the lateral fascia is usually quite thin and transparent. The lateral fascia is then incised at a point sufficiently anterior to preserve the neurovascular bundle, and the incision is carried cranially up to the area of the prostatic pedicle (Fig. 76–13). Recall that the neurovascular bundles are located dorsolateral to the prostate. In the past, this incision in the lateral fascia was made at random with blunt dissection. Although the neurovascular bundle was usually not removed with the specimen, it was injured during the dissection. With the technique described here, the incision in the lateral fascia can be made with precision and with knowledge of the location of the neurovascular bundle. If the induration on the side of the nodule appears to extend into the lateral pelvic fascia or neurovascular bundles, the fascia is divided at whatever point necessary to excise all evident tumor (see below). The primary objective of the surgical procedure is the removal of all tumor; in this setting, preservation of potency is of only secondary concern. Indeed, it may be necessary only to preserve the neurovascular bundles on one side to preserve potency (see further on).

Once the lateral fascia has been divided, the neurovascular bundles can be seen at the posterolateral edge of the prostate. Because the neurovascular bundles supply few vascular branches to the distal one third of the prostate, the bundles can usually be teased away from the prostate at this point. However, at the midpoint of the prostate, small arterial and venous branches are usually first visualized (Fig. 76–13). These first branches should be ligated individually using fine sutures or clips; mass ligatures should be avoided because they may produce inadvertent tenting of the bundle into

Fibromuscular attachments
to urogenital diaph.

Blad.

Rectum

Prostate

Rectourethralis
mus.

Lat. pelvic fascia

A

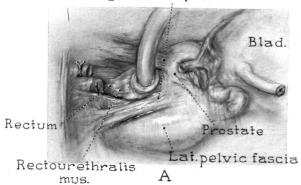

Divided rectourethralis mus.

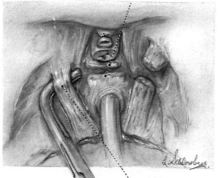

Division of fibromuscular
attachments in preparation apex
of prostate prior to division
of lat. pelvic fascia

B

Figure 76–11. Preparation of the apex of the prostate prior to division of the lateral pelvic fascia. *A,* The apex of the prostate is tethered to the urogenital diaphragm by fibromuscular bands that travel anteriorly, outside the lateral pelvic fascia. *B,* After the fibromuscular bands have been severed, the rectourethralis muscle fibers can be divided under direct vision.

Figure 76–12. The rectourethralis muscle has been divided, and the posterior plane between the anterior rectal wall and prostate has been developed. A right angle clamp is passed between the prostatic capsule and the transparent lateral pelvic fascia, identifying the site for the initial incision in the fascia, anterior to the neurovascular bundle.

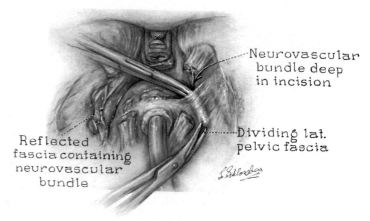

Neurovascular
bundle deep
in incision

Dividing lat.
pelvic fascia

Reflected
fascia containing
neurovascular
bundle

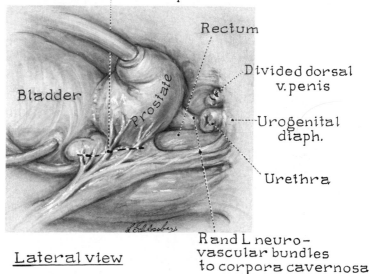

Division of lateral pedicle

Rectum

Divided dorsal
v. penis

Bladder

Prostate

Urogenital
diaph.

Urethra

R and L neuro-
vascular bundles
to corpora cavernosa

Lateral view

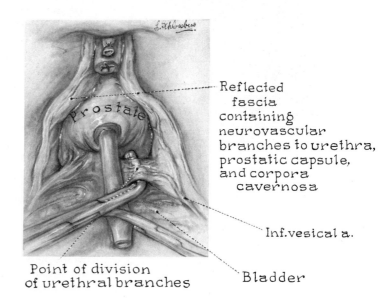

Prostate

Reflected
fascia
containing
neurovascular
branches to urethra,
prostatic capsule,
and corpora
cavernosa

Inf. vesical a.

Point of division
of urethral branches

Bladder

Figure 76–13. The upper figure illustrates that the lateral pelvic fascia has been divided bilaterally, releasing the apex of the prostate. The neurovascular bundles are intact. The site for ligation of the prostatic vascular pedicles, alongside the seminal vesicle and anterior to the neurovascular bundle, is identified by the dotted line. The lower figure illustrates the urethral branches of the prostatic artery being ligated.

the ligature, with subsequent injury. As one approaches the base of the prostate the bundles travel further posteriorly, and this is less of a problem. At this point the seminal vesicles with their overlying fascia are usually clearly identified. The lateral pedicles are divided on the lateral side of the seminal vesicles with interrupted 2-0 silk sutures (Fig. 76–13). The neurovascular bundles should be in full view; to avoid injuring these structures, the pedicles should not be ligated too far posteriorly.

Excision of the Lateral Pelvic Fascia and Neurovascular Bundle

Under certain circumstances it may be necessary to excise the lateral pelvic fascia and

neurovascular bundles completely on one or both sides. This decision may be made either preoperatively or intraoperatively based on a variety of clinical findings: (1) surgery on an impotent patient; (2) induration involving the lateral sulcus found on preoperative physical examination; (3) induration in the lateral pelvic fascia found intraoperatively after the endopelvic fascia has been opened; or (4) fixation of the neurovascular bundle to the capsule of the prostate, detected once the lateral pelvic fascia has been divided. In these situations the lateral pelvic fascia and neurovascular bundle can be isolated, ligated, and divided under direct vision out at the apex of the prostate lateral to the urethra (Fig. 76–14A). Next, the lateral pelvic fascia can be divided posterior to the neurovascular bundle on the posterolateral surface of the

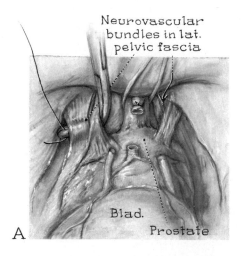

A

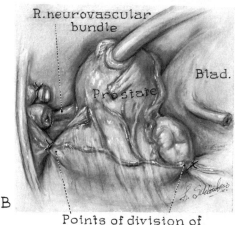

B

Points of division of neurovascular bundle

Figure 76–14. Steps in wide excision of lateral pelvic fascia and neurovascular bundle. *A,* Ligature placed around lateral pelvic fascia and neurovascular bundle at apex of prostate lateral to urethra. *B,* Points of division of neurovascular bundle at apex and tip of seminal vesicle. Lateral pelvic fascia will be divided posterior to neurovascular bundle on lateral surface of rectum.

rectum. Once again, this can be performed under direct vision with the dissection terminating at the tip of the seminal vesicle, where the neurovascular bundle is again ligated and divided (Fig. 76–14*B*). In this way the neurovascular bundle and lateral pelvic fascia can be excised under direct vision in a more complete way than was previously possible. Once this has been accomplished, the rectum is dissected free from the posterior surface of the prostate over to the lateral pelvic fascia on the contralateral side. Thus, that neurovascular bundle can be clearly delineated and skeletonized, enabling it to be preserved in its entirety. Indeed, it may be necessary only to preserve one neurovascular bundle to preserve potency (see further on).

Following a dissection such as this, the excised specimen demonstrates abundant soft tissue covering the lesion (Fig. 76–15*A*), wide excision of all soft tissue on the lateral ipsilateral side of the rectum, and preservation of the contralateral neurovascular bundle (Fig. 76–15*B*).

Division of the Bladder Neck and Excision of the Seminal Vesicles

At this point in the procedure the prostate has been almost completely mobilized. The anesthesiologist should now give the patient an ampule of indigo carmine dye to aid in identification of the ureteral orifices later. The bladder neck is incised anteriorly at the prostatovesicular junction (Fig. 76–16). There should be little fear that tumor is present at this site because the anterior fibromuscular stroma of the prostate contains little or no glandular tissue. The incision is carried down to the mucosa, the mucosa is incised, the Foley balloon is deflated, and the two ends of the catheter are clamped together to provide traction (Fig. 76–17*A*). The mucosa overlying the posterior bladder neck is incised next, and the plane between the posterior bladder wall and seminal vesicles is developed. Care must be taken to avoid inadvertent dissection within the layers of the trigone, which might result in ureteral injury. The correct plane of dissection can often be identified laterally, especially if the prostatic pedicles have been fully divided. In this case, it is fairly easy to develop a lateral plane between the bladder and seminal vesicles at the level of the prostatovesicular junction (Fig. 76–16). Once the plane has been established, the vasa deferentia are divided in the midline and the seminal vesicles are dissected free from surrounding structures (Fig. 76–17). Residual vascular pedicles along the lateral surface of the seminal vesicles are divided and ligated; this helps to expose the tips of the seminal vesicles. As the tips of the seminal vesicles are dissected free, the small arterial branch at each tip should be identified, divided, and ligated.

Previously, the lateral pedicles to the prostate were divided on the lateral surface of the seminal vesicles near their junction with the prostate. Thus, during the process of dissecting out the seminal vesicles they will be located in a pocket formed by the posterior wall of the bladder and the lateral pelvic fascia with the neurovascular bundle. Care should be exercised not to damage the neurovascular bundles during this step in the operation. Any residual attach-

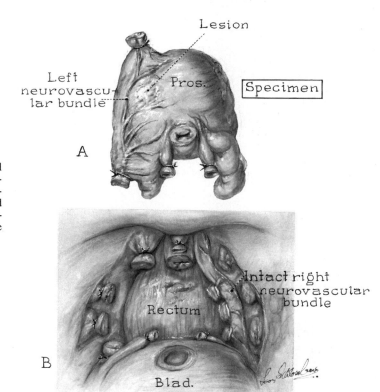

Figure 76–15. Appearance of radical prostatectomy specimen (A) and operative field (B) following unilateral complete excision of lateral pelvic fascia and neurovascular bundle. Note the well-delineated intact right neurovascular bundle (B).

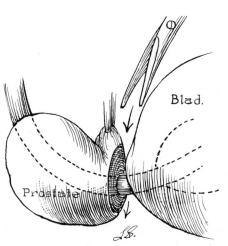

Figure 76–16. Schematic diagram of the technique for division of the bladder neck.

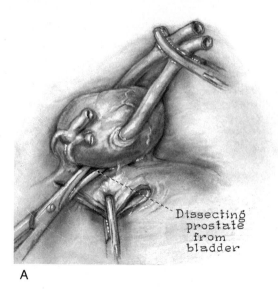

A

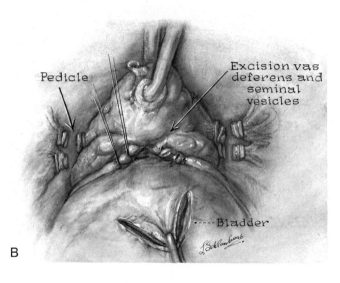

B

Figure 76–17. The bladder neck has been divided. *A,* An Allis clamp is used to elevate the posterior bladder neck during dissection of the plane between the posterior bladder wall and the seminal vesicles. *B,* Division of the vasa deferentia and excision of the seminal vesicles.

ments of Denonvilliers' fascia are divided, and the specimen is removed. The specimen is inspected carefully to identify any area in which the margin of resection is uncertain. If a questionable area is found, biopsies of the adjacent area or wider resection is indicated. The bulldog clamps are removed, and the operative site is inspected carefully for bleeding. Small bleeding vessels on the neurovascular bundle should not be cauterized for fear of coagulating the fine nerve bundles. Bleeding from these small vessels usually ceases spontaneously.

Bladder Neck Closure and Anastomosis

The bladder neck is reconstructed with interrupted sutures of 00 chromic catgut to ap-

proximate full-thickness mucosa and muscularis. This is usually accomplished by reapproximating the posterolateral margins of the bladder neck on both sides (Fig. 76–18). In cases in which the bladder neck has been resected more widely, the "tennis racket" closure may be used. The efflux of indigo carmine from the ureteral orifices is noted while placing these sutures; ureteral catheters are usually unnecessary. Care is taken to include the posterior vesical musculature that may have been dissected off the posterior wall of the bladder during excision of the seminal vesicles. The bladder neck is narrowed until it is approximately the diameter of the fifth finger. A new Foley catheter (20 F, 5-cc balloon) is placed through the urethra with the tip positioned just inside the pelvis (Fig. 76–18). To faciliate identification of the distal urethra, a sponge stick is used to displace the rectum

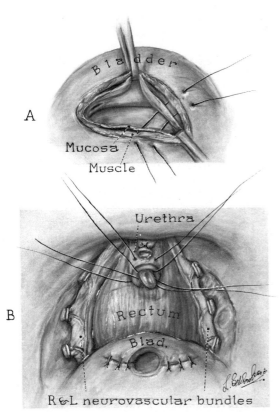

A

B

Figure 76–18. In the upper drawing, the bladder neck closure is performed using 2-0 chromic catgut. The closure is performed at the posterolateral margins of the bladder neck bilaterally. In the lower drawing, the vesicourethral anastomosis is performed using four 2-0 chromic catgut sutures. Care should be taken during placement of the posterior sutures to avoid injury to the neurovascular bundles.

posteriorly. A 00 chromic catgut suture on a ⅝ circle tapered needle is used to reapproximate the bladder neck to the urethra in four quadrants (the 1 o'clock, 5 o'clock, 7 o'clock, and 11 o'clock positions) (Fig. 76–18).

Initially, the two anterior sutures (1 o'clock and 11 o'clock) are placed by passing the needle from inside the urethral lumen (alongside the catheter) to the outside of the urethral stump without incorporating the striated pelvic floor musculature. If the sutures are placed deep in this musculature they may damage the branches of the pelvic plexus to the corpora cavernosa as they travel laterally through the striated musculature to innervate the corpora cavernosa. With traction on the two anterior sutures and with downward displacement on the sponge stick, it is usually quite easy to place the two posterior sutures. At this point, care should be taken to avoid incorporation of the neurovascular bundles in these two sutures. Next, using

a separate needle, the sutures are placed through the bladder neck in their respective quadrants. After the four sutures are placed, the balloon and valve on the catheter are tested, the catheter is positioned in the bladder, and the sutures are tied. The balloon is then inflated with 15 ml of saline, and the catheter is irrigated. Small, closed-suction catheters are placed, the operative site is irrigated vigorously with saline, and the incision is closed with absorbable sutures and skin clips. The catheter is carefully taped to the thigh.

Alternate Approaches

In 1959, Ansell and Campbell reported independently on a radical retropubic prostatectomy technique in which the procedure commences at the bladder neck. In 1978, Mittemeyer and Cox revived this concept, and recently this approach has gained popularity (Middleton, 1981; Lieskovsky and Skinner, 1983; Crawford and Kiker, 1983). Proponents of this technique emphasize the value of early ligation of the vascular and lymphatic supply of the prostate before manipulation; theoretically this early ligation may decrease dissemination of tumor cells. These surgeons also favor transection of the membraneous urethra at the completion of the procedure, thereby lessening blood loss from the dorsal vein complex. In addition, because division of the urethra occurs while it is held on traction at the completion of the operation, they feel that this is an ideal time to place sutures in the urethra.

APPLICATION OF THE POTENCY PRESERVING TECHNIQUE TO RADICAL CYSTOPROSTATECTOMY

Virtually all patients who undergo radical cystoprostatectomy are impotent postoperatively. The cause of impotence in this setting may be both vascular and neurogenic. However, if only the anterior branches of the hypogastric artery are ligated, blood flow through the internal pudendal artery should be undisturbed. Similarly, if the principles outlined in the foregoing material are adhered to, injury to the pelvic plexus can be avoided. I have been encouraged by my early experiences using this procedure and will outline the technique briefly.

The procedure is performed through a lower-midline transperitoneal abdominal incision. The space of Retzius is developed in the usual way, and the peritoneum overlying the bladder is divided so that it can be removed with the specimen. A bilateral pelvic lymph node dissection is performed; this dissection removes the lymphatics overlying the external and internal iliac vessels below the bifurcation of the common iliac artery, including the lymph nodes in the obturator fossa. The obliterated umbilical artery and superior vesical arteries are transected bilaterally (Fig. 76–19), and the ureters are divided. Next the plane between the bladder and rectum is developed by incising the peritoneum at the apex of the rectovesical cul-de-sac. Gentle blunt dissection is then used to free the rectum from the prostate down to the level of Denonvilliers' fascia (Fig. 76–20). During this procedure, some of the thin fascia and small vessels on the lateral surface of the bladder, inferior to the superior vesical pedicle, are transected. The lateral dissection, however, is not carried down as far as the lateral pedicles of the bladder. As mentioned earlier, the neurovascular bundles travel within this envelope of tissue.

At this point, the downward dissection stops, and the procedure proceeds as outlined for radical retropubic prostatectomy (see Figs. 76–6 to 76–13). Because most patients have not undergone a needle biopsy of the prostate and because bladder tumors rarely involve the prostate and lateral pelvic fascia, isolation of the prostate and preservation of the neurovascular bundles is much easier than in most radical retropubic prostatectomies performed for prostatic cancer. Once the membraneous urethra has been transected and the lateral pelvic fascia and pedicles to the prostate have been divided, the seminal vesicles are dissected away from the neurovascular bundles on either side (Fig. 76–21). As the seminal vesicles are dissected free from their posterior attachments to the rectum, a broad communication opens between the dissection from below and the posterior dissection from above. On either side laterally one can palpate the remaining pedicles to the bladder. These pedicles can be ligated and divided in the standard way, taking care to avoid injury to the neurovascular bundle. The intact neurovascular bundles can be visualized as the procedure is completed (Fig. 76–22).

When performing radical cystectomy, one must adhere to the usual principles designed for the radical removal of cancer. Any lateral fixation must be excised widely. Indeed, it may only be necessary to preserve the neurovascular bundles on one side to preserve potency (see later discussion).

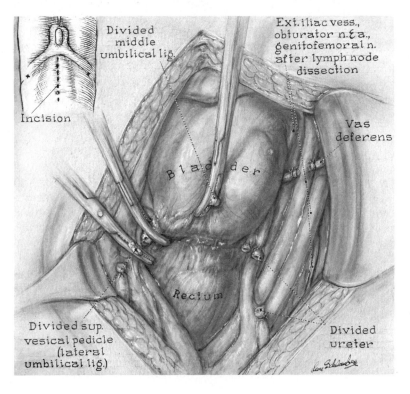

Figure 76–19. Steps in radical cystoprostatectomy. A bilateral pelvic lymph node dissection has been completed. The superior vesical arteries and lateral umbilical ligaments and ureters have been divided.

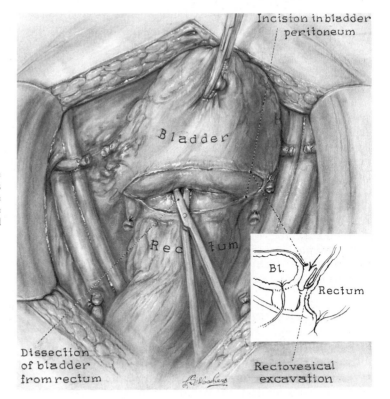

Figure 76–20. The peritoneum at the apex of the rectovesical cul-de-sac has been incised, and the plane between the bladder and rectum is developed. The next step in the procedure is illustrated in Figure 76–6.

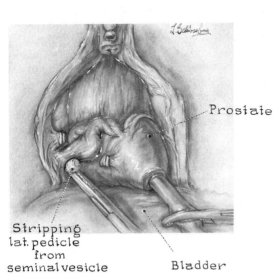

Figure 76–21. The steps illustrated in Figures 76–6 to 76–13 have been completed. Next, the seminal vesicles are released from the neurovascular bundles laterally and the rectum posteriorly.

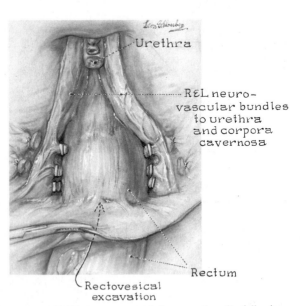

Figure 76–22. Appearance of the operative site following completion of the cystoprostatectomy, demonstrating the intact neurovascular bundles.

POSTOPERATIVE MANAGEMENT

The postoperative recovery of men who undergo radical retropubic prostatectomy is usually smooth, and the patients ambulate immediately. Intravenous fluids are administered until fluid intake can be tolerated by mouth, usually by the first or second postoperative day. The closed-suction tubes are left in place until they cease to function, usually on the third or fourth postoperative day. Occasionally patients will have moderate amounts of urinary extravasation for 7 to 10 days. This is usually of no consequence. Patients are discharged from the hospital with a Foley catheter in place usually within 7 to 10 days; they then return 3 weeks after the procedure for removal of the catheter. Initially most patients have significant amounts of stress incontinence, which generally resolves within the first or second postoperative month.

COMPLICATIONS

Radical retropubic prostatectomy is a well-tolerated procedure with minimal morbidity. Table 76–1 lists the complications from four reported series totaling 322 patients. The mortality rate is acceptably low (0 to 1.7 per cent). The complications can be divided into those occurring intraoperatively, early in the postoperative period, and late in the postoperative period. They will now be discussed in greater detail.

Intraoperative Complications

The most common intraoperative problem during radical retropubic prostatectomy is hemorrhage, usually from venous structures. Hemorrhage can occur during pelvic lymphadenectomy if one of the branches of the hypogastric vein is inadvertently torn. In this setting the use of fine cardiovascular silk suture ligatures is advised. Hemorrhage can also occur during the incision in the endopelvic fascia if the incision is made too close to the prostate, during division of the puboprostatic ligaments if the ligaments are not dissected free from the superficial branch of the dorsal vein, and during exposure of the apex of the prostate with transection of the dorsal vein complex. However, this bleeding can be satisfactorily controlled once the dorsal vein has been ligated and divided. It is imperative to obtain excellent hemostasis before approaching the apex of the prostate so that the anatomy can be viewed in a bloodless field. Most often, blood loss during the procedure occurs gradually from multiple small veins and results in an average accumulated loss of 1 to 3 units. This loss can be reduced through temporary occlusion of the hypogastric arteries by using bulldog clamps and through the use of spinal or epidural anesthesia. Three less common complications include injury to the obturator nerve during the pelvic lymph node dissection, rectal injury, and ureteral injury. If the obturator nerve is inadvertently severed, an attempt should be made to reanastomose the nerve with very fine nonabsorbable sutures. Rectal injury is an infrequent but serious complication. It can occur during dissection of the apex of the prostate and when the plane between the rectum and Denonvilliers' fascia is being developed. The rectum should be closed in two layers after freshening the edges of the incision. Interposing omentum between the rectal injury and the vesicourethral anastomosis reduces the possibility of a vesicourethral fistula. At the conclusion of the procedure the rectum

TABLE 76–1. COMPLICATIONS FOLLOWING RADICAL RETROPUBIC PROSTATECTOMY

	Kopecky et al., 1970	McDuffie, 1978	Middleton, 1981	Lieskowsky, 1983	Crawford, 1983
Number of patients	73	59	50	65	75
Mortality	0%	1.7%	0%	1.5%	0%
Intraoperative complications					
rectal injury	1.4%	3%	2%	3%	0%
ureteral injury	1.4%				
Early complications					
thrombophlebitis	6.9%		12%	3%	
pulmonary embolus	2.7%		2%	4.6%	
wound infection	16%			3%	5%
lymphocele			2%	3%	
urethrovesical dehiscence	4%			1.5%	
Late complications					
contracture of bladder neck	12%	5%	6%		2.6%
incontinence	1.4%	0%	4%	3%	1.3%
impotence	91%	92%	100%		

should be dilated widely. In addition one should probably perform a proximal diverting colostomy. Ureteral injuries occur secondary to inadvertent dissection within the layers of the trigone while attempting to identify the proper cleavage plane between the bladder and seminal vesicles. If this occurs, ureteral reimplantation should be undertaken.

Early Postoperative Complications

Thrombophlebitis and pulmonary embolism are two of the most common and potentially serious complications of the procedure. It has been reported that thrombophlebitis occurs in 3 to 12 per cent of patients and pulmonary emboli occurs in 2 to 5 per cent of patients (Table 76–1). Some authors have advocated postoperative anticoagulation therapy using either warfarin sodium (Lieskovsky and Skinner, 1983) or minidose heparin. However, the efficacy of minidose heparin has yet to be established, and the agent appears to be associated with an increase in the incidence of prolonged lymphatic drainage or lymphocele formation (Catalona et al., 1980). My own approach to the prevention of thrombophlebitis has been careful attention, both intraoperatively and postoperatively, to avoid venous stasis. During the operation, patients are placed in the Trendelenberg position to provide adequate venous drainage of the lower extremities. Patients are then ambulated on the first postoperative day, they are encouraged to perform dorsiflexion exercises 100 times every hour while awake, and they are discouraged from sitting with their legs in the dependent position for 3 to 4 weeks postoperatively. Our incidence of pulmonary emboli in over 100 consecutive cases is only 3 per cent with these measures.

Disruption of the urethrovesical anastomosis can lead to permanent incontinence. This complication occurs most frequently when the Foley catheter is inadvertently removed in the early postoperative period. To avoid this complication, the balloon and valve on the catheter should be tested immediately before the catheter is placed in the bladder. Some authors have advocated making a small cystotomy incision, passing a nylon suture through the eye of the catheter, and then tying the suture over a button on the anterior abdominal wall. The catheter should be taped carefully to the thigh, and the anchorage of the catheter should be examined each postoperative day. If the catheter happens to fall out prematurely, we usually make one attempt to pass a smaller-caliber catheter into the bladder. If this is not successful on the first attempt, the patient is cystoscoped, and the catheter is placed under direct vision.

Late Postoperative Complications

Contracture of the bladder neck has been reported to occur in 3 to 12 per cent of cases. It is usually caused by a lack of accurate mucosa-to-mucosa apposition of the bladder to the urethra at the time of the anastomosis, but it can also be caused by overzealous reconstruction of the bladder neck. Patients with bladder neck contracture usually complain of a dribbling stream; it may, however, be difficult to make the diagnosis if the patient's only complaint is overflow incontinence. A catheter should always be passed in any patient who complains of incontinence to make certain that there is no obstruction or significant residual urine. Bladder neck contractures usually respond to one or two dilations. If this does not work, I have found that dilation under anesthesia with injection of triamcinolone acetonide (200 mg) directly into the area of the stricture helps to resolve this complication permanently.

Fortunately, urinary incontinence is an infrequent complication of radical retropubic prostatectomy, occuring in only 0 to 4 per cent of reported series (see Table 76–1). However, incontinence is more frequent when a pubectomy is performed (Middleton, 1977) or when Vest sutures are used (Kopecky et al., 1970). There are several mechanisms of urinary continence in men: the vesical neck, the passive urethral mechanism, and the external sphincter-pelvic floor mechanism. All passive mechanisms, such as the bladder neck and the intrinsic urethral mechanism, are most effective when elevated by the tonic activity of the pelvic floor (Hinman, 1976). The incontinence that occurs in patients after radical prostatectomy can often be related to rigidity of the remaining posterior urethra and nonelevation of the bladder base after voluntary cessation of urination (Hinman, 1976). Consequently, to achieve continence after radical retropubic prostatectomy, it is mandatory to avoid injury to the pelvic floor mechanism, to reconstruct the vesical neck so that it will provide a passive mechanism of continence, and to avoid stricture formation by coapting the bladder neck to the urethra accurately. Recently the role of the external sphincter mechanism has come under greater scrutiny. This complex, now termed the "distal urethral sphincter" (DUS), is composed of two types of skeletal muscle (see Chapter 72). The "intrinsic" skeletal muscle is intimately attached to the underlying urethra and is composed of "slow-twitch" fibers that are innervated by the autonomic branches of the pelvic plexus. These fibers can maintain tonus for long periods without fatigue and thus are ideal for passive continence. The outer or "extrinsic" layer of skeletal muscle is similar to the surrounding pelvic floor muscles. It is attached to the urethra only on its posterior aspect and acts mainly as a sling. These "fast-twitch" fibers are innervated by the pudendal nerve, fatigue earlier, and contract on command. They contribute minimally to passive continence but are useful in interrupting the urinary stream during coughing or straining. With the nerve-sparing type of prostatectomy described in this chapter, the autonomic innervation to the intrinsic skeletal muscle should be preserved, and thus the incidence of postoperative incontinence should be lower.

Preservation of Potency

For years it was assumed that most if not all patients who underwent radical prostatectomy would be impotent postoperatively. For this reason, many patients and their physicians selected less effective forms of treatment. Recently we completed a study of the causes of impotence following radical prostatectomy. We concluded that impotence results from injury to the pelvic nerve plexus that provides autonomic innervation to the corpora cavernosa (Walsh and Donker, 1982). Based on these anatomic studies, injury to the pelvic plexus appears to occur in at least two ways: (1) most commonly during apical dissection by transection of the urethra and the adjacent lateral pelvic fascia, through which the branches to the corpora cavernosa travel and (2) during division of the lateral pelvic fascia and lateral pedicle. These conclusions led to the minor modifications of the procedure that have been outlined in great detail in this chapter. This modified technique of radical retropubic prostatectomy has now been used in operations on more than 100 men between the ages of 34 and 72 years of age with stages A2 and B adenocarcinoma of the prostate. Follow-up evaluation after 3 months or longer is available on 64 men who were potent preoperatively and who have sexual partners (Walsh and Mostwin, 1984). At 3 and 6 months after surgery, 30 to 40 per cent of patients are potent. At 9 months postoperatively 60 per cent of patients are potent, and after 1 year 86 per cent of patients have experienced the return of sexual function. In all surgical procedures, every attempt was made to excise all tumor; in some cases one neurovascular bundle was sacrificed.

The specimens have undergone careful pathologic evaluation for the extent of periprostatic tissue. From the surgical principles outlined in Figure 76–1, one would assume that the soft tissue margins of resection following radical retropubic prostatectomy should be wider than those achieved with radical perineal prostatectomy. Evaluation of the margins of specimens from radical perineal and the modified retropubic prostatectomy confirmed this assumption (Walsh et al., 1983). In the past, incisions in the lateral pelvic fascia were made at random; it is likely that the branches of the pelvic plexus were merely transected and not excised, thus leaving the transected neurovascular bundle in place on the lateral rectal wall (Middleton, 1981). However, through use of the anatomic approach to radical prostatectomy outlined in this chapter, one should be able to avoid unnecessary injury to the lateral pelvic fascia at the level of the distal urethra and make an informed decision about the extent of resection of the lateral pelvic fascia and lateral pedicles of the prostate.

The surgical margins in the first 100 consecutive patients who underwent this procedure have just been evaluated (Eggleston and Walsh, 1985). Of the first 100 patients, 41 per cent had established periprostatic tumor in soft tissue; yet the surgical margins of resection were positive in only seven patients. In all seven of those patients there was extensive extraprostatic involvement by tumor; in five of the seven there was involvement of the seminal vesicles; and in none were the surgical margins positive only at the site of the nerve-sparing modification. Based upon these findings, there is no indication that the modified surgical procedure compromises the adequacy of the removal of cancer, which is determined primarily by the extent of the tumor rather than by the operative technique.

In performing all procedures, the primary goal of surgery is to remove all tumor. Potency is of secondary concern. It is not clear how often patients will be potent if the neurovascular bundle is sacrificed on one side. Based upon my limited experience at this time, 3 patients in whom the neurovascular bundle was sacrificed on one side are potent (Walsh and Mostwin, 1984). In patients undergoing radical extirpation of tumors of the sacrum, it has been shown that sacrificing the sacral nerve roots on one side does not affect sexual performance adversely (Gunterberg and Petersen, 1976). Further experience may make it possible to sacrifice the neurovascular bundles routinely on one side with confidence and thus widen the margins of excision. The primary goal should be a reduction in the morbidity of radical prostatectomy without reducing its efficacy as the most effective form of treatment for localized prostatic cancer. It is hoped that these new techniques will encourage more urologists to take a greater interest in offering this option to the young, healthy, sexually active patient, who is often the ideal candidate for this procedure.

References

Albers, D.D., Faulkner, K.K., Cheatham, W.N., Elledge, E.F., and Coalson, R.E.: Surgical anatomy of the pubovesical (puboprostatic) ligaments. J. Urol., *109*:388, 1973.

Ansell, J.S.: Radical transvesical prostatectomy: Preliminary report of an approach to surgical excision of localized prostatic malignancy. J. Urol., *82*:373, 1959.

Campbell, E.W.: Total prostatectomy with preliminary ligation of the vascular pedicle. J. Urol., *81*:464, 1959.

Catalona, W.J., Kadmon, D., and Crane, D.B.: Effect of mini-dose heparin on lymphocele formation following extraperitoneal pelvic lymphadenectomy. J. Urol., *123*:890, 1980.

Chute, R: Radical retropubic prostatectomy for cancer. J. Urol., *71*:347, 1954.

Crawford, E.D., and Kiker, J.D.: Radical retropubic prostatectomy. J. Urol., *129*:1145, 1983.

Eggleston, J.C. and Walsh, P.C.: Nerve-sparing radical retropubic prostatectomy: Pathologic findings in the first 100 cases. American Urological Association Meeting Program, Abstract 511, 1985.

Fisher, H., Herr, H., Sogani, P., and Whitmore, W.F., Jr.: Modified pelvic lymph node dissection in patients undergoing I-125 implantation for carcinoma of the prostate. American Urological Association Meeting Program Abstract No. 299, 1981.

Flocks, R.H.: The arterial distribution within the prostate gland: Its role in transurethral resection. J. Urol., *37*:524, 1937.

Gunterberg, B., and Petersen, I.: Sexual function after major resections of the sacrum with bilateral or unilateral sacrifice of sacral nerves. Fertil. Steril., *27*:1146, 1976.

Hinman, F.: Male incontinence: Relationship of physiology to surgery. J. Urol., *115*:274, 1976.

Jewett, H.J., Eggleston, J.C., and Yawn, D.H.: Radical prostatectomy in the management of carcinoma of the prostate: Probable causes of some therapeutic failures. J. Urol., *107*:1034, 1972.

Kopecky, A.A., Laskowski, T.Z., and Scott, R., Jr.: Radical retropubic prostatectomy in the treatment of prostatic carcinoma. J. Urol., *103*:641, 1970.

Lich, R., Grant, O., and Maurer, J.E.: Extravesical prostatectomy: A comparison of retropubic and perineal prostatectomy. J. Urol., *61*:930, 1949.

Lieskovsky, G., and Skinner, D.G.: Technique of radical retropubic prostatectomy with limited pelvic node dissection. Urol. Clin. North Am., *10*:187, 1983.

Memmelaar, J.: Total prostatovesiculectomy—Retropubic approach. J. Urol., *62*:340, 1949.

Middleton, A.W., Jr.: A comparison of the morbidity associated with radical retropubic prostatectomy with and without pubectomy. J. Urol., *117*:202, 1977.

Middleton, A.W., Jr.: Pelvic lymphadenectomy with modified radical retropubic prostatectomy as a single operation: Technique used and results in 50 consecutive cases. J. Urol., *125*:353, 1981.

Millin, T.: Retropubic prostatectomy: New extravesical technique: Report on twenty cases. Lancet, *2*:693, 1945.

Millin, T.: Retropubic Urinary Surgery. Baltimore, The Williams & Wilkins Co., 1947.

Mittemeyer, B.T., and Cox, H.D.: Modified radical retropubic prostatectomy. Urology, *12*:313, 1978.

Paulson, D.F., Lin, G.H., Hinshaw, W., and Stephani, S.: The Uro-Oncology Research Group: Radical surgery versus radiotherapy for adenocarcinoma of the prostate. J. Urol., *128*:502, 1982.

Reiner, W.G., and Walsh, P.C.: An anatomical approach to the surgical management of the dorsal vein and Santorini's plexus during radical retropubic surgery. J. Urol., *121*:998, 1979.

Walsh, P.C.: Radical Retropubic Prostatectomy and Cystoprostatectomy: Surgical Technique for Preservation of Sexual Function. A film produced by Aegis Productions, Inc. and distributed by Norwich Eaton Pharmaceuticals, Inc., 1984.

Walsh, P.C.: Radical prostatectomy for the treatment of localized prostatic carcinoma. Urol. Clin. North Am., *7*:583, 1980.

Walsh, P.C., and Jewett, H.J.: Radical surgery for prostatic cancer. Cancer, *45*:1906, 1980.

Walsh, P.C., and Donker, P.J.: Impotence following radical prostatectomy: Insight into etiology and prevention. J. Urol., *128*:492, 1982.

Walsh, P.C., Lepor, H., and Eggleston, J.C.: Radical prostatectomy with preservation of sexual function: Anatomical and pathological considerations. Prostate, *4*:473, 1983.

Walsh, P.C., and Mostwin, J.L.: Radical prostatectomy and cystoprostatectomy with preservation of potency: Results utilizing a new nerve sparing technique. Br. J. Urol., *56*:694, 1984.

Weyrauch, H.M.: Surgery of the Prostate. Philadelphia, W.B. Saunders Co., 1959, p. 27.

Young, H.H., and Davis, D.M.: Young's Practice of Urology. Vol. 2. Philadelphia, W. B. Saunders Co., 1926, pp. 463–466.

CHAPTER 77

Perineal Prostatectomy

PERRY B. HUDSON, M.D.

Perineal prostatectomy is not a single operation. Several types of surgery fall into this category. Each is useful for a particular kind of patient whenever corrective surgery is sought. Judgements of the value of each procedure for individual patients can reasonably be made. A surgical operation that most closely meets the patient's needs is selected, without unwarranted risk, depending upon certain factors, such as the patient's age and general condition and his expressed subjective desires.

HISTORY OF PERINEAL SURGICAL APPROACH TO THE PROSTATE

More than 2000 years ago, surgeons devised and employed a median perineal incision for the removal of vesical calculi. In the first century A.D., a semielliptical incision in the perineum was used for partial removal of the prostate gland. Subsequently, there was little known use of this surgical approach for several hundred years.

Sporadic accounts of perineal removal of bladder stones or parts of the prostate have been noted from the seventeenth, eighteenth, and early nineteenth centuries. In 1867, both the recognition of carcinoma and the availability of anesthesia prompted the first perineal operation for prostatic cancer. A deliberate but blind enucleation operation for benign hyperplasia was described in 1873. Surgical records from the years 1882 and 1891 describe the earliest excision with urethral reconstruction and the first standardized perineal excision for benign prostatic enlargement.

Slightly later, a number of significant advances in technique were made by different surgeons. Modifications were made in the anatomic approach and instruments used for the excision of obstructing prostatic tissue and reconstruction of the operative site. Perineal prostatic surgery changed from crude, blunt dissections to precise surgical exercises performed under vision, with accurate hemostasis, identification of structures, and reconstitution of the urinary tract.

Weyrauch has summarized the documented evolution of this form of surgery (Table 77–1).

INDICATIONS FOR PERINEAL PROSTATIC SURGERY

One accepted indication for the perineal surgical route is carcinoma of the prostate that is amenable to total prostatovesiculectomy. The approach is also ideal for removal of large prostatic calculi, since calculi and obstructing glandular tissue may be removed under direct vision. When calculi occupy the entire gland, total perineal prostatectomy is the operation of choice, as it is for intractable infection of the prostatic cortex that fails to yield to treatment. This indication sometimes arises following one or several transurethral prostatectomies. Because of the advantage of dependent drainage, perineal prostatotomy is usually indicated for prostatic abscess.

Patients with a wide pelvic outlet and a thin perineum are especially good subjects for the perineal approach.

Since the mortality rate and postoperative cardiopulmonary morbidity is low, the perineal approach is particularly desirable for patients who are poor operative risks.

TABLE 77–1. LANDMARKS IN DEVELOPMENT OF PERINEAL PROSTATECTOMY

Contribution	Surgeon	Year
PRIMITIVE "BLIND" TECHNIQUES		
First perineal lithotomy: initial step in perineal approach to prostate	Ammonius Lithotomus	460–357 B.C.
Curved incision for perineal lithotomy	Celsus	25 A.D.
Accidental removal of prostatic lobe during perineal lithotomy	Covillard	1639
First perineal prostatectomy: median incision	Guthrie	1834
First perineal prostatectomy for carcinoma: median incision	Billroth	1867
Blind finger enucleation via median perineal urethrotomy	Gouley	1873
Curved incision of Celsus for excision of prostatic carcinoma: reconstruction of urethra	Leisrink	1882
Standardization of technique described by Gouley	Goodfellow	1891
Balloon to pull prostate toward perineum: inflated in bladder	Syms	1900
OPERATION PERFORMED UNDER VISION		
Median perineal prostatectomy under vision: a "perineal" table, prostatic tractor, and lobe enucleator	Proust	1901
Conservative perineal prostatectomy: curved skin incision, inverted Y incision for enucleation, preservation of verumontanum and ejaculatory ducts; perineal retractors, prostatic tractor, and lobe forceps	Young	1903
Radical perineal prostatectomy for carcinoma: removal of prostate, seminal vesicles, ampullae of the vasa, and surrounding fascia	Young	1905
Preservation of structures surrounding external sphincter; suture of vesical neck to stump of urethra	Hans Wildbolz	1906
Hemostatic bag for perineal prostatectomy: large drainage tube passing through center of bag	Edwin Davis	1924
Plastic closure: bleeding controlled by suture, obliteration of prostatic fossa	Gibson	1928
APPROACH WITHIN ANAL SPHINCTER		
Exposure via cleavage plane between external anal sphincter and longitudinal fibers of rectum	Haim	1936
Standardization of approach beneath anal sphincter	Belt	1939

(From Weyrauch, H. M.: Surgery of the Prostate. Philadelphia, W. B. Saunders Co., 1959.)

Indications for Biopsy

Perineal prostatic biopsy by the open surgical method may constitute the initial step in surgical therapy for patients, since, simultaneously, it constitutes the last step in diagnosis before selection of the definitive operation. It must be understood that the election of open surgical biopsy through a perineal incision does not commit the surgeon to performing a definitive operation through this incision. It is in the interest of the patient to elect definitive operation by transurethral, suprapubic, retropubic, or perineal approaches after initial perineal prostatic biopsy. In practice, open perineal biopsy is now rarely used, having been replaced by needle biopsy or transurethral biopsy.

If the microscopic examination of quick-frozen sections obtained from the perineal biopsy reveals no carcinoma, the conservative operation that is best suited to the patient's needs and desires is used to relieve the progressive effects and symptoms of benign prostatic obstruction. In contrast, if adenocarcinoma is detected in the quick-frozen specimen from per-ineal biopsy, a radical perineal prostatectomy is performed. If a mistaken false-negative impression of benign tissue is obtained and a conservative operation is performed, a secondary treatment may be required after the permanent paraffin sections of either the residue of the unfrozen biopsy specimen or the surgical specimen from conservative prostatectomy have been examined.

If prostatic cancer is detected by the quick-frozen section technique and if suspicious tissue lies outside the anatomic boundary delineated by the anterior layer of Denonvilliers' fascia, a second quick-frozen section is taken from the tissue in question. This type of local extension is a signal of incurability. Such patients are best treated by other means, such as radiation therapy or hormonal therapy.

Indications for Simple Perineal Prostatectomy

The principal indication for a simple perineal prostatectomy is extensive benign prostatic enlargement with obstruction of the urinary tract. The distribution of benign hyperplasia in the different prostatic lobes is not important. Middle lobes or subtrigonal extensions of benign prostatic enlargement are readily accessible through the perineal incision. Furthermore, the existence of hypertrophied interureteric ridges ("bar formation") and the presence of vesical calculi and diverticula that drain completely following voiding or bladder catheterization are not contraindications to simple perineal prostatectomy.

The main contraindication to this operation is in the younger patient, for whom sexual potency is extremely important. Any of the operations that relieve urethral obstruction by the removal of prostatic tissue may alter sexual potency. However, simple perineal prostatectomy probably interferes with an active sex life more frequently than do other techniques.

Simple perineal prostatectomy may also be undertaken simultaneously with abdominoperineal surgery for primary malignant disease in the large bowel. Under such circumstances, the perineal prostatectomy operation is performed rapidly, conveniently, and safely at the same surgical session with, and immediately following, removal of the perineal portion of the rectum.

An advantage of simple perineal prostatectomy is that it permits microscopic tissue examination of any portion of the dorsal prostate before enucleation is begun. The blood loss during this operation is the least of any of the open techniques than can be employed. Other advantages include the absence of a need for a general anesthetic or for postoperative narcotic sedation for pain, the possibility of immediate ambulation, and the lowest incidence of thromboembolic and other vascular complications. In addition, reoperation is required very rarely, and both postoperative stricture of the urethra and infection are similarly rare. Contracture of the vesical neck during the postoperative period is not encountered with the technique described in this chapter.

Indications for Subtotal Perineal Prostatectomy

The term *subtotal prostatectomy* is used by urologists to indicate that the entire "anatomic" prostate gland is removed, including both the benignly enlarged prostate gland and the entire posterior or dorsal prostate. The seminal vesicles and sections of the vas deferens that are removed in radical prostatectomy are left in situ.

Subtotal perineal prostatectomy is used principally for the removal of benignly enlarged prostate glands containing multiple calculi. These calculi characteristically are located between the posterior prostate and the benignly enlarged periurethral glandular tissue. The persistence of calculi after transurethral resection operations and after simple enucleation prostatectomy may result in the persistence of prostatic infection. Therefore, it is desirable to remove all the calculi; this can be best accomplished by subtotal perineal or subtotal retropubic prostatectomy.

One other indication for subtotal prostatectomy is an abscess that has clinical significance, as well as prostatic cysts that extend into the dorsal prostate.

Subtotal perineal prostatectomy is used for patients in whom an active sex life is not a serious consideration.

Indications for Radical Perineal Prostatectomy

The principal indications for radical perineal prostatectomy were cancer and tuberculosis. The latter condition rarely requires radical surgical removal today; tuberculosis of the male genital tract can be eradicated or suppressed by drug therapy.

Microscopic confirmation of cancer in a surgical specimen of a preoperatively palpated nodule or an indurated area in the prostate is an indication for radical perineal prostatectomy. When the biopsy has been achieved by the open surgical route, the biopsy incision is used for the excisional operation.

When patients are to undergo prostatic surgery of any sort, perineal prostatic biopsy may be performed and a quick-frozen section made. If cancer is found unexpectedly, it is feasible to continue with the radical prostatectomy.

In patients who have not been subjected to perineal prostatic biopsy prior to conservative transurethral, retropubic, or suprapubic prostatic surgery, the surgical specimens removed may contain microscopically detectable prostatic cancer. Radical perineal prostatectomy is one possible solution during the postsurgical period following these conservative operations, but most urologists today prefer to turn to more encompassing therapy at such times, such as radiation or hormonal therapy.

When compared with modern exenterative surgery in the pelvis, radical perineal prostatectomy is not a radical cancer operation; it is an operation in which the entire prostate gland, the intact seminal vesicles, the short segments of the vas deferens on each side, and the fascial covering of all these structures are removed en bloc. The continuity of the urinary tract is reestablished by direct end-to-end anastomosis of the bladder neck to the membranous urethra, which is severed proximal to the main urethral attachment of the external sphincteric muscles.

Total prostatectomy was performed originally through the perineal surgical approach. Precisely the same tissues are removed as in a total or "radical" retropubic prostatectomy. Approximately the same cure rate for cancer is to be expected from both operations. A principal disadvantage of the perineal route is that evaluation of the pelvic lymph nodes is not possible in the same operative field. However, some surgeons elect to do it as a sequel to negative results from lymphadenectomy.

However, the radical perineal prostatectomy operation has several advantages. It can be performed through the same incision used for perineal prostatic biopsy. This makes feasible the use of quick-frozen section techniques to verify the malignant character of the prostatic nodule palpated preoperatively, or to constitute the final portion of the appraisal for any patient undergoing prostatic surgery. Radical perineal prostatectomy affords an opportunity for more precise reconstruction of the urinary tract after the excisional portion of the operation has been completed, and it causes less blood loss than radical retropubic prostatectomy. Therefore, the final functional result is better, the mortality rate is lower, and the morbidity is of less consequence. In addition, use of the perineal surgical route for total prostatectomy makes the employment of either saddle spinal block or epidural regional anesthesia possible, a distinct advantage for the age group in which prostatic cancer occurs.

THE OPERATION

Preoperative Preparation

Urinary antisepsis is begun as soon as the decision is made to perform an operation. Ideally this program of urinary antisepsis is also started before cystoscopic or panendoscopic examination. The choice of drugs and dosages is wide and variable and is guided by urine culture and sensitivity testing.

If perineal prostatic surgery is to be performed in the morning, no food is taken orally after midnight on the day preceding the operation. When surgery is contemplated for the afternoon, the patient is permitted a clear liquid breakfast.

Although blood loss may be very small in perineal prostatic surgery, two 500-ml units of compatible whole blood should be reserved.

Preparation of the patient includes scrubbing with surgical soap and shaving the lower abdomen, pubis, scrotum, perineum, perianal region, both thighs, and the lumbosacral region. Preparation of the lumbosacral region may be omitted if regional anesthesia or spinal anesthesia is not to be used.

Bowel preparation consists of repeated enemas until a completely clear return is obtained. The use of laxatives and sterilization of the bowel by antibiotics is unnecessary.

Operating Surgical Team

Perineal prostatic surgery may be performed by two, three, or four members of the team, excluding the instrument nurse. Many of the operations are such that the surgeon and a single assistant will encounter awkwardness in their work. A team of three is better, but it is helpful to remember that the modern techniques were devised for a team of four. The reasons are simple. The rectal ("posterior") retractor must be held carefully to afford exposure without injuring the ventral rectal wall. Attempts to use weighted retractors produce unsatisfactory results. The third assistant stands on the patient's left side to hold both the rectal retractor and the left lateral retractor. The second assistant holds the curved urethral tractor and the right lateral retractor. The first assistant helps in the excisional and reconstructive surgical steps.

Employment of the team of four minimizes error, blood loss, and wasted time.

Surgical Instruments

The only essential surgical instruments that are peculiar to perineal prostatic surgery are the straight and curved prostatic tractors. The curved instrument is inserted urethrally at the start of every perineal operation. The straight tractor is inserted through a prostatotomy or through the transected urethra distal to the prostatic apex.

Position of the Patient (Fig. 77–1)

It is preferable to use an operating table that permits immediate raising and lowering of either the head or the perineum to a position that is convenient for the surgeon.

Precautions must be taken to bolster the patient's shoulders. In the extreme lithotomy position, the weight of the body rests mainly upon the shoulders; if they are not cushioned, pressure on the brachial plexus may lead to nerve palsy. Abduction of the arms on the shoulders is avoided for the same reason. Foam rubber is well suited to this purpose. Likewise, pivots for holding the legs should be bolstered with a soft material to prevent pressure on the legs. If foot cradles are not used, the legs are fixed to pivots by means of elastic bandages.

The perineum may be supported by a perineal elevator, sand bags, or folded towels. Since there is such wide variation in the size and contour of the sacral region from patient to patient, it is desirable to have an assortment of sand bags and towels on hand so that the proper height can be achieved. The common mistake in positioning the patient is to fail to pull the buttocks sufficiently far down to elevate the perineum to a plane parallel with the floor. When proper position is obtained, the perineum projects beyond the end of the operating table.

Intraoperative Therapy

During all perineal prostatic operations several measures are routinely taken.

Prophylactic Antihemorrhagic Therapy. Five gm of epsilon-aminocaproic acid are injected into the intravenous line during the first hour to suppress proteolytic enzymes in both blood and urine. This ensures a favorable reaction that permits firm clot formation and maintenance. Blood loss during and after surgery is thereby reduced.

Prophylactic Antibacterial Therapy. Therapeutic level doses of an intravenously administered antibiotic is begun 15 minutes before the surgical incision is made.

Techniques

Perineal Prostatic Biopsy. The surgical dissection is shown in Figures 77–2 to 77–11. It is a technique very similar to the Belt approach and requires minimal disturbance of nerves and blood vessels; it also provides clear vision and identification of each structure to be incised or preserved.

Simple Perineal Prostatectomy. The surgical dissection for exposure in this operation is identical to that employed for biopsy. During

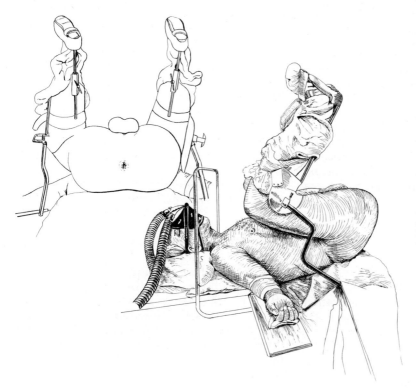

Figure 77–1. The lower section of the table is turned down in a vertical direction, and an instrument tray is affixed to this portion. The upper portion of the table is elevated at an angle of 30 degrees. The patient's position is maintained by the shoulder braces and by the pressure exerted on the foot by the stirrup mechanism. Note that the perineum is in an almost horizontal position. The upper extremity is extended at an angle that does not exceed 45 degrees with the long axis of the torso. Limitation of abduction in this way prevents temporary brachial palsy. Pronation of the arm also prevents brachial palsy.

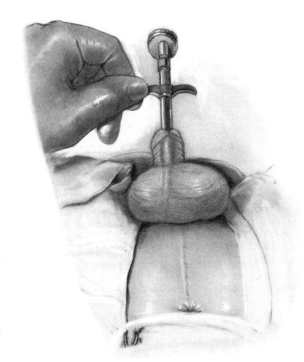

Figure 77–2. The curved urethral tractor has been inserted, rotated to determine that its tip is well within the lumen of the bladder, and the blades have been opened by clockwise rotation of the knob. Throughout the biopsy procedure this instrument is held firmly by the crosspiece. The assistant's wrist should rest upon the patient's thigh so that dangerous and unnecessary motion cannot injure the bladder from within. Sterile draping leaves the anus exposed.

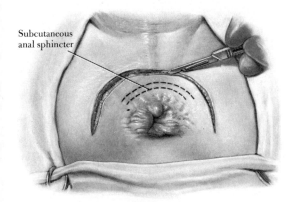

Subcutaneous
anal sphincter

Figure 77–3. The double dotted lines indicate the position of the subcutaneous anal sphincter. Topically, this is indicated by wrinkling or puckering of the skin external to the mucocutaneous junction.

Figure 77–4. The left index finger has been insinuated between the apex of the ventral rectal wall and the central tendon. The central tendon is actually an extension of the subcutaneous muscle fibers of the anal sphincter toward the bulb of the urethra. It varies greatly in both its width and its depth. It may reach and join with the fused leaves of the levator ani muscles. Such fusion is often termed erroneously the "rectourethralis muscle." Several small arterial vessels are encountered in the transection of the central tendon; these should be ligated.

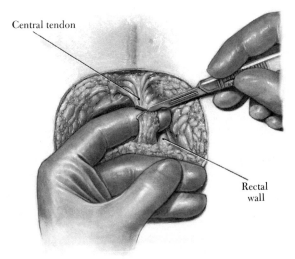

Central tendon

Rectal
wall

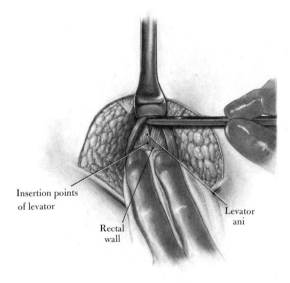

Insertion points
of levator

Levator
ani

Rectal
wall

Figure 77–5. The middle and index fingers of the left hand are still used in preference to a posterior or rectal retractor. It is seen that the slight midline separation in the leaves of the levator ani muscles has come into view. Notice is also taken of the insertion points of the levator on each side as it fuses directly with the external longitudinal smooth muscle of the ventral rectal wall.

Figure 77–6. With the posterior layer of Denonvilliers' fascia retracted out of view, the prostatic biopsy is performed with a scalpel. The lower (proximal) long limb of the biopsy incision is made first so that bleeding cannot obscure the field. Fulguration of blood vessels is deferred until the specimen is removed in order to preclude confusing morphologic findings during frozen section examination. Note the wide band of undisturbed true prostatic capsule (anterior Denonvilliers' fascia) included in the biopsy specimen. This sheet of tissue contains rich nerve networks, which are frequently invaded by cancer cells; it is therefore of diagnostic significance.

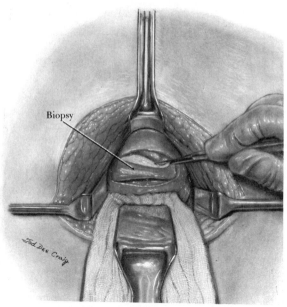

Biopsy

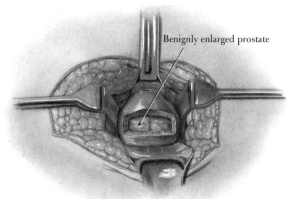

Benignly enlarged prostate

Figure 77–7. Penetration of the biopsy incision at least to the level of the periurethral benignly enlarged parts of the prostate is shown here. This guarantees that the full thickness of the "posterior" or cancer-forming part of the prostate is included in the specimen.

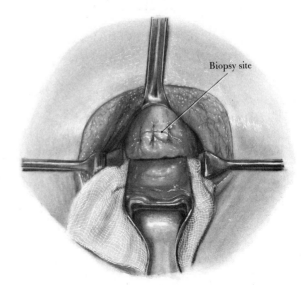

Figure 77–8. Interrupted sutures of 00 atraumatic chromic catgut are placed through the full thickness of the posterior prostatic tissue. Small bleeding vessels along the cut edge of the tissue are electrocoagulated before these sutures are tied. The edges of the biopsy site are approximated more easily for suture tying if the prostatic tractor is elevated to a vertical position. This maneuver releases pressure on the bladder neck and prostate and allows the wound edges to come together without tension.

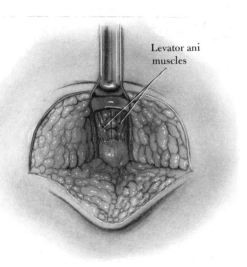

Figure 77–9. The second step in closing is the placement of interrupted sutures of 00 chromic catgut to reapproximate the levator ani muscles in the midline. These sutures are tied without tension on the muscle. They may be omitted.

Figure 77–10. Drainage of the perineal prostatic surgical incision is never carried out directly through the wound. Instead a small counterincision is made. The dotted lines indicate the pathway into the deep portion of the tissues previously exposed without entry into the superficial portions. Interrupted sutures of 00 chromic catgut are being placed to reapproximate the severed ends of the central tendon.

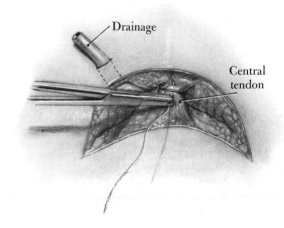

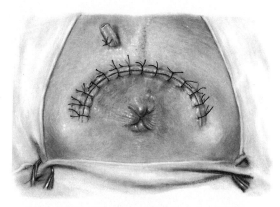

Figure 77–11. Skin closure with interrupted sutures.

biopsy, a prostatotomy is automatically made through the full thickness of the dorsal ("posterior") prostate. If the biopsy excision is centrally located and only benign tissue is seen by quick-frozen section examination, this site is developed for enucleation of obstructing prostatic tissue. When the biopsy site is eccentrically located it is sutured, and a location at the midpoint between the prostatic apex and base is chosen to commence enucleation. A similar location is chosen if the surgeon declines biopsy as a preliminary step. In Figures 77–12 to 77–31 a technique for simple perineal prostatic prostatectomy is sequentially delineated.

Subtotal Perineal Prostatectomy. This procedure is sometimes called total perineal prostatectomy. The word "total" would perhaps be better reserved as a synonymous term for radical perineal prostatectomy. The technique is described in detail in Figures 77–32 to 77–45.

It may be noted that the following variations are often utilized:

1. Puboprostatic ligaments are undermined rather than divided.

2. Apical dissection (transection of the membranous urethra) precedes dissection of the base of the prostate and bladder neck.

3. The apex of the prostate is divided 1 cm proximal to the proximal end of the membranous urethra.

The choice of detailed steps shown here is the result of experience with these and other considerations.

Radical Perineal Prostatectomy. Attention to the smallest details in the description of this operation (Figs. 77–46 to 77–67) simply reflects precisely what must transpire in the operating room if good functional results are to be obtained. Meticulous attention to Halsted's principles of surgery is rewarding here, both for the excision of cancer without iatrogenic, avoidable spread of malignancy and for the reconstruction of the urinary tract and its proper function postoperatively.

CARE AFTER PERINEAL PROSTATIC SURGERY

On the day of the perineal operation, the patient is kept at bed rest. He may sit up, read, and take a clear liquid diet. On the evening of the day of operation, 30 ml of mineral oil is given orally, and this dose is repeated for the 4 succeeding postoperative days. Postoperative antibiotics and epsilon aminocaproic acid are given according to the surgeon's choice.

No pain-relieving drugs are ordered routinely during the postoperative period for the patient recovering from perineal prostatic surgery, since there is very little pain.

The three-way indwelling Foley urethral catheter is attached to a closed, sterile continuous-drainage system with mannitol-sorbitol solution irrigation flowing at a rate of 125 ml per hour. The collected urine is measured, and the amounts are recorded at 2-hour intervals; orders are left to report any decrease in the urinary output.

Rectal treatments or temperature determinations and enemas are contraindicated during the first 5 postoperative days.

On the second postoperative day the patient is given a regular hospital diet, and at this point the patient is ambulatory.

Perineal surgical dressings are removed completely on the day after surgery, and no further surgical dressings are applied to the wound. Sterile towels, which are changed as frequently as required, are placed under the perineum.

Beginning on the first postoperative day and as soon as the perineal surgical dressing is removed, the following routine perineal care program is begun and is repeated four times daily:

1. Wash the perineum carefully with surgical soap.

2. Dry gently and spray with 1 per cent neomycin sulfate solution.

3. Apply a heat lamp for 20 minutes and protect the scrotum.

In the case of simple perineal prostatic biopsy, the perineal drain and urethral catheter are removed on the first day after operation; the perineal wound sutures are removed on the eighth postoperative day, and warm baths are begun as soon as the sutures have been re-

Text continued on page 2808

Figure 77–12. The lateral retractors on either side hold back the levator ani muscles. Very little traction is exerted upon the upper retractor. The lower one, under which a gauze sponge has been placed to protect the rectal wall, is also lightly held. With a scalpel, a line of cleavage is being started between the benignly enlarged periurethral prostatic tissue and the true dorsal prostate. This line of enucleation is begun on the proximal side of the biopsy site, which is now used for the incision. If this were not the case, blood might run downward later in the operation and obscure this particular area from perfect vision. To ensure a clean enucleation operation and to avoid tearing the posterior prostate, which later will be closed, the enucleation is begun with a scalpel.

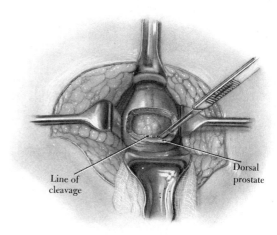

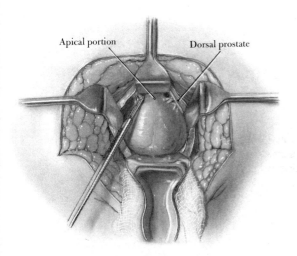

Figure 77–13. Both lateral right angle retractors are inserted between the periurethral glandular tissue and the dorsal prostate. The superior retractor is placed in such a way that it exposes the apical portion of the enlarged periurethral prostatic tissue that is being removed. Again, coagulation of adhesions is followed by division with the scalpel. The retractor shown most inferiorly in this view is also inside the dorsal prostatic tissue; such a maneuver is not necessary at this point in the dissection.

Figure 77–14. Under direct vision, the prostatic urethra is being divided with a scalpel. The curved metal prostatic urethral tractor is seen through the opening in the urethra.

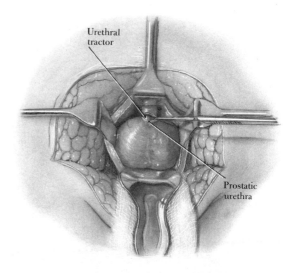

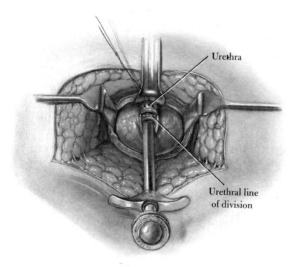

Urethra

Urethral line
of division

Figure 77–15. Note the position of the straight prostatic tractor. The blades are now open inside the bladder, and gentle traction on the handle of the instrument draws the "prostate" down into view. A single marking suture has been placed in the dorsal aspect of the distal end of the urethra. The dotted line indicates the remaining urethral line of division.

Figure 77–16. Adhesions on the ventral (abdominal) aspect of the prostatic specimen are divided. Care is taken here to coagulate the adhesions before they are divided. Otherwise retraction of bleeding vessels will make hemostasis unsatisfactory. Vigorous traction on retractors is not necessary throughout this operation. It is necessary only to alter the angle at which the instrument is held.

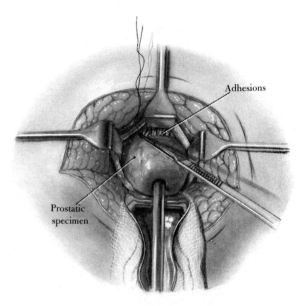

Adhesions

Prostatic
specimen

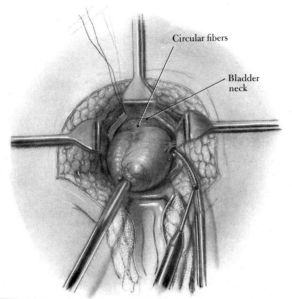

Circular fibers

Bladder
neck

Figure 77–17. Prompt clamping and subsequent coagulation of bleeding vessels that are injured inadvertently minimize blood loss. The anterior (ventral) aspect of the bladder neck is now freed of adhesions. Traction upon the prostatic tractor brings the gland well out into the surgical wound. Note the circular fibers. This is the anatomic internal sphincter, which is carefully preserved to prevent postoperative stress incontinence.

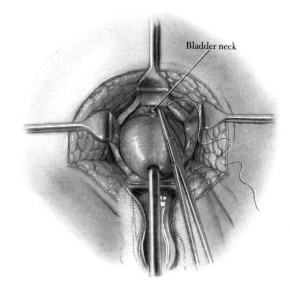

Figure 77–18. At this point in the operation, major steps for hemostasis commence. A 00 chromic atraumatic catgut suture is being placed at the most anterior (ventral) portion of the bladder neck. Circular fibers are distal to the point at which the suture is being placed. This suture should extend as deeply into the tissues as is consistent with the size of the semicircular needle and the thickness of the tissue in each individual situation.

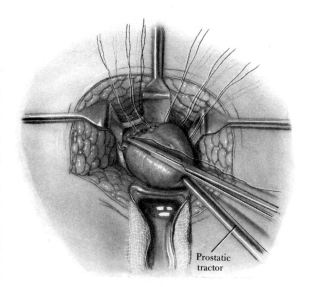

Figure 77–19. Careful examination of this and the foregoing illustrations will emphasize the use of the straight prostatic tractor to facilitate placement of sutures in the bladder neck. In this view the instrument is carried almost out to the patient's left thigh in order to expose the right posterolateral aspect of the bladder neck for suturing. Again, the right angle retractor nearest to the point at which the suture is to be placed is angulated to expose at least 1 cm of tissue.

Figure 77–20. The prostatic tractor has now been carried upward, and its handle points toward the patient's left knee. A right posterolateral hemostatic suture is being placed. For the first time the broad retractor that covers the gauze pad on the ventral rectal wall is brought into play.

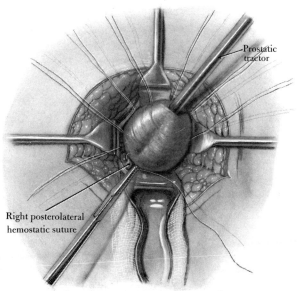

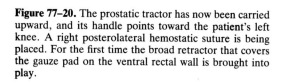

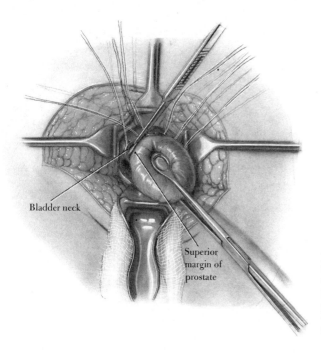

Bladder neck

Superior margin of prostate

Figure 77–21. At the right lateral aspect of the bladder neck, just distal to the hemostatic sutures, the scalpel is used to transect all layers of the bladder just above the superior margin of the prostate. Again, retraction is emphasized only on those right-angle retractors that are closest to the scalpel at any point in this part of the dissection.

Figure 77–22. In difficult exposures, two empty sponge forceps are utilized in this fashion. One blade of each instrument is placed in the prostatic urethra and the other is placed outside it. The tips of these instruments, seen here as the surgeon would hold them, are then depressed in such a way that the bladder neck region is exposed. This is sometimes necessary in order to be able to see the bladder neck clearly and to transect it at right angles to the external surface of the muscle coats.

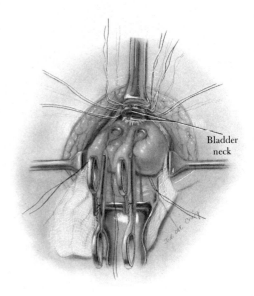

Bladder neck

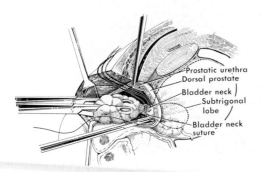

Prostatic urethra
Dorsal prostate
Bladder neck
Subtrigonal lobe
Bladder neck suture

Figure 77–23. This is a semisagittal view of the dissection and the problems yet to be encountered in the operation. This most superior retractor obscures the severed end of the prostatic urethra in that distal portion, which subsequently will be anastomosed with the bladder neck. This retractor is, therefore, inside the dorsal prostate ("surgical capsule"). On the far side, the right angle lateral retractor is seen on the patient's right side. The effect of traction on both the empty sponge forceps placed on the prostatic specimen to be removed is seen readily in this view. Note how the bladder neck is elongated by this traction. The left lateralmost bladder neck suture is being placed. It is often necessary to "back" the needle against soft tissues and then to bring it forward into a deep bite. This maneuver is of particular value when exposure is minimal. Of additional interest here is the dotted outline of the subtrigonal lobe of benignly enlarged prostatic tissue encountered in some patients. Obviously, simple amputation for 360 degrees at the bladder neck would leave this lobe in situ.

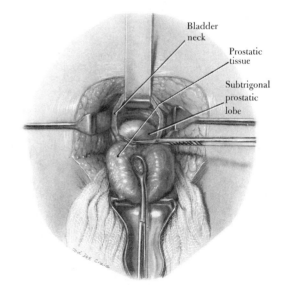

Figure 77–24. The most superior retractor has been inserted into the bladder neck. A malleable ribbon retractor or a narrow curved retractor suffices. Gentle elevation of this retractor in a vertical direction exposes to view the smooth, rounded epithelial covering of the subtrigonal prostatic lobe. The scalpel is being used to incise the transitional epithelial lining of the bladder neck without entering the subtrigonal lobe itself. The combination of elevation of the most superior tractor and gentle traction on the empty sponge forceps placed in the midline on the prostatic tissue that is being removed produces the exposure demonstrated here.

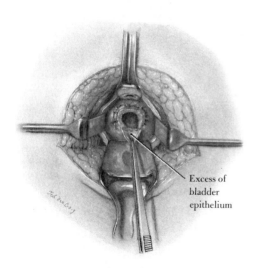

Figure 77–25. With the surgical specimen removed, it is seen that there is an excess of bladder epithelium on the trigonal side. This excess of tissue is excised with a scalpel across the dotted line shown here. The bladder neck is then ready to be anastomosed to the urethra.

Figure 77–26. The urethral catheter has been inserted from the urinary meatus through the membranous urethra and out of the severed distal prostatic portion. Gentle traction is exerted on the catheter in a vertical direction parallel to the handle of the most superior retractor. This facilitates visualization of the entire edge of urethra that is to be anastomosed to the bladder neck. The first anastomosing suture has been placed. It is advisable to place the bladder neck portion of this suture first. This minimizes the amount of traction that may be placed inadvertently on the suture after it has pierced the urethra. The urethra is a much more friable structure and is injured easily. Note that the knot in this suture has to be tied outside the lumen of the urinary tract. It should also be emphasized that it is best not to use the hemostatic sutures in the bladder neck for the anastomosis.

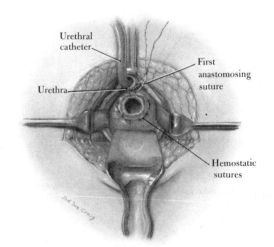

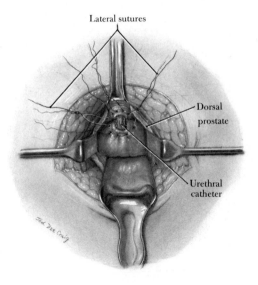

Lateral sutures

Dorsal prostate

Urethral catheter

Figure 77–27. With the lateral sutures placed but not tied for anastomosis, the tip of the urethral catheter is advanced into the bladder. With the bag of the catheter inflated to prevent accidental removal, the remaining sutures are placed to unite the urethra with the bladder neck. Clear exposure of the area is obtained by gentle traction on all four of the retractors that are still inside the dorsal prostate ("surgical capsule").

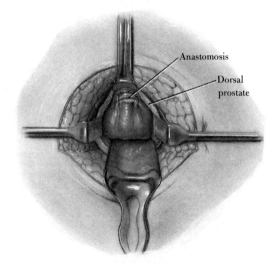

Anastomosis

Dorsal prostate

Figure 77–28. The anastomosis has been completed. This closure is usually watertight but need not be so. Following this stage, all four retractors are removed from their positions with tips inside the dorsal prostate.

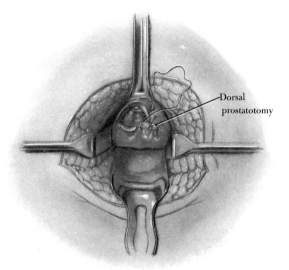

Dorsal prostatotomy

Figure 77–29. The lateral retractors here are simply holding back the separated edges of the levator ani muscles. The traction should be gentle on these lateral retractors because branches of the pudendal plexus on either side may be crushed against the rami of the ischial bone. With a running suture of 00 atraumatic chromic catgut, the dorsal prostatotomy is being closed. (This is the site of the biopsy.)

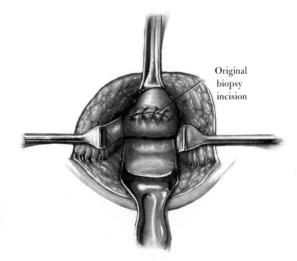

Figure 77–30. This closure is watertight. The running sutures serve to secure the reapposed edges of the original biopsy (prostatotomy) incision. They also serve to provide hemostasis. Prostatic capsular vessels can be sources of postoperative venous oozing.

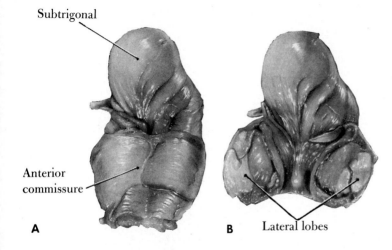

A **B** Lateral lobes

Figure 77–31. *A,* This is the surgical specimen from the foregoing perineal enucleation prostatectomy operation. The subtrigonal part is seen at the superior aspect of this illustration. The lower portion contains the anterior commissure, which covers the lateral lobular enlargements. *B,* Specimen with the anterior commissure divided to expose the prostatic urethra. The lateral lobes are now seen clearly on either side.

Figure 77–32. Prior to this stage in the operation, the routine perineal prostatic exposure has been carried out. It is assumed that the biopsy specimen from the posterior prostate will have been examined by the frozen section method and will have been found to contain no malignant tissue.

In this view the levator ani muscles are held behind each of the lateral retractors. The dotted line shows the line of incision that will be made in the anterior layer of Denonvilliers' fascia (anatomic prostatic capsule). The stay suture is placed in the membranous urethra just distal to the apex of the prostate gland.

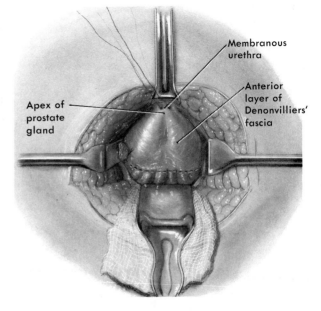

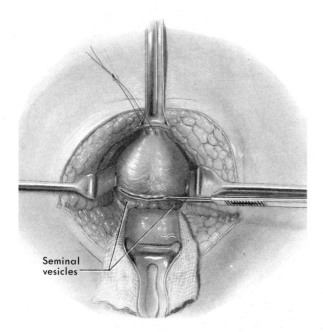

Figure 77–33. With the No. 15 scalpel blade, an incision is being made here through the anterior layer of Denonvilliers' fascia. This incision is placed at the upper border of the prostate at a point just distal to the bulge in the seminal vesicles. If this incision is placed too far proximally, the seminal vesicles will be entered unnecessarily. If the incision is placed too far distally, a portion of the prostate will not be excised with the surgical specimen.

Seminal vesicles

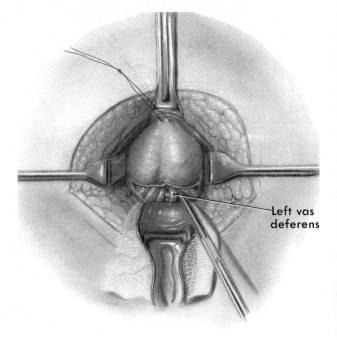

Figure 77–34. Separation of the cut edges of the anterior layer of Denonvilliers' fascia makes it possible to identify the left vas deferens, which is being elevated with a right-angle hemostatic forceps.

Left vas deferens

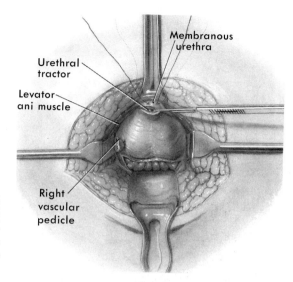

Figure 77–35. A 180-degree incision is made in the membranous urethra just proximal to the stay suture placed previously in the membranous urethra distal to the apex of the prostate gland proper. Note that the shiny surface of the curved urethral tractor is seen. The ligated right vascular pedicle to the prostate is seen on the left side of this illustration at the toe of the lateral retractor, which holds back the patient's right levator ani muscle.

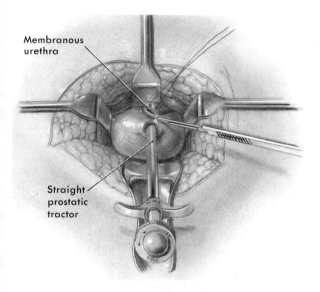

Figure 77–36. The curved urethral prostatic tractor has been removed, and in its stead the straight prostatic tractor has been introduced through the membranous urethra and the prostatic urethra and into the bladder. Its blades are opened, and it is being used for traction while the last portion of the urethra is transected.

Figure 77–37. Note the completely transected membranous urethra with the stay suture in place. Just above and proximal to this point the two puboprostatic ligaments are seen clearly, though the symphysis pubis is not visible. These ligaments are divided with the small scalpel blade between right angle clamps, as shown here. They are then secured with suture ligatures of chromic catgut. Downward traction on the straight urethral prostatic tractor toward the surgeon's feet facilitates bringing these ligaments into view. An increase in the vertical angle of the patient also facilitates visualization here.

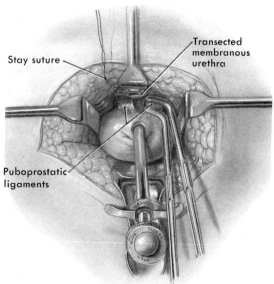

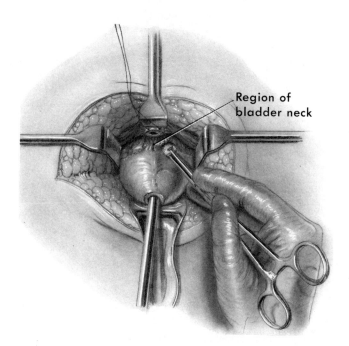

Region of
bladder neck

Figure 77–38. The precise region of the bladder neck is being identified and exposed by blunt dissection with the small gauze dissector. All blood vessels, regardless of size, are fulgurated or suture-ligated as they are encountered in this region. This minimizes blood loss and facilitates dissection in a clear, bloodless field.

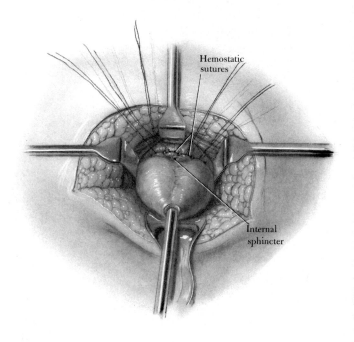

Hemostatic
sutures

Internal
sphincter

Figure 77–39. The hemostatic chromic 00 atraumatic sutures placed through all layers of the bladder wall are shown here. These are identical to the sutures placed in a radical perineal prostatectomy. The circular fibers of the internal sphincter or bladder neck are seen clearly here very much as they appear at the operating table.

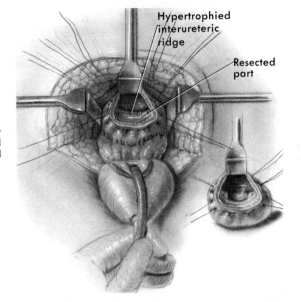

Figure 77–40. The dotted lines indicate the extent of resection of the hypertrophied interureteric ridge with the small scalpel blade. The inset in this illustration shows the resected part of the interureteric ridge.

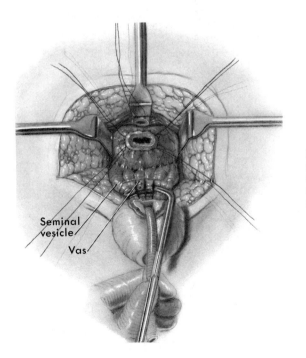

Figure 77–41. Right-angle clamps placed only on the proximal side are used prior to amputation of the vas and seminal vesicle on either side. They are secured with 00 chromic atraumatic catgut suture ligatures. This completes excision of the surgical specimen.

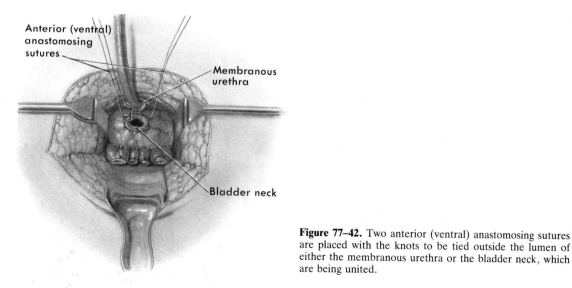

Figure 77–42. Two anterior (ventral) anastomosing sutures are placed with the knots to be tied outside the lumen of either the membranous urethra or the bladder neck, which are being united.

Figure 77–43. After the ventral sutures have been tied, an indwelling urethral catheter is advanced from the meatus and, under vision, through the anastomotic site and into the bladder. With the bulb inflated to hold the catheter securely in the bladder, the lateral anastomosing sutures are placed. Finally a mattress suture is shown to close the remaining gap in the urethra. Note that the knot in this mattress suture is placed proximally on the bladder neck rather than on the urethral side. Although a watertight closure is highly desirable, excessive suturing is not, for it increases the amount of scar tissue deposited in this critical zone, which is located just adjacent to the external sphincteric mechanism.

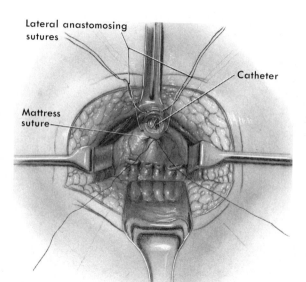

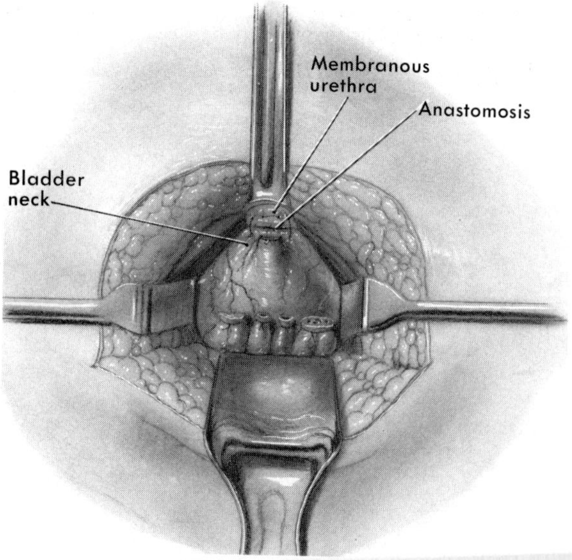

Figure 77–44. This figure shows completion of the anastomosis with the edges of the bladder neck drawn firmly adjacent to the cut edges of the membranous urethra. Excessive tension is not placed on these sutures, because devascularization will result with subsequent scar formation or fistula.

Figure 77–45. This is the excised surgical specimen. At the bottom of this illustration the cut edges of the two vasa deferentia (in the midline) are shown and, lateral to them, the cut stumps of the distal portions of the seminal vesicles. The lumen just above these four structures is that of the amputated bladder neck.

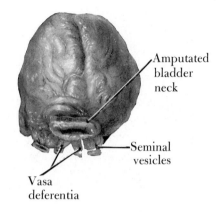

Amputated bladder neck

Seminal vesicles

Vasa deferentia

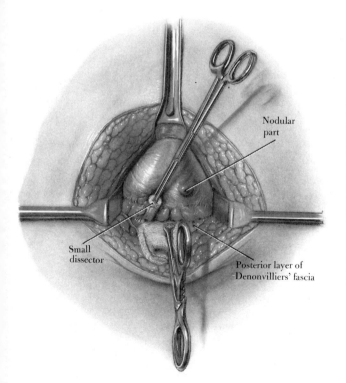

Nodular part

Small dissector

Posterior layer of Denonvilliers' fascia

Figure 77–46. The nodular part of the prostate, which has been thought clinically to be cancerous, is evident in the left posterior aspect of the prostate. Prior to excisional biopsy of this mass, the space between the two layers of Denonvilliers' fascia is developed by blunt dissection. The posterior layer of Denonvilliers' fascia is retracted. The lower (proximal) cut edge of this fascial layer is visible beneath the forceps sponge, which is used to retract it over the ventral surface of the rectal wall. During this portion of the dissection, the forceps sponge serves as a retractor; it is held almost immobile while the fascial plane is developed by an upward motion of the small dissector. In this way minimal pressure is exerted on the ventral rectal wall as the dissection progresses.

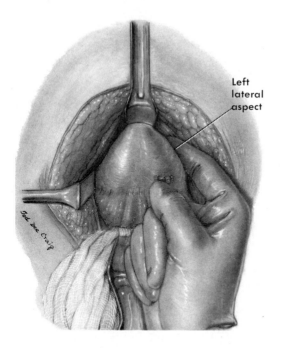

Left
lateral
aspect

Figure 77–47. The curved urethral tractor has now been returned to the original position used for the preliminary dissection and biopsy. This brings the prostate prominently into the surgical wound. The left lateral aspect of the prostate is freed by blunt dissection. Close following of the anatomic capsule (anterior Denonvilliers' fascia) ensures avoidance of the lateral venous plexuses as the dissection proceeds ventrally around the gland. After both lateral aspects of the prostate are freed, the finger is swept toward the rectum until it encounters resistance from the vascular pedicle and fascial folds over the arteries and veins as they enter medially to supply the prostate and bladder neck regions. The vessels in this pedicle are derived mainly from branches of the inferior vesical artery.

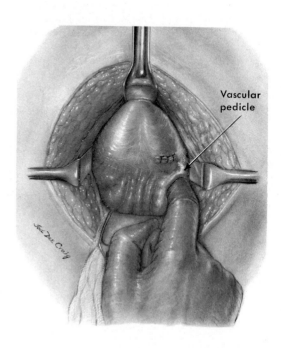

Vascular
pedicle

Figure 77–48. A space is developed by blunt dissection on the lower aspect of the left prostatic vascular pedicle.

Figure 77–49. Curved clamps are placed completely across the left prostatic vascular pedicle, and the scalpel is used to divide it.

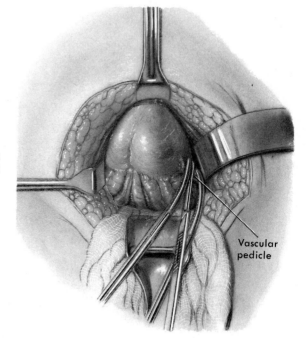

Vascular pedicle

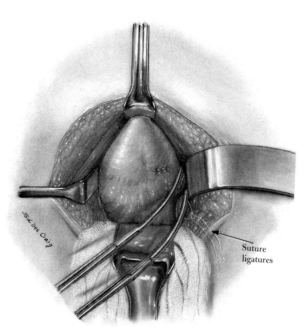

Suture ligatures

Figure 77–50. The severed ends of numerous blood vessels are clearly evident as the suture ligatures are being tied. This part of the operation greatly reduces the potential for bleeding during the rest of the procedure.

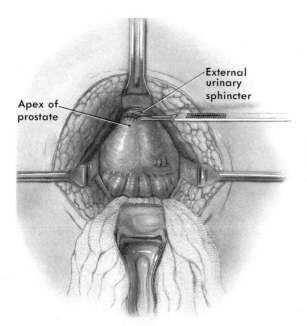

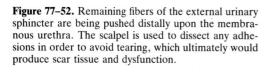

Figure 77–51. Fibers of the external urinary sphincter mechanism are often draped across the apex of the prostate. The scalpel blade is used to begin an atraumatic dissection designed to preserve these fibers.

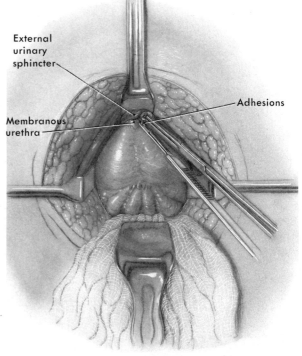

Figure 77–52. Remaining fibers of the external urinary sphincter are being pushed distally upon the membranous urethra. The scalpel is used to dissect any adhesions in order to avoid tearing, which ultimately would produce scar tissue and dysfunction.

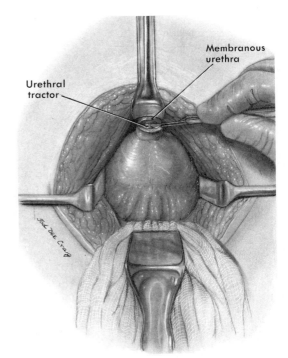

Figure 77–53. The membranous urethra is divided for 180 degrees. The curved urethral tractor is visible through this incision in the urethra. The tractor blades are then closed, and the instrument is withdrawn through the urethral meatus.

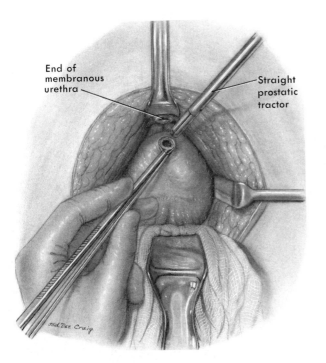

Figure 77–54. The straight prostatic tractor is inserted through the prostatic urethra and into the bladder, and the blades are opened. Care is taken to avoid unnecessary retraction pressure upon the severed end of the membranous urethra and the external urinary sphincteric fibers.

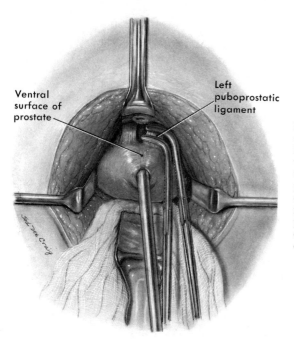

Ventral
surface of
prostate

Left
puboprostatic
ligament

Figure 77–55. Right-angled hemostatic forceps have been applied to the patient's left puboprostatic ligament. The lower clamp should be placed as close as possible to the ventral surface of the prostate. In order to get exposure of this sort, light traction is exerted downward (toward the patient's coccyx). This places the puboprostatic ligaments on tension as they come clearly into view. Excessive traction is avoided to preclude tearing of the ventral surface of the prostate. Following division of these ligaments, the severed ends of each are secured with suture ligatures of 00 chromic catgut.

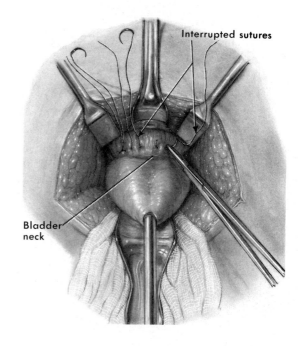

Interrupted sutures

Bladder
neck

Figure 77–56. Interrupted sutures of 00 chromic atraumatic catgut are placed around the circumference of the bladder neck for 180 degrees and are knotted securely. They are not used for the subsequent anastomosis between the bladder neck and the urethra but are placed for hemostatic purposes.

Figure 77–57. This is the surgeon's view when deep, through-and-through hemostatic sutures have been placed and tied across the ventral 180 degrees of the vesical outlet. The surgical blade is held at right angles to the cut surface of the bladder neck muscle. This incision is carried through the epithelial lining of the bladder.

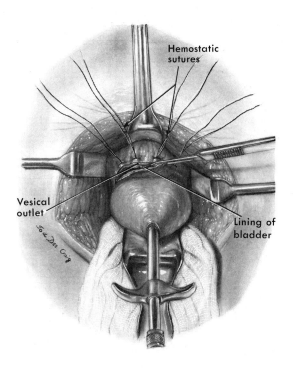

Figure 77–58. The straight tractor is swung toward the patient's left thigh, and the tip of the blade is used to elevate the bladder neck for placement of the far right lateral suture. The interureteric ridge is seen in this view because the surgeon has placed the ventral retractor inside the open bladder neck.

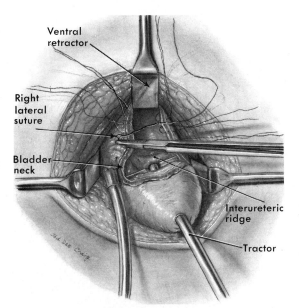

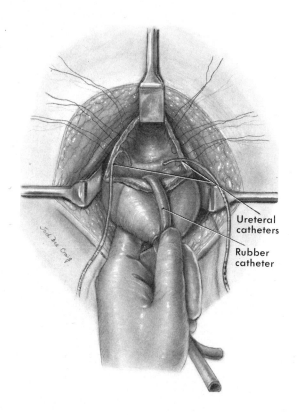

Figure 77–59. For a right-handed surgeon it is useful to replace the metal tractor with a rubber catheter folded upon itself, the index finger of the left hand being advanced to make the dorsal rim of the bladder neck taut. Ureteral catheters have been advanced on either side.

Ureteral catheters

Rubber catheter

Figure 77–60. With a scalpel, the dorsal bladder neck is incised distal to the ureteral orifices. Preferably a margin of 1 cm is left between the cut edge of the orifices. These layers of muscle include the trigonal muscle as well as the detrusor fibers laterally.

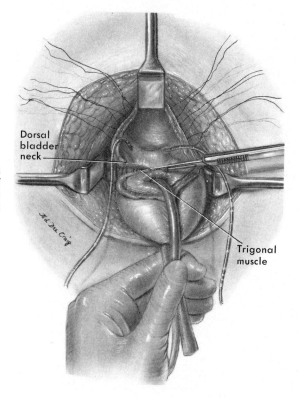

Dorsal bladder neck

Trigonal muscle

Figure 77–61. The index finger of the left hand is in the position shown by the broken line. It is used to elevate the right vas deferens so that the right vas deferens is grasped with the hemostatic forceps through a small opening made in the ventral surface of the anterior leaf of the genital fascia. The early, complete dissection between the two layers of Denonvilliers' fascia makes it possible to accomplish this step easily and promptly. The vas deferens is the remaining structure that holds the seminal vesicles firmly. After division of the vasa, traction on the specimen to be excised does not move the ureters down with it. There are no major blood vessels remaining. The bladder neck is hidden by the ventral retractor.

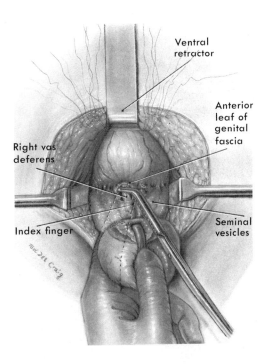

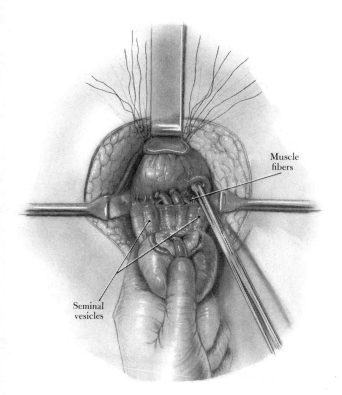

Figure 77–62. The few residual muscle fibers attached to the cephalad tip of the seminal vesicles are removed by blunt dissection.

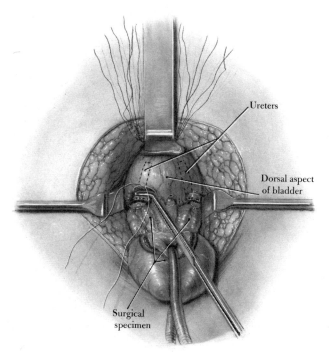

Figure 77–63. The ligature is being placed on the dorsal aspect of the bladder, and the position of the ureters is noted by the broken lines. Rarely can the ureter be seen at this point. Visualization is unwise because deprivation of the blood supply would be an inevitable consequence. This completes the dissection around the seminal vesicles required so that the surgical specimen can be removed.

Figure 77–64. After the surgical specimen has been removed, the urethral catheter is inserted through the urinary meatus and is brought out of the transected membranous urethra. The ends of this catheter are held together by hemostatic forceps so that the catheter is used for traction in a vertical direction. This traction exposes the ventral rim of the membranous urethra, which is then united with interrupted 00 chromic atraumatic sutures to the ventral rim of the vesical neck. The knots on these sutures are tied outside the lumen of the urinary tract. Note the dorsal hemostatic sutures in the bladder neck.

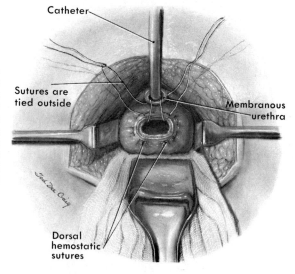

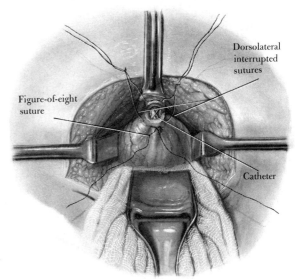

Figure 77–65. Two additional dorsolateral interrupted sutures have been placed and are ready to be tied. In addition, a figure-of-8 suture has been placed to complete the anastomosis. The knot on this suture is placed on the vesical rather than the membranous urethral side. The urethral bag catheter has been advanced into the bladder and inflated.

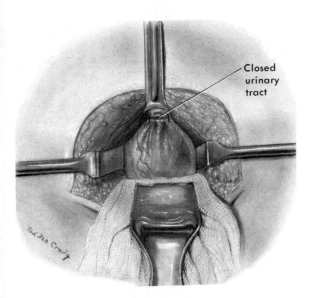

Figure 77–66. This is the appearance of the completely closed urinary tract.

Figure 77–67. This drawing shows the surgical specimen obtained by radical perineal prostatectomy. Note that the fascial coverings of the prostate, the seminal vesicles, and most of the vas deferens are intact.

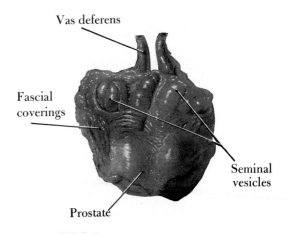

moved. As a matter of routine, the patient is discharged from the hospital on the seventh day after operation. The urinary antiseptic drug is continued when the patient is discharged from the hospital for 10 days.

In simple perineal prostatectomy, the perineal drain is removed on the third postoperative day if serous drainage has disappeared or is greatly decreased. A soap and water enema is administered on the fifth postoperative day if the patient has not had a spontaneous bowel movement. This enema should be administered by a registered nurse or a surgical orderly who is well trained in urologic techniques. The surgical incision sutures are removed on the eighth postoperative day in simple perineal prostatectomy patients. The patient can be discharged from the hospital with his catheter in place. The urethral catheter is allowed to remain until about the twelfth day after operation. The time and amount of each voiding after removal of the catheter are recorded carefully. If the patient has begun to void without dysuria, the urinary antiseptic drug may be discontinued 10 days after removal of the catheter.

Minimal routine follow-up visits after this operation are scheduled at 1 week, 1 month, 6 months, and every 6 months thereafter. An intravenous urogram with a post-voiding film and urine culture are performed whenever pyuria or dysuria develops following discharge from the hospital. Catheterization with determination of residual urine and the passage of metal sounds is contraindicated.

The program for radical perineal prostatectomy varies from that for simple perineal prostatectomy operations in that the urethral catheter is not removed until about the fourteenth postoperative day.

COMPLICATIONS

Inadvertent Removal of Indwelling Urethral Catheter

After simple biopsy, regardless of how soon the indwelling urethral catheter accidentally may be removed, it is not replaced. If the patient is watched carefully, voluntary voiding occurs. No attempt is made to restrict fluid intake. If it becomes evident that blood clots have accumulated in the bladder and are producing acute urinary retention, recatheterization is mandatory. Under such circumstances a straight urethral catheter without an inflatable bag is used.

The use of stylets or catheter guides is best avoided. Because there is no surgical reconstruction of the prostatic urethra in biopsy operations, no difficulty is encountered in recatheterization.

When simple perineal prostatectomy is performed according to the technique described and illustrated in this chapter, there is virtually no raw area left in the prostatic urethra. Instead there is a reconstitution of the urinary tract with its normal lining of transitional cell epithelium. The majority of patients whose catheters have been removed inadvertently, even in the first 12 hours postoperatively, will be able to void spontaneously. Medication with cholinergic drugs and warm baths and ambulation of the patient are helpful in inducing micturition. Even though the amount of the first voidings may be extremely small, the conservative program would not be abandoned until and unless gross, painful distention of the bladder supervenes. In this event two courses of action may be followed.

First, the urethral catheter may be replaced. This should be carried out by an experienced urologist. A well-lubricated catheter is placed upon a malleable metal stylet and is introduced with the right hand. The index finger of the left hand is inserted into the rectum to guide the tip of the catheter as it advances. This procedure minimizes the possibility of inserting the catheter beneath the bladder neck with perforation or undermining of the trigone. As soon as the stylet has been removed and if there is doubt concerning the proper placement of the catheter, especially if urinary return is not immediate, a small amount of radiopaque liquid, not more than 5 ml, is injected into the drainage lumen of the catheter, and a plain x-ray film is exposed. This procedure should be followed before irrigation of the catheter is undertaken. In this way one avoids the serious consequence of irrigating a catheter that is in an extravesical location.

The second course that may be followed is suprapubic insertion of a 14-gauge polyethylene tube through a long needle (see Chapter 8). In this instance the needle is used to aspirate the bladder and to provide a guide within which the polyethylene tube, which has multiple perforations in its terminal 2 cm, is inserted. This maneuver has been found quite safe provided that the bladder is greatly distended. If plastic tube drainage by needle aspiration is the method chosen, the tube is left indwelling until the patient voids spontaneously and without residual urine. This will occur within a week after the operation.

Accidental removal of the catheter after radical perineal prostatectomy should not be cause for alarm. Almost invariably the patient voids spontaneously. If spontaneous voiding does not occur, a considerable period of waiting is permissible, because there is small chance that clot formation will occur within the bladder lumen. The reason is that a direct anastomosis between the bladder neck and the urethra has been effected without a raw surface of any appreciable size. In addition, the prostatic fossa is removed.

If recatheterization is required following radical perineal prostatectomy, two courses are open to the surgeon. First, the polyethylene suprapubic tube may be placed. Second, a small-caliber indwelling urethral catheter can be inserted through a panendoscopic sheath. This sheath should be introduced by direct vision panendoscopy of the anterior and membranous urethra. It must be borne in mind that trauma to the line of anastomosis will cause separation of the bladder neck from the urethra. This is particularly true between the fourth and tenth postoperative days, at which time the absorbable sutures will have become weakened by enzymatic action. Separation of the anastomotic line is particularly undesirable following radical prostatectomy because it predisposes to formation of a narrow, hard stricture in the space between the bladder neck and the urethra.

Extravasation of Urine

Extravasation of urine following simple perineal prostatic biopsy is usually the result of inadvertent entry of the biopsy knife into the prostatic urethra. Dependent drainage is afforded lateral to the surgical incision by the rubber drain, which provides egress for the extravasation. The only unusual measure required for this complication is to allow the indwelling catheter and perineal drain to remain until evidence of extravasation has ceased. This program provides the quickest re-establishment of continuity of the urinary tract and guards against abscess formation or delayed healing of the perineum. If there is doubt concerning the differentiation between serous drainage from the perineum and continuing urinary leakage, an intravenous injection of 5 ml of 5 per cent indigo carmine is employed to make the distinction.

Urinary extravasation occurring early in the postoperative course of simple perineal prostatectomy patients may be ignored. It usually decreases with time when the patient assumes the vertical position for walking. Ambulation therefore should be encouraged. If extravasation becomes evident after the catheter has been removed, no immediate measures are taken unless the drainage site and perineal incisions have healed solidly. In this circumstance, a small-caliber straight rubber catheter is inserted into the reopened drain site to the depth necessary for tapping the extravasation. It is then left strapped in place until all evidence of extravasation has ceased.

Persistent extravasation of urine for 5 days with no indwelling catheter is treated by reinsertion of the urethral catheter. Reinsertion of a well-lubricated, small-caliber urethral catheter at this stage is not particularly dangerous. However, if recatheterization is elected, the catheter should remain indwelling for at least 5 days, even though evidence of extravasation may cease almost immediately. This usually precludes the necessity for multiple recatheterizations. If there is no distal obstruction, recatheterization is not required, since proper healing occurs spontaneously and without stricture formation.

Urinary extravasation occurring after radical perineal prostatectomy is not uncommon during the first postoperative week. The rubber drain lateral to the operative incision is simply left for a prolonged period of time, until all evidence of extravasation has ceased. If urinary extravasation occurs after the catheter has been removed on the fourteenth postoperative day, immediate recatheterization is indicated. The guiding metal stylet is not used for this purpose. The catheter is left inlying for an additional 5 to 7 days, and the free escape of extravasated urine is assured.

Improper Drainage or Occlusion of the Indwelling Catheter

If the urethral catheter becomes occluded after simple biopsy, irrigation with 20 ml or less of mannitol-sorbitol irrigating solution may be employed to clear the passage. If fluids will enter the bladder but will not return, the inflatable bag should be deflated. This often corrects angulation of the tip of the catheter so that it drains properly. If the lumen of the catheter is occluded and cannot be freed to drain adequately, a small urethral catheter with adequate lubrication is inserted through the drainage lumen of the double-lumen inlying catheter and is aspirated by piston syringe. If these measures fail, the indwelling cather is removed, according to the method already outlined, and is not replaced unless the patient fails to void.

Continuous routine postoperative bladder irrigations are employed after perineal enucleation prostatectomy. Reversal of input-outflow directions in the system usually dislodges small clots. Aggressive piston syringe irrigation will help further.

With a continuous irrigation system, one must never attempt to dislodge a clot by simply increasing greatly the inflow rate. This will seat the obstructing clot firmly in the eye of the catheter and guarantee an overdistended bladder, spasms, and more bleeding.

If occlusion occurs without evidence of intravesical clots in the immediate postoperative period, one must suspect that angulation of the tip of the catheter has occurred and is the cause of the occlusion. The catheter bag should be deflated, and as soon as adequate drainage is provided, the catheter is taped into place for the remainder of the early postoperative convalescence.

If hemorrhage has been sufficient to fill the urinary bladder with clotted blood, a piston-type syringe is employed to evacuate the clots. This can usually be done through the urethral catheter. In the event that this procedure fails, the catheter may be removed and replaced with a firm-walled catheter. In extreme cases or whenever there is doubt concerning entry of the catheter into the bladder, a panendoscope is advanced into the bladder for evacuation of the clots. After the clots have been evacuated, a small-caliber catheter is inserted through the panendoscope and is left inlying. The temptation to use a large-caliber catheter should be resisted because the likelihood of this condition recurring is small. Evacuation of the clots is almost always followed by clear urinary drainage.

After radical perineal prostatectomy, improper drainage from the indwelling urethral catheter is almost always the result of a proximally angulated catheter tip. Hemorrhage is rarely the cause. The gradual withdrawal of fluid from the catheter bag, with constant observation to determine the point at which drainage is re-established, constitutes the preferred method of management. If there is enough fluid remaining in the bag to retain the catheter at the point at which proper drainage is re-established, no further corrective measures are indicated. The clearing of clots from the bladder at the termination of the operation is almost always nearly complete after radical perineal prostatectomy.

However, gentle irrigation with 20 ml of irrigant is permissible. It is best not to use a piston-type syringe; undue hydrostatic pressure may cause leakage at the anastomatic line between the bladder neck and the membranous urethra.

Postoperative Hemorrhage

Postoperative hemorrhage is almost never encountered. When it is, one must suspect a blood dyscrasia that was not disclosed during the routine preoperative evaluation. Emergency hematologic consultation is required. If bleeding from the wound is excessive, local hemostasis under infiltration anesthesia should be undertaken promptly.

Urinary Tract Infection

Infection should be treated by changing the patient to a urinary antiseptic drug not previously employed immediately after the collection of an additional urine sample for culture and drug sensitivity testing. The catheter is removed as soon as possible in order to exclude the foreign body factor from the cycle of conditions that favor continuation of infection. An exception to this rule is made when there are copious amounts of viscous, purulent urethral discharge; bladder and urethral irrigation with a 2 per cent neomycin sulfate solution is then used for 48 hours prior to removal of the catheter. Whenever there is inadequate drainage around the catheter, a smaller-caliber catheter is substituted.

Urinary Fistula

Urinary fistula can be eradicated spontaneously by prolonging the time of urethral catheter drainage. Care should be taken to ascertain that the urinary drainage through the catheter is unobstructed.

Delayed Wound Healing and Wound Infection

The nonabsorbable sutures used to close the perineal skin are left for up to 2 weeks postoperatively, if partial dehiscence or gross infection develops. Infected areas are cultured, and drug sensitivity tests are performed on the

PERRY B. HUDSON   **2811**

organisms recovered. As soon as the catheter has been removed from the urethra, warm baths given twice daily will be beneficial. Because of idiosyncrasy in the anastomotic arterial supply, the apex of the lower lip of the incision may slough in an area of approximately 1 cm^2. This slough is almost invariably superficial, for it results from ischemic necrosis of the small area supplied by arteries that have been divided as they traverse longitudinally the "central tendon" projection of the subcutaneous fibers of the external rectal sphincter.

Epididymitis

Epididymitis may occur a few days to several weeks after all types of prostatic surgery. Indeed, epididymitis may be a sequel to urethral instrumentation or cystoscopy that is not accompanied or followed by prostatic surgery. Therefore, to prove effective, preventive measures—that is, urinary antiseptic or antibiotic drugs and vasectomy—must precede urethral instrumentation.

After epididymitis develops, it has a predictable course. General malaise, moderate to high fever, chills, anorexia, and severe scrotal pain herald the presence of this condition. The epididymis—unilaterally or bilaterally, simultaneously or not—becomes greatly swollen and exquisitely tender. Antibiotic drug therapy is often in progress when epididymitis develops.

Therapy consists of restricted ambulation, preferably bed rest. Scrotal support is maintained by bridge or suspensory. Ice packs early and heat later are applied locally in treating this bacterial infection. If an antibiotic drug is administered, it should be a different one from the drug previously given to the patient.

Local therapy hastens recovery, alleviates symptoms, reduces predisposition to recurrent attacks, and prevents scrotal abscess requiring surgical drainage.

Stress Urinary Incontinence

In the occasional patient with stress urinary incontinence or otherwise imperfect urinary control following simple perineal prostatectomy, the pre-existing obstruction will have required the development of very high intravesical pressures for micturition. There will be a period of reconditioning for the detrusor reflex arc while the bladder becomes accustomed to a reduced force of muscular contraction, both to initiate voiding and to serve as a level for "resting tone" of the detrusor. This fact should be explained to the patient carefully, and he should be prompted to continue the use of sphincteric voiding exercises.

Cystitis

Cystitis, often combined with urethritis or pyelonephritis, is most commonly a postoperative problem after transurethral resection or suprapubic prostatic enucleation. The condition is evident from dysuria and the presence of pus in the urine. Confirmation and a guide to therapy are best obtained by urinary bacterial culture and drug sensitivity studies on cultured pure strains of the isolated organisms. Immediate therapy is limited to methenamine mandelate, sulfa drugs, or other ordinary urinary antiseptics. This therapy is continued until the causative organism has been identified, which will permit rational antibiotic therapy.

Persistent or recurring cystitis suggests residual bladder urine, which makes cure nearly impossible. Postvoiding urogram x-ray films or urethral catheterization should not be delayed if cystitis is unresponsive to careful medicinal therapy.

In cases of highly viscous, purulent discharge, irrigation of the bladder with nonabsorbable antibiotics is most helpful.

In any event, therapy must be prompt and definitive if ascending pyelonephritis is to be prevented.

Fecal Fistula

Fecal fistula is treated by sterilization of the bowel, using neomycin sulfate in a dosage of 1 gm per hour for four doses, followed by 1 gm every 4 hours. This program is followed for 72 hours and is then discontinued. Simultaneously with the start of the bowel sterilization program, the patient is placed on parenteral feeding with vitamin supplementation. The rectal sphincter is dilated manually, and a soft rectal tube is inserted for a distance of 14 cm. This tube is never irrigated but when occluded is replaced. The drainage by indwelling urethral catheter is continued until the fecal fistula is closed. Warm baths, two or three times daily, in which the urethra and catheter are not submerged, assist in the healing process. Diligent adherence to this schedule prevents the formation of persistent fistulas.

Pyelonephritis

Parenchymal infection of the kidney is a disorder that requires prompt recognition and vigorous, persistent therapy. It may occur after all types of prostatic surgical operations. A principal consideration is to rule out obstructive uropathy. Either persistent residual urine or partial ureteral obstruction precludes eradication of pyelonephritis to the point of nonrecurrence. Therefore, intravenous urography with a postvoiding film is required before a second course of drug therapy is instituted or whenever the first course fails.

Ureteral Occlusion

Partial or complete ureteral occlusion is an uncommon postprostatectomy disorder, with the exception of the inflammatory type of occlusion that may follow any type of prostatic operation. If intolerable colic, complete nonvisualization by intravenous urography, or overwhelming kidney infection supervenes, relief by ureteral retrograde catheter intubation becomes mandatory. If catheterization fails, surgical relief is necessary. This type of secondary surgery depends upon individual circumstances, so generalizations on this topic are neither appropriate nor helpful.

Acute Urinary Retention Following Removal of the Catheter

When the patient is unable to void voluntarily after 12 days of catheter drainage, a single dose of a cholinergic drug is given in combination with warm baths and ambulation. If these measures are futile, a urethral catheter of small caliber (No. 16 F) is reinserted and is left indwelling for at least 3 days. Intermittent catheterization should not be employed. It is exceedingly rare that a patient is unable to void following 3 additional days of catheter drainage. When this situation does develop, panendoscopy of the lower urinary tract is indicated. In rare instances, a mechanically obstructing flap of tissue must be removed with a resectoscope. When there is no mechanical cause for the obstruction, cystometric studies should be carried out immediately following cystoscopy. In exceedingly rare instances, the cause of obstruction is neurologic.

SURGICAL TRAUMA OF THE RECTUM

The surgeon's fear and anticipation of urinary or fecal fistulas, or combinations of both, are unwarranted. This danger, like that of urinary incontinence, exists mainly in the imagination of surgeons who seldom or never employ perineal techniques for prostatic surgery. Precise surgical technique, prompt recognition of rectal injuries, and adequate surgical correction, combined with proper postoperative care, preclude persistent fistula. The preferred techniques for perineal surgery depicted here are such that quick inspection of the ventral rectal wall will either give assurance that rectal injury has not occurred or will permit immediate recognition of an injury that must be repaired.

Postoperative Care

The postoperative care of the patient with a rectal injury repaired during perineal prostatic surgery is as follows: Before the patient is removed from the operating table, the rectal sphincter should be dilated with the hand to a diameter of approximately 10 cm. This can be accomplished by gradual and persistent dilatation over a period of 5 minutes. The procedure causes a certain degree of paralysis, which may last for several days.

The patient should be started on a program of bowel sterilization medication at once. A soft rectal tube is inserted 15 cm and is left inlying.

Parenteral feeding is prescribed for 2 to 3 days, followed by 1 week of a nonresidue liquid oral diet. The drain in the perineum is removed 1 week after surgery. The urethral catheter is left indwelling for slightly longer than is usual. For example, in simple perineal prostatectomy, it is left indwelling for 2 weeks and is removed only if there is no evidence of rectocutaneous fistula formation. The rectal tube is removed 1 week after surgery, and is changed whenever it becomes occluded. The rectal tube is never irrigated.

References

Al-Ghorab, M. M.: Perineal prostatectomy: Results and evaluation. The Annual Congress of the Egyptian Urological Association, Cairo, 1973.

Belt, E.: Radical perineal prostatectomy in early carcinoma of the prostate. J. Urol., *40*:287, 1942.

Belt, E.: Total perineal prostatectomy in 398 patients with prostatic carcinoma. Urologe, 9:65, 1970.

Belt, E., and Schroeder, F. H.: Total perineal prostatectomy for carcinoma of the prostate. J. Urol., 107:91, 1972.

Belt, E., Ebert, C. E., and Surber, A. C., Jr.: A new anatomic approach in perineal prostatectomy. J. Urol., 41:482, 1939.

Berlin, B. B., et al.: Radical prostatectomy for carcinoma of the prostate: survival in 143 cases treated from 1935 to 1958. J. Urol., 99:97, 1968.

Byar, D. P., and Mostofi, F. K.: Carcinoma of the prostate: prognostic evaluation of certain pathologic features in 208 radical prostatectomies. Examined by the step-section technique. Cancer, 30:5, 1972.

Catalona, W. J., and Scott, W. W.: Carcinoma of the prostate. In Harrison, J. H., Gittes, R. F., Peremutter, A. D., Stamey, T. A., and Walsh, P. C., (Eds.): Campbell's Urology. 4th ed. Vol. 2. Ch. 31. 1978, pp. 1085–1124.

Colston, J. A. C.: The surgical treatment of carcinoma of the prostate. N. Engl. J. Med., 223:205, 1940.

Colston, J. A. C.: Carcinoma of the prostate: A study of the percentage of cases suitable for the radical operation. JAMA, 127:69, 1945.

Colston, J. A. C.: Radical perineal prostatectomy for early cancer: follow-up studies of 108 personal cases. JAMA, 169:700, 1959.

Colston, J. A. C., and Brendler, H.: Endocrine therapy in carcinoma of the prostate; preparation of patients for radical perineal prostatectomy. JAMA, 134:848, 1947.

Crabtree, E. G.: Surgery of the fibrous prostate; an operation for total excision of the gland. Am. J. Surg., 8:958, 1930.

Crabtree, E. G.: Total perineal prostatectomy for the small prostate. Am. J. Surg., 18:251, 1932.

Culp, O. S.: Metastases from occult carcinoma of the prostate. J. Urol., 40:530, 1938.

Culp, O. S.: Radical perineal prostatectomy; its past, present and possible future. J. Urol., 98:618, 1967.

Culp, O. S., and Meyer, J. J.: Proceedings: radical prostatectomy in the treatment of prostatic cancer. Cancer, 32:1113, 1973.

Davis, W. H., Scardino, P. L., and Carlton, F. E.: Radical perineal prostatectomy: a 20-year overview. J. Urol., 106:100, 1971.

Estrada, P. C., and Scardino, P. L.: Total perineal prostatectomy after cobalt 60 therapy: report of a case. J. Urol., 106:100, 1971.

Fiedler, U., et al.: Results of radical perineal prostatectomy: 14 years' experience (author's translation). Urologe (A), 16:56, 1977.

Gibson, T. E.: Improvements in perineal prostatectomy. Surg. Gynecol. Obstet., 47:531, 1928.

Hauri, D., Schauwecker, H., Schmucki, O., et al.: Urinary continence after radical prostatectomy: the urodynamic proof of an antomical hypothesis (author's translation). Urol. Int., 31:(3):145, 1976.

Henline, R. B.: Prostatic calculi: treatment by subtotal perineal prostatectomy. J. Urol., 44:146, 1940.

Hinman, F.: Principles and Practice of Urology. Philadelphia, W. B. Saunders Co., 1935.

Hinman, F.: Surgery in cancer of the prostate. JAMA, 119:6669, 1942.

Hinman, F., Jr.: Early diagnosis and radical treatment of prostatic cancer. California Med., 68:338, 1948.

Hodges, C. V.: Vesicourethral anastomosis after radical prostatectomy experience with the Jewett modification. J. Urol., 118:209, 1977.

Hudson, P. B.: Symposium on the prostate. Perineal prostatectomy. Urol. Clin. North Am., 2:69, 1975.

Hudson, P. B.: Perineal prostatectomy. In Campbell, M. E., and Harrison, J. H. (Eds.): Urology. 3rd ed. Vol. 3. Philadelphia, W. B. Saunders Co., 1970, p. 2427.

Hudson, P. B., and Stout, A. P.: An Atlas of Prostatic Surgery. Philadelphia, W. B. Saunders Co., 1962.

Hudson, P. B., and Stout, A. P.: Prostatic cancer. XVI. Comparison of physical examination and biopsy for detection of curable lesions. N.Y. State J. Med., 66:351, 1966.

Hudson, P. B., Ty, M., Jr., and Lilien, O. M.: Prostatic cancer. XV. Incurable cancer following conservative prostatic surgery for clinically benign obstruction. Ann. Surg., 152:308, 1960.

Inglis, J. M.: Premedication in the geriatric patients. Geriatrics, 22:115, 1967.

Jewett, H. J.: Radical perineal prostatectomy in early carcinoma of prostate: An analysis of 190 cases. J. Urol., 61:277, 1949.

Jewett, H. J.: Radical perineal prostatectomy for early cancer. Bul. N.Y. Acad. Med., 34:26, 1958.

Jewett, H. J.: The case for radical perineal prostatectomy. J. Urol., 103:195, 1970.

Jewett, H. J.: The present status of radical prostatectomy for stages A and B prostatic cancer. Urol. Clin. North Am., 2:105, 1975.

Jewett, H. J.: Radical perineal prostatectomy for palpable, clinically localized, non-obstructive cancer: experience at the Johns Hopkins Hospital 1909–1963. J. Urol., 124:492, 1980.

Jewett, H. J., Bridge, R. W., Gray, G. F., Jr., and Shelley, Wm.: The palpable nodule of prostatic cancer. Results 15 years after radical excision. JAMA, 203:403, 1968.

Johnson, C. M.: Perineal prostatectomy. J. Urol., 44:821, 1940.

Kimbrough, J. C., and Rowe, R. B.: Carcinomas of prostate. J. Urol., 66:373, 1951.

King, D. S.: Post-operative pulmonary complications: part played by anesthesia and shown by 2 years study at Massachusetts General Hospital. Anesth. Analg., 12:343, 1933.

Kischev, S.: New elements in the technique of perineal prostatectomy. Urologe (A), 11:130, 1972.

Kittbredge, W. E.: Perineal approach to the prostate. J. Med. Assoc. Ga., 46:467, 1957.

Kraus, C. T., and Persky, L.: Radical perineal prostatectomy in patients over age of seventy. Urology, 18(4):368, 1981.

Lee, L. W., Malashock, E. M., and Davis, N. B.: Experience with transurethral prostatic resection and perineal prostatectomy in one clinic: comparative review of 3400 patients. Nebr. Med. J., 43:47, 1958.

Lewis, L. G.: Carcinoma of the prostate: Young's radical perineal prostatectomy. J. Urol., 47:302, 1942.

Lowsley, O. S.: Total perineal prostatectomy. J. Urol., 43:275, 1940.

Lowsley, O. S., and Kirwin, T. J.: Clinical Urology. 2nd ed. Baltimore, The Williams & Wilkins Co., 1944.

Lucas, W. G.: Radical perineal prostatectomy for carcinoma of prostate. Med. J. Aust., 1:378, 1960.

McCullough, D. L., et al.: Morbidity of pelvic lymphadenectomy and radical prostatectomy for prostatic cancer. J. Urol., 117:206, 1977.

Murphy, G. P., et al.: Prostatic cancer evolution of treatment at a comprehensive center (1970–1974). Urology, 8:357, 1976.

Narshy, W., Zayed, H. and Bishara, A.: Anesthesia for perineal prostatectomy. M.E.J. Anesth., 4(3), 1974.

Rathore, A. H.: Perineal prostatectomy. JPMA, *30*:204, 1980.

Rich, A. R.: On the frequency of occurrence of occult carcinoma of the prostate. J. Urol., *33*:215, 1936.

Saadi, M. H.: Perineal retropubic prostatectomy. Br. J. Clin. Pract., *28*:331, 1974.

Scott, W. W., and Parlow, A. L.: Evaluation of hormonal therapy followed by radical perineal prostatectomy on selected cases of advanced prostatic carcinoma. J. Urol., *65*:1093, 1951.

Smith, G. G.: Total perineal prostatectomy. Pa. Med. J., *44*:1391, 1941.

Smith, G. G.: The treatment of carcinoma of the prostate. J. Urol., *64*:671, 1950.

Vest, S. A.: Radical perineal prostatectomy, modification of closure. Surg. Gynecol. Obstet., *70*:935, 1940.

Walsh, P. C., and Jewett, H. J.: Radical surgery for prostatic cancer. Cancer, *45*:1906, 1980.

Way, G. L., and Clarke, H. L.: Anesthetic technique for prostatectomy. Lancet, *4*:888, 1959.

Wheeler, J. S.: A modification of the Young procedure for radical perineal prostatectomy. J. Urol., *114*:419, 1975.

Young, H. H.: The early diagnosis and radical cure of carcinoma of the prostate: being a study of 40 cases and presentation of a radical operation which was carried out in 4 cases. Johns Hopkins Hosp. Bull., *16*:315, 1905.

Young, H. H.: Advantages of perineal route in treatment of various diseases of prostate. Proc. Roy. Soc. Med., *23*:65, 1930.

Young, H. H.: An exposition of perineal prostatectomy. JAMA, *103*:1085, 1934.

Young, H. H.: The radical cure of cancer of the prostate. Surg. Gynecol. Obstet., *64*:472, 1937.

Young, H. H.: Perineal prostatectomy. *In* Cyclopedia of Medicine. Philadelphia, F. A. Davis Co., 1940, pp. 576–593.

Young, H. H.: The cure of cancer of the prostate by radical prostatectomy (prostastoseminal vesiculectomy): History, literature and statistics of Young's operation. J. Urol., *53*:188, 1945.

Young, H. H., and Davis, D. M.: Young's Practice of Urology. Philadelphia, W. B. Saunders Co., 1926.

Zoedler, D., et al.: Report of 100 total prostatectomies (author's translation). Urologe (A), *16*:61, 1977.

CHAPTER 78

Transurethral Surgery

LAURENCE F. GREENE, M.D., PH.D.

TRANSURETHRAL PROSTATIC RESECTION

SELECTION OF PATIENTS

The decision as to whether transurethral prostatic resection (TURP) for benign prostatic hyperplasia is warranted should be made after evaluating the patient's symptoms, estimating the size of the prostate, and noting objective evidence of outlet obstruction.

Symptoms. Urinary symptoms that result from benign prostatic hyperplasia may be obstructive or irritative. The former includes decrease in caliber, loss of normal trajectory and interruption of the urinary stream, hesitancy, and straining to urinate. Acute retention may occur. These symptoms result from mechanical obstruction to passage of urine by the adenomatous mass in the prostatic urethra. The irritative symptoms, such as frequency, urgency, and urgency incontinence, in the absence of significant residual urine and infection, result from detrusor hyperreflexia (Turner-Warwick et al., 1973; Turner-Warwick, 1973; Cote et al., 1981). The latter condition is a simple reflex response initiated by stimulation of afferent sensory nerves entrapped or irritated by the enlarged prostate. This stimulation evokes a detrusor response.

Size of Prostate. An estimate of the size of the prostate is made after digital rectal examination, excretory urography (noting the prostatic filling defect), and endoscopy. Each of these examinations may yield false impressions. Thus, a significant median lobe enlargement may not be detected by digital rectal examination. Furthermore, if the examination is performed in the presence of a large amount of residual urine, the base of the distended bladder may be palpated and thus be misinterpreted as an enlarged prostate. In addition, during excretory cystography, the enlarged prostate may not cause a visible filling defect. Finally, endoscopic evaluation of the size of the prostate is made by noting the increase in length and height of the prostatic fossa and the intrusions of the prostatic lobes into the urethra. Unfortunately, the lateral extent of the prostate cannot always be accurately estimated endoscopically; therefore, the estimate of the size of the prostate may be incorrect. In general, however, estimates gained from these studies will indicate whether transurethral surgery is feasible.

Evidence of Obstruction. Some objective evidence of outlet obstruction should be sought. The urologist's observation of a poor stream, which the patient confirms to be typical, is important. Sophisticated urodynamic studies usually are not necessary, but a uroflow determination is advisable. Nomograms can be developed from such studies, and it has been demonstrated that in 98 per cent of the maximal flow measurements in patients with obstruction, the nomogram values are less than minus 2 standard deviations (Siroky et al., 1979, 1980).

Patients with significant symptoms, enlarged prostates, and poor uroflow tracings are surgical candidates. Those with mild symptoms, with or without enlargement of the prostate and normal uroflow values, can be treated conservatively. Patients with significant symptoms, without prostate enlargement but with uroflow values suggesting outlet obstruction, may be considered for transurethral incisions of the prostate.

PREOPERATIVE MANAGEMENT

Diseases that frequently affect men in the age group in which benign prostatic hyperplasia is common are coronary, valvular, and hypertensive heart disease; cerebrovascular disease;

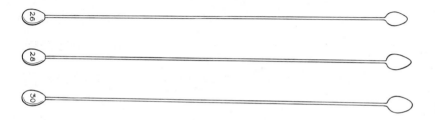

Figure 78–1. Otis bulbs.

chronic lung diseases; renal insufficiency; and diabetes mellitus; patients with prostatic carcinoma may experience intravascular coagulation and fibrinolysis. Preoperative measures to control these diseases are necessary.

ANESTHESIA

Regional anesthesia by subarachnoid block is the safest mode of administration and is thus employed most often. General anesthesia may be used, and local anesthesia has been suggested in selected cases.

EQUIPMENT

A variety of resectoscopes, with working elements that control the loop in different manners, and excellent telescopes are available. Resections can be performed with continuous flow resectoscopes, with suprapubic trocar cystostomy, or with conventional means. Proponents of each technique claim its superiority. The irrigant employed should be nonhemolytic and near-isotonic. A 1.5 per cent glycine solution, which is commercially available, is satisfactory.

TECHNIQUE

Calibration of the Urethra. The TURP commences with urethral calibration to prevent postoperative urethral strictures. Evidence is convincing that urethral trauma, resulting from the use of resectoscope sheaths too large for the caliber of the urethra, causes such strictures (Emmett et al., 1963). The caliber of the meatus and fossa navicularis in approximately 25 per cent of men undergoing transurethral surgery is 26F or smaller, and that of the anterior urethra in 10 per cent of these men is also 26F or smaller. The caliber of resectoscope sheaths usually employed for TURP, on the other hand, is 26F or larger. The repeated movements of such sheaths within the tight urethra produce significant trauma. It is not sufficient to dilate the urethra with sounds or to employ the smaller resectoscope sheath of 24F in such individuals. A meatotomy or internal urethrotomy, or both, may be necessary.

Calibration is performed by drawing the penis up at right angles to the patient's body, and an Otis bulb (bougie à boule) (Fig. 78–1) lubricated with sterile jelly is carefully and slowly passed through the meatus, fossa navicularis, and anterior urethra. Bulbs of 26, 28, and 30F are advanced successively, and resistance or "jump or hang" during their passage is an indication for meatotomy or urethrotomy.

MEATOTOMY. Meatotomy and incision in the fossa navicularis will be considered together. If possible, meatotomy is avoided because the normal meatus imparts the whirling nature to the urinary stream and thereby prevents spraying. If meatotomy is advisable to prevent meatal stricture, an Otis urethrotome is introduced into the urethra for a distance of 2 cm, with the dial and the knife slot pointing upward (12 o'clock position of the urethra). The wheel is turned until definite, but not severe, resistance is encountered. The knife handle is then slowly but deliberately withdrawn, thereby incising the meatus at the 12 o'clock position. Passage of a 30F Otis bulb is then attempted; if unsuccessful, the meatotomy is repeated until the bulb can pass easily.

Narrowing at the proximal end of the fossa navicularis is encountered more frequently than narrowing at the meatus. Incision at this site is accomplished by passing the Otis urethrotome approximately 2 cm into the urethra and performing the maneuvers already described; an effort is made to avoid meatotomy for the reasons mentioned.

INTERNAL URETHROTOMY. The penis is drawn up at right angles to the patient's body. An Otis urethrotome in the closed position is inserted into the urethra with the dial and knife slot pointing to the 12 o'clock position of the urethra (Fig. 78–2). The instrument is passed gently and slowly until the tip rests lightly in the bulbar urethra. An assistant stretches the penis along the length of the urethrotome while the surgeon expands the urethrotome by turning the wheel in a clockwise direction. Short, to-and-fro movements of the urethrotome are made while the wheel is turned; these movements

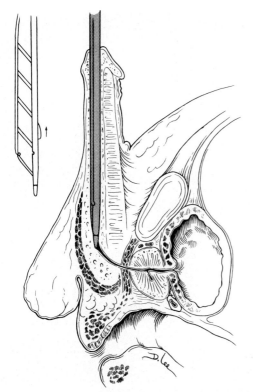

Figure 78–2. Otis urethrotome within urethra. *Inset,* Urethrotome expanded and knife blade traversing knife slot.

enable the operator to appreciate when the urethrotome is snug within the urethra. (Expansion of the urethrotome should not be measured by the numbers on the dial. These values are frequently inaccurate, particularly if the urethrotome has been employed for some time.)

The aim of the procedure is to make a clean, linear cut in the roof of the urethra (12 o'clock position) without tearing the urethra. The knife is withdrawn through the entire length of the urethra with a slow, steady, deliberate motion. The urethrotome is then closed and removed, and passage of a 30F bulb is attempted. If obstruction is still encountered, internal urethrotomy is repeated until a 30F bulb can be passed easily through the anterior urethra. Subsequent urethroscopy will reveal that only the narrowed areas of the urethra have been cut.

Preliminary Cystoscopic Examination. The bladder is examined and any abnormality or pathologic lesion is noted. Particular attention is paid to vesical diverticula, which should be entered, if possible, and examined. These diverticula must be examined at the end of the resection to make certain that they do not contain prostatic chips. The trigone, the position of the ureteral orifices, and their relationship to the prostatic enlargement should be determined. Hypertrophy of the trigone may be mistaken for prostatic hyperplasia, and resection of this structure may damage the ureteral orifices.

An estimate must be made of the size of the prostate to decide whether TURP is feasible. This assessment is accomplished by noting the distance from the most intravesical extent of the prostate to the verumontanum. This distance may be increased from a normal length of 2 to 3 cm to 4 or 6 cm in patients with significant prostatic hyperplasia. Similarly, with increasing enlargement of the lateral lobes, the distance between the roof and the floor increases. The extent of the lobular protrusion of the prostate into the prostatic urethra is noted, but the lateral extent of the prostate is difficult to estimate.

Surgical Plan. The goal of each operation is excision of the adenoma down to the surgical capsule. It is therefore imperative to recognize adenomatous tissue and to distinguish it from surgical capsule. Prostatic tissue covered by urethral mucosa is flesh-colored and granular and contains visible arteries and veins. Resection of the mucosa exposes coarse, white, granular, vascular adenomatous tissue (Fig. 78–3A). The surgical capsule appears as a firm, white, fibrous membrane (Fig. 78–3B).

The technique to be described for performing prostatic resection is one that "works for me." There is, however, no *one* right way to perform a resection. Expert resectionists offer convincing arguments as to why, for example, the resection must be started anteriorly, or at the median lobe, or at the 3 or 9 o'clock position, or at the most accessible position. Each resectionist, with increasing experience, develops a technique that is personally satisfactory.

My technique is influenced by three factors. First, inasmuch as tissue moves during a resection and it is easier to resect tissue from the floor of the prostatic urethra than from the roof or lateral walls, early maneuvers are designed to drop the tissue into the floor. Second, I seek to define the boundaries of the surgical field as early as possible. Finally, I make an earnest effort to maintain hemostasis throughout the operation.

Excision of Tissue. The goal when resecting prostatic tissue is to slice a fragment of tissue cleanly. The fragment then floats into the bladder, propelled by the irrigant. The inexperienced resectionist generally encounters two problems. First, the distal end of the chip of tissue remains attached; second, the excised tissue may stick to the loop. Experience gained

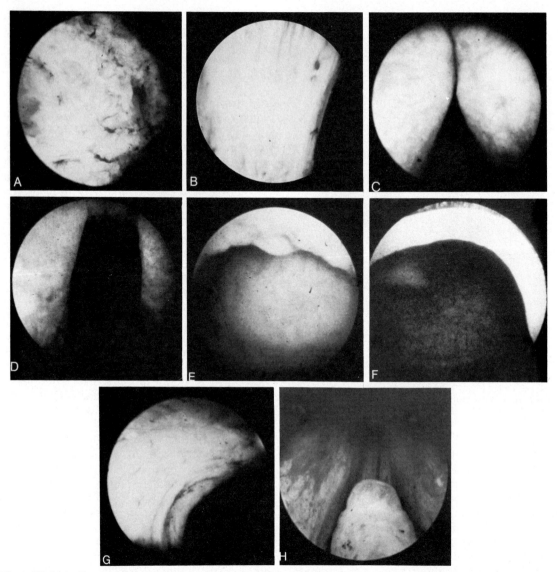

Figure 78–3. *A,* Coarse, white, meaty appearance of prostatic adenoma. *B,* Firm, white, fibrous appearance of prostatic capsule. *C,* Inverted V appearance of lateral lobes at 12 o'clock position, indicating intravesical extension of these lobes. *D,* Inverted U appearance of lateral lobes at 12 o'clock position, indicating intraurethral confinement of these lobes. *E,* Prostatovesical junction is poorly defined if bladder is empty. *F,* Prostatovesical junction is defined if bladder is partially filled. *G,* Circular fibromuscular fibers of vesical neck at 11 o'clock position. *H,* Apices of lateral lobes are flattened and spread apart if bladder is full.

with certain maneuvers minimizes both problems.

The excised chip of prostatic tissue should be shaped like a boat, and this can be accomplished by manipulating the loop in the same manner as a backhoe. The loop is extended and embedded in the prostatic tissue by activating the cutting current. The loop is drawn through the prostatic tissue for the desired distance, and the ocular end of the resectoscope is then elevated, carrying the loop out of the prostatic

tissue and thereby severing the distal end of the chip from the prostate. The loop excises tissue not by moving through the prostatic tissue in a straight line but by scooping out the chip of tissue. The chip should be cut off before the loop enters the sheath. Charring of the sheath is not desirable and is avoided by proper timing, so that the current is discontinued just as the loop enters the sheath.

Unduly slow passage of the loop through the tissue causes the latter to adhere to the loop, a difficulty that is eliminated with practice. The experienced resectionist will disengage tissue with a subsequent cut. Vision is obscured if a chip of tissue is adherent to a loop that is within the sheath. By extending the loop, the prostatic urethra is visualized and the site of the next cut can be selected. The loop with its adherent chip is moved into position, and the ensuing cut releases one or both chips of tissue. From time to time, however, it may be necessary to remove the working element and free the prostatic chip by moving the loop sideways through a plastic or suede brass brush. Tissue may adhere to a loop that is broken, carbonized, or coated with adherent tissue.

An additional movement of the resectoscope sheath may be employed to cut long chips of tissue during resection of large adenomas. The loop is extended to its limit and is maintained in that position. The extended loop is drawn through the prostate by sliding the sheath through the urethra antegrade. When the apex is approached, the sheath is held stationary and the loop is permitted to finish its excursion to cut off the prostatic chip. The sheath is then moved forward, and the loop is extended to send the cut chip into the bladder and to prepare for the next stroke.

This technique is applied only when resecting moderate- or large-sized glands. With this technique, the loop is visible as it enters and is drawn through the tissue, but the exact site of its emergence can only be estimated. Therefore, injury to the external sphincter is avoided if apical tissue is not excised while sliding the sheath of the resectoscope through the urethra. During resection of apical tissue, the sheath is placed and maintained in a position in which movements of the loop will not damage the external urethral sphincter. The length of the prostatic chip is then wholly dependent on the distance of excursion of the loop. Similarly, when excising small adenomas, it is sufficient to resect chips that are equal in length to excursions of the loop. Routine cuts are made antegrade toward the surgeon. Rarely, when fragments to be cut are close to the verumontanum, retrograde cuts may be needed.

RESECTION OF MODERATE-SIZED, BILATERAL PROSTATIC ADENOMAS. Bilateral, lateral lobe prostatic hyperplasia of moderate size is encountered most frequently. The resection of such a gland commences anteriorly at the vesical neck. If the lateral lobes form an inverted V at the vesical neck anteriorly (Fig. 78–3C), they extend intravesically and must be excised by directing the loop intravesically. If they form an inverted U (Fig. 78–3D), the lobes are entirely intraurethral, prostatic adenoma is not present at the neck of the bladder, and the resection should be limited to the prostatic fossa; resection of the normal vesical neck should be avoided.

The importance of bladder distention during the different stages of the operation must be understood, and the degree of distention is varied and regulated by the surgeon. The bladder should be moderately distended, particularly anteriorly, before proximal resection near the vesical neck is begun. If the bladder is empty or nearly empty, the vesical neck and prostatovesical junction will not be clearly defined, the prostatic fossa may merge imperceptibly with the lateral and anterior walls of the bladder, and, if flabby or atonic, the bladder may prolapse almost into the prostatic fossa (Fig. 78–3E). Resection under such circumstances carries the danger of resecting the walls of the bladder adjacent to the prostate, with possible perforation. Therefore, 75 to 100 ml of irrigant should be instilled into the bladder before resection is begun. Moderate distention of the bladder results in a clear definition of the vesical neck and the prostatovesical junction, causes the walls of the bladder to move out of the surgical field, and makes resection of these walls virtually impossible (Fig. 78–3F).

Resection is initiated at the 11 o'clock position, and successive cuts are made until the circular fibromuscular fibers of the vesical neck are exposed (Fig. 78–3G). These exposed fibers become the proximal boundary of the surgical field (Fig. 78–4). They should not be resected, however, because deep resection may result in postoperative contracture of the vesical neck. Furthermore, the prostatovesical junction is thin, and deep resection at this site may result in separation of the prostatovesical junction and perforation. Excision of prostatic tissue proceeds in a counterclockwise direction to the 9 o'clock position, exposing the prostatic surgical capsule distally. The purpose of this maneuver is to free the bulk of the right lateral lobe and to permit it to drop medially onto the floor of the prostatic fossa (Fig. 78–5).

Attention is then turned to the left lobe anteriorly. It may be noted that resection of the right lobe results in a shift of the left lobe. Thus, if an inverted V was present at the 12 o'clock position at the start of the resection, excision of part of the right lobe may cause the left lobe to shift downward; the apex of the V would thus be at the 1 or 2 o'clock position. Resection of the left lateral lobe is then started at the 1 or 2

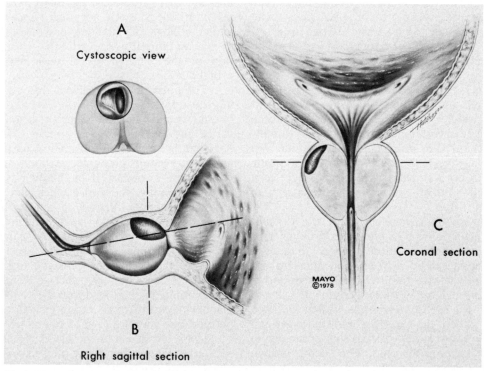

A
Cystoscopic view

C
Coronal section

MAYO
©1978

B
Right sagittal section

Figure 78–4. Exposure of circular fibromuscular fibers in region of vesical neck from 11 o'clock to 9 o'clock positions.

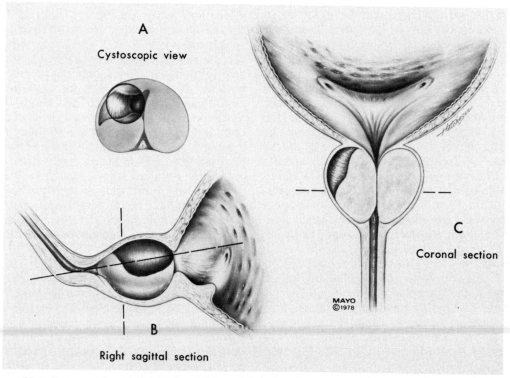

A
Cystoscopic view

C
Coronal section

MAYO
©1978

B
Right sagittal section

Figure 78–5. Exposure of prostatic capsule on right and dropping of right lateral lobe onto floor of prostatic fossa.

o'clock position and carried down to the 3 o'clock position in the region of the vesical neck, exposing the circular fibers of this structure. The resection is continued distally in a clockwise direction, causing the left lateral lobe to drop medially onto the floor of the prostatic fossa. When this excision is completed, the lateral lobes, which were separate at the start of the procedure, are often touching ("kissing laterals") (Fig. 78–6). Thus, the goal of dropping the lateral lobes onto the floor of the prostatic fossa, where they may be excised more easily, has been achieved. The 12 o'clock position near the vesical neck is then examined; usually, only a small amount of tissue need be excised from this site.

With the right lateral lobe lying on the floor of the prostatic fossa, resection of this fallen lobe is started at the 9 o'clock position proximally; the posterior portion—that lying on the floor of the prostatic fossa—is resected. Care must be taken not to resect too deeply in the region of the inferior aspect of the vesical neck, to prevent undermining of the trigone. The resection is carried directly to the right side of the verumontanum (Fig. 78–7). By this maneuver, the distal boundary of the resection, posteriorly adjacent to the verumontanum, is

quickly and accurately established. The apical portion of the right lobe that is attached laterally is not excised at this time but has been "undercut," which aids in its identification and distinguishes it from sphincter.

A similar procedure is carried out on the left lobe. Starting proximally at the 3 o'clock position, the posterior portion of the lobe is resected to the left side of the verumontanum (Fig. 78–8); the apical portion of the lobe attached laterally remains but is undercut. While resecting proximally, care is again taken not to undermine the trigone. At this stage, therefore, the posterior portions of the lateral lobes to the verumontanum have been excised. The adenoma that remains is situated anteriorly, laterally, and distally in the prostatic urethra. The apical portion of this tissue, that adjacent to the verumontanum, is excised (undercut).

The verumontanum, an easily identified landmark denoting the distal boundary of the resection posteriorly, renders excision of the posterior portion of the lateral lobes, as described, a safe procedure, and urinary incontinence is unlikely. Such a reassuring landmark is not visible as the resectoscope is turned to view the anterior and lateral distal boundaries of the resection. Undercutting the lateral lobes as de-

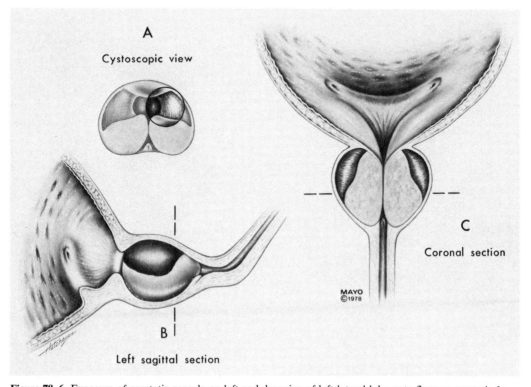

Figure 78–6. Exposure of prostatic capsule on left and dropping of left lateral lobe onto floor or prostatic fossa.

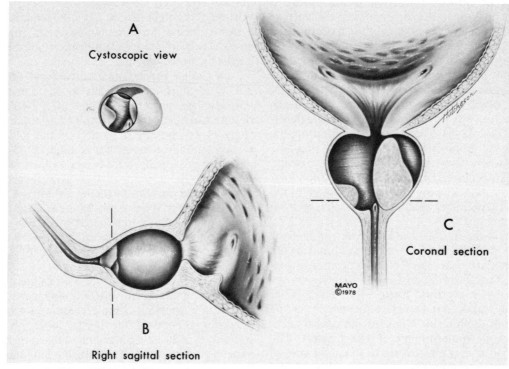

Figure 78–7. Excision of posterior portion of right lateral lobe to the verumontanum.

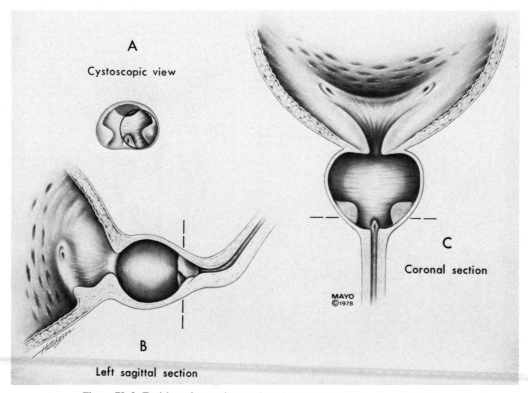

Figure 78–8. Excision of posterior portion of left lateral lobe to verumontanum.

scribed, however, makes them readily identifiable as masses projecting into the prostatic fossa, and they can be removed without fear of damage to the external sphincter.

Resection of the right apical mass is begun in the midline anteriorly and carried in counterclockwise fashion toward the site of the undercutting (Fig. 78–9). The procedure is then repeated on the left apical mass; the posterior portions of these masses may fall alongside or even over the verumontanum. Resection of these fragments completes the excision of the adenoma (Fig. 78–10).

Resection of adenoma on the floor of the prostatic fossa and about the verumontanum frequently may be aided by counterpressure from a finger in the rectum. The index finger inserted into an O'Connor sheath provides an estimate of the amount and site of prostatic adenoma and, by counterpressure, facilitates excision of tissue. In addition, the verumontanum, if obscured by fallen prostatic tissue, may be rendered visible by digital rectal pressure.

The degree of filling of the bladder is also of significance when resecting at the apex of the prostate. If the bladder is essentially filled, the vesical distention is transmitted to the prostatic fossa, resulting in spreading, flattening, and anterolateral displacement of the lateral lobes (see Fig. 78–3*H*). Resection of the apices of the lateral lobes under such circumstances is more difficult; the fragments are smaller, and rectal counterpressure, if necessary, is less effective. If, however, the bladder and prostatic fossa are not distended by irrigant, the apical tissue projects into the prostatic fossa about the verumontanum and is resected easily (Fig. 78–11*A*).

The external sphincter is slightly distal to the verumontanum and is identified simply as the site at which the urethra first assumes a circular shape. Others describe "a circular wrinkling of the overlying mucosa with movements of the instrument" or "transverse wrinkles in the urethral mucosa, something like a concertina." These nuances are difficult to appreciate.

RESECTION OF LARGE, BILATERAL PROSTATIC ADENOMAS. In resecting these tumors, the basic approach is the same as that described for moderate-sized adenomas, namely, dropping the lateral lobes onto the floor of the prostatic fossa for easier excision. This is accomplished in successive steps, however, and for descriptive purposes the operative field is divided into a vesical zone, which contains tissue proximal and distal to but near the vesical neck; a midprostatic

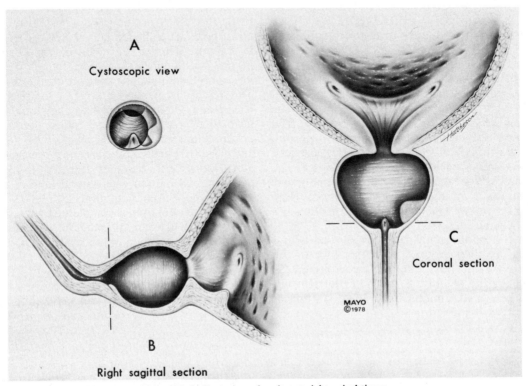

Figure 78–9. Resection of undercut right apical tissue.

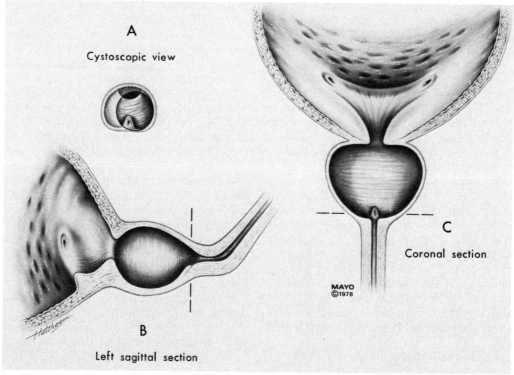

A

Cystoscopic view

B

Left sagittal section

C

Coronal section

MAYO
©1978

Figure 78–10. Completion of resection by excising undercut left apical tissue.

zone, which contains more distal tissue; and an apical zone, which consists of tissue at the apex of the prostate adjacent to the verumontanum (Fig. 78–12).

The resection is started anteriorly on the right lobe from the 11 to the 9 o'clock positions. The intravesical tissue is excised and the resection is then continued distally, exposing the fibromuscular vesical neck (Fig. 78–13). The result is the dropping of the proximal portion of the right lateral lobe—that in the vesical neck zone—onto the floor of the prostatic fossa. The process is repeated on the left lobe anteriorly from the 1 to the 3 o'clock positions (Fig. 78–14). Tissue remaining at the 12 o'clock position is then resected.

The midprostatic portions of the lateral lobes are then dropped onto the floor of the fossa. Again, this result is accomplished by resecting the anterior portions of the right lateral lobe in the midprostatic zone, starting at

the 11o'clock position and carrying the resection to the 9 o'clock position (Fig. 78–15); the anterior portions of the left lateral lobe are treated in a similar manner (Fib. 78–16). The portions of the lateral lobes that come to rest on the floor of the midprostatic zone are then resected. The resection of anterior tissue, followed by resection of tissue dropped to the floor, may have to be repeated several times, depending on the length of the lateral lobes (Figs. 78–17, and 78–18). Finally, the resection reaches the apical zone, and tissue is resected from the posterior portions of each lateral lobe at each side of the verumontanum (Figs. 78–19 and 78–20). The operation is completed by resection of tissue in the apical zone in the manner described for resection of moderate-sized, bilateral adenomas (Fig. 78–21).

RESECTION OF TRILOBAR PROSTATIC ADENOMAS. These adenomas usually consist of hyperplasia of each lateral lobe as well as the

Text continued on page 2831

Figure 78–11. *A*, Apices of lateral lobes approach one another if bladder is empty. Compare with Figure 78–3H *B*, Pulsatile or continuously bleeding artery. *C*, Sheetlike bleeding from venous sinus. *D*, "High-riding" vesical neck with no visible prostatic hyperplasia. *E*, Collings knife at 7 o'clock position at vesical neck. *F*, Start of incision at vesical neck. *G*, Incision deepened at vesical neck between right lateral and median lobes. *H*, Incision in floor of prostatic urethra approaching right side of verumontanum (sequence continued in Figure 78–23).

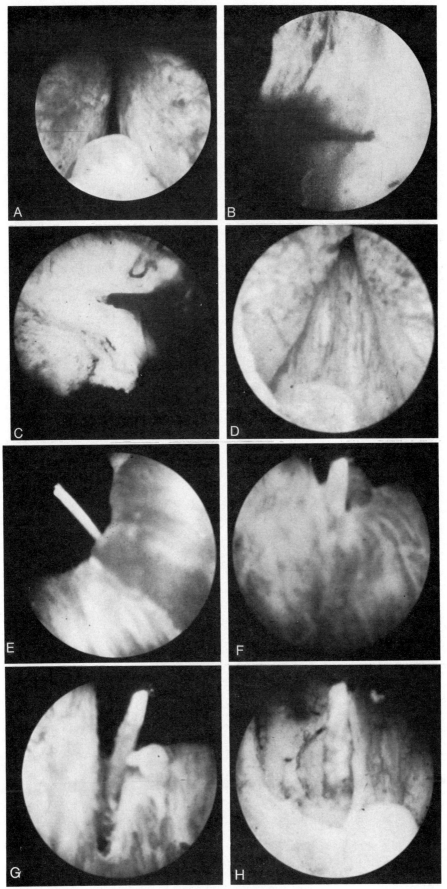

Figure 78–11. *See legend on opposite page*

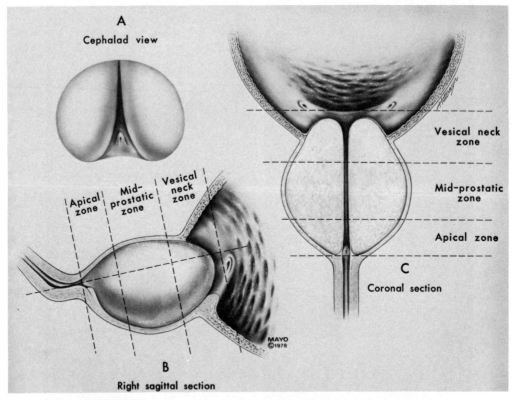

Figure 78–12. Large bilateral prostatic adenoma with intravesical extension.

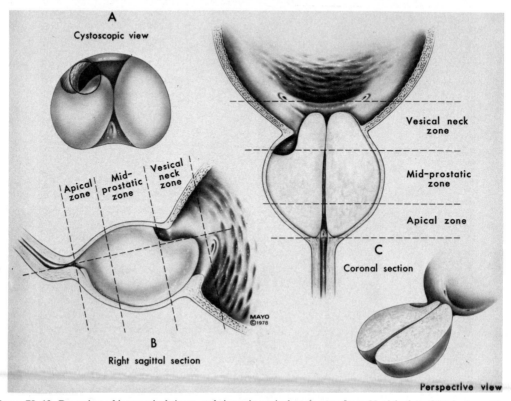

Figure 78–13. Resection of intravesical tissue and tissue in vesical neck zone from 11 o'clock to 9 o'clock positions.

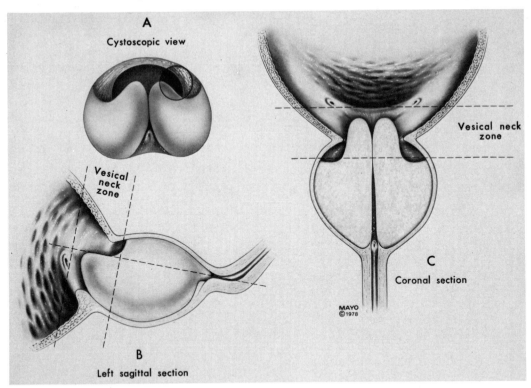

Figure 78–14. Resection of intravesical tissue, tissue in vesical zone from 1 o'clock to 3 o'clock positions, and anterior tissue.

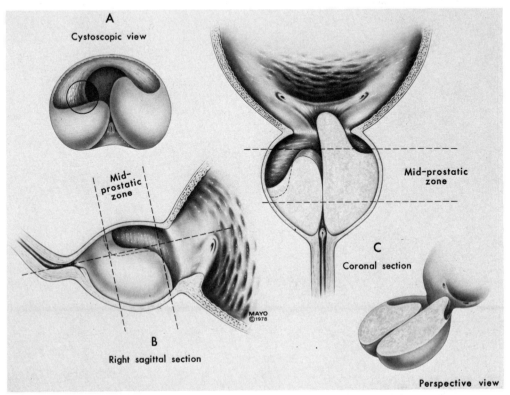

Figure 78–15. Resection of right anterolateral tissue in midprostatic zone, resulting in dropping of right lateral lobe onto floor of prostatic fossa.

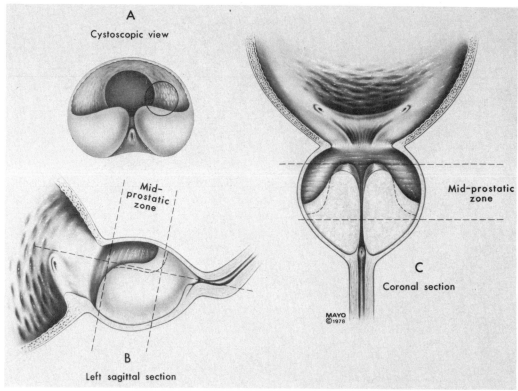

Figure 78–16. Resection of left anterolateral tissue in midprostatic zone, resulting in dropping of left lateral lobe onto floor of prostatic fossa.

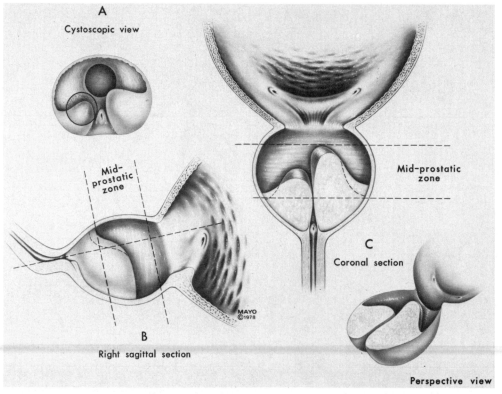

Figure 78–17. Resection of right anterolateral tissue more distally in midprostatic zone, dropping additional tissue onto floor of prostatic fossa.

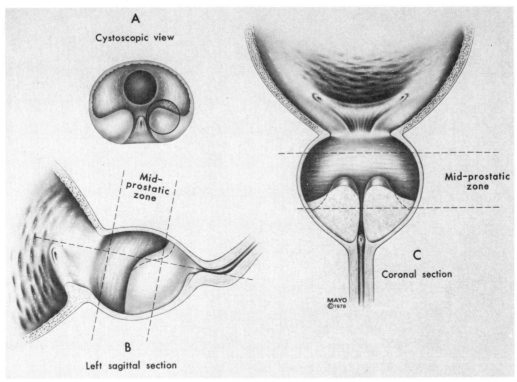

Figure 78–18. Resection of left anterolateral tissue more distally in midprostatic zone, dropping additional tissue onto floor of prostatic fossa.

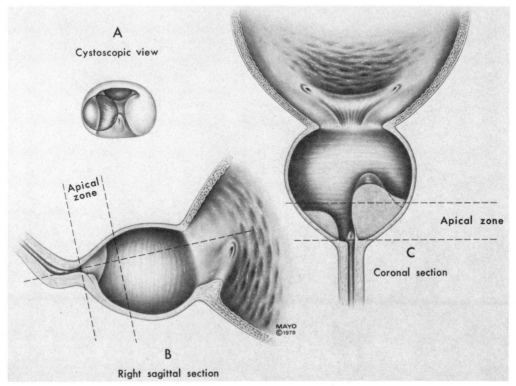

Figure 78–19. Resection of posterior tissue in apical zone to the right side of verumontanum.

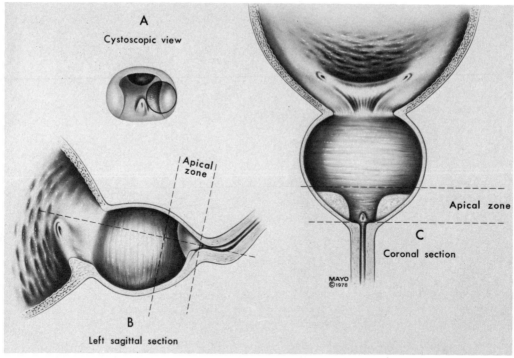

Figure 78–20. Resection of posterior tissue in apical zone to the left side of verumontanum.

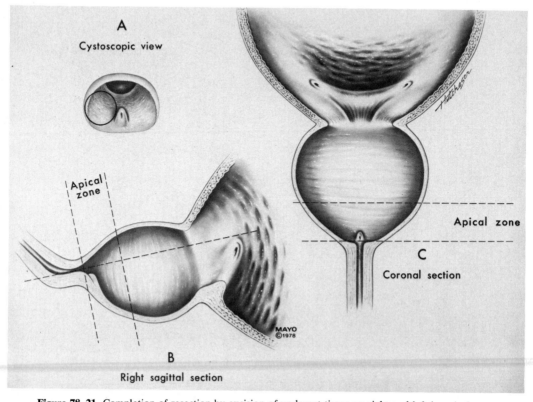

Figure 78–21. Completion of resection by excision of undercut tissue on right and left in apical zone.

median lobe. In such cases, the sequence followed when resecting the lateral lobes remains unchanged, but the presence of a large median lobe may require modifications in technique. Problems that may occur are interference with movements of the resectoscope from prostatic fossa to bladder, thereby hindering resection; deep excision of the lobe, resulting in undermining (separation) of the trigone; trauma to the ureteral orifices; and fragmentation of a large portion of the lobe that passes into the bladder but is too large to exit through the resectoscope sheath.

Resection of the median lobe should be delayed until a later phase or, if possible, the last phase of the resection, unless the enlarged lobe interferes with free movements of the resectoscope. In such a situation, only that portion of the median lobe that will allow free movement of the resectoscope should be resected. The purpose of incomplete resection of the median lobe at this stage is to prevent separation at the prostatovesical junction. Such separation or undermining of the trigone can be appreciated as a slit or crevice of variable depth and length that is parallel to the lower quadrant of the vesical neck. If such undermining occurs early in the surgical procedure, it is usually aggravated during resection of the lateral lobes and interferes with movement of the resectoscope from prostatic fossa to bladder.

Hemostasis. Bleeding during resection may be from arteries, from venous sinuses, and, less often, from veins; each requires separate management. Arterial bleeding may be pulsatile (coinciding with the patient's pulse rate) or continuous, and it persists even after the bladder is full and pressure within the prostatic fossa is high (see Fig. 78–11*B*). Generally, arterial bleeding is controlled easily by electrocoagulation. The degree of hemostasis sought is one that maintains a clear operative field and prevents excessive loss of blood. A single artery may be encountered repeatedly during resection of an area of adenomatous tissue. In this event, coagulation need not be repeated. Rather, the artery should be coagulated as it emerges from the surgical capsule.

A cardinal rule is that hemostasis should be secured in an area of resection before resection in another area is begun. If this is not done, bleeding from multiple sites will obfuscate the operative field.

Bleeding from an opened venous sinus may be difficult, or impossible, to stop by electrocoagulation, and loss of blood may be excessive. Furthermore, the pressure in the venous sinus, approximately 10 to 12 mm Hg, is lower than the pressure of the irrigant in the prostatic fossa. Irrigating fluid thereby may intravasate and produce hypervolemia, hyponatremia, and hemoglobinemia if hemolytic irrigant is employed; bacteremia may occur if the operative field is infected.

Venous sinus bleeding appears as bright, continuous, nonpulsatile, sheetlike welling of blood from an irregular dark cavity or slit (see Fig. 78–11*C*). Coagulation of the sinus should be attempted, but this effort usually results in enlargement of the opening and fails to stop the bleeding. At times, the open sinus may not be visible because the pressure of the irrigant in the prostatic fossa is greater than venous pressure, which prevents bleeding while the operative field is examined. However, while the bladder contents are evacuated through the resectoscope sheath, pressure in the prostatic fossa decreases and an outpouring of dark red blood, indicative of venous sinus bleeding, may be noted.

Persistent attempts to arrest sinus bleeding by electrocoagulation should not be made, because passage of irrigant into the blood stream occurs when the resectoscope with its issuing stream of irrigant is directed against the sinus during such attempts. The resection should be accomplished as rapidly and as carefully as possible. The bleeding venous sinus can be controlled by proper placement of the hemostatic bag of the catheter that is inserted at the completion of the surgical procedure.

Evacuation of Prostatic Chips. At the conclusion of the operation, all prostatic chips must be evacuated from the bladder. An Ellik evacuator, which is a piece of blown glass that permits the injection of irrigating fluid into the bladder, should be used to remove the bladder contents by suction (Fig. 78–22). The instrument is filled by immersing it in a deep vessel that

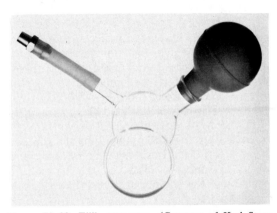

Figure 78–22. Ellik evacuator. (Courtesy of Karl Storz–Endoscopy America, Inc.)

contains irrigant, and the bulb is repeatedly compressed so that the receptacle and bulb are filled with irrigant and air is evacuated. Approximately 150 ml of irrigant is instilled in the bladder, and the filled evacuator is connected with the sheath of the resectoscope. The distal end of the sheath is directed toward the base of the bladder, and the bulb is compressed slowly so that the fragments, which are drawn into the evacuator, settle in the lower bulbous chamber. When the fluid in the upper chamber is free of fragments, it can be reinjected into the bladder, thereby repeating the process.

Insertion of Urethral Catheter. The TURP is completed by insertion of a 22F or 24F catheter that incorporates a hemostatic balloon of 30-ml capacity. "One-way" catheters are available for straight drainage, and "two-way" catheters may be used for simultaneous irrigation and drainage of the bladder. Catheters with balloons of larger capacity (75 ml) and different shapes are also available.

Most urologists prefer to have the distended balloon seated against the vesical neck. To achieve this, the catheter is passed and fluid in amounts of 20 to 50 ml is introduced into the balloon while it is in the bladder. The balloon is then "snugged up" against the vesical neck, and the resulting tamponade of the prostatic fossa secures hemostasis. Irrigation of the bladder is repeated until the irrigant returns clear or is only slightly blood-tinged.

Most surgeons avoid distending the balloon in the prostatic fossa because they believe this causes severe pain and spasms of the bladder, prevents contraction of the prostatic fossa, interferes with hemostasis, and results in postoperative urinary urgency and incontinence. I could not substantiate these claims in a controlled study of this problem (Greene, 1971). Furthermore, the study demonstrated that the balloon, distended in the prostatic fossa, is helpful in securing hemostasis.

If only fair hemostasis is achieved by electrocoagulation, excellent or acceptable hemostasis can be gained by distending the hemostatic balloon in the prostatic fossa. A 24F Foley catheter with a 30-ml hemostatic balloon is inserted, and 15 ml of water is instilled into the balloon while it is in the bladder. The balloon is then slowly and deliberately drawn into the prostatic fossa by gentle tugging on the catheter and is held in that position while an additional 15 ml of water is added to the balloon. If irrigation of the bladder indicates that adequate hemostasis has not been achieved, 10-ml increments of fluid are successively instilled into the balloon until hemostasis is acceptable.

Removal of Urethral Catheter. The urethral catheter is removed as soon as possible, usually 24 or 48 hours after insertion. This practice, however, has certain caveats, namely, that a good resection has been performed, the urethra is not compromised, the patient feels well, and the urine is reasonably clear.

Transurethral Incisions of Prostate. Transurethral incisions of the prostate (Orandi, 1978) are performed for patients with significant urinary obstructive symptoms, poor uroflow tests, and insignificant prostatic hyperplasia. The vesical necks in such instances appear "high-riding" (see Fig. 78–11D). Sophisticated urodynamic studies, including micturitional vesicourethral static pressure profiles, may be necessary to exclude detrusor hyporeflexia, isolated bladder neck obstruction, and dyssynergia of the external urethral sphincteric mechanism (Yalla et al., 1982).

The first incision, made with a Collings knife, is started at the 7 o'clock position at the vesical neck and is carried deep along the floor of the urethra to the right side of the verumontanum (Figs. 78–11E to H and Fig. 78–23A). It is not unusual to expose fat or to enter the seminal vesicles, and such occurrences have not produced problems. A similar incision is made at the 4 o'clock position at the vesical neck and is continued to the left side of the verumontanum. After bilateral incisions are completed, the vesical neck and prostatic urethra appear wide open (Fig. 78–23B).

A biopsy of the prostate is obtained from the midline with the loop of the resectoscope to exclude Stage A carcinoma (this may serve in large part to salve the conscience of the urologist). Hemostasis is secured by electrocoagulation, and a catheter is inserted. The balloon is distended in the prostatic fossa as a hemostatic device; experience has shown that significant bleeding may occur in the immediate postoperative period. Generally, the catheter is removed 24 hours after surgery.

COMPLICATIONS

Two significant operative complications of TURP are bleeding, which has been discussed, and perforation of the prostatic capsule. The latter may result in extravasation and intravasation of irrigating fluid if a venous sinus has been opened, and dilutional hyponatremia (TUR syndrome).

Perforation of Prostatic Capsule. Perforation results from failure to recognize the surgical capsule and cutting into this structure. If the capsule is incised deeply, it appears lacy and filmy (Fig. 78–23C). A perforation appears as

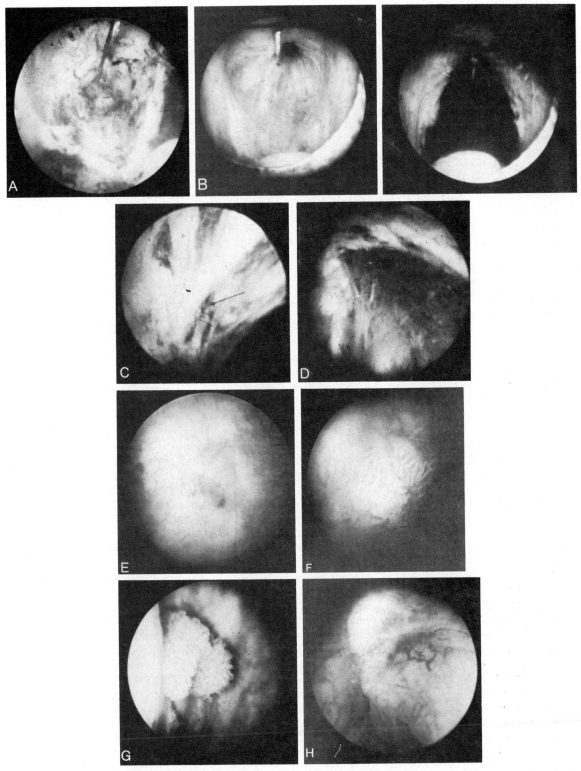

Figure 78–23. *A,* Incision completed (continued sequence from Figure 78–11). *B,* Preoperative appearance of prostatic urethra *(left)*; after bilateral incisions *(right)*. *C,* Deeply incised prostatic capsule appears lacy and filmy. *D,* Perforation of prostatic capsule appears as diaphanous cavity. *E,* Carcinoma in situ has appearance of an area of acute cystitis. *F,* Velvety appearance of carcinoma in situ when the bladder wall is viewed in profile. *G,* Villous appearance of low-grade, low-stage vesical neoplasm. *H,* Lateral border of solid nodular, high-grade infiltrating carcinoma of bladder.

an irregular, diaphanous cavity interspersed with fibrous bands; at times, fat may be visible (Fig. 78–23D).

EXTRAVASATION AND INTRAVASATION. Perforation and its resultant extravasation should be suspected from cystoscopic findings long before the patient shows signs or symptoms. The earliest signs of extraperitoneal extravasation result from irrigant entering the periprostatic and perivesical spaces, elongating the prostatic urethra, and elevating and compressing the lateral borders of the bladder. As a result, the resectoscope is grasped more tightly and its movements are restricted. In addition, the prostatic urethra appears more distant than at the start of the resection, the prostatovesical junction becomes less well defined, and the excision of adequate chips of tissue is more difficult. Finally, and most decisively, the bladder becomes more distant. Thus, the trigone, easily visible at the start of resection, is seen only if the resectoscope is pushed forward forcibly. Similarly, the posterior wall of the bladder either appears to be off in the distance or is not visible at all. A disparity between the amount of irrigant instilled and that recovered is not readily apparent, because only a small amount extravasates at each filling. A late sign of extravasation is compression of the bladder by the extravasated fluid, producing decreased vesical capacity, increased intravesical pressure, and rapid clouding of the visual field. Tenderness and rigidity of the abdominal wall and an abdominal mass are late signs of significant extravasation.

The earliest symptom of extraperitoneal extravasation is restlessness, followed by nausea, vomiting, and abdominal pain that develops despite spinal anesthesia. Pain is usually localized to the lower part of the abdomen or to the back. The patient pales and perspires, and the pulse rate increases. Dyspnea may be noted, and hypotension and shock may appear.

If extravasation or intravasation is suspected, the operation should be terminated as rapidly as possible, but hemostasis must first be secured. Bleeding must be controlled even if the extravasation is increased, because the simultaneous management of extravasation and hemorrhage is formidable. Furthermore, all chips of tissue must be removed from the bladder to avoid plugging of the catheter. Hemostasis is secured by electrocoagulation, and a one-way hemostatic bag catheter is inserted. Simple drainage into a drainage bag may be employed, or the catheter may be attached to a suction apparatus. Cystography should be performed to establish the diagnosis and to provide some measure of the extent of extravasation.

Dilutional Hyponatremia (TUR Syndrome). This term refers to a significant alteration in homeostasis produced by intravasation or extravasation of irrigating fluid during TURP. This complication results from the entrance of irrigating fluid into the vascular compartment through open venous sinuses or perforations in the prostatic capsule (Madsen and Madsen, 1965; Madsen and Naber, 1973).

The signs and symptoms of dilutional hyponatremia and its complications include elevation in systolic, diastolic, and pulse pressures, bradycardia, and eventual hypotension and cardiovascular collapse. Tachypnea, dyspnea, cyanosis, blindness, coma, and convulsions may develop. If general anesthesia has been employed, restlessness, nausea, and disorientation may not be observed; dyspnea and cyanosis may not be appreciated because of assisted ventilation. The only manifestations of dilutional hyponatremia in such circumstances may be increasing hypertension, an increase in pulse and central venous pressures, and abdominal distention.

In the opinion of some clinicians, mild degrees of extravasation can be managed conservatively as indicated, but moderate or significant extravasation demands suprapubic perivesical drainage. It is my opinion, however, that such drainage is rarely necessary. Antibacterial drugs should be administered.

Patients with dilutional hyponatremia require close monitoring of central venous pressure, blood gases, blood loss, urinary output, and cardiac status. Serum osmolality and sodium and potassium levels must be followed closely, particularly during the first few hours after onset of the syndrome, because changes in electrolyte levels may occur rapidly.

Specific treatment consists of producing a net loss of body water. If serum osmolality and plasma sodium are low, 40 to 100 mg of furosemide should be administered intravenously. The patient should be observed closely for signs of cardiovascular collapse with pulmonary or cerebral edema. Differing opinions exist concerning the use of hypertonic saline solution, but 250 to 500 ml of 3 to 5 per cent sodium chloride is frequently administered intravenously.

TRANSURETHRAL SURGERY OF VESICAL NEOPLASMS

Fortunately, the majority of vesical neoplasms can be treated transurethrally. Their management has been aided by improved technology. Furthermore, the urologist is helped immeasurably when expertise in urinary cytology and interpretation of frozen-tissue sections is available.

Carcinomas treated transurethrally for cure include carcinoma in situ; exophytic carcinomas, which are usually low in stage and grade; and carcinomas with limited infiltration into muscle, which usually are of higher grade. Carcinomas of advanced stage may be resected for symptomatic relief. The diagnosis of vesical neoplasms is discussed in Chapter 30. Suffice it to say here that bimanual digital abdominorectal examination in men or abdominovaginal examination in women while the patient is under anesthesia is helpful in diagnosis. Such examinations, by detecting a mass, fixation, rigidity, or hardness, help in estimating the size and stage of the carcinoma and in making decisions concerning treatment.

CARCINOMA IN SITU

It may be difficult to make a cystoscopic diagnosis of carcinoma in situ because its appearance is neither distinctive nor consistent and depends not on the changes in the mucosa, but rather on the alterations in the submucosa. It may appear as an area of acute or chronic cystitis, or its texture may be velvety or granular; the borders of the lesion are indistinct and fade imperceptibly into adjacent areas that are apparently normal (Fig. 78–23*E*). The lesion may be obvious, but in most instances one is seeking nuances. Therefore, the bladder must be examined with varying degrees of filling so its walls can be seen enface and in profile, with illumination of varying intensity and with telescopes of different viewing angles (Fig. 78–23*F*).

Biopsy, best performed with cold cup forceps, may permit definitive diagnosis from examination of frozen-tissue sections; even experienced pathologists, however, may also require fixed sections. Biopsy specimens used to diagnose carcinoma in situ or epithelial atypia are obtained from areas posterolateral to each ureteral orifice, trigone, lateral walls, base, posterior wall, and dome of the bladder, and from the prostatic urethra, or the urethra in women.

Carcinoma in situ can be destroyed by electrocoagulation, preferably with a ball electrode; regional or general anesthesia is advisable. Such treatment may be employed if the lesion is not too large, perhaps 5 cm or less in diameter, or if the lesions are limited in number (Utz et al., 1980). Inasmuch as it is generally not possible to determine the exact limits of the lesion, it is better to err by electrocoagulating an area too large than one too small. The success of such treatment can be determined only by subsequent urinary cytology, cystoscopy, and biopsy.

EXOPHYTIC CARCINOMAS

Exophytic carcinomas of the bladder may be single or may be so numerous as to indicate carcinomatosis. These lesions may be small or may be so large that the entire bladder appears to be filled with tumor. They may occur at any site in the bladder. Low-grade lesions usually have a fine, villous pattern and a small, thin pedicle (Fig. 78–23*G*). High-grade tumors have a more solid appearance and a thicker, more fibrous pedicle.

Some surgeons prefer to excise vesical neoplasms with a continuous-flow resectoscope rather than with a conventional resectoscope because the bladder contains smaller volumes of irrigant with the former; consequently, the wall of the bladder is thicker and perforation is less likely. Thin loops, such as Nos. 10 or 12, are advisable. Pure cutting current between 50 and 70 mA and coagulating current between 40 and 50 mA are employed. The use of water as an irrigant has the theoretical advantage that cancer cells can be destroyed by the hypotonic solution.

Exophytic lesions are excised by passing the activated loop through the most accessible parts of the lesion. Rarely, it is possible to resect the pedicle primarily and thereby remove the tumor in toto. It is difficult to secure hemostasis during resection of the frondular portions of the tumor, but this is easily accomplished when the pedicle is reached. Generally, one major bleeding artery is encountered that can be coagulated and the pedicle is excised, exposing normal muscle. The pathologist should be apprised of the site of the specimens submitted for examination. If additional, smaller lesions (less than 1 cm in diameter) are present, they can be destroyed by electrocoagulation.

Several other principles apply to excision of exophytic lesions. If the tumors are multiple, particularly those in the dome, the uppermost lesions in the bladder are excised first. If lower lesions are excised first, bubbles of gas formed during the excision rise and obscure lesions in the dome. These bubbles form even if tumors of the dome are resected initially. Gas can be removed by aspiration with a ureteral catheter.

Tumors situated in the dome may be difficult to reach. In such circumstances, minimal filling of the bladder and suprapubic pressure will help bring the tumor into the surgical field. Transurethral excision of extensive tumors in the dome of the bladder that are difficult to reach may be managed by placing the patient prone (Nachtsheim et al., 1981). This approach presents no problems in women but requires an external urethrotomy in men.

Neoplasms located on the lateral walls or base can be excised by advancing and retracting the loop into the sheath as it is employed in prostatic resection. The movement of the loop coincides with the concavity of the bladder. Tumors of the posterior wall, on the other hand, are excised by advancing the loop into a fixed position and moving the entire sheath up and down or side to side as one might manipulate a paint brush; "tennis racquet" loops have been devised for this purpose.

INFILTRATING CARCINOMAS

The consensus is that infiltrating carcinomas in which infiltration into muscle is only modest (Stage B1, T2) are suitable for transurethral resection. A minority of urologists believe cancers that infiltrate through the muscle are suitable for transurethral excision. Such lesions are usually of high grade and appear solid or ulcerative but may have exophytic elements (Fig. 78–23H).

Resection of the most accessible portion of the lesion is undertaken, and the bulk of the tumor is resected down to the level of the adjacent mucosa. Resection is continued by excising loop-wide segments starting at the edge of the tumor and moving centrally, from superficial to deep tissue layers, controlling the bleeding before moving to the next loop-wide segment. The resection is carried down to normal muscle. The site of resected specimens should be identified for the pathologist. Coagulation of the area of excision and a 0.5-cm diameter peripheral area is carried out with a ball electrode. Random biopsies of the bladder, as mentioned, complete the procedure.

Severe spasm of the adductor muscles of the thigh may complicate resection of tumors located in the lower lateral wall of the bladder. Such spasms result from stimulation of the obturator nerve and may lead to perforation of the bladder or incomplete resection of the tumor. Simple, but usually ineffective, measures to prevent such spasms include avoiding significant distention of the bladder, changing the site of the inactive electrode, or lowering the frequency of the current. Succinylcholine or D-tubocurarine may be administered, but general anesthesia and endotracheal intubation are then required. If spasms are a serious obstacle to definitive surgery, the obturator nerve can be blocked by the injection of lidocaine either transvesically or within the obturator canal (Augspurger and Donohue, 1980).

Perforation of the bladder is the most significant complication of transurethral resection of a vesical neoplasm. Preventive measures include minimal filling of the bladder during resection to prevent overdistention and thinning of the wall of the bladder. Extraperitoneal perforations are treated by catheter drainage and antibacterial drugs. There is an increasing tendency to treat intraperitoneal perforations in a similar manner; however, formal closure and copious irrigation of the peritoneal cavity are thus required.

VISUAL INTERNAL URETHROTOMY

Internal urethrotomy with the use of a cold-knife visual urethrotome has been effective in the treatment of urethral strictures (Kirchheim et al., 1978). At times the operation must be repeated to achieve a cure. Better results are obtained when treating short, traumatic strictures than long, inflammatory strictures. The procedure may be performed on an outpatient basis using local anesthesia.

Technique. A retrograde urethrogram depicting the number, location, extent, and severity of the stricture should be obtained. The urethrotome is passed to the stricture. If there is uncertainty as to its course, a small ureteral catheter advanced through the stricture serves as a guide for the incisions. The knife is extended and held in place, and the stricture is incised at the 12 o'clock position by moving the entire urethrotome antegrade in a series of short, arc-like motions, with the fulcrum approximately at the center of the instrument (Fig. 78–24A). It is necessary to incise the full extent of the stricture—deeply, distally, and proximally. Bleeding is usually insignificant.

After internal urethrotomy, calibration of the urethra with Otis bulbs is performed. If the urethra does not easily accept a 26 F bulb, deeper incisions of the stricture should be made. The operation is concluded by passage of a Silastic catheter, which may be removed the following day.

VESICAL LITHOLAPAXY AND LITHOTRIPSY

SELECTION OF PATIENTS

The process of selecting patients for litholapaxy has changed since the introduction of electrohydraulic and ultrasonic litholapaxy.

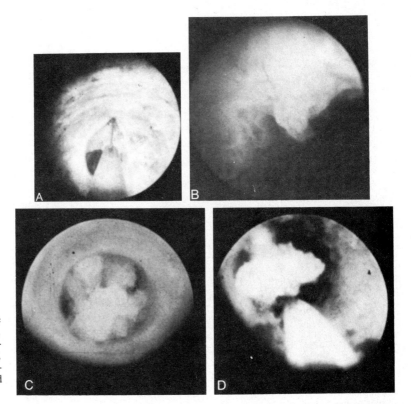

Figure 78–24. *A,* Urethral stricture is incised at 12 o'clock position. *B,* Ureteroscopic appearance of low-stage, low-grade ureteral tumor. *C,* Ureteroscopic view of ureteral calculus. *D,* Ureteral calculus engaged within stone basket.

When only mechanical lithotrites were available, calculi larger than 4 to 5 cm in diameter, particularly if multiple, were not suitable for litholapaxy. The use of electrical energy in litholapaxy has removed such limitations. Nevertheless, crushing very large calculi by hydraulic or sound waves can be a prolonged, tedious task, and suprapubic removal of such calculi is preferred.

Vesical calculi in association with prostatic hyperplasia can be crushed and TURP performed. Obviously, if the prostatic adenoma and the vesical calculi are large, an open operation to remove both is indicated. Calculi with a foreign-body nidus and dumbbell calculi formed in association with a vesical diverticulum may pose relative contraindications to litholapaxy.

TACTILE LITHOLAPAXY

Tactile litholapaxy, a "blind" procedure, is mentioned in passing for the sake of completeness. It is an excellent operation in the hands of the skilled, but unfortunately is rarely taught, is rarely practiced, and is all but a lost art. Indeed, the Bigelow lithotrite is not available in most operating theaters. Briefly, the lithotrite is passed into the bladder, the stone is blindly maneuvered between the opened jaws and

crushed, and the fragments are evacuated. An excellent description of the technique was prepared by DeWeerd (1979).

VISUAL LITHOLAPAXY

Stone Forceps. Stone forceps passed in the sheath of a cystoscope or resectoscope may be used to grasp and remove vesical calculi (Fig. 78–25). The caliber of the sheath limits the size of calculi that can be removed. Larger, soft stones can be crushed with this instrument or with a stone punch (Fig. 78–26), and the fragments are then evacuated.

Mechanical Litholapaxy. A variety of instruments that permit mechanical crushing of vesical calculi under vision are available (Fig. 78–27). The lithotrite is a powerful, potentially dangerous instrument, and the surgeon should be thoroughly familiar with its construction and use.

Preliminary urethral calibration and internal urethrotomy, if necessary, are performed so that a large resectoscope sheath can be employed to evacuate stony fragments. Cystoscopy is performed, and information regarding number, size, shape, and probable composition of the calculi is obtained. Sacculation or vesical diverticula, which may contain stones or in which stony fragments may lodge, are noted.

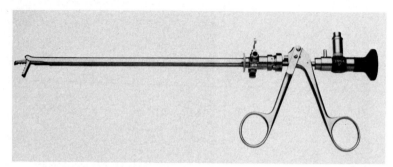

Figure 78–25. Stone forceps. (Courtesy of Karl Storz–Endoscopy America, Inc.)

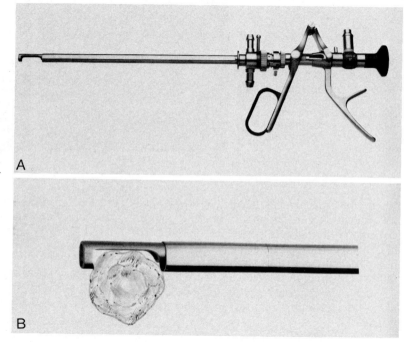

Figure 78–26. *A,* Stone punch. *B,* Fragment evacuated with punch. (Courtesy of Karl Storz–Endoscopy America, Inc.)

A

B

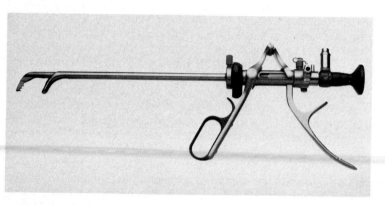

Figure 78–27. Visual lithotrite. (Courtesy of Karl Storz–Endoscopy America, Inc.)

Irrigant, approximately 150 ml, is introduced into the bladder and the cystoscope is withdrawn. The lithotrite in closed position is then passed. An assistant compresses the penis against the shaft of the lithotrite, or a tourniquet is applied to prevent escape of fluid from the bladder. When the calculus is in view, the jaws of the lithotrite are opened, with the tips of the blade directed posteriorly, and the calculus is engaged (Fig. 78–28). Alternatively, the calculus may be engaged by directing the jaws of the lithotrite anteriorly, depressing its distal end, and moving the female jaw back and forth. After the calculus is engaged, it is lifted from the base of the bladder while rotating and moving the lithotrite to be certain that mucosa has not been engaged. The calculus is viewed and the handles of the lithotrite are approximated, which causes the calculus to be crushed. If increased force is required, the screw spindle device, incorporated in the instrument, may be used. Larger fragments of calculus are then crushed, and the process is repeated until it is judged that the fragments are small enough to be evacuated through the selected sheath. The jaws of the lithotrite are closed, and after inspection shows that no stony spicules that could traumatize the urethra are evident, the lithotrite is removed.

A resectoscope sheath is passed and sand and stony fragments are washed out; the Ellik evacuator may be used to advantage. Fragments that do not wash out can first be extracted or crushed with stone forceps. Final inspection of the bladder usually reveals sandy material enmeshed in the mucosa by a fibrinous membrane; this can be dissolved by continuous irrigation of the bladder for 24 hours with an appropriate solution of Renacidin or bicarbonate of soda through a two-way irrigating catheter.

Electrohydraulic Lithotripsy. With this technique, a calculus is disrupted by a series of electrohydraulic shock waves (Bülow and Fröhmuller, 1981). Essentially, the apparatus consists of a pulse generator, which builds up electrical energy that can be discharged at intervals. An instrument panel permits the control of voltage. The generator is connected to a probe by a high-voltage cable, and the rate and duration of discharge are controlled by a foot switch. The probe that is positioned close to the calculus may be used with an operating cystoscope. If, in addition, TURP is contemplated, a resectoscope sheath may be substituted.

The procedure consists of bringing the probe into intimate contact with the calculus. A short series of 1- to 3-second electrohydraulic shocks are applied, interspersed by 5- to 10-

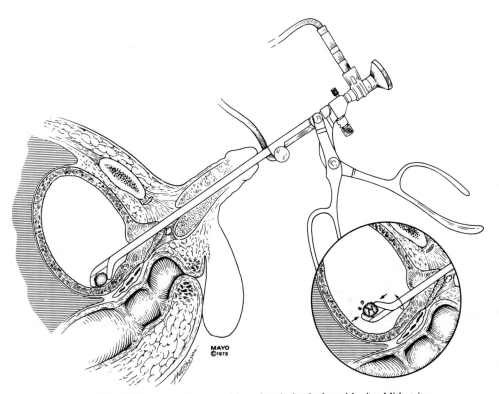

Figure 78–28. Engagement and crushing of vesical calculus with visual lithotrite.

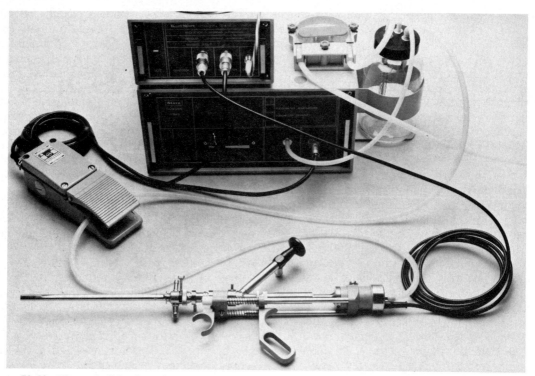

Figure 78–29. Ultrasonic lithotrite, ultrasonic generator, and suction apparatus. (Courtesy of Karl Storz–Endoscopy America, Inc.)

second intervals to permit the generator to build up energy. Inasmuch as stones are unequal in size, rigidity, and texture, it is necessary to determine the suitable type and intensity of current. In the case of hard calculi, such as mixed or oxalate stones, considerable exploration of the stone by the probe may be required until an adequate disruption point is found. Initial bursts of shock waves directed to the same spot on the stone will cause it to crack, and thereafter fragmentation is easily accomplished. Rough calculi are more easily disrupted than are smooth stones. Contact between the probe and bladder mucosa is to be avoided. Fragments are evacuated as described for visual litholapaxy.

Ultrasonic Lithotripsy. Disruption of calculi by ultrasound has been utilized more recently (Terhorst et al., 1972). A high-frequency generator is employed to produce electromagnetic oscillations and is connected by cable to a transducer. A drill is activated by oscillations of the ultrasonic transducer (Fig. 78–29). The drill is applied to the stone, and after a period of "hammering," the calculus is disrupted and the fragments are evacuated. Postoperative care after electrohydraulic and ultrasonic litholapaxy is similar to that described for visual litholapaxy.

TRANSURETHRAL MANIPULATIVE TREATMENT OF URETERAL CALCULI

The manipulative treatment of ureteral calculi by a cystoscopic approach is employed enthusiastically by some urologists, disregarded by others, and roundly condemned by a few. However, all are of the opinion that manipulation is a formidable procedure, which is potentially dangerous and therefore not undertaken lightly, and which requires a high degree of judgment and skill on the part of the surgeon. There is also agreement that, when accomplished successfully, this form of treatment serves the patient well.

The introduction of rigid and flexible ureteropyeloscopes, electrohydraulic and ultrasonic lithotripsy, and percutaneous endourologic procedures has influenced the management of ureteral calculi. It appears likely that increased experience with the newer endoscopic instruments will alter radically the indications and techniques for manipulating ureteral calculi. Conventional manipulative procedures will first be discussed in this section, and the subject will again be addressed under Transurethral Ureteropyeloscopy.

SELECTION OF PATIENTS

Spontaneous passage, if possible, is the most desirable method by which a ureter may rid itself of a calculus. If spontaneous passage appears unlikely or if repeated, severe renal colic, recurrent febrile illnesses, or progressive hydronephrosis and impairment of renal function result, the calculus should be manipulated, if certain requirements are met.

Manipulation should be limited to calculi that are less than 0.6 to 0.8 cm in greatest diameter. Such calculi may be extracted with confidence of success, whereas successful manipulation of calculi 1.0 to 1.5 cm in diameter is rare. Calculi more than 1.5 cm in diameter usually are not suitable for manipulation. In general, manipulation should be limited to calculi contained in the lower one third of the ureter inasmuch as the potential for ureteral trauma is greater if the calculus is located in the upper two thirds of the ureter. This limitation is less rigid since the introduction of ureteroscopes.

TECHNIQUE

The administration of a broad-spectrum antibiotic should be instituted before the procedure and continued postoperatively for 24 hours after the removal of all catheters. A plain film roentgenogram, to ascertain the position of the calculus, is obtained when the patient is placed on the operating table. An image intensifier is an invaluable aid in this procedure. Some surgeons believe maximal relaxation is important and recommend spinal anesthesia be used, while others believe that general anesthesia is sufficient.

It is not possible to detail the many and varied approaches to manipulation and the preferences for extractors. The following represents the technique I employ. An operating cystoscope is passed through the urethra, and the bladder is examined. A Davis stone extractor is advanced in the ureter that contains the calculus, and grating or obstruction, if present, is noted. If the catheter passes without much difficulty, manipulation may begin. If the Davis extractor cannot be passed by the calculus, an attempt to pass a whistle-tip or spiral-tip ureteral

catheter (4 F) should be made. If such a catheter can be passed beyond the calculus, it may be possible to pass the Davis catheter alongside the ureteral catheter or once the latter is removed.

At times, obstruction may be overcome by the use of two ureteral catheters. The two catheters are passed to the site of the calculus, and attempts are made to pass one and then the other by the calculus. After one catheter has been passed, it may be simple to pass a second catheter alongside the first. If considerable maneuvering was necessary to pass one or two ureteral catheters or if the catheter is grasped tightly between the calculus and the ureteral wall, manipulative procedures should be delayed. In such instances, the catheter is left indwelling, a urethral catheter is inserted into the bladder, and the patient is returned to his room. After 48 hours, the ureteral catheter has usually caused sufficient ureteral dilation to permit easy passage of the catheters or the extractor. Failure to pass a ureteral catheter past a calculus necessitates abandonment of any attempt at manipulation.

The Davis extractor is employed first because it is one of the safest extractors; if used properly, this device permits extraction of a high percentage of stones. The extractor (Fig. 78–30) consists of a ureteral catheter with a monofilament nylon thread passed through a slightly transverse hole (a) in the catheter 10 cm from the tip, with each end of the nylon thread passing back into the lumen of the catheter 15 and 17 cm distal to the tip (b), traveling down the lumen, and emerging at the butt of the catheter. Traction applied simultaneously on both ends of the nylon thread pulls points a and b toward each other, forming a three-point grasping snare at point a.

The technique of extraction consists of passage of the extractor, with or without a stylet, up the ureter, assuring that the snare segment is above the calculus or that 15 cm of extractor has been passed. While the catheter is passed alongside the calculus, grating or an obstruction that can be overcome may be perceived. As they emerge from the catheter, both ends of the nylon thread are wrapped about one jaw (rubber-covered) of a small hemostat, which is then locked. This hemostat helps to grasp the threads

Figure 78–30. Davis extractor.

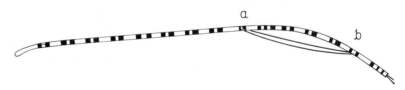

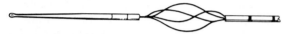

Figure 78–31. Dormia extractor.

and is a marker for the distance the threads have moved. The threads are retracted 1 cm or until firm resistance is encountered, and the ends of the thread are again grasped by the rubber-covered jaws of a second hemostat just as they emerge from the catheter. The aim is not to create a loop but rather to fashion a three-pointed snare. The extractor is slowly withdrawn, and engagement of the calculus is sensed by increased resistance to further movement. Firm, steady traction, limited to that which can be gained with only thumb and index finger, is applied to the extractor and the calculus within as it is drawn into the bladder. If the calculus cannot be engaged in two or three attempts, the Davis extractor should be replaced by the Dormia extractor.

The Dormia extractor is safe and effective. In the closed position, it looks like a 6 F ureteral catheter with a metal tip and a proximal handle. When the handle is pushed forward, a four-wire, helical coil basket is seen at the distal tip (Fig. 78–31). A long or short filiform tip may be used if desired.

The closed extractor is passed beyond the calculus. When the tip of the extractor is well beyond the calculus, the handle is pushed forward, opening the wire cage. The extractor is then slowly withdrawn, again employing only the amount of traction obtained from the use of the thumb and index finger. During withdrawal, the extractor is moved slightly in clockwise rotation to maintain the calculus within the cage. The cage should be observed closely as it emerges from the ureteral orifice to determine whether a calculus is enclosed. In some instances, the calculus will drop from the cage as soon as the latter reaches the bladder, and unless this is observed by the surgeon, further, fruitless attempts to extract the calculus from the ureter may be made.

Ultimately, if the calculus cannot be engaged, the Johnson extractor, a more formidable and potentially dangerous instrument, may be used. This extractor (Fig. 78–32) consists of a spindle-shaped arrangement of four flexible wires attached to a flexible wire shaft. A filiform bougie is attached to the distal end of the wires. The length of the spindle may vary from 2.5 to 3 cm, and its greatest diameter is about 8 mm. The calculus is engaged within this wire basket. In practice, the extractor is gently passed so that the basket reaches and surpasses the stone by several centimeters. In some instances, the passage may be so smooth that no inkling of the site of the calculus is obtained, and the level to which the basket should be passed must be estimated from study of the roentgenograms. In other instances, the passage of the basket alongside the calculus and its actual engagement within the basket will impart to the fingers of an experienced surgeon the sensation of a slight increase in resistance to movements of the extractor. Finally, it may be impossible to appreciate that the calculus has been engaged, and this information can be ascertained only after withdrawal of the basket into the bladder. The technique of engagement of the calculus and withdrawal of the extractor is similar to that described for the Dormia extractor.

POSTOPERATIVE CARE

After extraction from the ureter, the calculus is examined to see if it is intact, and its size is compared with that noted on the roentgenogram (the image is slightly magnified). The calculus, including its nucleus, should be analyzed to determine its chemical nature.

Immediately after extraction of the calculus, one or preferably two ureteral catheters are passed to the kidney and a urethral catheter is inserted. A daily urinary output of approximately 2500 ml is desirable; hence, parenteral fluids are required during the first 24-hour postoperative period. The catheters may be withdrawn after 24 or 48 hours, and the administration of broad-spectrum antibiotics is continued for 24 hours after withdrawal of the catheters.

After extraction of a calculus it may be impossible, although always desirable, to pass ureteral catheters to the kidney to secure drainage postoperatively. The passage of the catheter

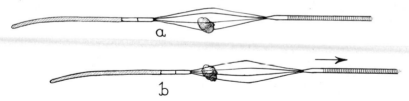

Figure 78–32. Johnson extractor. Calculus engaged within extractor *(a)*. Withdrawal of extractor (in direction of arrow) causes greater impaction of calculus in extractor *(b)*.

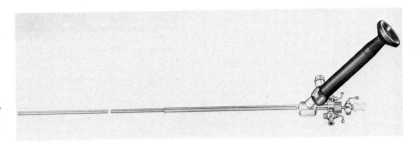

Figure 78–33. Operating uretero-pyeloscope, 9.5 F. (Courtesy of Karl Storz–Endoscopy America, Inc.)

may be obstructed at the torn ureteral meatus or at the previous site of the calculus. In such instances, the patient may experience renal pain and fever during the postoperative period, but such symptoms ordinarily disappear after conservative, symptomatic treatment.

COMPLICATIONS

Complications that may follow unsuccessful attempts at manipulation include hydronephrosis and pyelonephritis. Conservative treatment, including drainage of the kidney by catheter, if possible, and the administration of antibacterial drugs, will generally suffice. Perforation of the ureter by catheter or extractor may require ureterolithotomy and stenting of the ureter by catheter. Avulsion of the ureter demands immediate surgical exploration, the findings of which dictate the necessary treatment.

TRANSURETHRAL URETEROPYELOSCOPY

The introduction of ureteropyeloscopes has added a new dimension to transurethral diagnosis and treatment of lesions of the ureter and kidney. The state of the art is changing constantly because of the technological improvements in these devices and their accessories. The commonly employed ureteropyeloscopes vary in length from 38.5 to 41 cm and in diameter from 9.5 F to 12 F (Fig. 78–33). Some ureteropyeloscopes accept both forward and lateral viewing telescopes and have a working channel that allows passage of stone baskets, brushes, biopsy forceps, coagulating electrodes, and various other catheters (Fig. 78–34). Ureteropyeloscopy has been used in the management of tumors of the ureter (see Fig. 78–24*B*) and renal pelvis, ureteral obstruction,

and hematuria and positive cytology from the upper part of the urinary tract (Huffman et al., 1983). It has been employed most extensively, however, in the management of ureteral and pelvic calculi. The limiting factors of size and position of ureteral calculi described for "blind" endoscopic manipulation do not apply to ureteropyeloscopy. Lyon has removed calculi from all sites in the ureter and stones as large as 16 by 9 mm from the renal pelvis (Huffman et al., 1983).

Ureteroscopy or ureteropyeloscopy is started by dilating the ureteral orifice with metal dilating tips, a Grüntzig catheter, or Braasch bulbs. The ureteroscope is then gently introduced into the dilated ureteral orifice and advanced in the ureter carefully (Fig. 78–35). An effort is made not to overdistend the upper part of the urinary tract with irrigant. The calculus is visualized (see Fig. 78–24*C*) and the stone basket is passed (Fig. 78–36). The calculus may be engaged either during passage or withdrawal of the basket and is extracted under vision (see Fig. 78–24*D*).

Calculi that appear too large to be withdrawn through the ureter may be fragmented or disintegrated with the ultrasonic transducer. For this purpose, the telescope must be removed after the calculus has been secured within the stone basket. The ultrasonic transducer is inserted through the ureteropyeloscope and, with fluoroscopic guidance, is brought into contact with the calculus. Ultrasonic disintegration of the calculus is performed when good contact is established. Constant irrigation through the instrument is maintained to provide cooling and to allow removal of stone fragments by suction placed on the transducer. Larger fragments can be removed with the stone basket while under direct vision. Goodfriend (1984) has developed an ultrasonic transducer that permits disintegration of a calculus under direct vision.

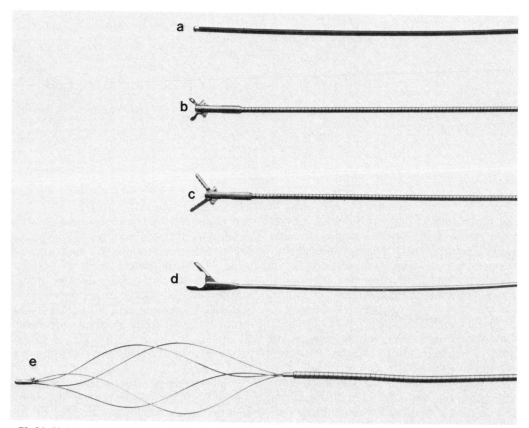

Figure 78–34. Ureteropyeloscopic operating instruments: *a*, coagulating electrode; *b*, biopsy forceps; *c*, grasping forceps; *d*, biopsy, cutting forceps; *e*, stone basket. (Courtesy of Karl Storz–Endoscopy America, Inc.)

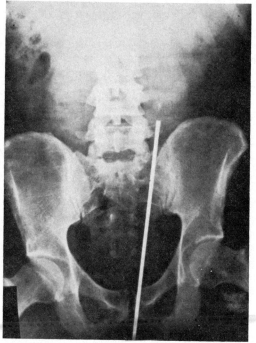

Figure 78–35. Calculus and ureteropyeloscope in mid left ureter.

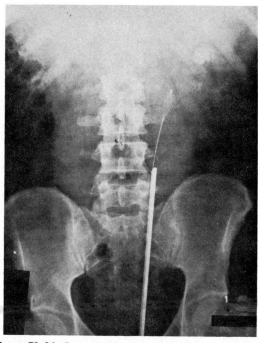

Figure 78–36. Stone basket passed beyond calculus preparatory to engagement of calculus.

References

Augspurger, R.R., and Donohue, R.E.: Prevention of obturator nerve stimulation during transurethral surgery. J. Urol., *123*:170, 1980.

Bülow, H., and Fröhmuller, H.G.W.: Electrohydraulic lithotripsy with aspiration of the fragments under vision—304 consecutive cases. J. Urol., *126*:454, 1981.

Cote, R.J., Burke, H., and Schoenberg, H.W.: Prediction of unusual postoperative results by urodynamic testing in benign prostatic hyperplasia. J. Urol., *125*:690, 1981.

DeWeerd, J.H.: Litholapaxy. *In* Greene, L.F., and Segura, J.W. (Eds.): Transurethral Surgery. Philadelphia, W.B. Saunders Co., 1979, p. 293.

Emmett, J.L., Rous, S.N., Greene, L.F., DeWeerd, J.H., and Utz, D.C.: Preliminary internal urethrotomy in 1036 cases to prevent urethral stricture following transurethral resection: caliber of normal adult male urethra. J. Urol., *89*:829, 1963.

Goodfriend, R.: Ultrasonic and electrohydraulic lithotripsy of ureteral calculi. Urology, *23*:5, 1984.

Greene, L.F.: Use of hemostatic bag after transurethral resection. J. Urol., *106*:915, 1971.

Huffman, J.L., Bagley, D.H., and Lyon, E.S.: Extending cystoscopic techniques into the ureter and renal pelvis. JAMA, *250*:2002, 1983.

Kirchheim, D., Tremann, J.A., and Ansel, J.S.: Transurethral urethrotomy under vision. J. Urol., *119*:496, 1978.

Madsen, P.O., and Madsen, R.E.: Clinical and experimental evaluation of different irrigating fluids for transurethral surgery. Invest. Urol., *3*:122, 1965.

Madsen, P.O., and Naber, K.: The importance of the pressure in the prostatic fossa and absorption of irrigating fluid during transurethral resection of the prostate. J. Urol., *109*:446, 1973.

Nachtsheim, D.A., So, E.P.H., and Greene, L.F.: Transurethral resection of lesions in the dome of the bladder. Urology, *18*:84, 1981.

Orandi, A.: Transurethral incision of the prostate. J. Urol., *12*:187, 1978.

Siroky, M.B., Olsson, C.A., and Krane, R.J.: Flow rate nomogram. I. Development. J. Urol., *120*:665, 1979.

Siroky, M.B., Olsson, C.A., and Krane, R.J.: The flow rate nomogram. II. Clinical application. J. Urol., *123*:208, 1980.

Terhorst, B., Lutzeyer, W., Cichos, M., and Pohlman, R.: Die Zerstörung von Harnsteinen durch Ultraschall. II. Ultraschall-Lithotripsie von Blasensteinen. Urol. Int., *27*:458, 1972.

Turner-Warwick, R.T.: Clinical problems associated with urodynamic abnormalities with special reference to the value of synchronous ciné/pressure/flow cystography and the clinical importance of detrusor function studies. *In* Lutzeyer, W., and Melchior, H. (Eds.): Urodynamics. New York, Springer-Verlag, 1973, p. 237.

Turner-Warwick, R.T., Whiteside, C.G., Arnold, E.P., Bates, C.P., Worth, P.H.L., Milroy, E.G.J., Webster, J.R., and Weir, J.: A urodynamic view of prostatic obstruction and the results of prostatectomy. Br. J. Urol., *45*:631, 1973.

Utz, D.C., Farrow, G.M., Rife, C.C., Segura, J.W., and Zincke, M.D.: Carcinoma in situ of the bladder. Cancer, *45*(Suppl.): 1842, 1980.

Yalla, S.V., Yap, W., and Fam, B.A.: Detrusor urethral sphincteric dyssnergia: micturitional vesicourethral pressure profile patterns. J. Urol., *128*:969, 1982.

CHAPTER 79

Surgery of the Seminal Vesicles

JOHN M. PALMER, M.D.

The seminal vesicles reside in one of the most well protected areas in human anatomy and rival the pineal body in surgical inaccessibility. Surgery of the seminal vesicles enjoyed great popularity in the late nineteenth and early twentieth centuries, when these organs were thought to be the source of infective foci leading to inflammatory rheumatism in the male. Perineal seminal vesiculotomy was the most common procedure performed, usually for nonspecific inflammation. Fuller, before 1900, managed 700 such cases by perineal incision and drainage. Nonspecific inflammation gave way to tuberculosis as the major indication for surgical intervention in the early part of this century. With the discovery of antibiotics, however, inflammatory diseases have largely subsided, and the modern urologist is called upon only infrequently to manage lesions of surgical significance involving these historically interesting paired organs. Malignancy is rare and is usually diagnosed when cure is already impossible. There are several intriguing congenital anomalies that do necessitate operative intervention, and the presence of these makes up the major indication for surgery of the seminal vesicles.

EMBRYOLOGY

Toward the end of the sixth week of embryonic development, the cloaca is divided by the urorectal septum into a dorsal anorectal canal and a ventral primitive urogenital sinus. The mesonephric duct, which empties first into the cloaca and subsequently into the evolving urogenital sinus, produces the ureteric bud at the end of the fourth week. The bud differentiates into the rudimentary collecting system as well as the ureter by reciprocal induction with the surrounding metanephric blastema; the latter leads to the excretory portion of the kidney.

The site of origin of the ureteric bud from the mesonephric duct, as well as the short transverse portion of the mesonephric duct between the bud and the urogenital sinus, normally becomes incorporated by differential growth into an expanded region identified later as the *trigone* and the *proximal urethra*. In this process, the ureteral orifices normally come to be craniolateral to the secondary terminal orifices of the mesonephric ducts, i.e., the *ejaculatory ducts*. By the end of the embryonic period (the beginning of the ninth week), the remaining portion of the mesonephric duct is well separated from the ureter; it later gives rise to the prostatic urethra, the ejaculatory ducts, the vas deferens, and part of the epididymis.

In fetuses of about 60 mm in length, the seminal vesicles originate from the *ampulla*, that portion of the lower end of the mesonephric ducts that dilates to about four times its original size. At the lower end of this vertical ampulla, just before the ducts angle to give rise to the short, narrow, transverse terminal segment, the *ejaculatory ducts*, two dorsicranial diverticula, appear. These diverticula of simple epithelium (not surrounded by layers of mesenchyme like the terminal ducts) are the paired primordia of the *seminal vesicles* (Gray and Skandalakis, 1972).

Because of the intimate relationship of the distal ureter to the mesonephric duct at the earlier stages of development, failure of relative craniolateral migration of a ureteral orifice can lead to profound alterations in structure. These include ureteral ectopy into any of the meso-nephric duct structures (most commonly the prostatic urethra or the seminal vesicle), result-ing in abnormal renal development. These con-genital abnormalities constitute the major rea-sons for seminal vesicle surgery in current urologic practice (Harbitz and Liavag, 1968). In 104 cases of ureteral ectopy reviewed by Burford and associates (1949), the most common site of entry was the prostatic urethra, and the second most common site was the seminal vesicle (Bur-ford et al., 1949). Ectopic ureteral drainage into the seminal vesicle was noted with greater fre-quency (22 out of 32 cases) by others (Riba et al., 1946). The latter found a normal ipsilateral kidney in only one patient, with 24 of the remaining 31 patients having either renal agen-esis (10) or only rudimentary renal development (14).

PATHOLOGIC ENTITIES

Congenital

URETERAL ECTOPY

Ectopic ureterocele in females is usually associated with a duplex collecting system. In the male, ectopic ureterocele often occurs with-out duplication, and this is particularly true when the ureter drains into a mesonephric duct structure (Cremin et al., 1975). Ectopic male ureters terminate most frequently in the pros-tatic urethra (54 per cent). The ureters may also enter the seminal vesicles (28 per cent), the vasa (10 per cent), or the ejaculatory ducts (8 per cent) (Schnitzer, 1965). When the latter three structures receive the ureter, there is usually associated renal dysgenesis with contralateral renal hypertrophy and an absent ipsilateral tri-gone. In the typical case, a soft, fluctuant mass is palpated on rectal examination. There is often perineal or testicular pain, which may be related to sexual intercourse. Epididymitis has been reported infrequently. Urinary symptoms may be entirely absent. Treatment consists of sur-gical excision or unroofing of the enlarged sem-inal vesicle, with appropriate management of the renal and ureteral abnormality. The best surgical exposure for such lesions is a lower abdominal incision that allows extension into the involved flank if upper tract surgery is also indicated.

CYSTS

Cyst of the seminal vesicle is a rare lesion, with only 13 cases reported prior to 1969, 4 of these with associated renal agenesis. The fifth, sixth, and seventh cases of agenesis were re-ported by Furtado (1973). Cysts of the seminal vesicle probably result from congenital obstruc-tion of the juncture between the vesicle and the ejaculatory duct. The ureteric bud arises in the 4-week-old embryo from a site of angulation of the mesonephric duct just before it enters the cloaca. The seminal vesicle arises from a similar angulation of the mesonephric duct, but at a much different site and at a much later time in development. Therefore, though the ureteric bud and the seminal vesicles have similar geo-metric origins with reference to the mesonephric duct, they are not closely related in time and space. For this reason, the relationship of sem-inal vesicle cysts to renal agenesis is embryo-logically unclear. Cysts are usually discovered in the third decade of life and are almost always solitary (Beeby, 1974). Seminal vesicle cysts may reach immense proportions. For example, 5000 ml of fluid was aspirated by Smith in 1874 in the first reported case of "hydrocele" of the seminal vesicle (Hart, 1961).

Seminal vesicle cysts must be differentiated from other cystic structures encountered in the male pelvic floor. These include:

1. Wolffian duct remnants—occur along the course of the vas deferens, on the lateral pos-terior surface of the bladder. Sperm are absent on aspiration.

2. Müllerian duct remnants—the largest of the cystic structures, present along the midline of the posterior aspect of the bladder. Sperm are absent on aspiration.

3. Prostatic cysts—usually adjacent to the prostate laterally. Sperm are absent on aspira-tion.

4. Diverticula of the ejaculatory duct—sperm are present on aspiration. Epididymides are normal on palpation, and findings on sem-inal vesiculography are also normal.

5. Seminal vesicle cysts—located lateral to and behind the bladder. They are usually three to four times the normal seminal vesicle in size but smaller than müllerian duct cysts. Sperm are present on aspiration. Frequently the ipsi-lateral epididymis is enlarged (Rieser and Grif-fin, 1964).

Neoplasia

Benign lesions of the seminal vesicle in-clude fibromas, myomas, and cystic adenomas. Of the malignancies, adenocarcinoma is by far the most common, with only four cases of sarcoma having been reported (Buck and Shaw, 1972). Although the first case of probable adenocarcinoma of the seminal vesicle was reported in 1883, Lyons (1925) deserves credit for recording the first well-documented lesion *not* involving the prostate. There have been 34 acceptable cases of adenocarcinoma reported up to 1973 (Goldstein and Wilson, 1973). Half the reported patients with cancer of the seminal vesicle are older than 60 years of age, but several cases have occurred in men in their thirties. Hematuria is a common symptom and often involves the initial portion of the urinary stream. Sometimes mucus is passed in the urine. Hemospermia is rare. Bladder outlet obstruction is common with advanced lesions. Obliteration, deformity, or filling defects, or any combination of the three, are noted in the vesicles or in the ampullae on seminal vesiculographic examination. A recent case demonstrated the value of the CT scan in defining the lesion (Benson et al., 1984). Early invasion of the urinary bladder or rectum is the rule, along with intraprostatic extension. Half the reported cases have demonstrable metastases at the time of diagnosis, with common involvement of lungs, bone, and neighboring organs (Banchieri and Cappa, 1968).

On cystoscopic examination, the verumontanum is generally abnormal, and the ejaculatory ducts are prominent. The bladder base may be elevated, and the ureters may be displaced or dilated. Rectal examination in most instances defines an enlarged, irregular mass (Smith et al., 1967).

The prognosis for neoplastic lesions of the seminal vesicles is poor. Surgical treatment must be radical if cure is to be accomplished. Prostatovesiculectomy with associated cystectomy is usually necessary. The standard retropubic approach is probably superior for this lesion, since it yields early and complete access to the bladder and prostate, and since pelvic lymphadenectomy can be added, if indicated.

Miscellaneous Lesions

CALCIFICATION

Calcification of the vasa is a pathognomonic sign of diabetes mellitus. It is usually seen in older diabetics with long-standing disease. Before the twentieth century, such calcification usually resulted from chronic suppurative inflammation or tuberculosis. Calcification of the seminal vesicles and vasa also has been reported with uremia (Silber and McDonald, 1971).

CONGENITAL ABSENCE

Young males born with mucoviscidosis have a high incidence of hypoplasia or absence of mesonephric duct derivatives, particularly the vas deferens. Olson and Weaver (1969) reported unilateral absence of the seminal vesicle in 4 of 18 infants who failed to survive this syndrome.

AMYLOID DEPOSITION

Deposition of amyloid in the seminal vesicle is not an unusual finding at autopsy. Amyloid deposits seem to occur with aging, and they are noted in 4 to 9 per cent of all autopsies; however, the incidence increases to greater than 30 per cent after the seventh decade of life. One symptomatic case of amyloidosis of the seminal vesicle cured by surgery has been reported (Krane et al., 1973).

Methods of Diagnosis

Vasoseminal vesiculography is a simple diagnostic tool that allows complete radiographic visualization of the seminal vesicle. Originally described by Belfield in 1913, it has varied little over the years. The procedure was commonly performed during and immediately following World War II, but with the advent of the "antibiotic era," indications for it have become relatively rare. Present indications for vasoseminal vesiculography include male sterility, suspicion of a congenital anomaly, a constant genital infection, and a palpable abnormality of the prostate or the seminal vesicle. Endoscopic catheterization of the ejaculatory ducts is possible but seldom successful. A more dependable method is to isolate the vas high in the scrotum with the patient under local anesthesia. It is not necessary to incise the vas deferens, although this causes no damage. A 23-gauge needle is introduced through the wall and into the lumen. One ml of methylglucamine diatrizoate (Renografin) affords excellent visualization of the vas, the seminal vesicle, and the ejaculatory duct. Films are initially obtained in the anteroposterior projection, followed by a view directed toward the feet with 30 to 35 degrees of cranial angulation. If desired, a few drops of contrast can be injected into the distal vas to define it as well as the epididymis.

The normal seminal vesicle fills easily on vasographic examination (Fig. 79–1). The contours are regular with sharp borders, and the organs are symmetric with the midline. Reflux into the bladder is common, but vasourethral

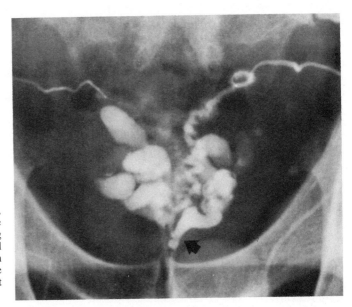

Figure 79–1. Normal vesiculogram. On the left, the ampulla of the vas deferens is seen to give origin to the seminal vesicle before continuing as the ejaculatory duct (arrow). Note the normal convoluted appearance of each vesicle, with sharp borders and midline symmetry. On the right, the distal vas deferens has emptied, but the ejaculatory duct is normal in appearance.

reflux is rare and suggests prostatic malignancy. Dilatation of the ampulla and the seminal vesicle is seen with urethral stricture (Mitty, 1971).

Alternative, noninvasive methods of estimating seminal vesicle volume include transurethral or transrectal ultrasonography and CT scan of the pelvis. Although these methods lack the resolution of vasograms for luminal defects, they offer better definition of the soft tissue of the seminal vesicles and complement vasography in evaluating cysts or mass lesions (Holm and Gammelgaard, 1981).

ANATOMY

The seminal vesicles are located anterior to Denonvilliers' fascia, which is thought to be a fused extension of both layers of the inferior peritoneum. This fascia separates the prostate, the seminal vesicles, and the ampullae from the rectum. The seminal vesicles are 5 to 6 cm long and 15 mm wide. The anterior superior surface of the vesicles lies under the inferior posterior surface of the bladder and the trigone. The medial border lies about 1 cm lateral to the ampullae of the vas deferens, and the lateral border is adjacent to vesical prostatic veins and to branches of the hypogastric nerve. The natural enlargement of the vas deferens where it forms the ampulla begins at about the level of the ureteral orifice. The venous drainage of the vesicle terminates in the vesicoprostatic venous plexus. The arterial blood supply is brought by

the artery of the ductus deferens, an offshoot from the umbilical branch of the internal iliac artery. In addition, branches from the inferior vesical and the middle rectal arteries supply the vesicle.

SURGERY

Ullman is credited with the first complete removal of the seminal vesicle in 1899. Early authors advocated an inguinal approach, tracing the vas deferens inferiorly to locate the seminal vesicle. Fuller popularized perineal vesiculotomy for removal of foci of infection in men suffering from inflammatory rheumatism. A variety of surgical approaches have been described subsequently, and at least ten different techniques were listed by de Assis in 1952. His article is recommended for both historical details and a good description of the suprapubic transperitoneal approach (de Assis, 1952).

Three general routes to the seminal vesicles are available to the surgeon: anterior (abdominal), perineal, and posterior. *Anterior* routes are either transvesical or paravesical. They include either suprapubic or inguinal incisions and either extra- or intraperitoneal surgery. In general, unilateral benign lesions are managed by retroperitoneal surgery, and bilateral or malignant lesions require the transperitoneal approach.

Perineal surgery affords good access to the juncture of the seminal vesicle with the ampullae, but if the vesicle is at all enlarged, access to the proximal portion is limited.

Posterior surgery includes the ischiorectal, coccygeal-perineal, inguinoperineal, median posterior, transischiatic, sacral, and transrectal approaches.

The variety of procedures described is testimony to the inaccessibility of these organs and also to the changing indications for surgery through the years. Antibiotics have largely eradicated chronic suppurative infections of the vesicles, and tuberculosis has been similarly controlled. Current indications for operation are congenital abnormalities and, rarely, neoplasia.

Surgical Approach

Two techniques are described: perineal and transvesical. The author advocates the perineal approach for smaller lesions, particularly if inflammation is present. For larger lesions, the transvesical approach provides superior exposure. Malignant lesions or large cysts, particularly if associated with ureteral anomaly or renal aplasia, will require a combined transperitoneal and retroperitoneal approach in most cases.

PERINEAL

As in all perineal surgery, a thoroughly emptied bowel is mandatory. In some instances, a complete bowel preparation with antibiotics may be advantageous if the risk of rectal injury is high. Correct positioning of the patient in the exaggerated perineal position is of primary importance in the approach to the seminal vesicle. The Young table, the Palmer perineal board, or a similar apparatus that allows caudal extension of hips and pelvis toward the surgeon is helpful. The surface plane of the perineum should be horizontal. A standard perineal incision is made, arching about 2 cm outside the moist perianal skin and staying just medial to the ischial tuberosities. The knife is held in a horizontal plane and advanced 6 or 8 cm into the lateral ischiorectal fossae, blade upward on each end of the incision, and rotated vertically to develop the fossae sharply (Fig. 79–2). This maneuver will allow insertion of each index finger into the ischiorectal fossa, where the rectum can be easily palpated. The fingers are gently worked through the deep tissues and then brought together in the midline anterior to the rectum (Fig. 79–2, *Inset*). The left index finger then traverses the entire incision (Fig. 79–3), allowing sharp division of the subcutaneous tissue and the central tendon. If this maneuver is

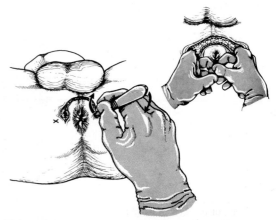

Figure 79–2. A standard perineal incision has been made. At the lateral portions the knife is inserted deeply, medial to the tuberosities and lateral to the rectum, into the ischiorectal fossae. The blade is rotated upward to create two spaces large enough to accept the surgeon's index fingers.
   Inset, The index fingers are inserted deeply into the lateral ischiorectal fossae. The rectum can be palpated in the midline. The fingers are bluntly worked back and forth anterior to the rectum until one finger can traverse the entire incision behind the central tendon.

performed correctly, the remainder of the dissection to Denonvilliers' fascia can be carried out bluntly, with a 4 × 4 inch sponge over the right index finger and the double-gloved left index finger in the rectum. The Lowsley retractor must be placed at this point to elevate the prostate toward the surgeon. The rectum knuckles in an anterior direction over the prostate gland and must be gently pushed inferiorly during this dissection. The natural tendency to go toward the easily palpable Lowsley retractor in the membranous urethra must be avoided, and a direction toward the flat prostatic surface must be maintained. The distinctive whitish, glistening surface of Denonvilliers' fascia is

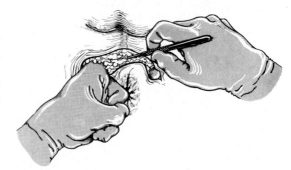

Figure 79–3. With the left index finger traversing the space between the two ischiorectal fossae and anterior to the rectum, the subcutaneous tissue and the central tendon are sharply divided.

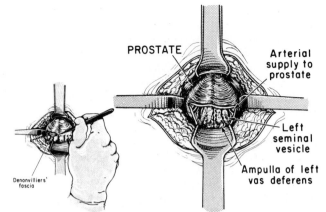

Figure 79–4. *Inset,* With the posterior retractor displacing the rectum deeply in a posterior direction, Denonvilliers' fascia is divided at the base of the prostate gland, directly exposing the ampullae and the seminal vesicles.

The final operative exposure is shown in the main figure. The layers of Denonvilliers' fascia have been displaced posteriorly by the retractor, affording full access to the seminal vesicles.

readily identified. The rectum is moved away from the prostatic surface in a posterior direction, and with persistence will completely fall away. Electrocautery division of the levator muscles facilitates exposure at this point. The seminal vesicles lie deep to both layers of Denonvilliers' fascia. The latter is incised transversely at the prostatic base (Fig. 79–4, *Inset*). The rectal retractor can then be used to displace this fascia in a deeply posterior direction, exposing the two medial ampullae of the vasa and, lateral to each of these, the seminal vesicles (Fig. 79–4). The arterial supply to the prostate gland courses between the layers of Denonvilliers' fascia and enters the prostatic base at its extreme lateral surface, outside the vesicles. Except in the presence of tumor (for which this approach is not advocated), the blood supply of the seminal vesicle is not a major source of intraoperative bleeding, and no unusual means need be taken for its control.

This approach is indicated primarily for inflammatory lesions or for minor cystic enlargement. Large cysts, particularly those with an associated ureteral or renal anomaly, should be managed by abdominal surgery.

TRANSVESICAL

This approach was originally described by Thompson Walker (de Assis, 1952). In 1968, Walker and Bowles utilized a transverse trigonal incision below the ureteral orifices in a patient with a seminal vesicle cyst. Politano et al. (1975) have described circumferential division of the entire bladder from the vesical neck to expose the seminal vesicles. In our experience, the vertical trigonal incision has always afforded adequate exposure, and it does not compromise the integrity of the subtrigonal musculature.

The bladder is exposed in the retroperito-

neal space and incised. The small initial incision is stretched until it is large enough to expose the entire bladder floor and the trigone. Exposure is maintained distally by the suturing of the bladder wall to the inferior margin of the skin incision; proximally, it is held by a pair of ribbon retractors positioned over two small laparotomy tapes. The trigone is divided vertically in the midline, beginning just inside the bladder neck. Full-thickness traction sutures placed along the extent of this incision greatly facilitate exposure (Fig. 79–5). Lateral dissection will disclose first the ampulla of the vas deferens and then the

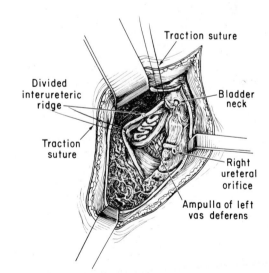

Figure 79–5. Transvesical approach to the seminal vesicles. The bladder has been opened anteriorly, and the trigone has been divided by a vertical incision. Note the divided interureteric ridge as a landmark. This exposes the medial ampullae of the vasa and, immediately lateral to these, the seminal vesicles. All four structures lie between the posterior surface of the trigone and the rectum. Traction sutures on the edges of the posterior vesical incision are extremely useful to obtain full exposure.

seminal vesicle. These two structures lie in the same anatomic plane but are easily differentiated. Utilization of this approach enables large cystic masses or inflammatory lesions to be totally excised or marsupialized into the bladder. Following definitive surgery, the vertical trigonal incision is reapproximated with interrupted 2–0 chromic sutures, and a lateral vesical drain is placed on the involved side.

CONCLUSION

Surgery of the seminal vesicle is challenging because of its infrequent application. Careful patient selection and firm operative indications are mandatory for satisfactory outcome. The actual operative technique is not difficult, however, and in correctly selected patients will afford good results.

References

de Assis. J. S.: Seminal vesiculectomy. J. Urol., *68*:747, 1952.

Banchieri, F. R., and Cappa, A. P.: Un cas de cancer de la vesicule seminale gauche. J. Urol. Nephrol. (Paris), *74*:890, 1968.

Beeby, D. I.: Seminal vesicle cyst associated with ipsilateral renal agenesis: A case report and review of the literature. J. Urol., *112*:120, 1974.

Benson, R. C., Clark, W. R., and Farrow, G. M.: Carcinoma of the seminal vesicle. J. Urol., *132*: 483, 1984.

Buck, A. C., and Shaw, R. E.: Primary tumors of the retrovesical region with special reference to mesenchymal tumors of the seminal vesicles. Br. J. Urol., *41*;47, 1972.

Burford, C. F., Glenn, J. E., and Burford, E. H.: Ureteral ectopia: Review of the literature and two case reports J. Urol., *62*:211, 1949.

Cremin, B. J., Friedland, G. W., and Kottra, J. J.: Ectopic ureterocele in single non-duplicated collecting system: Diagnosis by radiography. Urology, *5*:154, 1975.

Furtado, A. J. L.: Three cases of cystic seminal vesicle associated with unilateral renal agenesis. Br. J. Urol., *45*:536, 1973.

Goldstein, A. F., and Wilson, E. S.: Carcinoma of the seminal vesicle—with particular reference to the angiographic appearance. Br. J. Urol., *45*:211, 1973.

Gray, S. W., and Skandalakis, J. E.: Embryology for Surgeons (Chaps. 16 and 19). Philadelphia. W. B. Saunders Co., 1972.

Harbitz, T. B., and Liavag, I.: Urogenital malformation with cyst of the seminal vesicle, ipsilateral dilated ureter and renal agenesis. Report of a case and review of the literature. Scand. J. Urol. Nephrol., *2*:217, 1968.

Hart, J. B.: A case of cyst or hydrops of the seminal vesicle. J. Urol., *86*:137, 1961.

Holm, H. H., and Gammelgaard, J.: Ultrasonically guided precise needle placement in the prostate and the seminal vesicles. J. Urol., *125*:385, 1981.

Krane, R. J., Klugo, R. D., and Olsson, C. A.: Seminal vesicle amyloidosis. Urology, *2*:70, 1973.

Lyons, O.: Primary carcinoma of the left seminal vesicle. J. Urol., *13*:477, 1925.

Meiraz, D., Fischelovitch, J., and Lazebnik, J.: Agenesis of the kidney associated with congenital malformation of the seminal vesicle. Br. J. Urol., *45*:541, 1973.

Mitty, H. A.: Roentgen features of reflux into the prostate, seminal vesicles and vasa deferentia. Am. J. Roentgenol. Radium Ther. Nucl. Med., *112*:603, 1971.

Olson, J. R., and Weaver, D. K.: Congenital mesonephric defects in male infants with mucoviscidosis. J. Clin. Pathol., *22*:725, 1969.

Politano, V. A., Lankford, R. W., and Susaeta, R.: A transvesical approach to total seminal vesiculectomy: A case report. J. Urol., *113*:395, 1975.

Reddy, Y. N., and Winter, C. C.; Cyst of the seminal vesicle: A case report and review of the literature. J. Urol., *108*:134, 1972.

Riba, L. W., Schmidlapp, C. J., and Bosworth, N. L.: Ectopic ureter draining into seminal vesicle. J. Urol., *56*:332, 1946.

Rieser, C., and Griffin, T. L.: Cysts of the prostate. J. Urol., *92*:282, 1964.

Schnitzer, B. J.: Ectopic ureteral opening into seminal vesicle: A report of four cases. J. Urol., *93*:576, 1965.

Silber, S. J.: and McDonald, E. D.: Calcifications of the seminal vesicles and vas deferens in a uremic patient. J. Urol., *105*:542, 1971.

Smith, B. A., Jr., Webb, E. A., and Price, W. E.: Carcinoma of the seminal vesicle. Trans. Am. Assoc. Genitourin. Surg., *58*:128, 1966; J. Urol., *97*:743, 1967.

Tanahashi, Y., Watanabe, H., Igari, D., Harada, K., and Saitoh, M.: Volume estimation of the seminal vesicles by means of transrectal ultrasonotomography: A preliminary report. Br. J. Urol., *47*:695, 1975.

Walker, W. C., and Bowles, W. T.: Transvesical seminal vesiculostomy in treatment of congenital obstruction of seminal vesicles: Case report. J. Urol., *99*:324, 1968.

CHAPTER 80

Surgery of the Urethra

CHARLES J. DEVINE, JR., M.D.

ANATOMY

Anatomy of the penis and urethra has been described in Chapter 1; however, certain details must be emphasized in discussion of surgery of the urethra. The corpora cavernosa are distinct at their base, where each crus is attached to the adjacent inferior ramus of the symphysis pubis, and join at the level of the suspensory ligament of the penis. Distal to this point they are, in effect, one structure with a septum consisting of multiple strands extending from the dorsal midline to the ventral midline (Fig. 80–1). A third erectile body, the corpus spongiosum, encloses the urethra and lies in the ventral groove beneath the septum. At the distal end the corpus spongiosum expands to form the glans penis covering the tips of the corpora cavernosa. The urethral meatus is slitlike and ventrally aligned on the undersurface of the tip of the glans. As the corpus spongiosum continues into the perineum, it broadens to form the bulb, ending at the urogenital diaphragm.

The urethra maintains a constant lumen size through the penis, becomes larger in the bulb, and narrows again as it turns upward as the membranous urethra, penetrating the urogenital diaphragm to join with the urethra in the prostate. The fossa navicularis in the glans is lined with stratified squamous epithelium, as is the pendulous urethra in the penile shaft. In the bulb the lining cells gradually change through areas of pseudostratified columnar epithelium to a delicate transitional epithelium in the membranous urethra. There is a submucosal layer throughout, with an outer muscular layer in the prostatic and membranous portions. Numerous glands open into the urethral lumen, and the ducts of Cowper's glands opening into the bulbar urethra can cause confusing shadows during urethral x-ray studies.

Fascial Layers

The erectile bodies are closely contained by the deep fascia of the penis (Buck's fascia), a septum of which separates the corpus spongiosum from the corpora cavernosa. Extensions of Buck's fascia attach the three corporal bodies in the perineum to the structures with which they are in contact and form the fascial compartments of the perineum with Colles' fascia, which is the continuation in the perineum of the dartos or superficial fascial layer of the penis.

The blood supply of the penis is derived from branches of the pudendal artery. The urethral artery and the artery to the bulb of the urethra enter the bulb on each side and run in the corpus spongiosum in a lateral position; they might easily be injured when internal urethrotomy or sphincterotomy is being done in the 3 or 9 o'clock position. Just beyond the takeoff of these arteries the terminal branches of the pudendal arteries become the deep (profunda) arteries of the penis, entering the medial aspects of the corpora cavernosa near this termination; the dorsal arteries of the penis, which pass medial to the crus of the corpora cavernosa to run on the dorsal surface of the corpora cavernosa lateral to the deep dorsal vein, terminate in branches going to the glans penis. These terminal arterial branches to the glans give the corpus spongiosum and urethra a double-ended blood supply, allowing the urethra to be mobilized from the glans to the bulb without ischemia developing (McGowan and Waterhouse, 1964). In hypospadias there is no urethra or corpus

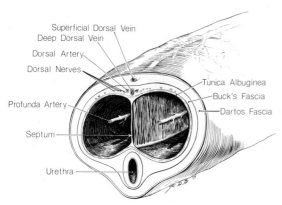

Figure 80–1. Anatomy of the penis illustrated in depth with a transverse section at about the junction of its middle and distal thirds. Note the configuration of the septum, which is not a solid sheet but is made up of multiple strands thickened at each end where they attach at the ventral and dorsal midlines of the tunica.

spongiosum to carry blood from the urethral arteries to the glans, so all of the blood supply to the glans comes from these terminal branches of the dorsal arteries.

URETHRAL MEATAL STENOSIS

In the newborn, a small urethral meatus probably will not be called to a urologist's attention unless the stenosis is associated with other congenital deformities (e.g., hypospadias) or causes voiding difficulties or a urinary tract infection (Allen and Summers, 1974). A full discussion of urethral meatal stenosis in boys can be found in Chapter 48.

If the urethral meatus of a boy appears very narrow and if there are associated symptoms, a meatotomy should be considered. To make this decision, voiding should be observed to see that the meatus opens as a full, forceful stream is passed. If the stream is narrow and excessively forceful, stenosis is probably present. The occluding skin is generally a thin layer that can be seen to pouch out with the opening in the center as the child voids. Figure 80–2 shows a voiding urethrogram of a boy with meatal stenosis. The pouching skin and the fine stream through the narrow meatus can be seen.

A urethral meatotomy can be done under local anesthesia, using the technique illustrated in Figure 80–3. It is important to insert the needle into the skin fold from the underside because the tip of the needle can then be observed and controlled. If insertion is done from the outside, the needle will pass through both layers of the fold, and a wheal cannot be

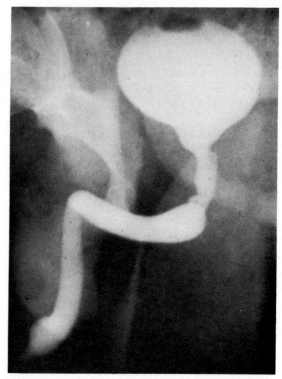

Figure 80–2. Voiding urethrogram of a child with meatal stenosis. Note that the entire urethra is dilated. The tiny stream distal to the meatus can be seen.

raised because of leakage of the anesthetic solution. After the meatotomy, the edges of the cut will seal together again unless they are kept open. The tip of an antibiotic ophthalmic ointment tube is the best instrument for this. The child's mother is instructed to separate the edges gently with the tip of the tube three times a day until they are healed—generally from 7 to 10 days. To be sure that the mother understands these instructions, one should watch her carry out the process, or she will be inclined to insert the tip of the tube only a little way in and squeeze out a glob of ointment. The ointment is used for lubrication; the wedge shape of the tip does the job.

In adolescents and adults, it is often necessary to place sutures to approximate the urethral mucosal edge to the glans epithelial edge to control bleeding (Fig. 80–4). Sometimes only one suture will be necessary at the apex of the incision. In adults, the tip of a ½-ounce Neosporin ointment tube can be used to keep the meatus open, using the technique described. Meatal stenosis occurs in adults following inflammation, specific or nonspecific urethral infections, either external or internal, and trauma (especially in association with indwelling catheters or urethral instrumentation).

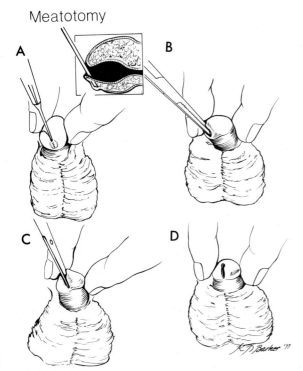

Meatotomy

Figure 80–3. Meatotomy. *A,* The needle is introduced into the obstructing leaf of tissue from the inside. This allows better control. About 0.5 ml of anesthetic material is used to form the wheal. *B,* The obstructing tissue is crushed with a mosquito clamp. *C,* The crushed tissue is incised. *D,* There is no bleeding, and the mother is instructed to keep the meatus open until it heals.

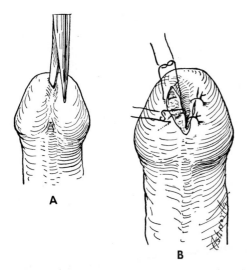

Figure 80–4. Meatotomy in normally developed penis. *A,* Incision in ventral aspect of glans. *B,* Closure of wound. (From Hand, J. R.: *In* Campbell, M. F. and Harrison, J. H. (Eds.): Urology, Vol. 3, 3rd Ed. Philadelphia, W. B. Saunders Co., 1970.)

BALANITIS XEROTICA OBLITERANS

Balanitis xerotica obliterans is the most common disease to cause stenosis. It affects the prepuce and the glans penis, causing white, thickened plaques that originate at the frenulum and involve the urethral meatus and, at times, the fossa navicularis. In uncircumcised men, the prepuce becomes edematous and thickened and often may be stuck to the glans (Bainbridge et al., 1971). The process may also involve segments of the distal urethra (Staff, 1970). Diagnosis is made by biopsy because of the similarity in appearance to other inflammatory conditions. When only the foreskin is involved, circumcision should be done. If urethral obstruction is present, a meatotomy by clamping and cutting or a meatoplasty by the advancing V-flap technique should be done. If there is associated urethral stricture, it is unlikely to be due to the balanitis xerotica obliterans process but probably has been caused by fibrosis secondary to chronic inflammation or possibly to previous attempts at dilation. In these circumstances I would proceed to a graft urethroplasty using full-thickness penile skin (Fig. 80–5).

We make a circumcising incision and reflect the skin on the ventral aspect of the penis to explore the extent of the urethra involved in the process. We next make an incision in the glans and urethra opening back to normal urethra. We excise the abnormal mucosa, leaving a raw area that is a good base for take of a graft. This area is measured and a full-thickness graft is obtained and applied to the opened glans, sewing around the edges but also placing sutures through the graft to secure it to the new bed. We then approximate the graft around a 24 F sound and close the glans tissue around it. We replace this sound with a smaller silicone catheter and leave it to divert the urine for approximately 10 to 14 days. This method has been successful. It makes a very normal-looking repair and carries an advantage over local flaps in that we move in skin that is less likely to be involved in the inflammatory process. Blandy and Tresidder (1967) devised a flap for this repair (Fig. 80–6) that we have used with success when the tissues are not so scarred.

REITER'S SYNDROME

Reiter's syndrome is characterized by inflammatory involvement of three membranes, producing urethritis, conjunctivitis, and arthri-

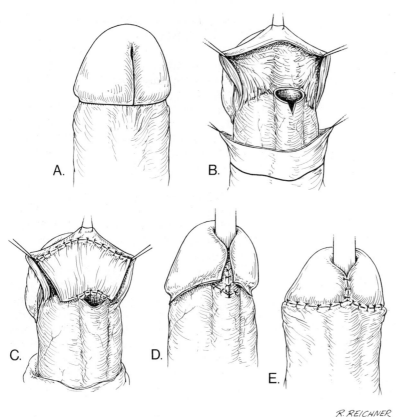

Figure 80–5. Patch graft meato-plasty with repaving of the fossa navicularis. *A,* The stenotic urethra is opened and a circumcising inci-sion made around the corona. *B,* The scarred mucosa has been re-moved from the fossa navicularis, and the normal-caliber urethra is mobilized and spatulated. The graft to be used is marked on the penile skin. *C,* The graft has been placed into the fossa navicularis secured by sutures in the midpart and to the edges of the glans epithelium and urethra. *D,* The urethral anasto-mosis is completed, and the graft has been tubed. *E,* The glans wings have been brought around and se-cured together and to the penile skin.

R. REICHNER

Figure 80–6. Advancing flap for meatoplasty. *A,* The strictured area is identified and a flap outlined that will fit into the defect. If the scarred meatus is too far proximal, it may be necessary to devise a transverse flap that can be elevated and turned into the defect. *B,* The urethra is dissected out and opened back to an area of normal caliber. *C,* The tip of the flap is sewn to the incised urethra and is turned into the defect with interrupted sutures on each side. *D,* When the caliber of the urethra is adequate, the sutures are placed fixing the skin flap to the epithelium of the glans. *E,* At the conclusion the opened meatus has been advanced back onto the glans.

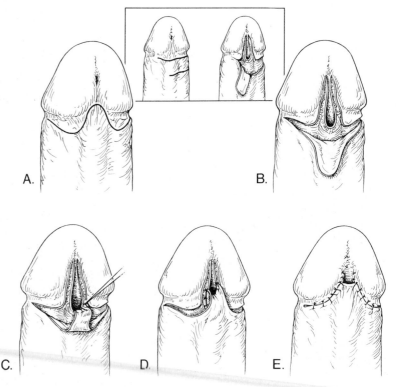

R. REICHNER

tis. In most cases the systemic effects of the disease far outweigh the local effects on the urethra. However, the urethritis may progress to severe inflammation with necrosis of the mucosa and severe stricture disease involving the full length of the urethra back to the prostate. Multiple tries at reconstruction only lead to further disease. Our attempts at excising the inflamed urethra and replacing it with a skin graft tube have not been successful. At present we create a perineal urethrostomy and excise the entire urethra distal to that area. We have laid in a wide skin graft from that point to the glans to await resolution of the inflammation before making a tube from it. These cases challenge a surgeon's ingenuity and patience.

MULTIPLE HEMANGIOMA

These lesions are exceedingly rare but, when seen, offer another challenge to the surgeon. All reported cases have been benign but have demonstrated a persistent nature if not totally controlled by local resection. Heman-

giomas will come to notice because of hematuria or a bloody urethral discharge, and on cystoscopy the dilated blood vessels can be seen. The urethral meatus is a common site, and the lesion will protrude, with bleeding from urination and blood on the underwear. The only reason for electrofulguration of this lesion is to control an acute episode of bleeding at a small isolated lesion. The lesion consists of vascular spaces lined by endothelial cells; the walls are thin and fragile, and the epithelium is usually squamous. Excision of the lesion with adequate margins will help to prevent recurrence. When the lesion is extensive or widely spaced, the entire involved urethra should be excised. Aggressive management will spare the patient prolonged morbidity (Fig. 80–7).

At the meatus the residual urethra can be sutured to the glans tissue, re-creating a functional meatus. When a segment of the more proximal urethra has been excised, it may be possible to mobilize the ends of the urethra and reanastomose them. If they do not reach, we reconnect the dorsal aspects of the cut ends and apply a patch graft. If the defect is too long for

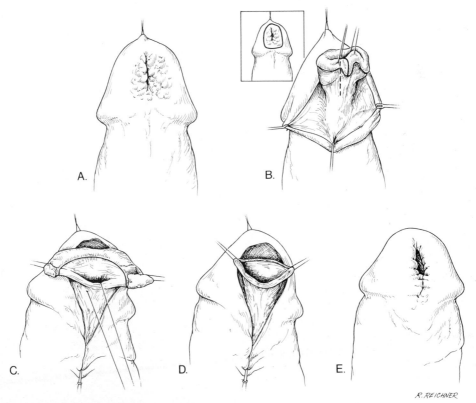

Figure 80–7. Excision of meatal urethral hemangioma. *A,* The hemangioma evident at the meatus involves the distal 1 1/2 cm of the urethra. *B,* A skin incision is planned to encompass the entire lesion. Dissection with strabismus scissors is carried out until normal urethra is encountered proximal to the lesion. *C,* The urethra is opened and the extent of the hemangioma marked. *D,* The hemangioma is resected. *E,* The urethra is reapproximated to the epithelium of the glans.

this, we insert a full-thickness tube graft or mobilize a pedicle of hairless skin to form a tube to bridge the gap. When the full length of the urethra must be replaced, we have found long tube grafts to work in about one half of the cases, but in the other half the tubes tend to contract in length and caliber. We therefore lay in the graft flat on the penile shaft and turn it into a tube about 6 months later (Roberts and Devine, 1983).

VERRUCAE ACUMINATA

Verrucae acuminata, or venereal warts, are villous lesions of the genitalia caused by a viral infection most probably transmitted by sexual intercourse. In men, they are common in the warm, moist areas under the prepuce or behind the corona of the glans and sometimes inside the urethra. They may involve the base of the penis and the scrotum. In women, they are commonly found at the introitus and around the urethral meatus. They also are sometimes found about the anus.

A large mass of verrucae involving the glans may be very difficult to differentiate from carcinoma of the penis. The entire mass of this Buschke-Löwenstein tumor must be excised, which usually requires removal of a part of the glans. We cover the defect with penile skin and excise the remainder of the prepuce. Small lesions on the skin may be handled by excision and fulguration of the bases, by simple electrofulguration, or by application of 25 per cent podophyllin in tincture of benzoin. The patient is given instructions in the use of this material at home, so newly apparent lesions can be treated before they become too large. Sexual partners of patients with verrucae should be examined, and any lesions discovered should be treated.

Verrucae in the urethra are a more serious problem. Those in the fossa navicularis can be managed by doing a wide meatotomy and excising the lesions and fulgurating their bases. Those farther up in the urethra are treated by cystoscopic electrofulguration or urethrotomy, with excision and fulguration for more extensive lesions. Rarely, verrucae involve the bladder (Bissada et al., 1974). Small areas may be resected, but with extensive involvement cystectomy and urinary diversion may be necessary. Whenever the mucosal surface is involved by verrucae, a regular program of cystoscopic evaluation must be set up, much as is done for transitional cell lesions.

URETHRAL DIVERTICULA

A diverticulum is an epithelium-lined pouch usually attached to the urethra by a narrow neck. A fistula is a tract lined with epithelium leading from the urethra to the skin.

Congenital urethral diverticula in the male result from incomplete development of the urethra, with a defect in only the ventral wall and subsequent stretching of this segment by the hydraulic force of the voiding stream. The downstream lip of the defect may serve as a valvular obstruction, increasing pressure in the lumen and the rate at which the diverticulum enlarges. Additional details regarding congenital urethral diverticula are found in Chapter 48. Injuries of the urethra may cause defects, such as a diverticulum or fistula, which are often associated with a urethral stricture (Fig. 80–8).

A congenital diverticulum in the prostatic urethra may be a large müllerian duct remnant associated with an intersex situation, although it often occurs in patients with a proximal hypospadias and represents an enlarged utricle (Devine et al., 1980). These diverticula may not be demonstrated on a voiding urethrogram but can be discovered by cystoscopy or by retrograde urethrogram. The tip of a urethral catheter will tend to catch in this opening, necessitating the use of a catheter guide; aside from this, however, they usually cause no problems and require no treatment. Occasionally, a large diverticulum will hold urine postvoiding and lead to dribbling, or it may be associated with recurrent infection. Surgical approach to this should be through the center of the trigone or transsacrally. Diverticula farther down in the urethra will cause obstruction and dribbling

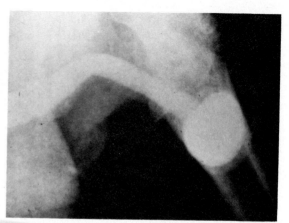

Figure 80–8. Voiding urethrogram demonstrating a diverticulum of the terminal urethra. This followed a hypospadias repair and was associated with a urethral meatal stricture.

because of delayed passage of contained urine and are often associated with infection or obstruction. We excise the diverticulum after exposing and dissecting its communication with the urethra. We then close this urethral opening after being sure that there is no distal obstruction to interfere with healing.

Diverticula of the female urethra may be due to dilatation of the periurethral glands or may be secondary to maternal birth trauma. They can cause severe pain when they become infected and distended with pus. Urethral discharge, dyspareunia, infection, and dribbling after voiding may be early findings. The diagnosis is made by palpation of a mass and expression of urine or infected material in some cases but in most cases requires x-ray confirmation. Sometimes a diverticulum will fill on voiding urethrogram, but demonstration of it may require the use of a special catheter that occludes the bladder neck and external meatus, with an opening in the side of the catheter that allows the urethra to fill with contrast material. A cancer may reside in a diverticulum. If so, a defect should be seen in the lumen of the structure.

Surgical procedures usually have as their objective removal of the diverticulum and closure of the urethra. This may be through a vertical incision in the vagina or through a curved incision across the vagina above the urethral meatus. In the latter case, a catheter in the urethra allows dissection between the vagina and the urethra in order to isolate the neck of the diverticulum (Sholem et al., 1974). After excision of the diverticulum and closure of the urethra, the intact vagina is replaced to cover the repair. A vertical incision made in the midline may be restricted to the segment just over the bulge of the diverticulum or may extend the length of the urethra from the meatus to the bladder neck. The urethra may be opened back to the neck of the diverticulum and a urethroplasty done after excision of the diverticulum. Spence and Duckett (1970) and O'Conor and Kropp (1969) have shown that it is possible to marsupialize a distal urethral diverticulum by incising the urethra and the wall of the diverticulum and allowing the tract to granulate. My experience with this procedure has not been good, and I would not use it unless the diverticulum were very small and very distal.

URETHRAL FISTULA

If the disruption after the trauma involves not only the urethra but also the covering structures, a fistula may result. This is a not infrequent complication of urethral surgery. As urine passes through the urethra there will be a leak to the outside. Unless there is obstruction downstream, scarring would tend to constrict the lumen of such a tract, but it is unusual for one to be obliterated by this process. Fistulas associated with inflammatory strictures and infected diverticula are more complex. Inflammatory tracts will develop parallel to the urethra and penetrate the tissues of the perineum and scrotum to open into multiple draining sinuses. Each time the patient voids, infected urine is forced into these tracts so that they persist and extend to become what is known as a watering-pot perineum.

Urethral fistulas may vary from pinpoint openings to large defects. Sometimes no problem will be seen immediately after urethral surgery, but later a leak will occur. When the meatus is stenosed or there is a stricture in the neourethra, voiding produces excess pressure proximal to this relative obstruction, causing a blowout and leakage of urine. If a fistula occurs after surgery, we replace the catheter for another 5 to 7 days, or, if the urinary diversion has been by a suprapubic tube, we reopen it to drainage. If the fistula is associated with a wound breakdown, no attempt should be made to close the defect with sutures, as they will not hold in the friable tissue and the defect will only be enlarged. The skin edges should be approximated with an adhesive (Steri-strip) bandage or Elastoplast secured on either side of the skin defect, with the edges of the tape being pulled together with sutures. If there is any question about the adequacy of the channel, a urethrogram should be made or a cystoscopic examination carried out. If the fistula is still present after the additional period of catheter drainage, it should be accepted and plans made to repair it in 6 months or more, when all the inflammation has resolved.

We close urethral fistulas in several ways. If the fistula is small and closure of the hole will not decrease the lumen of the urethra, a button of skin is incised around the fistula and its edges are cut even with the urethra. The urethra is then closed with interrupted 7-0 Vicryl sutures, turning the epithelium into the lumen. We test the suture line for watertightness and place a second row of sutures to bury this layer. A flap of the widely mobilized skin is swung over the repair, so that the suture lines are not apposed. A small silicone tube is used to divert the urine and is removed the next morning.

If the fistula is so large that simple closure will compromise the lumen of the urethra, we use a trap-door flap of penile skin left attached to one edge of the fistula while the other edges are incised even with the urethral mucosa. This flap is trimmed to fit exactly and is sewn in place with interrupted sutures of 6-0 or 7-0 Vicryl, which do not go through the epithelial edge but invert it completely into the lumen. Before a fistula or diverticulum is repaired, the urethra must be examined for obstruction distal to the obvious lesion. If a stricture is found, we repair it by a patch graft.

URETHRAL STRICTURE

The long-term result of urethral injury is a scar causing a decrease in the caliber of the urethra, i.e., a stricture. Strictures of the urethra may also result from inflammation, related either to gonorrhea or to other infections associated with indwelling urethral catheters or periurethral infection. Strictures caused by trauma commonly involve only the mucosal and submucosal tissues of the urethra, whereas inflammatory strictures also extend into the erectile tissue of the corpus spongiosum or the muscular layer of the membranous urethra.

Strictures cause obstruction to the flow of urine and produce symptoms associated with this obstruction, such as reduced caliber and velocity of the urinary stream and the necessity to exert force during urination. When the bladder begins to decompensate, symptoms typical of outlet obstruction will occur—nocturia, frequency, urgency, and stage voiding. Eventually the combination of obstruction and bladder decompensation will reach the point at which the patient is unable to void.

Strictures in Children

Strictures seen in childhood may or may not be congenital. When a child has a stricture, he or his parents may not be able to recall trauma sufficient to cause the stenosis. A diverticulum of the urethra may seem to be associated with a stricture, which is simply its downstream lip causing obstruction. Whenever a boy shows diminution in the flow of urine, a urethrogram should be done. It is probably not sufficient to do only a retrograde study; a small catheter should be passed and a voiding study obtained as well. Most of the time, stenosis of the urethra will be at the meatus. (We will not discuss urethral valves here.) The treatment of a meatal stenosis has been outlined.

In children, strictures after trauma are similar to adult strictures and may also follow the use of an indwelling catheter. Latex Foley catheters in the small sizes may contain unexpended plasticizer, which is irritating and can cause strictures. Silicone catheters are available in sizes as small as 8 F and should always be used when a catheter is going to be left in the urethra of a boy.

Inflammatory and Traumatic Strictures

Inflammatory strictures associated with urethritis are generally located in the pendulous and bulbous portions of the urethra, whereas those associated with instrumentation (following transurethral resection or use of an indwelling catheter) are found at the points where the urethral lumen is narrowest (the urethral meatus, the fossa navicularis, and the bladder neck) or where the urethra is fixed in position (at the penoscrotal junction by the suspensory ligament or in the membranous portion). In the past, gonorrhea was probably the most common cause of urethral stenosis. With modern treatment the inflammation associated with gonorrhea is unlikely to heal with fibrosis, so gonorrhea-related strictures are seen less frequently today.

Traumatic strictures may involve any portion of the urethra, but the segment beneath the symphysis pubis is most likely to be involved in a straddle-type injury, and the portion confined within or just above and below the urogenital diaphragm is most likely to be injured in an accident involving fracture of the pelvis.

The treatment of acute trauma, which is discussed elsewhere, has a marked effect on later treatment of the chronic lesions. The aim of acute treatment should be, if possible, to repair the defect so that there will be no need for further surgery. Often, however, the patient's condition will not permit such treatment, and a temporizing procedure must be done, accepting the necessity for further surgery.

A catheter should not be inserted until the injury has been defined. A retrograde urethrogram should be done using dilute intravenous contrast material. If fluoroscopic equipment is available, the inflow can be observed, limiting the volume of contrast used. In the anterior urethra a minimal tear with minimal extravasation requires only urinary drainage for 7 to 10 days. We insert a small silicone Foley catheter for this purpose and obtain a voiding urethrogram when we remove it. A suprapubic tube would serve as well for this, and the advent of the easily introduced percutaneous tubes has made this procedure more attractive than it was when a formal operation was necessary to install one.

When there is extensive extravasation of blood and urine, the area should be opened and drained. If the urethra is not transected, the injury can be handled as described. If it is transected, it should be mobilized and debrided and the ends spatulated with incisions 180 degrees apart. When the ends can be brought together without tension, we suture them with interrupted sutures of 5-0 PDS (polydioxanone)* over a 24 F catheter. We then remove this catheter and use a smaller silicone Foley for drainage. It is acceptable in this circumstance to put in a suprapubic tube and drain the extravasation (MacKinnon, 1975), but the patient should then be prepared for definitive repair in 3 to 6 weeks. When the lesion is longer or when there is concern about the viability of the urethra, the ends of the urethra are sewn down after spatulation and the edges of the skin attached, diverting the urine with a suprapubic tube.

It is important that the treatment of fractured pelvis and disrupted urethra fits both the anatomic situation and the skill and experience of the surgeon handling the repair. The puboprostatic ligaments firmly attach the prostate to the symphysis pubis, while the urogenital diaphragm fixes the urethra beneath the prostate. If the pelvic fracture has dislocated the symphysis, the prostate will go with it, plucked off the urethra like an apple from its stem. After injury, when the bladder with the prostate rides high, like "pie in the sky," it is likely that the ligaments have also been disrupted; if the prostate is still close to the pubic fragment, however, the puboprostatic ligaments will be intact. In either circumstance, if the patient is too ill or if the surgeon is unfamiliar with surgery of the prostate and urethra, a suprapubic tube should be inserted and repair left for a later day and a more experienced surgeon. If there is any question at all, this course will cause the patient the least harm and should be followed.

When the patient's condition allows it and the surgeon's ability and experience justify it, a primary urethral reapproximation can be carried out. This should not be a blind procedure, such as is implied by the "interlocking sounds" or the "railroad" procedures. Also, extensive, especially lateral, dissection to mobilize the blad-

*Ethicon, Inc., Somerville, New Jersey 08876.

der and prostate should not be carried out for fear of disrupting whatever nerves might still be intact. We suck clots out of the midline and pass a Robinson catheter up the urethra to emerge from its distal stump at the urogenital diaphragm. We enter the bladder and remove the urine by suction, after which we pass a Robinson catheter out through the prostatic urethra. We sew the tips of these two catheters together and pull the urethral tube into the bladder. The bell of this tube is cut off so that it will fit smoothly over the tip of a No. 24, 30-ml Foley catheter. After the tip of the Foley catheter is sewn to the Robinson catheter, the Foley is pulled smoothly into the bladder. The bag is distended, and a gentle pull should be all that is necessary to replace the prostate in its anatomic position. If the puboprostatic ligaments are still intact, this cannot be done without reducing the pelvic fracture. Most diagrams illustrating ruptured membranous urethras show these ligaments to be disrupted by the trauma (Pierce, 1972; Ragde and McInnes, 1969), but this has not been our experience (Devine, 1980, 1982).

The residual strands of the puboprostatic ligaments must be cut to allow the prostate to be replaced without tension (Fig. 80–9). We have not had to use Vest sutures (Vest, 1940) to do this. The catheter is left in place without traction to guide the prostate home, while the urine is diverted through a suprapubic tube. At the end of this time the urethral catheter is removed, and, when continuity of the urethra has been demonstrated by a voiding urethrogram, the suprapubic tube is clamped for 1 or 2 days and then removed.

Because of the well-known fragility of Foley catheter bags, a silk or nylon suture is left tied to the tip of the urethral catheter. This is secured to the skin of the abdomen.

Iatrogenic Strictures

Strictures in the urethra may result from the efforts of physicians during passage of instruments (e.g., sounds, cystoscopes, or catheters) or may follow transurethral procedures (e.g., resection of prostate or bladder tumors). They also follow other operations in which a urethral catheter has been left indwelling and inflammation with urethritis has developed. Long-term catheter drainage, such as in acute dysfunction of the bladder following spinal cord trauma, also may lead to stricture. We have seen other patients in whom there has been

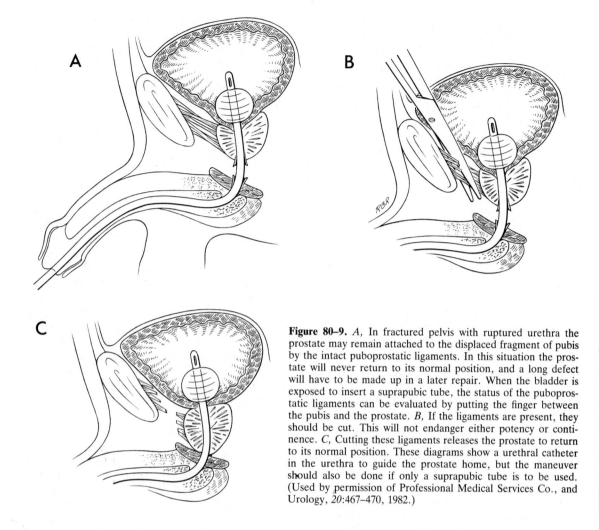

Figure 80–9. *A,* In fractured pelvis with ruptured urethra the prostate may remain attached to the displaced fragment of pubis by the intact puboprostatic ligaments. In this situation the prostate will never return to its normal position, and a long defect will have to be made up in a later repair. When the bladder is exposed to insert a suprapubic tube, the status of the puboprostatic ligaments can be evaluated by putting the finger between the pubis and the prostate. *B,* If the ligaments are present, they should be cut. This will not endanger either potency or continence. *C,* Cutting these ligaments releases the prostate to return to its normal position. These diagrams show a urethral catheter in the urethra to guide the prostate home, but the maneuver should also be done if only a suprapubic tube is to be used. (Used by permission of Professional Medical Services Co., and *Urology, 20*:467–470, 1982.)

extension of the stricture associated with long-term dilation of an existing short stricture. This is especially so in men with meatal stenosis caused by balanitis xerotica obliterans. Some believe that the extension of this stenosis in the urethra represents extension of the pathologic process, but, although characteristic inflammation is present, we feel that in many cases the extension up the urethra is secondary to the trauma of dilation rather than to extension of disease.

Inflammation of the urethra accompanies the use of an indwelling catheter. Because there is much less length at risk, this is less true in women than in men. It is probably more frequent in children, especially when small-sized latex catheters are used. The amount of inflammation is related to the size of the tube, the length of time the catheter is left indwelling, and the type of catheter care provided. We favor silicone catheters of the smallest practical size and leave them indwelling for the minimum

length of time. The drainage system should be closed so that infection is not introduced. This means that catheter irrigation should be used only for a clear indication and not as a routine measure, even after prostate surgery. In patients who will require long-term drainage of their bladder, intermittent catheterization or an indwelling suprapubic tube should be instituted as early as possible in the course of treatment.

Strictures associated with indwelling catheters usually occur at the same sites as those that follow instrumentation at the meatus, at the suspensory ligament, or in the membranous urethra, i.e., where the urethra is narrow or fixed. Inflammatory lesions associated with indwelling catheters are often full thickness, and these strictures do not respond well to simpler forms of treatment, such as dilation or internal urethrotomy.

In our practice we see patients with strictures related to previous urethral surgery. Many of these patients have had urethral construction in cases of hypospadias and epispadias, but others are failures of the treatment of a simpler stricture. We have analyzed the situation presented by these patients and have been able to identify some common factors responsible for these failures (Devine et al., 1978). We feel that an aggressive attitude is necessary in the proper performance of reconstructive surgery of the urethra. Lack of this attitude may be due to uncertainty as to what should be done and insecurity in carrying it out. This is just one of the reasons I feel that urologists interested in the repair of these defects should form a team, including an interested plastic surgeon, so that they can build on experience, each supporting the other. Although recurrent stenosis and urethral fistula are the most common complications of urethral repair, inadequate resection of chordee has been the most frequent problem in children we have seen who have failed hypospadias repair after multiple surgical procedures. We have termed these children "hypospadias cripples" (Horton and Devine, 1970). Scarring associated with multiple operations and that due to hematoma or infection may cause severe bending, which is difficult to repair. It is not possible to correct this bend without wide exposure. All the fibrotic tissue around the neourethra must be resected. If the urethra is not satisfactory, it should be excised; but if it is adequate and if the chordee cannot be corrected by resection of scar tissue, the dorsal aspect of the penis should be shortened by excision of an ellipse of tunica. If it is necessary to insert a dermal graft into the ventral side of the penile shaft, an island preputial flap will be necessary to reconstruct the urethra.

Although internal urethrotomy under vision is a satisfactory method for treating some strictures, it is not applicable to all. Often, the result of attempts to treat a stricture with this modality is a denser and more extensive stricture. It is difficult to evaluate the results of treatment in most of the series of patients treated by the newer techniques of endoscopic surgery, because in most reports the strictures are not characterized. Just as it was difficult to judge the results of treatment of carcinoma of the bladder until reporting surgeons agreed upon a common description of the character and extent of the tumors (stage and grade), it will not be possible to assess completely the usefulness of visual urethrotomy until this is done for urethral strictures. Location, length, depth, and density of strictures are factors affecting results; we have proposed that these be taken into account when results of treatment of strictures are discussed (Devine, 1983) (Fig. 80–10).

False Passage

During the course of treatment of a urethral stricture by the passage of instruments, one may

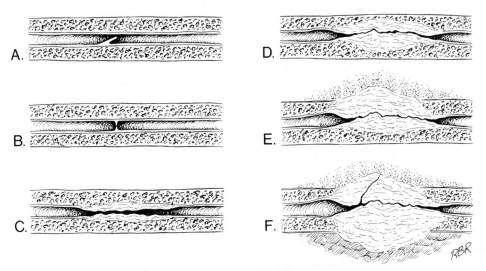

Figure 80–10. Diagrams of urethral strictures. *A,* Simple leaf of mucosa without deep involvement. *B,* Diaphragm of mucosa also without deeper involvement. *C,* Stricture involving only the mucosa and submucosa. This and the following lesions can be of any length and can involve any portion of the urethra. *D,* Stricture involving the mucosa, submucosa, and a portion of the spongy tissue. *E,* Stricture with scarring of the full thickness of the spongy tissue and involvement of the periurethral tissues. *F,* Complex stricture with total involvement of the urethra, spongy tissue, and periurethral tissue, complicated by a fistula. This can go on to formation of an abscess, or the fistula may open to the skin on the rectum. In many strictures, especially those associated with fracture of the pelvis, there will be no continuity between the two ends of the urethra.

well pass outside the lumen of the urethra, and, as the surrounding erectile tissue has little resistance to this trauma, a false passage may be created. Any instrument subsequently passed into the urethra may find its way into this tract, and this new tract may become epithelialized and persist. These tracts may be seen on x-ray studies and cause confusing shadows. Several patients seen in our institution have been found to be voiding through a false passage, which had required dilation at very frequent intervals. If a false passage is recognized at the time it first occurs, a filiform should be passed, under cystoscopic control if necessary, and the urethra dilated with followers so that an indwelling catheter may be passed. Leaving this catheter indwelling for several weeks will allow the false passage to heal, but there will always be more scar tissue present in this area.

Tumors may involve the urethra, and these are discussed in Chapter 31. One must always keep these in mind, as the obstruction caused by a tumor will be no different from that caused by a stricture. Also, strictures may cause hematuria. If the involved area in the urethra is irregular and if there is bleeding either during or after urination, a biopsy will have to be done. Whenever there is a mass lesion associated with inflammation or causing obstruction, it will have to be excised before an attempt at reconstruction can be carried out.

Diagnosis of Urethral Stricture

When a stricture has developed, the diagnosis is suspected by the history and confirmed by meeting obstruction when attempting to pass an instrument through the urethra. Urine flow rates will sometimes reveal more about how much trouble the patient is having than will his subjective symptoms (Cole et al., 1974). Cystoscopy is of help in differentiating the type of lesion (malignancies may masquerade as strictures), but retrograde and voiding urethrograms will be necessary to define the full extent of the stricture (Fig. 80–11). Flow of the medium will be diminished by the obstruction, and the urethra beyond the stricture (proximally with a retrograde urethrogram and distally with a voiding urethrogram) will not be properly delineated if only one technique is employed. Contrast medium suitable for intravenous injection should be used for these studies. The urethra involved in stricture disease is friable, and even with gentle introduction of the material, intravascular extravasation can occur (Fig. 80–12).

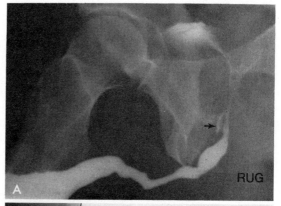

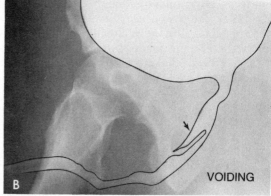

Figure 80–11. Retrograde *(A)* and voiding *(B)* urethrograms in a patient who has previously had a Johanson urethroplasty. This illustrates the necessity to do both studies. The strictured area in the bulb is quite apparent on each study, but the duplication of the lumen beginning in the membranous portion is only hinted at in the RUG, while the tremendously dilated penile urethra–the result of an older type hypospadias repair–can be seen only on the RUG. This dilatation caused no physiologic difficulty, but the valve action of the duplicated urethra was the major cause of the patient's continuing obstruction. This repair was effected by excision of the wall between the duplicated segments and the application of a patch graft.

Various clamps and devices are available for injection of contrast material so that the hands of the operator are not exposed to the x-ray beam. Some urologists introduce a Foley catheter into the urethra, distend the balloon with air, and inject through the lumen of the catheter. While this may be satisfactory, the distended balloon can obscure an important portion of the urethra. We have found the following simple technique quite useful. A gauze pad opened out to make a broad gauze band is placed around the penis behind the corona and secured with a large hemostatic clamp. A syringe with a catheter irrigation tip is used for the injection. The tip is placed into the urethra and the contents of the syringe gently introduced into the urethra. When this film has been made,

Treatment of Urethral Stricture

Treatment selected for a patient with a urethral stricture will depend upon the position, length, and density of the stricture and the general health of the patient. One or more of the following procedures may be used: (1) dilation; (2) internal urethrotomy; (3) external urethrotomy; (4) excision of the stricture with reanastomosis of the urethra; (5) marsupialization of the strictured urethra with subsequent urethroplasty; (6) repair with pedicle flaps; or (7) full-thickness skin graft urethroplasty.

DILATION

Dilation of the urethra must be a process of gradual stretching, because forceful disruption of the strictured area will lead to further scarring and subsequent worsening of the situation, with an increase in the length or density of the stricture. We never dilate a stricture in a male patient beyond 24 F, and sometimes it will take weeks of treatment to achieve that caliber. If the stricture is short and not especially dense, so that a small sound is easily passed, the patient is asked to return at weekly intervals; at each visit the next even-sized sound is passed until the 24 F instrument can be inserted with ease. The frequency of visits is decreased by doubling the time interval between visits. If dilation is going to be an acceptable modality, the eventual interval between visits will be every 6 to 12 months.

Because the tips of smaller sounds are sharp enough to penetrate the urethra and create a false passage, one must start with an 18 or 20 F instrument when first passing a sound in a patient with a stricture of the urethra. If the medium-sized sound will not pass, it becomes necessary to use filiforms and followers. The tip of the filiform may be straight or have a coudé or spiral curvature. One or several filiforms are passed into the urethra and manipulated until one passes through the stricture and into the bladder. We find that the coudé or spiral-tipped filiform will pass much more easily than the straight-tipped ones, so we generally begin with a spiral-tipped filiform and seldom have to use more than this one instrument. Filling the urethra with lidocaine (Xylocaine) lubricating jelly prior to manipulation makes the passage of any instrument considerably easier.

When the filiform has been passed, there are a number of instruments designed to attach by a male thread to the filiform and follow it through the urethra. The filiform is flexible enough to curl up in the bladder. For the initial

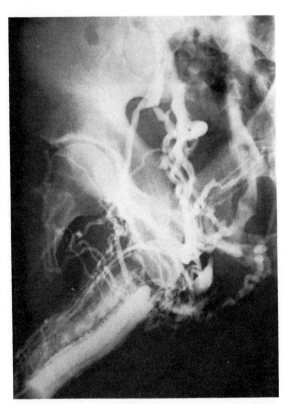

Figure 80–12. Venogram of the penis, pelvis, and inferior vena cava following gentle retrograde urethrogram. (From Horton, C. E., and Devine, P. C.: Strictures of the male urethra. *In* Converse, J. M. (Ed.): Reconstructive Plastic Surgery. Philadelphia, W. B. Saunders Co., 1977.)

a 5 or 8 F infant-feeding tube or a 10 plastic Tieman catheter is passed into the bladder. The bladder is filled, and an exposure is made while the patient is voiding as good a stream as he can generate. It is important that the urethra not have been dilated for 3 to 6 weeks prior to the radiologic investigation. If the patient has obstruction sufficient to cause urinary retention, a small percutaneous suprapubic tube, such as a Cystocath, should be placed for drainage prior to this evaluation and subsequent surgical therapy.

X-ray evaluation of a stricture that follows a fractured pelvis is often difficult. When the prostate and bladder lie high in the pelvis and there is marked distortion of the bony pelvis, an extensive urethroplasty will probably be needed. Often the prostate does come down into a reasonable position; however, if the bladder neck does not open during the cystogram, the prostatic and residual membranous urethra will not be visualized. It then will be necessary to do a cystoscopy through the cystostomy tract to look down the urethra from above to see how much of it is left.

dilation we prefer the flexible woven or plastic Phillips catheters. Urine can be obtained for culture and x-ray contrast medium instilled into the bladder for a voiding urethrogram. There may be an inclination at this point to proceed to dilate the urethra to its maximum by using one after another of these followers, but the urethra should not be stretched to more than a 12 or 14 F capacity. If the patient is not hurt, he will return for a regular series of dilations, and the urethra will ultimately remain open for a much longer time than if the dilations were all done at once.

If the stricture is too dense to respond to this regimen, a small catheter may be inserted and left indwelling. Sometimes it is necessary to leave the filiform and follower taped to the penis for 1 or 2 days to allow the stricture to soften for passage of a larger catheter. The Councill catheter (a Foley-type catheter with a hole at the very tip) may also be used. A special catheter guide is passed through the catheter, and the threaded tip of the guide passes through the hole. The tip is screwed to the filiform, and, after the catheter has been passed, the guide and filiform are withdrawn through the catheter. A catheter punch* can be used to put a hole in the tip of any silicone Foley, which then may be used with the Councill Stylette or passed over a guidewire. After a catheter has been in place for 2 to 3 days, the next even-sized catheter or one two sizes larger will pass with ease and can be left for another 3 to 4 days. We prefer silicone catheters for this process and do not progress above 24 F.

When it is difficult to pass dilating instruments, or when the stricture is of such a density that it is necessary to repeat the dilation procedure more than once every 6 months, or when the process of dilation is so painful that the patient returns for treatment only when he is in trouble, a surgical repair should be carried out. Occurrence of the complications of urethral stricture will also indicate the necessity for operative intervention. The fragility of the fibrotic strictured urethra can lead to extravasation of urine, which may collect outside the urethra and become infected or form single or multiple fistulas going to the perineal skin, scrotum, and suprapubic area. Also, with obstruction the frequency and severity of urinary tract infections will be increased; if these cannot be controlled, an operation will have to be done.

When there is a periurethral abscess or extravasation of urine, a suprapubic cystostomy should be established for urinary diversion, and the perineum should be widely drained. When multiple fistulas have been long established, there will be much associated inflammation. All of this tissue should be excised; when infection and inflammation have resolved, urethroplasty can be done.

INTERNAL URETHROTOMY

Internal urethrotomy may be done as a blind procedure using the Otis urethrotome, or under vision using a cold knife or a fulgurating electrode. With either procedure it is important to recognize that the incision should be made at only one site in the urethra. It is best done at the 12 o'clock position because of the urethral arteries that run in the bulb in the 3 o'clock and 9 o'clock positions. The incision must be through the full thickness of the stricture. It does not help to lacerate the urethral mucosa lightly in several directions, and one cut through the full thickness of the stricture is as good as several.

Otis Urethrotome. The urethra is dilated to a size that will accommodate the Otis urethrotome (Fig. 80–13), which is then attached to the filiform and passed into the urethra. The instrument is cranked open and the blade withdrawn. Since this blade is not knife-sharp, it cuts fibrotic stricture but not elastic normal urethra. The knife is replaced, and the instrument is opened further several times until it is

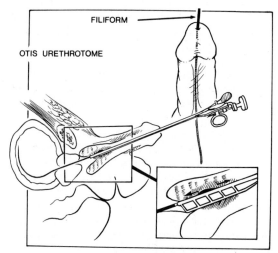

Figure 80–13. Otis urethrotome incising the urethral stricture with the blade elevated. (From Horton, C. E., and Devine, P. C.: Strictures of the male urethra. *In* Converse, J. M. (Ed.): Reconstructive Plastic Surgery. Philadelphia, W. B. Saunders Co., 1977.)

---

*V.P.I. Co., Cat. #053000, P.O. Box 227, Spencer, Indiana 47460.

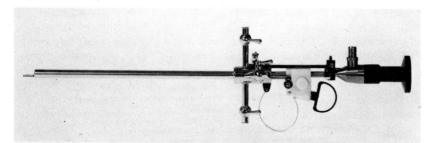

Figure 80–14. G-822 ACMI visual urethrotome. (Courtesy of American Cystoscope Makers, Inc., Stamford, Conn.)

opened to a 26 or 28 F. The instrument is withdrawn, and a silicone Foley catheter is inserted and left from 10 days to 6 weeks until re-epithelialization and healing have occurred.

Specialized instruments have been produced by a number of cystoscope manufacturers for internal urethrotomy under vision (Fig. 80–14). After passage of the instrument into the urethra, the area involved by the stricture is visualized (Fig. 80–15). We then pass a ureteral catheter through the strictured area. This serves as a guide for the cutting knife and to ensure

that the operator does not get lost as the cutting progresses. In the Olympus instrument the guide for this catheter passes through the stem of the knife blade, and we have found this to be a convenient feature. We then advance the knife into the stricture. This may cut its way in, but the procedure is not done simply by moving the knife back and forth like the cutting loop of a resectoscope. The knife blade is held extended, and, as the proximal end of the urethrotome is depressed the blade is elevated, cutting upward at 12 o'clock through the full depth of the

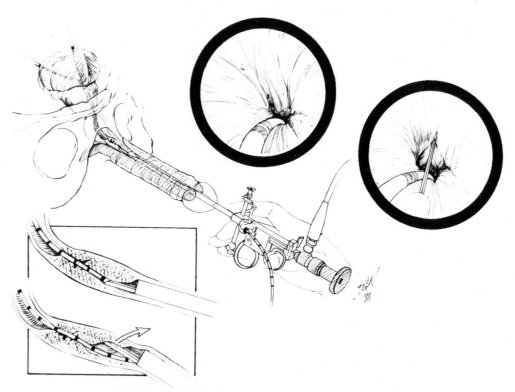

Figure 80–15. Internal urethrotomy under vision with a cold knife. A ureteral catheter is passed through the stricture, and the cold knife is advanced under vision into the stricture guided by this catheter. As the proximal end of the urethrotome is depressed, it cuts upward at 12 o'clock through the stricture. In short strictures, only one cut may be necessary, but in longer ones the ureteral catheter will allow the blade to be advanced farther and the incision to be elongated. The urethra is incised until a 24 F silicone catheter can be passed with ease in the adult or an appropriate smaller one in a child. (Used with permission from Devine, C. J., Jr., and Devine, P. C.: Operations for urethral stricture. *In* Stewart, B. H. (Ed.): Operative Urology. Baltimore, Williams & Wilkins Co., 1982, pp. 242–270.)

stricture. When the stricture is short, one pass may do the job; with longer and thicker strictures, however, the knife must be advanced, following the catheter farther through the lumen, and other cuts must be made to elongate the incision.

When the complete length of the stricture has been incised, the instrument should pass easily into the bladder, usually allowing a 24 F silicone catheter to pass with ease. The catheter should be left indwelling until the strictured area has healed and epithelium has covered the surface. The literature does not answer the question of how long this should be, because reports of the results of this procedure do not include a good description of the character of the lesion being treated. In some cases, 3 days seems to be long enough; in short strictures with only mucosal involvement this may be so, but when the stricture is long and the involvement deep with a great deal of fibrosis, removing the catheter on the third day would probably assure a recurrence. In these cases we leave the catheter for 6 weeks. In patients referred to us after unsuccessful treatment, we have been able to carry out a successful repeat internal urethrotomy by cutting deeper and leaving the catheter for a longer time. We will, at times, remove this 24 catheter after 7 to 10 days and replace it with a smaller silicone Foley for the full 6 weeks. In boys with short strictures, we have used the pediatric cystoscope and an electrode or cold knife to incise the stricture, similar to the manner in which urethral valves are handled today. We then pass a silicone Foley and leave it in place for at least 10 days.

When we remove the catheter, we fill the bladder with x-ray contrast and obtain a voiding urethrogram. Cystoscopy at that time also allows us to appraise the progress of regeneration of the mucosa. Prospective studies relating the character of the stricture and the length of catheter drainage to the success of the procedure should resolve this problem.

Urethrotomy instruments can also be used to treat contracture of the bladder neck, which may occur following even a well-done transurethral resection of the prostate. We make multiple incisions through the bladder neck at the 12, 4, and 8 o'clock positions. The Collings knife with the resectoscope can be used for the procedure, but it is important not to re-resect the entire bladder neck, as the contracture will probably recur.

The electroresectoscope has been used to treat stricture in the urethra. The use of the Collings knife for this purpose has mostly been supplanted by the cold knife; however, when

there is no continuity between the proximal and distal ends of the urethra yet x-ray studies demonstrate only a short defect, Lieberman and Barry (1983) claim excellent results from electroresection of the obstructing tissue. They pass a bright light, such as that with a flexible nephroscope, through the cystostomy and down the proximal urethra; they darken the light in the resectoscope and "cut for the light." We have not used this procedure.

When there is no continuity between the ends of the ruptured urethra, we plan open surgery. Also, many strictures will be so long or so dense that internal urethrotomy will not be successful, and strictures will recur after the procedure. It is possible to have a second or third attempt at the urethrotomy; however, when the mucosa has been so damaged by the disease that caused the stricture or by the trauma of the treatment of the injury, it will not regenerate to bridge the defect and an open surgical procedure will be indicated.

EXTERNAL URETHROTOMY

Exposing the urethra by an incision and cutting through the full thickness of the stricture, allowing it to regenerate over a catheter, has not proved to be more useful than internal urethrotomy; therefore, the former method is not used today to treat strictures. However, it is used when instruments are to be passed and the distal urethra is too small to accommodate them comfortably. We pass a sound and hold it against the perineum, incise the skin, and identify the urethra. We make an incision through the erectile tissue and urethra, catch the edges with black silk sutures, withdraw the sound, and pass the instrument. If a catheter is used after an operative procedure, it is not necessary to close this incision. For many years we used perineal urethrotomy for urinary diversion in patients with hypospadias, and the incisions closed spontaneously unless there was a distal obstruction.

EXCISION

A short urethral stricture may be treated by excising the affected area and reconstructing the cut ends. In order to do this, the urethra must be mobilized so that it can be stretched to fit the defect. The arterial supply of the urethra arises proximally and distally (McGowan and Waterhouse, 1964) from branches of the pudendal artery at the bulb and back perfusion derived from the glans at the distal end. Either supply is sufficient to sustain the entire length of the urethra. Although 1- to 2-cm defects may easily be bridged, even greater lengths can be covered by mobilizing the entire urethra (Zinman and Libertino, 1977). In the penis the corpus spongiosum is firmly attached by a leaf of Buck's fascia on each side of the ventral midline groove between the two corpora cavernosa. Once this space has been entered, incision of the septa of Buck's fascia will free the urethra, which will then be quite elastic. The incision should be made close to the tunica of the corpora cavernosa to avoid entering the thin wall of the vascular space surrounding the urethra. The blood vessels encircling the penile shaft should be electrofulgurated.

When the stricture has been excised and the proximal and distal ends of the urethra mobilized, we make dorsal and ventral incisions in the cut ends of the urethra 180 degrees apart, and construct a spatulated anastomosis over a small silicone Foley catheter, using interrupted sutures of 5-0 PDS (Fig. 80–16). When the repair is of the urethra in the perineum, we have not routinely used a suprapubic tube or urinary diversion, other than the inlying Foley catheter that is left for 10 days. This procedure is not as useful in the pendulous urethra because mobilization of the urethra in the penis may lead to chordee. Erections also create a problem in healing with any repair in the penile urethra. If a catheter transversing the repair is left to drain the urine, the area of repair will be traumatized as the penis changes in length with erection, and there is no medication that will obviate erections. We therefore leave a short stenting tube in the repair for 3 to 5 days and drain the urine through a percutaneous bladder tube, such as a Cystocath.*

---

*Dow Corning Corporation, Cat. #330-8, #330-12, Medical Products, Midland, Michigan 48640.

Figure 80–16. Stricture excised, urethra opened ventrally and dorsally, and urethra anastomosed. (From Horton, C. E., and Devine, P. C.: Strictures of the male urethra. *In* Converse, J. M. (Ed.): Reconstructive Plastic Surgery. Philadelphia, W. B. Saunders Co., 1977.)

If the urethra cannot be brought together without tension, the operation of Hamilton Russell (Russell, 1914) may be carried out. Matching spatulating incisions are made in the ventral aspect of the urethra, and the dorsal edges are sewn together with interrupted sutures of 5-0 chromic gut. The urine is diverted by a suprapubic tube, and the urethra is allowed to regenerate from this buried strip of epithelium. Denis Browne based his hypospadias operation upon his experience with this procedure (Johanson, 1953). It is also useful in trauma cases, when there is a large defect in the urethra or so much trauma that the viability of the urethra is in question (Fig. 80–17). The technique of allowing a strip of epithelium to form a tube was also used by Young and Hand (Hand, 1970; Young and Davis, 1926), who excised the ventral wall of the stricture and allowed the urethra to regenerate from a bridge of dorsal urethral wall.

In 1950, Badenoch reported exposing the membranous urethra through a perineal incision, excising a short stricture, and reanastomosing the ends of the urethra by a pull-through procedure. The bladder was opened and a catheter passed down through the prostatic urethra and into the end of the distal urethra, where it was secured by sutures. When the catheter was pulled back into the prostatic urethra, the two segments were intussuscepted. The catheter was secured to the abdominal wall, and urine was diverted by way of a suprapubic tube. This pull-through procedure had been reported by a Russian, Solovov, in 1935 but had been virtually unnoticed. Wiggishoff and Kiefer (1964) reported success with this technique. Occasionally, the pulled-through end of the urethra acts as a valve and must be resected away to allow free passage of urine. Today, with proper positioning and exposure this procedure is seldom

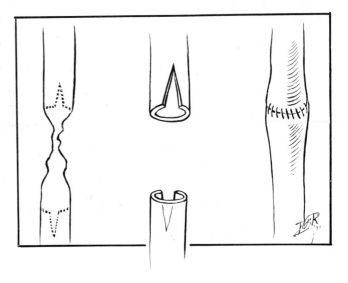

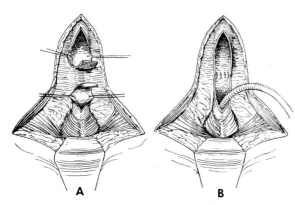

Figure 80–17. Hamilton Russell operation. *A,* Stricture and fibrous scar have been excised and the ends of the urethra mobilized. *B,* The urethra has been opened well into its normal lumen and the dorsal edges approximated with interrupted sutures. (From Hand, J. R.: *In* Campbell, M. F., and Harrison, J. H. (Eds.): Urology. Vol. 3, 3rd ed. Philadelphia, W. B. Saunders Co., 1970.)

necessary, as a suture anastomosis can usually be made.

If the urethra is not long or elastic enough to close the defect or if the penis is so distorted that it would require an inordinate length of urethra to accomplish this, we remove a portion of the lower part of the symphysis pubis with bone rongeurs to shorten the curve and accomplish the anastomosis. Waterhouse (1975) removed the entire symphysis in order to make a primary anastomosis.

This procedure has become popular for the repair of membranous urethral strictures, and the decision to proceed with resection of the bone as the first step is often made by evaluation of x-ray studies. Because of the difficulty in visualizing the urethra distal to the bladder neck, we feel that this should not be so and that in all cases the perineal dissection should be carried out first; then, if it is found necessary to resect the pubis, the suprapubic portion of the procedure can be carried out. We have not yet found it necessary to resect the entire pubis.

Transpubic Approach to Urethroplasty

Urologists have always recognized the difficulty of working on the prostate and membranous urethra, which lie behind the symphysis pubis. Walker (1921) described symphysiotomy (splitting the symphysis pubis) as an aid to removal of cancer of the prostate. In 1962, Pierce first described the use of this approach to repair a stricture in the membranous urethra following a fracture of the pelvis. The entire pubis was excised by cutting through the superior and inferior rami, staying close to the medial aspect of the obturator foramen. The excised pubis was discarded, and the urethral stricture was incised longitudinally and closed transversely through this "splendid exposure." Paine and Coombes (1968) raised a flap of pubis and replaced it. They did not state what happened to this flap, but it is now felt that the possibility of infection and sequestration of this bone obligates the surgeon to discard it and that no orthopedic problems have resulted from doing so (Morales et al., 1973; Patil and Yuan, 1983).

Ragde and McInnes (1969) reported using symphysiotomy for the immediate repair of urethral strictures in Vietnamese civilians who would be unwilling or unable to return for future care of urethral stricture. Their experience with this was good and possibly should be considered in our own civilian practice. Splitting of the symphysis is not the favored approach to this area today because of the orthopedic problems associated with springing the sacroiliac joints. Pierce (1972) has claimed that urethral continuity can and should be obtained in most patients with acute injury by direct suturing with chromic gut and has noted that removal of fragments of fractured pubic bone will allow a good view of the area for suturing. He no longer resects the entire pubic bone and has used free full-thickness tube grafts to bridge 3- to 4-cm gaps in the urethra. He notes that incontinence did not follow incision of the urogenital diaphragm anterior to the urethra.

Waterhouse et al. (1973) reported the use of pubectomy as an aid to surgical procedures on the lower urinary tract, including repair of membranous urethral strictures (Fig. 80–18). He made a midline incision to the base of the penis and carried it transversally as an L. The suspensory ligament of the penis is incised, and the dorsal vein of the penis is cut and tied. Others do not do this (Khan and Furlow, 1976). The retropubic dissection is difficult and is best carried out subperiosteally. A Gigli saw is used to cut out a wedge of bone, including the symphysis pubis. This should be wider at the top than at the bottom. The bone is discarded.

A sound is passed through the cystostomy opening to locate the proximal end of the strictured urethra by palpating the tip of the sound. Fibrous tissue in this area is excised until a wide opening has been made into the healthy urethra above the defect. Through a perineal incision the anterior urethra is dissected free, transected below the stricture, and mobilized as far as the glans penis. It is passed through an incision in the intercrural septum, spatulated, and anasto-

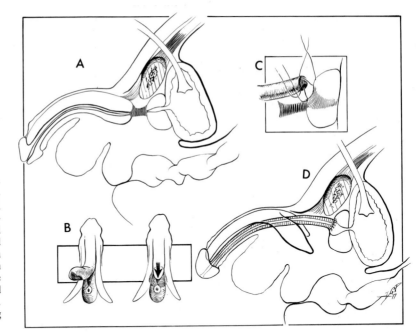

Figure 80–18. Waterhouse urethroplasty. *A,* Sagittal section illustrating membranous urethral stricture posterior to the symphysis pubis. *B,* With a perineal exposure, the urethra is freed from the urogenital diaphragm and passed up through an incision bypassing the stricture. *C,* The spatulated urethra is anastomosed to the opened prostatic urethra. *D,* Completed procedure showing the reconstituted urethra.

mosed from above to the opening in the prostatic urethra.

The description of the anastomosis of the urethra to an incision in the anterior aspect of the prostatic urethra above the stricture is an important contribution of this paper. This feature has had much to do with its success and should be adopted for all reanastomosis procedures. The anastomosis should not be made end-to-end. Waterhouse used 3-0 chromic sutures for this, over a 16 to 18 F silicone Foley catheter. Today we prefer 5-0 PDS. The wounds are closed with drains and a suprapubic tube. The patient was kept at bed rest for 5 days, then gradually ambulated. The urethral catheter was left for 10 days and a voiding urethrogram made prior to removing the suprapubic tube. Waterhouse noted that the additional exposure obtained by the pubectomy was more than he had expected to obtain by removing this narrow piece of bone. In children, we have found that the cartilaginous segment of the pubis can be excised with heavy scissors and that good exposure can be obtained by removing a very narrow piece of the symphysis.

Waterhouse reported 19 children in whom he repaired membranous urethral strictures. The transpubic approach was used in seven children, three patients had Turner-Warwick procedures, and nine had primary anastomoses that could be done from below. One of these patients had had a previous Turner-Warwick repair, and three had had transpubic procedures. One patient developed chordee because

of excessive shortening of the ventral surface of the penis by mobilization of the urethra. The only real failure was in a patient who had had previous injury to his anterior urethra. He now has had his urine diverted.

Further documentation of the usefulness of this approach to the repair of membranous urethral strictures has come from Allen (1975) and Khan and Furlow (1976). Allen is concerned that bypassing the sphincter with inlays from below or passing the urethra through the urogenital diaphragm will defunctionalize the external sphincter mechanism and place "the full burden of continence upon the bladder neck." He divided the symphysis pubis in his first three patients and, after incising the urethral stricture, put in a full-thickness patch graft of penile skin. In the next three patients the short stricture was excised, and the margins of the urethra were reapproximated. In the last patient the pubis was resected (Figs. 80–19 and 80–20). Khan and Furlow (1976) reported 11 patients and noted difficulty in recognizing and preserving the membranous urethral sphincter because it had usually been destroyed by the original accident.

Turner-Warwick, in his discussion of Waterhouse's paper, states that he rarely uses his inlay urethroplasty for short, traumatic strictures but prefers to do a spatulated end-to-end anastomosis (Turner-Warwick, 1975). The strictured area is identified and excised, and the resulting ends of the urethra are spatulated and reanastomosed with at least a 2-cm overlap. After supramembranous fracture-dislocation in-

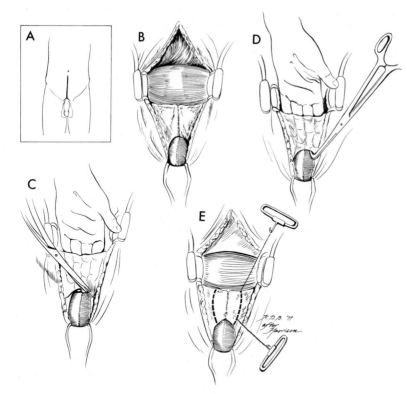

Figure 80–19. Pubectomy for urethroplasty. *A*, Diagram of the midline incision, which makes a T at the base of the penis. *B*, The symphysis pubis is exposed by retracting laterally and mobilizing the penis. *C*, Dissection is carried out behind the symphysis. When there is much scar, this will be done most easily in the subperiosteal plane. *D*, A right angle clamp is passed beneath the symphysis to grasp the Gigli saw. *E*, The saw is used to remove a trapezoidal segment of bone. (Adapted from Allen, T. D.: J. Urol., *114*:63, 1975.)

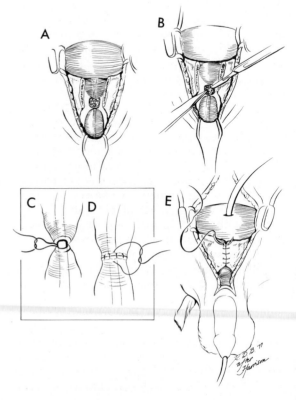

Figure 80–20. *A*, The stricture is exposed below the prostate and above the urogenital diaphragm. *B*, The scar is excised. *C, D,* The urethra is reapproximated. *E*, The periosteum of the symphysis is approximated, and the skin is subsequently closed. (Adapted from Allen, T. D.: J. Urol., *114*:63, 1975.)

juries, the 4 to 5 cm of elastic urethra available by mobilization of the bulb will allow a defect of 2 to 3 cm to be "resolved." The dislocated prostatic urethra is best left as a fixed point, as the extensive dissection necessary to free it from surrounding scar tissue will further compromise potency and increase the possibility of incontinence.

Short supramembranous strictures resulting from minor injury or well-treated major injury may be repaired by excision and reanastomosis through a perineal exposure. If this is not done well and fails, Turner-Warwick feels that a two-stage inlay procedure will be necessary to remedy the situation.

There is no question that the procedures for reanastomosis of the urethra should be done when feasible. Our own full-thickness skin graft procedure (to be discussed) can be used through a perineal approach to bridge any distance of destroyed urethra. However, when the prostate is above its normal position and cannot be reached from below, the transpubic approach should be used. This technique of exposing the prostate and membranous urethra is useful, as it is applied to other surgical problems and should be learned by all urologic surgeons.

MARSUPIALIZATION PROCEDURES

In 1960 Stewart converted a strictured urethra into hypospadias by incising the stricture and sewing the margins of the urethra to the skin. He repaired the urethra at a later stage by the technique of Ombrédanne. Johanson (1953)* also converted strictures to hypospadias but repaired them by the buried-strip technique of Denis Browne. In patients with particularly dense strictures of the penile urethra, Cecil excised the strictured portion of the urethra at the first stage and covered the defect with penile skin. He then closed the urethra by forming a Thiersch tube (Thiersch, 1869) and burying the penis in the scrotum as he did with hypospadias repairs.

In the Johanson procedure the strictured area of the urethra is incised, and 1.5 to 2 cm of the normal urethra on each end is opened. All defects of the urethra are excised, and the skin edges are sewn to the opened urethra with careful approximation of the skin to the mucosal edges. The urine was diverted for about 1 week.

At the second stage, at least 6 weeks later, an elliptical incision is made around the mucosa and bordering skin to form a strip that is allowed to form a tube for the new urethra. This strip should be as wide as two thirds of the circumference of the new urethra. The edges of the strip are not mobilized but are handled with care, so that injury will not impede symmetric growth. The lateral skin is undermined and closed in layers over the urethra, using the wire-and-stop technique of Denis Browne. Urine is diverted for 10 days by a perineal urethrostomy or a suprapubic tube.

In repair of the proximal urethra, Johanson attached a flap of scrotum to the membranous urethra, leaving the anastomosis in a deep scrotal depression, which made access to the proximal urethral opening difficult. Subsequent modifications of the technique have been directed mainly toward devising flaps that would allow easier access, so that necessary revision could be carried out with relative ease.

Leadbetter (1960) attached the tip of a posteriorly based V flap of perineal skin to the most proximal part of the urethral incision. Carefully placed sutures anastomosed the skin to the urethral mucosa without tension. Prior to the second stage the perineal skin was epilated by electrical coagulation. A three-layer closure was used at the second stage, closing the bulbocavernosus muscles but not attempting to approximate the skin of the neourethra. Colles' fascia and skin were then closed.

Pierce (1973) reported a series of patients with perineal urethral strictures repaired by the Leadbetter procedure. Because of the difficulty encountered in completing the urethral closure, older adults were encouraged to continue voiding through the perineal urethrostomy. McGuire and Weiss (1973) used the posterior-based perineal flap to establish a perineal urethrostomy in three infants with obstruction. Urethroplasty was not completed. Lapides (cited by Gerlaugh et al., 1959) used three layers of pull-out wire sutures for this closure. Fernandes, Orandi, and Draper (1966) closed the wound with one suture that included all layers and devised a perineal flap to be inserted into the posterior urethral opening to relieve stenosis at that point prior to the second stage. Gil-Vernet (1966) used a posterior perineal flap similar to the Leadbetter procedure but mobilized the scrotum and brought it posteriorly to attach to the lateral margins of the opened urethra. When he closed the defect, he brought epithelial edges together to form the neourethra.

The Turner-Warwick operation has been

---

*This paper by Johanson contains a masterly discussion of the history of surgical procedures used for repair of urethral strictures and should be read for that, as well as for its description of his technique and the philosophy of his approach to reconstructive surgery.

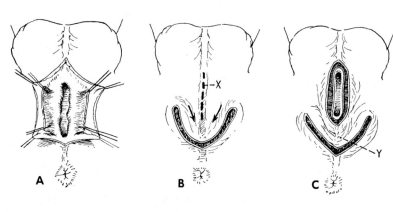

Figure 80–21. First stage of Turner-Warwick urethroplasty. *A,* Bulb has been exposed and incised. Urethral stricture and adjacent normal urethra have also been incised. *B,* Scrotal skin has been brought over open urethra in preparation for approximation of superior and inferior apex of primary incision. Broken line indicates position of second incision. *C,* Re-exposed urethra; note perineal bridge (Y). (From Hand, J. R.: *In* Campbell, M. F., and Harrison, J. H. (Eds.): Urology. Vol. 3, 3rd ed. Philadelphia, W. B. Saunders Co., 1970.)

characterized as a two-stage procedure and as the most versatile of the various urethroplasties designed to repair strictures in the membranous and supramembranous urethra up to the verumontanum (Hand, 1970). Turner-Warwick has pointed out that the most important stages of the repair are the five or six procedures done in the interval between the marsupialization and the final closure of the neourethra. At present he does not use this procedure routinely for membranous or supramembranous stricture associated with closed injuries but prefers to mobilize the urethra, excise the stricture, and anastomose the distal urethra to the prostatic portion. For large supramembranous strictures the transpubic approach is the procedure of choice.

The steps in the procedure are as follows. A midline incision is made in the scrotum, and the strictured urethra is opened. Excessively scarred tissue is removed, but some urethra is left for attachment of the scrotal inlay (Fig. 80–21). The mobilized scrotum is moved posteriorly, and a new incision is made over the opened urethra. The scrotal edges will be approximated to the urethral edges, with the posterior bridge between the original and the secondary scrotal incisions serving as the scrotal inlay. The deep sutures are placed, using a nasal speculum and a Turner-Warwick modified Reverdin-type needle holder with fine nylon suture material (Fig. 80–22), the tails being left long to make later removal easier. The lateral mattress sutures catch the full thickness of the bulb to furnish hemostasis (Fig. 80–23). A catgut suture is placed in the posterior angle of the incision in the bulb deep to the inlay, also for hemostasis. The original longitudinal scrotal in-

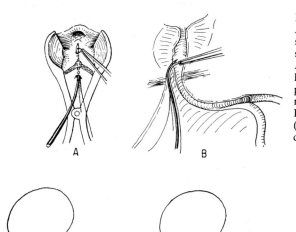

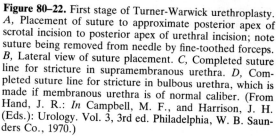

Figure 80–22. First stage of Turner-Warwick urethroplasty. *A,* Placement of suture to approximate posterior apex of scrotal incision to posterior apex of urethral incision; note suture being removed from needle by fine-toothed forceps. *B,* Lateral view of suture placement. *C,* Completed suture line for stricture in supramembranous urethra. *D,* Completed suture line for stricture in bulbous urethra, which is made if membranous urethra is of normal caliber. (From Hand, J. R.: *In* Campbell, M. F., and Harrison, J. H. (Eds.): Urology. Vol. 3, 3rd ed. Philadelphia, W. B. Saunders Co., 1970.)

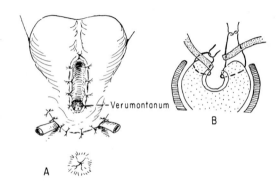

Figure 80–23. First stage of Turner-Warwick urethroplasty. *A,* Lateral margins of scrotal incision are being sutured to bulbous urethra with interrupted nylon mattress sutures; note approximation of scrotum to perineum. *B,* Detail of vertical nylon mattress sutures. (From Hand, J. R.: *In* Campbell, M. F., and Harrison, J. H. (Eds.): Urology. Vol. 3, 3rd ed. Philadelphia, W. B. Saunders Co., 1970.)

cision is closed transversely with a drain. Urine is diverted by a suprapubic tube.

Drains are removed on the second or third day, and the nonabsorbable urethral mattress sutures are removed on the fifteenth day. The deep sutures are removed under light anesthesia, using the nasal speculum and traction on the long tails of the sutures. The urethra is dilated. If stenosis has occurred, the epithelial surface behind the meatus will be disrupted and must be resurfaced by mobilizing the inlay and setting it into the defect. Hairs must be epilated. Since all living hair follicles do not have a hair present simultaneously, the dilation and resurfacing procedure must be repeated as often as necessary; sometimes a more formal flap must be elevated and set into the defect.

Before going to the final stage, enough time should be allowed for all the inflammation to have resolved from the scrotal flap, for the flap to have become fixed in its new location, and for the meatus to stricture down as much as it is going to. This usually requires 3 to 6 months. The "second stage" should not be done if the

meatus will not stay open without continued dilation.

To close the urethra the inlay is circumcised, with care taken that enough skin is left so that the urethra will close easily over a 24 or 26 F sound (Fig. 80–24). The surgeon should leave a generous amount of tissue and trim it as necessary. The bulb is freed up, and closure is accomplished with sutures that include the full thickness of the bulb and the urethral skin edge. The bulbocavernosus muscle is closed in the second layer and the skin and subcutaneous tissue in the third. A suprapubic cystostomy is favored for urine drainage, although a fenestrated Foley catheter through the repair can be used.

Waterhouse (1975) has used the Turner-Warwick procedure for repair of membranous urethral strictures in children when there has been damage to the anterior urethra, either by infection or by previous surgical procedures. These situations require the introduction of new tissue into the area. Our own choice in these instances is the full-thickness skin graft proce-

Figure 80–24. Second stage of Turner-Warwick urethroplasty. *A,* Incision to circumscribe scrotal inlay. *B,* Approximation of bulbar tissue. *C,* Approximation of bulbocavernosus muscle. *D,* Skin and subcutaneous tissue are closed loosely without drains by dead space encircling vertical mattress 3-0 nylon sutures. (From Hand, J. R.: *In* Campbell, M. F., and Harrison, J. H. (Eds.): Urology. Vol. 3, 3rd ed. Philadelphia, W. B. Saunders Co., 1970.)

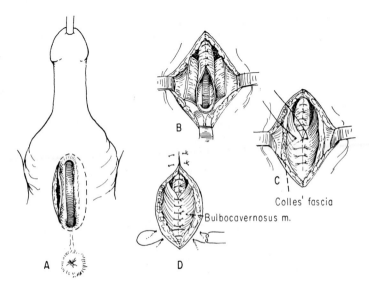

dure, as either a patch or a tube. It is rare not to be able to obtain enough tissue from the penis and, if necessary, we will take the required amount of skin from the penis and cover any penile defect with a split-thickness graft obtained from the groin. Devereux and Williams (1972) reviewed their procedures performed in children and concluded that urethroplasty should be done for all but minor strictures. Four of their patients had strictures of traumatic origin in the posterior urethra. When the bladder base was elevated, they mobilized the bladder neck and prostate to bring the prostatic urethra down into a more normal location. Continuity was then achieved by the Turner-Warwick procedure.

SKIN FLAPS

Multiple-stage procedures are still useful for complicated situations, but many surgeons have not been able to duplicate the results of the contributors of the procedures. Many patients decide not to have further surgery after the perineal urethrostomy has been established and must continue to have the meatus dilated. Restricture or diverticulum formation may complicate the second stage. At this date there is not much question that a single-stage operation that is relatively uncomplicated and carries a high success rate is the procedure of choice.

In order to reduce the number of operations, the scrotal flap procedure has been modified by Blandy and Singh (1975) to make it a one-stage procedure (Fig. 80–25). The tip of the V-shaped scrotal flap is incised, leaving a triangle of skin that is mobilized to develop an island flap based on a pedicle of dartos fascia and muscle. The tip of the flap is trimmed and is sewn to the deepest point in the open urethra proximal to the urethral stricture, using a 3-0 chromic suture. It can be placed just distal to the verumontanum. The pedicle is mobilized without tension, as this would imperil the blood supply to the flap.

The flap is then trimmed into an elliptical shape and used as a patch to reconstruct the urethra, the edges being approximated with running sutures of chromic gut. The bladder is drained by a small Foley catheter or by a suprapubic tube. The bulbocavernosus muscles are approximated loosely over the pedicle of the island flap, and the scrotal flap is used to close the perineum, using interrupted nylon sutures that are left for 10 days. The catheter is also left for 10 days. Hairs are not removed from the patch of scrotal skin used in this procedure; sensation remains, as patients have

complained that the scrotum felt wet. Blandy (1980) defended this procedure as he reported his experience with repair of urethral strictures. This is a valuable contribution and should be read by anyone venturing into this field of urologic surgery. Other pedicle flaps of local tissue, e.g., tunica vaginalis, perineal, scrotal, and penile skin, have been devised for urethroplasty (Kishev, 1971; Leadbetter, 1960; Orandi, 1972). With Duckett's introduction of the transverse island preputial flap for hypospadias repair (Duckett, 1981) there has been regenerated interest in the use of flaps of skin with pedicles long enough to reach more proximal areas of the urethra for repair of urethral strictures. Quartey (1983) has mapped the vascular supply of areas of the penis and has been successful in developing penile flaps that will reach the bulbous and membranous urethra.

A flap carries its own blood supply; a graft must acquire a new blood supply from the area where it is placed; a free flap has an artery and vein that must be anastomosed to a new vascular supply in the area to which it has been moved. Neurotized free flaps also carry a nerve that can be attached to a nerve, supplying sensation in the recipient area. These have become useful in reconstruction of the penis. When this chapter is rewritten for the next edition, these techniques will have assumed a much more prominent place in our surgical armamentarium.

SKIN GRAFTS

Embryologically, the urethra is derived from the same tissue as the skin of the penis and throughout most of its length is lined by squamous epithelium (Devine and Horton, 1977). Our long-term success with the use of full-thickness grafts for urethroplasty in hypospadias (Devine and Horton, 1961, 1978) led us to the consideration of its use in the repair of urethral strictures (Devine et al., 1963, 1968, 1976). Full-thickness skin grafts do not contract but continue to grow as the patient grows (Baran and Horton, 1972). The ideal donor site is the penis. Penile skin is full-thickness skin and is thin, soft, pliable, tough, hairless, accessible, and, in most circumstances, abundant. We have obtained a graft 19 cm long and 2 cm wide from an uncircumcised patient and still had enough penile skin to close comfortably (Devine et al., 1976). If the patient has been circumcised, we would choose to use penile skin and cover the penis with a split-thickness skin graft if acquisition of enough skin for the urethroplasty left a deficiency of penile skin.

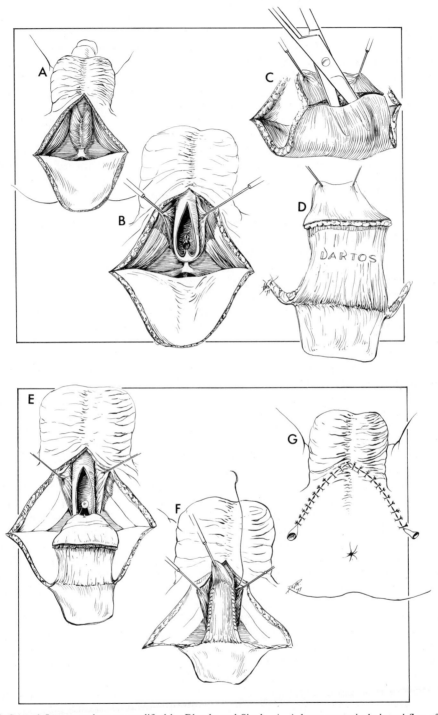

Figure 80–25. Scrotal flap procedure as modified by Blandy and Singh. *A,* A large posteriorly based flap of perineal and scrotal tissue is developed, exposing the bulbocavernosus muscles. *B,* The strictured area of the urethra is opened, exposing the verumontanum. *C,* The distal portion of scrotal skin is incised. *D,* The pedicle of dartos is developed. *E,* The tip of this flap is sewn to the tip of the incision in the urethra with a chromic suture. *F,* The flap is trimmed and sewn to the edges of the opened urethra with running chromic suture. *G,* The perineal-scrotal flap is used to re-cover the area. (Adapted from Blandy, J. P., and Singh, M.: Br. J. Urol., *47:*83, 1975.)

After excising the skin we remove all of the subcutaneous material from the graft, leaving the dermis and epidermis as a full-thickness skin graft. To do this, we stick the skin side of the graft to the bottom of a sterile pan on a piece of double-faced Paget dermatome tape.* We lift the dartos fascia layer with fine forceps and trim the tissue off with sharp scissors. In this process the dermis should not be thinned, as this would convert it to a split-thickness graft that would shrink as it matured. It is difficult to judge just how much tissue should be removed, but usually the subcutaneous tissue to be removed is pink, whereas the dermis is white.

If necessary, skin may be obtained from the inner surface of the arm, lateral chest, above the crest of the ileum, or other hairless area. This skin is much thicker than penile skin, and problems with graft contracture have been more frequent. When using nonpenile skin we use a strip of 3.5-cm width for a 24 F tube. The area is marked and cut with a knife. One end is elevated and all the fat trimmed off with a knife. If this nonpenile skin is very thick, it is proper to remove some dermis in this process.

Skin graft survival depends upon rapid acquisition of a new blood supply adequate for nutrition and disposal of products of metabolism (Converse et al., 1977). Fluid absorbed from the host bed maintains the cells of the graft. New vascular anastomoses depend upon (1) a favorable and well-vascularized host bed, (2) rapid absorption of serum soon after placement of the graft, (3) adequate immobilization of the graft on the host site to reduce disruptions of the delicate vascular communication as they form, and (4) rapid vascularization from the host site. Host capillary sprouts invade the graft, develop anastomoses with the graft vasculature, and are conducting blood within 48 hours.

Graft failures result from the following:

1. *Bleeding and hematoma beneath the graft.* Therefore, hemostasis must be complete before the graft is applied, and we use the mini–suction drains to be sure there is no build-up from oozing or exudate.

2. *External mechanical factors* that would prevent a tight apposition of the graft to its host bed. Prevention of this requires stenting of the graft and limitation of motion of the patient for at least the 24 to 36 hours required to form the new vascular connections, but preferably for 5 days, until the graft is firmly fixed by the healing process.

3. *Necrosis in the bed.* Prevention of necrosis requires that the tissues to which the graft is applied be appropriate. Fat, exposed bone, or avascular scar tissue is not a good bed for a graft, and what arterioles would grow into the graft would be insubstantial and prone to loss from one of the other causes.

4. *Infection.* In the region of the perineum and the urethra, the possibility of infection is always present. We use prophylactic antibiotics and watch carefully for inflammation, especially the strains of streptococci, which will rapidly lyse a graft.

Contracture of a graft involves not only the tissue placed as a graft but also the bed upon which it is placed. The penis offers no resistance to contracture, so grafts placed in the penis are more likely to contract, shortening and reducing the lumen of the neourethra. This has not happened, however, in the full-thickness tube grafts we have used in young boys for correction of hypospadias.

If the urethra is stenotic in the area of the stricture but appears to be healthy, we incise through the strictured area and leave the urethra in place, applying a full-thickness graft as a patch (Fig. 80–26). When the stricture is short, it is best to excise it rather than leave it in place; with long areas of stricture, however, it is best to leave the opened urethra as the dorsal wall to the grafted urethra to afford some stability to the repair and to diminish postoperative contracture, which can lead to shortening or constriction of the neourethra. If, after resecting the stricture and mobilizing the urethra, we are still unable to do a primary anastomosis, we will bring the ventral aspect of the two ends of the urethra together and complete the circumference of the urethra with a patch graft. When the stenosis is at the penoscrotal junction, it is important to remember that the bulb can be mobilized in a proximal direction. Thus, the very troublesome stricture seen there following a TUR and several attempts at internal urethrotomy can be excised, allowing the more normal proximal and distal ends of the urethra to be brought together. If the urethra and the surrounding erectile tissue are very fibrotic and inflamed, they must be excised. This defect can then be made up by applying a tube of full-thickness skin after fixing the spatulated ends of the urethra to the underlying erectile bodies.

I measure the defect to determine how much skin will be needed for the graft. The graft is applied loosely and not stretched at any

---

*3M Medical Products Division, Minnesota Mining & Manufacturing Co., 3M Center, St. Paul, Minnesota 55101.

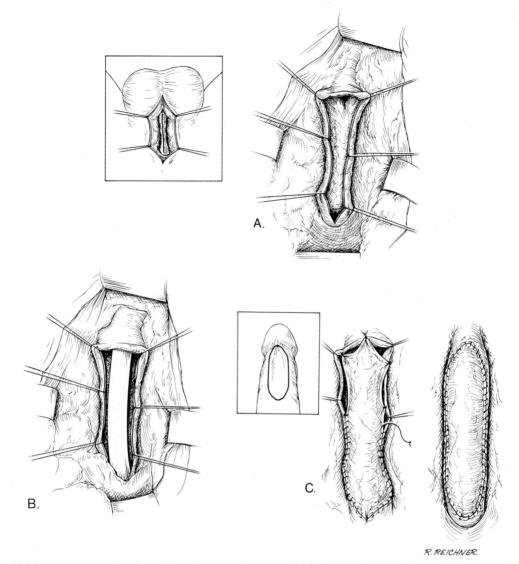

R. REICHNER.

Figure 80–26. Patch graft urethroplasty. After the area to be repaired is identified, an incision is made through the length of the stricture and for 1-1/2 to 2 cm into each normal end of the urethra. *A,* The edges are secured with black silk sutures. *B,* A 24 F silicone catheter is passed through the defect, which is measured, and a patch of penile skin is marked and excised. It may be possible to raise this on an island pedicle. *C,* The patch is sewn into the defect, first by interrupted sutures to ensure its smooth placement and then by running sutures of 5-0 P.D.S. to make a watertight closure. Subcutaneous fascia and skin are then closed over a mini–suction drain.

point in the repair. So that the final lumen will be 24 to 26 F in an adult, the combined width of the urethra and the graft should be 3 cm.

After the graft has been prepared, we place it in the defect with the epithelial surface into the lumen over a 24 F silicone Foley catheter as a mold. I tack the graft at each end and at several places along the margins with interrupted sutures: 5-0 chromic if it is necessary to place them inside the lumen, or 5-0 PDS if the epithelial edges are turned in. I then close the edge of the graft to the edge of the urethra with a running suture of 5-0 PDS. We use a cutting needle or the tapered RB-1 needle, which is

excellent for this. After the graft is in place, we use other PDS sutures to spread out the graft so that it will be fixed in place and be better exposed to the vascular tissues of the perineum. We then take the molding catheter out and test the suture lines by instilling methylene blue–dyed saline solution into the urethra and closing any leaks that may be revealed. If the repair is in the perineum, we put a smaller silicone Foley into the bladder and leave it as a drain. If the repair is in the penis, we place a suprapubic tube into the bladder and leave a section of the 24 F silicone tube in the urethra as a stent for 5 days.

TUBE GRAFT

The approach to the urethra is the same as with other strictures. If, after opening the urethra, the mucosa is scarred and the urethra is fibrotic and inflamed, a patch graft will not do well, and the stricture must be excised. If the ends of the urethra cannot be brought together, we will bridge the gap with a tubed graft of full-thickness skin (Fig. 80–27). If the spongy tissue can be preserved, it will make a good bed for the graft. If it is scarred, it must be removed; unless there is marked inflammation and scarring around it, these tissues will support a graft. This is one area where the tubed island flaps of penile skin described by Quartey (1983) will be very useful. The following description of constructing the tube applies to these flaps as well as to the grafts we use at present.

We spatulate the ends of the urethra and fix them to the deeper tissues with 4-0 to 5-0 PDS. There are several ways we can construct a tube to fit this gap. We can pass a 24 F silicone catheter through the distal urethra, form a tube around it, and attach the ends of the tube to the ends of the urethra. However, we prefer to lay the graft in the defect and fix it in place with several mattress sutures up the midline. Then we form the anastomosis at the proximal and distal ends with interrupted 5-0 PDS. After passing the 24 F catheter into the bladder, we complete the tube around it. As with other skin grafts in the urethra, we place lateral sutures to flatten the graft, fixing it and getting more exposure to vascular tissue. We may leave this 24 F catheter for 5 days and replace it with a smaller tube at that time, or, if we have inserted a suprapubic tube, we may remove the stenting catheter at that time.

We keep the patient at bed rest for 5 days during the immediate postoperative period while the graft is acquiring its blood supply. We then allow him to be up and about with his catheter attached to closed drainage. There is no way to prevent erections during the postoperative period, but large doses of Valium will help, and, if the patient is awakened at night by an erection, amyl nitrite pearls will help dissipate it. In 10 to 14 days we obtain a pericatheter urethrogram by passing a small feeding tube alongside the catheter in the urethra, or, if a suprapubic tube is in place, we obtain a voiding cystourethrogram. If extravasation is present, we leave the catheter for a longer time or reopen the suprapubic tube.

We follow these patients with repeated x-ray studies in 4 to 6 months and again in a year. If complications are going to happen, they usually will be seen by that time. If the neourethra does become stenotic, it will not respond well to an internal urethrotomy. We reopen the urethra and insert a patch graft. In several patients I have had to incise the full length of the tube to lay in a full-length patch graft, which should be 2 cm wide. We have put in a full-length tube graft urethra—30 cm or so in length—in a number of patients. These have worked well in some, but in others, in whom an inordinate amount of inflammation developed, they have not. We have had success with some of these patients by excising the full length of the urethra and laying a strip of skin 4 cm wide

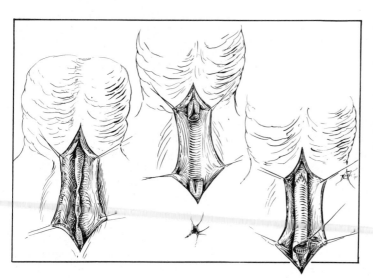

Figure 80–27. Perineal urethral stricture exposed, excised, and replaced with a full-thickness (tubed) skin graft. The molding catheter is not shown. If the substance of the bulb is healthy, we open the erectile tissue and excise the strictured mucosal tube. We then insert the graft and close the bulb around it. (From Horton, C. E., and Devine, P. C.: Strictures of the male urethra. *In* Converse, J. M. (Ed.): Reconstructive Plastic Surgery. Philadelphia, W. B. Saunders Co., 1977.)

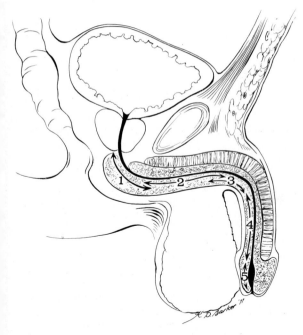

Figure 80–28. Diagram of a sagittal section illustrating the area discussed in the treatment of urethral strictures. 1. The deep bulb and the membranous portions of the urethra. 2. The area of the bulb. 3. The penoscrotal junction. Access to this area is usually by an incision bivalving the scrotum. 4. Penile lesions are approached by making a circumcising incision and reflecting the skin of the penis to the base, or, if a flap is to be used for the repair, by a longitudinal incision over the strictured area. 5. Glanular strictures are amenable to internal urethrotomy or a V flap of glans tissue.

corona of the glans and developing the subcutaneous plane, freeing up the loose layer of dartos fascia. The entire length of the shaft of the penis can be exposed by this maneuver. If, however, we intend to use a local flap of skin to repair the penile urethra, we make a midline incision on the ventral aspect of the penile shaft and dissect out the urethra.

Strictures in the region of the penoscrotal junction may be exposed by making a ventral incision in the midline at the penoscrotal junction; if the stricture extends into the bulb, a midline incision is made in the perineum. The plane beneath the scrotum is easily opened, and the procedure may be carried out beneath the scrotum. Alternatively, we divide the scrotum in the midline through the septum, retracting its contents to each side.

For strictures in the bulb we make a ventral incision off the midline of the perineum, beginning just behind the scrotum and swinging sharply across the midline near the perineal body to the ischial tuberosity on the other side. This gives excellent exposure and is placed so that the skin closure will not overlie the urethral repair.

For penile lesions the patient is placed supine; for penoscrotal lesions the position is modified by flexing the hips and knees into the "frogleg" position. Perineal exposure requires the lithotomy position, and, as the urethral

the full length of the defect. We cover this with a bolster and have had good results. Six months to a year later, after the inflammation has resolved, we bring the patient back and form a tube from this now mature and healthy tissue. This method has not yet stood the test of time but seems promising for these otherwise unsolvable problems.

The proper incision depends upon the area of the urethra involved by the stricture (Fig. 80–28). The anteriorly based V flap of glans tissue that we have developed for hypospadias repair is useful for strictures in the glans (Fig. 80–29). A V-shaped incision is marked on the glans, with the apex at the urethral meatus. This flap is elevated and advanced into an incision on the dorsal aspect of the urethra, widening the strictured area. If the stricture extends too far proximal for this to bridge it completely, we use the meatoplasty described earlier (Fig. 80–5) or handle the lesion as a penile stricture. Penile lesions are approached by making a circumcising incision 1 to 1.5 cm proximal to the

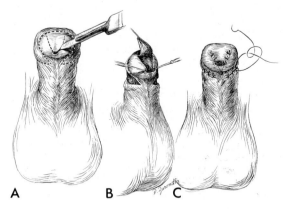

Figure 80–29. Author's procedure for urethral meatotomy. *A*, Skin incisions are outlined by the dotted line. The V-shaped flap of glans is incised and elevated. *B*, The flap has been elevated and an incision made on the dorsal surface of the urethra. Circumcision has been accomplished, removing the excess preputial hood in this child with glanular hypospadias. *C*, The flap of glans has been advanced into the urethra. The circumcision is then closed. (From Horton, C. E., and Devine, C. J., Jr.: Hypospadias. *In* Converse, J. M. (ed.): Reconstructive Plastic Surgery. Philadelphia, W. B. Saunders Co., 1977.)

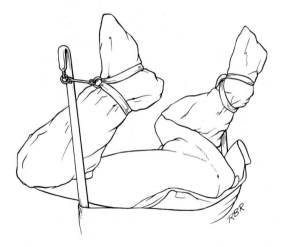

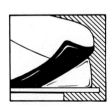

Figure 80–30. Patient in the deep lithotomy position. He has been given a general anesthetic. The insert shows the black Vac Pac, which has been molded to his contour before it is evacuated. This supports him and is elevated on a wedge-shaped sandbag supported by a board on the operating table. The patient's legs are held flexed by the stirrups, which do not exert pressure on the hip or knee joints.

incision may have to be carried into the membranous portion, the exaggerated lithotomy position is mandatory.

When the stricture in the membranous urethra has been caused by trauma associated with fracture of the pelvis, the prostate will probably be high-lying, and sometimes no patent urethra will be present between the apex of the prostate and the attachment of the bulb of the urethra.

We put the patient in the deep lithotomy position, such as we use for radical perineal prostatectomy (Fig. 80–30). From this position we can dissect the anterior aspect of the urethra and prostate well above the genitourinary diaphragm. Several things help with this: We use general anesthesia for complete relaxation and good control of the patient by the anesthesiologist. We place the patient on a Vac Pac,* with his hips low at the break of the foot piece of the table, his legs suspended by his feet in stirrups,† and his hips and knees flexed. The upper extensions of the Vac Pac are held to cradle his shoulders as the Vac Pac is evacuated, forming a stiff support for the patient. We now elevate his hips on sandbags, and the stirrups are rotated backward, placing his perineum parallel with the floor.

We make an incision in the midline extending from the scrotum and deviating to one ischial tuberosity as it nears the perineal body. Another incision from the other ischial tuberosity forms a Y (Fig. 80–31). We incise Colles' fascia (Fig. 80–31A) and expose the bulbocavernosus muscles. Lateral dissection is not necessary and, as it would open up tissue planes, should not be carried out. When the central tendon between these muscles is identified (Fig. 80–31B), we incise in this line to expose the bulb of the urethra (Fig. 80–31C). We do dissect the bulb of the urethra from the muscles. We continue the midline incision through the junction of the transverse perinei muscles and retract them posterolaterally to dissect the bulb of the urethra up to the genitourinary diaphragm (Fig. 80–31D). It is possible, and I feel preferable, to do this dissection without getting into the erectile tissue of the bulb. We then place a Denis Browne retractor* with the deep blades that my

*Olympic Medical Corporation, 4400 7th Street South, Seattle, Washington 98108.

†Lithotomy Leg Holders, American Sterilizer Co. (AMSCO), 2424 West 23rd Street, Erie, Pennsylvania 16514.

*Denis Browne retractor, Devine modification, American Hospital Supply Co., V. Mueller, 6600 West Touhy Avenue, Chicago, Illinois, 60648.

Figure 80–31. Diagram of perineal repair of membranous urethral stricture. An inverted Y incision extends from the midline of the scrotum to the ischial tuberosities. *A,* Colles' fascia has been opened to expose the bulbocavernosus muscles. *B,* The scissors are introduced to develop the space between the muscle and the bulb of the urethra. *C,* An incision is made, with the scissors in the midline, exposing the length of the bulb. *D,* We incise the transverse perinei muscles to expose the full extent of the bulb. *E,* The self-retaining retractor is placed to expose the genitourinary diaphragm. *F,* The strictured urethra is incised, freeing the bulb. *G,* The urethra is opened, showing an adequate lumen and the proximal overhang of the bulb. *H,* The circular sound has been passed through the suprapubic cystostomy; dissection of the scar has allowed it to pass into the perineum. *I,* The scar tissue has been removed from the anterior aspect of the prostate, and the urethra opened for the anastomosis. *J,* The proximal and distal segments of the urethra. *K,* The catheter has been passed and the ventral sutures are about to be tied. *L,* Anastomosis completed, with the reinforcing sutures in place.

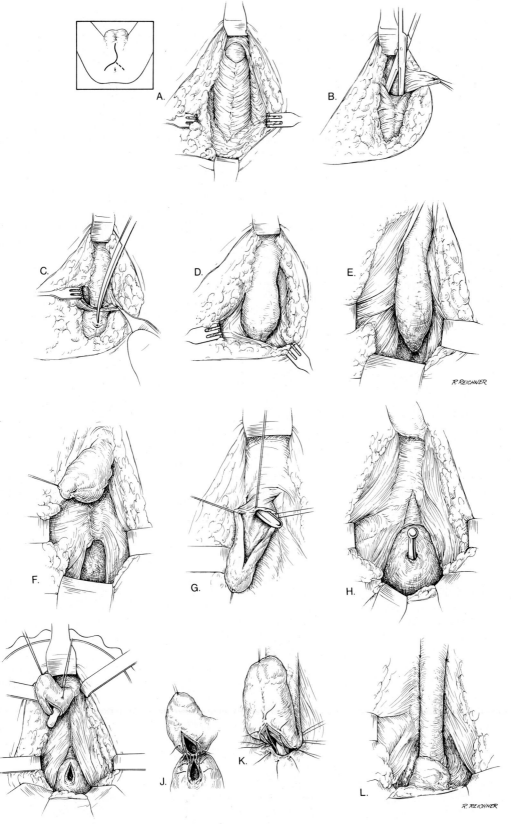

Figure 80–31. *See legend on opposite page*

brother, Dr. Patrick Devine, developed for this instrument (Fig. 80–31E).

We can now visualize the entire length of this segment of the urethra. We incise the urethra at the genitourinary diaphragm and free up the bulb (Fig. 80–31F). We spatulate the opening of the urethra in the bulb and place a red rubber catheter through it to retract it out of the field (Fig. 80–31G). We clean the genitourinary diaphragm and manipulate a semicircular urethral sound through the cystostomy incision into the prostatic urethra, advancing it until the tip can be felt. At times the posterior urethra may be so bound in scar tissue that this sound will not pass easily. We then pass a cystoscope or flexible nephroscope in through the suprapubic cystostomy site so that we can be certain that we are in the correct location. We incise the diaphragm, freeing the sound or scope so that it can be passed into the perineum (Fig. 80–31H). Note that the stricture is still present, and further dissection will be needed to free up the anterior aspect of the membranous and prostatic urethra before a primary anastomosis can be accomplished. We incise the genitourinary diaphragm toward the symphysis pubis until we are able to dissect out these structures (Fig. 80–31I). It is important to confine this dissection to the anterior aspect of the prostate so that the nerves involved in potency (Walsh et al., 1983) are spared.

In many cases the end of the proximal urethra can be mobilized easily; when a 30 F bougie à boule will pass with ease, we are ready for the anastomosis. We always pass a cystoscope into the bladder to identify the structures of the prostatic urethra, bladder neck, and ureteral orifices. We mobilize the bulb of the urethra by incising its attachments to the genitourinary diaphragm. These include the arteries to the bulb and the urethral arteries, but it is safe to proceed with this dissection because the vascularity of the urethra is such that blood flow from the glans is sufficient to supply the full length of the urethra (McGowan and Waterhouse, 1964). If it is necessary to continue onto the penis to get sufficient length, the entire urethra must be mobilized. It is best not to dissect onto the penis because of the possibility of creating chordee, and in most cases it is not necessary.

When the urethra has been mobilized, we place 5-0 PDS sutures through the dorsal edge of the spatulated distal urethra and the anterior lip of the opened proximal urethra. Another set of sutures is placed in the posterior lip of the proximal portion of the urethra (Fig. 80–31J).

After tying the anterior sutures, a 24 F silicone catheter is passed through the urethra and into the bladder. The posterior sutures are placed in the urethra and tied down to complete the primary repair (Fig. 80–31K). In placing these sutures we attempt to avoid the epithelial margins, turning the sutures into the lumen. We place further sutures of 5-0 PDS to secure the bulb of the urethra to the diaphragm and the underlying erectile bodies, taking tension off the repair (Fig. 80–31L). We close the muscle layers of the perineum and leave a small suction drain. We then close Colles' fascia and the skin with interrupted sutures.

If the elasticity of the urethra is not sufficient for this repair, or if there is so much scar tissue together with the complexities that might accompany a stricture associated with a fractured pelvis, we will remove a segment of the symphysis in order to make a primary anastomosis. However, if there were not a lot of scar and the tissues seemed vascular enough to nourish a graft, my preference would be to place a full-thickness graft tube to make up the defect rather than to excise the entire symphysis (Fig. 80–32).

Webster and Selli (1983) have reported excellent results with their procedure, which is very similar to this. Turner-Warwick (1983) opens the posterior aspect of the bulb of the urethra as a flap, cuts across the urethra distal to the stricture, and spatulates it on its anterior and posterior aspects. He excises the stricture, opening up the normal urethra proximal to it. The anterior aspect of the urethra is anastomosed to this—usually to the prostatic portion—by placing five sutures in the prostate, bringing them through the urethra, and tying down as the urethra is "pushed" into position. The posterior anastomosis is made and the urethra closed. The flap of bulb is closed to relieve tension. A fenestrated catheter and a suprapubic tube are left for 2 weeks, and large urethral sounds are passed from time to time during healing to prevent cross-urethral adhesions.

Turner-Warwick notes that severe fracture-dislocation injuries may result in long strictures with loss of continuity because of fibrosis resulting from the hematoma and failure to reduce the prostatic dislocation. Urinary extravasation into this periurethral hematoma may result in formation of a diverticulum, which would preclude a simple anastomosis between the bulb of the urethra and the prostate. In this case, exposure may be increased by resecting the posterior part of the pubis, leaving the anterior cortex intact, and by suprapubic resection of the

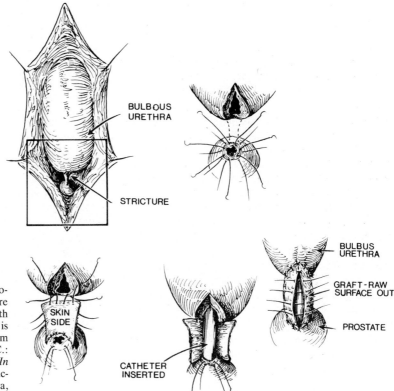

BULBOUS
URETHRA

STRICTURE

BULBUS
URETHRA

GRAFT-RAW
SURFACE OUT

PROSTATE

SKIN
SIDE

CATHETER
INSERTED

Figure 80–32. Tube graft urethroplasty: membranous urethral stricture exposed, excised, and replaced with a full-thickness skin graft that is wrapped around a catheter. (From Horton, C. E., and Devine, P. C.: Strictures of the male urethra. *In* Converse, J. M. (Ed.): Reconstructive Plastic Surgery. Philadelphia, W. B. Saunders Co., 1977.)

fibro-osseous scar tissue and diverticula. The mobilized urethra brought up through this tunnel is anastomosed to the anteriorly spatulated prostatic urethra. An omental pedicle flap mobilized from the transverse colon is used to bolster the repair and isolate the urethra from the fibrous tunnel in the area of the stricture. A fenestrated catheter is left through the repair for 3 weeks, and a suprapubic tube is retained until satisfactory voiding is established.

Distal to the membranous urethra the principles of the surgical procedure are similar, whatever the location of the stricture. We instill methylene blue into the urethra by syringe prior to the incision. This material stains the urethra sky-blue. The staining is deeper in color in the area of abnormal mucosa involved by the stricture, so that this area is easily identified and may be followed through a very densely fibrotic area. A large sound passed in the distal urethra to the stricture identifies its location. We make an incision in the urethra over the tip of the sound and secure the edges with stay sutures of black silk placed through the full thickness of the urethra and erectile tissue. These sutures keep the urethra open and help to control bleeding; for retraction, they are looped over

the ring of the self-retaining retractor. The sound is withdrawn, and a red rubber catheter is passed through the opening as an aid in retraction. The incision is continued through the full length of the stricture. One of three techniques is used at this point, depending upon the nature of the stricture (Devine and Horton, 1977; Devine et al., 1977*b*).

In most cases the urethra will appear to be relatively healthy and will require simply an increase in the caliber of the lumen at that point; therefore, a patch graft can be applied. The strictured area may be short or long. An incision is made into the normal urethra proximally and distally until a 30 F bougie à boule will pass without hang-up in an adult. This usually requires an incision of 1 to 1.5 cm. In children a proportionately smaller instrument will be used. A catheter (24 F in adults, smaller in children) is passed through the urethra to serve as a mold for the graft. The defect is measured, and a skin graft is measured and marked on the penile shaft. If a circumcising incision has been made, the distal end of the penile skin is used. If a long piece is required, it is obtained by a spiraling incision around the penile shaft.

In perineal procedures, if the bulb has been involved in an inflammatory process and is fibrotic, there will not be much bleeding from it, and we make no attempt to close it over the graft. If, however, it will close easily, we do so. The bulbocavernosus muscles are closed, interrupted sutures are placed in Colles' fascia, and the skin is closed with absorbable sutures. In the penile urethra the corpus spongiosum will be included in the closure of the urethra, and the retracted skin is replaced and attached with multiple chromic sutures at the corona. We leave a small suction drain in these patients and remove it on the first postoperative day.

With the marsupialization procedures it is usual, although exasperating, to have to open further strictured areas of the urethra between the first and "second" stages. This probably happens because (1) the full extent of the stricture was not recognized, and (2) there was difficulty in getting scrotal or perineal flaps high enough in the membranous urethra. If the entire strictured area is not corrected in a one-stage operation, the result can be much more serious than with the multiple-stage procedures.

References

Allen, J. S., and Summers, J. L.: Meatal stenosis in children. J. Urol., *112*:526, 1974.

Allen, T. D.: The transpubic approach for strictures of the membranous urethra. J. Urol., *114*:63, 1975.

Badenoch, A. W.: A pull-through operation for impassable traumatic stricture of the urethra. Br. J. Urol., *22*:404, 1950.

Bainbridge, D. R., Whitaker, R. H., and Shepheard, B. G. F.: Balanitis xerotica obliterans and urinary obstruction. Br. J. Urol., *43*:487, 1971.

Baran, N. K., and Horton, C. E.: Growth of skin grafts, flaps, and scars in young minipigs. Plast. Reconstr. Surg., *50*:487, 1972.

Bissada, N. K., Cole, A. T., and Fried, F. A.: Extensive condylomas acuminata of the entire male urethra and the bladder. J. Urol., *112*:201, 1974.

Blandy, J. P.: Urethral stricture. Postgrad. Med. J., *56*:383, 1980.

Blandy, J. P., and Singh, M.: The technique and results of one-stage island patch urethroplasty. Br. J. Urol., *47*:83, 1975.

Blandy, J. P., and Tresidder, G. C.: Meatoplasty. Br. J. Urol., *39*:261, 1967.

Boxer, R. J.: Reconstruction of the male external genitalia. Surg. Gynecol. Obstet., *141*:939, 1975.

Cole, A. T., Peterson, D. D., Biddle, W. S., and Fried, F. A.: Uroflowmetry: A useful technique in the management of urethral strictures. J. Urol., *112*:482, 1974.

Converse, J. M., McCarthy, J. C., Brauer, R. O., and Ballantyne, D. L., Jr.: Transplantation of skin: grafts and flaps. In Converse, J. M. (Ed.): Reconstructive Plastic Surgery. 2nd ed. Philadelphia, W. B. Saunders Co., 1977, pp. 157, 179–180.

Devereux, M. H., and Williams, D. I.: The treatment of urethral stricture in boys. J. Urol., *108*:489, 1972.

Devine, C. J., Jr., and Devine, P. C.: Urethral strictures (Editorial). J. Urol., *123*:506, 1980.

Devine, C. J., Jr., and Devine, P. C.: Operations for urethral stricture. In Stewart, B. H. (Ed.): Operative Urology. Baltimore, Williams & Wilkins Co., 1982, pp. 242–270.

Devine, C. J., Jr., Devine, P. C., Felderman, T. P., and Burns, C. N., Jr.: Classification and standardization of urethral strictures. Presented at American Urological Association, 78th Annual Meeting, Las Vegas, Nevada, April 1983.

Devine, C. J., Jr., Devine, P. C., and Horton, C. E.: Anterior urethral injury: etiology, diagnosis, and initial management. Urol. Clin. North Am., *4*:125, 1977*a*.

Devine, C. J., Jr., Franz, J. P., and Horton, C. E.: Evaluation and treatment of patients with failed hypospadias repair. J. Urol., *119*:223, 1978.

Devine, C. J., Jr., Gonzalez-Serva, L., Stecker, J. F., Jr., and Devine, P. C.: Utricular configuration in hypospadias and intersex. J. Urol., *123*:407, 1980.

Devine, P. C., and Devine, C. J., Jr.: Posterior urethral injuries associated with pelvic fractures. Urology, *20*:467, 1982.

Devine, P. C., and Horton, C. E.: Strictures of the male urethra. In Converse, J. M. (Ed.): Reconstructive Plastic Surgery. Philadelphia, W. B. Saunders Co., 1977, pp. 3883–3895.

Devine, P. C., Devine, C. J., Jr., and Horton, C. E.: Anterior urethral injuries: Secondary reconstruction. Urol. Clin. North Am., *4*:157, 1977*b*.

Devine, P. C., Fallon, B., and Devine, C. J., Jr.: Free full thickness skin graft urethroplasty. J. Urol., *116*:444, 1976.

Devine, P. C., Horton, C. E., Devine, C. J., Sr., Devine, C. J., Jr., Crawford, H. H., and Adamson, J. E.: Use of full thickness skin grafts in repair of urethral strictures. J. Urol., *90*:67, 1963.

Devine, P. C., Sakati, I. A., Poutasse, E. F., and Devine, C. J., Jr.: One stage urethroplasty: repair of urethral strictures with a free full thickness patch of skin. J. Urol., *99*:191, 1968.

Duckett, J. W.: The island flap technique for hypospadias repair. Urol. Clin. North Am., *8*:3, 1981.

Fernandes, M., Orandi, A., and Draper, J. W.: Urethroplasty: a new method of closure. J. Urol., *96*:779, 1966.

Gil-Vernet, J. M.: Un traitement des stenoses traumatiques et inflammatoires de l'uretre posterieur. Nouvelle methode d'uretroplastie. J. Urol. Nephrol., *72*:97, 1966.

Hand, J. R.: Surgery of the penis and urethra. In Campbell, M. F., and Harrison, J. H. (Eds.): Urology. 3rd ed. Philadelphia, W. B. Saunders Co., 1970, p. 2592.

Horton, C. E., and Devine, C. J., Jr.: A one-stage repair of hypospadias cripples. Plast. Reconstr. Surg., *45*:425, 1970.

Horton, C. E., McCraw, J. B., Devine, C. J., Jr., and Devine, P. C.: Secondary reconstruction of the genital area. Urol. Clin. North Am., *4*:133, 1977.

Johanson, B.: Reconstruction of the male urethra in strictures. Application of the buried intact epithelium technic. Acta Chir. Scand. (Suppl.), *176*:3, 1953.

Khan, A. U., and Furlow, W. L.: Transpubic urethroplasty. J. Urol., *116*:447, 1976.

Kishev, S. V.: A new "thumb" urethroplasty. J. Urol., *106*:231, 1971.

Lapides, J.: Cited by Gerlaugh, R. L., Ratner, W. H., and Murphy, J. J.: Late results of urethroplasty for stricture. J. Urol., *81*:763, 1959.

Leadbetter, G. W., Jr.: A simplified urethroplasty for stricture of the bulbous urethra. J. Urol., *83*:54, 1960.

Lieberman, S. F., and Barry, J. M.: Direct vision internal urethrotomy for traumatic obliteration of membranous urethra. AUA Annual Program Brochure, Las Vegas, 1983.

MacKinnon, K. J.: Lower urinary tract trauma. *In* Glenn, J. F. and Boyce, W. H. (Eds.): Urologic Surgery. 2nd ed. New York, Harper & Row, 1975.

McGowan, A. J., and Waterhouse, K.: Mobilization of the anterior urethra. Bull. N.Y. Acad. Med., *40*:776, 1964.

McGuire, E. J., and Weiss, R. M.: Scrotal flap urethroplasty for strictures of the deep urethra in infants and children. J. Urol., *110*:599, 1973.

Morales, P., Littmann, R., and Golimbu, M.: Transpubic surgery: a new approach to difficult pelvic operations. J. Urol., *110*:564, 1973.

O'Conor, V. J., Jr., and Kropp, K. A.: Surgery of the female urethra. *In* Glenn, J. F., and Boyce, W. H. (Eds.): Urologic Surgery. 1st ed. New York, Harper & Row, 1969, p. 572.

Orandi, A.: One-stage urethroplasty; four year follow-up. J. Urol., *107*:977, 1972.

Paine, D., and Coombes, W.: Transpubic reconstruction of the urethra. Br. J. Urol., *40*:78, 1968.

Patil, U. B., and Yuan, H. A.: Gait study in patients with transpubic prostatomembranous urethroplasty. AUA Annual Program Brochure, Las Vegas, 1983.

Pierce, J. M., Jr.: Exposure of the membranous and posterior urethra by total pubectomy. J. Urol., *88*:256, 1962.

Pierce, J. M., Jr.: Management of dismemberment of the prostatic-membranous urethra and ensuing stricture disease. J. Urol., *107*:259, 1972.

Pierce, J. M., Jr.: Urethroplasty for anterior urethral stricture. J. Urol., *109*:422, 1973.

Quartey, J. K. M.: One-stage penile/preputial cutaneous island flap urethroplasty for urethral stricture: A preliminary report. J. Urol., *129*:284, 1983.

Ragde, H., and McInnes, G. G.: Transpubic repair of the severed prostatomembranous urethra. J. Urol., *101*:335, 1969.

Roberts, J. W., and Devine, C. J., Jr.: Urethral hemangioma: Treatment by total excision and grafting. J. Urol., *129*:1053, 1983.

Russell, R. H.: The treatment of urethral stricture by excision. Br. J. Surg., *2*:375, 1914–1915.

Schulman, M. L.: Reanastomosis of the amputated penis. J. Urol., *109*:432, 1973.

Sholem, S. L., Wechsler, M., and Roberts, M.: Management of the urethral diverticulum in women: a modified operative technique. J. Urol., *112*:485, 1974.

Spence, H. M., and Duckett, J. W., Jr.: Diverticulum of the female urethra: clinical aspects and presentation of a simple operative technique for cure. J. Urol., *104*:432, 1970.

Staff, W. G.: Urethral involvement in balanitis xerotica obliterans. Br. J. Urol., *47*:234, 1970.

Stewart, H. H.: Reconstruction of the urethra for the treatment of severe urethral strictures. Br. J. Urol., *32*:1, 1960.

Thiersch, K.: Ueber die Enstehungsweise und Operative Behandlung der Epispadie. Arch Heilkunde, 20, 1869.

Turner-Warwick, R. T.: Urethral stricture. *In* Glenn, J. F., and Boyer, W. H. (Eds.): Urologic Surgery. 2nd ed., New York, Harper & Row, 1975, p. 697.

Turner-Warwick, R. T.: Urethral stricture surgery. *In* Glenn, J. F. (Ed.): Urologic Surgery. 3rd ed. Philadelphia, J. B. Lippincott Co., 1983, pp. 710–711.

Vest, S. A.: Radical perineal prostatectomy: modification of closure. Surg. Gynecol. Obstet., *70*:935, 1940.

Walker, G.: Symphysiotomy as an aid to the removal of cancer of the prostate. Ann. Surg., *73*:609, 1921.

Walsh, P. C., Lepor, H., and Eggleston, G. C.: Radical prostatectomy with preservation of sexual function. Anatomical and pathologic considerations. Prostate, *4* (5):473, 1983.

Waterhouse, K.: The surgical repair of membranous urethral strictures in children. Trans. Am. Assoc. Genitourin. Surg., *67*:81, 1975.

Waterhouse, K., Abrahams, H. G., Hackett, R. E., and Peng, B. K.: The transpubic approach to the lower urinary tract. J. Urol., *109*:486, 1973.

Webster, G. D., and Selli, C.: Management of traumatic posterior urethral stricture by one stage perineal repair. Surg. Gynecol. Obstet., *156*:620, 1983.

Wiggishoff, C. C., and Kiefer, J. H.: Pull-through reconstruction of the posterior urethra. Trans. Am. Assoc. Genitourin. Surg., *56*:23, 1964.

Young, H. H., and Davis, D. M.: Young's Practice of Urology. Philadelphia, W. B. Saunders Co., 1926.

Zinman, L., and Libertino, J. A.: The dismembered one-stage urethroplasty with an end-to-end primary anastomosis for bulbomembranous urethral strictures. Presented at the Seventy-Second Annual Meeting of the American Urological Association, Inc., Chicago, Ill., April 24–28, 1977.

CHAPTER 81

Surgery of the Penis

TERRENCE R. MALLOY, M.D.
ALAN J. WEIN, M.D.

This chapter will consider the surgical treatment of certain acquired disorders of the penis as well as prosthetic surgery for impotence. Specifically excluded will be hypospadias and epispadias, urethral stricture disease, trauma to the penis, vascular reconstruction for impotence, and cancer, all of which are covered elsewhere in this text.

RELEVANT GROSS ANATOMY

The penis comprises an anchored portion and a free or pendulous portion. The bulk of each is composed of three cyindrical masses of tissue—two corpora cavernosa and a single ventral corpus spongiosum. Each corporal body is made up of a loose trabecular meshwork of muscular and connective tissues surrounded by a dense fibrous covering, the tunica albuginea (Fig. 81–1). The corpora cavernosa share a common septum in the pendulous portion of the penis with many perforations that allow free passage of blood from one side to the other, allowing the two to function essentially as a single unit (Wagner, 1981). The corpus spongiosum is unpaired and lies in the ventral groove formed by the two larger cavernosal bodies. The corpus spongiosum contains the urethra and enlarges at its distal end to form the glans penis. The corpora cavernosa indent the proximal part of the glans, with their distal ends actually extending into the glans beyond the corona. All of the corporal bodies are surrounded by another dense fascial sheath, Buck's fascia, from which thin fibrous septa extend between the paired corpora cavernosa and the corpus spongiosum. Buck's fascia is an important structure in anchoring the anterior aspect of the penis to the symphysis pubic, as it fuses with the suspensory ligament and as it joins with Colles' fascia posteriorly at the triangular ligament. More superficially lies the dartos fascia, or Colles' fascia of the penis, which is just beneath the skin and is continuous with Scarpa's fascia of the abdomen.

The proximal or anchored portions are the crura of the corpora cavernosa. These are firmly attached to the ventral aspects of the ischial rami and therefore diverge and separate from each other at the level of the inferior aspect of the symphysis pubis. Each crus is covered by the ischiocavernosus muscle. The corpus spongiosum is attached proximally to the ventral aspect of the urogenital diaphragm and is covered by the bulbocavernosus muscle. This dilated, rather bulbous portion is pierced by the urethra after the latter traverses the urogenital diaphragm. The urethra is then surrounded by the corpus spongiosum to the meatus.

The blood supply of the penis is ultimately derived from the hypogastric arteries, which continue into the deep pelvis and perineum as the internal pudendal arteries via the lesser sciatic foramen and Alcock's canal. Each internal pudendal artery gives off a perineal branch and a bulbar and urethral artery before continuing as the artery of the penis. The urethral artery and the artery of the bulb enter at the level of the bulbous urethra on each side and run in the corpus spongiosum in a lateral position. Just beyond the takeoff of these arteries, the artery of the penis branches into the deep artery of the penis, which enters the medial aspect of the corpus cavernosum near its termination, and the dorsal artery to the penis, which passes medial to the crus of the corpus cavernosum to run in the groove between the

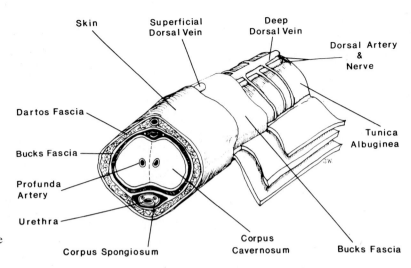

Figure 81–1. Gross anatomy of the penis.

two corpora cavernosa lateral to the deep distal veins, and which terminates in branches going to the glans penis.

The dorsal arteries run from the suspensory ligament to the glans beneath Buck's fascia, but superficial to the tunica albuginea. The deep arteries course longitudinally as one to three major branches within the substance of the corpus cavernosum. They are the only structures within this tissue that are not friable, and they are located closer to the midline cribriform septum of the corpus rather than being centrally located (Newman and Reiss, 1982). The paired arteries of the bulb and urethra also continue longitudinally to the glans, where they anastomose freely with the terminal branches of the dorsal artery (Deysach, 1939). Multiple large anastomotic channels connect all three major pairs of arteries along their entire course and freely pass through the tunica albuginea.

The venous drainage of the penis is more complex. One of the clearest and best illustrated discussions of the venous drainage of the penis is contained in the review by Newman and Northup (1981). According to these authors, three major divisions of veins are noted at separate levels—superficial, intermediate, and deep—as well as unnamed emissary, circumflex, and communicating vessels that allow such vast anastomoses that contrast material injected under sufficient pressure will fill all veins and spaces. The superficial level of veins includes the multiple subcutaneous veins that run deep to the dartos fascia but superficial to Buck's fascia; these contribute to forming the superficial dorsal vein of the penis in this same plane. This major vessel usually forms posteriorly and

empties into the scrotal veins. The intermediate veins lie deep to Buck's fascia but superficial to the tunica albuginea; they include the venae comitantes of the dorsal arteries and the most important vessel at this level, the deep dorsal vein. The major contributions forming the deep dorsal vein are 6 to 15 short, straight vessels from the glans as well as emissary and circumflex veins from the corpora cavernosa. The deep dorsal vein, therefore, drains both the glans and the corpora cavernosa under normal conditions. It passes beneath the arcuate ligament and terminates in the pudendal plexus in the pelvis.

The deep veins of the penis (different from the deep dorsal vein) include the bulbar veins that empty directly into the pudendal vein or pelvic plexus, the anterior and posterior urethral veins, and the deep veins of the corpora cavernosa. The anterior urethral veins join with the posterior emissary veins to produce the circumflex veins that travel around the circumference of the penis superficial to the tunica albuginea and empty into the deep dorsal vein. The posterior urethral veins anastomose with the bulbar veins and empty with the latter. The deep veins of the corpora cavernosa are often overlooked; they consist of four to five large vessels that leave the proximal end of each crus and drain into the pudendal plexus. All tissues superficial to Buck's fascia drain through the superficial dorsal veins into the saphenous, femoral, or scrotal veins. Proximally, the corpus spongiosum drains into the bulbar and urethral veins while the distal portion and glans empty into the deep dorsal vein as well. The crura of the corpora cavernosa drain into the deep veins of the penis, while the corpora cavernosa distal to

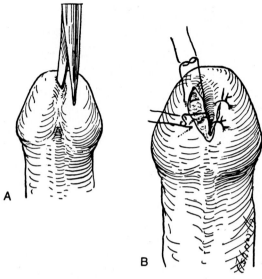

Figure 81–2. Meatotomy in normally developed penis. *A,* Incision in ventral aspect of glans. *B,* Closure of wound. (From Hand, J. R.: *In* Campbell, M. F., and Harrison, J. H. (Eds.): Urology. 3rd ed. Philadelphia, W. B. Saunders Co., 1970.)

the arcuate ligament empty through both the deep dorsal vein and the deep veins of the penis.

The dorsal arteries of the penis, the deep

dorsal vein, most of the nerves to the glans penis, and the lymphatics of the penile shaft run within, or just beneath, Buck's fascia. These structures can be lifted off the tunica albuginea by mobilizing Buck's fascia, thus allowing access to the dorsal part of the tunica albuginea of the corpora cavernosa without injury to them.

MEATOTOMY

In older children and adults, urethral meatotomy in a normally developed penis is generally carried out by making an incision in the ventral aspect of the glans (Fig. 81–2). Absorbable fine sutures are placed to approximate the urethral mucosal edge to the glans epithelial edge. Antibiotic ointment is generally applied, primarily to keep the edges from agglutinating, and the patient is asked to gently spread the meatus periodically. In children, when the meatal obstruction consists of a thin layer of occluding skin that pouches out as the child voids, the technique shown in Figure 81–3 can be used. The mother should be instructed to gently separate the edges of the meatus periodically during the day until they are healed. The tip of an antibiotic ophthalmic ointment tube may be used as an adjunct (Devine, 1979).

Meatotomy

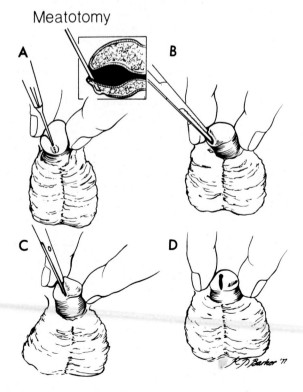

Figure 81–3. Meatotomy in infants. *A,* The needle is introduced into the obstructing leaf of tissue from the inside. This allows better control. About 0.5 ml of anesthetic material is used to form the wheal. *B,* The obstructing tissue is crushed with a mosquito clamp. *C,* The crushed tissue is incised. *D,* There is no bleeding, and the mother is instructed to keep the meatus open until its heals. (From Devine, C. J., Jr.: *In* Harrison, J. H., et al. (Eds.): Campbell's Urology. Philadelphia, W. B. Saunders Co., 1979.)

CIRCUMCISION

It is not the purpose of this chapter to discuss the arguments in favor of and against prophylactic or cosmetic circumcision. One of the few things agreed upon is that routine circumcision should never be carried out in the presence of hypospadias or any penile abnormality that is apt to require the use of the foreskin in subsequent reconstruction. Most circumcisions done just after birth are performed with the Gomco or a similar type of disposable clamp. When using such an instrument, it is important to first retract the foreskin and break any adhesions between the foreskin and the glans. The appropriate size of clamp bell is placed over the glans, and the foreskin is drawn forward over the bell and clamped in position. It is important to use the correct amount of tension to advance the foreskin and thereby prevent the excision of a too generous or an inadequate portion of prepuce. The clamp is applied as tightly as possible, and compression is maintained for several minutes to ensure adequate hemostasis. A scalpel is then used to excise the foreskin distal to the junction of the clamp and the bell.

The larger vessels usually present in older males are not easily sealed by this type of compression, and a more formal type of circumcision is required. An adequate and easily taught technique for this is pictured in Figure 81–4. After the foreskin has been retracted proximally over the glans to free any adhesions, it is drawn distally past the tip of the glans and the edges are grasped in the 3 o'clock and 9 o'clock positions with Allis clamps or hemostats. A vertical incision is made from the tip of the foreskin along the midline of the dorsal surface to a point just proximal to the corona. It is useful to first clamp the line of this incision with a hemostat to minimize bleeding. Through-and-through incisions through both sides of the foreskin are carried circumferentially and obliquely around both sides of the penile shaft. These parallel the corona and join at the frenulum. Retraction of the proximal penile skin edge exposes the bleeding points, which are controlled by cautery or ligatures of small-gauge catgut. The skin edges are then approximated with interrupted 4-0 absorbable sutures. It is generally helpful for the purpose of orientation to place the frenular suture first, in the manner shown; this also provides additional hemostasis for the vessels generally found in that area. A strip of Vaseline or antibiotic ointment gauze is then wrapped around the penis over the suture

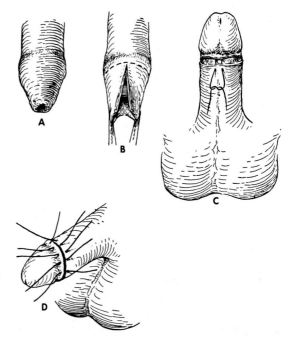

Figure 81–4. Technique of circumcision. See text for description. (From Hand, J. R.: *In* Campbell, M. F., and Harrison, J. H. (Eds.): Urology. 3rd ed. Philadelphia, W. B. Saunders Co., 1970.)

line and covered with gauze. An ice pack is useful to reduce postoperative pain and swelling.

Complications from this procedure should be few. Hyperesthesia of the glans is common for a short time, and patients should be informed that this may occur. Likewise, minor cosmetic imperfections, functionally insignificant, may occur, and these may be more bothersome to some patients than to others. Patients should be informed of this possibility preoperatively. The most common complication in the immediate postoperative period is a subcutaneous hematoma, which can reach quite large proportions. Evacuation of the hematoma should be performed and the bleeder ligated, if possible. If not, a firm compression dressing around the distal penis for a limited period of time will generally prevent further hemorrhage.

Occasionally, it may be necessary to carry out a dorsal slit procedure alone to correct an irreducible paraphimosis. To do so, the edges of the foreskin are secured with two clamps at the dorsal midline, and the foreskin is divided between them from its free end to within a few millimeters of the corona. The severed edges are then approximated with interrupted absorbable suture. Circumcision may be performed electively after the inflammation and edema have resolved.

CURVATURE OF THE PENIS

Devine (1979, 1982, 1984) has been responsible for the most comprehensive current summaries and descriptions of surgical procedures to correct penile curvature. The best known curvatures are probably those associated with hypospadias and epispadias, both of which are discussed elsewhere in this text. Abnormal bending of the penis may, however, also be produced by scarring of any of the tissue layers of the penis that occurs in such a way as to prevent adequate expansion during corporal engorgement, and by congenital disproportion of the corpora themselves. Peyronie's disease is an inflammatory condition of unknown etiology, which, if unremitting, results in fibrotic and nonexpansile thickenings of relatively discrete areas of the corporal tunica ("plaques").

The artificial erection (Gittes and McLoughlin, 1974) is an extremely useful technique to document penile curvature and to aid in its correction. A small catheter or Penrose drain is placed around the base of the penis and tightened with a hemostat. Physiologic saline is injected through a butterfly needle (18 to 20 gauge for an adult, 23 gauge for a child) into one corporal body. Corporal interconnections permit expansion of both erectile bodies, reproducing the patient's complaint.

Erectile curvature secondary to corporal disproportion and to lateral chordee of any cause may be corrected by the Nesbit tuck procedure (Fig. 81–5). The tunica albuginea in the area of maximum convex bend is exposed through a circumcision incision or by a simple longitudinal incision over the area; the entire area of curvature is exposed, with care taken to avoid any vascular and neural structures. Elliptical segments are outlined on the corporal tunica, each about 1 cm in width and about one-fourth the circumference of the corporal bodies in length. These are sharply dissected down to the corporal tissue, and the edges of the tunica are reapproximated. Sutures were described originally as interrupted 3-0 silk, but we and others have found 4-0 Prolene or running Vicryl, or a combination, just as suitable, as lone as a watertight closure is achieved. Checking the degree of straightening with an artificial erection after each ellipse is resutured ensures a maximally cosmetic result with the appropriate number of tucks. Subcutaneous tissue and skin are then closed with five interrupted absorbable sutures and fluffs. A moderate pressure dressing is applied, leaving the glans visible to permit prevention of strangulation secondary to over-

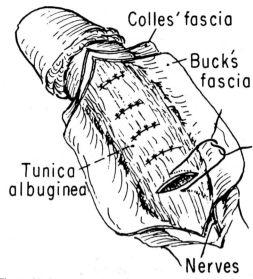

Figure 81–5. Nesbit straightening procedure. See text for description. (From Hand, J. R.: *In* Campbell, M. F., and Harrison, J. H. (Eds.): Urology. 3rd ed. Philadelphia, W. B. Saunders Co., 1970.)

zealous compression. Intercourse is prohibited for at least 1 month.

Multiple nonsurgical regimens have been used to treat Peyronie's disease. Success attributable to these therapies is sometimes difficult to separate from improvement consequent to the 20 to 50 per cent spontaneous resolution rate (Devine, 1979). This potential for improvement makes it mandatory that all possible efforts be made to delay attempts at surgical correction for at least 6 to 12 months after the patient is first seen. The only exceptions to this are patients whose plaques are calcified—improvement does not occur when tunical changes have progressed to this state—and patients who are totally incapable of sexual activity because of their disease.

When surgical therapy is performed, excision of the plaque with placement of a dermal graft, originally devised and popularized by Devine and Horton (1974), is the most common technique employed (Fig. 81–6). The exposure incision may be a circumcision type, as pictured, or may be simply a curvilinear incision over the dorsal midline of the penis. It is critically important with dorsolateral or dorsal plaques to carefully dissect the plane between Buck's fascia and the tunica; this exposes the plaque directly and permits elevation and retraction of the neurovascular bundle. As little erectile tissue as possible should be excised, but sometimes the fibrotic plaque seems to extend into the corporal tissue for a short distance. The dermal graft is

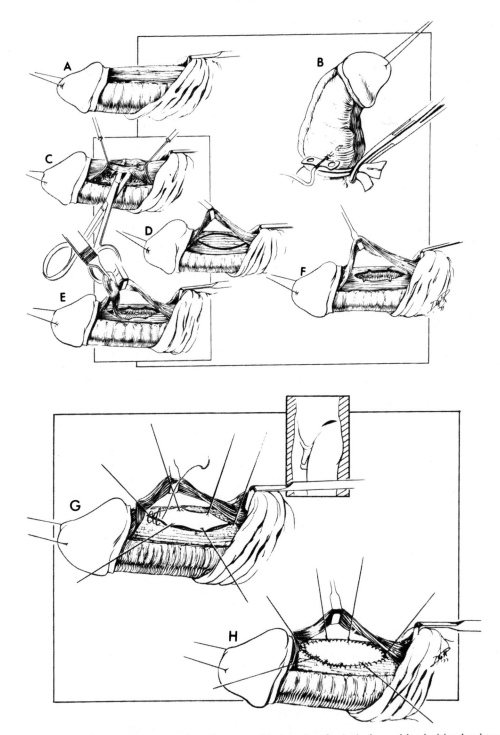

Figure 81–6. Excision of Peyronie's plaque and replacement with dermal graft. *A,* A circumcising incision has been made and the skin of the penis reflected to the base. If the prepuce is redundant, the excess is removed. *B,* An artificial erection discloses the curvature and allows assessment of the extent of the fibrotic plaque. *C,* An incision has been made in Buck's fascia, and the dorsal tissue is being dissected free of the plaque. *D,* The dorsal tissue containing the dorsal arteries and the deep dorsal vein and nerves has been dissected free and elevated, and the plaque of Peyronie's disease has been outlined on the tunica albuginea. *E,* The plaque is almost excised. The cut ends of the strands of the septum can be seen in the midline. *F,* Incisions have been made in the periphery of the defect to be sure that there will not be a straight line scar, which might contract, and that all diseased tissue has been excised. *G,* Prolene stay sutures have been placed as the graft is trimmed. *H,* Watertight closure; another artificial erection will now ensure that the penis is straight. (From Devine, C. J., Jr.: *In* Harrison, J. H., et al. (Eds.): Campbell's Urology. 4th ed. Philadelphia, W. B. Saunders Co., 1979.)

obtained from the groin over the iliac crest. The corporal defect should be stretched vertically and horizontally to determine the size of the graft, which should be slightly larger than the defect itself. The graft should be about 1 mm thick and mostly defatted; it should be placed fat side down. Approximately 12/1000 of an inch of epidermis is removed using either a knife or a dermatome. The graft is tacked into place with stay sutures of 4-0 or 3-0 Prolene, and suturing is finished with running 4-0 or 5-0 Vicryl. Buck's fascia and subcutaneous tissue are closed with fine absorbable suture, as is the penile skin. A moderate pressure dressing with fluffs is applied. The donor site is closed, after undermining of the skin edges with 4-0 Vicryl dermal sutures and with a running nylon or subcuticular Vicryl suture to approximate the skin.

Attempts should be made to decrease erections in the immediate postoperative period with sedation or amyl nitrate capsules, or both. Intercourse should be prohibited for 4 to 6 weeks.

Substances other than dermis have been used for this procedure. It would seem inadvisable to utilize any inelastic material for this expansile area. Das (1980) has described the use of tunica vaginalis for this purpose, and although some have expressed reservations about its strength, we have found it satisfactory and very easy to work with.

If the patient exhibits no or totally inadequate erectile activity, it is perfectly reasonable to place a penile prosthesis. Areas of deformity will become apparent with either the semi-rigid rod or the inflatable variety, and they should be corrected by incision or removal with grafting (Malloy et al., 1981). If a graft is placed primarily and erectile function adequate for intercourse is not regained, a penile prosthesis may then be placed. Fibrosis at the graft site may make the corporal dissection more difficult than usual.

Patients undergoing corrective surgery for penile curvature must be informed that a decrease in erectile ability is a potential complication. Our patients with Peyronie's disease are told that there is an approximately one in three chance of their intercourse ability being overall the same or worse after plaque excision and grafting. The possibility of partial loss of penile shaft or glans sensation, although unlikely, should also be mentioned. Pre- and postcorrection photographs, made either operatively or by the patient himself, may be useful to document cosmetic improvement.

PRIAPISM

Surgical management of priapism is indicated when the more conservative methods of therapy have failed to restore functioning venous drainage to the corpora cavernosa. Since the pathologic events involve primarily the corpora cavernosa while relatively sparing the corpus spongiosum and glans, most surgical maneuvers attempt to utilize the normal venous outflow routes of these latter two structures.

Simple needle aspiration of the corpora is usually the first aggressive type of therapy attempted (Harrow, 1969). A large-bore needle (as from a large intracath set) is inserted into the base of each corpus either through the dorsal glans or through the lateral penile shaft. With suction placed on the syringe, manual compression of the corpora is used in an attempt to remove all the dark venous blood and sludge. Saline irrigation with aspiration and manual massage will often result in detumescence, but rapid corporal filling generally recurs in spite of all makeshift mechanical methods to prevent it. The method we have found most helpful is to apply a moderate pressure dressing around the catheterized penis, bending the penis under the scrotum by bringing the catheter tubing up between the buttocks.

When detumescence is not achieved or maintained by aspiration and irrigation, a shunting procedure is considered. The Winter procedure, the simplest of these, attempts to establish three or four fistulas between the glans and the distal cavernosal tissue (Fig. 81–7) (Winter, 1978). Following corporal aspiration and irrigation, a Travenol prostatic biopsy needle is introduced in the closed position through the glans to the coronal septum, with care taken to avoid the urethra. The obturator blade is forced through the septum into the cavernosal body by opening the biopsy needle, and the needle is then closed by pushing the sheath over the fenestrated blade, trapping a button of septum and cavernosal tissue within the needle. The needle is then twisted in a circle and removed. This is repeated until two fistulas are created into each corpus. Brisk bleeding should occur from the glans puncture sites, and these require closure with a figure-of-eight absorbable suture. Effehoj (1975) had actually reported a procedure with a similar rationale some 3 years earlier. He incised the glans with a narrow knife and simply twisted a hole through the coronal septum.

The El-Ghorab procedure (Fig. 81–8) also

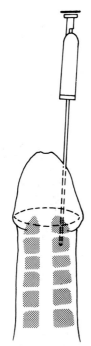

Figure 81–7. Winter procedure (cavernosal-glandular shunt). See text for description.

creates a cavernosal glanular shunt, but one of larger size (Wendel and Grayhack, 1981). An incision is made in the dorsal glans 1 cm distal to the coronal sutures and deepened to expose the tips of both corpora cavernosa. The tips are grasped with a Kocher clamp, and a circular core of tissue 5 mm in diameter is excised from each. The penis is massaged and irrigated, if necessary, to obtain arterial bleeding through these areas. The glans incision is closed superficially with absorbable suture so as to not

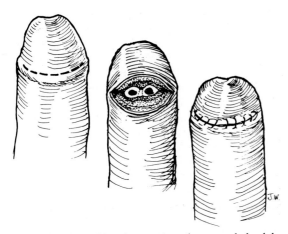

Figure 81–8. El Ghorab procedure (cavernosal-glandular shunt). See text for description.

obliterate the area of the shunt. A moderate pressure compression dressing is applied to the penile shaft. Some find intermittent compression with an appropriate-sized blood pressure cuff to be a useful postoperative adjunct. The cuff is inflated to mean arterial pressure for about 20 seconds every 15 minutes for the first 3 hours and then every 30 to 60 minutes for the next 12 to 24 hours.

If a distal shunt is not successful, the next simplest procedure is the construction of a shunt between the cavernosum and spongiosum bodies. This was described originally in 1964 by Quackels. This is shown (Fig. 81–9) as being done through an incision at the ventral-lateral penile base. To minimize the chance of a urethral fistula we recommend that this be done, with the patient in the lithotomy position, through a vertical perineal incision at the level where the corpora cavernosa begin to separate, as the spongiosum is thicker at this point. With a catheter in the urethra, a site is selected just distal to the bulb; two ellipses, approximately 2 cm long by 1 cm wide, are outlined on the adjoining surfaces of the corpus spongiosum and the corpus cavernosum. A continuous absorbable 4-0 suture is placed through what is to become the common back wall, and the ellipses are excised. After aspiration and injection of the corpora cavernosa (through sites elsewhere) have established free arterial bleeding, the anastomosis is completed with interrupted or running 4-0 absorbable suture. If a one-sided shunt is not successful in maintaining detumescence, a contralateral procedure should be done. The contralateral shunt should be done at a slightly different level to minimize tension on the spongiosum suture lines.

The cavernosal saphenous shunt was first described by Grayhack and associates in 1964 (Fig. 81–10). This is carried out through two incisions, one at the base of the penis and one over the saphenous vein in the groin. The vein is mobilized and divided about 8 to 10 cm from its femoral junction. The free end of the vein is led through a subcutaneous passageway between the two incisions. A 1-cm ellipse of corporal tunica is excised near the base of the penis, and, after irrigation of the corpora, the saphenous vein is spatulated and anastomosed to the tunical defect with 5-0 vascular sutures. Care must be taken not to twist the vein in the subcutaneous passage. If both corpora are not detumesced, the shunt may be done bilaterally. A moderate pressure dressing on the penile shaft with periodic compression by a blood pressure

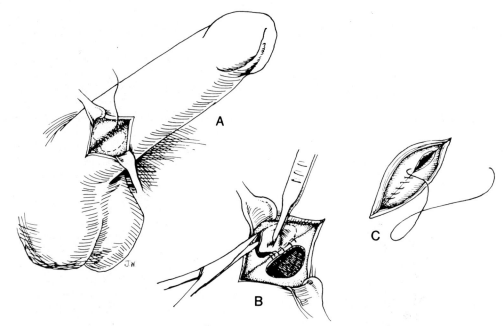

Figure 81–9. Quackels procedure (cavernosal-spongiosum shunt). See text for description.

cuff and heparinization help maintain an adequate shunt flow.

It is important to remember that all these shunts ultimately thrombose, hopefully after priapism has ceased to be a problem. If erectile dysfunction exists after a successful cavernosal-saphenous shunt and a Doppler study or flows show the shunt to be open, surgical closure of the shunt may be necessary.

Of critical importance for patients, family, and physician is a frank discussion of the goals of any procedure for priapism and the likelihood of their being satisfactory. It is unfortunate that successful detumescence is not accompanied by subsequent normal erectile function in up to 50 per cent of cases. When it occurs, this permanent damage to the erectile mechanism is a pathophysiologic result of the disease and not of the shunt procedure itself.

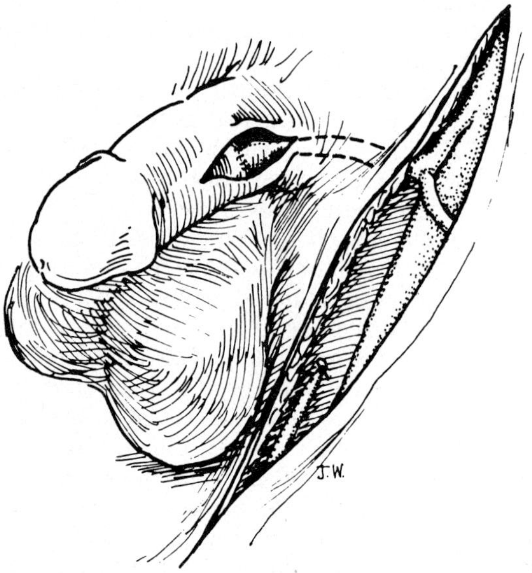

PENILE PROSTHESES

It was not until the middle of the twentieth century that penile prostheses were first used to treat erectile impotence. Early results were unsuccessful owing to prosthetic design, materials, and anatomic location. In the early 1970s, Scott, Bradley, and Timm developed the twin-cylinder implantable inflatable penile prosthesis (Scott et al., 1973), while Small and Carrion (1975) developed a twin-rod rigid prosthesis (Fig. 81–11). These two silicone prostheses allowed for more natural-appearing erections with better function. Finney (1977) developed a hinged flexi-rod prosthesis that enabled improved flexibility of the penis (Jonas and Jacobi, 1980) (Fig. 81–12). Jonas produced a semi-rigid rod prosthesis with a malleable silver wire core (Fig. 81–13). This permitted improved concealment for the penis and the ability to manipulate the

Figure 81–10. Grayhack procedure (cavernosal-saphenous shunt). See text for description.

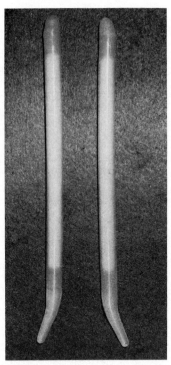

Figure 81–11. Small-Carrion twin rod prosthesis.

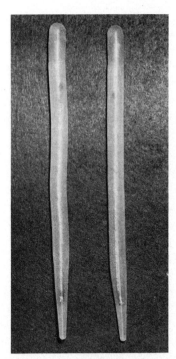

Figure 81–13. Jonas malleable silver wire prosthesis.

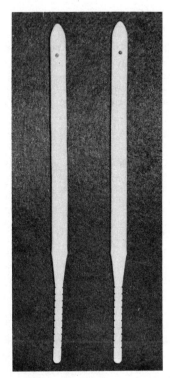

Figure 81–12. Finney hinged prosthesis.

device into an erect position. American Medical Systems in 1983 developed a flexible semi-rigid rod prosthesis with rear tip extenders for more exact sizing of the prosthesis to the patient's penis. In 1983 the Mentor Company produced an inflatable penile prosthesis featuring a polyurethane cylinder with mechanical tube connectors (Fig. 81–14). In the same year American Medical Systems developed an improved Scott model inflatable prosthesis (Model 700) to improve prosthesis survival (Fig. 81–15). All these prostheses have significantly broadened the surgical options available to urologists for treating patients with erectile dysfunction.

The choice of type and specific model of prosthesis to use depends on the patient's expectations and desires. The relative advantages and disadvantages of each type must be carefully explained to all patients so that they may participate in the choice (Malloy et al., 1980).

The initial aspect of all therapy for patients with impotence should be the expeditious and effective diagnosis of the etiologic factors. Categorization of the problem as primarily organic or psychogenic is important so that needless and expensive sex therapy is not wasted on patients

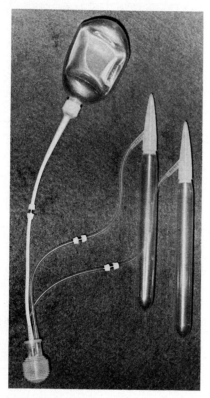

Figure 81–14. Mentor inflatable prosthesis.

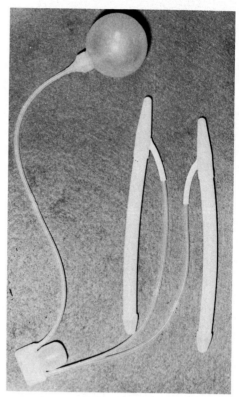

Figure 81–15. American Medical Systems M700 inflatable prosthesis.

who will be benefited only by a penile prosthesis and so that other patients who might benefit from conservative medical or psychiatric therapy will not immediately undergo surgery. The pathophysiology of erectile dysfunction and its evaluation have been discussed elsewhere in this text. Different philosophies of management prompt differences in emphasis on various points in the overall evaluation, however, and should be noted (Wein et al., 1984; Van-Arsdalen et al., 1983). We continue to consider nocturnal penile tumescence a most reliable screening study to differentiate psychogenic from organic impotence. Psychologic testing or consultation should be employed in all patients in whom emotional problems seem to be present and in those patients without a clear organic etiology for their impotence. Formal evaluation and counseling are not, however, mandatory in all cases.

The preoperative preparation for patients receiving penile prostheses is the same for rigid, semi-rigid, and inflatable devices. The particular operative approach to be used should be carefully chosen. For rigid and semi-rigid rod prostheses, operative techniques using suprapubic, scrotal, and penile approaches have been described. Penile incisions should be done with caution. Postoperative constrictive scars, neuromas, and glandular anesthesia have been reported, especially in diabetic patients. Penile incisions are avoided in plastic surgical procedures for similar reasons. The inflatable penile prothesis may be inserted by means of a suprapubic or scrotal approach.

Factors influencing site selection include the following: (1) experience of the surgeon; (2) abdominal stomas or areas of contamination; (3) scars from previous surgical incisions; (4) perineal scars, fistulas, or contaminated areas; and (5) coexistent conditions requiring simultaneous correction, such as hernias, hydroceles, bladder calculi, and the like.

The surgeon should choose the surgical approach with which he can best perform the surgery consistent with past experience while assuring the maximum functional satisfaction for the patient.

Preoperative preparation should include the following:

1. Broad-spectrum antibiotic prophylaxis beginning the day prior to surgery.

2. Surgical showers with povidone-iodine the night prior to surgery.

3. Signing of an informed surgical consent outlining all the potential risks and benefits of the surgery.

4. Surgical shave in operating area just prior to surgery.

5. Surgical scrub of patient's skin for a full 10 minutes with appropriate cleansing agent.

6. Surgeons and all assistants should scrub vigorously for 10 minutes. The operative suite should be carefully maintained for sterility. All unnecessary traffic should be avoided.

Surgical Insertion of Semi-Rigid Rod and Rigid Rod Prostheses

PERINEAL APPROACH (Fig. 81–16)

The perineal approach has proved to be very satisfactory for the insertion of any twin rigid or semi-rigid rod prosthesis. The patient is placed in the lithotomy position with the legs abducted. The midline perineal incision is made. The bulbous urethra is identified, as are the corpora cavernosa and crus on each side. A 2-cm vertical incision is made in the tunica albu-

ginea of each crus approximately 1 cm from the bifurcation of the crura. Traction sutures are placed on the tunica albuginea, and the corporal tissue is separated to form a tunnel distal to the glans penis and proximal to the crus. This tunnel is dissected laterally under the tunica albuginea. The tunnel is dilated from a number 7 to 10 cervical dilator. The dilation is carried distally to the glans penis and proximally to the crus. When the tunnel easily accepts the 10 dilator, a measuring device provided by the manufacturer or the Furlow inserter tool is used to measure the length of the tunnel.

The appropriate-sized prosthesis should be chosen so that there will be a comfortable fit from the crus out to the glans penis. The tunnel and wound are copiously irrigated with antibiotic solution prior to installation of the prosthesis. The length of the prosthesis to be implanted should be determined according to the directions of the manufacturer. The AMS Model 600 semi-rigid rod prosthesis comes in three sizes with rear tip extenders. Rear tip extenders are added to the prosthesis to determine the exact size required. The Finney flexi-rod pros-

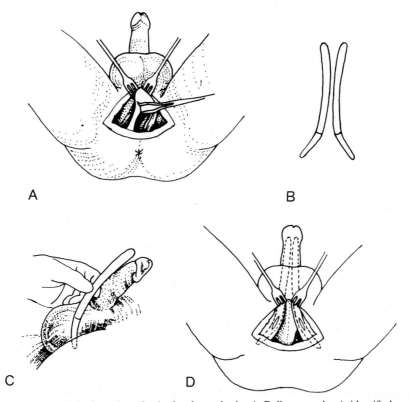

A

B

C

D

Figure 81–16. Perineal approach for insertion of paired rod prosthesis. *A,* Bulbous urethra is identified, as are the corpora cavernosa and crura. *B* and *C,* Appropriate-sized prosthesis is chosen so that there will be a comfortable fit from the crus to the glans penis. *D,* Prosthesis is inserted into the corpus cavernosum and advanced distally to the glans and proximally into the crus.

thesis is trimmed at the proximal tip to make the appropriate size. No matter what type of prosthesis is chosen, accurate measurement is essential so that the device will not migrate proximally with time. If this happens, the so-called SST deformity will develop; this has been one of the principal criticisms of the rigid rod prostheses.

The appropriate prosthesis is inserted into the corpus cavernosum and advanced distally to the glans and proximally into the crus. This can usually be accomplished by flexing the proximal end of the prosthesis to allow it to be inserted into the incision into the crus. The AMS Model 600 prosthesis has a hole in the distal end into which a traction suture may be placed. This traction suture may then be put through a Keith needle and inserted with the Furlow inserter tool. The Keith needle is pushed distally through the glans of the penis, bringing the traction sutures with it. With gentle traction on the sutures, the prosthesis can be guided into the proper position in the glans penis. When both prosthetic rods have been inserted, the tunica albuginea is closed with interrupted or running 3-0 PDS sutures. The subcutaneous tissue is closed with a continuous 3-0 chromic catgut suture, and the skin is closed with a subcuticular suture. This is used to obtain an early seal of the skin edges to prevent contamination from the rectum. Ice is used for 24 hours to prevent swelling.

SUPRAPUBIC APPROACH

Suprapubic surgical incisions may be transverse (infrapubic) or vertical, depending on the condition of the patient's abdomen and the presence of any previous surgical incisions. The transverse incision is made below the inferior border of the symphysis pubis in order to expose the bases of the corpora cavernosa. A vertical incision should be carried from the base of the penis to above the symphysis. Similarly, the incision should be deepened so that the most proximal portions of the corpora cavernosa can be exposed easily.

The corpora cavernosa are visualized, and 2-cm incisions are placed dorsolaterally in the tunica albuginea. The tunica is retracted with traction sutures so that dissecting scissors can carefully separate cavernosal tissue to form a tunnel distal to the glans penis and proximal to the crus. The tunnel is dilated from a number 7 to 10 cervical dilator. This should be done with care to avoid damaging or perforating the distal tunica albuginea, or corpus spongiosum urethra. Once the tunnel is established, measurements

are made with the manufacturer's measuring device or the Furlow inserter tool, as described for perineal insertion of prostheses. The appropriate length of prosthesis is determined, and the device is inserted after the wound has been copiously irrigated with antibiotic solution. The distal end of the prosthesis is inserted initially and placed into the area beneath the glans penis. A traction suture may be placed through the tip of the prosthesis and the Furlow inserter tool used to guide the tip of the prosthesis into the proper location. The proximal end of the prosthesis should fit snugly into the crus against the pubic ramus. There should not be excessive movement of the prosthesis, which would allow proximal migration in the postoperative period. An overly large prosthesis that has to be forced into the tunnel should not be used. This could cause undue pressure on the glans and urethra in the postoperative period, which could produce permanent pain or perforation. Accurate sizing is essential for optimum postoperative results. The tunica albuginea is closed with interrupted or continuous 3-0 PDS sutures. The subcutaneous tissue is closed with a continuous 3-0 chromic suture, and the skin is closed with a subcuticular suture to promptly seal the wound. Ice is applied to the operative area for 24 hours to prevent swelling.

PENILE SHAFT APPROACH

Incisions on the penile shaft for inserting rigid and semi-rigid rod prostheses must be made with considerable caution. Care must be taken not to damage the neurovascular bundle. If this surgical approach is used, a transverse incision is made on the dorsum of the penis approximately 2 cm proximal to the corona. The incision is carried down through the skin and subcutaneous tissue. The neurovascular bundle is identified and avoided. Two transverse incisions are made dorsolaterally in the tunica albuginea. Traction sutures are placed on the tunica so that dissecting scissors can be used to separate cavernosal tissue. The tunnel is dissected proximal to the crus and distal to the glans penis. The tunnel is dilated from a number 7 to 10 cervical dilator. The appropriate length for the tunnel is determined and the prosthesis selected according to manufacturer's instructions. In this approach the proximal portion of the prosthesis is inserted initially. Then by bending the distal portion, the implant is guided into the tunnel to its position underneath the glans penis. The tunica albuginea is closed with interrupted or continuous 3-0 PDS sutures. The subcutaneous space is closed with a continuous

3-0 chromic catgut suture, and the skin is closed with a subcuticular suture. Care must be taken in skin closure to prevent constricting scars or neuromas. Ice should be used on the area for 24 hours to prevent swelling.

Inflatable Penile Prosthesis

SUPRAPUBIC OR INFRAPUBIC APPROACH
(Figs. 81–17 to 81–21)

The American Medical Systems inflatable penile prosthesis and the Mentor inflatable prosthesis can be inserted in essentially the same manner. A transverse incision beneath the symphysis approximately 2 inches in length or a vertical midline incision from the base of the penis to 2 inches above the symphysis is used. The incision is carried through the subcutaneous tissue. A small 1-inch transverse incision is made in the anterior rectus fascia and carried down between the rectus muscles. Using the index finger, a space is developed in the perivesical space for the insertion of the reservoir. The tubing from the reservoir is either brought out through the incision in the rectus fascia or drawn through Hesselbach's triangle on the side in which the inflate-deflate mechanism will be in-serted. The reservoir is then placed in the proper position in the perivesical space. The collar of the reservoir should be positioned snugly against the floor of Hesselbach's triangle or just adjacent to the incision. The reservoir is then filled with a sterile isotonic solution. The surgeon may wish to put radiopaque dye into the system so that the device will be radiopaque. The reservoir should be filled with the appropriate amount of fluid according to the manufacturer's instructions. The anterior rectus sheath is closed with interrupted or continuous 0 Prolene sutures.

The corpora cavernosa are then identified bilaterally along with the midline neurovascular bundle. An incision is made dorsolaterally in the tunica albuginea of each corpus cavernosum. This is made in the most proximal portions of the corpora, close to the symphysis pubis. Traction sutures are placed on each border of the tunica so that dissecting sutures may separate cavernosal tissue distal to the glans and proximal to the crus. The tunnel created is dilated from a number 7 to a number 10 or 11 with a cervical dilator. The tunnel should not be dilated larger in order to avoid damage to the tunica albuginea. Overdilation might cause aneurysmal weakness of the tunica in the postoperative period. The Furlow inserter tool or Scott Dila-

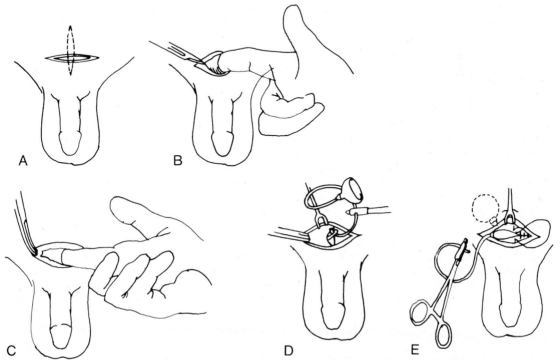

Figure 81–17. Suprapubic or infrapubic approach for insertion of inflatable penile prosthesis. *A,* Transverse infrapubic or vertical suprapubic incision. *B,* Index finger dissects space in perivesical area for reservoir. *C,* Space is dissected for tubing from reservoir. *D* and *E,* Unfilled reservoir and tubing are positioned in the perivesical space.

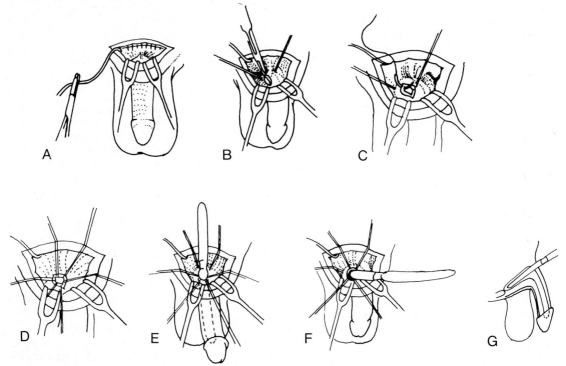

Figure 81–18. *A,* Closure of anterior rectus sheath. *B,* Incision is made dorsolaterally in the corporal tunica. *C* and *D,* Traction sutures are placed in the corporal tunical borders. *E* to *G,* Dilation of corporal tunnel proximally and distally from 7 to 10 or 11 F.

mez insert tool is used to measure the length of the tunnel distally and proximally. These added values are then used to determine the total cylinder length required plus rear tip extenders. Rear tip extenders are utilized to allow the input tube to exit in the middle of the incision. This prevents contact between the input tube and the inflatable portion of the cylinders (Malloy et al., 1983). Direct contact of two silicone surfaces can result in input tube wear. The new models of the AMS prosthesis have circumvented this with a Teflon coating on the input tube. The Mentor prosthesis similarly utilizes Silastic coating. Rear tip extenders added to the proximal end of the inflatable cylinder allow proper location of the input tube through the center of the incision. The size of the inflatable cylinder plus the length of the rear tip extenders should equal the length of the tunnel.

Proper selection of the appropriate cylinder size plus rear tip extenders should be determined by the manufacturer's instructions. For example, if the overall length of the tunnel in the corpora cavernosa is 17 cm, the total length of the cylinder plus rear tip extenders should be 17 cm. Measuring from the center of the incision distally to the glans, the distance is 10 cm.

Therefore, a cylinder should be selected such that the distance from the inlet tube to the distal end will be 10 cm. A 14-cm cylinder is the appropriate size (all cylinders measure 4 cm from the inlet tube to the proximal tip). Since a 14-cm cylinder is being used, a 3-cm rear tip extender is added to make the appropriate 17-cm length to fill the corpora cavernosa.

Preset 3-0 PDS sutures are placed through the borders of the tunica albuginea incisions prior to the insertion of the cylinders. This is done so that no inadvertent needle damage will be done to the inflatable portion of the cylinder during closure. The wound is copiously irrigated with antibiotic solution. The traction suture from the distal end of the cylinder is inserted into a Keith needle, which is placed in the central distal hole of the Furlow inserter tool. The inserter tool is passed distally to the glans penis. The cylinder is then drawn into the tunnel by traction on the sutures. The proximal end of the cylinder with rear tip extenders is placed proximally into the crus. The tunica albuginea is then closed. The procedure is carried out in both corpora cavernosa.

The space is fashioned for the inflate-deflate mechanism in the subcutaneous tissue of the

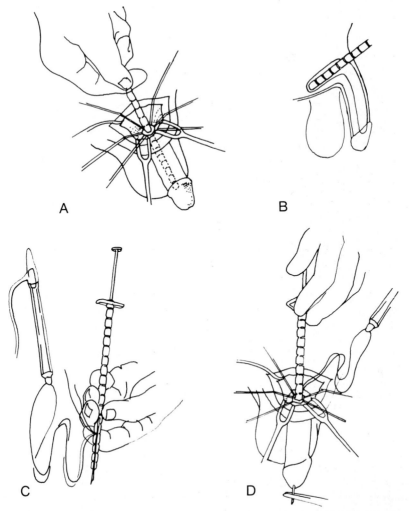

Figure 81–19. *A* and *B,* Furlow inserter tool is used to measure length of the corporal tunnel proximally and distally. *C* and *D,* Furlow inserter tool is used to place Keith needle, attached by a suture to the distal tip of the prosthesis, through the glans penis.

hemiscrotum that is appropriate for the patient. If the patient is right-handed, the right hemiscrotum is generally used. The scrotum is inverted into the wound with two fingers so that the subcutaneous tissue can be separated from the skin. Electrocautery is used to coagulate all small bleeding veins. The inflate-deflate mechanism is inserted with the deflate button located laterally. It should be inserted into the scrotum so that it is in the most dependent portion, well separated from the testicle. Once in place, the inlet and exit tubing are clasped with Babcock clamps over the skin. This maintains the inflate-deflate mechanism in the proper location while the connections are made. The tubing from the reservoir is connected to the inlet tubing of the inflate-deflate mechanism according to manufacturer's instructions. The outlet tubings from the

inflate-deflate mechanism are connected with right angle connectors to the tubing exiting from the cylinders in each corpus cavernosum.

The Mentor prosthesis uses mechanical connecting devices, whereas the American Medical Systems' connections are tied with 3-0 Prolene sutures. The tubing must be carefully trimmed to eliminate excess in the wound that can be palpated by the patient. The tubing should not be shortened unduly, however, since this will retract the inflate-deflate mechanism up toward the external inguinal ring. In this position the prosthesis may be difficult or painful to operate. With all the connections completed, the pump is activated several times. The cylinders are tested for uniform distention and proper placement beneath the glans penis. The sutures in the tunica albuginea are checked to

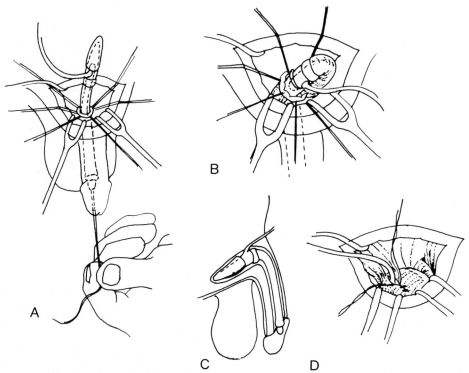

Figure 81–20. *A,* Cylinder is drawn into the corporal tunnel by traction on the suture. *B* and *C,* Proximal portion of the cylinder with rear tip extender(s) is inserted into the proximal crus. *D,* Tunical incision is closed by tying together the corresponding preset sutures from each side.

be sure there is no rupture with inflation. Excess bleeding from the incision should not be present after the sutures are tied. The prosthesis is then deflated. A suction type drain is left in the subcutaneous tissue and exited lateral to the wound. The subcutaneous space is closed with continuous 3-0 chromic catgut sutures. The skin incision is closed with a subcuticular 3-0 Prolene or Vicryl suture. The Jackson-Pratt suction drain may be employed for 18 to 72 hours, depending on the amount of drainage and the preference of the surgeon. A Foley catheter is inserted and removed on the first postoperative day.

SCROTAL APPROACH
(Figs. 81–22 and 81–23)

The patient is placed in a modified lithotomy position as previously described. An incision is made in the median raphe from the base of the penis down into the scrotum for approximately 3 cm. The incision is carried into the subcutaneous tissue. The urethra is identified, and a Foley catheter is inserted so that it can be retracted out of the operative field. The corpora cavernosa are identified, and the tunica albuginea is incised ventrolaterally with a 2-cm vertical incision. This incision should be in the most proximal portions of the corpora cavernosa. Traction sutures are employed to allow dissection distal to the glans and proximal to the crus. Cervical dilators, number 7 to 10 or 11F, are used to dilate the tunnel from the crus proximal to the glans penis. The selection of the appropriate cylinder plus rear tip extenders is done in the exact manner described for the infrapubic insertion of the inflatable prosthesis. The wound is copiously irrigated with antibotic solution. Preset 3-0 PDS sutures are placed in the tunica albuginea prior to the implantation of the cylinder. The traction sutures on the distal end of the cylinder are placed through a Keith needle, which is inserted into the Furlow inserter tool. The inserter tool is then placed into the tunnel and extended to the area under the glans penis. The obturator is inserted, pressing the Keith needle distally through the glans penis. The needle is grasped and removed, drawing the traction sutures out through the glans. Using the traction sutures, the cylinder is gently guided into the proper position beneath the glans penis. The rear tip extenders are carefully placed into the region of the crus. After both cylinders are inserted, antibiotic so-

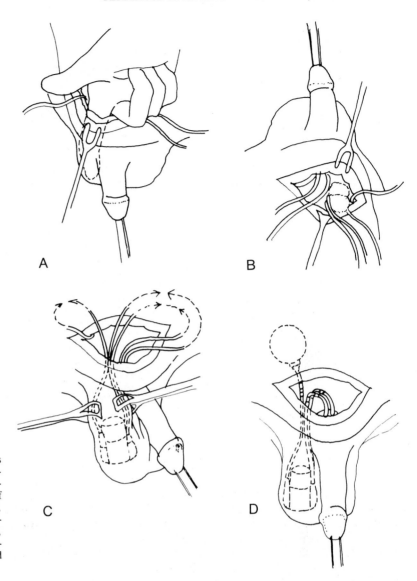

A

B

C

D

Figure 81–21. *A,* A subcutaneous pouch is dissected in the appropriate hemiscrotum for the inflate-deflate mechanism. *B,* Insertion of the pump into the scrotum. *C,* Inlet and exit tubing of pump secured with Babcock clamp. *D,* Tubings from reservoir and cylinders are connected to the inlet and exit tubings of the pump.

lution is used to irrigate the wound. The tunica albuginea is closed with the previously inserted 3-0 PDS sutures.

The reservoir may be inserted with a separate incision in the suprapubic area, as previously described. However, most surgeons prefer the following technique. The appropriate external inguinal ring is palpated with the finger. Using a nasal speculum, the floor of the inguinal canal is visualized and dissecting scissors gradually separate the transversalis fascia on the floor of the inguinal canal. With a number 6 or 7 cervical dilator the perivesical space is entered. The space is enlarged so that the surgeon's finger can palpate the area over Cooper's ligament into the perivesical space. The reservoir tool supplied by the manufacturer assists in guiding

the reservoir through the defect in the transversalis fascia and positioning it into the perivesical space. The reservoir is inflated with isotonic solution according to the manufacturer's instructions. The reservoir is pulled down against the floor of Hesselbach's triangle. If the defect appears large, the inguinal canal can be reinforced with interrupted 3-0 Prolene sutures.

The inflate-deflate mechanism is positioned in the ipsilateral hemiscrotum with the deflation button in the lateral position. The method of dissecting this space in the hemiscrotum is similar to that used for the infrapubic approach. Once the inflate-deflate mechanism is in the proper position, Babcock clamps are used to keep the tubing against the skin in the appropriate position. The tubing from the reservoir is

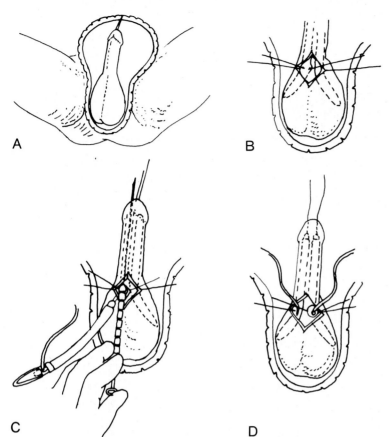

Figure 81–22. Scrotal approach for insertion of inflatable prosthesis. *A,* Midline vertical incision. *B,* Vertical ventrolateral incision is made in proximal corpora cavernosa. *C,* Furlow inserter tool places the cylinder traction sutures through glans penis. *D,* Closure of corporal tunica with preset sutures.

connected to the inlet tubing of the inflate-deflate mechanism. The outlet tubings from the inflate-deflate mechanism are connected to the appropriate tubing from each corpus cavernosum. The tubing from the contralateral corpus cavernosum is brought through the intrascrotal septum prior to connection with the inflate-deflate mechanism. When all connections are completed, the pump is activated several times to ascertain the proper position of the cylinders. The suture lines in the tunica albuginea are checked to rule out rupture of cylinders and inadvertent bleeding. The wound is copiously irrigated throughout the procedure with antibiotic solution. A Jackson-Pratt type suction drain is left in the subcutaneous space and exited through a stab wound laterally in the inguinal region. The subcutaneous space is closed with a continuous 3-0 Vicryl suture. A Foley catheter is placed and removed on the first postoperative day.

POSTOPERATIVE CARE

Rigid and Semi-Rigid Rod Prostheses. A Foley catheter is left indwelling until the first postoperative day. Ice is applied to the wound for 24 hours to prevent swelling and pain. Three intravenous doses of an aminoglycoside antibiotic are used as well as an appropriate broad-spectrum antibiotic during the hospital stay. The patient may be discharged whenever he is voiding well and his wound appears to be healing satisfactorily. He is maintained on an oral broad-spectrum antibiotic for 2 weeks, until the first postoperative visit. He is cautioned to avoid strenuous physical exercise and sexual activity. He is cautioned to use loose-fitting underclothing so that there is no pressure on the penis or the glans. Sexual activity can usually be resumed within 4 to 6 weeks. The patient is warned not to attempt sexual activity until there is no pain or tenderness over the penis. He should be followed periodically by the surgeon to guarantee that the prosthesis is working properly and is not causing problems in the penis or urethra. The patient should be told to report this situation if it develops.

Inflatable Penile Prosthesis. The patient is maintained in a true Trendelenburg position for approximately the first 18 hours after surgery

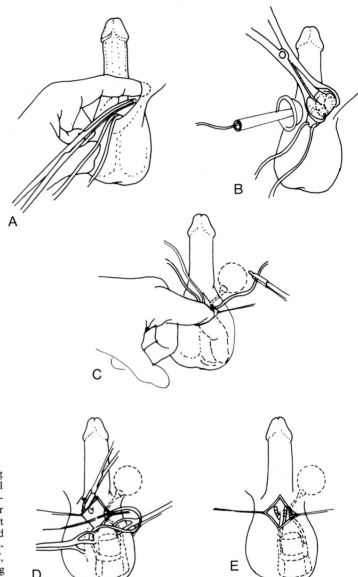

Figure 81–23. *A*, External inguinal ring is palpated with finger. *B*, Reservoir tool positions the unfilled reservoir in perivesical space. *C*, Subcutaneous pouch for pump dissected in ipsilateral scrotum (left shown here). *D*, Pump tubings secured with Babcock clamps to maintain dependent pump position in scrotum. *E*, Connections are secured prior to testing device.

to minimize swelling. Ice packs are applied to the penis and scrotum. A Foley catheter is left in for the same time period. The suction drain is maintained for at least 18 hours; if drainage is copious, it may be kept in place for 72 hours and (rarely) longer if necessary. The patient receives three doses of an aminoglycoside antibiotic and is maintained on broad-spectrum antibiotics for 2 weeks. The inflate-deflate mechanism is examined each day in the immediate postoperative period so that gentle traction can be used to maintain the position in the most dependent portion of the scrotum. The patient is discharged when he is voiding well and when

postoperative discomfort can be tolerated with only the use of oral analgesics. He is cautioned against strenuous exercise and sexual activities for 3 weeks. Tight underclothing is avoided. On the initial postoperative visit (2 to 3 weeks after discharge) the patient is instructed in the techniques of inflating and deflating the prosthesis. He is given an instruction sheet and advised to practice daily for the next 2 weeks. When he can use the device easily (usually 4 to 5 weeks postoperatively), he may resume sexual intercourse. Vigorous intercourse should be avoided for at least 4 more weeks to allow proper healing of the incision in the tunica albuginea.

MALE TO FEMALE TRANSSEXUAL SURGERY

Transsexual surgery was initially publicized in 1953, when Hamburger et al. reported the case of Christine Jorgenson. This surgery produced controversy in both the medical and the lay press as to its suitability for gender dysphoria. In the ensuing years many responsible medical centers have established gender identity clinics to diagnose and screen transsexuals. As of 1984 there are more than 40 such centers in the Western Hemisphere.

Patients requesting sexual reassignment surgery have increased in number over the past 30 years. However, the rationale under which such treatment is offered has become extremely complex. In an effort to standardize a program of care, the Harry Benjamin Internal Gender Dysphoria Association (Berger et al., 1978) has issued a publication entitled "Standards of Care: The Hormonal and Surgical Sex Reassignment of Gender Dysphoric Persons."* Physicians and surgeons contemplating treating transsexuals and recommending surgery for this condition should familiarize themselves with standards of care proposed in this monograph.

Gender dysphoria, i.e., transsexualism, is a psychologic state whereby a person demonstrates dissatisfaction with his or her sex of birth and the sex role, as socially defined, that applies to that sex, and who requests hormonal and surgical sex reassignment. Transsexualism is not an organic condition or problem but is definitely a psychologic condition. The diagnosis and screening must be done by psychiatrists and related personnel with assistance from urologists, gynecologists, plastic surgeons, endocrinologists, and social workers. The diagnostic procedure and preoperative treatment are extensive, and surgery should be considered only as the last step in a progressive program of medical-psychiatric therapy. Surgeons should never undertake the therapy of transsexuals on an individual basis. These patients are best treated with a team approach and should have extensive preoperative diagnostic tests and therapy before surgery is undertaken. Patients should be screened by psychiatrists and other professionals in the mental health field who have experience in working with patients exhibiting gender dysphoria.

The diagnostic criteria for transsexualism should be based on the following (American Psychiatric Association, 1978):

1. There is a persistent sense of discomfort and inappropriateness about one's anatomic sex.

2. There is a persistent wish to be rid of one's own genitals and to live as a member of the other sex.

3. The disturbance has been continuous (not limited to periods of stress) for at least 2 years.

4. There should be an absence of physical intersex or genetic abnormality.

5. The disturbance is not symptomatic of mental disorder, such as schizophrenia or depression.

Psychiatrists and psychologists making the recommendation in favor of sexual reassignment should have known the patient in a psychotherapeutic relationship for at least 6 months prior to such recommendation. It is advised that other sources of information about the patient (relatives, friends, employers) be interviewed to confirm the patient's statements of persistent gender dysphoria. Psychologic testing is mandatory to further document the diagnosis. The surgeon who is contemplating performing sexual reversal should have the written recommendation of such surgery by at least two behavioral scientists, one of whom is a psychiatrist.

The proposed surgical candidate should also be followed by an endocrinologist so that hormonal sex-reassignment therapy can be instituted after appropriate medical screening. The proposed surgical candidate should be on hormonal therapy for a minimum of 6 months and preferably 1 year prior to surgery. The potential benefits, medical side effects, and potential hazards must be carefully explained to the patient as well as the necessity for ongoing medical care. Hormonal therapy should never be initiated until a complete physical examination has been performed with appropriate laboratory tests, including liver enzyme studies and fasting blood sugar levels. Undiagnosed medical or endocrinologic conditions may be a contraindication to therapy or may preclude a modified hormonal regimen. The patient must understand that hormonal treatment can cause irreversible damage to the testicles even if it is stopped at some time in the future. The side effects of this therapy should be carefully documented for the patient and for his medical record. Hormonal therapy is both diagnostic and therapeutic in that patients report satisfaction or dissatisfaction with the sexual characteristics produced by such therapy.

Another important step in the screening of transsexual patients is the requirement that the individual be living full time in the social role of the desired sex for at least 12 months prior

---

*Available through the Janus Information Facility, 1952 Union Street, San Francisco, Calif. 94123.

to the surgery. The response and acceptance of coworkers, relatives, and friends are essential to evaluate the patient's ability to cope with the desired new lifestyle. At times, exceptions are made in this cross-dressing rule, e.g., in cases in which individuals cannot cross-dress at work. However, cross-dressing should be mandatory at all other times and in all social situations.

Persons being considered for sexual reassignment should be 21 years of age or older. Reaching maturity is essential for the legal and moral ramifications associated with such drastic and irreversible surgery. The patient should not be married at the time of surgery. If a patient is divorced, the surgeon, for his own protection, should receive legal documentation of the divorce.

A thorough urologic evaluation should be undertaken to rule out pre-existing genitourinary disorders that might complicate transsexual surgery. Because the urinary tract is drastically altered in this surgery, an intravenous urogram, urinalysis, SMA-12, and urine cultures are the minimal studies required. If the patient has a history of genitourinary voiding difficulties, urodynamic and cystoscopic studies should be done before consent to perform surgery is given.

Essential to postoperative success is the patient's thorough understanding of the surgical procedure. A detailed, specific, informed operative consent should be explained to and executed by the patient. Figure 81–24 displays the operative consent form used for male-to-female patients at the Pennsylvania Hospital Gender Identity Center. The terminology must be explained to the patient in basic words, so that no doubts exist as to the potential complications and the irreversibility of the surgery.

The final decision to perform transsexual surgery must be based on a thorough and complete diagnosis of gender dysphoria. The surgeon is the last member of a broad-based psychiatric-medical team, and he must consider the surgery as the last step in a complicated diagnostic and therapeutic program. To intervene with surgery before the proper diagnostic and therapeutic program has been completed could lead to tragic results. To circumvent any of the proposed steps, tests, and therapies would leave the surgeon in a potentially disadvantageous medicolegal position.

The patient is generally admitted to the hospital 2 days prior to surgery. He is started on a 2-day mechanical bowel preparation with a clear liquid diet. An intravenous pyelogram, chest x-ray, and electrocardiogram are obtained, plus the usual laboratory studies associated with major surgery. An electroencephalogram is performed if there is any history of neurologic disorders. Enemas are ordered to evacuate the colon and rectum in case the rectum is inadvertently damaged or entered during the surgery. A Betadine scrub preparation is used on the abdomen and perineum twice daily prior to surgery. The patient receives a detailed explanation of the previously described operative permit. If the patient should have any hesitation or misgivings about the surgery, he should be discharged from the hospital to be given more time to consider the proposed course of therapy. All potential complications should be explained to him.

Surgery to create female genitalia in a male transsexual consists of a radical penectomy, bilateral orchiectomy, urethroplasty, perineal dissection with a creation of a neovaginal vault, vaginoplasty, and vulvoplasty. The optimal surgical procedure to construct female genitalia should be a one-stage procedure and produce a vagina adequate for intercourse and one having a cosmetic appearance that is virtually indistinguishable from that of a normal genetic female. Our experience (Malloy et al., 1976) with an anterior-based penile pedicle graft procedure fulfills these requirements and has produced gratifying results. Pandya and Stuteville (1973), Granato (1974), Meyer and Kesselring (1980), Rubin (1980), and Glenn (1979), have also reported similar success with anterior-based pedicle flaps. Foerster and Reynolds (1979) have reported a one-stage procedure that utilized a split-thickness skin graft to line the neovagina rather than an anterior pedicle graft. Edgerton et al. (1970) described a two-stage posterior-based penile pedicle graft operation. They felt that this was necessary owing to a lack of mobility of an anterior-based flap to give sufficient vaginal depth. Our experience and that of others seem to indicate that this is not the case.

Whichever surgical technique is used, a thorough understanding of the perineal anatomy is essential. Those not familiar with the perineum, bladder, prostate, and rectum should not undertake this surgery. Meticulous and precise surgical technique is mandatory to prevent damage to adjacent organs.

The procedure takes between 3½ and 4 hours to perform. The patient needs complete relaxation of the lower abdomen and perineum. Therefore, general anesthesia or a continuous caudal anesthesia is required to maintain proper relaxation. It is essential during the perineal dissection that the patient be relaxed and not move; otherwise, damage could easily be done to the rectum or to the urethra, prostate, or bladder.

Operative Consent to Construct Female Genitalia in Male Transsexual

Patient_____ Age _____Date_____ Time_____ A.M.
                                                                                              P.M.

1. I hereby authorize Doctors_____ and/or such associates or assistants as may be selected by them to perform the following operations and/or medical procedures: Total Penectomy (removal of my penis), a bilateral orchiectomy (removal of both my testicles), fashion a vagina in the area where my scrotum now exists, and fashion a new urethra.

2. I understand that during the course of the operation and/or medical treatment unforeseen conditions may be revealed that may necessitate an extension of the original procedures or different procedures than those set forth above. I therefore authorize and request that the above named physicians, assistants and/or their designees perform such surgical procedures or render such medical treatment as are necessary and desirable in the exercise of professional judgment. The authority granted under this paragraph shall extend to treating the conditions that are both known and unknown to Doctors_____ at the time the operation is commenced.

3. I UNDERSTAND THIS OPERATION IS *TOTALLY IRREVERSIBLE* AND THAT I NO LONGER WILL BE ABLE TO HAVE INTERCOURSE AS A MALE OR TO CONCEIVE CHILDREN. I ALSO UNDERSTAND THAT THE ABOVE NAMED PHYSICIANS DO NOT GUARANTEE ANY SEXUAL PLEASURE OR FUNCTION AS A RESULT OF THE ABOVE STATED PROCEDURES.

4. I UNDERSTAND THAT BECAUSE OF THE NATURE OF THE ABOVE PROCEDURES IT IS IMPOSSIBLE FOR THE ABOVE NAMED SURGEONS TO PREDICT ALL THE POSSIBLE PSYCHIATRIC AND PHYSIOLOGICAL RESULTS OF THIS PROCEDURE. SOME OF THE POSSIBLE COMPLICATIONS EXPLAINED TO ME WHICH ARE INVOLVED IN THESE PROCEDURES INCLUDE IN ADDITION TO THOSE SET FORTH ABOVE, BUT NOT BY WAY OF LIMITATION ARE THE FOLLOWING: SEVERE LOSS OF BLOOD, INFECTION, CARDIAC ARREST, POOR COSMETIC RESULTS, PERMANENT PAIN AND DISCOMFORT, ADVERSE EFFECTS FROM ANESTHESIA, AND PSYCHIATRIC DISORDERS.

5. I consent to the administration of such anesthetics as may be considered necessary or advisable by the physician responsible for this service.

6. I am aware that the practice of medicine and surgery is not an exact science and results cannot always be anticipated. I acknowledge that no guarantee or assurance has been given to me by anyone as to the results that may be obtained in the operation to be performed upon me and of any medical, surgical, or therapeutic procedures in the Hospital. I understand that complete restoration of function will not be achieved (I will not be able to conceive children) as a result of this operation or procedure.

7. I certify that I am not presently married and will not be married prior to the operation contemplated herein.

8. I certify that I have read and fully understand this Consent Statement which has been preceded by an explanation by Doctors_____ and that their explanations in no way vary from the contents of this Consent Statement and are understood by me and I agree not to revoke, limit or alter this Consent except in writing delivered to Doctors_____ prior to commencement of the operation or procedures described hereto.

_____
PATIENT

_____
Signature of Witness

_____
Signature of Witness

_____
NOTARY's Signature

Figure 81–24. Operative consent form for male to female transsexual surgery.

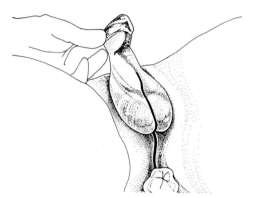

Figure 81–25. Male to female transsexual surgery. Incision made from base of penis through median raphe of scrotum to anal verge.

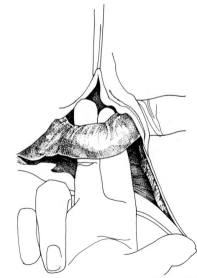

Figure 81–26. Suspensory ligament of penis divided so that corpora cavernosa and spongiosum urethra can be inverted posteriorly.

After anesthesia induction, the patient is placed in an exaggerated lithotomy position. A preparation is done in the operating room, followed by a rigorous surgical scrub of the abdomen, penis, scrotum, perineum, and thighs. Betadine surgical scrub and solution are recommended to prevent sepsis. At the completion of the preparation a sterile rectal shield is placed into the rectum and sutured in place so that the rectum can be palpated during surgery.

A midline incision is made from the base of the penis through the scrotum in the midline to the anal verge (Fig. 81–25). The subcutaneous tissue is excised to expose the corpus spongiosum and corpora cavernosa. The testicles and spermatic cord structures are freed to the external inguinal ring. The spermatic vessels and vas deferens are ligated separately and severed. The cord structure is then retracted into the inguinal canal, and the external inguinal ring is closed bilaterally with wire sutures to prevent possible future inguinal hernias. The testicles and distal spermatic cords are removed.

The suspensory ligament of the penis is severed. Dissection around the base of the corpora cavernosa and corpus spongiosum urethra is accomplished in the dorsal and ventral plane distal to the pubic ramus (Fig. 81–26). This procedure permits posterior retraction of these structures, which will invert the skin of the penis. The inverted penile skin is dissected to the glans penis, which is severed from the corpus spongiosum and corpora cavernosa (Fig. 81–27). The glans is left attached to the penile skin. The penile skin becomes the pedicle flap that will serve as the lining for the neovagina, and the glans penis will simulate the cervix.

The corpus spongiosum is separated from the corpora cavernosa. The corpora cavernosa

are separated in the midline and ligated at the base of each crus (Fig. 81–28). Hemostatic sutures are placed through the base of the crura prior to dissection to eliminate the chance of hemorrhage. All corpora cavernosa tissue should be excised to prevent painful erections in the proximal stumps during future sexual excitement. Various authors have reported leaving the bases of the corpora cavernosa and suturing them in the midline to form a neoclitoris. We feel that this tissue is bulky and often protrudes into anterior vaginal wall, causing problems and pain with intercourse. It should be entirely removed. The bulbospongiosus muscle is excised, and the corpus spongiosum is mobilized. The central tendon of the perineum is severed, and the rectourethralis muscle is

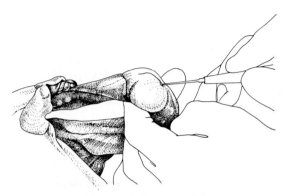

Figure 81–27. Glans penis is separated from corpora cavernosa and corpus spongiosum urethra.

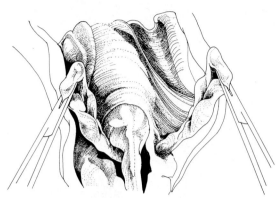

Figure 81–28. Proximal remnants of corpora cavernosa are divided so that the individual crus may be removed at the pubic ramus.

transected. An 18 Foley catheter is inserted into the urethra for guidance so that a plane can be dissected between the apex of the prostate and the rectum. Denonvilliers' fascia is identified and split transversely. This avascular plane allows deep dissection between the prostate and the anterior wall of the rectum. The dissection is carried posteriorly under the trigone of the

bladder and the posterior wall of the bladder to the peritoneal reflection. Adequate width for the vagina is assured by transecting the medial fibers of the levator ani muscles. With blunt dissection and gentle pressure a wide vaginal cavity is fashioned that extends posteriorly and cephalad through the endopelvic fascia to the peritoneal reflection. Dissection to this level is imperative for long-term vaginal depth and successful intercourse.

The subcutaneous space under the hypogastrium is freed to the level of the umbilicus. This is an extremely important step to allow the mobility of the anterior-based penile pedicle skin flap into the depths of the perineal dissection to the level of the peritoneal reflection. With caudal retraction on the mobilized lower abdominal skin, two heavy traction sutures are placed through the skin into the periosteum of the symphysis to keep the mobilized skin in the proper position. The inverted penile skin tube is distended with a silicone rubber vaginal stent. Subcutaneous fibrous bands and tissue are removed to allow maximum distensibility of the inverted penile pedicle graft. The inverted tube

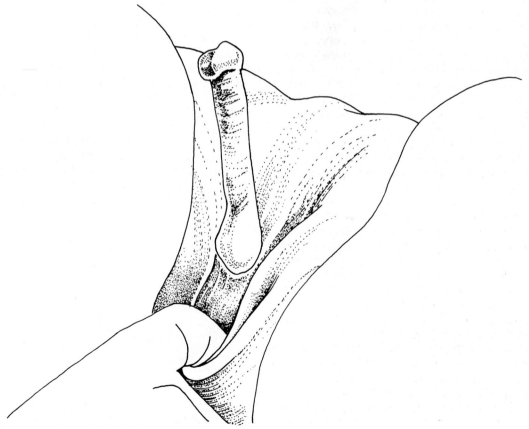

Figure 81–29. Urethra is brought through the anterior aspect of the penile pedicle skin flap.

with stent is placed into the perineum. Adequate depth and width should be present. If lack of depth is noted, further dissection is required. A depth of at least 18 cm should be present. The traction sutures are tied over gauze packings to prevent lacerations of the mobilized skin.

An elliptical 1.5 cm incision is made on the anterior wall of the inverted penile skin tube in a position beneath and proximal to the symphysis pubis. This site will be the meatus of the neourethra. The urethra is severed after the Foley catheter is removed. It is cut at an appropriate length and drawn through the hole in the pedicle graft with a traction suture (Fig. 81–29). The urethra is sutured to the skin with interrupted 4-0 chromic and 4-0 PDS sutures. There should be no tension on this anastomosis. There should also be no evidence of bleeding from the spongiosum tissue. The posterior aspect of the penile pedicle skin graft is sutured to the posterior aspect of the midline incision at the anal verge. This is done with 3-0 chromic sutures. At this point the scrotal tissue is drawn up so that appropriate labia majora may be fashioned. It is imperative to judge how much skin will be required to make normal-looking labia. Excess scrotal skin is severed, and imbricating chromic sutures are used to fashion the labia bilaterally. This step should be taken with considerable care so that the labia are symmetric and the introitus has a normal appearance.

With the completion of the labia a 16 Foley catheter remains in the urethra. The vaginal stent is placed deep into the vagina to prevent hematoma formation or stenosis of the vaginal cavity that has been created (Fig. 81–30). Gentle pressure ensures proper healing of the pedicle graft. Compression dressings are applied to the perineum, with the Foley catheter exiting anteriorly.

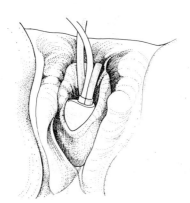

Figure 81–30. Vaginal stent is placed into the neovagina and inflated to ensure adequate depth and width.

The patient is kept NPO for the first 3 days after surgery. This is done to prevent bowel movements, which would soil the dressings and necessitate removing the bulky compression dressing. Antibiotic coverage with broad-spectrum antibiotics is instituted for a 14-day period. Total liquid diets are started on the fourth postoperative day. The dressings are changed on the sixth postoperative day and the catheter removed. The vagina and labia are carefully inspected. If the wound is healing well and the vaginal depth is adequate, the patient commences tub baths three times per day. She is instructed in the use of the silicone rubber vaginal stent, which is maintained in the vagina at all times except when urinating or bathing. The patient is customarily discharged on the seventh or eighth postoperative day and continues the same regimen at home. All antibiotics are maintained for a 2-week period. The vaginal stent is used continuously for 3 months to prevent vaginal stenosis or retraction. Special emphasis must be placed on the continuous use of the stent with all patients. If the stent is neglected or not properly placed, vaginal stenosis may result. Sexual relations are permitted after 8 weeks, depending on the status of the vagina and the degree of wound healing.

Since 1969, 68 male transsexuals had their initial surgery performed at Pennsylvania Hospital with the operative procedure described. The follow-up period has been from 1 year to 14 years, with the average being 5½ years. None has regretted having the surgery. There have been no serious psychiatric problems. All state that sexual activity has been satisfactory.

Table 81–1 lists the complications in this group of patients. One patient developed a colovaginal fistula when she used an electric stimulator for dilatation 5 weeks postoperatively. A colostomy for 6 weeks produced healing with no secondary problems. Osteitis pubis developed in another patient who engaged in sexual intercourse 12 days postoperatively. There were no other major complications.

TABLE 81–1. COMPLICATIONS IN 68 MALE
TRANSSEXUALS 1969–1984

Complications	No. Patients	Treatment
Osteitis pubis	1	Antibiotics, rest, analgesics
Colovaginal fistula	1	Colostomy for 6 weeks with subsequent closure
Psychiatric complications	0	

Foerster and Reynolds (1979), utilizing the one-stage procedure with skin graft, reported satisfactory results in 35 patients followed from 6 months to 5 years. Using a similar operative technique Pandya and Stuteville (1973) had satisfactory results in 18 of 19 patients.

References

American Psychiatric Association: Diagnostic and Statistical Manual. 3rd ed. Washington, D.C., 1978.

Berger, J.C., Green, R., Laub, D.R., Reynolds, C.L., Walker, P.A., and Wollman, L.: Standards of Care: The Hormonal and Surgical Sex Reassignment of Gender Dysphoric Persons. San Francisco, Janus Information Facility, 1978.

Das, S.: Peyronie's disease: excision and autografting with tunica vaginalis. J. Urol., *124*:818, 1980.

Devine, C.J., Jr.: Surgery of the penis and urethra. *In* Harrison, J.H., Gittes, R.F., Perlmutter, A.D., Stamey, T.A., and Walsh, P.C. (Eds.): Campbell's Urology. Philadelphia, W.B. Saunders Co., 1979, pp. 2390–2437.

Devine, C.J., Jr.: Operation for Peyronie's disease. *In* Stewart, B.H. (Ed.): Operative Urology, Lower Urinary Tract, Pelvic Structures and Male Reproductive System. Baltimore, The Williams & Wilkins Co., 1982, pp. 367–373.

Devine, C.J., Jr.: Surgery of penile curvature. *In* Paulson, D. (Ed.): Genitourinary Surgery. New York, Churchill Livingstone, 1984, pp. 607–628.

Devine, C.J., Jr., and Horton, C.E.: Surgical treatment of Peyronie's disease with a dermal graft. J. Urol., *111*:44, 1974.

Deysach, L.J.: The comparative morphology of the erectile tissue of the penis with especial emphasis on the probable mechanism of erection. Am. J. Anat., *64*:111, 1939.

Edgerton, M.T., Knoff, J.J., and Callison, J.R.: The surgical treatment of transsexual patients: Limitations and indications. Plast. Reconstruct. Surg., *45*:38, 1970.

Effehoj, J.: A new operation for priapism. Scand. J. Plast. Reconstruct. Surg., *8*:241, 1975.

Finney, R.P.: New hinged silicone penile implant. J. Urol., *118*:585, 1977.

Fishman, M.D., Scott, F.B., and Light, J.K.: Experience with inflatable penile prosthesis. Urology, *123*:86, 1984.

Foerster, D.W., and Reynolds, C.L.: Construction of natural appearing female genitalia in the male transsexual. Plast. Reconstruct. Surg., *64*:306, 1979.

Gittes, R.F., and McLoughlin, A.P.: Injection technique to induce penile erection. Urology, *4*:473, 1974.

Glenn, J.R.: One-stage operation for male transsexuals. Trans. Am. Assoc. Genitourin. Surg., *71*:130, 1979.

Granato, R.C.: Surgical approach to male transsexualism. Urology, *3*:792, 1974.

Grayhack, J. T., McCullough, W., O'Conor, V., Jr., et al.: Venous bypass to control priapism. Invest. Urol., *1*:509, 1964.

Hamburger, C., Sturup, G.K., and Dahl-Iverson, E.: Transvestism: Hormonal, psychiatric and surgical treatment. JAMA, *152*:391, 1953.

Harrow, B.R.: Simple technique for treating priapism. J. Urol., *101*:71, 1969.

Jonas, U., and Jacobi, G.H.: Silicone-silver penile prosthesis: description, operative approach and results. J. Urol., *123*:865, 1980.

Malloy, T.R., Noone, R.B., and Morgan, J.A.: Experience with the one stage surgical approach for constructing female genitalia in male transsexuals. J. Urol., *116*:335, 1976.

Malloy, T.R., Wein, A.J., and Carpiniello, V.L.: Comparison of the inflatable penile and the Small-Carrion prostheses in the surgical treatment of erectile impotence. J. Urol., *123*:678, 1980.

Malloy, T.R., Wein, A.J., and Carpiniello, V.L.: Advanced Peyronie's disease treated with the inflatable penile prosthesis. J. Urol., *125*:327, 1981.

Malloy, T.R., Wein, A.J., and Carpiniello, V.L.: Revised surgical technique to improve survival of penile cylinders for the inflatable penile prosthesis. J. Urol., *130*:1105, 1983.

Merrill, D.: Mentor inflatable penile prosthesis. Urology, *22*:504, 1983.

Meyer, R., and Kesselring, U.K.: One-stage reconstruction of the vagina with penile skin as an island flap in male transsexuals. Plast. Reconstruct. Surg., *66*:401, 1980.

Nesbit, R.M.: Congenital curvature of the phallus: report of three cases with description of corrective procedure. J. Urol., *93*:230, 1965.

Newman, H.F., and Northup, J.D.: Mechanism of human penile erection: an overview. Urology, *17*:399, 1981.

Newman, H.F., and Reiss, H.: Method for exposure of cavernous artery. Urology, *19*:16, 1982.

Pandya, N.J., and Stuteville, O.H.: A one-stage technique for constructing female external genitalia in male transsexuals. Br. J. Plast. Surg., *26*:277, 1973.

Quackels, R.: Cure of a patient suffering from priapism by cavernospongiosa anastomosis. Acta Urol. Belg., *32*:5, 1964.

Rubin, S.: A method of preserving the glans penis as a clitoris in sex conversion operations in male transsexuals. Scand. J. Urol. Nephrol., *14*:215, 1980.

Scott, F.B., Bradley, W.E., and Timm, G.W.: Management of erectile impotence: Use of implantable inflatable prosthesis. Urology, *2*:80, 1973.

Small, M.P., Carrion, H.M., and Gordon, J.A.: Small-Carrion penile prosthesis. Urology, *5*:479, 1975.

VanArsdalen, K.N., Malloy, T.R., and Wein, A.J.: Erectile physiology, dysfunction and evaluation. Part II: Etiology and evaluation of erectile dysfunction. Monogr. Urol., *4*:165, 1983.

Wagner, G.: Erection anatomy. *In* Wagner, G., and Green, R. (Eds.): Impotence. New York, Plenum Press, 1981, pp. 7–24.

Wein, A.J., Malloy, T.R., Lief, H.T., Hanno, P.M., and VanArsdalen, K.N.: Evaluation of the impotent man: University of Pennsylvania approach. *In* Barrett, D.M., and Wein, A.J. (Eds.): Controversies in Neuro-Urology. New York, Churchill Livingstone, 1984, pp. 481–488.

Wendel, E.F., and Grayhack, J.T.: Corpora cavernosa—glans penis shunt for priapism. Surg. Gynecol. Obstet., *153*:586, 1981.

Winter, C.C.: Priapism cured by creation of fistulas between glans penis and corpora cavernosa. J. Urol., *119*:227, 1978.

CHAPTER 82

Surgery of Penile and Urethral Carcinoma

JOSEPH T. SPAULDING, M.D.
HARRY GRABSTALD, M.D.

Successful management of any disease is based on a complete familiarity with its natural history and a precise delineation of the disease stage. Such descriptions of the natural histories of penile and urethral carcinoma, along with current staging systems, have been presented in preceding chapters (Chapters 31 and 34). Diagnostic criteria for clinical staging, which define as accurately as possible the extent of the disease in the individual case, have also been outlined. With these facts at his disposal, the clinician should then be able to apply an effective treat- ment plan, maximizing therapeutic benefit while minimizing morbidity.

MANAGEMENT OF THE PRIMARY TUMOR

Anatomic Considerations

The lymphatic anatomy of the penis and its cutaneous envelopes has been thoroughly stud- ied in the past (Rouviere, 1938). The lymphatics of the prepuce and penile skin converge on the dorsum of the penis and coalesce into several trunks. Coursing together toward the base of the penis, these trunks then separate to termi- nate bilaterally in the superficial inguinal nodes, particularly the superomedial group. The freely anastomotic nature of these channels disrupts any initial laterality of drainage, and thus lesions arising unilaterally on the penis may metastasize contralaterally or bilaterally to the regional nodes.

The network of lymphatics arising from the glans penis is somewhat more complex. All the lymphatics of the glans initially converge on the frenulum and then ascend along the corona to pass onto the dorsum of the penis as one to four larger collecting trunks. In the region of the suspensory ligament of the penis, these trunks are said to anastomose to form a presymphyseal lymphatic plexus that may include one or two small intercalating nodules. The presence of this presymphyseal plexus has been invoked to ex- plain the occasional recurrence of carcinoma in this site following penectomy (Pack and Rekers, 1942; Spratt et al., 1965), although the existence of a clinically significant repository in this region is doubted by others (Whitmore, 1975; Cabanas, 1977).

The termination of these trunks continuing from the presymphyseal area is a matter of some debate. The superomedial group of superficial inguinal lymph nodes on either side can act as the first lymphoid echelon for lymphatics origi- nating in the glans penis (Cabanas, 1977). Rou- viere (1938) described alternate pathways that terminate in nodes of the deep inguinal, external iliac, or hypogastric region. More recently, the existence of a direct lymphatic route from the penis to the pelvic lymph nodes has been ques- tioned (Riveros et al., 1967; Sen et al., 1967).

The corporal bodies are drained by lym- phatic trunks that course beside the dorsal vein of the penis to the region of the presymphyseal plexus. There they anastomose and may thus join the previously described pathway to the inguinal region. Additionally, direct drainage to the deep inguinal and external iliac regions has been demonstrated.

The lymphatic anatomy of the male urethra includes a rich mucosal network that extends throughout the length of the urethra and is particularly abundant in the region of the fossa navicularis. This network is continuous posteriorly with that of the prostate and bladder and anteriorly with that of the penis. Collecting ducts spring from the mucosal plexus to join with those from the glans and shaft in the anterior urethra and pass to the superficial inguinal nodes via the presymphyseal plexus. Those collecting ducts of the bulbomembranous urethra course through the urogenital diaphragm to join prostatic and bladder lymphatics and terminate in the obturator and medial external iliac nodes.

The scrotum has abundant lymphatic channels that anastomose freely along the median raphe. Superiorly, trunks arise in the region of the median raphe and course around the base of the penis to terminate in the superomedial group of the superficial inguinal nodes. Inferiorly, the trunks initially pass transversely and upward and then along the genitofemoral sulcus to the inferomedial group of superficial inguinal nodes. The abundance and free intercommunication of the scrotal lymphatics necessitates a very wide local excision of a primary carcinoma involving the scrotum.

In the female, the lymphatics of the proximal urethra course to the external iliac, hypogastric, and obturator nodes with the collecting ducts from the bladder and vagina. Lymphatic channels of the distal urethra and meatus freely communicate with vulvar lymphatics and course toward the mons veneris to then terminate in the superomedial group of the superficial inguinal nodes.

While clitoral lymphatic pathways to both the inguinal and external iliac groups are described, primary vulvar malignancy with clitoral extension does not involve the pelvic nodes without concomitant inguinal metastases. Such clinical correlation with urethral carcinoma extending to the clitoris is lacking.

The occasional presentation of distant metastatic disease in patients with penile carcinoma, with or without regional lymphatic involvement, suggests an additional mode of spread. Batson (1942) injected dye into the dorsal vein of the penis at the symphysis and noted that the dye coursed into the prostatic venous plexus, the lateral pelvic wall vessels, and the common iliac veins. Communication via the lateral sacral veins with the bony pelvis and lumbar spine was also demonstrated. Spread along this vertebral venous plexus has been invoked to explain the occurrence of isolated brain metastasis in penile carcinoma. Other sites of apparent hematoge-nous spread include the lung, liver, bone, and spleen (Melicow and Ganem, 1946). Similar vascular considerations apply to hematogenous spread from urethral tumors. Blood-borne metastasis is uncommon, however, despite the rich enveloping spongy tissue that affords ready vascular access.

Histologic Correlates

The pattern of progression of a particular malignancy can vary with its individual histologic character, and these differences may impact upon specific therapeutic considerations. Squamous carcinoma of the penis slowly enlarges, invades, produces significant local destruction, and embolizes through the local lymphatics to the regional lymph nodes of the groin in an orderly fashion. Pathologic evaluation of the resected primary tumor fails to show permeated lymphatic channels justifying the separate management of the primary tumor and its regional drainage. This approach is supported by wide clinical experience.

Early hematogenous and lymphatic dissemination is characteristic of melanoma, which may originate from the penis or urethra. Melanoma of the male and female urethra generally arises distally, but the ominous unpredictable nature of the tumor mandates its wide extirpation if clinically localized. Bracken and Diokno (1974) cite the high local/regional failure rate in patients with clinically localized penile and male urethral melanoma managed with conservative penectomy or without regional lymphadenectomy and recommend aggressive surgery to include radical penectomy and *simultaneous* bilateral ilioinguinal lymphadenectomy. Experience with melanoma at other sites demonstrates its propensity for secondary satellite lesions and in transit metastases. Wide local excision en bloc with regional lymphadenectomy has significantly reduced the incidence of local recurrence of extremity melanoma (Fortner et al., 1975). The single incisional en bloc resection of the primary and regional lymphatics described by Young (1931) is worthy of consideration for genital or urethral melanoma. Whether carefully selected small superficial lesions may be managed conservatively is unclear (Weiss et al., 1982).

Sarcoma of the penis usually presents as a circumscribed subcutaneous nodule, and in contradistinction to sarcomas at other sites exhibits little tendency to metastasize. Local recurrence is common (35 per cent) and repeated attempts at local control may be necessary. Fibrosarcoma and leiomyosarcoma are usually more bulky and the fibrosarcoma may metastasize early.

The management of metastatic lesions to the penis is usually palliative, since they arise most commonly in association with widespread dissemination from prostate, bladder, and rectal primaries. Rarely, isolated metastases to the penis have been encountered, however, and successfully excised.

Adenocarcinoma of the female urethra may on occasion arise within a urethral diverticulum, a location that may allow successful local excision.

Routine en bloc urethrectomy is advised at the time of cystectomy for transitional cell bladder cancer because it removes current or future sites of new tumor formation; it may improve local control by obviating tumor cell spillage with transection of the membranous urethra; it only slightly increases operative time, morbidity, and blood loss; and it simplifies postcystectomy follow-up.

Nonsurgical Treatment Options

The therapeutic alternatives in carcinoma of the penis and of the male and female urethra are varied and depend on disease stage. They have previously been discussed in Chapters 31 and 34, and detailed description here will be limited to surgical therapy. For a given stage of disease, the application of a particular modality will depend upon factors such as available soft tissue margin, patient acceptance, previous therapy, general condition of the patient, and personal bias of the treating physician.

PENIS CANCER

In situ lesions of the penis may be effectively controlled with topical chemotherapy (Goette, 1976). Excisional biopsy may provide both diagnosis and cure in selected cases of such lesions. Radiotherapy has also been successfully applied to in situ carcinoma of the penis (Mantell and Morgan, 1969; Kelley et al., 1974). Prophylaxis, however, is not afforded by any of these modalities, and careful follow-up is mandatory.

Radiotherapy for penis cancer has obvious psychologic and cosmetic advantages over surgery, particularly for invasive lesions. Many forms of delivery have been successfully applied, including radium and iridium mould, and interstitial, orthovoltage, and megavoltage external-beam techniques. Whereas local control is higher with external-beam therapy compared

with mould techniques, morbidity increases as well, e.g., meatal stenosis, urethral stricture, penile pain, and radionecrosis. Pretreatment circumcision and generous meatotomy are mandatory to minimize acute inflammatory complications such as phimosis, paraphimosis, and balano-ophisthitis. Therapy is more morbid if there is associated infection. Tumor persistence after irradiation is much more common than new tumor formation (Grabstald and Kelley, 1980) in locally recurrent penile carcinoma and ranges from 10 to 50 per cent, depending upon lesion size, depth of invasion, and radiation technique. Salvage penectomy is often successful therapy for patients failing primary irradiation (El-Demiry et al., 1984) or with debilitating complications (radionecrosis, pain).

Time to regression of a penile cancer treated by irradiation may be prolonged. Up to 12 months of observation may be required to verify local control (Pointon, 1975). With palpable inguinal adenopathy, a more expedient form of primary therapy, namely surgery, is appropriate.

Cryosurgery has been successfully utilized for verrucous carcinoma of the penis with anatomic and functional preservation of the penis (Carson, 1978; Hughes, 1979).

CANCER OF MALE URETHRA

Intraurethral instillation of multiple agents, including 5-fluorouracil, podophyllin, thiotepa, Clorpactin, colchicine, and bleomycin, has been reported for extensive condylomata acuminata (Danoff et al., 1981). Thiotepa or 5-fluorouracil provides high local concentrations with minimal morbidity and is advocated as an adjunct for low-grade superficial urethral cancer arising primarily or secondarily after successful bladder cancer management (Konnak, 1980; Leissner and Johansson, 1980). Concomitant transurethral resection probably plays the primary role, particularly with lesions of the posterior urethra where prostatic tissue may be safely sacrificed.

According to published experience, radiotherapy for this lesion has been palliative in intent. Bulbomembranous tumors are often sizable, regionally metastatic, and usually incurable at presentation. Some early distal urethral cancers have been controlled with external-beam irradiation alone or judiciously combined with intraurethral radium (Raghavaiah, 1978; Ellingwood and Million, 1983).

CANCER OF THE FEMALE URETHRA

Radiotherapy is a proven modality in female urethral cancer arising in the distal segment. External-beam, intracavitary, and interstitial or combination radiotherapy techniques have been effective (Grabstald et al., 1966; Prempree et al., 1984). Distal urethral tumors are controlled equally satisfactorily by simple excision. Lesions of the entire urethra are difficult to eradicate by either surgery or radiotherapy, prompting radiation trials as a preoperative adjunct (Bracken et al., 1976; Johnson and O'Connell, 1983).

Adjuncts to Surgical Treatment

Cytotoxic agents with demonstrated activity, alone or in combination, in metastatic penile carcinoma include bleomycin (Ichikawa et al., 1969; Yagoda et al., 1972; Kyalwazi et al., 1974), methotrexate (Garnick et al., 1979; Sklaroff and Yagoda, 1980), and *cis*-platinum (Sklaroff and Yagoda, 1979). Adjuvant chemotherapy trials in carcinoma of the penis have not yet been initiated but would seem logical for patients with poor prognostic features, such as multiple metastatic lymph nodes. Remarkable responses to combined treatment with irradiation and bleomycin have been reported and allowed on occasion subsequent conservative surgery for local control (Ichikawa, 1977). Preoperative radiation is commonly recommended for urethral cancer arising proximally in view of the dismal results of single modality therapy (Levine, 1980; Johnson and O'Connell, 1983; Klein et al., 1983).

Surgical Options—Primary Tumor

TISSUE CONFIRMATION

Histologic verification of the malignant nature of the lesion in question is an essential first step to staging and the formulation of a treatment plan. Tumors of the penis lend themselves to convenient incisional or dermal punch biopsy and adjacent normal tissue should be included to provide demonstration of invasion and infiltration—a critical differential point with small and low-grade lesions. Urethral tumors not presenting at the meatus can be sampled by transurethral resection or by curettage. Urethral washings may provide cytologic confirmation of malignancy. A large periurethral mass can be biopsied by needle or incisional biopsy techniques.

PENIS CANCER

Superficial lesions of the prepuce can be successfully excised primarily by circumcision with adjustment for adequate margins. These patients are prone to local recurrence by persistent tumor and by new tumor formation and must be followed closely (Hardner et al., 1972; Jensen, 1977; Narayana, 1982). Carefully selected superficial lesions of the skin of the penile shaft can also be simply excised. Excisional biopsy of lesions of the glans penis has not been uniformly successful and may result in diminished prognosis on recurrence (Ekstrom and Edsmyr, 1958; Hanash et al., 1970).

Invasive penile cancer not suitable for irradiation, by virtue of its size, location, or depth of invasion, is best managed by partial or total penectomy. Attainment of a 2 cm gross tumor margin affords excellent local control (Dean, 1952). Penile length sufficient to permit upright and directable micturition may be retained after sufficient partial penectomy. At least 3 cm of proximal shaft should be available for consideration of this technique. In selected cases where the residual stump is of inadequate length (< 2 cm from penoscrotal junction), its mobilization from the suspensory ligament and transposition to the perineum can supply additional length to allow directed voiding (deSouza, 1976). Total penectomy is necessary when adequate tumor margin precludes conservative resection.

Penile reconstruction is feasible following partial and total penectomy. Sexual, urinary, and cosmetic considerations need to be evaluated. Both single and multistage (Mukherjee, 1980) techniques have been described for reconstruction following total penile loss.

For more extensive or more proximal invasive lesions or with involvement of the scrotum, perineum, abdominal wall, or pubis, it may be necessary to perform emasculation, incontinuity cystectomy, or resection of the pubic arch (Shuttleworth and Lloyd-Davies, 1969), pubic symphysis (Mackenzie and Whitmore, 1968), or portions of the abdominal wall (Arconti and Goodwin, 1956; Skinner, 1974; Bracken and Grabstald, 1975).

MALE URETHRAL CANCER

Transurethral resection can be effective therapy for low-grade and superficial lesions of the penile or prostatic urethra (Mullin et al., 1974; Konnak, 1980). For isolated lesions of similar low stage and grade, a segmental urethrectomy with reanastomosis has occasionally been successful (Kaplan et al., 1967; Grabstald, 1973). Invasive lesions of the distal penile urethra are surgically managed by appropriate penectomy, although in selected cases the corporal bodies may be spared if the invasion seems superficial and limited within the corpus spongiosum. Proximal bulbomembranous lesions are prone to local recurrence, and preoperative radiotherapy with extended excision including the pubic arch or symphysis is recommended to try to achieve primary control (Bracken, 1982; Klein et al., 1983) and may be considered the treatment of choice.

Invasive transitional cell carcinoma of the prostatic urethra is a rare but aggressive tumor. Rational management would consist of radical cystourethrectomy following preoperative radiotherapy (Grabstald, 1973; Levine, 1980).

FEMALE URETHRAL CANCER

Therapy is based primarily on tumor extent and to a lesser degree on histologic type. Anterior or distal lesions are predominantly squamous cell type and, if of limited size, can be effectively controlled by partial urethrectomy alone. Urethral pressure profilemetry may allow careful case selection for radiotherapy where operative resection might jeopardize continence (Asmussen and Ulmsten, 1982). Urethral tumors arising in association with urethral diverticula, particularly adenocarcinoma, can also be successfully managed by local excision (Cea et al., 1977; Evans et al., 1981). Local recurrence is then subjected to wide extirpation. Restriction to superficial lesions, pathologic assessment of surgical margins, excision without violation and spillage, and careful follow-up would be features essential to the successful application of this conservative option. Radiotherapy followed by radical excision with anterior transvaginal pelvic exenteration is recommended for cancer involving the proximal or entire female urethra. Pubic arch or symphyseal resection has been suggested as a surgical adjunct to improve soft tissue margin and local control (Klein, 1983).

Specific Surgical Techniques

PARTIAL PENECTOMY

Successful local control by partial penectomy (Fig. 82–1) depends on division of the penis 2 cm proximal to the gross tumor extent. After the lesion is excluded by a towel secured along the proposed line of amputation, a tourniquet is applied at the base of the penis. The skin is incised circumferentially and the cavernous bodies are divided sharply to the urethra. The dorsal vessels are ligated and the urethra is then dissected proximally and distally to attain a 1 cm redundancy. The urethra is divided without sacrifice of the tumor margin and the

corpora are secured with interrupted sutures opposing the margins of the tunica albuginea. The tourniquet is removed, and additional hemostasis is attained as necessary. After a dorsal urethrotomy, a skin-to-urethra anastomosis is performed, and the redundant skin is approximated dorsally to complete the closure (Pack and Ariel, 1963). Alternatively, a guillotine amputation (Dean, 1952) may be performed with simple skin-to-urethra approximation to create the meatus. A small urinary catheter is placed and a light dressing applied, both of which may be removed in 3 to 4 days.

MODIFIED PARTIAL PENECTOMY

When the penile stump after partial penectomy would be too short for directing the urinary stream, further length can be attained by releasing the corpora from the suspensory ligament, dividing the ischiocavernosus muscle, and partially separating the crura from the pubic rami. The scrotum is incised along the raphe and skin flaps are fashioned for penile coverage. The testes are sutured to the symphysis and the scrotum is reconstructed cephalad to the transposed phallus (deSouza, 1976).

TOTAL PENECTOMY

The urethra is transposed to the perineum (Fig. 82–2) if the size of the primary lesion precludes a partial penectomy owing to insufficient residual penile length to direct the urinary stream. After appropriate draping of the primary lesion, a vertical elliptical incision is made around the base of the penis. Dissection along the corpora is performed with division of the suspensory ligament and dorsal vessels. The urethra is dissected sharply from the corpora to the bulbar region, this dissection being aided by distal division of the urethra and its ventral traction. The corpora are then divided and ligated.

A 1 cm ellipse of skin is removed from the region of the perineal body and a tunnel created bluntly in the perineal subcutaneous tissue. The urethra is grasped and transposed to the perineum without angulation. Spatulation of the urethra and a skin-to-urethra anastomosis are performed. The primary incision is then closed with drainage transversely to elevate the scrotum away from the new meatus. A urethral catheter is placed and the wound dressed.

EXTENDED EXCISION

With proximal urethral lesions or large genital tumors extensively involving the perineum, additional soft tissue clearance is recommended to maximize local control. In addition to en bloc

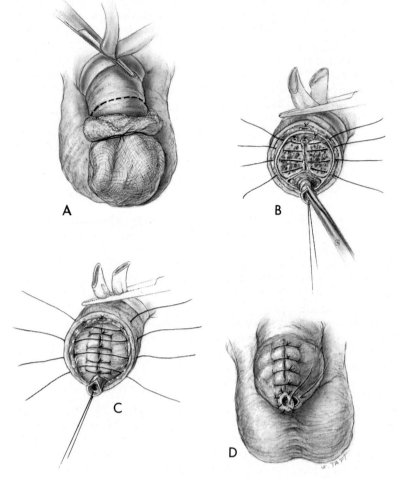

Figure 82–1. Partial penectomy. *A* and *B,* After exclusion of the lesion from the field, the corpora are divided with a 2 cm gross margin. *C,* The dorsal vessels are ligated, the cut margins of the tunica albuginea approximated, and the urethra spatulated. *D,* Simple skin closure and urethral meatus formation complete the procedure.

cystectomy, excision of the entire pubic arch or its subsymphyseal segment has been utilized as a surgical adjunct in these circumstances (Mackenzie and Whitmore, 1968; Shuttleworth and Lloyd-Davies, 1969; Bracken, 1982; Klein et al., 1983).

With the patient in a low lithotomy position to allow perineal access, the standard abdominal mobilization of the bladder is completed, except for preservation of the endopelvic fascia and the anterior pubic attachments. In the male, an inverted U-shaped perineal incision is initiated, based just medial to the ischial tuberosities, with the apex in the midperineum. The ischiorectal fossae are developed as in perineal prostatectomy and a tunnel is bluntly dissected just anterior to the rectum extending from one fossa to the other. The inferior skin flap is mobilized by sharply dividing the intervening subcutaneous tissue.

The superior flap is mobilized by sharply incising the subcutaneous tissue to the superficial fascia (Colles'). The dissection is continued bilaterally to the adductor musculature at the inferior pubic rami. Anteriorly the dissection is carried along the phallus to the penoscrotal junction. Wider exposure, if necessary, results from dividing the scrotum in the midline. Bulky tumors may necessitate sacrifice of portions of the scrotum or perineal skin. The testicles may still be preserved and sutured to the symphysis or placed in thigh pouches.

For small bulbomembranous urethral tumors, it is reasonable to consider preservation of the distal phallus for cosmetic and psychologic reasons. The corpora are divided and the stump is closed and anchored to the symphysis. Viability is maintained by the cutaneous blood supply. Larger lesions will necessitate a wider margin and perhaps the entire symphysis, precluding phallic preservation.

The perineal incision in the female is similar to but wider than that for standard transvaginal anterior pelvic exenterations. The labia majora are retracted and the introital incision is initiated anterior to the clitoris. It continues inferiorly to

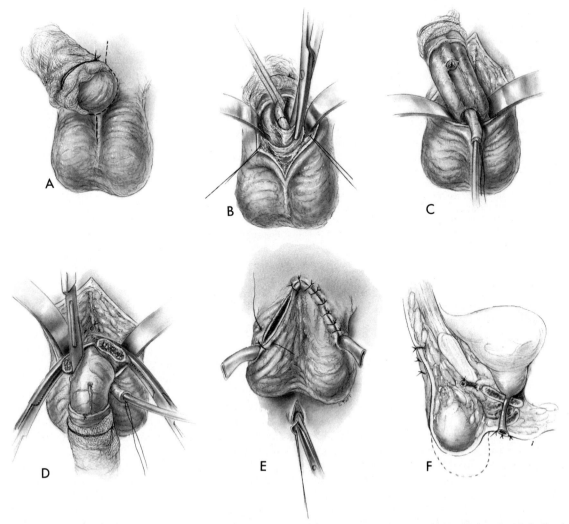

Figure 82–2. Total penectomy. *A,* A vertical elliptical incision encircles the base of the penis. *B,* The urethra is isolated at least 2 cm proximal to the gross lesion. *C,* The suspensory ligament has been divided. The urethra is transected and dissected from the corpora. *D,* The dorsal vessels are ligated, and the crura are transected with the stumps ligated. *E,* A button of perineal skin is excised, and the urethra is then transposed and spatulated to form the perineal urethrostomy. *F,* Horizontal closure of the primary incision with drainage serves to elevate the scrotum away from the urinary stream.

include the labia minora to the lower mid-vagina, where it joins the vaginotomies initiated from the pelvis. Dissecting anteriorly, the symphysis is cleared, while lateral dissection exposes the fascia overlying the origins of the adductors along the inferior pubic rami.

To complete the pubic arch resection, the adductor musculature is sharply divided bilaterally from the length of the inferior pubic ramus along the medial margin of the obturator foramen. A Gigli saw is then passed along the inferior ramus just posterior to the origins of the transverse perineal muscles. An inferiorly beveled transection is made bilaterally. The bevel is important for ease in perineal delivery

of the specimen. The entire symphysis is resected for bulky penile or urethral lesions involving the presymphyseal tissues and is accomplished by division of the superior rami at their junction with the symphysis (Fig. 82–3). The Gigli saw is introduced and laterally beveled osteotomies are completed (Fig. 82–4). For smaller lesions, the bulk of the symphysis can be preserved with resection of just the subsymphyseal arch. The Gigli saw is passed through the obturator foramina to incise the symphysis transversely, joining the foramina with an upward beveled osteotomy (Fig. 82–5). The specimen is then delivered en bloc. After hemostasis is secure, the omentum is mobilized to cover

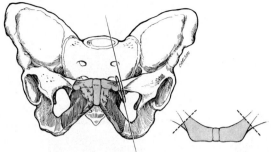

Figure 82–3. The shaded area is excised; beveling as shown facilitates removal of the bony segment. Total symphyseal excision should be considered for all bulky penile and proximal urethral (male and female) lesions. (From Bracken, R. B.: *In* Johnson, D., and Boileau, M. (Eds.): Genitourinary Tumors: Fundamental Principles. New York, Grune & Stratton, 1982. Used by permission.)

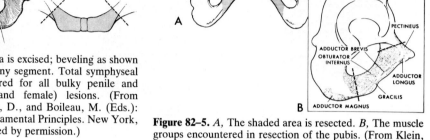

Figure 82–5. *A,* The shaded area is resected. *B,* The muscle groups encountered in resection of the pubis. (From Klein, F. A., et al.: Cancer, *51*:1241, 1983. Used by permission.)

the bowel. Myocutaneous flaps based on the gracilis muscle can be fashioned to close large perineal defects (Larson and Bracken, 1982).

MANAGEMENT OF REGIONAL DISEASE

Anatomic Considerations

The inguinal lymph nodes are divided into superficial and deep groups, which are anatomically separated by the deep fascia of the thigh, the fascia lata. The superficial group of nodes is composed of four to 25 glands (average, eight), which are situated in the deep membranous layer of the superficial fascia of the thigh, Camper's fascia (Daseler et al., 1948). The superficial group drains to the deep inguinal nodes, which,

two or three in number, lie along the femoral vessels within the femoral sheath, an extension into the thigh of the extraperitoneal fatty-areolar tissue in which the external iliac vessels run. The node of Cloquet, or Rosenmüller, is the most cephalad of this deep group and is usually situated within the femoral canal. The external iliac lymph nodes receive drainage from the deep inguinal, obturator, and hypogastric groups. In turn, drainage progresses to the common iliac and para-aortic nodes.

The blood supply to the skin of the inguinal region derives from branches of the common femoral artery, namely the superficial external pudendal, the superficial circumflex iliac, and the superficial epigastric arteries. Complete inguinal dissection necessitates ligation of these branches, and thus the viability of the skin flaps

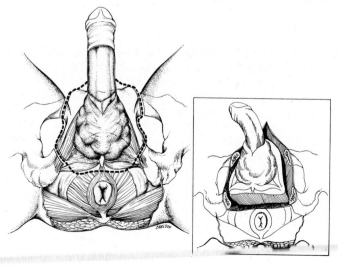

Figure 82–4. The anatomic relationships involved in such a resection. (From Bracken, R. B.: *In* Johnson, D., and Boileau, M. (Eds.): Genitourinary Tumors: Fundamental Principles. New York, Grune & Stratton, 1982. Used by permission.)

raised during the dissection depends on anastomotic vessels in the superficial fatty layer of Camper's fascia that course parallel to the natural skin lines. This is the anatomic basis for the superiority of the single oblique incision in regional node dissection, since it least disrupts these collaterals (Spratt et al., 1965). The cutaneous venous anatomy parallels the arterial branches.

The femoral nerve lies deep to the iliacus fascia and supplies motor function to the pectineus, quadriceps femoris, and sartorius muscles, and in addition provides cutaneous sensation to the anterior thigh. Division of the former branches would result in significant morbidity, but some of the latter sensory branches are commonly sacrificed in the regional node dissection. The obturator nerve is dissected in the course of pelvic node dissection and provides medial thigh cutaneous sensation and adductor motor function. Ordinarily this nerve escapes injury but its sacrifice is not incapacitating.

The genitofemoral nerve is commonly injured during the course of pelvic lymphadenectomy as it runs in intimate relationship with the iliac vasculature exiting the femoral canal to supply cutaneous sensation to the inguinofemoral region and a portion of the genitalia.

The femoral triangle, the area that contains the pertinent lymphatic groups, is bounded by the inguinal ligament superiorly, the sartorius laterally, and the adductor longus medially. The floor of the triangle is composed of the pectineus medially and the iliopsoas laterally.

Clinical Correlates

PENIS CANCER

The controversy regarding the timing of regional lymphadenectomy in the management of penile carcinoma has been well stated in Chapter 34 and elsewhere (Grabstald, 1980). In summary:

1. Approximately 30 to 60 per cent of patients with penile carcinoma will present with palpable inguinal lymphadenopathy. After treatment of the primary and resolution of lymphadenitis, half of these patients will have metastatic deposits at node dissection. The likelihood of metastatic deposits within palpable adenopathy is increased when the primary lesion is uninflamed, sizable, or high grade, when it shows stromal, vascular, or lymphatic invasion, or when the regional adenopathy is massive (Bassett, 1952; Marcial et al., 1962; Johnson et al., 1973).

2. Five to 20 per cent of patients with initially uninvolved nodes will develop metastatic adenopathy or will be found to harbor metastases at prophylactic lymphadenectomy (Beggs and Spratt, 1964; Hardner et al., 1972).

3. At primary dissection, if positive nodes are detected ipsilaterally, metastases are present contralaterally in 60 per cent of cases (Ekstrom and Edsmyr, 1958).

4. When delayed dissection is performed for subsequent adenopathy, metastatic deposits are usually found (85 per cent), and if the contralateral groin is clinically negative, subsequent metastatic deposits in that location are rare (< 10 per cent) (Ekstrom and Edsmyr, 1958).

5. There is no survival advantage for patients subjected to prophylactic dissection compared with those having secondary dissection for delayed lymphadenopathy (Ekstrom and Edsmyr, 1958; Beggs and Spratt, 1964; Johnson et al., 1973).

6. A "sentinel node" concept has been advanced based upon the observations of Cabanas (1977): When the superior medial superficial inguinal lymph node is negative, all nodes are negative at dissection; when only one node is positive, it is the "sentinel node"; when multiple nodes are positive, the sentinel node is always involved as well. This concept needs further clinical confirmation, since a patient with negative "sentinel node" biopsies who developed extensive regional metastases has been reported (Perinetti et al., 1980).

7. Stratification of treatment results based on the anatomic extent of ilioinguinal nodal involvement by metastatic carcinoma of the penis shows a 90 per cent survival rate with uninvolved nodes that falls to 70 per cent, 50 per cent, and 20 per cent with metastases to solitary (sentinel) inguinal, multiple inguinal, and pelvic nodes, respectively (Cabanas, 1977). Patients with common iliac or para-aortic nodal metastases have not been surgically salvaged. A minimal therapeutic dissection should clear the superficial and deep inguinal as well as the external iliac and obturator regions to the common iliac bifurcation.

MALE URETHRAL CANCER

The incidence of metastatic inguinal adenopathy from distal male urethral cancers is 50 to 60 per cent (Riches and Cullen, 1951; Ray et al., 1977). In contradistinction to penile primaries, there is little inflammation associated with these lesions and clinical adenopathy in this setting is a highly reliable sign of metastasis. Therapeutic dissection has been successful but there is no documented advantage to prophylactic surgery (Ray et al., 1977).

Tumors arising from the bulbomembranous and prostatic urethra drain primarily to the external iliac, obturator, and hypogastric nodes. Involvement of the inguinal nodes may result from retrograde filling from extensive pelvic adenopathy or directly from invasion of the perineum or genitals. While the incidence of metastatic pelvic or inguinal adenopathy is undefined, it carries an ominous prognosis. Only an occasional survivor has been reported following therapeutic lymphadenectomy (Marshall, 1957).

FEMALE URETHRAL CANCER

Inguinal metastases are more common with entire than distal urethral cancer (Antoniades, 1969) and are evident in 28 per cent overall (Grabstald, 1973). Palpable adenopathy accurately denotes metastasis (Grabstald, 1973), and survival is enhanced by therapeutic lymphadenectomy. Again, prophylactic dissection is not advised (Grabstald, 1973; Peterson et al., 1973; Bracken et al., 1976; Ray and Guinan, 1979). The incidence of pelvic nodal involvement is not well documented but may be low (20 per cent) (Peterson et al., 1973). Lymphangiography may allow preoperative recognition and consideration of a palliative approach in view of the serious prognostic impact (Bracken et al., 1976).

Nonsurgical Treatment Options

Although a variety of nonsurgical techniques is applicable to low-stage lesions of the penis and urethra, treatment of regional nodal disease is primarily surgical. Radiotherapy has been used as a palliative measure, as an adjunct to surgical excision, and as primary therapy with scattered favorable claims (Lenowitz and Graham, 1946; Staubitz et al., 1955; Ekstrom and Edsmyr, 1958; Murrell and Williams, 1965). The efficacy of this modality in regional disease is unproved primarily owing to the lack of histologic documentation in large numbers of patients undergoing such therapy. Not infrequently, an excised node proves on subsequent regional dissection to have been the only one involved (Cabanas, 1977), an additional factor to be considered in evaluating nonsurgical man-

agement. The induration that may follow radiotherapy to the groin makes clinical examination for recurrent disease more difficult and increases the local morbidity should surgery subsequently become necessary for uncontrolled regional disease. Recent reports support the implied advantage of surgery over irradiation (Williams, 1975; Jensen, 1977; Narayana et al., 1982). Presumably, these results can be extrapolated to inguinal deposits from urethral primaries as well (Antoniades, 1969; Ray et al., 1977; Prempree et al., 1984).

Surgical Options

Ilioinguinal lymphadenectomy has been associated with a significant incidence of lymph collection, lymphedema, skin slough, and infection (Table 82–1). In view of this morbidity, many clinicians are reluctant to advise routine groin dissection for penile or urethral carcinoma (Bracken et al., 1976; Ray and Guinan, 1979; Grabstald, 1981; Johnson and Lo, 1984).

Others (Fegen and Persky, 1969; Hardner et al., 1972; Gonzalez-Flores and Rodriguez-Rivas, 1976) advocate routine prophylactic dissection and feel that this approach will eradicate subclinical disease early and thereby improve the survival rate in this metastatic group.

Some (Edwards and Sawyers, 1968; Hanash et al., 1970) have performed percutaneous aspiration or excisional biopsy of suspicious adenopathy or even clinically negative nodes

TABLE 82–1. ILIOINGUINAL NODE DISSECTION

Complication	Incidence	Perioperative Countermeasures
Skin flap necrosis	14–65%	Oblique inguinal incision Skin flap thickness Care in tissue handling Transposition of sartorius muscle Excision of ischemic flap margins
Wound infection	10%	Interval resolution of region inflammation Mechanical bowel preparation Prophylactic antibiotics
Seroma/ lymphedema	19–50%	Ligation of transected lymphatics Transposition of sartorius muscle Closed catheter suction drainage Immobilization of dissected extremity Elastic support stockings

(DeKernion et al., 1973) to obtain histologic verification before proceeding with regional lymphadenectomy. Cabanas (1977) has routinely excised a "sentinel node" or nodes bilaterally from the superomedial region regardless of its clinical status. This approach combines the theoretical advantage of early detection of regional disease with the practical consideration of limiting treatment morbidity by appropriate case selection. While this concept has not been expanded to urethral cancer, clinical experience is warranted.

When regional disease has been proved by preliminary biopsy (N_1, N_2), surgical dissection of the ilioinguinal lymph nodes should follow. For penile cancer, if metastatic adenopathy is present in either groin at the time of presentation, bilateral regional node dissections should be done in view of the high incidence of bilateral deposits in this setting. On the other hand, if the regional nodes are judged initially free of disease, the delayed appearance of metastatic adenopathy should prompt ipsilateral dissection alone (Ekstrom and Edsmyr, 1958). For urethral cancer, lymphadenectomy is reserved for clinical adenopathy.

Intimate adherence of advanced inguinal disease (N_3) to the femoral vessels may require en bloc resection with vascular reconstruction. Autogenous tissue is preferable in this repair in view of the potential for suppurative complications. A prosthetic graft may replace the contralateral iliac system and provide a suitable autograft for the resected iliofemoral segment. Alternatively, bypass grafting through the obturator foramen can successfully revascularize the leg (Dardik et al., 1980; Cockburn et al., 1982). Resection of the femoral nerve, if necessitated by tumor extension, allows for maintenance of a useful extremity (Whitmore, 1970; Cockburn et al., 1982). If the soft tissue is extensively involved, hemipelvectomy may offer a reasonable chance for control of disease, although muscle invasion seems to denote incurability (Block et al., 1973).

Bilateral disease of this magnitude (N_3) is usually also distantly metastatic, but if localized it would require translumbar amputation for excision. This latter modality has not yet been applied to penile or urethral carcinoma, and consideration of such a step should prompt careful thought. Preliminary laparotomy with biopsy of the common iliac and para-aortic lymph nodes should be performed in order to exercise proper case selection in these advanced cases. A palliative dissection should be considered if the regional adenopathy is judged likely

to ulcerate prior to death even in the presence of distant metastasis. This prophylactic measure can obviate the development of significant pain, sepsis, and hemorrhage from uncontrolled disease.

Specific Surgical Techniques

SENTINEL NODE BIOPSY

The location of the saphenofemoral junction is estimated to be at a point two fingerbreadths lateral and inferior to the pubic tubercle. An incision through this point exposes the fossa ovalis and the greater saphenous vein with its medial tributaries, the superficial epigastric and the external pudendal veins (Fig. 82–6).

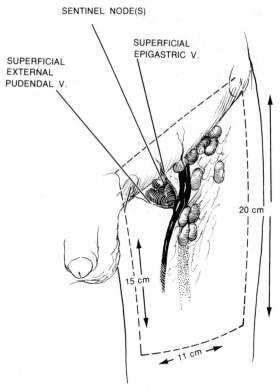

Figure 82–6. Sentinel node(s) biopsy. An incision is centered over a point two fingerbreadths lateral and inferior to the pubic tubercle. The saphenous vein and its medial tributaries are isolated at the fossa ovalis. All fibroadipose node-bearing tissue is then removed from this region and submitted for pathologic study. This figure also depicts the topography and dimensions of the quadrangle within which all inguinal nodal tissue is predictably situated. This area can be marked after positioning and draping in order to avoid excessive dissection and excessive compromise of collateral blood supply to the skin flaps. (From Spaulding, J.: *In* Javadpour, N. (Ed.): Principles and Management of Urologic Cancer. 1st ed. Baltimore, The Williams & Wilkins Co., 1979.)

Within the space bounded by these branches, the tissue is excised and submitted for microscopic examination. The superomedial area may contain several nodes and all should be removed to assure complete sampling. With histologic confirmation of metastatic involvement, complete dissection should be undertaken.

The surgeon should anticipate the direction of the preferred incision for groin dissection so that the biopsy incision may be included with the specimen if the biopsy result should dictate further surgery.

ILIOINGUINAL NODE DISSECTION

A 6-week interval following treatment of the penile lesion allows reduction of any inflammatory component of the regional adenopathy and minimizes the incidence of wound suppuration. Preliminary preparations for regional node dissection include mechanical preparation of the bowel, elastic support wraps or stockings for the legs, and preoperative antibiotics.

The patient is positioned with the involved thigh slightly abducted and externally rotated and the slightly flexed knee is supported with a pillow as necessary. A urethral catheter is placed and the scrotum positioned or sutured out of the operative field. A fungating tumor is excluded from the field by suturing a formalin-moistened sponge to the skin around the lesion prior to the routine skin preparation.

Various incisional approaches to the regional nodes in carcinoma of the penis have been described (Fig. 82–7). For cases requiring bilateral dissection, an oblique incision 5 cm below and parallel to the inguinal ligament is commonly used for excision of the superficial and deep inguinal nodes (Baronofsky, 1948). Addition of a lower midline extraperitoneal incision allows access to the pelvic nodal component and is recommended for bilateral management. The convenient access to preliminary laparotomy afforded by this approach needs no emphasis (Williams and Butcher, 1961; Whitmore and Vagaiwala, 1984).

Single incisions for ipsilateral excision of the ilioinguinal nodes may be vertical (Kuehn and Roberts, 1953), oblique (Woodhall, 1953; Spratt et al., 1965), or S-shaped (Gray and Bailey, 1957; Byron et al., 1962). A double incisional unilateral approach has been promoted with reportedly decreased wound morbidity (Wagner et al., 1971; Fraley and Hutchens, 1972). The inability to conveniently excise a previous biopsy scar or areas of cutaneous involvement is a limitation of the double incision technique. The single oblique incision is recommended for cases requiring unilateral dissection.

Application of Young's (1931) single incision en bloc removal of both the primary lesion and the regional nodes has been associated with a high incidence of suppurative complications that are presumably due to inflammatory seeding of the regional nodes from the commonly infected primary lesion. The use of separate incisions in the simultaneous treatment of a genital primary and the regional nodes has led to a reduction in suppurative complications compared with a single incision en bloc approach (Ballon and Lamb, 1975). Advanced local and regional disease may necessitate con-

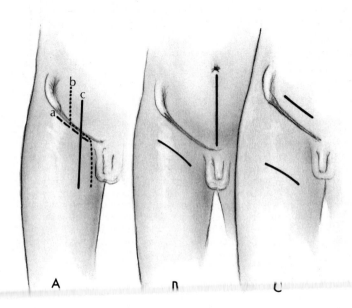

Figure 82–7. *A,* Single incisional approaches include (a) oblique, (b) S-shaped, and (c) vertical techniques. *B,* Double incisional techniques may combine a lower midline with an inguinal incision. *C,* Alternatively, an oblique abdominal incision may provide unilateral access to the pelvic nodes.

A   B   C

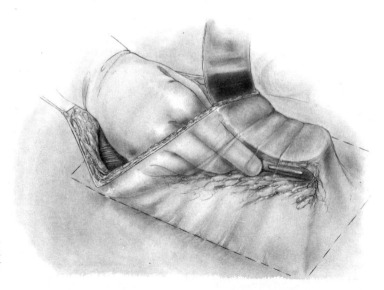

Figure 82–8. After a single oblique inguinal incision, superior and inferior flaps of 3- to 4-mm thickness are raised throughout the extent of the previously marked area of dissection.

sideration of an extended en bloc procedure. Otherwise, consideration of an in-continuity dissection should be reserved for cases of genital melanoma (Hovnanian, 1967).

The area to be dissected should encompass only potentially involved tissue to minimize morbidity. Based on anatomic study of 450 inguinal dissections, Daseler et al. (1948) defined a quadrilateral area within which all inguinofemoral lymph nodal tissue could be expected to lie. Bounded superiorly by a line 1 cm above and parallel to the inguinal ligament and extending laterally 12 cm from just above the pubic tubercle, this quadrilateral area is further delimited medially and laterally by perpendicular lines of 15 and 20 cm respectively, which also serve to define the inferior extent of the dissection. These boundaries can be marked out on the skin (Figs. 82–6 and 82–8) for convenient reference during the dissection.

After the skin incision has been made, skin flaps are fashioned throughout the entire premarked area of proposed dissection (Fig. 82–8). Tissue trauma may be minimized by the use of skin hooks and protective saline-moistened gauze sponges. The superficial fatty portion of Camper's fascia, approximately 3 to 4 mm in thickness, contains anastomotic cutaneous blood vessels and should be left adherent to the flaps. The thickness of the flaps is a critical factor in their viability and thus influences the likelihood of primary healing. Any suggestion of involvement by tumor should prompt elliptical excision of that skin segment rather than further thinning of the flap. Immediate skin grafting is preferable to both delayed grafting or late local recurrence.

The superior margin of the dissection is incised to the external oblique fascia and the tissue dissected inferiorly therefrom, clearing the inguinal ligament to the deep fascia of the thigh, the fascia lata. The fascia lata is then incised laterally just below the inguinal ligament overlying the sartorius muscle. In this plane and including both the deep fascia and the overlying subcutaneous tissue, the lateral, inferior, and medial margins are progressively divided and ligated with absorbable suture in order to occlude the ascending lymphatic channels and minimize lymph flow into the postoperative wound. The greater saphenous vein will be initially encountered along the inferomedial margin and must be specifically ligated. Medial mobilization of the nodal block is begun from the lateral margin with sacrifice of cutaneous branches of the femoral nerve only as necessary. The femoral artery and vein encompassed by the femoral sheath are dissected circumferentially free of the few deep inguinal nodes from the inguinal ligament to the apex of the femoral triangle. The superficial branches of the femoral artery and vein are divided, including the greater saphenous vein, which is doubly ligated at the saphenofemoral junction (Fig. 82–9). The inguinal tissue block is dissected from the medial and inferior margins so that it remains attached only by communications with the pelvic component at the femoral canal.

The pelvic nodal component is best accomplished through the lower midline extraperitoneal approach familiar to most urologic surgeons and will not be reviewed here. For unilateral dissection, however, there are three basic routes to this region through the recommended single oblique inguinal incision described by Spratt et

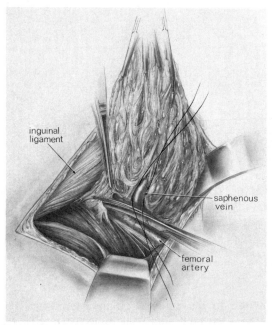

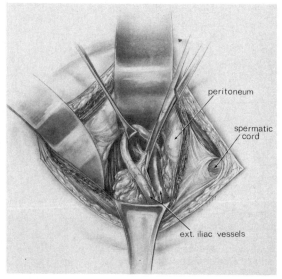

Figure 82–9. The flaps having been dissected, the entire circumference of this area is divided and the ascending lymphatics are ligated. The tissue is then mobilized from lateral to medial with exposition and skeletonization of the femoral vessels. Branches and tributaries are sacrificed, including the greater saphenous vein, which is double-ligated at its junction with the common femoral vein.

Figure 82–10. When only the ipsilateral pelvic component is to be addressed, access is readily gained to the retroperitoneum through an abdominal incision 4 to 5 cm above and parallel to the inguinal ligament. Nodal tissue is dissected from the iliac vessels, specifically including the external iliac and obturator groups.

al. (1965). The inguinal ligament can be divided vertically over the vessels or at the anterior superior iliac spine. Second, incision of the external oblique fascia and, reflecting the spermatic cord cephalad, division of the inguinal floor from the internal ring to the pubic tubercle with ligation of the inferior epigastric vessels will allow retroperitoneal access. Additionally, an incision in the anterior abdominal musculature 4 to 5 cm above and parallel to the inguinal ligament, with medial mobilization of the peritoneum, will expose the iliac region for nodal dissection (Fig. 82–10). The pelvic lymphadenectomy should minimally include the external iliac and obturator groups of nodes (Spratt et al., 1965). No further therapeutic benefit will be gained from common iliac or para-aortic dissection, but it can provide significant prognostic data. Some routinely extend their dissection to the aortic bifurcation (Daseler et al., 1948; Kuehn and Roberts, 1953; Skinner et al., 1972).

The specimen can then be delivered from the pelvis en bloc through the femoral canal (Fig. 82–11). The specimen should be carefully labeled or the inguinal and pelvic components submitted separately so that the extent of regional disease can be accurately determined.

Closure is begun with repair of the access to the retroperitoneum without drainage. Repair of the divided inguinal ligament is difficult and tenuous and it may be preferable to resect it. If the inguinal ligament has been resected, the anterior abdominal wall is sutured to the iliacus fascia and iliopsoas. Large abdominal wall defects are repaired with mesh if necessary (Karakousis, 1982). If entry has been through the floor of the inguinal canal, repair is analogous to standard herniorrhaphy. Regardless of the approach to the retroperitoneum, the iliopubic tract is sutured to Cooper's ligament to tighten the femoral canal. The sartorius muscle is then divided at the iliac spine and transposed to cover the femoral vessels; it is sutured to the inguinal ligament, the adductor longus, the iliacus, and the pectineus muscles. This maneuver (Baronofsky, 1948) serves to eliminate dead space, provide support for skin flaps, and protect the underlying femoral vessels from suppurative wound complications (Fig. 82–12).

Closed suction catheters are introduced into the area of dissection from a point peripheral to the skin flaps to obliterate dead space and prevent seroma formation (Raffl, 1952; Macdonald et al., 1958). This eliminates the need for compressive dressings over skin flaps that may be of marginal viability. The catheters may require irrigation and are usually removed after 5 to 7 days, when the aspirate volume is negligible and good flap adherence is evident (Silvis et al., 1955).

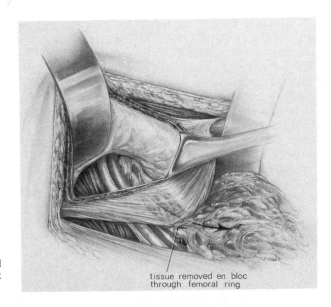

Figure 82–11. The entire specimen may be removed en bloc with delivery of the pelvic nodal component through the femoral canal.

tissue removed en bloc
through femoral ring

A continuous subcuticular skin closure with fine absorbable suture is effective. Evident ischemic margins should be excised primarily. Intravenous fluorescein has been shown to be a reliable predictor of skin flap viability (Smith and Middleton, 1979). Tension along the suture line should be avoided, and immediate skin grafting should be undertaken preferentially. Scrotal flaps may be fashioned to cover some residual groin skin defects (Arconti and Goodwin, 1956). Rotational skin flaps from the abdomen or anterolateral thigh can also be used to provide primary healing (Lee, 1955; Johnson et al., 1975; Airhart et al., 1982). Dressing the incision with collodion allows daily observation of the wound margins. Postoperative prophylactic antibiotics are prescribed; a broad-spectrum agent with antistaphylococcal and streptococcal activity (cephalosporin) is recommended.

Efforts should be made to minimize lymph flow during the initial postoperative period. A pillow splint around the lower leg and knee or the application of a posterior plaster splint deters hip flexion. Elastic wraps or stockings should be maintained, and with the bed flat, the foot of the bed is elevated on 3- to 6-inch blocks.

Figure 82–12. Closure of the wound includes repair of the access to the retroperitoneum, transposition of the sartorius muscle, placement of closed suction catheter drainage, and approximation of the skin edges without tension.

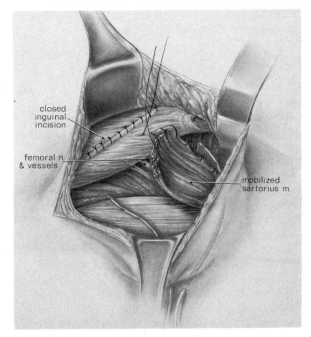

closed
inguinal
incision

femoral n.
& vessels

mobilized
sartorius m.

Because the patient should be kept at bed rest for 6 to 8 days, Coumadin anticoagulation has been recommended (Skinner et al., 1972). The incidence of clinical phlebitis and embolism after this procedure is low; Fortner et al. (1964) noted thrombophlebitis and nonfatal pulmonary embolism in only nine and four cases, respectively, among 206 patients with groin dissections. Prophylactic low-dose heparin therapy has also been recommended, but may increase postoperative complications (Hindsley et al., 1980; Sogani et al., 1981) and should probably be reserved for high-risk patients (Coon, 1976).

A low-residue diet is introduced to minimize fecal contamination, and the urinary catheter is retained until full urinary control can be expected. When primary healing appears well established, ambulation can be resumed. Prophylactic application of elastic fitted stockings and limb elevation reduce the incidence and severity of lymphedema following groin dissection (Karakousis et al., 1983).

HEMIPELVECTOMY

The technique of hemipelvectomy (Phelan and Nadler, 1964; Block et al., 1973) entails preliminary ligation of the ipsilateral iliac arteries and their major branches, medial mobilization of the bladder, ureter, rectum, and peritoneal contents, division of the bony pelvis at the pubic symphysis and the ipsilateral sacroiliac joint, and division of the intervening musculo-ligamentous attachments. The ipsilateral common iliac nodes are dissected and included with the specimen as well. The skin incision extends circumferentially from the iliac crest to the pubic tubercle and then along the genitocrural and gluteal folds, forming a posterior flap.

MANAGEMENT OF RECURRENT DISEASE

Local recurrence is generally the result of inadequate initial therapy with progression of persistent tumor. Following primary therapy, treatment of locally recurrent cancer of the penis is primarily surgical and penectomy is the most effective technique (Murrell and Williams, 1965). Likewise, radiotherapy has been successfully applied to local recurrence of penis cancer following primary surgery (Marcial et al., 1962). Identification of microscopic tumor at the margin of resection warrants immediate adjunctive therapy (Fegen and Persky, 1969). Cases of local recurrence after ilioinguinal lymphadenectomy must be individualized. If isolated and limited, the residual disease can be aggressively resected.

If more widespread, perhaps the result of tumor spillage, radiotherapy may be more appropriate. Chemotherapy can be expected to play an enlarging role in the advanced disease setting (Abratt et al., 1984; Ahmed et al., 1984).

References

Abratt, R. P., et al.: The treatment of bilateral ulcerated lymph node metastases from carcinoma of the penis. Cancer, *54*:1720, 1984.

Ahmed, T., et al.: Sequential trials of methotrexate, cisplatin, and bleomycin for penile cancer. J. Urol., *132*:465, 1984.

Airhart, R. A., DeKernion, J. B. and Guillermo, E. O.: Tensor fascia lata myocutaneous flap for coverage of skin defect after radical groin dissection for metastatic penile carcinoma. J. Urol. *128*:599, 1982.

Antoniades, J.: Radiation therapy in carcinoma of the female urethra. Cancer, *24*:70, 1969.

Arconti, J. S., and Goodwin, W. E.: Use of scrotal skin to cover wound defects in the groin and pubic area. J. Urol., *75*:292, 1956.

Asmussen, M., and Ulmsten, U.: The role of urethral pressure profile measurement in female patients with urethral carcinoma. Ann. Chir. Gynaecol., *71*:122, 1982.

Ballon, S. C., and Lamb, E. J.: Separate inguinal incisions in the treatment of carcinoma of the vulva. Surg. Gynecol. Obstet., *140*:81, 1975.

Baronofsky, I. D.: Technique of inguinal node dissection. Surgery, *33*:886, 1948.

Bassett J. W.: Carcinoma of the penis. Cancer, *5*:530, 1952.

Batson, O. V.: The role of the vertebral veins in metastatic disease. Ann. Intern. Med., *16*:38, 1942.

Beggs, J. H., and Spratt, J. S.: Epidermoid carcinoma of the penis. J. Urol., *91*:166, 1964.

Block, N. L., et al.: Hemipelvectomy for advanced penile cancer. J. Urol., *110*:703, 1973.

Bracken, R. B.: Exenterative surgery for posterior urethral cancer. Urology, *19*:248, 1982.

Bracken, R. B., and Diokno, A. C.: Melanoma of the penis and the urethra: 2 case reports and review of the literature. J. Urol., 111:198, 1974.

Bracken, R. B., and Grabstald, H.: Bladder carcinoma involving the lower abdominal wall. J. Urol., *114*:715, 1975.

Bracken, R. B., et al.: Primary carcinoma of the female urethra. J. Urol., *116*:188, 1976.

Bryon, R. L., et al.: Radical inguinal node dissection in the treatment of cancer. Surg. Gynecol. Obstet., *114*:401, 1962.

Cabanas, R. M.: An approach for the treatment of penile carcinoma. Cancer, *39*:456, 1977.

Carson, T. E.: Verrucous carcinoma of the penis. Arch. Dermatol., *114*:1546, 1978.

Cea, P. C., et al.: Mesonephric adenocarcinomas in urethral diverticula. Urology, *10*:58, 1977.

Cockburn, A. G., et al.: Bypass graft for femoral artery involvement by metastatic carcinoma of the penis. J. Urol. *127*:1191, 1982.

Coon, W. W.: Risk factors in pulmonary embolism. Surg. Gynecol. Obstet., *143*:385, 1976.

Danoff, D. S., et al.: New treatment for extensive condylomata acuminata: External radiation therapy. Urology, *18*:47, 1981.

Dardik, H., et al.: Remote profunda femoral bypass for limb salvage. Surg. Gynecol. Obstet., *151*:625, 1980.

Daseler, E. H., et al.: Radical excision of the inguinal and iliac lymph glands. Surg. Gynecol. Obstet., *87*:679, 1948.

Dean, A. L.: Conservative amputation of the penis for carcinoma. J. Urol., *68*:374, 1952.

DeKernion, J. B., et al.: Carcinoma of the penis. Cancer, *32*:1256, 1973.

deSouza, L. J.: Subtotal amputation for carcinoma of the penis with reconstruction. Ann. R. Coll. Surg., *58*:398, 1976.

Duncan, W., and Jackson, W. M.: The treatment of early cancer of the penis with megavoltage X-rays. Clin. Radiol., *23*:246, 1972.

Edwards, R. H., and Sawyers, J. L.: The management of carcinoma of the penis. South. Med. J., *61*:843, 1968.

Ekstrom, T., and Edsmyr, F.: Cancer of the penis. Acta. Chir. Scand., *115*:25, 1958.

El-Demiry, M. I. M., et al.: Reappraisal of the role of radiotherapy and surgery in the management of carcinoma of the penis. Br. J. Urol., *56*:724, 1984.

Ellingwood, K. E., and Million, R. R.: Carcinoma of the male urethra. Personal communication, 1983.

Evans, K. J., et al.: Adenocarcinoma of a female urethral diverticulum: A case report and review of the literature. J. Urol., *126*:124, 1981.

Fegen, P., and Persky, L.: Squamous cell carcinoma of the penis. Arch. Surg., *99*:117, 1969.

Fortner, J. G., et al.: Results of groin dissection for malignant melanoma in 220 patients. Surgery, *55*:485, 1964.

Fortner, J. G., et al.: En bloc resection of primary melanoma with regional lymph node dissection. Arch. Surg., *110*:674, 1975.

Fraley, E. E., and Hutchens, H. C.: Radical ilioinguinal node dissection—skin bridge technique. J. Urol., *108*:279, 1972.

Garnick, M. B., Skarin, A. T., and Steele, G. D.: metastatic carcinoma of the penis: Complete remission after high dose methotrexate chemotherapy. J. Urol., *122*:265, 1979.

Goette, D. K.: Review of erythroplasia of Queyrat and its treatment. Urology, *8*:311, 1976.

Gonzalez-Flores, B., and Rodriguez-Rivas, R.: The treatment of carcinoma of the penis. Personal communication, 1976.

Grabstald, H.: Tumors of the urethra in men and women. Cancer, *32*:1236, 1973.

Grabstald, H.: Controversies concerning lymph node dissection for cancer of the penis. Urol. Clin. North Am., *7*:793, 1981.

Grabstald, H., and Kelley, C. D.; Radiation therapy of penile cancer. Urology, *15*:575, 1980.

Grabstald, H., et al.: Cancer of the female urethra. JAMA, *197*:835, 1966.

Gray, D. B., and Bailey, H. A.: A new technic for radical ilio-inguinal lymph node dissection. Ann. Surg., *145*:873, 1957.

Hanash, J. A., et al.: Carcinoma of the penis: A clinicopathologic study. J. Urol., *104*:291, 1970.

Hardner, G. J., et al.: Carcinoma of the penis: Analysis of therapy in 100 consecutive cases. J. Urol., *108*:428, 1972.

Hindlsey, J. P., et al.: Mini-dose heparin therapy in pelvic lymphadenectomy and I-125 implantation of localized prostatic cancer. Urology, *15*:272, 1980.

Hovnanian, A. P.: The evolution and present status of pelvi-inguinal lymphatic excision. Surg. Gynecol. Obstet., *124*:851, 1967.

Hughes, P. S. H.: Cryosurgery of verrucous carcinoma of the penis. Cutis, *24*:43, 1979.

Ichikawa, T.: Chemotherapy of penis carcinoma. Recent results. Cancer Res., *60*:140, 1977.

Ichikawa, T., et al.: Bleomycin treatment of the tumors of the penis and scrotum. J. Urol., *102*:699, 1969.

Jensen, M. S.: Cancer of the penis in Denmark 1942–1962. Dan. Med. Bull., *24*:66, 1977.

Johnson, D. E., and Lo, R. K.: Complications of groin dissection in penile cancer. Urology, *24*:312, 1984.

Johnson, D. E., and O'Connell, J. R.: Primary carcinoma of female urethra. Urology, *21*:42, 1983.

Johnson, D. E., et al.: Carcinoma of the penis. Urology, *1*:404, 1973.

Johnson, D. E., et al.: Rotational skin flaps to cover wound defect in groin. Urology, *6*:461, 1975.

Kaplan, G. W., et al.: Carcinoma of the male urethra. J. Urol., *98*:365, 1967.

Karakousis, C. P. Exposure and reconstruction in the lower portions of the retroperitoneum and abdominal wall. Arch. Surg., *117*:840, 1982.

Karakousis, C. P., et al.: Lymphedema after groin dissection. Am. J. Surg., *145*:205, 1983.

Kelley, C. D., et al.: Radiation therapy of penile cancer. Urology, *4*:571, 1974.

Klein, F. A., et al.: Inferior pubic rami resection with en bloc radical excision for invasive proximal urethral carcinoma. Cancer, *51*:1238, 1983.

Konnak, J. W.: Conservative management of low grade neoplasms of the male urethra: A preliminary report. J. Urol., *123*:175, 1980.

Kuehn, C. A., and Roberts, R. R.: Amputation and radical lymph gland dissection in carcinoma of the penis; an operative technique. J. Urol., *69*:173, 1953.

Kyalwazi, S. K., Bhana, D., and Harrison, N. W.: Carcinoma of the penis and bleomycin chemotherapy in Uganda. Br. J. Urol., *46*:689, 1974.

Larson, D. L., and Bracken, R. B.: Use of gracilis musculocutaneous flap in urologic cancer surgery. Urology, *14*:148, 1982.

Lee, E. S.: Ilio-inguinal block dissection with primary healing. Lancet, *2*:520, 1955.

Leissner, K. H., and Johansson, S.: Topical application of 5-fluorouracil cream: A therapeutic alternative in the treatment of urothelial tumours of the distal urethra. Scand. J. Urol. Nephrol., *14*:115, 1980.

Lenowitz, H., and Graham, A. P.: Carcinoma of the penis. J. Urol., *56*:458, 1946.

Levine, R. L.: Urethral cancer. Cancer, *45*:1965, 1980.

Macdonald I., et al.: Exposure and suction drainage in the management of major dissective wounds. Surg. Gynecol. Obstet., *107*:532, 1958.

Mackenzie, A. R., and Whitmore, W. F.: Resection of pubic rami for urologic cancer. J. Urol., *100*:546, 1968.

Mantell, B. S., and Morgan, W. Y.: Queyrat's erythroplasia of the penis treated by beta particle irradiation. Br. J. Radiol., *12*:855, 1969.

Marcial, V. A., et al.: Carcinoma of the **penis. Radiology**, *79*:209, 1962.

Marshall, V. F.: Radical excision of locally **extensive** carcinoma of the deep male urethra. J. Urol., *78*:252, 1957.

Melicow, M. W., and Ganem, E. J.: Cancerous and precancerous lesions of the penis; a clinical and pathological study based on twenty-three cases. J. Urol., *55*:486, 1946.

Mukherjee, G. D.: Reconstruction of penis with urethra from groin and midthigh flap. J. Indian Med. Assoc., *75*:124, 1980.

Mullin, E. M., Anderson, E. E., and Paulson, D. F.: Carcinoma of the male urethra. J. Urol., *112*:610, 1974.

Murrell, D. S., and Williams, J. L.: Radiotherapy in the treatment of carcinoma of the penis. Br. J. Urol., *37*:211, 1965.

Narayana, A. S., et al.: Carcinoma of the penis. Cancer, *49*:2185, 1982.

Pack, G. T., and Ariel, I. M. (Eds.): Treatment of tumors of the penis. *In* Treatment of Cancer and Allied Diseases: Tumors of the Male Genitalia and the Urinary System. 2nd ed. New York, Harper & Row, 1963, p. 15.

Pack, G. T., and Rekers, P.: The management of malignant tumors in the groin; a report of 122 groin dissections. Am. J. Surg., 1942.

Perinetti, E., et al.: Unreliability of sentinel lymph node biopsy for staging penile carcinoma. J. Urol., *124*:734, 1980.

Peterson, D. T., Dockerty, M. B., Utz, D. C., and Symmonds, R. E.: The peril of primary carcinoma of the urethra in women. J. Urol., *110*:72, 1973.

Phelan, J. T., and Nadler, S. H.: A technique of hemipelvectomy. Surg. Gynecol. Obstet., *119*:311, 1964.

Pointon, R. C. S.: Carcinoma of the penis: External beam therapy. Proc. R. Soc. Med., *68*:779, 1975.

Prempree, T., et al.: Radiation therapy in primary carcinoma of the female urethra. Cancer, *54*:729, 1984.

Raffl, A. B.: The use of negative pressure under skin flaps after radical mastectomy. Ann. Surg., *136*:1048, 1952.

Raghavaiah, N. V.: Radiotherapy in the treatment of carcinoma of the male urethra. Cancer, *41*:1313, 1978.

Ray, B., and Guinan, P. D.: Primary carcinoma of the urethra. *In* Javadpour, N. (Ed.): Principles and Management of Urologic Cancer. Baltimore, Williams & Wilkins, 1979; pp. 445–473.

Ray, B., et al.: Experience with primary carcinoma of the male urethra. J. Urol., *117*:591, 1977.

Riches, E. W., and Cullen, T. H.: Carcinoma of the urethra. Br. J. Urol., *23*:209, 1951.

Riveros, M., et al.: Lymphadenography of the dorsal lymphatics of the penis. Cancer, *20*:2026, 1967.

Rouviere, H.: Anatomy of the Human Lymphatic System. Tobias, M. J. (transl.), Ann Arbor, Mich., Edwards Brothers, Inc., 1938.

Sen, A. K., et al.: Study of the lymphatic drainage from the growth in the penis by radioactive colloidal gold. Indian J. Cancer, *4*:295, 1967.

Shuttleworth, K. E. D., and Lloyd-Davies, R. W.: Radical resection for tumours involving the posterior urethra. Br. J. Urol., *41*:739, 1969.

Silvis, R. S., et al.: The use of continuous suction negative pressure instead of pressure dressing. Ann. Surg., *142*:252, 1955.

Skinner, D. G.: Management of extensive, localized neoplasms of the lower abdominal wall. Urology, *3*:34, 1974.

Skinner, D. G., et al.: The surgical management of squamous cell carcinoma of the penis. J. Urol., *107*:273, 1972.

Sklaroff, R. B., and Yagoda, A.: Cis-diaminedichloride platinum II (DDP) in the treatment of penile carcinoma. Cancer, *44*:1563, 1979.

Sklaroff, R. B., and Yagoda, A.: Methotrexate in the treatment of penile carcinoma. Cancer, *45*:214, 1980.

Smith, J. A., Jr., and Middleton, R. G.: The use of fluorescein in radical inguinal lymphadenectomy. J. Urol., *122*:754, 1979.

Sogani, P. C., et al.: Lymphocele after pelvic lymphadenectomy for urologic cancer. Urology, *17*:39, 1981.

Spratt, J. S., et al.: Anatomy and Surgical Technique of Groin Dissection. St. Louis, C. V. Mosby, 1965.

Staubitz, W. J., et al.: Carcinoma of the penis. Cancer, *8*:371, 1955.

Wagner, D. E., et al.: A new approach to radical retroperitoneal iliac and femoral node dissection. Arch. Surg., *103*:681, 1971.

Weiss, J., et al.: Melanoma of the male urethra: Surgical approach and pathological analysis. J. Urol., *128*:382, 1982.

Whitmore, W. F., Jr.: Tumors of the penis, urethra, scrotum and testis. *In* Campbell, M. F., and Harrison, J. H. (Eds.): Urology, Philadelphia, W. B. Saunders Co., 1970, p. 1201.

Whitmore, W. F., Jr.: Personal communication, 1975.

Whitmore, W. F., Jr., and Vagaiwala, M. R.: A technique of ilioinguinal lymph node dissection for carcinoma of the penis. Surg. Gynecol. Obstet., *159*:573, 1984.

Williams, J. L.: Carcinoma of the penis: Surgical treatment. Proc. R. Soc. Med., *68*:31, 1975.

Williams, K., and Butcher, H. R.: A technique for inguinal and iliac lymphadenectomy. Am. Surg., *27*:55, 1961.

Woodhall, J. P.: Radical groin surgery with particular reference to postoperative healing. Surgery, *33*:886, 1953.

Yagoda, A., et al.: Bleomycin, an antitumor antibiotic. Clinical experience in 274 patients. Ann. Intern. Med., *77*:861, 1972.

Young, H. H.: A radical operation for the cure of cancer of the penis. J. Urol., *26*:285, 1931.

CHAPTER 83

Surgery of Testicular Neoplasms

WILLET F. WHITMORE, JR., M.D.
MICHAEL J. MORSE, M.D.

Among the principal urologic cancers, testis tumors best conform to the traditional concept of primary tumor progressing to regional spread progressing to distant dissemination. The surgery of testis tumors can logically be discussed relative to each of these categories. Inguinal orchiectomy satisfies the criterion of adequate cancer surgery for the primary tumor and is accomplished with minimal risk and functional sacrifice. Retroperitoneal irradiation cures the majority of patients having seminoma and small-volume retroperitoneal lymph node metastasis. Retroperitoneal lymph node dissection (RPLND) cures the majority of those with small-volume regional lymph node metastasis from nonseminomatous germ cell testis tumors (NSGCTT) and offers the epitome of clinical staging accuracy for such patients. RPLND has been embraced by most urologic oncologists in North America as part of the treatment for patients with Stage I or II NSGCTT.

During the last 10 years, successful multidrug chemotherapy regimens have evolved for the treatment of advanced disease. Appropriate integration of surgery and chemotherapy has reduced the overall mortality rate for testis cancer to less than 15 per cent. The rationale and results of RPLND have been discussed in Chapter 33. This chapter provides a discussion of relevant anatomy and surgical technique.

PRIMARY TUMOR

Surgical Technique

Inguinal orchiectomy plays an unchallenged role in the treatment of testicular cancer regardless of cell type or clinical stage. Orchiectomy has several practical advantages, including (1) control of local disease with virtually 100 per cent effectiveness; (2) determination of histologic diagnosis and extent of local disease (P category); (3) cure of some patients with disease confined to the testis; and (4) little risk of side effects or complications and virtually no operative mortality.

The surgical principles and techniques of orchiectomy have been detailed elsewhere in the text.

Pathologic Characterization

The accuracy of pathologic staging is dependent upon the surgical specimen, the adequacy of the processing, and the interpretation thereof. Microscopic evaluation of the tunica, testicular appendages, and spermatic cord, in addition to the testis proper, provides relevant clinical information. The local growth patterns of testis tumors should all but ensure the adequacy of inguinal orchiectomy for local control.

The tunica albuginea provides a naturally resistant barrier to the local growth of testis tumors. Invasion of the epididymis or spermatic cord is uncommon (10 to 25 per cent) and involvement of the scrotum rare. Penetration of the tunica vaginalis is associated with a higher rate of distant metastasis but is not a prerequisite to such an event. In studying the relationships between P, N, and M categories in a series of 208 patients with nonseminomatous germ cell testis tumors (NSGCTT) treated at Memorial Sloan-Kettering Cancer Center (MSKCC) between 1975 and 1978, the local extent of the

TABLE 83–1. NSGCTT: Relationships Between Local Extent of Disease (P Category) and Nodal (N Category) and Distant (M Category) Metastases

Primary Tumor*	Clinical/Pathologic Stage			
	I	IIA	IIB,C	III
P1	46 (42%)	23 (21%)	26 (24%)	15 (14%)
P2	7 (25%)	1 (4%)	8 (29%)	12 (43%)
Px	26 (37%)	9 (13%)	19 (27%)	16 (23%)

*P1 = tumor confined to testis; P2 = invasion of tunica vaginalis, appendages, or spermatic cord
Modified from Whitmore, 1982.

primary tumor (many processed elsewhere) was unknown (Px) in one third of cases. The frequency and extent of metastasis (N and M categories) at the time of presentation were directly related to the P category of the primary testis tumor (Table 83–1). Roughly two thirds of those with a P1 primary lesion had either no (Stage I) or minimal (Stage IIA) evidence of retroperitoneal or distant disease after completion of surgicopathologic staging. In contrast, nearly three quarters of patients with a locally advanced primary tumor (P2, or invasion of the tunica vaginalis, appendages, or spermatic cord) harbored more extensive nodal disease or distant dissemination. During subsequent follow-up of 154 patients with disease that was deemed surgically resectable (some received "minimal" adjuvant chemotherapy), recurrence rates were higher in those with advanced primary lesions (Table 83–2). In patients with pathologic Stage I or II disease, invasion of the epididymis, testicular appendages, or spermatic cord was associated with an overall metastatic failure rate of greater than 50 per cent following apparently complete locoregional control (orchiectomy plus RPLND). When the primary tumor was con-

TABLE 83–2. Recurrence in Stages I and II Nonseminoma Related to P Category of the Primary Tumor

Primary Tumor*	Number of Patients with Recurrence		
	Surgical Stage (N Category)		
	I	II†	Total
P1	3/46 (6%)	5/44 (11%)	10/90 (11%)
P2	3/7 (43%)	4/6 (67%)	7/13 (53%)
Px	2/26 (7%)	3/25 (7%)	5/51 (10%)
Total	8/79 (10%)	12/75 (16%)	22/154 (14%)

*P1 = tumor confined to testis; P2 = invasion of tunica vaginalis, appendages, or spermatic cord.
†Adjuvant chemotherapy used in selected patients with Stage II disease.
Modified from Whitmore, 1982.

fined to the testis, recurrence was less likely (6 per cent in Stage I, 11 per cent in Stage II).

Although the experience is limited, the apparently higher rate of failure in patients with locally invasive testis tumors has led to the exclusion of such patients from trials involving surveillance (versus RPLND) for those with no clinical evidence of disease beyond the primary site (see also Chapter 33).

Inadequate or Inappropriate Surgery

Despite medical education on the subject of testis cancer, the frequency of physician-related delay or inappropriate treatment is considerable. Markland et al. (1973) reported that 19 of 36 patients referred to the University of Minnesota from 1965 to 1972 had undergone inadequate or inappropriate surgical excision of the primary tumor. They documented a risk of wound implantation or inguinal node metastasis subsequent to inadequate orchiectomy or transscrotal biopsy in 6 of 19 (32 per cent) cases and recommended hemiscrotectomy and inguinal node dissection in such patients. Roughly 25 per cent of patients referred to MSKCC with a diagnosis of testicular germ cell tumor over the last 30 years have undergone prior transscrotal exploration for the purpose of orchiectomy or biopsy, but the incidence of inguinal nodal involvement in such patients is very low (Klein et al., 1984). The M.D. Anderson Hospital and Tumor Institute (MDA) experience indicates that 32 of 224 (14 per cent) patients with testicular cancer seen between 1977 and 1979 were referred for treatment with a "tumor-contaminated scrotum"; yet the risk of subsequent local recurrence or spread to inguinal lymph nodes was small when appropriate cord excision and hemiscrotectomy were performed without inguinal lymph node dissection (Johnson and Babaian, 1980; Boileau and Steers, 1984).

Although the risk of local recurrence following transscrotal surgery is small, extension of the radiation portal to include the ipsilateral scrotum and groin is advised for patients with seminoma. The currently recommended treatment for patients with NSGCTT following such a misadventure is either removal of the retained spermatic cord segment in conjunction with excision of the previous scrotal incision or hemiscrotectomy (Fig. 83–1). Simple excision of the retained cord and previous incision site eliminates most, if not all, risk of local recurrence. Such is easily performed by a racquet-shaped

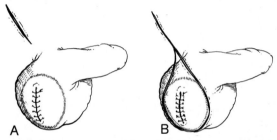

Figure 83–1. En bloc excision of residual spermatic cord and "contaminated" scrotum following transscrotal orchiectomy or biopsy. *A,* Two separate incisions. *B,* Racquet-shaped incision.

extension of the standard inguinal incision to encompass the scrotal site. Hemiscrotectomy involves a wider excision—to the midline raphe medially and inguinal skin crease laterally. If re-excision is planned in conjunction with simultaneous RPLND, the latter should be completed prior to the scrotal procedure to lessen the risk of tumor or bacterial contamination in the abdominal wound from the scrotal site. A small latex drain may be electively left in the scrotum if infection is suspected, but this is not a routine measure.

Sayegh et al. (1966) demonstrated that prior inguinal or scrotal surgery could alter the normal lymphatic drainage of the testis by establishing direct communications to ipsilateral inguinal lymph nodes. The majority of patients with inguinal node metastasis have a history of cryptorchidism (corrected or uncorrected), prior inguinal or scrotal surgery (hernia, varicocele repair, or tumor contamination), or massive retroperitoneal disease (with resultant retrograde spread). Reviews by Klein et al. (1984) and others indicate that the rate of metastasis to inguinal lymph nodes is exceedingly small. Although advocated in the past by some (Markland et al., 1973), prophylactic inguinal lymph dissection in patients with NSGCTT is not currently recommended, for the following reasons: (1) The overall incidence of groin metastasis from testis cancer is low regardless of prior history; (2) the operative morbidity of groin dissection (infection, peripheral edema) is high; (3) retrograde dissemination from bulky retroperitoneal disease is the most probable cause of spread to the groin; (4) multidrug chemotherapy may be effective in controlling retroperitoneal nodal metastasis (and would presumably have similar effects on nodal deposits elsewhere); and (5) the inguinal lymph nodes can usually be monitored closely by palpation, and biopsy readily done if metastasis is suspected. In the event of proved inguinal lymph node metastasis,

cisplatin-based chemotherapy is justified as the primary management, reserving groin dissection for residual disease.

Chemotherapy and the Primary Tumor

The evidence for a blood-testis barrier stems from two established observations: (1) Drug concentrations are generally lower in the seminiferous tubules than in the blood or other extravascular spaces; and (2) the testis represents a common site of relapse in childhood leukemia (Forrest et al., 1981; Stoffel et al., 1975). Fowler et al. (1979) reported second testicular germ cell tumors in three patients who either were receiving or had just completed chemotherapy for metastasic disease from a contralateral testis tumor. They also reported two patients with persistent, viable tumor in the testis following chemotherapy for metastasic NSGCTT (Fowler and Whitmore, 1981). Calvo et al. (1983) found viable tumor in three of five patients receiving chemotherapy as primary treatment for disseminated NSGCTT. Greist et al. (1984) noted persistent cancer (3/20) or residual teratoma (6/20) within the testis of patients treated initially with chemotherapy for metastasic disease. These observations emphasize the necessity for orchiectomy despite chemotherapy when the latter is delivered prior to surgical excision of the primary testicular tumor. If a palpable testis tumor responds completely to primary multidrug chemotherapy, inguinal orchiectomy is currently advocated. If, however, physical examination and testicular ultrasound study are normal prior to and following chemotherapy for a presumed extragonadal primary lesion, surveillance only of the testes appears justified (Fig. 83–2).

REGIONAL SPREAD

In 1898 Chevassu and Picque reported a mortality rate of 80 per cent in patients with testis cancer treated by orchiectomy alone. This and other similar clinical experiences (Kober, 1899) stimulated anatomic studies of the testicular lymphatics by Most (1898) and Cuneo (1901). These and later studies by Jamieson and Dobson (1910) and by Rouviere (1932) established the rationale for surgical excision of the primary tumor and regional lymph nodes. Cuneo is credited with performing the first successful retroperitoneal lymph node dissection in

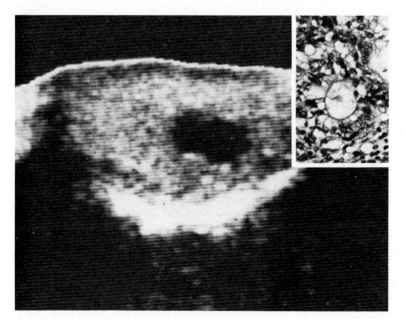

Figure 83–2. Testicular ultrasound study of a 28-year-old man who presented with back pain and an abdominal mass but clinically normal testes. At diagnostic laparotomy, an incisional biopsy of an unresectable retroperitoneal mass revealed embryonal carcinoma. Cyclic multidrug chemotherapy resulted in a 90 per cent reduction of the abdominal mass on serial CT scans. Persistent endodermal sinus tumor was detected in the testis (inset) despite chemotherapy, but no histologically viable elements were noted in lymph nodes excised simultaneously during RPLND.

1906, although Roberts (1902) had performed a similar procedure in a patient who died of postoperative complications. Between the world wars, few advocated lymphadenectomy over retroperitoneal irradiation for regional lymph node metastasis. Following World War II, the procedure gained favor in the United States. Lewis (1948) reported a large series of patients treated successfully by RPLND via the lumboinguinal approach, while Cooper et al. (1950) demonstrated the utility of the thoracoabdominal incision. Mallis and Patton (1958) later emphasized the transabdominal bilateral dissection of the retroperitoneal nodes. Ray et al. (1974) defined the limits of a modified lymphadenectomy for patients with Stage I NGSCTT in an attempt to reduce the extent of the surgical dissection and the frequency of ejaculatory dysfunction. Donohue (1977) added a suprahilar lymphadenectomy to the conventional bilateral lymph node dissection.

The rationale of retroperitoneal lymph node dissection in patients with testis cancer is based upon the following considerations: (1) Retroperitoneal lymph node metastasis is usually the first and frequently the sole site of metastasis spread. Survival rates in patients with retroperitoneal lymph node metastasis treated by orchiectomy and RPLND are in the range of 50 to 65 per cent. Patients whose regional nodes are pathologically free of metastasis following orchiectomy are generally cured (85 to 95 per cent), treatment failures in this group being most commonly identified by pulmonary metastasis. The logical inference is that the majority of testis tumors spread initially to retroperitoneal lymph nodes and that early vascular dissemination is uncommon. (2) Retroperitoneal lymph node dissection provides the most accurate assessment of regional lymph node spread. Despite progressive improvement in clinical staging procedures, lymphadenectomy will identify metastasis in approximately 10 to 15 per cent of patients with clinically negative staging evaluations. As clinical staging methods improve, the false negative staging error can be expected to diminish, thus weakening the argument for RPLND as a staging procedure. Although variability in the initial site of lymph node metastasis discourages random surgical biopsy, fine-needle aspiration of suspicious lymph nodes identified by lymphangiography (LAG) or computerized tomography (CT), or both, may provide pathologic confirmation without formal RPLND.

Retroperitoneal Lymphatics

The retroperitoneum is rich in lymphatics that form a chain from the inguinal ligaments to the diaphragm. Many nodes and vessels are grouped about the larger vascular trunks, uniting the lymph drainage from the extremities, pelvis, testes, and abdomen. Lymphatics from the lumboaortic (and mesenteric) nodes converge at the cisterna chyli, which is an inconstant saclike dilatation approximately 5 cm long situated in front of the bodies of L1 and L2 immediately medial to the abdominal aorta. The thoracic duct begins at the upper end of the cisterna chyli at the lower border of T12 and enters the thorax through the aortic hiatus behind the diaphragmatic crura.

The lymphatics of the testis drain to the area of its embryologic origin within the retroperitoneal space, while the epididymis drains into the pelvic lymph nodes. Accumulated experience from anatomic studies (Most, 1898; Cuneo, 1901; Jamieson and Dobson, 1910; Rouviere, 1932), radiologic procedures (Busch and Sayegh, 1963; Busch et al., 1965; Chiappa et al., 1966; Sayegh et al., 1966; Wahlquist et al., 1966), and surgical explorations (Whitmore, 1960, 1968; Ray et al., 1974; Donohue et al., 1982) has provided considerable data regarding the primary and secondary lymphatic drainage of the testis, which may be summarized as follows:

1. Four to eight collecting lymphatics emerging from the testicular mediastinum accompany the spermatic vessels upward through the inguinal canal and continue cephalad into the retroperitoneal space. As the spermatic vessels cross the ureter, the accompanying lymphatic channels fan out in concave arches to the lymph nodes distributed around the aorta and vena cava. Subsequent drainage occurs by way of the cisterna chyli and thoracic duct into the left supraclavicular nodes and subclavian vein. Anatomic variations of the thoracic duct permit metastasis to mediastinal and supraclavicular lymph nodes and, infrequently, to those of the cervical or axillary regions. Major lymphatic trunks, communicating with the thoracic duct, occasionally (approximately 10 per cent) drain to the right supraclavicular nodes. Numerous other potential lymphaticovenous communications may become manifest with lymphatic obstruction or trauma, explaining the observed variations in metastasic sites.

2. The lymphatics of the epididymis drain into the pelvic nodes, while those of the scrotum drain into the inguinal nodes. Metastasis in inguinal lymph nodes may be a consequence of prior iliac, inguinal, or scrotal surgery, with resultant disruption of the usual lymphatic pathways of the testis, or of retrograde lymphatic spread from disease in the retroperitoneal or pelvic lymph nodes.

3. The primary lymphatic drainage from the right testis is to the interaortocaval, precaval, preaortic, paracaval, right common iliac, and right external iliac nodes, in that order. Subsequent drainage is to the para-aortic, left common iliac, and left external iliac nodes (Ray et al., 1974) and to the supahilar nodes (Donohue, 1977).

4. The primary lymphatic drainage from the left testis is to the para-aortic, preaortic, left common iliac, and left external iliac nodes, in that order. Subsequent drainage is to the interaortocaval, precaval, paracaval, right common iliac, and right external iliac nodes (Ray et al., 1974) and to the suprahilar nodes (Donohue, 1977).

5. Most, but not all, lymph nodes draining the testicle are filled when pedal lymphangiography is performed; additional lymph nodes are visualized when adjunctive testicular or funicular lymphangiograms are performed (Busch and Sayegh, 1963; Busch et al., 1965; Chiappa et al., 1966; Sayegh et al., 1966; Wahlqvist et al., 1966).

6. Lymphangiographic crossover from the right to the left is apparently common and may be immediate, whereas crossover from the left to the right is apparently rare and seems to occur only after the primary nodes are filled.

Extent of Lymphadenectomy

One would need to know the details of the lymphadenectomy, including site, size, and number as well as the microscopic pathology of metastasic nodes in patients receiving no further form of therapy, to precisely define the relationships between methods of RPLND and survival, and such data are not available. Experiences from various major treatment centers for testis tumors (Indiana, California, Italy, London, MSKCC, MDA, and others), wherein differences in RPLND and in chemotherapy routines may or do exist, indicate that such differences have little, if any, demonstrable impact on end results.

BILATERAL LYMPH NODE DISSECTION

Mallis and Patton (1958) documented the rationale for a bilateral retroperitoneal lymph node dissection in patients with regional nodal disease from NSGCTT, although the same field of dissection was defined earlier by Hinman (1914). The limits of this dissection extend to the renal pedicles superiorly, to a point 2 cm below the common iliac bifurcation inferiorly, and to the ureters laterally (Fig. 83–3). All the spermatic lymphatics and blood vessels on the tumor-bearing side and the upper one third of the contralateral spermatic vessels are included in such dissection. All apparent lymphatic and perivascular tissues are removed from the lateral, anterior, posterior, and medial aspects of the major vessels thus defined.

Surgicopathologic correlations from

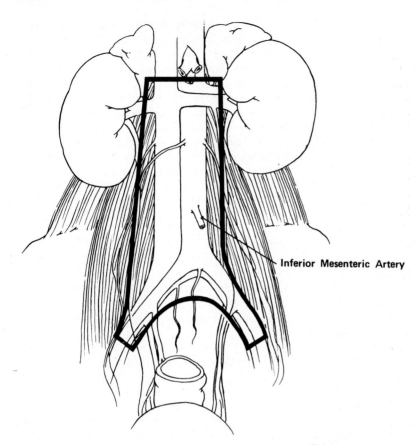

Inferior Mesenteric Artery

Figure 83–3. Bilateral retroperitoneal node dissection.

RPLND have suggested that a "modified" bilateral dissection would encompass the sites of retroperitoneal lymph node metastasis in the majority of instances in which the disease proved resectable. Such a modified dissection is usually employed at MSKCC for patients with clinically and surgically negative lymph nodes, a complete bilateral extirpation being reserved for those with positive lymph nodes, documented by preoperative or intraoperative staging (Ray et al., 1974). While only the extent of the modified bilateral dissection is defined herein, the conventional complete bilateral dissection will be accomplished by combining the approaches described for tumors originating in the right or left testis, respectively, and basically includes the area of bilateral dissection described by Patton and Mallis (1959) and earlier by Hinman et al. (1923).

MODIFIED BILATERAL LYMPH NODE DISSECTION

For a right-sided tumor, the dissection includes removal of all lymphatic, fatty, and areolar tissue from (1) the lateral, anterior, posterior, and medial aspects (interaortocaval) of the inferior vena cava from the renal vessels

above to the aortic bifurcation below; (2) the anterior aspect of the aorta from the left renal vein above the aortic bifurcation below, usually preserving the inferior mesenteric artery; (3) the lateral aspect of the aorta for 3 to 4 cm below the level of the angle between the aorta and the left renal vessels (i.e., to the level of origin of the inferior mesenteric artery) as far laterally as the termination of the left spermatic vein; and (4) the aortic bifurcation distally, the right common iliac vessels, and the proximal 2 cm of the right external iliac vessels (Fig. 83–4).

For a left-sided tumor, the dissection includes removal of all lymphatic, fatty, and areolar tissue from (1) the lateral, anterior, posterior, and medial aspects (interaortocaval) of the aorta from the renal vessels above to the aortic bifurcation below; (2) the anterior aspect of the inferior vena cava from the renal vessels above to the aortic bifurcation below; and (3) the aortic bifurcation distally and the left common iliac vessels and proximal 2 cm of the left external iliac vessels (Fig. 83–5).

The renal vessels are usually cleanly dissected within 3 to 4 cm of the aorta and vena cava but are not dissected into the renal hilum. The ipsilateral boundary of dissection is the

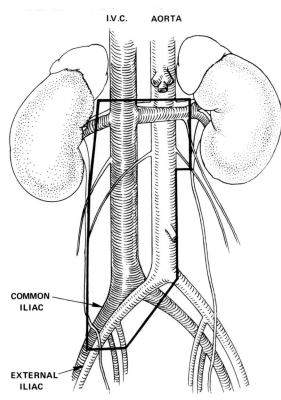

Figure 83–4. Modified bilateral dissection for right-sided tumor.

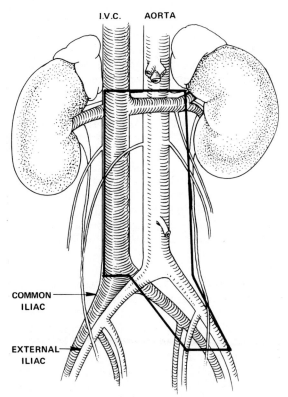

Figure 83–5. Modified bilateral dissection for left-sided tumor.

ureter. The ipsilateral main sympathetic trunk is usually preserved, although its communicating rami are sacrificed from the level of L1 to L3. The inferior mesenteric artery and vein and the various lumbar arteries and veins may or may not be sacrificed, depending upon the size and distribution of metastasis. The area between the common iliac arteries in front of the left common iliac vein (interiliac) has commonly been dissected, whether the tumor is on the right or on the left side.

The ipsilateral spermatic vessels down to the internal ring and the proximal 8 to 10 cm of the contralateral spermatic vessels are removed along with various amounts of adjacent fat. Invasion of the epididymis or spermatic cord by the primary tumor is an indication for extending the dissection inferiorly along the ipsilateral external iliac vessels to Poupart's ligament, including the obturator nodes.

SUPRAHILAR LYMPHADENECTOMY

The rationale of a suprahilar dissection has been largely developed from the experiences of Donohue (1977, 1982) (Fig. 83–6). In a preliminary communication concerning 28 patients with resectable retroperitoneal lymph node metastasis, Donohue documented suprahilar disease in approximately one quarter of those with infrahilar metastasis (Donohue, 1977). A later surgicopathologic study indicated that in patients with negative nodes below the renal hilum, isolated suprahilar metastasis was rarely encountered (1 in 100 patients). In 40 patients with limited infrahilar disease (fewer than five positive nodes and no nodes larger than 2 cm in diameter), only three had positive suprahilar nodes. In two of these patients, suprahilar disease was documented in tissues apparently contiguous with or adjacent to the involved infrarenal lymph nodes, suggesting that such metastasis could be excised during an appropriately executed "conventional" bilateral RPLND (see earlier). In 43 patients with a moderate infrahilar tumor burden (five or more positive nodes or node(s) exceeding 2 cm in diameter), 16 (37 per cent) had suprahilar metastasis. With massive retroperitoneal disease, involvement of lymph nodes above the renal vessels was frequently documented (14 of 17, or 85 per cent).

Donohue's observations clearly demonstrate that spread to regions adjacent to the primary site of nodal metastasis becomes more likely as the burden of regional node involvement increases. However, because the primary lymphatic drainage of the testis is not to suprahilar lymph nodes, in the absence of bulky disease these lymph nodes rarely contain metas-

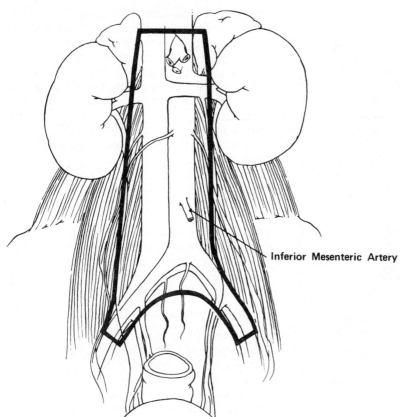

Figure 83–6. Bilateral retroperitoneal lymph node dissection "extended" to include suprahilar regions.

Inferior Mesenteric Artery

tasic disease. Furthermore, because most suprahilar lymph nodes are located *behind the aorta between the crura of the diaphragm,* these lymph nodes are difficult, if not impossible, to resect and are not included in the usual suprahilar dissection (Schmeller et al., 1981; Crawford, 1984) (Fig. 83–7).

COMMENT

Uncertainty regarding the optimal extent of the lymphadenectomy is attributable to the lack of consistent definitions of unilateral and bilateral dissections, to variations in the thoroughness with which such dissections are performed, to undefined differences in the site, size, number, and microscopic pathology of resected nodes, to variations in the extent of pathologic study and interpretations of dissection specimens, and to the beneficial and nullifying effects of chemotherapy. (For example, if all patients with suprahilar lymph node involvement were destined to fail with distant metastases, their survival might depend more on response to chemotherapy than on whether a suprahilar dissection was performed. Retrocrural supradiaphragmatic metastasis is a case

in point.) At MSKCC a preoperative ipsilateral lymphangiogram gives an indication of lymph node distribution and metastasis that is materially useful in planning the extent of dissection. Based on a less than 10 per cent error in operative clinical impression of the status of the retroperitoneal lymph nodes (Ray et al., 1974), it is suggested that when the nodes are judged negative clinically and at exploration, a modified bilateral lymph node dissection should be performed for either right- or left-side tumors. When the lymph nodes are suspect or are grossly positive, a bilateral lymph node dissection is recommended, suprahilar dissection of any palpable nodes being included.

Indications for Retroperitoneal Lymphadenectomy

Uncertainties relating to the optimal management of the retroperitoneal lymph nodes (surgery, irradiation, or chemotherapy, or a combination of these) are presented in Chapter 33; the indications for RPLND may be summarized as follows:

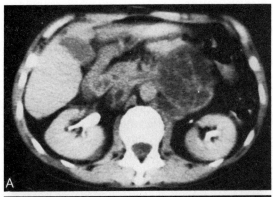

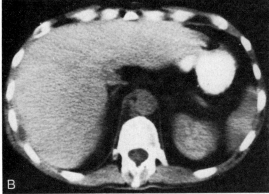

Figure 83–7. Representative pretreatment CT scans obtained from a 34-year-old male with a nonseminomatous testis tumor and a bulky retroperitoneal metastasis *(A)*. An enlarged retrocrural node is demonstrated *(B)*. Retrocrural lymphadenopathy is common in patients with suprahilar lymph node metastasis (Schmeller et al., 1981). Boundaries of a transabdominal retroperitoneal lymphadenectomy with or without an additional suprahilar dissection fail to encompass such retrocrural metastasis unless the diaphragmatic crura are incised. This maneuver is more readily accomplished through a thorocoabdominal exposure, wherein the entire diaphragmatic leaflet can be divided. (The overall impact of extended excisions remains undefined and debatable, considering the effectiveness of current chemotherapy regimens. The demonstration of suprahilar or retrocrural metastasis justifies initial treatment with platinum-based multidrug chemotherapy.)

1. Nonseminomatous germ cell neoplasms
   a. Clinical Stage I or II.
   b. Clinical Stage III after downstaging by chemotherapy or radiotherapy, or both.
2. Seminomatous germ cell neoplasms
   a. Clinical Stage I or II with elevated alpha fetoprotein.
   b. Clinical Stage II with progressive radiographic (CT, LAG) abnormality following "curative" doses of irradiation to the retroperitoneum or multiagent chemotherapy, or both.
   c. Clinical Stage II with persistent elevations of the beta subunit of human chorionic gonadotropin following "curative" doses of irradiation to the retroperitoneum or systemic combination chemotherapy, or both.

Perioperative Management

PREOPERATIVE CARE

Investigation. In addition to the standard clinical (electrocardiogram), laboratory (complete blood count; determinations of serum electrolytes and acid-base balance, proteins, albumin, calcium, and glucose; renal and liver studies; tumor marker levels; urinanalysis), and radiologic investigations (chest x-ray, intravenous pyelogram, lymphangiogram, computerized tomography of abdomen and pelvis, including or excluding the chest) outlined in Chapter 33, patients scheduled for a retroperitoneum lymphadenectomy should have a coagulogram (platelets, partial thromboplastin time, and prothrombin time determinations). In selected cases, a barium enema study, an upper gastrointestinal series, an inferior vena cavogram, or an aortogram with selective visceral studies may be indicated.

PREOPERATIVE PREPARATION

Chest. To ensure optimal postoperative care, the patient should be familiarized before surgery with chest physiotherapy, deep breathing and coughing exercises, and bedside mechanical rebreathing devices. Patients should refrain from smoking for at least 2 weeks preoperatively. Patients pretreated with bleomycin should have a determination of arterial blood gas levels and pulmonary function. Immediate preoperative baseline Swan-Ganz catheter determinations are also advisable in patients with compromised pulmonary reserve.

Bowel. A proper mechanical bowel preparation technically facilitates the dissection and may minimize the extent and duration of postoperative ileus. Patients are placed on a low-residue diet 48 hours and on clear fluids 24 hours prior to operation. Citrate of magnesia (250 ml) is given orally 36 hours prior to surgery, and cleansing enemas are given 36 and 12 hours preoperatively. Castor oil (30 to 60 ml given 24 hours before surgery) greatly diminishes the intraluminal content of the small bowel. Such bowel preparation undoubtedly causes some preoperative dehydration, but this has not been a recognized problem in young adults, who are hydrated intravenously for 8 hours preoperatively. Determination of the serum potassium levels 12 hours prior to surgery is advisable, since bowel preparation may result in hypokalemia.

Patients should be advised of the probable loss of seminal emission and of the availability (and expectations) of sperm-banking facilities. General anesthesia should not be administered within 48 hours after lymphangiography (because of pulmonary toxicity). Prophylactic antibiotics are not routinely used.

INTRAOPERATIVE CARE

A rapid reduction in the effective circulating blood volume may occur during retroperitoneal lymphadenectomy. Continuous oscilloscope monitoring of the electrocardiogram to detect cardiac irritability is advisable. Insensible fluid losses related to third-space sequestration consequent to bowel manipulation and those related to lymphadenectomy are unavoidable. Technical misadventure may result in sudden, rapid blood loss. At least two large veins should be cannulated preoperatively with large plastic needles (not in the lower extremities).

During prolonged procedures, serial hematocrit measurements provide a rough guideline as to the type of infusion required. Hematocrits above 45 are an indication for colloid and/or crystalloid administration and those below 30 for whole blood administration. Central venous pressure monitoring is more a reflection of right-sided cardiac competence than of blood volume and therefore can be misleading unless the overall clinical picture is taken into account. The urine ouput should be maintained at a minimum of 40 to 60 ml per hour.

Periodic hyperinflation of the lungs may decrease the risk or severity of atelectasis. Patients who have received bleomycin require more intensive pre- and postoperative monitoring. Bleomycin toxicity, which is usually dose-related, may occur after total doses of 100 mg or more. It consists of an interstitial fibrosis that may be clinically silent but is reflected in moderate obstructive lung disease and an impairment of carbon dioxide diffusion. Goldiner et al. (1978) suggested that the alveolar membrane lesion caused by bleomycin may be severely aggravated by levels of oxygen that would normally be safe and possibly may be aggravated by overhydration with crystalloid. These findings have led to the adoption of the following guidelines for patients who have been heavily pretreated with bleomycin and who are undergoing general anesthesia: (1) The concentration of oxygen in the inspired air (FI_{O_2}) should not exceed 24 per cent, either intraoperatively

or during the postoperative period, and (2) a somewhat negative fluid balance is sought. These objectives are most precisely achieved by Swan-Ganz catheter monitoring of the pulmonary artery pressure, cardiac output, arterial blood gas levels, pulmonary shunt fraction, and total body oxygen consumption. The variation in alveolar-arterial oxygen gradient before and after surgery is significantly lower in patients so treated, and there appears to be a parallel reduction in postoperative morbidity and mortality.

POSTOPERATIVE CARE

Proper postoperative care is contingent upon an appreciation and anticipation of postoperative complications. In the immediate postoperative period, serial monitoring of the vital signs (pulse, blood pressure, temperature, and respiration), of the urine output, and of hematocrit levels is indicated. Fluid management should be tailored to the static and dynamic losses and to the overall clinical picture. Attention should be given to the extent of abdominal pain; serial abdominal examinations are performed to detect inordinate peritoneal irritation. A nasogastric sump drainage instituted at the time of laparotomy should be continued until small bowel peristalsis returns. Ambulation is encouraged within the first postoperative day, and the urethral catheter is usually removed the morning following surgery. During the first 4 to 5 postoperative days, serial examination of the chest, abdomen, and lower extremities will aid in the early detection of potential complications in these areas.

Operative Technique for Lymphadenectomy

The usual retroperitoneal lymph node dissection (RPLND) may be accomplished through a variety of approaches, including the extraperitoneal lumboinguinal approach (Chevassu, 1910; Lewis, 1948), the extrapleural extraperitoneal approach (Nagamatsu, 1959), the chevron approach (Chute et al., 1967), the thoracoabdominal approach (Cooper et al., 1950), or the transabdominal transperitoneal approach (Mallis and Patton, 1958). Various other incisions (Fraley et al., 1977; Catalona and Rubenstein, 1978) provide wide exposure to retroperitoneal structures without entering the peritoneal cavity. The extraperitoneal lumboinguinal approach (Chevassu, 1910; Hinman, 1914; Lewis, 1948) provides less exposure than other approaches, not only for dissection across the midline but also for dissection at the level of the renal vessels and above. The transabdominal and thoracoabdominal approaches are the most widely used at present (Fig. 83–8).

TRANSABDOMINAL APPROACH

The midline or paramedian transabdominal approach was first utilized by Roberts in 1902 and was reported by Mallis and Patton in 1958. This has been the usual approach in the last 800 RPLND's at MSKCC. Usually it permits facile dissection on either side of the midline to the upper margins of the renal vessels. Higher exposures can be obtained by costal extensions into the eighth or ninth interspace but are necessary in less than 5 per cent of the procedures. This approach permits rapid opening and closure of the wound, affords optimal access to the great vessels, and is associated with little postoperative morbidity.

THORACOABDOMINAL APPROACH

The thoracoabdominal approach described by von Mikulicz in 1896 was first reported for RPLND by Cooper et al. in 1950 and later was discussed in detail by Skinner and Leadbetter (1971). The patient is placed in the lateral position, the body being torqued 10 degrees posteriorly. The incision begins in the posterior axillary line over the tenth rib and is continued anteriorly and inferiorly into the right lower quadrant just lateral to the rectus muscle. The tenth rib is resected, the pleural and retroperitoneal spaces are opened, and the diaphragm is divided dorsolaterally. A right-sided incision permits satisfactory exposure across the midline up to the level of the superior mesenteric artery and above, whereas with a left-sided exposure, dissection across the midline is hampered by the superior and inferior mesenteric arteries. The inferior mesenteric artery may be divided to facilitate exposure.

TECHNIQUE FOR RETROPERITONEAL LYMPHADENECTOMY BY A MIDLINE TRANSABDOMINAL APPROACH

The patient is placed in the supine position, and the skin of the chest wall, abdomen, pubis, genitalia, and upper thighs is suitably prepared. A Foley catheter is inserted and connected to continuous drainage. A midline incision is made from the xiphicostal junction to a point midway between the umbilicus and the symphysis pubis. This incision may be extended to the symphysis pubis if a pelvic lymph node dissection is necessary.

Upon opening the peritoneum it is important to obtain complete muscular paralysis and to institute sump nasogastric suction. Division of the falciform ligament allows for upward displacement of the liver, as the wound edges are spread by two self-retaining Balfour retractors. Preliminary palpation and inspection of the liver, spleen, pancreas, kidneys, bowel, and retroperitoneal lymph nodes are carried out to determine operability and the presence of metastases. When large retroperitoneal tumors are encountered, it is advisable to palpate the aorta

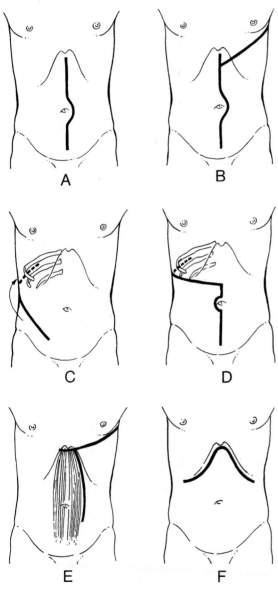

Figure 83–8. Surgical approaches to retroperitoneal lymphadenectomy. *A,* Midline incision. *B,* Midline incision with costal extension. *C,* Thoracoabdominal approach. *D,* Thoracoabdominal midline incision. *E,* Thoracoabdominal paramedian incision. *F,* Chevron incision.

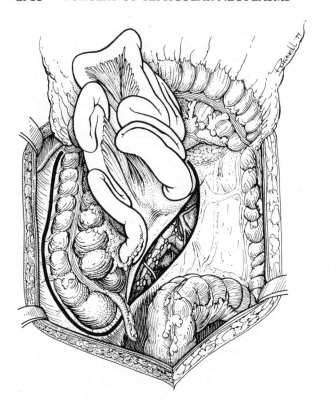

Figure 83–9. Incision of the posterior parietal peritoneum over the aorta. This incision extends from the ligament of Treitz along the left side of the root of the small bowel mesentery to the ileocecal region. It may be electively extended superiorly and medially to the duodenojejunal flexure and inferolaterally around the cecum and ascending colon.

near the diaphragmatic hiatus to locate a "tumor-free" area in the event that rapid temporary occlusion becomes necessary. The greater omentum and the transverse colon are then reflected superiorly onto the chest between warm moist packs.

The small bowel is displaced to the right or exteriorized between warm moist packs, and an incision is then made in the posterior parietal peritoneum, medial to the inferior mesenteric vein (Fig. 83–9). This incision is continued cephalad to the ligament of Treitz and is extended superiorly and medially to the duodenojejunal flexure, allowing for superior mobilization of the fourth portion of the duodenum and pancreas. At this point, condensations of the ligament of Treitz and several large intestinal lymphatic trunks draining into the retroperitoneal lymphatics will be encountered; it is best to secure their divided ends with hemoclips or ligatures. The incision in the posterior parietal peritoneum is continued inferiorly along the medial aspect of the small bowel mesentery and extended across the right gonadal vessels, ureter, and common iliac vessels, around the cecum, and up the right paracolic gutter along the white line of Toldt. The duodenum is then kocherized, allowing cephalad reflection and exterioration of the small bowel, cecum, and ascending colon onto the chest wall, where they are protected by moist laparotomy pads or a

bowel bag, or both (Fig. 83–10). Retraction superiorly of the exteriorized viscera may be further facilitated by a stationary Gallagher retractor or large Deaver retractors.

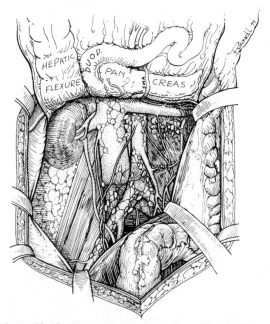

Figure 83–10. The retroperitoneal space. The duodenum has been kocherized; its second, third, and fourth portions have been reflected superiorly along with the pancreas and superior mesenteric artery. The entire right colon has been mobilized and exteriorized.

Injury to important structures is best avoided by defining the limits of dissection prior to proceeding with lymphadenectomy. The surgeon should be cognizant of the following structures by means of inspection and palpation: the superior and inferior mesenteric arteries, the ureters, the renal vessels, and the pancreas. The origin of the superior mesenteric artery from the aorta should be defined. Undue traction or retractor compression of this vessel must be avoided; periodic inspection for pulsations and small bowel color is important. The celiac axis is not visualized by this approach unless a costal extension is added and the left paracolic gutter incised to allow medial reflection of the spleen and stomach (Fig. 83–11). In the latter case, the celiac axis is more readily approached from the left side of the aorta.

The right ureter may be located beneath the spermatic vessels and retracted laterally with a soft rubber tape to protect it from injury. To isolate the left ureter, a plane is bluntly developed between the left leaf of the incised posterior parietal peritoneum, with the colonic mesentery arterior and the retroperitoneal lymphatic space posterior. The origins of the inferior mesenteric artery, the left ureter, and the left psoas muscle are specifically exposed. The inferior mesenteric artery may need to be sacrificed to improve exposure but can be preserved in most instances.

The actual lymphadenectomy is electively begun in the left hilar region (Fig. 83–12). Attention is directed first to the left renal vein, and the renal perivascular lymphatic tissue is mobilized inferiorly. The adrenal (with or without the inferior phrenic), spermatic, and lumbar venous tributaries are tied with 3–0 silk and then divided. The left renal artery(ies) is (are) identified at the origin from the aorta and dissected free of areolar and lymphatic tissue. The perivascular tissue in the immediate infrarenal aorta is then cleared, remaining as close as possible to the vessel wall without developing a subadventitial plane. The spermatic arteries will be encountered, and early ligature of these vessels prevents the subadventitial hematoma that often results when they are avulsed from the aorta.

Inferior traction on the renal hilar lymphatics and superior countertraction on the renal vessels by means of a vein retractor expose the posterosuperior terminations of the hilar lymphatics. Frequently, the short lumbar tributary to the left renal vein courses through these hilar lymphatics, and the vein should be secured close to the medial border of the psoas muscle. The ureteropelvic junction constitutes the lateral limit of dissection and may become visible at this point. The left spermatic vein often has small renal capsular communications that are easily secured and divided.

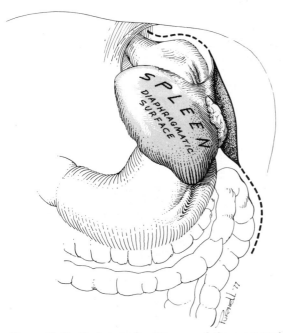

Figure 83–11. Technique for exposure of the suprarenal aorta. The incision in the left paracolic gutter along the white line of Toldt is extended superiorly to include the splenophrenic ligament and the parietal peritoneal attachments of the greater curvature, fundus, and gastroesophageal junction. The proximal descending colon, splenic flexure, spleen, body and tail of the pancreas, greater curvature of the stomach, fundus, and gastroesophageal junction are then reflected "en bloc" medially. This provides easy access to the suprarenal aorta (see Figure 83–15).

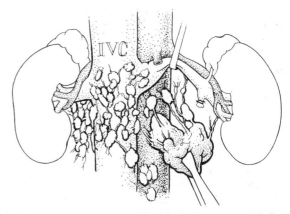

Figure 83–12. Left renal hilar lymphadenectomy. Inferior traction on the renal hilar lymphatics and superior countertraction on the renal vessels expose the terminations of the hilar lymphatics, which may be secured by ligature or hemoclip. It is important to remain as close as possible to the wall of the major vessels without developing a subadventitial plane.

The hilar lymphatics are then reflected medially against the aorta, the plane of dissection proceeding immediately anterior to the psoas fascia. Close to the aorta, the posterior layer of Gerota's fascia will be encountered and should be incised at its musculovertebral attachment to facilitate mobilization of the retroaortic nodes. Following skeletonization of the left renal vessels, the fibrofatty and lymphatic tissue anterior to the aorta may be divided from the origin of the superior mesenteric artery to the aortic bifurcation. The spermatic arteries are secured with ligatures and divided. (Throughout the procedure it is important to ligate or clip the cut ends of visible lymphatic channels, as this lessens postoperative lymphatic leakage. Hemoclips are generally not advisable on the aorta or vena cava, since they are so easily avulsed during the maneuvers of dissection.) The inferior mesenteric artery is then skeletonized for a distance of about 3 cm, including the immediately adjacent descending colon mesenteric nodes with retroperitoneal lymph node specimen. When necessary, this artery can be sacrificed without apparent untoward effects, provided that the marginal colonic artery is present and intact.

The para-aortic tissue may be reflected laterally to expose the lumbar vessels. The lumbar arteries can usually be preserved without compromising the extent or quality of the dissection. The lumbar sympathetic trunk is preserved, but numerous small communicating rami adherent to the lymph node mass are sacrificed. The lateral retroaortic tissues are mobilized during this phase of dissection, a step that facilitates later dissection of the interaortocaval region. Lymph node dissection then proceeds along the anterior and lateral aspects of the aorta, care being taken not to injure any lower pole renal vessels, which should always be anticipated. As the lymphatic tissue is cleared from the anterior psoas fascia and lateral aspect of the aorta, the fossa of Marcille will be encountered inferiorly, and care must be taken not to avulse the iliopsoas vessels and any small muscular branches from the left common iliac vessels. The common iliac artery and the proximal 2 cm of the left external iliac artery are then clearly dissected.

Attention is directed next to the precaval, paracaval, and lateral retrocaval nodes, and a similar dissection is carried out. The right spermatic vein is ligated at the vena cava, and the right renal vein and artery are skeletonized. Communications between the ureteral and right spermatic vessels are secured close to the ureter, allowing for lateral mobilization of the ureter from the area of dissection. The right common

iliac and the proximal 2 cm of the right external iliac artery are then dissected.

The interaortocaval and medial retrocaval and retroaortic lymph node dissection is then carried out. This will be facilitated by prior mobilization of the great vessels and lateral retraction of each by means of a vein or brain retractor. The right renal artery is isolated and cleaned throughout its retrocaval course. Care must be taken to secure all proximal lymphatic communications, as tributaries to the cisterna chyli are located in this region. The correct plane of dissection is immediately anterior to the anterior spinal ligament, which should be cleanly exposed in its entirety. It may be necessary during this part of the dissection to sacrifice one or more lumbar arteries and/or veins.

During the interiliac dissection, injury to the left common iliac vein is avoided by anterior reflection of the right common iliac artery and early ligature of the venous tributaries, which may otherwise be avulsed as traction is applied to the interiliac nodal tissue. Finally, on the side of the testicular tumor, the spermatic vessels are traced to the internal inguinal ring and dissected en bloc, sometimes with a surrounding cuff of peritoneum and properitoneal fat. The previously ligated ends (from orchiectomy) are then gently avulsed from the inguinal canal.

At the completion of a bilateral dissection, the great vessels should be skeletonized (Fig. 83–13). The anterior spinal ligament is easily

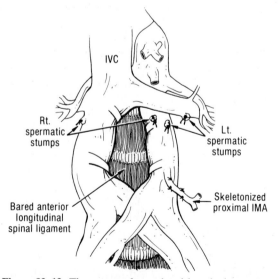

Figure 83–13. The extent of completed lymphadenectomy. The aorta and vena cava have been mobilized and can be retracted laterally. The interaortocaval nodes have been removed, uncovering the anterior spinal ligament. All perivascular tissue about the great vessels and major tributaries have been excised, leaving the stumps of the spermatic vessels and exposing the skeletonized proximal inferior mesenteric artery.

recognized, as are the stumps of the right and left spermatic vessels and the skeletonized proximal inferior mesenteric artery. The area of dissection is thoroughly irrigated with water, a maneuver that may or may not have a carcinostatic effect but that facilitates detection of residual bleeding. The bowel and mesentery are then inspected for injury, and the posterior parietal peritoneum is loosely repaired with interrupted 2–0 silk sutures (approximately 1 cm apart) to permit peritoneal access of any retroperitoneal accumulations. Careful retroperitonealization diminishes the risk of small bowel obstruction. At this stage an "elective" appendectomy may be performed. (In more than 1000 lymph node dissections at the MSKCC, "routine" appendectomy has not been associated with a recognizable morbidity.)

APPROACH FOR LARGE RETROPERITONEAL TUMORS

When dealing with large retroperitoneal tumors or when contemplating re-explorations, it may be advisable to include the following in the preoperative work-up: (1) inferior vena cavography and aortography to evaluate possible anomalies of the vasculature and their relationships to the tumor, (2) an upper gastrointestinal contrast series to assess duodenal invasion, and (3) a barium enema to detect colonic encroachment. At laparotomy, if the aortic pulsation can be felt only through the tumor mass, it is advisable to control the aorta (preferably below the renal vessels or, alternatively, below the superior mesenteric artery) and the common iliac arteries with umbilical tapes. This maneuver may be lifesaving if the aorta is entered. One can avoid a major pitfall when dealing with large retroperitoneal tumors by appreciating their tendency to be intimately involved with, and at times to invade, the adventitia of the aorta and the inferior vena cava and their major tributaries. For this reason, the plane that is most readily dissectible between the aorta and the tumor may be subadventitial. Dissection in such a plane, however, creates a problem in aortic repair should injury occur, since conventional suture repair of an aorta stripped of adventitia is unsatisfactory, if not impossible. Accordingly, in situations in which a plane between tumor and adventitia cannot be identified, it is generally preferable to leave tumor capsule on the great vessels rather than vascular adventitia on tumor capsule. Direct invasion that compromises the aortic wall integrity may occasionally necessitate graft replacement. With the exception of caval thrombosis (by tumor penetration), deliberate efforts to perform major vessel excisions (Mathisen and Jaradpour, 1980) confer little or no therapeutic gain (versus the operative risks). In such cases, reliance on chemotherapy or radiotherapy for tumor control may be preferable (Fig. 83–14).

With large left-sided tumors, especially those causing lateral displacement of the left kidney with stretching and superior bowing of the renal vessels, massive suprahilar infradiaphragmatic extension is common. In this situation, good exposure of the periaortic area above the left renal artery at the level of the aortic diaphragmatic hiatus becomes necessary and is achieved by a costal extension of the abdominal incision with medial mobilization of the splenic flexure of the descending colon and of the spleen, pancreas, and stomach. This is accomplished by incision of the peritoneum of the left lumbar gutter along the white line of Toldt, of the splenophrenic ligament, and of the parietal peritoneal attachments of the stomach (see Fig. 83–11). This permits medial reflection of the descending colon, spleen, stomach, and tail of the pancreas, exposing the aorta at the diaphragmatic hiatus. The celiac axis and the superior mesenteric artery will then be deflected medially along with their visceral distributions.

With massive right-sided tumors, the bulk of nodal metastases will be in the interaortocaval region, and further exposure by a costal extension is often not helpful. Additional exposure is gained by mobilizing the entire right colon and kocherization of the duodenum with anterosuperior reflection of its second, third, and fourth portions. Such efforts will fall short of exposing lymph nodes in the posterior mediastinum above the right diaphragmatic crus. Exploration of the lesser sac after division of the gastrocolic omentum is advisable to ascertain the uppermost extension of the tumor and to assess resectability. Tumor involvement of the small bowel mesentery, superior mesenteric artery, celiac axis, or porta hepatis precludes resection.

Postoperative Complications

MORTALITY

The operative mortality of retroperitoneal lymph node dissection has declined steadily since the turn of the century. Hinman's (1914) historical review of 51 patients with operable testis cancer indicated a surgically related mortality rate of 9 per cent. Lewis (1948) reported no operative deaths in 169 consecutive patients following RPLND. Prior to the introduction of multidrug chemotherapy regimens, there was no operative (hospital) mortality in more than 450

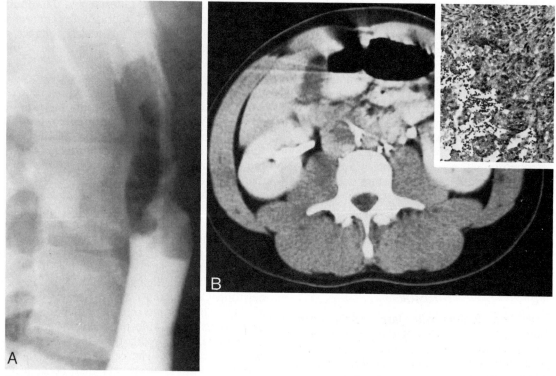

Figure 83–14. Inferior vena cavogram *(A)* and abdominal CT scan *(B)* (the latter following pedal lymphangiography) performed on a 30-year-old patient who presented with bilateral pedal edema, backache, and gynecomastia. An elevated B-hCG was noted, but physical examination and testicular sonography were unremarkable. Cytologic examination of aspirated blood clot obtained during caval contrast study substantiated the diagnosis of a primary extragonadal germ cell tumor. Following chemotherapy-induced seroconversion of B-hCG and partial remission on serial CAT scans, a bilateral retroperitoneal lymphadenectomy with caval resection was performed. Inset shows persistent embryonal carcinoma within the excised caval segment. Eighteen months after completion of two additional adjuvant cycles of multiagent chemotherapy, the patient is alive with no evidence of disease.

lymphadenectomies performed at MSKCC. The successes of chemotherapy have encouraged more aggressive surgery and radiotherapy for recurrent or persistent metastases. Such an approach exposes a greater number of patients, with lesions previously deemed inoperable or unresectable, to the cumulative risks of multimodal approaches. Despite these considerations, the reported operative mortality remains exceedingly low, less than 1 per cent (Table 83–3). Not surprisingly, at present the major cause of death associated with RPLND appears to be chemotherapy-related.

MORBIDITY

Many of the postoperative complications of retroperitoneal lymphadenectomy are similar to those attending any intra-abdominal operative procedure (Table 83–3).

Wound Complications. Wound infection occurs in 1 to 8 per cent of patients and is treated in conventional fashion. Dehiscence is exceedingly rare with proper abdominal closure,

even in the presence of large tumors or prior chemotherapy or radiotherapy. Predisposing factors include wound hematoma, infection, devascularizing wound closures (poor technique), atelectasis, and prolonged ileus.

Respiratory Complications. These are probably the most common but often the least well documented postoperative complications. Bleomycin pneumonitis is certainly the exception since the report of Goldiner et al. (1978). Five fatal cases of postoperative respiratory insufficiency were documented in patients with metastatic testis cancer and prior bleomycin administration. All five developed respiratory distress in the immediate postoperative period, characterized by severe hypoxia, decreased lung compliance, and diffuse interstitial pulmonary edema on serial chest radiographs. Despite the rapid and appropriate deployment of all available life support facilities and intensive medical care, all patients died of "adult respiratory distress syndrome" within 2 weeks of operation. Autopsy studies revealed the destruction of

TABLE 83–3. Complications of Retroperitoneal Lymph Node Dissection

Author	Staubitz	Johnson	Pizzocaro	Schmucki	Vahlensiek	Whitmore
Number of Patients	72	152	155	152	242	333
Bowel obstruction	—	—	3	—	3	7
Lymphocele/ascites	—	3	3	2	3	—
Vascular injury	—	—	2	—	1	—
Hemorrhage/hematoma	1	—	—	2	2	—
Ureteral injury	1	—	1	—	3	—
Nephrectomy (secondary)	1	—	—	1	1	—
Wound infection/sepsis	2	5	1	1	3	28
Dehiscence	1	—	—	—	—	—
Ventral hernia	1	—	—	—	—	—
Atelectasis/pneumonitis	—	—	—	2	—	11
Thromboembolic events	—	—	—	3	—	3
Hepatitis	—	—	1	1	—	—
Gastrointestinal bleeding	1	—	—	—	—	—
Pancreatitis	—	—	—	—	—	—
Operative mortality	—	—	—	1	1	—*

*Patients reviewed by Whitmore did not include five patients who died postoperatively of bleomycin toxicity (Goldiner et al., 1978) and one other who died apparently from an ischemic necrosis of the cecum while on postoperative chemotherapy (Vugrin et al., 1981).

Types I and II pneumatocytes, interstitial fibrosis, damaged alveolar-capillary membranes, and negative cultures.

In a prospective study of 12 closely matched patients who survived RPLND and who had similar doses of bleomycin for disseminated testis cancer, three important contributing factors were suggested: (1) The inspired oxygen concentration was significantly lower in survivors; (2) survivors received more colloid and less crystalloid than nonsurvivors; and (3) the mean alveolar-arterial oxygen pressures, higher than normal in both groups preoperatively, were significantly greater postoperatively in those who died. This study suggested that perioperatively the inspired oxygen concentration and crystalloid:colloid ratio should be reduced in bleomycin-treated patients. Prior to this report the total dose of bleomycin in the VAB regimen used at MSKCC (see Chapter 33) had already been markedly reduced, and the present VAB-6 regimen has eliminated bleomyin from the third induction. The cumulative bleomycin dose in VAB-6 is roughly one half of that given in the PVB schedule. Patients receiving bleomycin should undergo pre- and postinduction pulmonary function studies during the VAB-6 regimen to detect subtle changes in performance. Since 1974 there have been no anesthetic-related deaths in the MSKCC series.

Atelectasis is a less well documented complication, which, to a certain extent, probably accompanies almost every major abdominal operative procedure. It is commonly held that artificial ventilation (constant tidal volumes) causes a reduction in alveolar surfactant, which results in a decreased lung compliance progressing to decreased ventilation (but normal perfusion), progressing to hypoxia. Clinically, atelectasis is manifested within the first 24 hours postoperatively and is characterized by temperature and pulse elevation, rales, decreased breath sounds, and bronchial breathing. Prophylactic measures include the cessation of smoking 2 weeks preoperatively, periodic manual hyperinflation of the lungs intraoperatively, and early ambulation and the use of a rebreathing apparatus to stimulate hyperventilation postoperatively. Expectorants and the inhalation of mucolytics and bronchodilators are helpful once atelectasis has been diagnosed.

In 58 patients undergoing thoracoabdominal RPLND, Skinner and Leadbetter (1971) noted postoperative pneumothorax or hemothorax in eight (14 per cent), seven of whom had no chest tube inserted at surgery. Low-suction chest drainage for 24 hours or more virtually eliminates such an occurrence.

Intra-abdominal Complications. Significant hemorrhage is usually manifested in the immediate postoperative period and is rarely encountered 12 to 24 hours following surgery. Delayed hemorrhage may occur when a major vascular injury has been repaired. Pancreatic injuries are rarely reported, although Sago et al. (1979) noted severe pancreatitis in three patients undergoing suprahilar lymphadenectomy. When a pancreatic injury is detected intraoperatively, the pancreas should be sutured with nonabsorbable material and the area adequately drained.

Vascular anomalies, multiple renal vessels

or duplicated collecting systems, and horseshoe kidney may pose a threat to the unwary and should always prompt appropriate attention to surgical detail. Renal pedicle injury occurs infrequently but, when recognized, should be repaired by a surgeon who is comfortable with vascular reconstruction.

Postoperative paralytic ileus is common up to 3 to 4 days postoperatively. A prolonged ileus (especially when accompanied by peritoneal irritation) may be associated with mechanical obstruction or, less commonly, with retroperitoneal hematoma, pancreatitis, urinary extravasation, renal pedicle injury, bowel infarction, mesenteric hematoma, or an appendiceal stump leak. With proper retroperitonealization the incidence of postoperative mechanical obstruction caused by adhesions or internal herniation is low. Most mechanical obstructions will respond to conservative measures; however, when they are persistent or recurrent, operative intervention becomes necessary.

Chylous ascites is an exceedingly rare complication (Selli et al., 1984). Marked abdominal distention in the early postoperative period, sometimes with an associated pleural effusion, raises the possibility of a chylous leak. Diagnosis is confirmed by abdominal ultrasound and paracentesis. Conservative measures (bed rest, diuretics, dietary restriction of long-chain fatty acids, total parenteral nutrition) will generally resolve the situation (Herz et al., 1978). When massive or persistent accumulation occurs, a closed loop obstruction with lymph leakage through obstructed intestinal lacteals or a proximal thoracic duct obstruction (by clinically unrecognized mediastinal lymph node involvement) should be suspected. In such cases a peritoneovenous shunt may obviate the need for re-exploration and ligation of the disrupted lymphatics.

Sexual Dysfunction. Sexual dysfunction is a common, if not uniform, side effect following bilateral retroperitoneal lymphadenectomy. Libido, potency, and orgasm remain unaltered, but ejaculatory function and fertility are impaired following RPLND in the vast majority of patients. Complete excision of the retroperitoneal lymph nodes disrupts the thoracolumbar sympathetic outflow (T12–L3) but generally has no effect on parasympathetic innervation (S2–S4) of the pelvic viscera. A brief consideration of the pertinent functional neuroanatomy provides some insight regarding therapy of the sexual disturbances following RPLND.

Parasympathetic fibers from pelvic splanchnic (from the nervi erigentes) and pudendal nerves mediate or contribute to (1) erectile function of the penis, (2) contraction of the pelvic floor muscles, and (3) closure of the bladder neck sphincter mechanism. Bilateral RPLND (see earlier), done with or without ipsilateral pelvic lymphadenectomy, does not disrupt the pelvic parasympathetic nerve supply, which originates deep in the presacral space. Orgasm follows the transmission and perception of afferent stimuli from the pelvic floor and internal sex organs to cortical centers. Similar to parasympathetic efferent fibers, these sensory pathways are, by virtue of their location, not subject to injury during RPLND.

The thoracolumbar sympathetic outflow (T12–L3) to the pelvic viscera reaches the hypogastric plexus via the paravertebral ganglia, the aorticomesenteric plexus, and the ureteral plexus. Sympathectomy as a result of either a "modified" or a conventional bilateral lymphadenectomy (with or without suprahilar dissection) may be associated with permanent ejaculatory dysfunction; as a consequence, following RPLND, patients produce little or no seminal fluid. Ejaculation is a coordinated act consisting of (1) seminal emission, (2) bladder neck closure and relaxation of the external sphincter, and (3) antegrade propulsion of seminal fluid. Seminal emission—smooth muscle contractions of the vas deferens, ejaculatory ducts, ampullae, seminal vesicles, and prostatic urethra, resulting in deposition of seminal fluid into the urethra—is mediated by thoracolumbar sympathetics. Bladder neck closure is regulated by both sympathetic and parasympathetic neural pathways. Clonic contractions of the pelvic floor are controlled by pelvic parasympathetics. Lymphadenectomy necessarily interrupts the T12–L3 sympathetics and may logically disturb normal seminal emission and closure of the bladder neck.

Some postulate that lack of seminal emission is responsible for the disturbed ejaculatory function following RPLND (Kom et al., 1971). Others believe that the main dysfunction stems from sympathetic denervation of the bladder neck, which results in retrograde ejaculation (Kedia et al., 1977). There is circumstantial evidence that following RPLND, ejaculation is diminished or absent, owing to a combination of both defects. Nijman et al. (1982) implicated retrograde ejaculation as the cause of post-RPLND sexual dysfunction, by demonstrating spermatozoa in postcoital urine specimens of patients following surgery. Antegrade ejaculation with the production of viable spermatozoa was achieved in the majority of patients treated with an alpha-sympathomimetic agent, imipramine (25 to 50 mg). Lange et al. (1984) reported success in restoring ejaculatory function in patients following RPLND by using alpha-adrenergic drugs—pseudoephedrine hydrochloride (two 90-mg doses 1 hour apart before coitus) or the combination of brompheniramine maleate (12 mg) plus phenylephrine hydrochloride (15 mg) plus phenylpropylamine hydrochloride (15 mg) once every 12 hours for 2 weeks.

Narayan and coworkers reported the spontaneous return of antegrade ejaculation in 25 of 55 (45 per cent) patients who had undergone "extended" RPLND 3 months to 3 years previously. Nine of the 25 patients with restored function fathered children. The authors attributed the return of sexual function to the modified limits of their "extended" lymphadenectomy (Fig. 83–15). In patients with clinical Stage I disease and with no apparent lymphadenopathy at exploration, RPLND included a bilateral suprahilar and a bilateral infrahilar node dissection inferiorly to the origin of the inferior mesenteric artery. The dissections were completed by removal of ipsilateral nodal tissue along the common iliac vessel but without removal of contralateral iliac nodes or the preaortic, precaval, and interaortal nodes below the level of the inferior mesenteric artery (Fraley et al., 1977). The thoracolumbar sympathetic ganglia, which are located on either side of the vertebral column under the edges of the great vessels, are not routinely resected. Such a dissection, which spares the contralateral hypogastric plexus and probably portions of the aorticomesenteric plexus, may preserve sympathetic pathways important in normal ejaculatory function (Lange et al., 1984).

Fossa et al. (1984) have noted that ejaculation is preserved in the majority of patients following unilateral infrahilar lymphadenectomy. Based on prospective anatomic-histopathologic correlations, Hermanek and Sigel (1982) recommend frozen-section biopsies of the resection margins to determine the feasibility of performing a limited infrahilar RPLND. Macroscopic retroperitoneal lymph node metastasis, a history of previous scrotal violation, and extragonadal extension of the primary tumor were listed as factors necessitating a bilateral RPLND.

The value of preoperative semen cryopreservation is unquantified but appears questionable; semen quality and quantity immediately following orchiectomy may be poor and therefore unsuitable for preservation (Bracken and Johnson, 1976). More study in this area, however, appears warranted; it is currently the posture at MSKCC to have patients with a testis tumor submit specimens for semen analysis and cryopreservation, if appropriate, prior to chemotherapy and surgery.

DISTANT SPREAD

The evolution and success of cisplatin-based multiagent chemotherapy have extended the indications for surgery in patients with advanced testicular cancer. Modern chemotherapy regimens induce complete remissions (CR) in 60 to 70 per cent of patients with bulky Stage II or Stage III disease. The addition of appropriate surgical excision for residual disease has augmented the clinical CR rate (chemotherapy alone) by roughly 20 per cent, increasing the overall CR rate (chemotherapy plus surgery) to between 80 and 90 per cent. The rationale for cytoreductive surgery has been established (as discussed in Chapter 33) mainly by four clinical observations: (1) Following chemotherapy for advanced disease, persistent cancer has been detected within the surgically resected specimen. (2) Complete excision of residual cancer results in survival rates comparable to those achieved when chemotherapy alone has induced a pathologic CR (no tumor in the excised specimen). (3) No other means of detecting residual cancer currently exists. (Serum tumor markers may be normal despite active disease). (4) Surgical excision surpasses other available means of treatment in such situations.

Although cytoreductive surgery has been applied to metastatic disease in the neck, inguinal regions, brain, and liver, the most common indications are pulmonary and retroperitoneal metastases. The indications for surgery

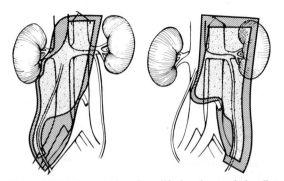

Figure 83–15. Boundaries of modified and extended unilateral lymphadenectomy for right- and left-sided clinical Stage A tumors. (From Lange, P. H., Narayan, P., and Fraley, E. E.: Semin. Urol., 2:264, 1984. Used by permission.)

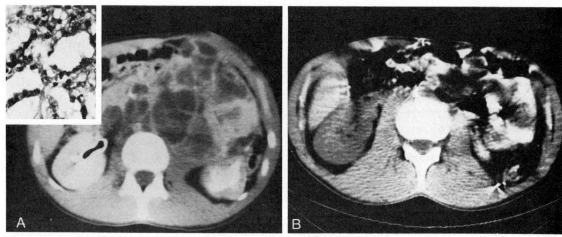

Figure 83–16. Abdominal CT scans of a 23-year-old male who presented with a left testis tumor, a palpable abdominal mass, and an elevated AFP. Following multidrug chemotherapy the level of AFP normalized, but a large complex retroperitoneal mass persisted. *A,* Inset demonstrates a microfocus of endodermal sinus tumor in wall of mass deemed surgically unresectable elsewhere. *B,* Representative scan taken 2½ years following bilateral retroperitoneal lymph node dissection (plus thoracotomy to remove suprahilar, retrocrural, and posterior mediastinal nodes) and following two additional cycles of platinum-based chemotherapy.

in the chest and the retroperitoneum differ slightly. For pulmonary lesions, surgery is not considered until after a trial of chemotherapy. Surgical intervention is reserved for persistent or enlarging nodules despite chemotherapy but is ill advised unless serum tumor markers normalize. Seroconversion of marker status from positive to negative enhances, but does not assure, the possibility that mature teratoma or fibrosis is present. The same considerations generally apply to retroperitoneal metastasis when distant disease is also present. Surgical intervention in such cases is delayed until a trial of chemotherapy has been completed—usually 1 month after three cycles of VAB-6 or four cycles of PVB.

When only bulky Stage II disease exists, two approaches have been utilized: (1) immediate surgical "debulking" followed by adjunctive chemotherapy or (2) preliminary chemotherapy followed by surgical exploration. Few studies have addressed this question. Javadpour et al. (1981) reported the results from a randomized trial that compared primary surgery plus adjunctive chemotherapy with primary chemotherapy plus additional surgery, if necessary. The overall CR rate was slightly higher in the primary chemotherapy group (52 per cent versus 44 per cent), while one operative fatality was recorded in the surgery-first group. Given the favorable effects of chemotherapy, even upon large metastases, chemotherapy initially is preferred by most surgeons, especially when the feasibility of surgical excision appears remote.

The probability of detecting residual cancer following chemotherapy for large metastases (roughly 30 per cent), the uncertain natural history of "benign" teratoma, and the current inability to discriminate either from tumor necrosis-fibrosis, encourage surgical efforts to resect persistent masses following chemotherapy (Fig. 83–16). In general, such efforts following chemotherapy fail unless serum tumor markers are negative; normal serum marker levels, however, do not guarantee complete remission by chemotherapy, which further encourages surgical exploration in such instances.

In patients with disease in both the retroperitoneum and the chest, response to chemotherapy may differ. Clinically, pulmonary metastases often respond immediately and completely to multiagent chemotherapy, whereas bulky retroperitoneal disease generally remains apparent post chemotherapy. A clinical CR in the chest is usually durable and does not necessitate surgical confirmation. Experience with follow-up only in patients with pulmonary metastasis and minimal or "nonbulky" retroperitoneal disease treated primarily with chemotherapy is small; it does not permit firm conclusions regarding the capacity of chemotherapy alone to control these presumptive metastatic deposits.

If disease persists radiographically in the chest and abdomen following chemotherapy, histologic examination of removed tissue does not consistently reveal identical findings in lung and retroperitoneal deposits. Studies at MSKCC and by Mandelbaum and coworkers indicate that roughly one third of patients harboring residual disease in both the chest and the abdomen display dissimilar histology when surgical specimens from each area are compared. In the majority of cases the least favorable histology was identified in the retroperitoneal tissues. Another study by Koops et al. (1984) indicated that malignant elements were more frequently documented in persistent pulmonary lesions. While the observed discrepancies may be ascribed to differences in initial tumor volumes in the respective sites, it may be speculated that tumor heterogeneity is a potential contributing factor. Based on such observations, surgical excision of all residual masses is favored following primary multiagent chemotherapy if preoperative serum tumor marker levels are normal. Metastatic disease in brain, liver, and bone are, in general, excepted because of inaccessibility and the lack of documented benefit.

CONCLUDING REMARKS

The evolution of successful chemotherapy and of increasingly accurate clinical staging has altered the indications for surgery in testicular cancer. The need for routine retroperitoneal node dissection in patients with clinical Stage I disease is under investigation. The indications for surgery in patients with advanced disease, however, have been extended by improvements in chemotherapy. Patient acceptance, cost effectiveness, and the relative long-term toxicities of chemotherapy versus surgery, quite apart from cancer control, are important considerations in addressing these and other issues.

References

Boileau, M. A., and Steers, W. D.: Testis tumors: The clinical significance of the tumor-contaminated scrotum. J. Urol., *132*:51, 1984.

Bracken, R. B., and Johnson, D. E.: Sexual function and fecundity after treatment for testicular tumors. Urology, *7*:735, 1976.

Brenner, J., Vugrin, D., and Whitmore, W. F., Jr.: Cytoreductive surgery for advanced nonseminomatous germ cell tumors of the testis. Urology, *19*:571, 1982.

Busch, F. W., and Sayegh, E. S.: Roentgenographic visualization of human testicular lymphatics: A preliminary report. J. Urol., *89*:106, 1963.

Busch, F. W., Sayegh, E. S., and Chenault, O. W., Jr.: Some uses of lymphangiography in the management of testicular tumors. J. Urol., *93*:490, 1965.

Calvo, F., Hodson, N., Barrett, A., and Peckham, M. J.: Chemotherapy of primary (in situ) testicular tumors: Response in advanced metastatic disease. Br. J. Urol., *55*:560, 1983.

Catalona, W. J., and Rubenstein, M. A.: An incision for extended suprahilar retroperitoneal lymphadenectomy. J. Urol., *119*:316, 1978.

Chevassu, M.: Tumeurs du testicule. Bull. Soc. Chir. (Paris), *36*:236, 1910.

Chiappa, S., Uslenghi, C., Bonadonna, G., Marono, P., and Ravai, G.: Combined testicular and foot lymphangiography in testicular carcinoma. Surg. Gynecol. Obstet., *123*:10, 1966.

Chute, R., Baron, J. A., and Olsson, C. A.: The transverse upper abdominal "chevron" incision in urological surgery. Trans. Am. Assoc. Genitourin. Surg., *29*:14, 1967.

Cooper, J. F., Leadbetter, W. F., and Chute, R.: The thoracoabdominal approach for retroperitoneal gland dissection: Its application to testis tumor. Surg. Gynecol. Obstet., *90*:486, 1950.

Cuneo, B.: Note sur les lymphatiques du testicle. Bull. Soc. Anat. (Paris), *76*:105, 1901.

Donohue, J. P.: Retroperitoneal lymphadenectomy. The anterior approach including nonseminomatous testicular cancer in adults. Urol. Clin. North Am., *4*:509, 1977.

Donohue, J. P., and Rowland, R. G.: Complications of retroperitoneal lymph node dissection. J. Urol., *126*:338, 1981.

Donohue, J. P., Zachary, J. M., and Maynard, B. R.: Distribution of nodal metastases in nonseminomatous testis cancer. J. Urol., *128*:315, 1982.

Drasga, R. E., Einhorn, L. H., Williams, S. D., Patel, D. N., and Stevens, E. E.: Fertility after chemotherapy for testicular cancer. J. Clin. Oncol., *1*:179, 1983.

Forrest, J. B., Turner, T. T., and Howards, S. S.: Cyclophosphamide, vincristine and the blood-testis barrier. Invest. Urol., *18*:443, 1981.

Fossa, S. D., Klepp, O., Ous, S., Lien, H. H., Stenwig, A. E., Abyholm, T., and Kaalhus, O.: Unilateral retroperitoneal lymph node dissection in patients with nonseminomatous testicular tumor in clinical stage I. Eur. Urol., *10*:17, 1984.

Fowler, J. F., and Whitmore, W. F., Jr.: Intratesticular germ-cell tumours: Observations on the effect of chemotherapy. J. Urol., *126*:412, 1981.

Fowler, J. F., Vugrin, D., Cvitkovic, E., and Whitmore, W. F., Jr.: Sequential bilateral germ-cell tumours of the testis despite interval chemotherapy. J. Urol., *122*:421, 1979.

Fraley, E. E., Markland, C., and Lange, P. H.: Surgical treatment of Stage I and II nonseminomatous testicular cancer in adults. Urol. Clin. North Am., *4*:455, 1977.

Goldiner, P. L., Carlson, G. C., Cvitkovic, E., Schweizer, O., and Howland, W.: Factors influencing postoperative morbidity and mortality in patients treated with bleomycin. Br. Med. J., *1*:1664, 1978.

Goldstein, M., and Waterhouse, K.: When to use the Chevassu maneuver during exploration of intrascrotal masses. J. Urol., *130*:1199, 1983.

Greist, A., Einhorn, L. E., Williams, S. D., Donohue, J. P., and Rowland, R. G.: Pathologic findings at orchiectomy following chemotherapy for disseminated testicular cancer. J. Clin. Oncol., *2*:1025, 1984.

Hermanek, P., and Sigel, A.: Necessary extent of lymph node dissection in testicular tumours; a histopathological investigation. Eur. Urol., *8*:135, 1982.

Herz, J., Shapiro, S. R., Konrad, P., and Palmer, J.: Chylous ascites following retroperitoneal lymphadenectomy: Report of 2 cases with guidelines for diagnosis and treatment. Cancer, *42*:349, 1978.

Hinman, F.: The operative treatment of tumors of the testicle. JAMA, *63*:2009, 1914.

Hinman, F., Gibson, T. E., and Kutzmann, A. A.: The radical operation for teratoma of testis. Surg. Gynecol. Obstet., 37:429, 1923.

Jamieson, J. K., and Dobson, J. F.: The lymphatics of the testicle. Lancet, 1:493, 1910.

Javadpour, N., Ozols, R. F., Barlock, A., Anderson, T., and Young, R. C.: A randomized trial of cytoreductive surgery versus chemotherapy alone in bulky Stage III (poor prognosis) testicular cancer (Abstract C-549). Proc. Am. Soc. Clin. Oncol., 22:473, 1981.

Johnson, D. E.: Retroperitoneal lymphadenectomy: Indications, complications and expectations. Rec. Res. Cancer Res., 60:221, 1977.

Johnson, D. E., and Babaian, R. J.: The case for conservative surgical management of the ilioinguinal region after inadequate orchiectomy. J. Urol., 123:44, 1980.

Kaswick, J. A., Blomberg, S. D., and Skinner, D. G.: Radical retroperitoneal lymph node dissection: How effective in removal of all retroperitoneal nodes? J. Urol., 115:70, 1976.

Kedia, K., and Markland, C.: The effect of pharmocological agents on ejaculation. J. Urol., 114:569, 1975.

Kedia, K., Markland, C., and Fraley, E. E.: Sexual function after high retroperitoneal lymphadenectomy. Urol Clin North Am., 4:523, 1977.

Klein, F. A., Whitmore, W. F., Sogani, P. C., Batata, M., Fisher, H., and Herr, H. W.: Inguinal lymph node metastases from germ cell tumors. J. Urol., 131:497, 1984.

Kober, G. M.: Sarcoma of the testicle. Am. J. Med. Sci., 117:535, 1899.

Kom, C., Mulholland, S. G., and Edson, M.: Etiology of infertility after retroperitoneal lymphadenectomy. J. Urol., 105:528, 1971.

Koops, H. S., Oldhoff, J., Slejfer, D. T., Oosterhuis, J. W., and Homan van der Heide: The role of surgery after remission-induction chemotherapy in non-seminoma Stage III testicular tumors. In Progress and Controversies in Oncological Urology. New York, Alan R. Liss, 1984, pp. 233–238.

Lange, P. H., Narayan, P., and Fraley, E. E.: Fertility issues following therapy for testicular cancer. Semin. Urol., 2:264, 1984.

Lewis, L. G.: Testis tumors: Report on 250 cases. J. Urol., 59:763, 1948.

Lewis, L. G.: Testis tumors. In Advances in Surgery. Vol. 2. New York, John Wiley & Sons, 1949, pp. 419–493.

Mallis, N., and Patton, J. F.: Transperitoneal bilateral lymphadenectomy in testis tumor. J. Urol., 80:501, 1958.

Markland, C., Kedia, K., and Fraley, E. E.: Inadequate orchiectomy for patients with testicular tumors. JAMA, 224:1025, 1973.

Mathisen, D. J., and Javadpour, N.: En bloc resection of inferior vena cava in cytoreductive surgery for bulky retroperitoneal metastatic testicular cancer. Urology, 16:51, 1980.

Most, H.: Uber Maligne Hdengeschwulste und ihre Metastaden. Virchows Arch. (Pathol. Anat.), 154:138, 1898.

Nagamatsu, G. R.: New extraperitoneal approach for bilateral retroperitoneal lymph node dissection in testis tumor. J. Urol., 90:457, 1959.

Nijman, J. M., Jager, S., Boer, P. W., Kremer, J., Oldhoff,

J., Schraffordt, L., and Koops, H.: The treatment of ejaculation disorders after retroperitoneal lymph node dissection. Cancer, 50:2967, 1982.

Parkinson, M. C., and Chabrel, C. M.: Clinicopathological features of retroperitoneal tumours. Br. J. Urol., 56:17, 1984.

Patton, J., and Mallis, N.: Tumors of the testis. J. Urol., 81:457, 1959.

Pizzocaro, G., Durand, J. C., Fuchs, W. A., Merrin, C. E., Musumeci, R., Schmucki, O., Vahlensiech, W., Whitmore, W. F., Jr., and Zvara, V. L.: Staging and surgery in testicular cancer. Eur. Urol., 7:1, 1981.

Ray, B., Hajdu, S. I., and Whitmore, W. F., Jr.: Distribution of retroperitoneal lymph node metastasis in testicular germinal tumors. Cancer, 33:340, 1974.

Roberts, J. B.: Excision of the lumbar lymphatic nodes and spermatic vein in malignant disease of the testicle. Ann. Surg., 36:539, 1902.

Rouviere, H.: Anatomie des Lymphatiques de l'Homme. Paris, Masson et Cie, 1932.

Sago, A. L, Ball, T. P., and Novicki, D. E.: Complications of retroperitoneal lymphadenectomy. Urology, 13:241, 1979.

Sayegh, E., Brooks, T., Sacher, E., and Busch, F.: Lymphangiography of the retroperitoneal lymph nodes through the inguinal route. J. Urol., 95:102, 1966.

Schmeller, N. T., Siegelman, S. S., and Walsh, P. C.: Anatomical consideration in suprahilar lymph node dissection for testicular tumors. Urol. Int., 36:341, 1981.

Selli, C., Carini, M., Mottola, A., and Barbaghi, G.: Chylous ascites after retroperitoneal lymphadenectomy: Successful management with peritoneovenous shunt. Urol. Int., 39:58, 1984.

Signel, A., and Krieger, F.: Scrotal operation or biopsy of testicular tumors—a fatal mistake? Recent Results. Cancer Res., 60:212, 1977.

Skinner, D. G., and Leadbetter, W. F.: The surgical management of testis tumors. J. Urol., 106:84, 1971.

Staubitz, W. J., Early, K. S., Magoss, I. V., et al.: Surgical management of non-seminomatous germinal testis tumors. Cancer, 32:1206, 1973.

Stoffel, T. J., Nesbit, M. E., and Levitt, S. H.: Extramedullary involvement of the testis in childhood leukemia. Cancer, 35:1203, 1975.

Vugrin, D., Whitmore, W. F., Jr., Sogani, P. C., Bains, M., Herr, H., and Golbey, R. B.: Combined chemotherapy and surgery in treatment of advanced germ cell tumors. Cancer, 47:2228, 1981.

Wahlqvist, L., Hulten, L., and Rosencrantz, M.: Normal lymphatic drainage of the testis studied by funicular lymphangiography. Acta Chir. Scand, 132:454, 1966.

Whitmore, W. F., Jr.: Treatment of testis neoplasms. In Proceedings of the Fourth National Cancer Conference. Philadelphia, J. B. Lippincott Co., 1960.

Whitmore, W. F., Jr.: Germinal tumors of the testis. In Proceedings of the sixth National Cancer Conference. Philadelphia, J. B. Lippincott Co., 1968.

Whitmore, W. F., Jr.: Surgical treatment of adult germinal testis tumors. Semin. Oncol., 6:55, 1979.

Whitmore, W. F., Jr.: Patterns of failure following surgical treatment of urologic neoplasms. Cancer Treat. Symp., 2:41, 1983.

CHAPTER 84

Surgery of the Scrotum and Its Contents*

STUART S. HOWARDS, M.D.

In this chapter, the surgical procedures of choice for pathologic conditions of the scrotum and its contents are described and illustrated. For some conditions, alternative approaches are also illustrated, and for most lesions, additional reasonable procedures are briefly described and referenced. The surgical correction of the undescended testis is described in Chapter 46. The indications for procedures to improve male fertility are discussed in Chapter 12. The indications for other operations are briefly reviewed in this chapter.

SURGERY OF THE SCROTAL WALL

REPAIR OF SCROTAL INJURIES

Superficial scrotal injuries can be repaired with the use of local anesthesia, whereas deeper, more extensive wounds should be treated with the patient under regional or general anesthesia. Initially, the scrotum is carefully examined aseptically, with sterile gloves and a face mask used to avoid contamination. The depth of the wound is usually uneven. All dirt should be washed away with sterile saline and a mild antiseptic solution, such as povidone-iodine (Betadine). Wounds treated within 4 to 6 hours of trauma can be closed primarily; the older, contaminated wound should first be drained. The area to be repaired is infiltrated with 0.5 or 1.0 per cent lidocaine. A lidocaine block of the spermatic cord may also be useful. Careful debridement of necrotic and ischemic tissue is absolutely essential. Meticulous care to obtain hemostasis is also critical for all scrotal surgery; intrascrotal bleeding often results in large hematomas because of the lack of tissue pressure in the scrotal sac. Deeper structures can be approximated with 4-0 absorbable sutures. The skin is closed with interrupted, 4-0 chromic catgut or a running, subcuticular absorbable 4-0 suture. A pressure dressing and a scrotal support are applied. The use of an ice pack during the first 12 hours after surgery will reduce edema.

Injuries with loss of up to 50 per cent of the scrotal skin can usually be primarily repaired without grafting or the creation of flaps. Even when only small scrotal remnants remain viable, regeneration will usually result so that large denuded areas are eventually covered. Meshed split-thickness grafts can be used to fill open areas. Avulsed scrotal skin also can be used as a full-thickness free graft (Gibson, 1954). Treatment of total avulsion of the scrotal skin depends on the degree of contamination and the time that has elapsed since the injury. In massive, clean injuries less than 18 hours old, debridement and closure by split-thickness skin grafting (Manchanda et al., 1967) or thigh flaps (Tiwari et al., 1980) are reasonable options. The formation of a single scrotum is preferable, although some technical difficulties necessitate the creation of a bifid scrotum.

The thick split-thickness technique requires a 1½–1 meshed graft, which is of sufficient length to allow for the contracture that occurs in the early postoperative period. Split-thickness

---

*This work is based on the excellent contribution of Bruce Stewart to the fourth edition of *Campbell's Urology*. The text relating to several conditions for which the author's approach is similar to that of Dr. Stewart has been utilized without alteration. A few of the illustrations from the fourth edition have also been retained, although the majority of the figures are new.

grafts will not succeed if the tunica vaginalis is absent. Meshed grafts are preferred because they tolerate more movement and give a corrugated appearance to the neoscrotum. One end of the graft is sutured to the posterior margin of the perineal wound. The graft is then folded upward around the testes, and the other end is sutured to the anterior margin of the wound, adjacent to the base of the penis (Fig. 84–1). The lateral margins of the skin graft are then brought together to complete the formation of a scrotal pouch. The midportion of the graft is sutured to the bed of the wound to produce two separate scrotal compartments (Fig. 84–1). Some of the sutures are left long to aid in anchoring a fluff-gauze pressure dressing, which is applied to the anterior and posterior surfaces of the newly formed scrotum.

If it is not possible to obtain a skin graft large enough for the formation of a single scrotal sac, construction of a bifid scrotum is necessary. A smaller graft is used to cover each testis individually. The graft is initially sutured to the base of the scrotal wound and is then brought over and around the testis to form an individual pouch. Sutures are again left long to secure fluff dressings that wrap each newly formed scrotal pouch individually (Conley, 1956). The two sacs can be joined as a second-stage procedure after complete healing has taken place.

When there is tissue infection or, as mentioned, the loss of the tunica vaginalis, free grafts will not take. In addition, immediate grafting exposes the donor sites to infection. In infected patients, all of the infected skin, often including the penile and perineal areas, must be debrided to control infection. The testicles are then dressed and allowed to granulate. McDougal (1983) recommended a two-stage approach that has a higher success rate and involves a shorter hospital stay when compared with split-thickness grafting. After the infection is controlled, the testicles are placed superficially beneath the skin in the midst of the areas that eventually become flaps (Fig. 84–2a). These flaps, which are based superiorly and laterally, receive their blood supply from the external pudendal and the medial circumflex femoral arteries, and remain innervated. If required, the penile shaft and perineum are covered with split-thickness skin grafts. Six weeks later, the flaps are incised as shown in Figure 84–2b. The medial aspect of the flap is the perineal wound; the inferior margin is curved. The incision for the flaps extends to the superficial fascia of the thigh, and care is taken that no subcutaneous tissue overlies the testicle. The flaps are rotated medially and joined at the midline (Fig. 84–2c). The thigh wounds can be closed primarily, avoiding a grafting procedure. Drains are placed beneath the flaps (Fig. 84–2c). McDougal (1983) reported excellent cosmetic results in three patients. Many other techniques have been recommended to treat total avulsions and extensive infections of the scrotum (Stewart, 1979; Furnas and McCraw, 1980). Tiwari et al. (1980) described a one-stage technique in which superiorly based thigh flaps and split-thickness skin

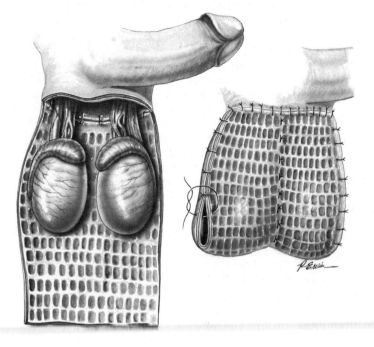

Figure 84–1. Bilateral meshed split-thickness graft for total scrotal avulsion.

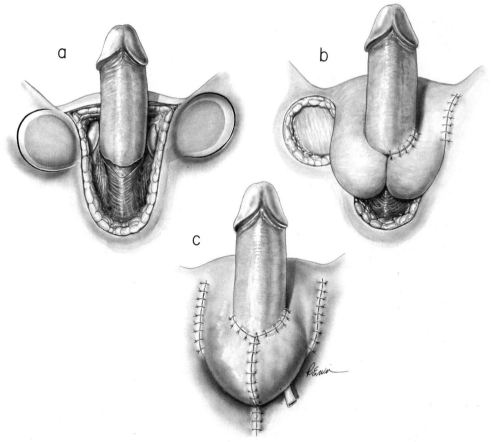

Figure 84–2. Delayed full-thickness superior-lateral pedicle grafting procedure for the correction of scrotal avulsion. Testes were placed beneath skin of thigh at first stage*(a)*. One lateral incision is closed, and one has yet to be closed *(b)*. If split-thickness is required, skin grafts are applied to the penis *(c)* and perineum.

grafts are used to cover the donor areas. This method might be useful for patients with extensive, traumatic loss of scrotal skin.

Although most scrotal defects are best treated with the methods described, injuries with extensive loss of substance, particularly if penile reconstruction is necessary, may require the use of anterior thigh musculocutaneous flaps. These flaps, based primarily on the profunda femoris artery through its medial and lateral circumflex femoral branches, allow the transfer of viable, bulky muscle tissue to the perineum and groin. As illustrated in Figure 84–3, the available muscle includes the gracilis, sartorius, rectus femoris, vastus lateralis, and tensor fascia lata. The two most useful muscles for reconstruction of the male perineum and genitalia are the gracilis and tensor fascia lata. The gracilis flap is best for penile reconstruction, whereas the tensor fascia lata flap is much wider, enabling superior groin coverage. A detailed description of the anatomy and surgical technique related to these flaps is presented in the surgical atlas edited by Mathes and Nahai (1979).

MANAGEMENT OF SCROTAL INFECTIONS

Infected abrasions should be cleaned, debrided, and treated with wet to dry, fine-mesh gauze dressing that is changed every 4 to 6 hours. Localized intrascrotal infections can usually be drained in the outpatient clinic with the use of local anesthesia; however, extensive abscesses may require an aggressive debridement, which necessitates the use of regional or general anesthesia.

Severe infections may progress to extensive suppuration and scrotal gangrene. Fournier's disease is a fulminating, necrotizing cellulitis of the perineum that spreads rapidly and destroys the full thickness of the scrotal wall, sometimes involving penile and sacral skin. The disease is caused by a synergistic polymicrobial infection, which results in obliterative endarteritis and thus necrosis (Lamb and Juler, 1983). Perirectal abscesses can spread and lead to gas gangrene

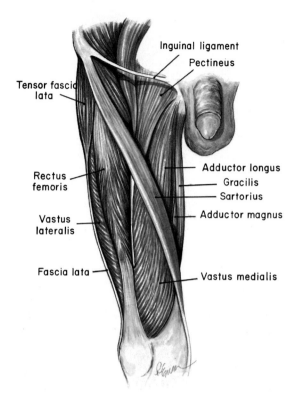

Inguinal ligament

Pectineus

Tensor fascia lata

Rectus femoris

Vastus lateralis

Fascia lata

Adductor longus

Gracilis

Sartorius

Adductor magnus

Vastus medialis

Figure 84–3. Muscles available for myocutaneous flaps to repair extensive injuries of the scrotum, penis, and perineum. The gracilis and tensor fascia lata are most frequently used.

with necrosis of the entire scrotal skin and lower abdominal wall. Periurethral abscesses may also progress to the development of scrotal gangrene with extensive scrotal skin loss.

In all these conditions, active debridement of necrotic skin is necessary to provide drainage and to prevent the development of further skin loss. General supportive measures must be employed, with the use of appropriate broad-spectrum antibiotics as well as wet to dry, fine-mesh gauze dressing. After the disease process has been arrested and the subcutaneous tissues are granulating cleanly, delayed primary closure of scrotal skin may be accomplished. If the defect involves virtually all of the scrotal skin, as in the case of extensive Fournier's disease or scrotal gas gangrene, the secondary reconstructive procedures should be employed.

Tuberculous infections of the scrotal wall secondary to complicated tuberculous epididymitis are seldom seen, owing to the availability of adequate drug therapy. These infections respond well to systemic antituberculous therapy. Excision of the involved scrotal wall is seldom required.

EXCISION OF SCROTAL WALL LESIONS

Benign Tumors. Sebaceous cysts are the most common benign tumors of the scrotal wall.

These lesions, as well as fibromas, lipomas, and myxomas, can be excised locally, often in an outpatient setting. The use of an antibacterial skin preparation is necessary before excision, and meticulous hemostasis is essential after removal of the lesion. The subcutaneous tissues and the skin are then closed in layers with fine catgut sutures. A subcuticular closure is often desirable. The patient should wear a scrotal support until all pain and tenderness have dissipated.

Malignant Tumors. Malignant tumors of the scrotal wall, which are rare, occasionally result from exposure to known carcinogens. The vast majority of these tumors are squamous cell carcinomas. The primary lesion should be treated by wide excision with a 2- to 3-cm margin and primary closure. Resection of the scrotal contents is rarely necessary. Treatment of the regional nodes is controversial. Ray and Whitmore (1977) recommend careful observation if the nodes are not clinically suspicious. If the nodes are palpable, they prefer an ipsilateral ilioinguinal dissection, reserving bilateral lymphadenectomy for the occasional patient with documented bilateral resectable metastatic disease. Fine-needle aspiration biopsy is a useful diagnostic technique in these patients.

Scrotal Elephantiasis. Elephantiasis may involve the skin of the scrotum and the base of the penis; in some cases, it may reach heroic proportions. In North America and the European countries this condition is rare; simple edema of the scrotum due to lymphatic obstruction constitutes a more common indication for resection and scrotal plasmic reconstruction (Dickson and Hofsess, 1959).

If scrotal involvement is not extensive, simple resection of the redundant scrotal skin with primary closure is all that is necessary (Bunce, 1975). However, when the condition massively involves the scrotum and the penis, preventing palpation of the underlying testes and cord structures, it is advisable to begin the dissection at the base of the scrotum and to identify and exteriorize cord structures and testes (Desai and Williams, 1959). The dissection can then be carried downward and laterally over the base of the scrotum, completely resecting the edematous tissue (Fig. 84–4a and b). Small, medial thigh flaps may then be raised (see Fig. 84–2a and b), and remnants of relatively normal scrotum can be brought across anteriorly in the

midline to cover cord structures and testes. The base of the incision is closed by mobilization of perineal skin, bringing it up to appose the midline closure. Should extensive involvement of the penile skin coexist, this area can be entirely resected and covered with a split-thickness graft. The graft should be anastomosed to itself anteriorly to avoid superimposition of suture lines. The tube of normal mucous membrane extending from the glans penis to the margin of the foreskin should be preserved and should be brought down as a cuff to cover the distal penile shaft (Fig. 84–4c). A fluff-gauze pressure dressing is applied after repair. Perioperative systemic, broad-spectrum antibiotics are recommended. Because the majority of the scrotal blood supply enters the scrotal wall superiorly and laterally, it is usually best to incise the scrotum transversely or in slightly oblique fashion whenever possible. During scrotal surgery, it is usually possible to identify the direction and location of major scrotal blood vessels and to avoid transecting them.

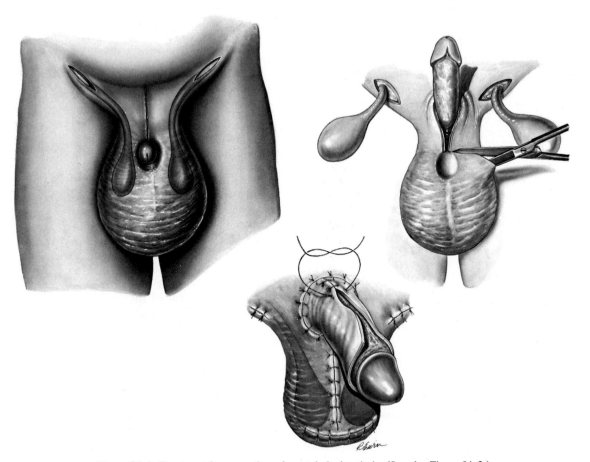

Figure 84–4. Treatment for correction of scrotal elephantiasis. (See also Figure 84–2.)

SURGERY OF THE TESTIS

TESTICULAR RUPTURE AND HEMATOCELE

Testicular rupture occurs after penetrating injuries or severe blunt trauma during which the tunica albuginea is torn. A hematocele is first recognized as a painful scrotal mass surrounding the testis. It does not transilluminate. The differential diagnosis includes torsion of the spermatic cord, cord torsion of an appendage, and epididymitis. If bloody fluid is obtained by aspiration of the mass, surgical exploration is indicated. Testicular radionuclide scanning may be helpful if the diagnosis is not clear (McConnell et al., 1982; McCormack et al., 1966). All equivocal cases should be explored. A scrotal incision is made through the tunica vaginalis. The wound is then debrided, including resection of necrotic seminiferous tubules if the testis has been ruptured. After hemostasis is obtained, the tunica albuginea (if torn) is closed with a running suture. If contaminated, the wound is drained.

INGUINAL RADICAL ORCHIECTOMY

The inguinal approach is indicated in all patients in whom malignancy of the scrotal contents has not been ruled out. We also use this approach in all pediatric cases. We prefer a transverse incision in the skinfold above the inguinal ligament to the standard inguinal incision (Fig. 84–5). The fascia of the external oblique muscle is incised in the direction of its fibers, upward from the external ring; the ilioinguinal nerve is identified; and the cord is isolated. If the diagnosis is in doubt, a rubber shod or vascular clamp is placed across the vascular pedicle before the testis is delivered from the scrotum (Fig. 84–5). If an intratesticular mass is present, immediate orchiectomy rather than biopsy is usually indicated. The vessels and the vas deferens are clamped individually at points as high as possible, and the cord structures are divided between the clamps. We prefer suture ligations and leave one long, permanent suture so that the end of the spermatic cord can be easily identified during retroperitoneal lymphadenectomy, if indicated. The operative specimen is draped out of the area of the incision, particularly if a biopsy is performed.

SCROTAL (SIMPLE) ORCHIECTOMY

Scrotal orchiectomy is utilized to treat recurrent epididymo-orchitis not responsive to medical therapy, and for castration, which is most often indicated for palliation in prostatic carcinoma. Orchiectomy for idiopathic intract-

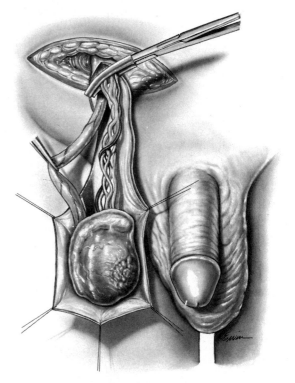

Figure 84–5. Inguinal orchiectomy through transverse incision. Rubber-shod clamp (illustrated) or vascular clamp is placed on vessels. Tunica vaginalis is not routinely opened as illustrated.

able orchialgia should be performed only as a last resort and only in those few patients who have had documented pain relief from regional blocks and whose extensive psychiatric evaluation indicates there are definite potential benefits from surgery.

The incision for a scrotal orchiectomy is made between the major blood vessels. A bilateral orchiectomy can be performed through a single transverse scrotal incision. When orchiectomy is done because of inflammatory disease, the spermatic cord should be delivered completely into the incision and divided between hemostats at levels as high as possible on the cord. After removal of the testis and the cord structures, the vessels and the vas deferens are secured individually with ligatures. Reabsorbable sutures are used, and the wound is drained for several days. We prefer a total bilateral epididymo-orchiectomy when the procedure is performed to eliminate testicular androgen secretion, such as in patients with prostatic cancer. Some authors have recommended a subepididymal orchiectomy (Fig. 84–6) (Stewart, 1979) or an intracapsular orchiectomy, enucleating the testicular parenchyma from the tunica albuginea (Roen, 1967). We find these are not usually

Care should be taken to avoid injury to the epididymis. The incision is continued to the tunica vaginalis. When this tunic is incised, there is a characteristic efflux of several drops of clear fluid (Fig. 84–7b). It is helpful to place two 4-0 chromic stay sutures in the tunica vaginalis for retraction and to aid closure. Two additional stay sutures are placed through the tunica albuginea, and a small ellipse of the tunica with adjacent tubules is resected with a sharp scalpel or razor blade, shaving the bulging tissue with the use of a no-touch technique (Fig. 84–7c). The specimen is immediately placed in Bouin, Zenker, or similar fixative without being handled by forceps or by gauze. Most authorities believe that formalin should be avoided, as it distorts the germinal epithelium. If the pathologist is not familiar with special fixatives, however, it may be better to use formalin. The tunica albuginea, vaginalis, and skin are closed in three separate layers of running 4-0 catgut

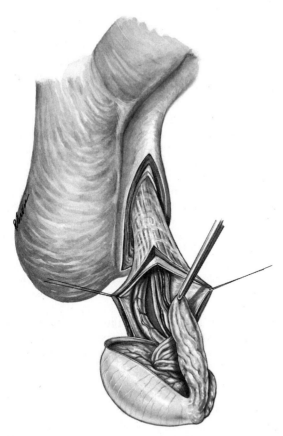

Figure 84–6. Scrotal subepididymal orchiectomy. Epididymis is sharply dissected from testis.

necessary. If the patient desires a normal-appearing scrotum, we insert a testicular prothesis. Although many authors recommend drainage for 1 or 2 days, we do not drain clean scrotal wounds. We always use a scrotal support until the pain and tenderness have resolved and an ice pack for the first 24 hours after surgery.

TESTIS BIOPSY

The indications for testis biopsy in infertile men are discussed in Chapter 12. The scrotum should be shaved and prepared with an antiseptic solution. General, regional, or local anesthesia may be used. Local technique involves infiltration in the area of the incision with 1 per cent lidocaine. The addition of a 0.25 per cent bupivacaine block of the spermatic cord decreases intra- and postoperative discomfort. The testis should be held firmly on its posterior aspect, thus allowing the scrotal skin on the anterior surface to stretch tightly in the area of incision. This stretching forces the epididymis to remain posterior and allows the scrotal skin to part without the need for retraction. A 1- to 2-cm vertical skin incision is made (Fig. 84–7a).

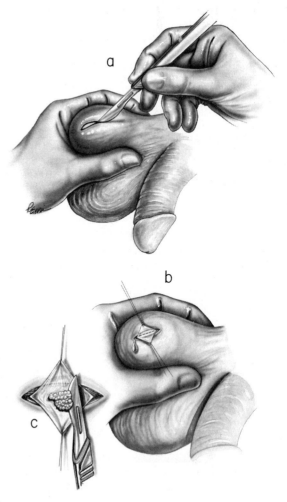

Figure 84–7. Testis biopsy. Note guide sutures on tunica vaginalis in b and c.

sutures; a subcuticular closure may be used. The patient should wear a scrotal support for 3 to 5 days.

SURGERY OF THE CORD STRUCTURES

TORSION OF THE SPERMATIC CORD, APPENDIX TESTIS, AND APPENDIX EPIDIDYMIS

Torsion of the spermatic cord may be intravaginal or extravaginal. The extravaginal form is uncommon and usually is noted as a round, firm, discolored scrotal mass in newborns. Although some authorities do not perform surgery in these infants, we recommend orchiectomy, especially in view of recent data that are suggestive of an adverse effect of a retained necrotic testis on the contralateral gonad (Harrison et al., 1981). There is also disagreement as to the need to repair the contralateral side in newborns with extravaginal torsion (Allen, 1976; Johnson, 1982). Intravaginal torsion is due to an absence of the usual attachment of the posterior aspect of the testis to the scrotal wall such that the tunica vaginalis covers the epididymis and testis (the "bell clapper" deformity). Twisting of the vascular pedicle, which causes pain, usually occurs at puberty or in early adulthood.

The physical findings suggestive of spermatic cord torsion include a high-riding, swollen, tender testis, a supratesticular mass, and an anterior epididymis (180 or 270 degree torsion).

The scrotal wall may be red and edematous as in epididymitis, but elevation of the scrotum does not relieve the pain as is often the case in the latter condition (Prehn's sign). Normal urinalysis results suggest torsion rather than epididymitis. We frequently detort the testis manually, with or without anesthetizing the cord. This manipulation confirms the diagnosis and dramatically relieves the pain. Occasionally, when the diagnosis is equivocal, we obtain a radionuclide scan. All patients should be surgically explored if the diagnosis of torsion of the cord cannot be absolutely excluded. We sometimes delay surgery after successful detorsion and perform an elective bilateral orchiopexy. Torsion of an appendix usually occurs in pre- or peripubertal boys. Discomfort can be severe, but frequently the pain and tenderness are localized to the area of the ischemic tissue. Often a blue-black necrotic appendix can be seen through the scrotal skin (Dresner, 1973). If the diagnosis is unequivocal, the patient may be treated nonoperatively (Allen, 1976; Johnson, 1982), although it is often more expeditious to correct the problem surgically.

Torsion of the spermatic cord should be repaired as soon as possible through a scrotal incision. The incision is carried through the tunica vaginalis (Fig. 84–8a), and the cord is untwisted. The testis is observed, and if normal color returns, it is then anchored by three nonabsorbable sutures through the tunics and into the scrotal wall (Fig. 84–8b). We prefer to place these sutures through the median septum, but sometimes it is more convenient to use the

Figure 84–8. Exposure and repair for torsion of the spermatic cord.

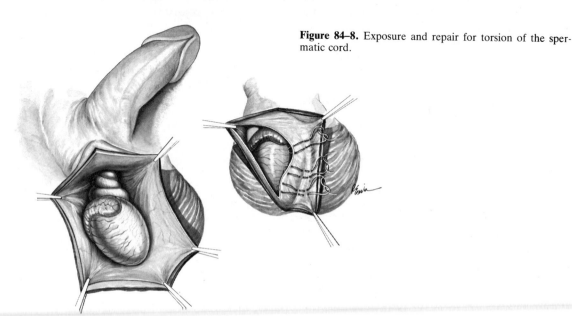

scrotal wall. Late detorsion has been described after orchiopexy with reabsorbable sutures. Should extravaginal torsion be present, a more extensive dissection of the cord structures is necessary to ensure that detorsion is complete and that normal circulation is restored to the testis.

If obvious, complete necrosis of the testis has occurred, orchiectomy is advisable, especially in view of the results of work by Harrison (1981). If, however, there is reasonable doubt regarding the future viability of the testis, it should be left in situ. Testes with apparently irreversible ischemia may remain viable and support Leydig cell function. Sepsis and abscess formation are rare, even if a totally infarcted testis is left in place.

Upon completion of detorsion and fixation of the ipsilateral testis, the contralateral scrotal compartment must be opened and the testis should be firmly affixed to surrounding structures to prevent future torsion on this unaffected side, which does occur and can result in anorchia.

The surgical approach to torsion of the appendices is similar to that already outlined. The twisted appendix testis or appendix epididymis is swollen and erythematous in most cases; treatment consists of simple excision. Some authorities recommend excision of the contralateral appendix, but we do not do this excision routinely.

VASECTOMY

Vasectomy remains that most practical method of male fertility control. Patients should be emotionally stable, mature, and well motivated. Careful informed consent should be obtained, including a discussion of possible recanalization, irreversibility, and the animal data suggesting acceleration of atherosclerosis in monkeys that have undergone vasectomy (Alexander and Clarkson, 1978; Clarkson and Alexander, 1980). Because to date all of the carefully done studies in man have shown no adverse cardiovascular effects, we still perform vasectomies when appropriate. Several informative brochures are available that augment the physician's explanation of the procedure to the patient.

The patient should be examined during the initial interview to determine whether the procedure can be done under local anesthesia. This is almost always the case. The midportion of the vas deferens is palpated between the thumb and fingers and is elevated by digital compression to lie just beneath the anterior scrotal skin

(Fig. 84–9a). To facilitate future vasovasostomy, vasectomy should be performed above the convoluted portion of the vas. The skin, the subcutaneous tissue, and the fascia surrounding the vas deferens at the level selected are infiltrated with a local anesthetic agent in an amount sufficient to anesthetize a 3- or 4-cm segment of the vas deferens. A 1- to 2-cm skin incision is made longitudinally over the exposed vas and is carried down to the level of the sheath. The procedure can also be done through a single 3- to 4-cm transverse incision. The vas is then firmly grasped with a towel clamp and is delivered into the operative field. A longitudinal incision is then made through surrounding fascia to expose the vas (Fig. 84–9b). With the vas still held in the towel clamp, the muscular wall of the vas deferens is carefully dissected free from surrounding structures with a hemostat, with care to deliver only the vas deferens and not to include its adjacent blood vessels. After a 2- or 3-cm segment has been exposed by blunt dissection, the midportion of the exposed vas deferens is grasped with a hemostat and is elevated farther into the operative field; the towel clamp is then removed (Fig. 84–9c).

Firm, downward traction on this hemostat places the distal vas under tension as it courses upward toward the inguinal ring. Palpation of the entire vas at this time confirms the side on which vasectomy is performed. Repeating this maneuver on both sides will avoid the technical error of ligating the vas deferens twice on the same side. The distal segment of the vas is then grasped with a second hemostat, and the vas is transected with the scalpel about 5 mm from the ends of the clamps, removing a segment that is sent for pathologic examination (Fig. 84–9 d and e). The abdominal end of the vas is ligated with permanent suture material (Fig. 84–9f). After checking it for bleeding, the abdominal end is released and the perivasal fascia is approximated over it with 4-0 chromic suture to create a fascial barrier between the two ends of the vas (Fig. 84–9g). The lumen of the testicular end of the vas is fulgurated with a needle electrode (Fig. 84–9g). Bleeding can be controlled with cautery or ligatures. Dartos muscle and the skin are closed with 4-0 and 3-0 chromic sutures, respectively.

We believe that careful hemostasis and the interposition of fascia between the ends of the vas are important. Our technique of suture-ligating one end and cauterizing the other is arbitrary. Ligating, clipping, or cauterizing both ends of the vas are reasonable alternatives. Whichever technique is used, care should be

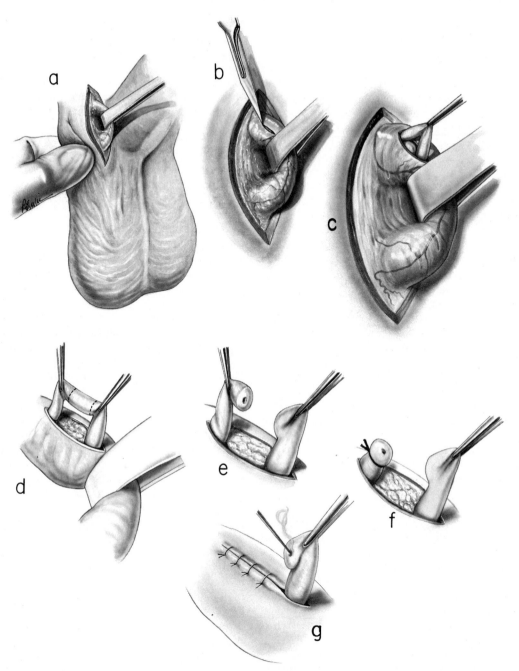

Figure 84–9. Vasectomy incision and removal of vas from its sheath *(a to c)*. We usually use a towel clamp rather than the illustrated instrument to grasp the vas in its sheath. Removal of a segment of vas *(d and e)*. Permanent suture ligature of abdominal end of vas *(f)*. Electrocauterization of testicular end of vas and interposition of fascia *(g)*.

exercised to avoid necrosing the ends of the vas, which increases the chance of recanalization.

VASOGRAPHY

Radiographic evaluation of the vas deferens and seminal vesicles is indicated in azoospermic men with normal spermatogenesis. Only after definite localization of the site of obstruction can reparative surgery be undertaken. If a site of obstruction is obvious, as in patients who have had a vasectomy, formal vasography is not necessary (see further on). In addition, vasography may aid in the identification of distal wolffian duct structures in patients without ambiguous genitalia. Contrast is injected either directly into the vas or in a retrograde fashion via the ejaculatory ducts. The latter method is technically difficult and will not be discussed.

If the patient is azoospermic and has not had previous testis biopsy, this is done initially as described and a frozen section is sent for analysis. After normal spermatogenesis has been demonstrated, the vas deferens is isolated. A spaghetti loop is placed around the vas for traction. The vas is placed on a flat tongue depressor and a 23- or 25-gauge needle is inserted cephalad into the vas (Fig. 84–10). A lymphangiogram needle may also be employed. Contrast material used for intravenous urography is diluted with two parts sterile saline, and 2.5 ml of the mixture is injected. Supine radiographs are obtained (see Fig. 7–26, Chapter 7). Oblique films often help to demonstrate the ejaculatory ducts, which are obscured by contrast within the proximal urethra. We have not encountered stricture formation using this technique. One also can document patency without using radiography by injecting methylene blue dye in the vas and checking the urine for the dye. In fact, if more than 3 or 4 ml of saline can be freely injected, the system is almost certainly open. The needle is removed and, if indicated, reinserted at a point caudad; 0.5 ml of contrast is then injected, demonstrating the convoluted vas and epididymis.

VASOVASOSTOMY

The frequency with which vasovasostomy is performed has increased dramatically because a significant percentage of the millions of men who underwent vasectomy in the last two decades are now seeking to regain their fertility.

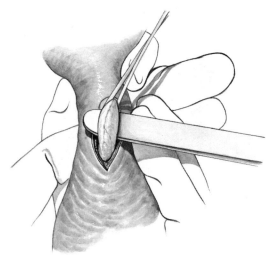

Figure 84–10. Isolation and stabilization of vas for vasography.

The most common reason for requesting a reversal is remarriage, although religious conversion or an altered attitude toward family size also motivates many of these individuals. Improved operative techniques and results have also contributed to the recent popularity of vasal reanastomosis (Owen, 1977; Silber, 1978a; Belker et al., 1978; Lee and McLoughlin, 1980; Howards, 1980; Sharlip, 1981). Considerable controversy exists regarding the most effective surgical method (Middleton and Henderson, 1978; Schmidt, 1975; Stewart, 1979; Lee and McLoughlin, 1980; Sharlip, 1981). We believe that (1) surgeons who perform the procedure regularly obtain better results than those who do it occasionally; (2) the use of optical aids *probably* increases the success rate; (3) the use of stents is not advantageous if the anastomosis is watertight; and (4) a formal two-layer anastomosis (Silber, 1978a) is no more effective than a modified two-layer anastomosis (Howards, 1980). This view is reinforced but not unequivocally proved correct by the clinical studies of Sharlip (1981) and the animal experiments of Lamesch and Dociu (1981), the results of which show equal fertility rates with the two techniques.

Our bias is that a more precise operation can be performed with the aid of a microscope, and that the standard two-layer anastomosis is unduly tedious and is not cost-effective. Therefore, we perform a modified, microscopic, two-layer anastomosis. The following equipment is used: (1) a zoom operating microscope with foot pedals to control focus, magnification, and position; (2) microsurgical instruments, including a needle holder, scissors, two straight-toothed forceps, two straight smooth forceps, and polished, J-shaped jeweler's forceps; (3) a vas deferens clamp; (4) Ethicon 10-0 Ethilon suture (1711G) on a GS-16 needle and any 8-0 monofilament suture; (5) an operating table that allows the surgeon to sit comfortably with his knees under the field; (6) bipolar microdiathermy; and (7) a small syringe and needle for irrigation.

With the patient under general or continuous epidural anesthesia, a vertical scrotal incision is made, and the testicle, epididymis, and proximal vas deferens are removed from the scrotum (Fig. 84–11a). The surgeon's hands should rest on a platform of towels for stabilization during the microsurgical phases of the operation. The site of the vasectomy is identified (Fig. 84–11b). The scarred area is placed on a tongue blade and is sharply excised with a scalpel. The proximal end of the vas is then cut

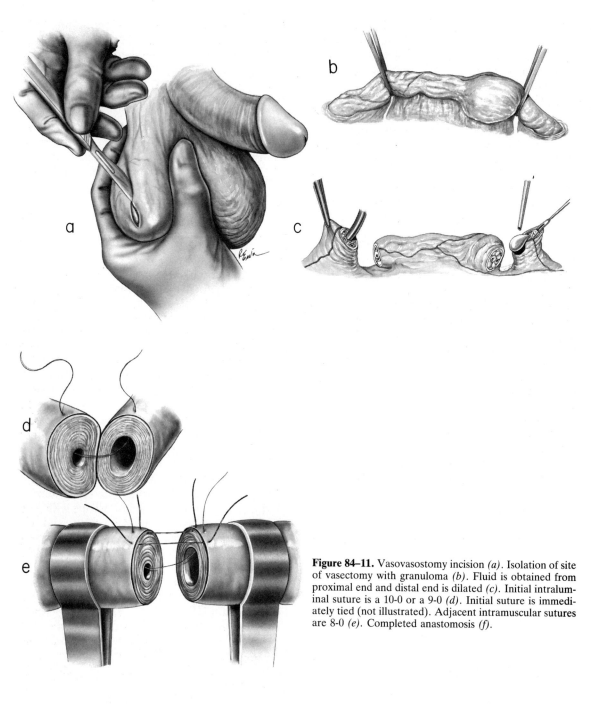

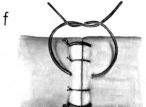

Figure 84–11. Vasovasostomy incision *(a)*. Isolation of site of vasectomy with granuloma *(b)*. Fluid is obtained from proximal end and distal end is dilated *(c)*. Initial intraluminal suture is a 10-0 or a 9-0 *(d)*. Initial suture is immediately tied (not illustrated). Adjacent intramuscular sutures are 8-0 *(e)*. Completed anastomosis *(f)*.

back until fluid is seen (Fig. 84–11c). The fluid is collected by capillary action in a small capillary tube. The fluid is viewed under a microscope; a better prognosis is associated with the presence of spermatozoa. If no spermatozoa are seen in the fluid, we proceed unless inspection of the epididymis reveals an obvious proximal obstruction. Although the chance of success is reduced in this setting, we feel there is no way to ascertain whether fertility will result. If these patients remain azoospermic postoperatively, we then perform a testis biopsy; if spermatogenesis is normal, we explore the epididymis. If an epididymal obstruction is identified, an epididymal vasostomy is done.

During vasovasostomy, the distal end of the vas is resected until a normal lumen and a well-vascularized wall are seen. The distal lumen is gently dilated with curved jeweler's forceps (Fig. 84–11c). The patency of the distal segment may be confirmed quickly and easily by passing a 4-0 suture into the lumen. Bleeding is carefully controlled with bipolar cautery. Devascularization of the vas has not been recognized as a problem.

The two ends of the vas are then placed in a vas deferens approximator clip (Fig. 84–11e). If a formal two-layer anastomosis is to be done, the folding vas clamp and the technique described by Belker (1984) may be useful. If the outer diameter of the vas deferens is small, it is helpful to place a sterile piece of rubber tubing over one arm of the clip. A sterile piece of blue plastic material is then cut from a surgical drape, or any other inexpensive material, and is placed under the two ends of the vas. This sheet provides an excellent background, and its puncture with a fine needle at multiple sites allows the blood and irrigating fluid to drain, thus maintaining a clear surgical field. A 10-0 suture is then passed through the entire thickness of the vas deferens, puncturing, in order of occurrence, the serosa of the proximal segment, its mucosa, the mucosa of the distal end, and finally the distal serosa (Fig. 84–11d). The suture is tied. Two 8-0 sutures are then placed through the muscle, one on either side of the 10-0 suture (Fig. 84–11e). These sutures, which do not enter the lumen, are tied and thereby stabilize the anastomosis. Three or four additional through-and-through 10-0 sutures are then placed, so a suture is in place in each of the four quadrants. It is often easier to place the last two sutures before tying them. The anastomosis is reinforced with one or two 8-0 sutures between each of the original stitches (Fig. 84–11f). The second layer of sutures does not enter the lumen. If the

anastomosis is made to the proximal convoluted vas deferens or to the epididymal tubule itself, it is often easier to use six to eight through-and-through sutures in a single layer. The testis and epididymis are then returned to the scrotum, and the dartos muscle and skin are closed in layers.

The procedure can be done on an outpatient basis, or the patient may be hospitalized the night of surgery and discharged the following morning. He is able to return to work within a day or two but is advised to wear a scrotal support and to avoid heavy lifting and ejaculation for 2 weeks. Aspirin is sufficient for pain relief. Three months postoperatively, semen analysis often reveals a good sperm count with poor motility. After 6 months, the count is usually stable or slightly improved and the motility is significantly improved.

If spermatozoa were present in the fluid obtained from the distal vas deferens at surgery, more than 90 per cent of the patients will have spermatozoa in their postoperative ejaculate. The subsequent pregnancy rate is approximately 40 to 70 per cent. The reasons for the discrepancy between incidence of patency and fertility are unknown. Possible factors include testicular malfunction secondary to the previous vasectomy, abnormal epididymal function, delayed transport of spermatozoa, immunologic abnormalities, and female infertility. The fertility rate after vasovasostomy slowly decreases as the interval between vasectomy and reanastomosis increases. The consensus is that the preoperative presence of serum antisperm antibodies does significantly affect the prognosis; however, there is strong evidence that the presence of seminal antisperm antibodies postoperatively does decrease fertility (Linnet et al., 1981).

There are many other techniques of vasovasostomy currently in use. Acceptable modifications include local anesthesia to reduce the cost (Fuchs, 1982; Kaye et al., 1982) and nonmicroscopic repairs incorporating many of the principles outlined previously. The experience of the surgeon is often more important than the details of the technique.

EPIDIDYMOVASOSTOMY

Epididymal obstruction is likely to be the cause of azoospermia in a man whose testicular biopsy demonstrates normal spermatogenesis, who has seminal fluid that yields positive results when tested for fructose, and in whom vasographic examination is normal. Most commonly these patients have postinflammatory obstructive lesions, a congenital blockage, or acquired secondary obstruction after a vasectomy.

Microscopic anastomosis of the vas deferens to a single epididymal tubule is conceptually the ideal procedure (Silber, 1978b). Although this new technique has not been proved to yield more pregnancies than the macroscopic method, it certainly is more physiologic. The equipment and general techniques necessary for microscopic surgery are described in the section on vasovasostomy. A vertical incision is made in the hemiscrotum and is carried through the parietal layer of the tunica vaginalis. The testis, epididymis, and vas are delivered out of the scrotal compartment. Visual inspection of the epididymis often reveals dilated epididymal tubule segments. In the absence of obviously dilated segments, the microscope is used at low magnification to localize tubular dilatation.

After identification of the site of probable obstruction, the epididymis is dissected distally, freeing it from the testis. An elastic loop is placed around this portion of the epididymis. To be certain that no vasal obstruction is present, the vas is dissected free just distal to the convoluted portion, and vasography is performed (Fig. 84–12a).

After vasal patency is confirmed, the vas is divided distal to the convoluted area. A single tubule above the suspected level of obstruction is then transected (Thomas, 1983) (Figs. 84–12b and 84–13a). If no obvious site of obstruction is identified, an arbitrarily chosen distal location is incised. The transected tubule is examined

for egress of luminal fluid. When fluid is seen effluxing from a tubule, it is sampled with a capillary tube and examined microscopically for the presence of sperm. If sperm are not evident, a more proximal tubule segment is transected. The presence of sperm confirms that the incision is proximal to the site of obstruction. If we cut a tubule within 1 cm of the ductuli efferentes and still do not find any spermatozoa, we transect the epididymis at this site and remove a 5-mm transverse section of the epididymis on the distal side of the transection and examine this tissue microscopically (Turner and Howards, 1981). If sperm are present in that section, we perform the anastomosis at this level. We do not perform an anastomosis closer than 5 to 7 mm to the ductuli efferentes, because fertility is unlikely if the anastomosis is in such close proximity (Schoysman and Stewart, 1980), although Silber (1980) reported success with proximal anastomoses. An end-to-end or end-to-side anastomosis is made to the epididymal tubule from which the sperm-containing fluid is egressing. It is helpful to stain the cut epididymal tubule with a drop of methylene blue dye (Belker, 1984). If the entire epididymis has been transected, the tubule from which fluid is effluxing is best identified by applying pressure to the proximal epididymis, swabbing the transected surface, and microscopically observing the cut surface.

The tubule is anastomosed to the vas, using the vas-approximating clamp, by placing four to six 10-0 nylon sutures. The sutures pass through

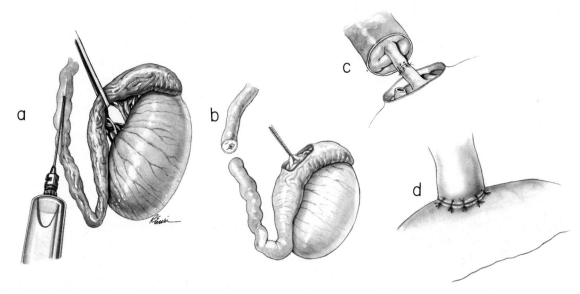

Figure 84–12. Epididymovasostomy: vasogram to rule out distal obstruction *(a)*. Tongue blade and elastic are used as shown in Figure 84–10. End-to-end anastomosis of vas to single epididymal tubule *(b to d)*.

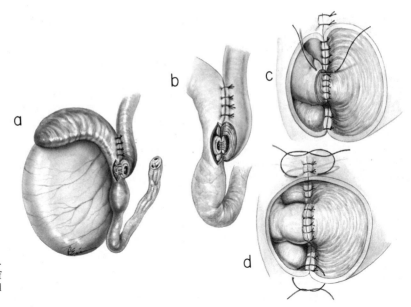

Figure 84–13. Epididymovasostomy: end-to-end anastomosis of vas deferens to single epididymal tubule.

the individual epididymal tubule and the vas (Fig. 84–12c). Six to ten 8-0 nylon sutures are used to approximate the seromuscular layer of the vas to the tunica of the epididymis (Fig. 84–12d). An alternative to the end-to-end anastomosis is an end-to-side anastomosis. The vas is sutured to the epididymal capsule with 5-0 sutures (Fig. 84–13a), and a posterior row of 8-0 sutures is placed between the epididymal capsule and the seromuscular layer of the vas (Fig. 84–13a). Then, the epididymal tubule, which has been incised longitudinally, is sutured to the lumen of the vas with 10-0 sutures (Fig. 84–13b). The anterior portion of the anastomosis is complete in the same two layers (Fig. 84–13c and d). After completion of either anastomosis, the testis is returned to the scrotum, which is closed in separate layers by using chromic sutures.

Postoperative care is similar to that described for vasovasostomy. Although convincing data are insufficient at this time regarding the advantages of microscopic vasoepididymostomy, we believe the direct tubular anastomosis is physiologically and anatomically the preferred procedure.

Other options include the end-to-end microsurgical anastomosis after transection of the epididymis (Silber, 1978b) (described earlier) and the classic procedure used to perform vasoepididymostomy, which is macroscopic and involves an incision in the body of the epididymis, transecting multiple lumina. A longitudinal incision is made in the vas, which is sewn side-to-side with the epididymal tunic (Fig.

84–14). The success of the procedure is dependent upon formation of a sperm fistula between these two structures.

EPIDIDYMECTOMY

Epididymectomy for recurrent epididymitis is rarely indicated. An occasional patient with chronic recurrent or indolent suppurative epididymitis may require epididymal excision for complete relief of symptoms. In some instances, a complete epididymo-orchiectomy is necessary. We do not hesitate to perform an epididymo-orchiectomy in elderly patients with suppurative epididymal orchitis that has not responded promptly to nonoperative therapy. Tuberculous epididymitis, with extension into surrounding scrotal structures and the development of cutaneous sinus tracts, is extremely uncommon and

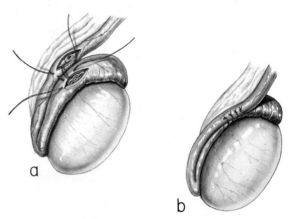

Figure 84–14. Macroscopic epididymovasostomy.

usually responds adequately to antituberculous drug therapy. Partial epididymectomy is occasionally indicated for adenomatoid tumors or for cases in which focal epididymal induration presents a problem in differential diagnosis.

Epididymectomy for the relief of chronic pain of undetermined cause should rarely, if ever, be performed. Certainly this procedure is not indicated unless pain relief has been documented after blocking the cord with local anesthesia and a competent psychologist or psychiatrist has evaluated the patient and recommends excision.

If the epididymectomy is done because of infection, appropriate antibacterial therapy is begun at least 12 hours before surgery. The testis with its tunics is delivered through the anterior scrotal incision, as for simple orchiectomy, and the tunica vaginalis is opened to allow adequate inspection of the epididymis and the lower vas deferens. The vas deferens is isolated

(Fig. 84–15a) and transected at as high a level in the cord as is technically possible, and the distal lumen of the vas is cauterized with a needle electrode or is suture-ligated. Small vessels in this area may require separate electrocoagulation or suture ligation. The vas deferens is then dissected downward, including its convoluted portion and the tail of the epididymis. Care is taken to avoid surrounding vascular structures during this dissection. The epididymis is then separated from the testis, beginning at the lower pole, with a combination of sharp and blunt dissection (Fig. 84–15b). As the dissection is carried upward, the vascular pedicle is encountered near the junction of the middle and upper thirds of the testis. Extreme care must be taken at this point to preserve the blood supply to the testis. With the vascular pedicle kept between thumb and forefinger behind the epididymis, the epididymis can be elevated anteriorly, and the testicular blood supply can be

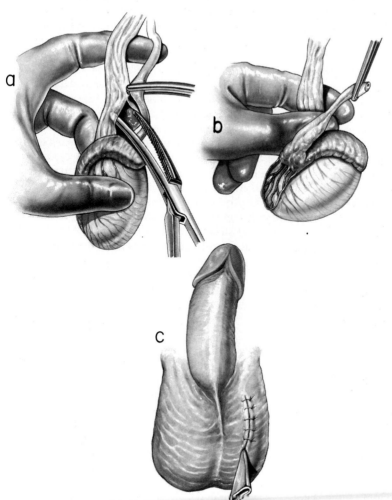

Figure 84–15. Epididymectomy. Isolation of the vas *(a)*. Removal of the epididymis from the testis *(b)*. Closure *(c)*.

more easily preserved (Fig. 84–15*b*). Small vascular branches to the epididymis are divided and secured, and the remainder of the epididymis is then separated from the testis. The ductuli efferentes attaching the caput to the testis should be ligated. Hemostasis is completed with light electrocautery or fine suture ligatures, and the incision is closed in layers after a small Penrose drain has been brought out separately through the scrotal wall in a dependent position (Fig. 84–15*c*). If the underlying inflammatory condition has caused rupture through the tunics and has involved the skin, excision of contiguous skin with wide scrotal debridement must be carried out along with total epididymo-orchiectomy. After surgery, a scrotal pressure dressing is applied, and appropriate antibacterial therapy is administered until healing is complete.

VARICOCELE REPAIR

The indications for varicocele repair in infertile men with suboptimal semen quality are discussed in Chapter 12. Varicoceles are also occasionally corrected in boys and fertile men for cosmetic reasons or to eliminate symptoms. There are three distinct approaches to the ligation of the internal spermatic vein: scrotal, inguinal, and retroperitoneal. The scrotal approach is used infrequently because it is difficult to be certain that all of the numerous veins in the pampiniform plexus are ligated, and it is also possible to damage one or more of three arteries (spermatic, differential, and cremasteric) that supply the testis and epididymis. The theoretical advantage of a scrotal incision is that all veins, even those that do not anastomose to the internal spermatic vein, can be ligated. The inguinal and the retroperitoneal approaches are both widely used and accepted. The inguinal approach is described by Dubin and Amelar (1977) and Lipshultz and Howards (1983). The eponyms Ivanissevich and Palomo are often used to refer to the inguinal and retroperitoneal approaches. This terminology is confusing, however, because Ivanissevich described both techniques. Indeed, the retroperitoneal approach, which we prefer and subsequently describe, is more similar to the operation Ivanissevich (1960) described in his article on the subject than it is to the higher, Palomo approach.

High Ligation. Under suitable anesthesia, the patient is prepared and draped and is placed in reverse Trendelenburg position to fill the veins. A short transverse incision is made just medial to the anterior superior iliac spine, approximately at the level of the internal ring (Fig. 84–16*a*). The external oblique fascia is incised

in the direction of its fibers (Fig. 84–16*b*). The internal oblique muscle is retracted caudad with an abdominal retractor (Fig. 84–16*c*). The dilated vein is usually identified easily without any further dissection (Fig. 84–16*c*). The vein is then freed from the surrounding fat by using blunt or, preferably, sharp dissection. The dissection is continued toward the renal vein to as high a level as is convenient to look for anastomosing collateral vessels. The vein is ligated and a segment is removed (Fig. 84–16*d*). The area is inspected for additional veins (Fig. 84–16*d*). At this level, there are usually only one or two veins, although multiple veins are occasionally encountered. Care is taken to avoid dividing the artery or lymphatic channels. The use of a Doppler probe makes identification of the artery easy, and we routinely use this technique. Although interruption of the internal spermatic artery at this level probably does not significantly injure the testis, we nevertheless preserve the vessel. The vas deferens can be seen at the lower medial aspect of the incision as it curves into the pelvis (Fig. 84–16*d*). The internal oblique muscle is tacked back in position, and the external oblique is closed with nonreabsorbable sutures. A subcuticular skin closure is used for aesthetic reasons and to eliminate the need for suture removal. The patient is discharged the next day. The procedure can also be done on an "in-and-out" or day-surgery basis. We do not think it is necessary to visualize the ureter, as some surgeons advocate. Performed in the manner described, this technique is simple and does not, as has been asserted, convert an easy procedure into a major operation.

The incision for the inguinal approach is indicated by the dashed line in Figure 84–16*a*. The external oblique muscle is incised to the external ring to expose the spermatic cord, which is mobilized. Then the spermatic fascia is incised and the veins are ligated. At this level, there are usually two or three veins and occasionally there are many veins. As with the higher approach, care is taken to preserve the artery and lymphatic vessels.

SPERMATIC CORD TUMORS

Most tumors of the spermatic cord are benign, including lipomas, hydroceles of the cord, fibromas, and adenomatoid tumors of the vas deferens. Perhaps the most common benign "tumor" found in the spermatic cord is sperm granuloma after vasectomy. Unless significantly symptomatic, these lesions do not require definitive therapy. Local excision is usually curative. Malignant tumors of the spermatic cord are

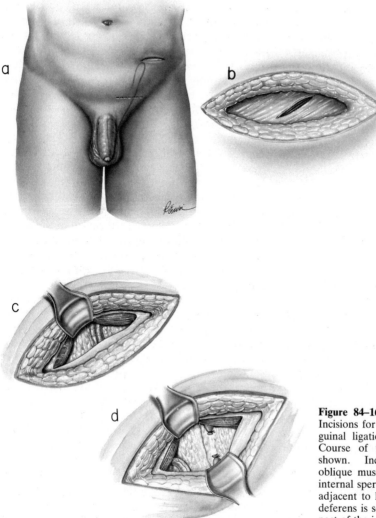

Figure 84–16. Varicocele repair. Incisions for high ligation and inguinal ligation (dashed line, *a*). Course of the vas deferens is shown. Incision of external oblique muscle *(b)*. Exposure of internal spermatic vein *(c)*, artery adjacent to ligated vein. The vas deferens is seen in the medial aspect of the incision *(d)*.

relatively rare and can occur at all ages. The most common tumor in the younger age group is embryonal rhabdomyosarcoma; fibrosarcomas, leiomyosarcomas, and liposarcomas occur more typically in the older age groups. The treatment of sarcomas of the cord is complex, often involving multiple modes of therapy with surgery and drugs.

Treatment should include inguinal orchiectomy as described, with high ligation of cord structures at the inguinal ring in all cases. If the scrotum is involved or if previous biopsy has been done on the lesion through a scrotal incision, a partial or hemi-scrotectomy may be indicated. Initial spread of these tumors is by both lymphatic and vascular channels. In many instances, supplemental retroperitoneal node dissection after orchiectomy is advisable. Groin dissection should also be performed if inade-

quate local excision or local recurrence of tumor in the inguinal nodes is evident (Malek et al., 1972).

SURGERY OF THE TUNICS

HYDROCELECTOMY

A hydrocele of the testis is an excess collection of fluid between the tunica vaginalis and the tunica albuginea. Infants in whom the processus vaginalis has not sealed may develop a hydrocele. These fluid collections will often seal and disappear spontaneously in the first few months of life. Therefore, hydrocele repair should be delayed until age 9 to 12 months. In adults, hydrocelectomy should be considered only if the lesion is of sufficient size to cause significant discomfort or embarrassment to the patient. Before electing conservative management of hydroceles, however, the clinician should be certain that serious underlying disease is not present. Hydroceles can occur secondary to tumors or inflammatory conditions of the testis and epididymis. Therefore, particularly in younger men, the hydrocele should be aspirated to allow adequate palpation of these structures before a diagnosis of idiopathic hydrocele is made. The aspirated fluid can be sent for cytologic diagnosis. Sclerotherapy with several different agents, including 5 to 10 ml of 2.5 per cent phenol in water (Nash, 1979) and 3 per cent sodium tetradecyl sulfate (Macfarlane, 1983), has been reported to have a high success rate. One to three treatments are required. To date, we have reserved this approach for patients who are poor surgical candidates.

Hydrocele can be repaired through a transverse or oblique scrotal incision (Fig. 84–17a). Meticulous hemostasis is important in all scrotal surgery to reduce the incidence of postoperative hematomas. The hydrocele is delivered through an adequate scrotal incision. Bleeding is reduced and the procedure is facilitated if the surgeon dissects through the multiple layers of fascia to the plane just outside the tunica vaginalis before excising the hydrocele. The hydrocele at first looks like a bluish cyst. After dissection, the sac is opened anteriorly and the testis and the epididymis are carefully inspected. Redundant sac is then excised, and all bleeding vessels are secured by cautery or with suture ligature (Fig. 84–17b). At this point, there are several options. The sac may be entirely or partially excised. In either case, the surgeon may merely place a running, locked suture along the entire length of the remaining sac. A second option, which we prefer, is to leave 2 or 3 cm of hydrocele sac attached to the testis and the epididymis, to bring these edges behind the testis, and to complete the closure with a running, locked reabsorbable suture (Fig. 84–17c). This method eliminates raw, oozing surfaces and prevents reformation of hydrocele as a result of inversion and reapposition of the edges of the hydrocele sac. The surgeon must avoid closing the sac too tightly at its upper end, which could adversely affect the blood supply to the testis.

Additional alternative procedures include the Lord (1964) operation and the simple extrusion procedure (Solomon, 1955; McGown and Howley, 1969). These procedures are said by their advocates to be quicker and are less frequently followed by hematoma formation. The extrusion involves suturing the incised edge of the hydrocele sac to the epididymotesticular junction without dissecting or excising the sac. The Lord procedure consists of reefing the redundant hydrocele sac with multiple plicating suture.

Regardless of the method used to eliminate the hydrocele, the testis is then replaced in the scrotum, which is loosely closed in layers. We do not drain the scrotum, although this is advocated by other authors (Stewart, 1979). We place ice on the scrotum for the first 12 to 24 hours after surgery and use a firm scrotal support.

SPERMATOCELECTOMY

A spermatocele is a cyst of the rete testis, ductuli efferentes, or epididymis that is filled with fluid and spermatozoa. These cysts are outside the tunica vaginalis and usually transilluminate. Spermatoceles are usually small and do not require surgical treatment; they should be treated surgically only if they cause pain or embarrassment to the patient or in those rare cases in which they cannot be differentiated

Figure 84–17. Hydrocelectomy. Incision (a), excision of excess tunica vaginalis (b), and suturing of tunica around epididymis (c).

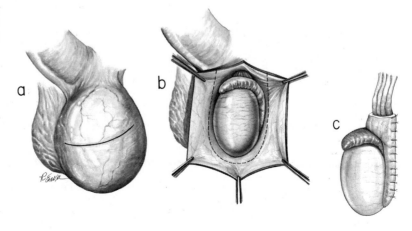

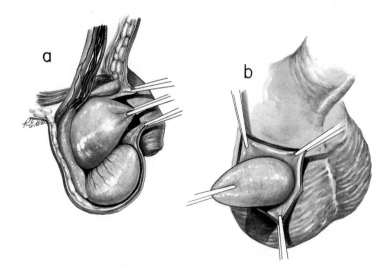

Figure 84–18. Spermatocelectomy. Exposure and excision.

from adenomatoid tumors or focal inflammatory conditions of the epididymis.

The spermatocele is approached through an anterior scrotal incision, with just enough exposure to circumscribe the lesion adequately. The dissection is carried down to the thin wall of the spermatocele itself. Many spermatocele may simply be "shelled out" intact, without extensive mobilization of the epididymis or of the adjacent testis (Fig. 84–18). In the case of larger spermatoceles, the few small blood vessels and fascial attachments arising from the epididymis may be transected and ligated by sutures individually. After excision of the spermatocele and complete hemostasis, it is usually possible to secure a layer of adjacent fascia over the epididymal defect and to close the wound in layers without the need for drainage. Ice and a scrotal support are used postoperatively, as after hydrocelectomy.

References

Alexander, N. J., and Clarkson, T. B.: Vasectomy increases the severity of diet-induced atherosclerosis in *Macaca fascicularis*. Science, *201*:538, 1978.

Allen, T.: Disorders of the male external genitalia. *In* Kelalis, P. P., King, L. R., and Belman, A. B. (Eds.): Clinical Pediatric Urology. Philadelphia, W. B. Saunders Co., 1976.

Belker, A. M.: Microsurgical repair of obstructive causes of male infertility. Semin. Urol., *2*:91, 1984.

Belker, A. M., Acland, R. D., Sexter, M. S., et al.: Microsurgical vasovasostomy: laboratory use of vasectomized segments. Fertil. Steril., *29*:48, 1978.

Bunce, P. L.: Scrotal Abnormalities. New York, Harper & Row, 1975, p. 783.

Clarkson, T. B., and Alexander, J. N.: Long term vasectomy—effects on the occurrence and extent of atherosclerosis in rhesus monkeys. J. Clin. Invest., *65*:15, 1980.

Conley, J. J.: A one-stage operation for the repair of the denuded penis and testicles. N. Y. State J. Med., *56*:3014, 1956.

Desai, H. C., and Williams, H. W.: Treatment of elephantiasis by wide excision and grafting. Ind. J. Surg., *21*:369, 1959.

Dickson, R. W., and Hofsess, D. W.: Nontropical genital elephantiasis. J. Urol., *82*:131, 1959.

Dresner, M. L.: Torsed appendage: diagnosis and management; blue dot sign. Urology, *1*:63, 1973.

Dubin, L., and Amelar, R. D.: The varicocele and infertility. *In* Amelar, R. D., Dubin, L., and Walsh, P. C. (Eds.): Male Infertility. Philadelphia, W. B. Saunders Co., 1977.

Fuchs, E. F.: Cord block anesthesia for scrotal surgery. J. Urol., *128*:718, 1982.

Furnas, D. W., and McCraw, J. B.: Resurfacing the genital area. Clin. Plast. Surg., *7*:236, 1980.

Gibson, T.: Traumatic avulsion of skin of scrotum and penis: use of avulsed skin as free graft. Br. J. Plast. Surg., *6*:283, 1954.

Harrison, R. G., Lewis-Jones, D. I., Moreno, M. J., and Connolly, R. C.: Mechanism of damage to the contralateral testis in rats without ischemic testis. Lancet, *2*:723, 1981.

Howards, S. S.: Vasovasostomy. Urol. Clin. North Am., *7*:165, 1980.

Ivanissevich, O.: Left varicocele due to reflux: experience with 4,470 operative cases in 42 years. J. Int. Cell. Surg., *34*:742, 1960.

Johnson, J. H.: Acquired lesions of the penis, the scrotum, and the testis. *In* Williams, D. I., and Johnston, J. H. (Eds.): Paediatric Urology. London, Butterworth, 1982.

Kaye, K. W., Lange, P. H., and Fraley, E. E.: Spermatic cord block in urologic surgery. J. Urol., *128*:720, 1982.

Lamb, R. C., and Juler, G. L.: Fournier's gangrene of the scrotum. A poorly defined syndrome or a misnomer. Arch. Surg., *118*:38, 1983.

Lamesch, A. J., and Dociu, N.: Microsurgical vasovasostomy. Eur. Surg. Res., *13*:299, 1981.

Lee, L., and McLoughlin, M. G.: Vasovasostomy. A comparison of macroscopic and microscopic techniques at one institution. Fertil. Steril., *33*:54, 1980.

Linnet, L., Hjort, T., and Fogh-Anderson, P.: Association between failure to impregnate after vasovasostomy and sperm agglutinins in semen. Lancet, *1*:117, 1981.

Lipshultz, L., and Howards, S. S.: Surgical treatment of male infertility. *In* Lipshultz, L., and Howards, S. S. (Eds.): Infertility in the Male. London, Churchill Livingstone, 1983.

Lord, P. H.: A bloodless operation for the radical cure of idiopathic hydrocele. Br. J. Surg., *51*:914, 1964.

Macfarlane, J. R.: Sclerosant therapy for hydroceles and epididymal cyst. Br. J. Urol., *55*:81, 1983.

Manchanda, M. S., Singh, R., Keswani, R. K., and Sharma, C. G.: Traumatic avulsion of scrotum and penile skin. Br. J. Plast. Surg., *20*:97, 1967.

Mathes, S. J., and Nahai, F.: Clinical Atlas of Muscle and Musculocutaneous Flaps. St. Louis, C. V. Mosby Co., 1979, p. 519.

McConnell, J. D., Peters, P. C., and Lewis, S. E.: Testicular rupture in blunt scrotal trauma: a review of 15 cases with recent application of testicular scanning. J. Urol., *128*:309, 1982.

McCormack, J. L., Kretz, A. W., and Tocantis, R.: Traumatic rupture of the testicle. J. Urol., *96*:80, 1966.

McDougal, W. S.: Scrotal reconstruction using thigh pedicle flaps. J. Urol., *129*:757, 1983.

McGown, A. J., and Howley, T. F.: Experiences with the extrusion operation for hydrocele. J. Urol., *101*:366, 1969.

Melek, R. S., Utz, D. C., and Farrow, G. M.: Malignant tumors of spermatic cord. Cancer, *29*:1108, 1972.

Middleton, R. G., and Henderson, D.: Vas deferens reanastomosis without splints and without magnification. J. Urol., *119*:763, 1978.

Nash, J. R.: Sclerotherapy for hydrocele and epididymal cysts. Br. J. Surg., *66*:289, 1979.

Owen, E. R.: Microsurgical vasovasotomy: a reliable vasectomy reversal. Aust. N.Z. J. Surg., *47*:305, 1977.

Ray, B., and Whitmore, W. F.: Experience with carcinoma of the scrotum. J. Urol., *117*:741, 1977.

Roen, P. R.: Atlas of Urologic Surgery. New York, Appleton-Century Crofts, 1967.

Schmidt, S. S.: Principles of vasovasostomy. Contemp. Surg., 7:13, 1975.

Schoysman, R., and Stewart, B. H.: Epididymal causes of male infertility. Monogr. Urol., *1*:1, 1980.

Sharlip, E. D.: Vasovasostomy: comparison of two microsurgical techniques. Urology, *17*:347, 1981.

Silber, S. J.: Vasectomy and its microsurgical reversal. Urol. Clin. North Am., *5*:573, 1978*a*.

Silber, S. J.: Microscopic vasoepididymostomy: specific microanastomosis to the epididymal tubule. Fertil. Steril., *30*:565, 1978*b*.

Silber, S. J.: Vasoepididymostomy to the head of the epididymis: recovery of normal spermatozoal motility. Fertil. Steril., *34*:149, 1980.

Solomon, A. A.: The extrusion operation for hydrocele. N.Y. State J. Med., *55*:1885, 1955.

Stewart, B. H.: Surgery of the scrotum and its contents. *In* Harrison, J. H., et al. (Eds.): Campbell's Urology. 4th ed. Philadelphia, W. B. Saunders Co., 1979.

Tiwari, I. H., Seth, H. P., and Mehdiratta, K. S.: Construction of the scrotum by thigh flaps. Plast. Reconstr. Surg., *66*:605, 1980.

Turner, T. T., and Howards, S. S.: Microscopic vasoepididymostomy: examination of epididymal lumen content for presence of spermatozoa. Fertil. Steril., *36*:533, 1981.

CHAPTER 85

The Adrenals

ROBERT G. DLUHY, M.D.
RUBEN F. GITTES, M.D.

INTRODUCTION

The adrenal glands have attained a great importance in urologic and general surgery since the advent of life-preserving substitution therapy, which makes bilateral, total adrenalectomy feasible. The increased knowledge of the pathologic physiology of the adrenal cortex and medulla and the continuing progress in radiographic, biochemical, and radioisotopic techniques in research and clinical investigation have increased both diagnostic and therapeutic accuracy. There has been a greater appreciation of the influence of adrenocortical disorders on sexual differentiation. More insight has been gained from experience and knowledge of the renal-adrenal interrelations serving to regulate blood pressure. Progress in anesthesiology has contributed extensively to the advances in the surgery of the adrenal and has made possible the safe removal of tumors of the cortex and medulla.

ANATOMY, EMBRYOLOGY, AND ANOMALIES

The adrenal glands are small, yellowish brown flattened, somewhat triangular structures lying retroperitoneally within the perinephric fascia and in close proximity to the upper pole of each kidney. Their size varies considerably even in normal subjects and is importantly influenced by the condition of the individual; infection and other types of stress often produce a significant increase in adrenal size. The average adrenal gland weight is 4 gm, and each gland is usually 4 to 6 cm long and 2 to 3 cm wide (Neville and Mackay, 1972).

The adrenal glands are composed of cortex and medulla (chromaffin tissue). The cortex in man constitutes approximately 90 per cent of the gland by weight. On section, the medulla is soft and grayish tan, developing a dark brownish color upon exposure to chromates. The medullary tissue is completely surrounded by cortical tissue, so that the medullary cells are bathed by high concentrations of steroids. This anatomic relationship promotes the N-methylation of norepinephrine to epinephrine, since the enzyme phenylethanolamine-N-methyltransferase (PNMT) is inducible by high levels of glucocorticoids.

The adrenal glands have an extraordinarily rich blood supply, estimated to be 6 to 7 ml per gm of tissue per minute. The lymphatics of the glands drain into lateral aortic nodes. The nerve supply is derived primarily from the splanchnics, and the fibers are medullated, preganglionic, and cholinergic in type. Stimulation of the adrenal nerves results in a prompt discharge of medullary hormones.

Microscopically, the adrenal cortex is divided, from without inward, into three zones: the zona glomerulosa, zona fasciculata, and zona reticularis (Fig. 85–1). The cortex is composed of large, lipid-laden epithelioid cells arranged in irregular cords around sinusoids. It is clear that active regeneration of a partially destroyed or resected adrenal cortex can occur if cells of the capsule and zona glomerulosa survive. Zonation of the cortex is functional as well as structural. The zona glomerulosa produces aldosterone and is regulated by angiotensin II and potassium; the inner layers, which secrete cortisol and sex steroids, are dependent on pituitary corticotropin (ACTH) for control of growth and secretions.

The adrenal gland develops from two separate antecedents that remain functionally and

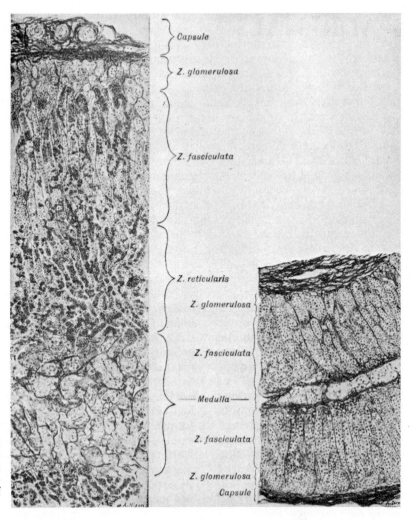

Figure 85–1. Section of an adrenal (left) of a man and (right) of a 6-month-old infant. Mallory azan stain. About 105 ×. (From Maximow and Bloom: Textbook of Histology.)

structurally distinct as cortex and medulla (Soffer et al., 1961). During the fourth week of embryonal life, mesothelial buds appear at the level of the upper third of the mesonephron and project into the celom at each side of the root of the dorsal mesentery. Eventually, they coalesce to form a compact mass of cells, the adrenal cortex, lateral to the aorta. Cortical buds that do not join the main cellular mass disappear or form accessory adrenal tissue in the region of the adrenal, kidney, celiac plexus, spermatic vessels, testis, broad ligament, or ovary. The medulla is of ectodermal origin and is derived from the primitive cells (sympathogonia) of the sympathetic nervous system. These cells ultimately give rise to sympathoblasts (which develop into mature ganglion cells) and pheochromoblasts (which develop into chromaffin cells). The sympathochromaffin cells migrate to the region of the adrenal cortical mass and penetrate the latter to form, at approxi-

mately the seventh week of fetal life, the adrenal medulla. Numerous small groups of chromaffin cells are also found in association with the prevertebral sympathetic ganglia and the celiac, mesenteric, renal, adrenal, and hypogastric plexuses. A larger collection above the aortic bifurcation is called the organ of Zuckerkandl. In the bladder, chromaffin cells are found with the sympathetic nerve fibers.

During intrauterine life the adrenal glands attain a relatively enormous size, owing to rapid growth of the fetal cortex (Villee, 1972). At the fourth fetal month they are actually larger than the kidneys; at birth they are approximately one third as large. In adult life the normal ratio of adrenal to kidney size is approximately 1:28. During the first 3 weeks of postnatal life, the adrenal loses appoximately half its weight, owing almost entirely to degeneration of the fetal cortex. Absolute adrenal size changes little during early childhood, and birth weight is not regained until puberty. There is evidence that the fetal adrenal cortex is an important endocrine organ during intrauterine life, serving as the primary source of steroid precursors utilized by the placenta for the formation of estriol and related compounds during pregnancy.

Anomalies. Accessory adrenal tissue may consist of cortical or medullary tissue alone or may contain both. Although it is generally recognized that accessory cortical bodies are frequently present in infants, their persistence in adults was formerly considered uncommon. However, it is now recognized that they may be found in a significant number of adults, frequently being located in the neighborhood of the adrenal glands themselves or near the celiac axis, or, less commonly, along the genitourinary tract, in the pelvis, or even embedded in other organs such as the pancreas or liver. In rare instances, tumors arise in these ectopic bodies.

The anomalies of the adrenal gland of surgical importance include bilateral absence (in unviable monsters) and unilateral agenesis, often in association with unilateral renal agenesis or hypoplasia. Heterotopia (developmental inclusion of the entire gland in or beneath the renal capsule) occurs more often in males, is frequently bilateral, and may be accompanied by adrenal hypoplasia. Although its occurrence is rare, careful examination of the adrenal in all cases of surgery on a single kidney is warranted, in addition to detailed study of all kidneys that have been removed. Benign adrenal cysts with or without adrenal insufficiency may be congenital or may develop following adrenal hemorrhage. The variety and incidence of anomalies were reported in 51,088 autopsies studied by Campbell (1970).

SURGICAL ANATOMY

The adrenal glands exhibit certain important anatomic similarities on the right and left sides. Each gland is attached by a vascular supply that is more independent of the kidney than has been commonly emphasized, although each lies in a superior extension of the perinephric fascia of Gerota. Each lies superior and medial to the upper pole of the kidney and may be described as a low pyramid, surrounded by adipose tissue and containing convolutions to which are attached multiple fibrous septa from the perinephric fascia. A deeper yellow color and firmer consistency enable one to differentiate the gland from fat. The basal surface is often concave, and the superior convexity extends upward along the aorta on the left and between the liver and vena cava on the right. The glands are much more inaccessible in obese or heavily muscled patients. Exposure is ordinarily easier in the female patient than in the male, owing to the lighter and less well developed musculoskeletal structures.

Knowledge of the blood supply and delicate architecture of these well-hidden glands greatly facilitates their surgical removal (Netter, 1965). Arterial blood reaches the adrenals through channels derived from the inferior phrenic artery (one or more) superiorly, from the aorta mesially, and from the renal arteries inferiorly (Fig. 85–2). One is impressed surgically by the great vascularity of these relatively small glands. Blood from the cortex drains into capillary networks that ultimately pass into the very well developed venous system of the medulla. The largest adrenal vein on the right side is quite short and enters directly into the vena cava; on the left these veins are longer and there are also branches to the renal vein. Each vein is quite thick-walled and muscular. On each side veins accompany branches of the phrenic artery (Fig. 85–2). On the left, venous channels leave the cortex to join the vena cava and the splanchnic, splenic, and pancreatic veins to reach the portal system. Each gland has multiple fibrous attachments around the entire periphery, which must be severed by sharp dissection in order to avoid tearing the septa of the fragile cortex. The nerve supply is from the splanchnic chain and is on the mesial aspect accompanying the larger vessels. The lymphatics run in the fibrous trabeculae and form a plexus about the central vein of the medulla.

SURGICAL APPROACHES

Various surgical approaches to the adrenal have been utilized with success. The transabdominal approach has the advantage of simultaneous bilateral exploration but the disadvantage of requiring transperitoneal displacement of viscera. Excellent exposure is accomplished by the transthoracic approach (Chute et al., 1949) but carries the limitation of a unilateral operation. The bilateral posterior subcostal approach of Young, with the patient in the prone position, is a direct route that permits exploration of each gland simultaneously with minimal disturbance of other viscera. It is obvious that simultaneous bilateral exposure was of particular value when an adrenal tumor was suspected but had not been localized preoperatively. However, the posterior approach has the limitation of a small operative field with somewhat re-

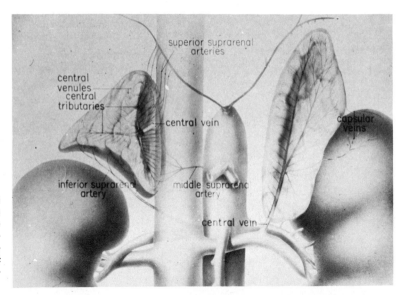

Figure 85–2. Arterial and venous anatomy of the adrenal glands. The venous structures are relatively constant and very important in the performance of selective catheterization for sampling and for diagnostic venography. (Courtesy of J. Bookstein, M.D.)

stricted visualization, and such blind exploration is now precluded by modern imaging techniques (Fig. 85–3).

A flank approach affords a wider field of operation with direct access to the gland on one side at a time and is extremely useful when an adrenal tumor has been accurately localized prior to operation. In the case of suspected tumor, palpation of the opposite adrenal can be accomplished with this approach by opening the peritoneum but must be done with reservations as to accuracy. The approach to the *left* adrenal is easily made by subperiosteal resection of the eleventh rib, entering the perinephric space through the bed of the rib.

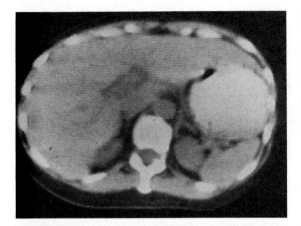

Figure 85–3. Imaging by computerized tomography has revolutionized the localization of adrenal tumors. Shown here is an example of a patient with pheochromocytoma whose left adrenal is seen on this section. It has a normal wishbone shape well outlined by radiolucent fat. The resolution of the normal adrenal is at the 0.5 cm level in high-quality scans (see Chapter 7).

The kidney is completely mobilized by sharp dissection, displaced inferiorly to the iliac fossa, covered with a gauze pad, and held in place out of the operative field, usually with a hand or a Deaver retractor. The adrenal is drawn down by the traction on the renal fascia and is identified by palpation and inspection. The left adrenal is usually lower than the right and is in less intimate contact with the aorta than is the right gland with the vena cava. The lower one third of the adrenal is always in close proximity to and attached to the left renal artery. The renal vessels are carefully observed during the entire dissection of the left adrenal gland.

The splenic vessels cross the field laterally and superiorly in the anterior peritoneal covering. The adrenal is best dissected free along its periphery laterally until one can palpate its anterior surface freely from upper to lower pole. Next, the vessels from the phrenic artery entering the superior pole are divided between clamps or clips. Usually these can be ligated. Electrocoagulation is useful in controlling the smaller vascular branches. Next, the larger vessels leaving the mesial aspect and, finally, the inferior vascular attachments of the gland are secured and divided.

The *right* adrenal is ordinarily less accessible than the left, and its removal is somewhat more hazardous because of its intimate relationship with both the liver and the vena cava high in the subdiaphragmatic angle (Figs. 85–4 and 85–5). In all but thin patients, it is best to resect the eleventh rib and the operation is greatly facilitated by the flank position rather than the prone position. After careful subperiosteal re-

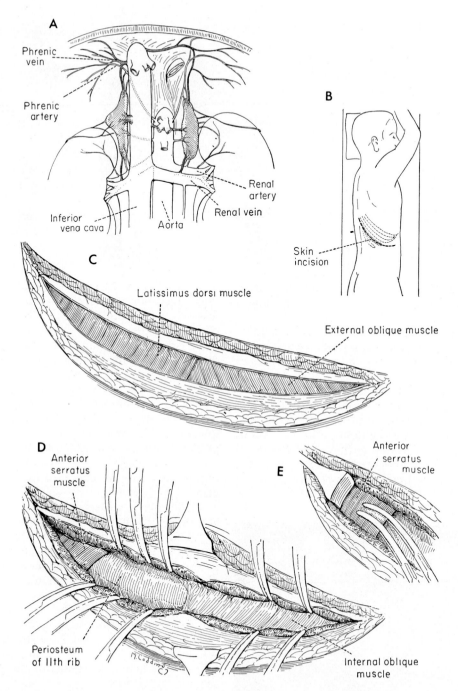

Figure 85–4. The flank approach to the right adrenal. *A,* Anatomic diagram of the adrenal glands, showing the relation of the right and left adrenals to the vena cava and aorta as well as to the kidneys. The definitive blood supply derived from the renal vessels and from the aorta and vena cava and the superior branches from the phrenic vessels are each shown and designated. One of the more important features of surgery of the right adrenal is the short-vein entering the vena cava, which one must carefully secure by a ligature before dividing it close to the gland. *B,* Position of the patient as he lies on his left side and the direction of the incision over the eleventh rib for the approach to the right adrenal. *C,* The incision has been made, showing exposure of the latissimus dorsi and external oblique muscles. *D,* The external oblique muscle has been divided to expose the internal oblique and periosteum over the eleventh rib. The anterior serratus muscle is exposed. *E,* The anterior serratus muscle is being clamped before division.

Illustration continued on opposite page.

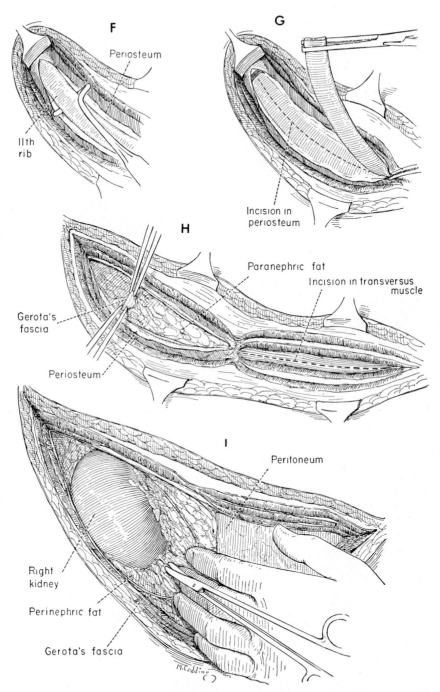

Figure 85–4 *(Continued).* The flank approach to the right adrenal (continued). *F,* Subperiosteal exposure of the eleventh rib has been accomplished, and the rib is being freed from its bed. *G,* Subperiosteal resection of the eleventh rib in its distal two thirds has been accomplished. Incision in the underlying periosteum is indicated. *H,* Incision in the periosteum has been completed, and Gerota's fascia of the false renal capsule is being lifted to be opened. Internal oblique muscle has been divided, and the incision to be made in the transversus muscle is indicated. *I,* Gerota's fascia has been opened and dissection of the kidney for mobilization is being carried out. The transversus muscle has been incised. Complete and free mobilization of the kidney is desirable in order that it may be displaced inferiorly without distortion of the vascular pedicle or the parenchyma.

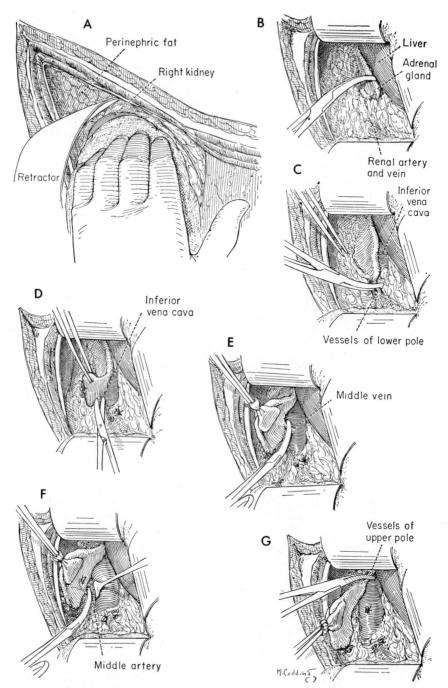

Figure 85–5. Flank approach to the right adrenal (continued). *A,* The kidney has been completely freed in its entire circumference superiorly and inferiorly by sharp dissection and is now being displaced down into the iliac fossa, where it will be protected by a gauze pad and held in place by a Deaver retractor. *B,* The suprarenal fossa is adequately exposed; the liver is seen anterosuperiorly, and the adrenal below it is still encased in the perinephric fat. *C,* The lower polar vessels of the adrenal coming from the renal vessels have been exposed and are being clamped before division and ligation. *D,* The lower pole of the adrenal is being lifted, and the gland is being dissected free from fascial attachments to the vena cava. *E,* The gland is being lifted from the vena cava. The large adrenal vein emptying into the vena cava is exposed and is being clamped prior to ligation. *F,* The vena cava is being retracted mesially to expose small vascular branches that are pursuing a posterior course and are being clamped. These are often secured with silver clips. *G,* The entire adrenal gland has been freed from the vena cava, and the upper vessels from the phrenic vessels are exposed and are being clamped prior to ligation. This completes the right adrenalectomy. All these anatomic relationships and the details of the definitive procedure of adrenalectomy must be remembered in the removal of small or large tumors of the adrenal.

section of the eleventh rib, the pleura can be adequately protected and retracted, unopened, from the operative field. After displacement of the kidney, the gland is dissected free from its attachments to the infrahepatic fascia.

The vena cava is identified and exposed, and the relations of the gland to this structure are studied. The gland is freed along its periphery as dissection progresses, and the inferior blood supply from the renal vessels is isolated, clamped, divided, and ligated. The lower pole of the gland can now be lifted to expose the main adrenal vein as it enters the vena cava; the former is doubly ligated and divided or is clamped with an atraumatic Satinsky hemostat and divided. Finally, the superior blood supply from the phrenic vessels is secured and adrenalectomy is completed by their division.

The transperitoneal approach to the adrenals by an upper abdominal transverse incision is illustrated in Figures 85–6 and 85–7. This approach to both renal and adrenal surgery has gained popularity in the last decade and has been modified as an inverted U or "frown" incision extending obliquely down to the iliac crest on each side. This approach is particularly applicable for pheochromocytoma because of the potential this tumor has for multiple origin. It is not desirable for the obese patient with Cushing's syndrome. The thoracoabdominal approach is desirable for large tumors.

PHYSIOLOGY OF THE ADRENAL CORTEX

STEROIDOGENESIS

Adrenal steroids are synthesized from acetate, via cholesterol. Scission of the cholesterol side chain forms Δ^5-pregnenolone (Fig. 85–8); the transformation involves several enzymic steps (Brooks, 1979). Evidence indicates that the action of corticotropin in stimulating steroidogenesis may well occur at this point. Two enzymes, 3β-hydroxysteroid dehydrogenase and a Δ^5-3-ketosteroid isomerase, catalyze the conversion of Δ^5-pregnenolone to progesterone (Fig. 85–9), which is then hydroxylated at C-17 to form 17-hydroxyprogesterone. Δ^5-pregnenolone also undergoes 17α-hydroxylation to 17-hydroxypregnenolone, which in turn is converted by the dehydrogenase-isomerase system into 17-hydroxyprogesterone. (These alternate pathways from cholesterol to 17-hydroxyprogesterone are common to the synthesis of steroid hormones in the adrenal cortex, testis, ovary, and placenta.) Progesterone and 17-hydroxy-progesterone are hydroxylated at C-11, C-21, and C-18 to form the major corticosteroid hormones—cortisol, corticosterone, and aldosterone. The dehydrogenases, isomerases, and hydroxylases are complex enzyme systems with multiple components, and the conversions outlined may involve several intermediates.

It has long been recognized that the adrenal gland secretes androgenic steroids. The established pathways for androgen synthesis in the adrenal cortex follow the same routes as those established for the testis. As shown in Figure 85–10, C-21 steroids hydroxylated at the C-17 position can undergo oxidative removal of the C-20-21 side chain, resulting in the formation of 17-ketosteroids; 17-hydroxy-Δ^5-pregnenolone gives rise to dehydroepiandrosterone, and 17-hydroxyprogesterone to Δ^4-androstenedione. The latter is hydroxylated at C-11 to form 11β-hydroxy-Δ^4-androstenedione. All three of these 17-ketosteroids have been isolated from adrenal venous blood. In the testis, Δ^4-androstenedione is further reduced to testosterone. It has been shown that adrenal homogenates can also carry out this reaction, but in the intact adrenal gland most of the androstenedione is converted by C-11-hydroxylation into the 11β-hydroxy derivative. The 17-ketosteroid formed in the largest quantity by the adrenal cortex is dehydroepiandrosterone sulfate.

Although estrogens have not been demonstrated in normal adrenal venous blood, it is clear that the levels are elevated in certain states of adrenocortical hyperfunction (e.g., adrenal carcinoma). Estrogens appear to be produced in the adrenal cortex or in the periphery from testosterone or Δ^4-androstenedione by aromatization of the A ring (Fig. 85–10).

The fetal adrenal has long been of great interest to endocrinologists, primarily because of its relatively great size (Villee, 1972). The activity of the 3β-hydroxysteroid dehydrogenase system is relatively low. It has been postulated that the partial deficiency of this enzyme system effectively reduces the output of cortisol, leading in turn to increased secretion of corticotropin by the fetal hypophysis and hypertrophy of the cortex sufficient to restore cortisol production. The result is progressive enlargement of the fetal cortex and a high output of Δ^5-steroids, including dehydroepiandrosterone sulfate, which is converted to 16α-OH-dehydroepiandrosterone sulfate in the fetal liver. Their secretion as sulfate conjugates apparently protects the fetus from the potential masculinizing effects of these weak androgens. Placental microsomes plus supernatant can aromatize 16α-OH-dehydroepiandrosterone sulfate to estriol,

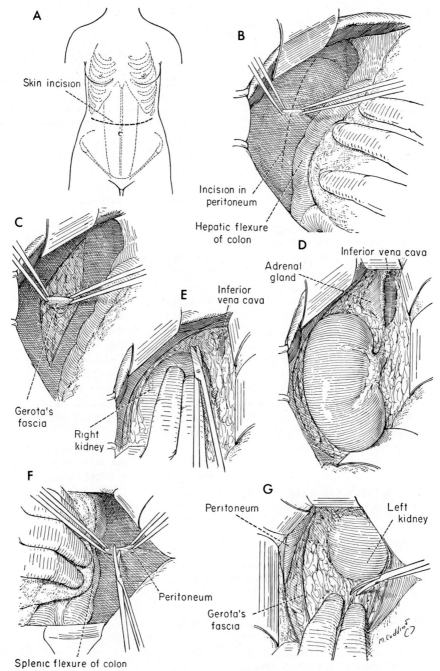

Figure 85–6. Bilateral transabdominal approach to the adrenals and retroperitoneal sympathetic chain. *A,* Diagram indicating the transverse abdominal incision that divides both rectus muscles and, laterally on each side, the external oblique, internal oblique, and transversalis muscles extending out below the costal margin when necessary. *B,* After careful transabdominal exploration, the intestines are walled off and the right retroperitoneum is approached, the ascending colon and hepatic flexure of the colon being displaced mesially and covered with wet gauze pads. The incision in the posterior layer of the peritoneum overlying the kidney is indicated. *C,* Incision has been made in the posterior layer of the peritoneum, exposing the false renal capsule of Gerota's fascia. *D,* The right kidney is exposed and is freed by sharp dissection until it can be completely mobilized. *E,* The right kidney has been completely freed up; its vascular pedicle is exposed. The vena cava is shown, and the adrenal lying superiorly is exposed. Exploration of the adrenal, as well as the lumbar sympathetic chain, can now be carried out with excision of any tumors of the lumbar sympathetic chain on this side or of the adrenal itself, as shown in Figure 85–5. *F,* The intestines have been walled off mesially from the left pararenal gutter; the posterior layer of the peritoneum is being opened for exploration on the left side. *G,* The retroperitoneum has been opened and the lower pole of the left kidney exposed. Dissection of the perinephric tissues has begun.

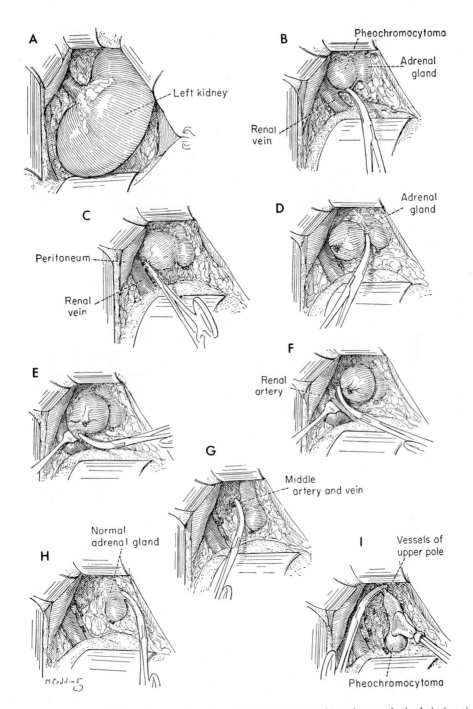

Figure 85–7. The bilateral transabdominal approach to the adrenals and retroperitoneal sympathetic chain (continued). *A,* The left kidney and its vascular pedicle are exposed and ready to be displaced inferiorly. *B,* The kidney has been displaced inferiorly, and a clamp is being placed on the vein to the lower pole of the left adrenal. A pheochromocytoma in the extra-adrenal tissues has also been exposed. *C,* A branch from the renal vein to the extra-adrenal tumor is being clamped before ligation. *D,* Dissection is being carried out between the adrenal, which contains a tumor in its lower pole, and the extra-adrenal tumor that lies between the adrenal and the renal vein. *E,* Dissection between the pheochromocytoma and the renal vessels is being carried out. *F,* An artery to the extra-adrenal tumor from the renal artery is being clamped before division and before ligation preceding removal of the tumor. *G,* Lateral attachments of the adrenal gland are being dissected free and clamped before division. *H,* Mesial vascular attachments of the adrenal are being secured before incision and ligation. *I,* The superior attachments derived from the phrenic vessels are being divided betwen clamps prior to division, which will complete the adrenalectomy and the removal of the adrenal gland containing a pheochromocytoma.

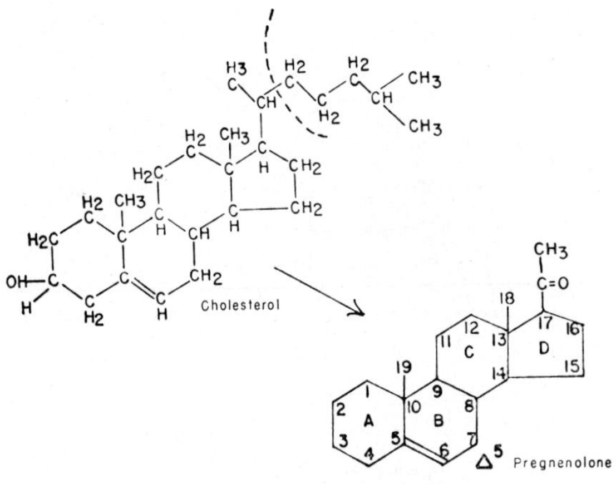

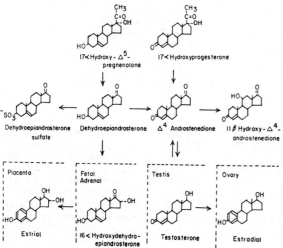

Figure 85–8. Conversion of cholesterol to pregnenolone. The cholesterol formula shows the complete steroid structure; the pregnenolone formula shows the conventional representation of the steroid molecule with the rings designated by letter and the carbon atoms numbered.

Figure 85–9. Corticosteroid synthesis in the adrenal cortex. Enzyme systems are numbered: (1) β-hydroxysteroid dehydrogenase:Δ5-oxosteroid isomerase complex, (2) C-17-hydroxylase, (3) C-21-hydroxylase, (4) C-11-hydroxylase, (5) C-18-hydroxylase. Δ signifies a double bond, and the attached number shows its position in the nucleus.

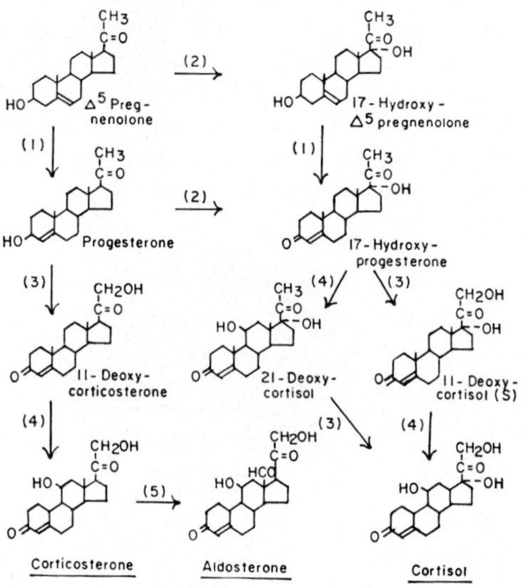

Figure 85–10. Sex hormone synthesis. The upper portion of the scheme shows the synthesis of adrenal androgens. The lower panel shows conversion of androstenedione to testosterone (testis, adrenal cortex, and, to a small degree, the liver); 16 α-hydroxylation of dehydroepiandrosterone by the fetal adrenal and conversion to estrogen in the placenta; and conversion of androgen to estrogen in the ovary. Note that the initial steps in sex hormone synthesis are the same in all these organs.

the predominant urinary estrogen in pregnant women (Ryan, 1959). Thus, it would appear that the estrogens characteristically produced in large quantity during pregnancy by the maternal placenta are formed from precursors supplied by the fetal adrenal cortex (Fig. 85–10).

HORMONE SECRETION

The major secretory product in man that has glucocorticoid action is cortisol. Corticosterone has been isolated, but only in small amounts. Aldosterone is the major mineralocorticoid. Quantitatively, dehydroepiandrosterone sulfate is the main androgen. Smaller amounts of 11β-hydroxy-Δ^4-androstenedione, Δ^4-androstenedione, and dehydroepiandrosterone are also secreted. Although compounds having estrogenic and progestational activity may be released in minute amounts by normal adrenals, the contribution is so small that they are not ordinarily classified as adrenocortical hormones. However, in certain abnormalities of biosynthesis these steroids may be secreted in relatively large amounts and cause hormonal disturbances.

STEROID METABOLISM

The major circulating glucocorticoid is cortisol. Most of the circulating cortisol is bound to a specific alpha-2 globulin, transcortin or cortisol-binding globulin (CBG) (Sandberg and Baunwhite, 1971). The bound cortisol is in reversible equilibrium with a small moiety in free solution, and in all likelihood it is the latter fraction that is directly involved in the biologic actions of the hormone. When the binding sites of CBG become saturated at plasma cortisol levels of 25 to 27 μg per dl, the quantity present in free solution rises significantly. One effect of protein-binding is to reduce the glomerular filtration of cortisol; in contrast, the hormonally inactive metabolites of cortisol, conjugated mainly as water-soluble glucuronides, are not protein-bound and are excreted much more efficiently by the kidneys.

The half-life of free cortisol in plasma, measured with C-14–labeled tracer quantities, is 80 to 100 minutes (Peterson, 1971). This comparatively rapid rate of removal is accomplished largely by the liver. Cortisol and cortisone are interchangeable via reversible reduction-oxidation at C-11. Reduction of the 3-ketone group and of the double bond at C-4-5 forms tetrahydrocortisol; further reduction of the C-20 ketone group produces cortol. Similarly, reduction of cortisone produces tetrahydrocortisone and cortolone. The enzyme glu-

curonosyl transferase couples the 3α-hydroxy group of these metabolites with uridine diphosphate–glucuronic acid to form glucuronides, which are excreted in the urine. In addition, approximately 5 per cent of cortisol undergoes oxidative removal of the C-20-21 side chain to form 17-ketosteroids (the 11β-hydroxy- and 11-keto- derivatives of etiocholanolone and androsterone). Only a very small fraction of cortisol is excreted unchanged into the urine: 20 to 100 μg per day (Beisel et al., 1964).

The metabolic turnover of aldosterone is more rapid, because it is only weakly bound to protein (Brooks, 1979). Aldosterone undergoes hepatic reduction to tetrahydro derivatives and conjugation with glucuronic acid. However, a small fraction appears in the urine as an acid-labile 3-oxo compound (probably a glucuronide, conjugated at C-18); it is the latter fraction that is usually estimated in the clinical laboratory and, on the average, amounts to 5 to 25 μg per day on a normal dietary sodium intake (Luetscher et al., 1965).

Dehydroepiandrosterone and Δ^4-androstenedione are reduced to androsterone and etiocholanolone (Fig. 85–11). These 17-ketosteroids are also conjugated at the C-3 position in the liver and are excreted in the urine as sulfates or glucuronides (Migeon, 1972).

Testosterone is the most important androgen in man. In normal males, testosterone output primarily reflects testicular secretion; accordingly, plasma testosterone levels are an excellent index of Leydig cell function. Similar to cortisol, testosterone is tightly bound to a specific sex steroid–binding globulin. In most

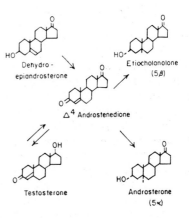

Figure 85–11. Metabolism of androgens. Some dehydroepiandrosterone is directly excreted in the urine; most is converted to androstenedione. The latter is reduced to 17-ketosteroids (e.g., etiocholanolone and androsterone); a small amount is reversibly changed to testosterone in the adrenal.

instances, measurement of the total testosterone level correlates with the clinical situation. On the other hand, mild androgen abnormalities correlate best with the free hormone concentration, which is assessed by the measurement of both the total testosterone concentration and the per cent testosterone bound. In some adrenal disorders overt virilization occurs, reflecting potent androgen activity. This is secondary to peripheral (hepatic) metabolism of normal adrenal cortical products to testosterone rather than from adrenal secretion of testosterone (Camacho and Migeon, 1966). Dehydroepiandrosterone and its sulfate ester can be converted by the liver to testosterone but only in minute amounts; Δ^4-androstenedione is the main peripheral precursor (Korenman and Lipsett, 1964), forming both testosterone glucuronide (which is excreted in the urine) and free testosterone (Fig. 85-11), some of which re-enters the circulation and is hormonally active. In normal females, as much as 50 per cent of circulating testosterone is derived peripherally from androstenedione of adrenal and ovarian origin (Tait and Horton, 1965). It is known that testosterone is metabolized in certain tissues (e.g., prostate, epididymis, skin) to 5α-dihydrotestosterone (DHT) (Wilson, 1980).

FUNCTIONS OF THE ADRENAL CORTEX

The physiologic actions of cortical hormones are diverse and complex and, in all probability, influence the function of all body cells. Both electrolyte and intermediary metabolism are affected. The electrolyte functions comprise sodium retention and increased excretion of potassium and hydrogen ions (Ludens and Fanestil, 1979). Steroids controlling these functions have been called mineralocorticoids (primarily aldosterone). The functions related to the control of carbohydrate, fat, and protein metabolism are controlled by glucocorticoids (primarily cortisol) (Baxter and Forsham, 1972). Although originally defined by their metabolic actions, glucocorticoids and mineralocorticoids are best defined by specific cytosolic receptors in target tissues that mediate the actions of the hormones (Baxter and Rousseau, 1979). After binding to cytosolic receptors, the steroid-receptor complex enters the nucleus and interacts with nuclear receptors. Specific genes are then expressed with transcription of specific messenger RNA's, and ultimately new protein synthesis results. These proteins mediate the steroid response and may be inhibitory or stimulatory in the specific tissue that is influenced. The distinction between mineralocorticoids and gluco

corticoids is by no means complete; for example, cortisol has a significant effect on electrolyte metabolism in addition to its other actions. Besides their primary functions, glucocorticoids exhibit a "permissive effect," whereby other hormones exhibit their full actions only in the presence of small amounts of glucocorticoid; fat mobilization by epinephrine and vasoconstriction by norepinephrine are good examples, because both actions require the presence of small amounts of cortisol (Granner, 1979).

Electrolyte Metabolism. Regulation of electrolyte excretion is influenced predominantly by aldosterone, acting on the ion-exchange mechanism of the distal renal tubule subsequent to binding to a specific mineralocorticoid receptor. Severe mineralocorticoid deficiency results in sodium, chloride, and water loss, leading to hyponatremia, dehydration, a reduction of plasma volume, hypotension, and, in extreme cases, vascular shock. In addition, renal excretion of potassium and hydrogen ions is impaired, with resulting hyperkalemic acidosis. On the other hand, excessive mineralocorticoid secretion results in lower blood and tissue levels of potassium that can be severe enough to produce characteristic abnormalities of neuromuscular and cardiac function. Hypokalemia is often accompanied by a depletion of hydrogen ions and the characteristic hypochloremic alkalosis.

Intermediary Metabolism. Adrenocortical failure results in difficulty in maintaining normal blood glucose concentrations during fasting. The defect results primarily from a decrease in hepatic gluconeogenesis (the production of glucose from amino acid precursors), which is normally regulated by cortisol (Exton, 1979). Aldosterone is devoid of this action at physiologic levels. An excess of cortisol produces an insulin-resistant state and hyperglycemia (steroid diabetes) in some patients. The tendency to develop diabetes under the influence of glucocorticoids is probably inversely related to the reserve capacity of the islets of Langerhans to augment the secretion of insulin.

The regulation of gluconeogenesis depends primarily upon the influence of insulin, glucagon, and cortisol on the balance between synthesis and degradation of proteins; cortisol diminishes the synthesis of proteins from amino acid precursors while accelerating the breakdown of cellular proteins. The amino acid residues are deaminized in the liver, with a resultant increase in the production of urea and in the formation of liver glycogen. The net result is a deviation of body proteins to available carbohydrate. Glucocorticoids also accelerate gluco-neogenesis by directly stimulating the synthesis of specifc hepatic enzymes, such as tryptophan pyrrolase and tyrosine amino transferase. Finally, glucocorticoid-induced hyperaminoacide-mia indirectly facilitates gluconeogenesis by stimulating glucagon secretion.

Effects of Excessive Concentrations of Glucocorticoid. The protein catabolic actions of excess cortisol have profound functional structural effects. Body growth may be impaired; interference with the formation of osteoid tissue results in osteoporosis; inhibition of granulation may interfere with wound healing; and muscular strength is reduced because of proximal muscle wasting.

Cortisol excess produces a neutrophilic leukocytosis, eosinopenia, and lymphopenia. Cortisol does not produce lysis of lymphocytes; lymphopenia results from redistribution of circulating lymphocyte pools. T-cells or the small lymphocytes derived from the thymus are most profoundly influenced. Antibody production is not altered unless glucocorticoids are administered at high dosage over long periods of time. Cortisol opposes the increase in capillary permeability that is seen in acute inflammation and impedes endothelial sticking of leukocytes and diapedesis through the capillary wall. The structure of all connective tissue elements, including reticular cells, fibrils, and ground substance, may be affected. As a result of these effects on both fixed and migratory cellular defensive elements and on the microvasculature, the inflammatory response is reduced (the so-called anti-inflammatory actions of glucocorticoids) (Baxter and Rousseau, 1979). The ability to withstand injury, and particularly infection, may also be seriously deranged.

Elevated levels of cortisol lower the threshold for electrical excitation of the brain. Psychiatric disturbances may occur when cortisol is present in excess.

Cortisol may produce peptic ulceration by increasing gastric acidity and/or reducing the mucosal barrier to the back-diffusion of hydrogen ions.

The production of angiotensinogen is stimulated by cortisol, leading to higher levels of angiotensin II, which is an extremely potent vasoconstrictor and a specific stimulant of aldosterone production (Stockigt et al., 1979). In addition, cortisol sensitizes the arterioles to the pressor effects of norepinephrine.

Glucocorticoids suppress the pituitary secretion of ACTH. Accordingly, primary adrenal failure is associated with increased levels of ACTH and hyperpigmentation. The increased pigmentation is due to elevated plasma levels of ACTH or of other pituitary peptides, such as beta-lipotropin, which are secreted in a parallel fashion with ACTH. The hyperpigmentation was initially believed to be the result of elevated levels of melanocyte-stimulating hormones (α-MSH and β-MSH), which share common amino acid sequences of the ACTH peptide. However, recent evidence suggests that neither α-MSH nor β-MSH exists in man; the previously reported MSH levels were thought to be produced artifactually from larger peptides during the sample extraction process (Hoffman, 1974).

Sexual Effects. The adrenal cortex secretes steroids that are weakly androgenic, primarily Δ^4-androstenedione and dehydroepiandrosterone. The growth of axillary and pubic hair in females appears to be controlled primarily by adrenal androgens. It is possible that in females adrenal androgens also have a weak anabolic effect, enhancing protein synthesis from amino acids (Migeon, 1972).

The Adrenal Cortex and Stress. The extensive studies of many investigators have shown that the adrenal cortex plays a significant role in normal responses to major stress (Selye, 1947). The importance of an adequate adrenal response to changes in the external environment and to dislocations of the internal milieu is best demonstrated by the marked vulnerability of patients with adrenocortical insufficiency to stress of all types.

The hormone primarily implicated in the metabolic phenomena occasioned by acute stress is cortisol. The manner in which cortisol confers its protective effects is largely unknown. However, the relationship is roughly quantitative, in that the more severe the stress, the larger the quantity of cortical hormone required to protect the organism. Thus, as demonstrated by Ingle (1949), a normal circulating level of cortisol may be adequate to resist brief stresses of moderate intensity. However, with prolonged or severe insults the pituitary-adrenocortical system is activated, primarily as a result of neurohormonal stimuli involving the hypothalamus, with a resultant acceleration of cortisol production. For example, it has been repeatedly demonstrated in man that major surgical procedures constitute a serious stress, eliciting a marked increase in ACTH and adrenocortical secretion (Moore, 1953). Therefore, it is evident that activation of the pituitary-adrenocortical system is requisite to the safe conduct of major surgery; that patients with adrenocortical insufficiency cannot be safely subjected to surgical procedures unless adequate quantities of cortisol are administered; and that patients undergoing surgery for removal of functioning adrenal tumors or total adrenalectomy require preoperative corticosteroid preparation and postoperative hormone maintenance.

SYNTHETIC ANALOGS OF CORTISOL

Cortisol is the naturally secreted glucocorticoid of the adrenal cortex. Glucocorticoid hormones have been widely used in clinical medicine for replacement therapy but more frequently have been utilized for their anti-inflammatory actions in certain diseases, such as rheumatoid arthritis and bronchial asthma. Since glucocorticoid hormones also possess protein-wasting properties, attempts have been made to synthesize cortisol analogs with heightened anti-inflammatory and reduced catabolic properties. The "side effects" of these analogs should be looked upon as the expected catabolic actions of nonphysiologic concentrations of glucocorticoid hormones.

Substitutions at various sites of the cortisol molecule have produced a number of synthetic analogs with altered biologic properties. In general, these synthetic compounds have an increased affinity for glucocorticoid receptors. As a result, the biologic properties of synthetic analogs differ from those of cortisol in three fundamental ways. First, synthetic analogs are more potent anti-inflammatory agents than cortisol on a per milligram basis. However, synthetic analogs do not dissociate the anti-inflammatory from the protein-wasting actions of glucocorticoid hormones. Thus, equipotent

doses of cortisol and its analogs share similar propensities for producing the undesirable side effects of glucocorticoids. Second, most synthetic analogs have diminished sodium-retaining activities, and this may be clinically important in patients predisposed to sodium retention. Finally, modifying the structure of cortisol leads to altered steroid metabolism, usually prolonging both blood and tissue half-lives. Since synthetic analogs have long half-lives and are ordinarily less tightly bound to cortisol-binding globulin, they have a greater propensity for producing iatrogenic Cushing's syndrome, especially if administered in divided doses.

As with the use of insulin preparations, the physician must select certain representative glucocorticoids and master their individual properties. Table 85–1 presents the most commonly used adrenal preparations. The glucosteroids are divided into three groups according to the duration of biologic activity. Short-acting preparations have a biologic half-life of less than 12 hours; long-acting preparations, greater than 48 hours; and intermediate preparations, between 12 and 36 hours.

CONTROL OF ADRENOCORTICAL FUNCTION

Growth and maintenance of normal adrenocortical structure are controlled by adrenocorticotropin (ACTH) released from the anterior pituitary gland. In addition, ACTH regulates the synthesis and secretion of cortisol and the adrenocortical sex steroids. There is evidence that ACTH stimulates the generation of membrane-bound 3'-5' cyclic adenosine monophosphate (AMP), which in turn activates ad-

TABLE 85–1. ADRENAL PREPARATIONS*

	Anti-inflammatory Potency	Equivalent Potency (mg)	Sodium-Retaining Potency
Short-acting			
Hydrocortisone	1	20	2+
Cortisone	0.8	25	2+
Intermediate-acting			
Prednisone	3.5	5	1+
Prednisolone	4	5	1+
Methylprednisolone	5	4	0
Triamcinolone	5	4	0
Long-acting			
Paramethasone	10	2	0
Betamethasone	25	0.60	0
Dexamethasone	30	0.75	0

*The steroids are divided into three groups according to the duration of biologic activity. Short-acting preparations have a biologic half-life of less than 12 hr; long-acting, greater than 48 hr; intermediate, between 12 and 36 hr. Triamcinolone has the longest half-life of the intermediate-acting preparations. (From Dluhy, R. G., Lauler, D. P., and Thorn, G. W.: Med. Clin. North Am., 77 1155, 1973.)

renocortical protein kinase enzymes (Gill, 1979). This leads to phosphorylation of proteins that subsequently activate steroid biosynthesis.

ACTH is a polypeptide with 39 amino acids and a molecular weight of 4500. Certain basophilic cells in the anterior pituitary gland are the source of ACTH, because fluorescein-labeled antibodies to ACTH are bound by these cells. Recent evidence also indicates that β-lipotropin and ACTH are probably secreted by the same pituitary cell from a larger precursor molecule, pro-opiomelanocortin (Miller et al., 1980).

Corticotropin-releasing hormone (CRH) is a recently identified hypothalamic peptide (41 amino acids), first isolated from sheep. It is secreted into the pituitary-portal blood system, where it effects the release of ACTH from the anterior pituitary gland (Vale et al., 1981). Three major factors control CRH and ACTH release: plasma cortisol levels, the sleep-wake cycle, and stress (Krieger, 1979). The latter two control mechanisms influence CRH via neural pathways. Hypothalmic monoaminergic neurotransmitters (e.g., serotonin and dopamine) are also known to modify CRH, and consequently ACTH, release.

Finally, a sensitive mechanism exists for the self-regulation of pituitary-adrenocortical function by cortisol (Ganong, 1963) via a negative feedback loop. Cortisol probably decreases the responsiveness of the anterior pituitary adrenocorticotropic cells to CRH. A fall in plasma cortisol levels leads to a rise in ACTH output; conversely, a rise in cortisol levels inhibits ACTH secretion. This so-called servomechanism maintains the level of plasma cortisol within relatively stable limits. One practical consequence of this mechanism is of great importance: Protracted administration of cortisol (or its congeners) may so effectively inhibit hypothalamic-pituitary function that adrenocortical atrophy ensues.

The control of aldosterone output differs markedly from that of cortisol (Williams and Dluhy, 1972) (Fig. 85–12). Several mechanisms have been recognized: (1) ACTH does increase aldosterone secretion, but the effect is far less than that on cortisol output and is not sustained, so that the secretion rate returns to previous levels despite continued ACTH administration. (2) Potassium appears to lead directly to increased aldosterone secretion. Since aldosterone also facilitates potassium excretion, potassium and aldosterone can be viewed as another feedback loop. (3) The primary mechanism for the control of aldosterone production appears to reside in a feedback system involving the kidney, with the sensor apparatus residing in the juxtaglomerular apparatus. In the presence of decreased renal perfusion pressure, the juxtaglomerular cells, which cuff the afferent arterioles, release an increased amount of renin, an enzyme that acts on the α_2-globulin angiotensinogen to produce the decapeptide angiotensin I. Angiotensin I is enzymatically converted to angiotensin II by an enzyme found primarily in pulmonary tissue (so-called converting enzyme). Angiotensin II is a potent stimulator of the zona glomerulosa of the adrenal cortex, resulting in increased aldosterone output. Angiotensin II is also the most potent pressor compound in the body and exerts this action by directly constricting arteriolar smooth muscle. It is now apparent that stimuli such as sodium restriction, reduction in intravascular volume, hemorrhage, and dehydration exert their effects by way of this feedback system. The macula densa cells in the distal convoluted tubule, which are in close apposition to the juxtaglomerular cells, may also control renin release by monitoring the sodium load in the tubular fluid. Renin release is influenced by extrarenal mechanisms as well, such as the sympathetic nervous system and potassium (Gordon et al., 1967). (4) Recent studies also support a role for dopamine on the regulation of the renin-angiotensin-aldosterone system. The primary effect seems to be a tonic, direct inhibition of aldosterone secretion by dopamine (McKenna et al., 1979).

Figure 85–12. Control of aldosterone secretion by means of interrelationships between the potassium and renin-angiotensin feedback loops.

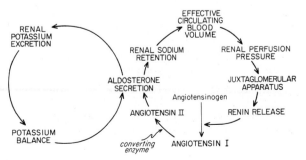

LABORATORY EVALUATION OF ADRENOCORTICAL FUNCTION

Adrenal Androgens

URINARY 17-KETOSTEROIDS, PLASMA DHEA, TESTOSTERONE

The procedure for measuring 17-ketosteroids is not specific for adrenal androgen production, since it reflects the output of steroids with androgenic activity from all sources, including the testis and ovary. Moreover, the implied correlation with androgenicity is often lacking. For example, testosterone is the most potent androgen but is not a 17-ketosteroid, whereas eitocholanolone, one of the major urinary 17-ketosteroids, is devoid of androgenic activity. On the average, the normal range for 17-ketosteroid levels in adult males is 10 to 25 mg/24 hr and for females 5 to 15 mg/24 hr. Over the age of 50 years, excretion gradually declines. One third or less of the urinary 17-ketosteroids in males arise in the testis.

The preferred and specific assessment of adrenal androgen production can be accomplished by measuring in plasma the principal adrenal androgen, dehydroepiandrosterone (DHEA) sulfate (Brooks, 1979). Owing to its prolonged metabolic clearance rate, this steroid has a long half-life in blood and does not exhibit a diurnal rhythm. Therefore, a randomly obtained sample is representative of adrenal androgen production.

In general, disorders associated with decreased adrenal secretion of cortisol show a low output of adrenal androgens, but an important exception is the adrenogenital syndrome (see Chapter 41). Thus, adrenal androgen levels do not provide a good index of adrenal function in hypo- or hyperadrenocorticism. In adrenal tumors producing virilizing effects in the female, such as adrenal carcinoma, adrenal androgen production and testosterone levels are usually greatly elevated.

The most potent naturally occurring androgen is testosterone from the testis. However, in certain virilizing disorders, significant quantities of this hormone or its immediate precursors (which can be converted to testosterone in the liver) are secreted from the adrenal. Methods involving radioimmunoassay or competitive protein-binding are available for the measurement of testosterone in plasma or urine. The plasma concentration appears to be the most useful method, since it reflects the quantity of free testosterone available for tissue activity. As discussed previously, the total (predominantly protein-bound) testosterone level usually correlates with the clinical status of the patient. However, a more specific assessment of the unbound concentration can be made by measuring the total testosterone concentration as well as the per cent free (unbound) testosterone by dialysis techniques (Moll and Rosenfield, 1979). In this way, errors in interpretation due to changes in the concentration of sex steroid–binding globulin can be avoided. Urinary values may be deceptive because of the conversion of other steroids to urinary conjugates of testosterone, without appreciably influencing the level of free testosterone in the plasma. In most studies, in normal adult males plasma testosterone has ranged from 300 to 1000 ng/dl, and in normal females from 30 to 100 ng/dl. Urinary values for testosterone glucuronide vary according to the methodology employed, but most authors have found 30 to 150 µg/24 hr in adult males and 4 to 15 µg/24 hr in normal females.

Adrenal Glucocorticoid Assessment

17-HYDROXYCORTICOIDS (17-OHCS); 17-KETOGENIC STEROIDS (17-KGS)

17-Hydroxycorticoids mainly measure tetrahydrocortisone and tetrahydrocortisol, which normally represent 25 to 35 per cent of the total urinary metabolites of cortisol (Silber and Porter, 1954). They also detect tetrahydro-11-deoxycortisol, the main metabolite of 11-deoxycortisol (compound S) (see Fig. 85–9). Normal values are 4 to 12 mg/day in adult males and 2 to 10 mg/day in females. Although the excretion of urinary 17-hydroxycorticoids does not reflect the plasma cortisol level (see further on), the correlation in most circumstances is high. The method also shows some degree of correlation with the cortisol secretion rate and therefore affords a reasonably good guide to adrenocortical activity. Low values are not sufficient for the diagnosis of adrenocortical insufficiency. For example, patients with other diseases (such as myxedema or chronic debilitating illness) frequently have low values of urinary 17-hydroxycorticoids, even though the adrenal glands are intact. Their plasma cortisol levels are normal if the metabolic disposal of the hormone is decreased in proportion to the secretion rate. In such cases, the low urinary corticoid level accurately reflects the low adrenal secretion of cortisol, and the normal plasma cortisol level accurately reflects an intact adrenocortical structure. In contrast, patients with true adrenal insufficiency show a significant decrease in both urinary cortisol metabolites and plasma cortisol. Patients with hyperadrenocorticism leading to increased cortisol secretion (Cushing's syndrome) show, in most instances, elevated levels of urinary 17-hydroxycorticoids. Very obese patients and muscular individuals may also show an increase in urinary corticoid levels, but plasma cortisol values are often normal, reflecting an increased rate of cortisol catabolism. Adjustments for body size can be made; 3 to 7 mg of 17-hydroxycorticoids are excreted by normal subjects per gm of creatinine (Streeten et al., 1969).

Urinary 17-ketogenic steroids are less commonly measured to estimate cortisol secretion. In addition to determining the Porter-Silber cortisol metabolites, these methods measure cortol and cortolone, 17-hydroxypregnenolones, and the pregnanetriols. Since this method measures a larger fraction of cortisol metabolites than 17-hydroxycorticosteroids, the normal values are higher (8 to 20 mg/24 hr).

URINE FREE CORTISOL

A highly sensitive and specific method for estimating cortisol hypersecretion, which has frequently replaced the measurement of the urinary metabolites of cortisol, is the measurement of unchanged or so-called free cortisol in the urine. This reflects the unbound, biologically active cortisol in the blood that has been filtered and has escaped renal tubular reabsorptive mechanisms. Normal subjects excrete less than 100 μg per day as free cortisol (Murphy, 1968).

PLASMA CORTISOL; ACTH

The plasma cortisol level is an important index of adrenocortical activity. A number of methods have been developed, but it is recommended that radioimmunoassays that specifically measure cortisol only be employed (Ruder et al., 1972).

In the evaluation of the relationship between the amount of cortisol in plasma and the biologic activity of the hormone, at least two factors must be considered. First, plasma cortisol levels show diurnal fluctuation, with highest values in the morning and lowest levels at bedtime. Plasma cortisol levels at 8 A.M. in normal subjects range from 5 to 15 μg/dl. Recent studies also indicate that cortisol is secreted in an episodic pulsatile fashion, with a peak secretory activity between 4 A.M. and 8 A.M., with few

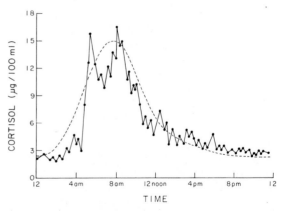

Figure 85–13. Diurnal pattern of plasma cortisol levels illustrating the episodic, pulsatile nature of secretion.

secretory episodes late in the evening (Fig. 85–13) (Weitzman et al., 1971). An alteration in the diurnal pattern may be important in interpreting the physiologic significance of plasma hormone levels. Thus, a bedtime cortisol level greater than 10 μg/dl is distinctly unusual and probably reflects an abnormality in the regulation of cortisol secretion. Second, cortisol exists in the blood in two different physiochemical states—in free (5 per cent) aqueous solution and bound (95 per cent) to a protein (cortisol-binding globulin [CBG]). In all likelihood, only the non–protein bound steroid is biologically active (free to diffuse into tissue spaces). Assay techniques measure both moieties. Since CBG is nearly saturated at normal cortisol concentrations, elevated hormone levels produce a disproportionate increase in the concentration of free cortisol. Thus, it is clear that the extravascular (tissue) concentration of cortisol depends on the concentration of the binding protein as well as on the concentration of steroid. As an example of this relationship, CBG binding is normally increased during pregnancy, resulting in an elevated total plasma cortisol level but not with associated clinical hyperadrenocorticism, since free or unbound cortisol values remain normal.

Plasma ACTH levels, measured by radioimmunoassay, are becoming increasingly available and can often be of major diagnostic importance (Berson and Yalow, 1968). Normal levels at 8 A.M. range from 20 to 100 pg/ml. As with plasma cortisol, one must take into account the fact that ACTH is secreted diurnally, episodically, and in response to stress.

SECRETION (PRODUCTION) RATE

It is clear that the concentration of plasma cortisol does not always reflect the rate of secretion by the adrenal cortex. For example, a normal plasma cortisol level in the presence of a decreased rate of disposal suggests decreased secretion of steroid, whereas a normal level in the presence of an increased rate of degradation suggests increased secretion. In order to resolve such uncertainties, isotopic cortisol can be utilized to obtain a more quantitative measure of adrenocortical secretion. Two methods have been employed: (1) the kinetic method (Peterson, 1959); and (2) the dilution method (Tait and Horton, 1965). Using these methods, the cortisol production rate in normal adults is 16 ± 6 mg/24 hr or 10 to 12 mg/m²/24 hr. Although laborious and costly, isotopic methods of estimating actual production rates of steroids can be very informative and are specific diagnostic techniques.

Adrenal Mineralocorticoid Assessment

ALDOSTERONE; PLASMA RENIN ACTIVITY (PRA)

Plasma levels of aldosterone and plasma renin activity may be accurately measured by radioimmunoassay techniques, but values must be related to time of day, posture, and dietary sodium and potassium intake (Ito et al., 1972). Supine plasma aldosterone levels based on a 100 mEq sodium–100 mEq potassium intake range from 1 to 5 ng/dl, while PRA levels range from 2 to 6 ng/ml/hr. Upright plasma aldosterone and PRA levels after 60 minutes of ambulation are usually two- to fourfold greater than supine values. Aldosterone secretion can also be estimated by measuring urinary aldosterone metabolites. For example, the 3-oxo or acid labile conjugate normally represents approximately 10 per cent of the aldosterone secreted daily; normal values range from 5 to 25 μg per day. Using isotopic aldosterone, secretion rates can be determined by the dilution methods; normal values range from 50 to 250 μg per day on a 100 mEq sodium–100 mEq potassium intake.

It is important to remember that sodium depletion and potassium loading stimulate the secretion of aldosterone (conversely, sodium loading and potassium depletion suppress aldosterone output); thus, evaluation of aldosterone levels requires knowledge of both sodium and potassium intakes (see further on and Figure 85–24 for diagnostic use of saline loading in suspected hyperaldosteronism) (Williams and Dluhy, 1972). PRA levels are influenced primarily by dietary sodium intake. Stimulation of PRA can be achieved by restriction of sodium intake. Assumption of the upright posture is an additional stimulus for the release of PRA and is often coupled to a volume-depleting maneuver (such as sodium restriction or diuretic administration). Dietary potassium also has a modest effect on PRA levels, with potassium loading suppressing the release of PRA and vice versa.

Dynamic Testing

ADRENOCORTICAL STIMULATION; ACTH TEST

The response to ACTH is a specific test of adrenocortical reserve function. ACTH is given intravenously (250 μg, 25 units, of synthetic α1-24 ACTH in 500 ml normal saline over 8 hours). Synthetic α1-24 ACTH has replaced lyophilized ACTH because of its greater purity and a lack of animal protein contaminants. Normal subjects show the following responses to an 8-hour ACTH infusion: Levels of 17-hydroxycorticosteroids rise to 15 to 30 mg/24 hr, and plasma cortisol levels increase to a range of 35 to 50 μg/dl. A rapid screening test can be done, using plasma cortisol values 30 to 60 minutes after the intramuscular or intravenous administration of 25 units (250 μg) of α1-24 ACTH (Dluhy et al., 1974). Normally, cortisol levels double or increase 7 to 11 μg/dl above basal levels within 30 to 60 minutes (see Fig. 85–15A).

ADRENOCORTICAL ENZYME INHIBITION: METYRAPONE TEST OF ACTH RESERVE

The compound metyrapone (Metopirone) produces a selective partial inhibition of 11β-hydroxylase activity (see Fig. 85–9). Cortisol synthesis is effectively blocked and 11-deoxycortisol (compound S), the immediate precursor, is secreted. The compound S has little or no effect on ACTH release; the secretion of corticotropin increases, and the adrenal cortex responds with a greater output of 11-deoxycortisol. The latter is metabolized to tetrahydro-11-deoxycortisol (tetrahydro-S) and is excreted in the urine. Tetrahydro-S is also measured by the 17-hydroxycorticosteroid procedure. Metyrapone is usually given orally, 750 mg every 4 hours for six doses. The normal response is a rise in urinary corticosteroid values to at least twice the baseline value, maximal values being reached during the 24-hour period following drug administration. Collection of urine can be avoided by obtaining plasma samples for the measurement of 11-deoxycortisol and cortisol prior to and following the metyrapone administration (Staub et al., 1979). The expected normal response is a reversal of the normal 11-deoxycortisol:cortisol ratio, with the former steroid rising to a level of greater than 10 µg/dl. An increment in ACTH levels is even more definitive and is confirmatory of normal pituitary-ACTH reserve. Thus, the metyrapone test specifically measures pituitary reserve function (when the adrenal cortex is intact); there is no response in pituitary disorders in which ACTH output is lost (Liddle et al., 1959). The metyrapone test will not reflect ACTH reserve if subjects are ingesting glucocorticoids or compounds that accelerate the metabolism of metyrapone, e.g., phenytoin (Dilantin).

INSULIN-INDUCED HYPOGLYCEMIA TESTING OF ACTH RESERVE

Pituitary ACTH reserve can be tested by insulin-induced hypoglycemia. Crystalline or regular insulin is given as a bolus (0.1 to 0.15 units/kg body weight) in order to acutely lower blood glucose levels below basal (usually within 30 to 45 minutes) (Jacobs and Nabarro, 1969). Coincident with the hypoglycemic nadir, ACTH and cortisol levels promptly increase. Owing to the difficulty in obtaining accurate ACTH assays, an increment in cortisol above control of greater than 7 to 10 µg per dl is generally used to define the normal response of the pituitary-adrenal axis.

PITUITARY ADRENOCORTICAL SUPPRESSION; DEXAMETHASONE SUPPRESSION TEST

Elevated levels of plasma cortisol suppress pituitary secretion of ACTH; as a result, adrenocortical function falls to a low level. Similarly, the administration of very potent synthetic glucocorticoids inhibits adrenal activity but will not contribute significantly to the results of corticosteroid measurements. Dexamethasone is usually used, because its ACTH-suppressing activity is approximately 30 times that of cortisol. Dosage is 0.5 mg orally every 6 hours for 2 days; on the second day, 17-hydroxycorticoids normally fall below 3.0 mg/24 hr and plasma cortisol drops to levels under 5.0 µg/dl. A more rapid procedure has also proved very useful: 1.0 mg of dexamethasone is given orally at midnight; plasma cortisol, drawn between 8 and 9 A.M. the following morning, is normally less than 5 µg/dl and is usually less than 3.0 µg/dl (Crapo, 1979) (Fig. 85–14).

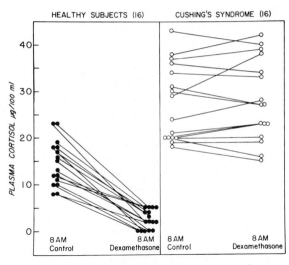

Figure 85–14. The rapid dexamethasone suppression test separates patients with Cushing's syndrome from healthy subjects or other obese subjects. Note the overlap in cortisol levels between the two groups before suppression. The patients with very high basal cortisol levels were those with ectopic ACTH production by a nonendocrine tumor as the underlying cause. (From Melby, J.: N. Engl. J. Med., 285:735, 1971.)

ADRENOCORTICAL INSUFFICIENCY

The modern study of the adrenal glands (and of clinical endocrinology) was begun by the English clinician Thomas Addison, who described chronic adrenal insufficiency in 1855. Until 1950 the prognosis of patients afflicted with adrenocortical insufficiency was dismal. However, with the isolation and synthesis of crystalline adrenal steroid hormones, the outlook has been completely altered.

PRIMARY ADRENOCORTICAL INSUFFICIENCY

Addison's disease is relatively rare, the death rate in the United States being approximately 0.3 per 100,000 population. It is predominantly a disease of adult life and affects males and females with equal frequency. The underlying event is the destruction of functioning adrenocortical tissue. There are two major causes: fibrocaseous tuberculosis and a process of bilateral adrenocortical necrosis (usually called adrenal atrophy), which appears to be the result of an autoimmune process. Tuberculosis is a rare cause of primary adrenal failure today. Pathologically autoimmune (idiopathic) atrophy is associated with lymphocytic infiltration of the adrenal glands (Rabinowe et al., 1984). Idiopathic adrenocortical failure also occurs in association with other primary endocrine organ failure syndromes, such as Type I diabetes mellitus, primary hypoparathyroidism, and chronic thyroiditis (Hashimoto's disease). In approximately 2 per cent of patients, various other causes of primary adrenal failure are encountered, including bilateral metastatic tumor, amyloidosis, histoplasmosis, and blastomycosis.

The disease is usually insidious in onset, but occasionally the first evidence of adrenal failure is the development of crisis, usually precipitated by an acute infection or other stress. In the approximate order of frequency, the following symptoms and signs are observed: muscular weakness, easy fatigability progressing to exhaustion, weight loss, increased pigmentation of the skin and mucous membranes, hypotension, gastrointestinal complaints (including anorexia, nausea, vomiting, diarrhea, and abdominal pain), and episodes suggestive of hypoglycemia. Emotional instability and periods of depression are common. Hyperpigmentation (secondary to elevated ACTH and lipotropin levels) usually occurs early and is the most striking physical evidence of the disease. It is most marked over exposed parts and pressure points, and the color of normally pigmented areas becomes darker. In approximately 10 per cent of cases, irregular areas of vitiligo appear. Arterial hypotension is a cardinal sign. Abnormalities of gastrointestinal function are very common and constitute the primary complaint of many patients. Secondary sex characteristics are usually little affected, except for a reduction in growth of axillary and pubic hair in female patients.

Hyponatremia and hyperkalemia are frequently, but not invariably, encountered. Hypoglycemia rarely occurs except during prolonged fasting. Twenty to 25 per cent of patients reveal suprarenal calcification by x-ray. Although this finding is not pathognomonic, calcification in the presence of documented adrenal insufficiency suggests an infectious etiology, such as tuberculosis or histoplasmosis. Plasma cortisol levels and the urinary output of 17-ketogenic steroids, 17-hydroxycorticoids, and 17-ketosteroids are all low, but values within the lower range of normal do not rule out the diagnosis.

Diagnosis. The diagnosis of adrenocortical failure depends upon the demonstration of inadequate adrenal hormone reserve following ACTH stimulation. The availability of potent preparations of ACTH made possible the development of highly specific tests (Thorn et al., 1951). In normal individuals the administration of ACTH produces a significant rise in plasma and urinary corticosteriods. Patients with primary adrenal insufficiency exhibit no response or, at most, a slight subnormal increase (Table 85–2). ACTH levels are also persistently elevated (greater than 150 pg/ml) in the presence of low circulating levels of cortisol. A simple screening test is the measurement of blood aldosterone and cortisol levels 30 to 60 minutes after the intramuscular or intravenous injection of 25 units (250 μg) of α1-24 corticotropin (cosyntropin) (Dluhy et al., 1974). The normal response is a doubling of cortisol levels or an absolute increment above control greater than 7 to 10 μg/dl. Blood aldosterone levels usually increase 5 to 15 ng/dl above control at 30 minutes (Fig. 85–15A). In patients with primary adrenal insufficiency, plasma aldosterone and cortisol levels both fail to rise following ACTH stimulation, since there is total loss of adrenocortical function. A rise in plasma aldosterone levels in association with a subnormal cortisol response suggests a diagnosis of secondary (pituitary) adrenocortical failure, since aldosterone secretion is maintained by the renin-angiotensin system (Fig. 85–15B).

Indirect tests of adrenocortical function (delayed water diuresis following an acute water load, deficient renal regulation of electrolyte excretion demonstrated by the use of low-salt diet, and induction of hypoglycemia by prolonged fasting) should no longer be used.

Treatment. Therapy is based upon specific hormone replacement. The primary steroid in substitution treatment is cortisol (cortisone can be used interchangeably); synthetic corticoste-

TABLE 85–2. URINARY 17-HYDROXYCORTICOSTEROIDS IN ADRENAL INSUFFICIENCY*

	Control	ACTH†			Metyrapone‡	
		DAY 1	DAY 2	DAY 3	DAY 1	DAY 2
Normal subject	0–10	20	30	35	12	18
Primary failure (Addison's disease)	0–4	3	4	3	—	—
Secondary failure (hypopituitarism)	0–5	5	10	14	2	3

*Mg/24 hr.
†Cortrosyn (synthetic α1–24 ACTH) 250 μg by 8-hour intravenous infusions on days 1, 2, and 3.
‡Metyrapone, 750 mg orally every 4 hours, for six doses on day 1.

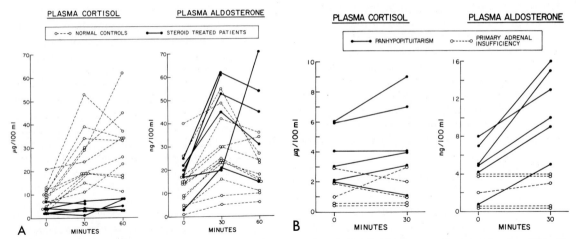

Figure 85–15. Rapid ACTH test (0.25 mg α1-24 corticotropin IM) with blood aldosterone and cortisol levels at 30 to 60 minutes in normal subjects *(A)* and in patients with primary and secondary adrenocortical failure *(B)*. In normal subjects, ACTH produces a rise in aldosterone and cortisol levels; in patients with primary adrenal failure, both hormones respond subnormally. A rise in aldosterone levels with a subnormal cortisol response indicates a diagnosis of secondary (pituitary) adrenocortical failure, since aldosterone secretion is maintained by the renin-angiotensin system.

roid derivatives generally are not employed owing to their prolonged biologic half-lives. For maintenance treatment, an average daily dose of 20 to 30 mg of cortisol (or 25 to 37.5 mg of cortisone) is generally effective. Dosage should be divided into two or three oral doses. The administration of cortisol results in a restoration of appetite, muscular strength, body weight, and a general feeling of well-being. The pigmentation is considerably lightened. Most important, the capacity to withstand exogenous stress is greatly enhanced. Indeed, the ultimate survival of a patient with Addison's disease depends upon the proper adjustment of cortisol therapy during periods of significant stress. Dosage should be increased to 75 to 150 mg per day. When oral administration is precluded by vomiting, cortisol should be given by intravenous infusion or intramuscularly, using the rapidly absorbed hemisuccinate or phosphate preparations.

In those patients with primary adrenal insufficiency, the use of a mineralocorticoid is also required. The preparation of choice is fluorocortisol, an extremely potent synthetic mineralocorticosteroid with effects on electrolyte metabolism equal to those of aldosterone. It is active when given orally. Maintenance dosage ranges from 0.05 to 0.1 mg daily or every other day.

The combined administration of cortisol and fluorocortisol has resulted in the complete rehabilitation of these patients. However, it should be emphasized that the success of maintenance treatment largely depends upon the successful education of the patient concerning the potential threat of intercurrent stress and the necessity of taking increased quantities of cortisol during these periods. These patients should be registered with a medical alerting system; they should also be provided with an emergency kit that contains injectable glucocorticoid and mineralocorticoid, which should be used when they are unable to take their medications orally.

HYPOALDOSTERONISM

Hypoaldosteronism has been reported in association with normal cortisol production and hyporeninism, postoperatively following removal of an aldosteronoma, and as a congenital biosynthetic defect. In mild cases, excessive sodium wastage occurs during salt restriction; in severe cases, however, excessive urinary sodium loss occurs on a normal sodium salt intake.

Isolated hypoaldosteronism occurs most commonly in adult patients in association with hyporeninism, hyperkalemia, and abnormal renal function (so-called hyporeninemic hypoaldosteronism) (Schambelan et al., 1972). Most patients present with significantly elevated serum potassium levels in the setting of normal or minimally impaired renal function. The majority of these patients also have glucose intolerance. Plasma renin and aldosterone levels fail to rise following sodium restriction; cortisol secretion rises normally following ACTH stimulation, excluding a diagnosis of Addison's disease or primary adrenocortical insufficiency. In another syndrome, patients have a biosynthetic defect and are unable to transform the C-18 methyl group of corticosterone to the aldehyde grouping because of a deficiency of the enzyme 18-hydroxysteroid dehydrogenase. Aldosterone secretion is low, while the secretion of corticosterone and 18-hydroxycorticosterone and the levels of plasma renin activity are elevated. Reversal of salt wasting and hyperkalemia can be achieved in these syndromes by mineralocorticoid therapy (0.1 to 0.3 mg of 9α-fluorohydrocortisone).

SECONDARY ADRENOCORTICAL INSUFFICIENCY

The most common cause of secondary adrenal failure is suppression of the pituitary-adrenal axis as a side effect of chronic high-dose glucocorticoid therapy for a number of medical illnesses, such as bronchial asthma or chronic active hepatitis. In this circumstance, suppression of ACTH is "isolated," as the secretions of the remaining hormones are preserved.

Generalized failure of anterior pituitary gland function (panhypopituitarism) is commonly due to tumors; a chromophobe adenoma or craniopharyngioma is usually found. Extensive destruction can result from pituitary infarction, most often secondary to post-partum hemorrhage with vascular shock (Sheehan's syndrome). The functional reserve of the anterior pituitary is such that clinical manifestations are usually absent until 75 to 90 per cent of the gland has been destroyed. In some cases, complete failure ensues; more frequently, some functions are maintained. Deficiency of gonadal function usually dominates the clinical picture.

Adrenocortical insufficiency secondary to pituitary failure (inadequate corticotropin production) results in adrenocortical atrophy. It differs from primary insufficiency in certain ways. Cutaneous hyperpigmentation is not encountered, since ACTH and lipotropin levels are reduced. Electrolyte abnormalities differ from those seen in primary adrenocortical failure, since aldosterone secretion is maintained. Dilutional hyponatremia may be seen because of impaired free-water clearance secondary to cortisol insufficiency. On the other hand, hyponatremia and hyperkalemia suggest mineralocorticoid insufficiency.

The response of the atrophic gland to ACTH is typically delayed, although, in contrast to primary failure, adrenocortical activation does ensue following prolonged stimulation (Table 85–2). A more specific test of the capacity of the pituitary gland to secrete corticotropin depends on the use of metyrapone or insulin-tolerance testing (see earlier). Failure to respond to metyrapone or insulin-hypoglycemia testing (in a patient who does respond to corticotropin) provides a specific diagnostic approach to adrenal insufficiency secondary to pituitary failure.

Treatment of secondery adrenal insufficiency involves the use of cortisol as described; fluorocortisol is rarely required. In addition, thyroidal and gonadal replacement therapy should be employed as indicated.

ACUTE ADRENOCORTICAL INSUFFICIENCY

Adrenal Crisis. An adrenal crisis is an acute, severe exacerbation of adrenocortical insufficiency. It is a medical emergency and, if not properly and energetically treated, is often fatal. The onset of acute stress, such as infection, trauma (including minor as well as major surgery), and gastrointestinal upsets, in patients with adrenal insufficiency must be considered an indication for an immediate increase in cortisol dosage. Acute adrenal insufficiency is characterized by fever, anorexia, nausea, vomiting, headache, diarrhea, abdominal pain, dehydration, hypotension progressing to vascular shock, marked weakness and extreme lethargy, and, rarely, hypoglycemia. Laboratory study often reveals hyponatremia, hyperkalemia, and azotemia, especially in patients with vomiting or diarrhea; in patients previously maintained on mineralocorticoid substitution therapy, serum electrolyte determination may be normal. Patients with secondary adrenal insufficiency (those maintained on chronic glucocorticoid therapy and those with pituitary insufficiency) may not exhibit severe dehydration, since mineralocorticoid secretion is usually preserved.

Treatment. Treatment of adrenal crisis requires the immediate provision of high levels of cortisol. In addition, support of the cardiovascular system with intravenous sodium and water may be life-saving in patients with primary adrenal insufficiency, who are usually severely dehydrated. Vasopressor agents also may be required.

A soluble cortisol preparation (hemisuccinate or phosphate) is given by rapid intravenous injection (100 mg), followed by a continuous intravenous infusion of an additional 100 to 200 mg of cortisol over a period of 12 to 24 hours. Thereafter, 50 to 100 mg of cortisol succinate is given by intramuscular injection every 8 hours until the patient is fully awake and able to eat. Cortisol may then be given orally and dosages gradually tapered (approximately 20 to 30 per cent per day) to maintenance levels. At that time, fluorocortisol administration is resumed.

Water, sodium, and glucose must be provided; 5 per cent dextrose in normal saline solution is commonly used. One to 3 liters will be required depending upon the degree of dehydration and hyponatremia. If crisis was preceded by prolonged nausea, vomiting, and diarrhea and dehydration is severe, several liters of saline may be required within the first few hours.

Evidence of infection is diligently sought, and appropriate antibiotic therapy is employed. If hypotension is profound, vasopressors may be added to the intravenous infusion and the rate adjusted to maintain optimal blood pressure levels.

ADRENAL HEMORRHAGE

Adrenal apoplexy is usually associated with overwhelming sepsis. Meningococcemia has been encountered in approximately 75 per cent of the cases reported; other organisms (staphylococci or streptococci) have been involved less frequently. The outstanding post-mortem finding is extensive bilateral adrenal destruction due to hemorrhage, involving mainly the zona reticularis and zona fasciculata. Rarely, the hemorrhage ruptures through the capsule of the adrenal into the peritoneal cavity. Other systemic changes are those of fulminant sepis.

The disease is characterized by the manifestations of septic shock. Extensive cutaneous purpura usually occurs. Cyanosis is intense. Fever appears early and may reach extreme levels. Death often comes within 24 to 48 hours. Blood cultures are usually, but not always, positive; Gram-stained smears taken from cutaneous lesions may also reveal the organism.

Specific treatment must not await the interpretation of blood cultures. Since control of sepsis is critical, antibiotic chemotherapy is indicated. Second, vascular shock must be overcome if treatment is to be successful; whole blood transfusion and vasoconstrictors may be needed. The routine use of high-dose steroids is recommended, but since there is insufficient time for diagnostic testing, there is little evidence to support an increased survival rate. If total adrenal destruction has occurred, replacement therapy with cortisol will eventually be required. However, in most cases survival depends upon the control of infection and the reversal of vascular shock. Until recently, the disease had been considered uniformly fatal, but with early diagnosis and vigorous treatment, recovery can be achieved in some cases.

Adrenocortical insufficiency due to bilateral adrenal hemorrhage has been encountered occasionally in patients receiving anticoagulant therapy (e,g,. heparin treatment after myocardial infarction or during the early postoperative period). The occurrence of unexplained hypotension, dehydration, and a declining serum sodium:potassium ratio in the presence of excessive urinary sodium chloride excretion is an indication for diagnostic work-up and replacement therapy (as outlined for Addison's disease).

ADRENAL INSUFFICIENCY ASSOCIATED WITH SURGERY OF THE ADRENAL AND PITUITARY GLANDS

Adrenal insufficiency secondary to ablative surgery has two different causes: the removal of hyperfunctioning adrenocortical tissue (tumor or bilateral adrenal hyperplasia), and adrenalectomy or hypophysectomy as a therapeutic approach to systemic disease (e.g., metastatic carcinoma of breast).

Unilateral tumors of the adrenal cortex that secrete excessive quantities of cortisol are associated with contralateral adrenocortical atrophy because of pituitary suppression via the negative feedback control system. The inability of the atrophic gland to compensate for the increased hormone requirement imposed by resection of the tumor can result in adrenal crisis. Therefore, *all patients undergoing unilateral or bilateral adrenalectomy require treatment with cortisol.* It is essential that hormone therapy for adrenal or pituitary surgery be prophylactic as well as substitutive; once a severe crisis of adrenal insufficiency has occurred, the condition of the patient may deteriorate rapidly, and sudden death during acute cardiovascular collapse may occur. The aim of therapy is to provide a high circulating level of cortisol. Corticosteroid treatment during adrenalectomy is outlined under the section on Cushing's syndrome.

In the event that adrenal crisis occurs in a patient who has not received prophylactic adrenocortical steroids, immediate treatment is essential. The plan of fluid, electrolyte, and hormone therapy described for acute adrenal insufficiency should be promptly instituted.

ADRENOCORTICAL HYPERFUNCTION

The adrenal cortex secretes cortisol, aldosterone, and other corticosteroids, androgens, and progesterone. In various clinical disorders the gland may secrete an excess of one or more of these compounds. Consequently, a variety of clinical syndromes may occur. The causative adrenal lesion may be bilateral cortical hyperplasia or tumor, either benign or malignant.

The clinical features of Cushing's syndrome reflect the metabolic phenomena resulting from excessive levels of cortisol. The clinical manifestations of the adrenogenital syndrome are primarily sexual and are, in large part, dependent upon the sex of the patient as well as the age of onset. Female patients, especially those with adrenocortical tumors, may present both the metabolic alterations characteristic of cortisol excess and masculinization resulting from the overproduction of androgens. The changes of aldosteronism are primarily due to abnormalities of electrolyte metabolism.

CUSHING'S SYNDROME

Cushing's syndrome, properly defined, refers to the clinical picture described in 1932 by Harvey Cushing. The disease is comparatively rare, occurs most frequently in young adults, and is three to five times more common in females.

Pathogenesis. Cushing's syndrome is due to a chronic excess of cortisol. In about 25 to 30 per cent of the cases an adrenocortical neoplasm is found; somewhat more than half of these tumors are benign. Malignant and most benign tumors are autonomous and independent of ACTH control. In fact, when an adrenal tumor is the primary source of excess cortisol, pituitary ACTH output is suppressed and nontumorous adrenal tissue is atropic. Rarely, an adrenal rest tumor arises in ectopic adrenocortical tissue, most commonly located in the perinephric area but also found near the celiac axis, ovaries, testis, or elsewhere.

In 70 to 75 per cent of the patients with Cushing's syndrome, an adrenal neoplasm is not present. Cushing postulated that in these cases the disorder arises from a pituitary basophilic adenoma (Cushing's disease). Although early studies failed to confirm pituitary basophilic tumors as an important cause of the disease, it is now clear that the anterior pituitary gland is significantly involved. In rare cases, an obvious basophilic or chromophobe pituitary adenoma is found and the sella turcica is enlarged. Liddle (1967) postulated that the majority of patients with adrenocortical hyperplasia and a radiographically normal sella turcica have increased and inappropriate secretion of pituitary ACTH. In most cases, plasma ACTH levels are moderately elevated; in others, the concentration is

in the upper normal range. However, in patients with increased levels of circulating cortisol, any measurable quantity of plasma ACTH is "inappropriately" high. In addition, patients with Cushing's disease do not show a normal decline in plasma ACTH levels late in the day (explaining a lack of diurnal variation in plasma cortisol). Thus, it would appear that an increased pituitary production of ACTH leads to adrenocortical hyperplasia and increased secretion of cortisol. It has been demonstrated that a reduction in cortisol output (e.g., adrenalectomy) results in further elevation of ACTH, whereas the administration of additional cortisol produces some fall in the secretion of plasma ACTH. Therefore, it has been suggested that the primary defect in Cushing's disease may reside in the pituitary-hypothalamic axis, whereby ACTH secretion is "reset" to respond to higher than normal levels of circulating cortisol. However, recent studies suggest that a significant number of patients with bilateral hyperplasia have ACTH-secreting pituitary microadenomas that often can be demonstrated by high-resolution CT scanning of the pituitary gland (Tyrrell, 1980). The role of corticotropin-releasing hormone (CRH) in such cases is unsettled.

Paraendocrine tumors (malignant neoplasms of nonendocrine tissues, which secrete polypeptides that exert hormone activity) also may be responsible for Cushing's syndrome. These neoplasms synthesize polypeptides that are biologically, chemically, and immunologically indistinguishable from ACTH. They also secrete melanocyte-stimulating hormones (such as β-lipotropin), and as a consequence patients are frequently hyperpigmented. Ectopic ACTH production leads to bilateral adrenocortical hyperplasia, and pituitary corticotropin is suppressed by the hypercortisolism. "Oat cell" bronchogenic carcinomas have most frequently been responsible, but many other tumors have been implicated (malignant thymoma, pancreatic carcinoma, bronchial carcinoid tumor) (Singer et al., 1978).

Signs and Symptoms. Cushing described a syndrome including obesity of characteristic truncal distribution, amenorrhea in females or impotence in males, hypertrichosis in females, purplish cutaneous striae, plethora, hypertension, muscular weakness, glycosuria, and osteoporosis (Fig. 85–16). In some cases, cutaneous ecchymoses, erythremia, edema, albuminuria, and a marked susceptibility to infection occur.

Obesity is ususally moderate in degree. The typical redistribution of adipose tissue produces

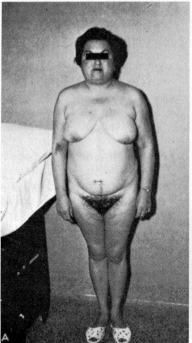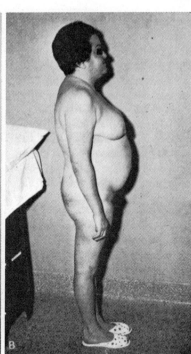

Figure 85–16. *A,* A 34-year-old female with Cushing's syndrome; the steroid studies in this patient are shown in Table 85–3. The patient shows truncal obesity and mild hirsutism. *B,* Note that cutaneous striae and ecchymoses are absent, in contrast to most cases shown in textbooks.

the classic "moon" facies and prominent fat deposits in the dorsal, cervical, supraclavicular, and suprascapular areas (Fig. 85–17). Plethora may be marked, but true erythremia occurs only rarely. Suppression of gonadal function is common. Hirsutism occurs in many females, but true virilization is unusual. Arterial hypertension is frequently present and sometimes persists in long-standing cases despite cure of other signs and symptoms. The effects of excess cortisol produce muscle weakness, osteoporosis, easy bruisability, and ecchymoses. Purplish striae are found in about two thirds of the patients. Mental disturbances, ranging from emotional lability to major psychoses (usually of the depressive or paranoid type), appear frequently. Many distinctive physical features associated with Cushing's syndrome are often absent in patients with paraendocrine tumors. On the other hand, hypokalemic alkalosis and hyperglycemia are characteristic findings.

Associated Laboratory Findings. A moderate neutrophilic leukocytosis is often found. The hematocrit is usually within the normal range, but mild elevation is occasionally present. Hypokalemia, sometimes accompanied by hypochloremia and metabolic alkalosis, is usually restricted to those patients with markedly elevated levels of cortisol secretion. About three fourths of the patients exhibit mild glucose

intolerance following a standard glucose load, but overt diabetes occurs in a much smaller number, and diabetic ketoacidosis is rare. There is an increased incidence of nephrolithiasis, probably as a result of increased urinary calcium excretion secondary to progressive osteoporosis. When osteoporosis is found, it is usually most marked in the axial skeleton (spine and pelvis), but in severe and long-standing cases even the skull (including the lamina dura) may be involved. Fractures of vertebrae, ribs, and pelvis can follow relatively mild trauma.

Diagnosis. The diagnosis of Cushing's syndrome primarily requires evidence of loss of normal pituitary-adrenocortical feedback control. Thereafter, it is necessary to identify the underlying lesion—bilateral adrenocortical hyperplasia or neoplasia.

The best screening test demonstrating that the feedback control of adrenocortical function is abnormal is the overnight dexamethasone suppression test. In patients with Cushing's syndrome, a single oral dose of dexamethasone (1 mg), given at midnight, fails to elicit the normal degree of pituitary-adrenocortical suppression; plasma cortisol levels measured the following morning are above 5 μg/dl and are often above 10 to 20 μg/dl (Fig. 85–14). The diagnosis is then confirmed with the low-dose dexamethasone suppression test. Although cortisol pro-

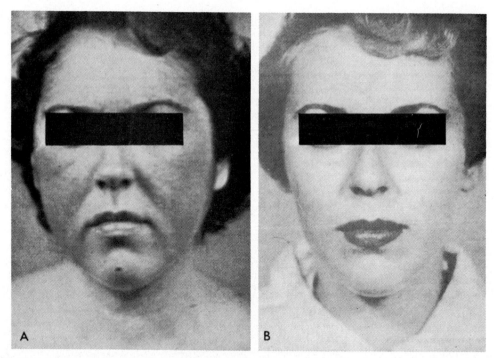

Figure 85–17. *A,* Woman, aged 23 years, 6 months after the development of moon face and other early signs of Cushing's syndrome due to an adrenocortical adenoma on the left side. *B,* Same patient 6 months after surgical removal of adenoma of the adrenal cortex. (From Harrison, J. H.: Surgery of the adrenals. *In* Davis, L. [Ed.]: Christopher's Textbook of Surgery. Philadelphia, W. B. Saunders Co.)

duction is regularly suppressed in normal subjects given small doses of dexamethasone (0.5 mg every 6 hours for 48 hours), little or no suppression occurs in patients with Cushing's syndrome (Little, 1960). A normal response on the second day is a decrease of urinary 17-hydroxycorticoids to less then 3 mg per day; plasma cortisol levels are less than 5 μg/dl after 2 days of dexamethasone administration. A normal response demonstrates that the hypothalamic-pituitary system responds appropriately to an increase in plasma glucocorticoid levels.

Increased adrenocortical production of cortisol can also be confirmed by measurement of free cortisol in the urine with a carefully timed 24-hour collection. Values in excess of 100 μg per day are found. However, it is stressed that abnormal suppression of cortisol secretion is the most specific and definitive test (Table 85–3).

Having established evidence for an excessive production of cortisol, it is most desirable to determine the etiology of the glucocorticoid excess. Indirect evidence may be obtained from additional pharmacologic testing. When larger doses of dexamethasone are employed (2 mg every 6 hours for 48 hours), the so-called high-dose dexamethasone test, suppression of urinary

corticosteriod excretion to values less than half the baseline can be demonstrated in patients with adrenal hyperplasia (Aron et al., 1981). This is consistent with the "reset" hypothesis, indicating that when high enough glucocorticoid values in plasma are attained, suppression of ACTH production does occur. It is to be recalled that a major proportion of these patients have been found to have ACTH-secreting pituitary microadenomas. On the other hand, patients with adrenal neoplasms (either benign or malignant) and those with ACTH-producing paraendocrine tumors fail to show a significant fall of plasma or urinary steroids even with large doses of dexamethasone. An intermediate syndrome is bilateral cortical nodular hyperplasia, in which variable suppression is seen following high-dose dexamethasone administration. In this entity, a mixture of autonomously functioning nodules and ACTH-stimulated hyperplastic tissue is seen.

While the response to ACTH stimulation is of interest, it is of little diagnostic value. Patients with adrenocortical hyperplasia usually demonstrate increased reactivity to exogenous ACTH. The response of benign adenomas is variable; hyperreactivity to corticotropin may or may not occur, depending on whether the

TABLE 85–3. STEROID STUDIES IN A CASE OF CUSHING'S DISEASE*

	Urine			Plasma
	17-OHCS (MG/24 HR)	17-KS (MG/24 HR)	FREE CORTISOL (µG/24 HR)	CORTISOL (µG/DL)
Control	15	19	242	23; 19†
"	18	20	249	24; 23
ACTH‡	51	40	1200	71
Dexamethasone				
2.0 mg/day	18			
"	14			21
Dexamethasone				
8.0 mg/day	14			
"	10	Baseline cortisol secretion rate: 47 mg/day		
"	7			8
Metyrapone§	24			
"	42			

*Thirty-four-year-old female (Fig. 85–16).
†Morning and evening cortisol plasma values.
‡ACTH, 20 USP units via 8-hour IV infusion.
§Metyrapone, 750 mg every 6 hours orally for 24 hours. All studies in this patient were consistent with a diagnosis of idiopathic adrenocortical hyperplasia, and this was the lesion found at operation. Total adrenalectomy was performed.

adenoma is functioning in an autonomous manner. Adrenocortical carcinoma is usually resistant to ACTH stimulation, reflecting the autonomy of the tumor tissue and atrophy of the contralateral gland.

Certain other studies are often useful in making the diagnosis of an adrenocortical tumor. A malignant lesion is always suggested when urinary 17-ketosteroids are elevated to very high values (greater than a threefold elevation above normal); a gross increase in plasma dehydroepiandrosterone sulfate parallels the 17-ketosteroid urinary excretion elevation. Another reliable indicator of malignancy is the excessive excretion of certain biosynthetic precursors of cortisol; the measurement of urinary tetrahydro-S (tetrahydro-11 deoxycortisol) or plasma 11-deoxycortisol has proved particularly valuable.

Benign adrenocortical adrenal tumors usually are pure cortisol-producing and lead to suppression of ACTH secretion and atrophy of the surrounding normal as well as contralateral adrenal gland. As a consequence, plasma ACTH levels are usually undetectable, and adrenal androgen levels (e.g., dehydroepiandrosterone sulfate) are subnormal.

In cases of paraendocrine origin (nonendocrine tumors producing ACTH), baseline plasma cortisol and urinary steroid values are often markedly elevated. Hypokalemic alkalosis is very common, in contrast to cases of Cushing's syndrome from other causes and this finding should always stimulate attempts to demonstrate the paraendocrine disorder. These patients usually exhibit no suppression of cortisol production

with dexamethasone, at low- and high-dosage levels. Plasma ACTH and β-lipotropin levels are usually extremely high (greater than 250 pg/ml), this is in contrast to patients with pituitary ACTH overproduction, in whom the ACTH levels are in the normal range or are modestly elevated (Besser and Edwards, 1972). Nonendocrine tumors also produce biologically inactive ACTH fragments as well as the inactive large molecular weight ACTH precursor or prohormone pro-opiomelanocortin.

Identification of the lesion responsible for Cushing's syndrome is ultimately a radiographic diagnosis, usually involving CT imaging of the suspected abnormal tissue (see Chapter 7). Generally, the laboratory data direct the investigation: Suppression of cortisol with high-dose dexamethasone testing in association with modestly elevated levels of ACTH should lead to CT imaging of the pituitary in an attempt to find a microadenoma. Markedly elevated levels of ACTH and adrenocortical secretion suggest a paraendocrine or ectopic lesion; careful inspection of the chest x-ray should be the first step in this situation. On the other hand, if the hormonal profile suggests an adrenal neoplasm (and ACTH levels are low or undetectable), the first study would logically be radiographic CT imaging of the adrenal glands (Figs. 85–18 and 85–19).

Differential Diagnosis. The major difficulty arises in patients with obesity, hypertension, and diabetes mellitus, especially in females with these disorders accompanied by hirsutism. Extreme obesity is uncommon in Cushing's syndrome, and in exogenous obesity the distribu-

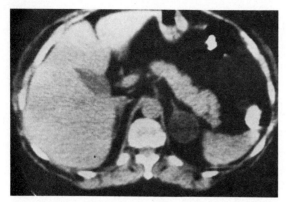

Figure 85–18. Computerized tomography of left adrenal in a patient with Cushing's syndrome. The racquet-shaped image demonstrates a 2-cm adenoma and its appended portion of normal gland (compare with Figures 85–3 and 85–19).

tion of excess fat is generalized. It should be recognized that baseline 17-hydroxycorticoid excretion values in patients with exogenous obesity are often moderately elevated, but diurnal variation and urinary free cortisol levels are normal. Finally, the application of the overnight dexamethasone suppression test is decisive in most patients with obesity or hirsutism.

Iatrogenic Cushing's syndrome that is induced by the administration of glucocorticoids or ACTH may be clinically indistinguishable from the naturally occurring disorder. If the question of diagnosis arises, the exogenous glucocorticoid should be stopped and the patient placed on dexamethasone at a dosage level of 2.0 mg per day. Patients with the iatrogenic disorder will demonstrate low baseline steroid excretion and plasma cortisol values, owing to

prolonged suppression of the hypothalamic-pituitary system. Patients with endogenous Cushing's syndrome will exhibit the usual findings of elevated urinary and plasma corticosteriod values.

Hyperpigmentation in patients with Cushing's syndrome points to a neoplasm producing excessive quantities of ACTH and lipotropin. The responsible lesion may be a paraneoplastic tumor or a pituitary neoplasm—most commonly a chromophobe adenoma. In the latter circumstance the sella turcica may be enlarged, depending upon the size of the lesion (Fig. 85–20). In some cases, these tumors produce severe headaches and visual disturbances (field losses and ophthalmoplegia). In patients with paraneoplastic or ectopic production of ACTH, the onset of Cushing's syndrome tends to be acute, and the progress of the disease may be so rapid that patients often fail to develop the classic manifestations of the disease. In particular, obesity is usually absent, while hypokalemic alkalosis is often severe.

Treatment of Cushing's Syndrome. When an accurate diagnosis has been established, treatment should be undertaken, because the 5-year mortality of patients with untreated Cushing's syndrome approaches 50 per cent (Plotz et al., 1952).

Following adrenal resection or successful removal of a pituitary microadenoma, the signs and symptoms of the disease gradually regress

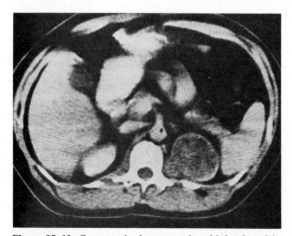

Figure 85–19. Computerized tomography of left adrenal in a patient with Cushing's syndrome. The large mass of heterogeneous density suggests an adrenal carcinoma, which indeed it was (compare with Figure 85–18).

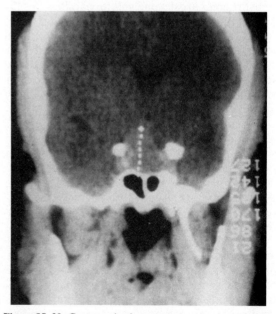

Figure 85–20. Computerized tomography of a chromophobe adenoma in the sella turcica of a patient with Cushing's syndrome presenting with hyperpigmentation, headaches, and a visual field defect.

(Fig. 85–21). Hypertension usually subsides, but in long-standing cases it may persist. When overt diabetes is present, its postoperative course is variable, but a reduction in insulin requirement is common. Osteoporosis ceases to progress; unfortunately, it rarely shows a significant degree of healing, although return of bone structure toward normal has been observed in children. The mental status of the patient usually undergoes marked improvement.

Treatment of Adrenal Tumor. The treatment of a benign, primary adrenocortical tumor is complete surgical resection. In almost all cases the condition is unilateral, so that the involved adrenal gland can be removed and the contralateral (atrophic) gland left intact; the ultimate recovery of normal adrenocortical function in the remnant gland eliminates the need for permanent hormone replacement therapy. If the patient has congestive heart failure, potassium depletion, or infection, appropriate measures must be taken to deal with these complications before surgery is undertaken.

Once surgical treatment has been elected, the following considerations are fundamental:

1. It is imperative that all patients subjected to the extirpation of adrenocortical tissue be firmly supported intra- and postoperatively by glucocorticoid hormone replacement. Full-scale hormone treatment should be employed regardless of the extent of adrenal resection, because the incidence of complications attributable to proper hormone therapy is negligible. Adequate quantities of cortisol are necessary both during and following surgery. Water-soluble preparations of cortisol (hemisuccinate or phosphate) should be given intravenously, as a continuous infusion of hydrocortisone at a rate of 10 mg per hour, beginning with preoperative medications and continuing for 24 hours postoperatively. Over the ensuing 5 to 7 days the total daily dosage is gradually reduced in 20 to 30 per cent decrements toward physiologic levels. Continuous intravenous infusion of hydrocortisone can usually be discontinued 36 to 48 hours after surgery, and the doses can then be intermittently administered every 6 to 8 hours intramuscularly or orally.

2. When preoperative studies are indicative of tumor and the tumor has been localized, unilateral adrenal resection is usually carried out through a lateral incision. In most cases the

Figure 85–21. *A,* Full-face view of patient with hyperadrenocorticism, 1954, treated by total adrenalectomy at that time. *B,* Photograph of same patient 6 months after total adrenalectomy, showing striking improvement. All symptoms and signs of Cushing's syndrome had disappeared. *C,* Deep pigmentation, headache, and failing vision supervened in 1957; emergency craniotomy was necessary after radiation therapy. *D,* Disappearance of pigmentation after removal of chromophobe adenoma of pituitary by Dr. Donald Matson is shown in the facial view. (From Rothenberg, R. E. [Ed.]: Reoperative Surgery. New York, McGraw-Hill Book Company, 1969.)

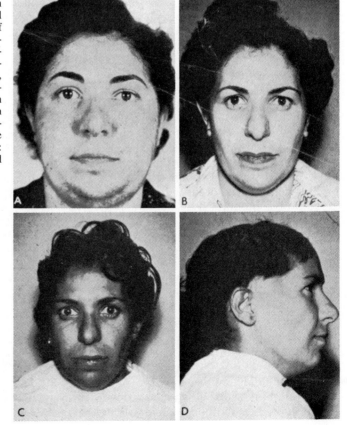

CT scan is sufficient radiologic preparation for large tumors, and a thoracoabdominal approach is preferred. In instances of large adrenal tumors, selective arteriography is sometimes used as a road map for surgery (see Fig. 85–27). Some malignant tumors can be completely resected, and their management is then identical with that of benign adenoma. If total resection of an adrenal carcinoma cannot be accomplished, subtotal removal may be performed, and subsequently chemotherapy is employed (see further on).

3. Postoperatively the patient is maintained on doses of cortisol sufficient to prevent symptoms of adrenocortical insufficiency. With the doses of cortisol employed for maintenance treatment, symptoms very similar to those of adrenal insufficiency may appear in patients with long-standing hyperadrenocorticism (postadrenalectomy syndrome). Weakness and lassitude, headache, depression, anorexia, nausea, vomiting, diarrhea, and joint pains often occur. Therefore, it is essential that the dose of cortisol be gradually tapered from the high levels employed in the immediate postoperative period. Should symptoms of the postadrenalectomy syndrome appear, elevation of the cortisol dose relieves these symptoms; thereafter, gradual tapering of dosage is resumed. As complaints of weakness, anorexia, and muscular aching decrease, the dosage of cortisol is slowly and gradually decreased until supportive therapy is no longer necessary. Ordinarily, hormone treatment can be withdrawn in approximately 3 to 6 months. The first step in a withdrawal schedule designed to gradually reactivate adrenocortical function is to administer cortisol replacement therapy as a single morning dose (Byyny, 1976). A gradual reduction in this dose (e.g., 5-mg decrements) is then accomplished every 2 to 4 weeks as the patient is stabilized at each dose level. If major illness occurs during the succeeding 6 to 12 months, it is necessary to give supplemental cortisol.

Treatment of Adrenocortical Hyperplasia. In patients with Cushing's disease there is excessive secretion of ACTH from the anterior pituitary gland. In most instances the sella turcica is radiographically normal, but a small microadenoma (less than 10 mm in size) may be visualized by high-resolution CT scanning. In a small number of patients with excess ACTH secretion (5 per cent or less), the sella turcica is found to be obviously enlarged by a pituitary tumor at the time the diagnosis is made. These tumors are usually chromophobe adenomas and may produce neighborhood signs and symptoms

owing to compression of adjacent neural structures (see Fig. 85–20). In a third group of patients whose symptoms are usually marked by very high cortisol and ACTH levels, there is ectopic ACTH production by a nonendocrine tumor, usually malignant. In these patients the characteristic physical features of Cushing's syndrome are absent, but excessive mineralocorticoid secretion (with severe hypokalemia) dominates the clinical presentation.

Treatment of Patients with Obvious Pituitary Tumor (Cushing's Disease). Tumors that are not neurologically aggressive (and those that have been incompletely removed) may be treated with irradiation, using a telecobalt source to deliver 4500 rads (tumor dose) to the pituitary through multiple ports. However, as a primary therapy it is effective in only 15 per cent of adults (Orth and Liddle, 1971). With alpha particles delivered by a linear accelerator, it it possible to deliver 8000 rads to the pituitary gland with reasonable safety (Linfoot, 1979). Internal pituitary irradiation has also been employed, using stereotactic implantation of yttrium-90 by the transsphenoidal route; use of this procedure appears to be limited by potential deleterious effects of irradiation of perisellar structures. Tumors exhibiting progressive expansion and producing visual field defects, ophthalmoplegia, and other signs should be surgically removed or decompressed generally via the transsphenoidal approach. With more extensive involvement, the transfrontal approach may be necessary. Postoperatively, these patients require adrenocortical substitution therapy and may need gonadal and thyroid replacement treatment as well.

Treatment of Patients With Microadenomas or Normal Pituitary Glands. If a pituitary tumor is imaged by high-resolution CT scanning of the pituitary gland, transsphenoidal microdissection is the initial treatment of choice in most centers to correct the pituitary ACTH hypersecretion. Transsphenoidal surgery is successful in correcting the hypercortisolism in 85 per cent of patients with microadenomas (Tyrrell et al, 1978). However, radiographic studies may be normal and a microadenoma may still be present. Controversy exists as to whether these patients should be "explored." It is also unclear as to whether removal of these pituitary microadenomas will lead to permanent cure, since these neoplasms may recur over time if the fundamental abnormality is hypothalamic dysfunction. In some centers, pituitary radiation is the treatment of choice (either conventional external irradiation or alpha-particle therapy).

The remission rate, however, is less than 50 per cent; moreover, there is a long lag time between treatment and remission in responsive patients. Finally, owing to the long lag time, use of external pituitary irradiation may be contraindicated in the presence of rapidly progressing or severe Cushing's disease.

Chemotherapy has also been employed with variable success in bilateral hyperplasia. The serotonin antagonist cyproheptadine blocks the stimulating effect of hypothalamic serotonin on the release of CRF, thereby secondarily reducing pituitary ACTH secretion. A medical or chemical adrenalectomy may also be accomplished by the administration of ortho,para' DDD (mitotane) (2 to 3 gm/day), aminoglutethimide (1 gm/day) and/or metyrapone (2 to 3 gm/day) (Lutton et al., 1979; Child et al., 1976).

Patients who present with severe Cushing's syndrome (e.g., psychosis, severe osteoporosis, and so forth) are candidates for bilateral total adrenalectomy. Although this is a definitive cure of the hypercortisolemia, at least a tenth of these patients develop pituitary tumors after surgery (Nelson's syndrome).

NELSON'S SYNDROME. Prior to the introduction of transsphenoidal pituitary surgery, bilateral adrenalectomy had been performed for more than 20 years in the treatment of Cushing's syndrome. During this time a complication had appeared: Approximately 10 to 20 per cent of these patients with normal sella turcicas preoperatively developed pituitary tumors over the subsequent postoperative months to years (so-called Nelson's syndrome) (see Fig. 85–21). Almost all these tumors have been chromophobe adenomas that secrete very high levels of ACTH. Patients usually present with progressive hyperpigmentation or symptoms or signs of pituitary tumor, such as headache or visual disturbances. Since these tumors can appear as late as 10 to 15 years postoperatively, all adrenalectomized patients should be followed indefinitely with ACTH levels and periodic high resolution CT scanning of the sella turcica (Moore et al., 1976). Rising levels of ACTH or an obviously elevated value in an adrenalectomized patient on adequate glucocorticoid replacement therapy should always lead to careful radiographic evaluation of the sella turcica by computerized tomography.

Treatment of ACTH-Producing Paraendocrine Tumors. Although the most satisfactory treatment of Cushing's syndrome due to ectopic secretion of ACTH is the surgical removal of the neoplastic source of ACTH, this can rarely be accomplished. Occasionally such an isolated tumor is identified by CT scanning, and its removal cures the patient. Most tumors that secrete ACTH are malignant and have metastasized by the time the diagnosis has been established. In such cases, metyrapone or ortho-para'DDD can be used in an effort to control the excess secretion of cortisol and the consequent metabolic abnormalities, such as hypokalemia and hyperglycemia.

PRIMARY ALDOSTERONISM

In 1955, a new syndrome was described, characterized by arterial hypertension, hypokalemia and alkalosis, muscle weakness, and vasopressin-resistant polyuria. Conn (1955) demonstrated the cause to be an overproduction of aldosterone by an adrenocortical adenoma. The major clinical manifestations (and the keys to diagnosis) stem from two major changes produced by excessive aldosterone:potassium depletion and arterial hypertension.

Etiology. Aldosterone-secreting adrenocortical adenomas characteristically are small, yellow tumors that may be indistinguishable on gross examination from the relatively common nonfunctioning cortical nodules. Almost three fourths of these tumors have measured less than 3 cm in diameter, and in some cases the diameter has been less than 0.5 cm.

In most series the ratio of female-to-male cases is about 2:1. Approximately 80 per cent of patients have been between the ages of 30 and 60 years. Rarely, an adrenal carcinoma has been encountered.

The term "primary aldosteronism" refers specifically to the syndrome produced by autonomous hypersecretion of aldosterone. The etiologic lesion is usually a solitary adenoma (70 per cent), but in the remaining patients aldosterone hypersecretion is the result of bilateral cortical nodular hyperplasia (also termed idiopathic hyperaldosteronism). When diffuse or nodular cortical hyperplasia is present, it is possible that the zona glomerulosa cells have undergone a primary metabolic derangement, leading to autonomous oversecretion of aldosterone. Alternatively, the zona glomerulosa may be responding to an undetected stimulus. Since cortisol production is normal and plasma renin levels are low, elevleted levels of neither ACTH nor angiotension II can be implicated. However, one hypothesis suggests that there is enhanced sensitivity of the zona glomerulosa to low circulating levels of angiotension II. Alternatively, increased levels of another, as yet unidentified, pituitary factor that stimulates aldosterone production have been reported (so-called aldosterone-stimulating factor). Unlike the favorable prognosis of most patients with solitary adenoma, patients with bilateral nodular hyperplasia and associated hypertension are often not benefited by adrenalectomy, even if bilateral.

Pathophysiology. Aldosterone in excess increases the distal renal tubular reabsorption of sodium and the excretion of potassium, hydrogen, ammonium, and magnesium ions. Sodium retention leads to expansion of extracellular and plasma volumes, followed by an increase in glomerular filtration rate and renal plasma flow and a decrease in renin production. Eventually the kidney "escapes" from the sodium-retaining action of aldosterone, but potassium-wasting persists. As a result, a progressive depletion of total body potassium ensues. The decreased intracellular potassium is partially compensated for by a movement into cells of hydrogen ions, leading to systemic alkalosis. The latter, particularly in the presence of hypokalemia, may cause paresthesias and even tetany. Chronic potassium wastage also produces significant changes in neuromuscular function, ranging from mild weakness to frank paralysis. In addition, a hypokalemic tubular nephropathy occurs, leading to poor concentrating ability and a reduced capacity to acidify the urine. The urine is relatively alkaline and contains more ammonium than is usual at that pH. There is an exaggeration of the normal postural sodium diuresis; in some patients this is sufficient to reverse the normal nocturnal sodium retention and results in a marked sodium diuresis and nocturia. These changes appear to be secondary to an expanded extracellular fluid volume in the presence of hypertension.

The exact mechanism(s) by which excess aldosterone causes hypertension is not known. However, in all species (including man) that develop high blood pressure in response to large quantities of mineralocorticoids, the hypertension appears to be secondary to changes in sodium metabolism, since salt restriction prevents the rise in blood pressure. Because the administration of aldosterone and salt decreases plasma renin levels, it appears that a mechanism other than the renin-angiotensin system must be involved. Tobian (1960) has suggested that the increased sodium and water content of the arteriolar wall that follows mineralocorticoid administration may increase peripheral vascular resistance and thereby raise the blood pressure.

Signs and Symptoms. Muscular weakness, the most common symptom, affects mainly the trunk and lower extremities and in severe cases may progress to transient paralysis. However, the actual incidence of paralysis appears to be well below that recorded in the early history of the syndrome when, as expected, advanced cases were recognized first. Paresthesias of the face, hands, and feet attributable to alkalosis and hypokalemia may occur, and even tetany may result. Persistent frontal or central headaches are frequent. Polyuria occurs commonly, but severe nocturia is the specific complaint of some patients.

The physical findings in the 145 cases collected by Conn et al. (1964b) are listed in Table 85–4. All patients had hypertension. Typically, the elevation of blood pressure is moderate in degree and benign in course and often has been present for years. However, a major elevation of diastolic blood pressure may be present, and, rarely, malignant hypertension has been encountered. Postural changes in blood pressure are sometimes marked. About half the patients exhibit a mild to moderate retinopathy. In the early stages heart size is normal; later, cardiomegaly and then heart failure may appear. The electrocardiogram often reflects hypokalemia with flattened or inverted T waves, large U waves, sagging ST segments, and a prolonged P-R interval. Cardiac arrhythmias and premature contractions are common. Loss of deep tendon reflexes, paralysis, or other signs of profound potassium depletion have occurred in far advanced cases. Tetany has appeared when hypokalemic alkalosis is present but may be noted only with hyperventilation or compression of an artery (Trousseau's sign). Edema is characteristically absent, attesting to the escape from sodium retention. However, in cases of long duration, congestive heart failure may develop or the hypertensive nephropathy may progress to azotemic failure; in these patients, edema does occur.

Laboratory Findings. Table 85–5 lists the major biochemical abnormalities encountered. Demonstration of hypokalemia has been the most widely used screening test for primary

TABLE 85–4. SIGNS IN PRIMARY ALDOSTERONISM

	Per Cent
Hypertension	100
Retinopathy	50
Cardiomegaly	41
Positive Trousseau's sign	17
Tetany	9
Paralysis	4

TABLE 85–5. LABORATORY ABNORMALITIES IN
PRIMARY ALDOSTERONISM

Blood	Urine
Hypokalemia	Decreased concentrating ability
Alkalosis	Decreased ability to acidify
Hypernatremia	Increased potassium excretion
Hypomagnesemia	(high urinary excretion of
Increased plasma	potassium, 40 mEq/24 hr or
volume	greater, at low plasma potas-
Increased plasma	sium levels)
aldosterone	Normal 17-OHCS and 17-KS
Decreased plasma	Increased aldosterone excretion
renin level	and secretion rates

aldosteronism. It is emphasized that serial measurements of serum potassium may be necessary in order to demonstrate hypokalemia. Furthermore, when the hypertension of these patients is treated by salt restriction, the decreased sodium load presented to the distal tubular ion-exchange mechanism reduces the tubular secretion and urinary excretion of potassium, and serum potassium levels may rise to normal. In this case, the resumption of a normal salt intake or even salt-loading may be required to uncover the hypokalemia. Serum potassium levels may also be within the normal range in patients treated with potassium-sparing diuretics, such as amiloride or the aldosterone antagonist, spironolactone. In most cases, potassium levels will be consistently below normal. In a very rare early case, serum potassium concentration may be consistently normal. However, in severe disease or in patients treated with potassium-wasting diuretics, the decrease in serum potassium may be marked (to less than 2.5 mEq per liter), reflecting a marked loss of total body potassium. Serum bicarbonate values are increased, but in mild or early disease, normal levels are sometimes found. Serum magnesium concentrations may also be reduced.

Serum sodium levels are usually in the upper range of normal, occasionally slightly elevated. Total exchangeable sodium is usually increased, but to a lesser degree than in states of gross edema. The extracellular and plasma volumes are expanded in most cases (Biglieri and Forsham, 1960). The rise in plasma volume is in contrast to the decline seen in patients with essential hypertension marked by high diastolic pressure (Tarazi et al., 1968).

In many patients, urine osmolality is low, and an overnight concentration test or a vasopressin test reveals impaired ability to concentrate the urine. A mild degree of proteinuria is found in a similar proportion of cases, some-

times in association with pyuria and bacilluria. Urine pH is neutral to alkaline, with a low titratable acidity and a relatively high output of ammonia and bicarbonate ions.

Urinary potassium wastage is a common characteristic of the disease. It is important that the 24-hour urinary excretion of potassium be evaluated in relation to simultaneous serum potassium measurements. This should be assessed in the absence of diuretic therapy or potassium supplementation. Most patients with non–mineralocorticoid mediated etiologies of potassium depletion (e.g., chronic diarrhea, thiazide diuretics, and so forth) are capable of definite, although imperfect, renal conservation of potassium. Renal excretion of potassium usually continues at a level of 10 mEq per day in the absence of dietary intake. Consequently, urinary potassium output is less than 20 mEq per day. In contrast, in patients with primary aldosteronism, urinary potassium excretion is above 30 mEq per day and usually is greater than 40 mEq per day in the face of hypokalemia.

Urinary glucocorticoid and androgen levels are normal in patients with primary aldosteronism. Occasionally these indices have been elevated when the disease is caused by adrenal carcinoma. It should also be recalled that patients with ectopic ACTH secretion primarily present with a potassium-depletion syndrome. In this situation, aldosterone secretion is not elevated, but potassium-wasting is a consequence of the increased secretion of deoxycorticosterone by the greatly elevated ACTH levels.

Indices of aldosterone output are elevated for the level of dietary sodium in patients with primary aldosteronism. In a normal subject on a normal salt intake (150 mEq sodium/day), recumbent plasma aldosterone is usually 20 to 100 ng/dl, urinary aldosterone 25 to 150 μg/day, and aldosterone production rates 250 to 1200 μg/day. In addition to dietary sodium, these values can be importantly influenced by other factors. For example, potassium loading may cause aldosterone levels to rise; more importantly, severe potassium depletion has been shown to depress a previously elevated value to within the normal range. Moreover, since basal plasma aldosterone levels are variable, failure of sodium loading to suppress secretion is a more definitive test to document autonomy of aldosterone output (see further on).

As described previously, there exists a renal-adrenal mechanism for the normal maintenance of sodium balance and systemic renal perfusion (see Fig. 85–12). When its perfusion is reduced, the kidney releases renin through

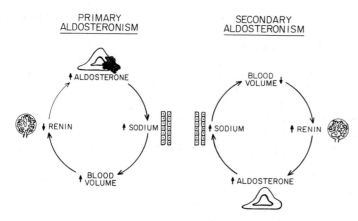

Figure 85–22. Hyperaldosteronism may be seen in association with elevated (secondary) or depressed (primary) levels of plasma renin activity. In primary aldosteronism an adrenal neoplasm or bilateral hyperplasia is the initiating event. Secondary aldosteronism is most commonly seen in edematous disorders (e.g., cirrhosis, renal failure), in which the elevated renin levels are a physiologic adjustment to a contracted blood volume; it is also present in renal artery stenosis, secondary to the stimulus of elevated levels of renin and angiotensin II.

the juxtaglomerular apparatus. Renin is an enzyme that acts on the substrate angiotensinogen to form the decapeptide angiotensin I; angiotensin I is then enzymatically converted to the octapeptide angiotensin II by a converting enzyme located primarily in the lung. Angiotensin II stimulates aldosterone secretion which causes retention of sodium and tends to restore renal perfusion. In 1964, Conn suggested that this system, functioning through feedback mechanisms, might result in subnormal plasma renin activity (PRA) in primary aldosteronism (Fig. 85–22) and that this finding could provide an additional diagnostic criterion (Conn et al., 1964a). It now has been amply confirmed that when aldosterone is secreted autonomously, plasma renin activity is low. Futhermore, procedures that are known to stimulate a significant rise in plasma renin levels in normal subjects (the maintenance of upright posture and sodium deprivation) are ineffective in patients with primary aldosteronism. Samples are drawn after the patient has been upright for 3 to 4 hours on the fourth or fifth day of a low-sodium diet (10 mEq/day); in addition, a diuretic such as furosemide may be given on the first day of dietary restriction in order to hasten sodium depletion. Under these conditions, plasma renin activity in normal recumbent subjects on a 10 mEq sodium intake ranges between 2.5 and 8 ng/ml/hr and rises to 6 to 20 ng/ml/hr after 3 hours of ambulation. Alternatively, on a normal dietary sodium intake, stimulation of renin may be accomplished by the administration of a potent diuretic (40 to 80 mg furosemide) followed by 2 to 3 hours of ambulation (Ferriss et al., 1978a). The normal response is a rise in plasma renin to 8 to 15 ng/ml/hr. Stimulated renin levels below 1 ng/ml/hr are found in most patients with primary aldosteronism. Confusion sometimes occurs because approximately 20 per cent of patients with essential hypertension have diminished renin responsiveness to volume depletion and upright posture, so-called low-renin essential hypertension. These patients, however, are rarely spontaneously hypokalemic, and as a group their PRA levels are higher than in those with primary aldosteronism.

Diagnosis. The autonomous secretion of aldosterone by the adrenal gland(s) is indicated by an *inappropriately* elevated urinary secretion rate (or plasma level) of aldosterone on a liberal intake of sodium. At the same time, the excess hormone leads to sodium retention and suppresses renal renin secretion (Fig. 85–22). These two changes provide the major contemporary criteria for the diagnosis of primary aldosteronism; failure to suppress aldosterone output during sodium loading and subnormal plasma renin levels in the face of salt deprivation (Conn et al., 1964a).

Expansion of plasma volume suppresses aldosterone secretion in normal subjects but not in patients with primary hyperaldosteronism. This can be accomplished by dietary salt loading, using a diet containing at least 200 mEq of sodium per day (with potassium intake held at normal levels of 60 to 90 mEq per day). In normal subjects, the aldosterone secretion and urinary excretion rates are significantly reduced within 3 to 5 days. Because aldosterone output declines, urinary potassium excretion may fall somewhat and serum potassium concentration shows little change. However, in patients with primary aldosteronism, the output of aldosterone is not suppressed, and, because of the increased amount of sodium delivered to the ion-exchange apparatus of the renal distal tubule, urinary potassium excretion increases and hypokalemia develops or becomes more severe. Conversely, severe sodium restriction (10 to 20 mEq per day) leads to a fall in urinary potassium levels and a rise in serum potassium levels in patients with aldosteronism.

In a diagnostic setting, aldosterone secretion may be suppressed by oral or intravenous saline loading. A simple but easily accomplished study is the intravenous saline infusion test (Fig. 85–23). In the recumbent position, the patient receives an infusion of 2 liters of normal saline (500 ml per hr over a 4 hour period) with a measurement of plasma potassium and aldosterone levels at the beginning and end of the infusion (Kem et al., 1971). In normal subjects, post-infusion plasma aldosterone levels are always less than 10 ng/dl and are commonly less than 5 ng/dl. An alternative, more elaborate suppression study is the infusion of 2 liters of saline over a 4-hour period on each of 2 consecutive days. Measurement of urinary aldosterone secretion or excretion is obtained on the day before and on each of the 2 infusion days. On the second day of saline infusion, aldosterone secretion is less than 150 μg/day. In patients with primary aldosteronism, minor or no change in aldosterone levels is seen during these suppression studies.

Biglieri et al. (1972) have also devised a stringent suppression study. Patients are given a sodium intake of at least 120 mEq per day throughout. After a control period, the potent mineralocorticoid deoxycorticosterone acetate is given intramuscularly, 10 mg every 12 hours for 3 days. Aldosterone excretion is measured before and on the third day of deoxycorticosterone administration. Urinary aldosterone declines more than 70 per cent below control levels in normal subjects and in patients with essential hypertension. Patients with primary aldosteronism show little change. The procedure has been especially useful in the diagnosis of those cases with borderline aldosterone values. An alternative suppression test using an oral mineralocorticoid is the administration of fluorohydrocortisone acetate (fluorinef, 0.5 mg twice daily) for 3 days with subjects on a 200 mEq sodium intake (Biglieri et al., 1970a). Plasma or urinary aldosterone levels are measured before and after fluorinef administration.

A recently introduced screening test for primary aldosteronism involves the use of the converting enzyme inhibitor captopril. Twenty-five mg of captopril is given to the recumbent hypertensive subject, and plasma aldosterone levels are obtained prior to and 2 hours following administration of captopril. The rationale for this test is that in patients with primary aldosteronism, angiotensin II levels are suppressed; accordingly, no change in plasma aldosterone levels is obtained pre- or postadministration of captopril. In all other patients with essential hypertension, lowering of the angiotensin II levels with captopril results in lowering of plasma aldosterone levels.

In summary (Fig. 85–24), the major criteria for the diagnosis of primary aldosteronism are as follows: hypertension; hypokalemia that persists when potassium-wasting diuretics have been discontinued; increased aldosterone output that does not suppress despite high sodium intake or mineralocorticoid administration; and suppressed plasma renin levels that fail to rise normally under conditions of upright position and restricted sodium intake. Most patients with aldosterone-producing adenomas become normotensive and normokalemic when they receive the aldosterone antagonist spironolactone in a dose of 50 to 100 mg every 6 hours over a 2- to 5-week period. This therapeutic response is not

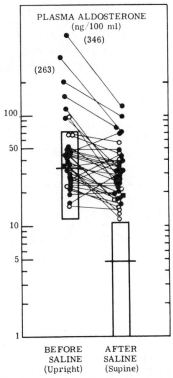

Figure 85–23. Intravenous saline loading test. The patient receives an infusion of 2 liters of normal saline over a 4-hour period. Aldosterone and potassium levels are drawn at the beginning and end of the infusion. In normal subjects (bar graphs) postinfusion plasma aldosterone levels are less than 10 ng/μ and commonly less than 5 ng/dl. Patients with hyperaldosteronism (circles) fail to suppress normally and are segregated out by the test. Open circles represent patients with bilateral hyperplasia; closed circles are patients with adenomas. (From Weinberger, M. H., et al.: Ann. Intern. Med., 90:386, 1979.)

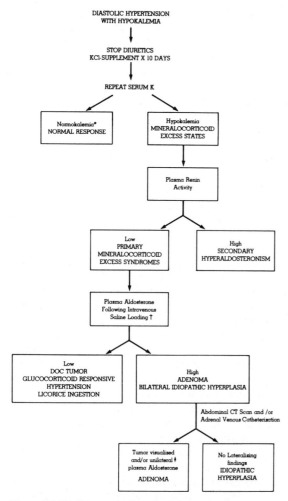

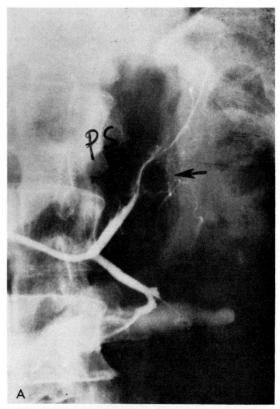

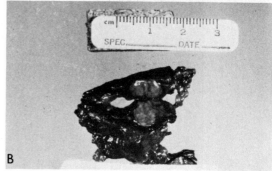

Figure 85–24. Diagnostic flow chart for evaluating patients with suspected primary aldosteronism.

*Serum K$^+$ may be normal in some patients with hyperaldosteronism who are taking potassium-sparing diuretics (spironolactone, triamterene) or ingesting low sodium–high potassium intakes.

†This step should not be taken if hypertension is severe (diastolic > 115 mm Hg) or if cardiac failure is present. Also, serum potassium levels should be corrected before the infusion of saline. Alternative methods producing comparable suppression of aldosterone secretion include oral sodium loading (200 mEq per day for 3 days) or 10 mg deoxycorticosterone acetate (DOCA) intramuscularly every 12 hours for 3 days. (From Petersdorf, R. G., and Adams, R. D. (Eds.): Harrison's Principles of Internal Medicine. New York, McGraw-Hill Book Co., 1983. Used by permission.)

Figure 85–25. Selective left venogram *(A)* outlining a 5-mm adenoma (arrow) in a patient with primary hyperaldosteronism. He had undergone renal artery surgery years earlier at another institution without relief of hypertension. A hemiadrenalectomy was performed *(B)*, and the patient was cured.

diagnostic of primary aldosteronism, since some patients with essential hypertension may also show a positive blood pressure lowering response. On the other hand, patients with accelerated hypertension and patients with idiopathic hyperplasia often experience correction of hypokalemia but persistence of hypertension.

Since aldosteronomas are often small, roentgenographic studies aimed at visualization are frequently unrewarding. Current techniques include computerized tomography imaging, adrenal venography, and iodocholesterol scanning. Iodocholesterol scanning (Beierwaltes et al., 1971) and computerized tomographic techniques (Linde et al., 1979) have been reported to be effective in the preoperative localization of aldosterone-producing adenomas; however, their main limitation is failure to image the not uncommon adenoma that is under 1 cm in size. At venography, a small tumor missed by CT is usually visualized by the stretching or distortion of the normal venous network (Fig. 85–25). Venography permits radiologic localization, and, in addition, adrenal vein sampling may demonstrate a two- to threefold increase in plasma aldosterone concentration on the side bearing the tumor (Nicolis et al., 1972). In patients with hyperaldosteronism secondary to idiopathic or cortical nodular hyperplasia, plasma aldosterone levels will be elevated bilaterally. It is important that bilateral venous samples be obtained simultaneously, as spurious unilateral localization may occur if the secretion of aldosterone is intermittently stimulated by ACTH during the stress of the procedure. Thus, cortisol levels in the adrenal venous effluents should also be measured. Comparable cortisol levels from both sides exclude a stress response if samples were not obtained simultaneously and also ensure that both catheters were in the adrenal veins.

Differential Diagnosis. Primary aldosteronism must be considered in the differential diagnosis of hypertension, hypokalemia, and situations in which aldosterone output is abnormally elevated. However, at the onset it should be remembered that primary aldosteronism is rare, ranging between 1 and 2 per cent in an unselected hypertensive population.

The greatest difficulties in differential diagnosis arise in those conditions marked by both high blood pressure and hypokalemia. A low serum potassium concentration due to excessive urinary potassium excretion is a frequent finding in certain types of hypertension; these are listed in Table 85–6. However, by far the most frequent cause of hypokalemia in hypertensive patients is the therapeutic use of diuretic agents (especially agents with long biologic half-lives, such as chlorthalidone). In patients in whom hypokalemia is solely a consequence of diuretic therapy, plasma renin levels and aldosterone are elevated (secondary hyperaldosteronism). In addition, patients with either primary or secondary hyperaldosteronism are susceptible to hypokalemia during diuretic therapy. Moreover, since the sodium depletion secondary to diuretic treatment also increases aldosterone output, it is important that the work-up of these patients be properly designed. Diuretics should be stopped for at least 1 week, and potassium replacement (potassium chloride) should be given. Thereafter, potassium administration is stopped, and the patient is allowed a normal salt intake. Persistence of hypokalemia favors a diagnosis of hyperaldosteronism, and further studies are indicated (Fig. 85–24).

Measurement of stimulated plasma renin activity is useful, since a number of diagnostic possibilities are excluded if the levels are normal or elevated. When plasma renin levels are found to be suppressed, the most common problem in the differential diagnosis is between solitary adenoma and idiopathic hyperplasia. These diagnoses cannot be distinguished on biochemical grounds, since suppressed renin levels and hyperaldosteronism are characteristic of both diseases. CT scanning or simultaneous cannulation of the adrenal veins, or both, may be necessary

TABLE 85–6. HYPOKALEMIC STATES IN THE DIFFERENTIAL DIAGNOSIS OF PRIMARY ALDOSTERONISM

	Aldosterone Production	Plasma Renin
HYPERTENSION		
Primary aldosteronism		
Idiopathic nodular hyperplasia or solitary adenoma	↑	↓
Secondary aldosteronism:		
Malignant hypertension	↑	↑
Renovascular hypertension	↑ or N	↑ or N
Renin-secreting renal tumor	↑	↑
Diuretic therapy of hypertension	↑ initially	↑ initially
Defects of corticosteroid biosynthesis with associated mineralocorticoid excess:		
17-Hydroxylase deficiency	↓	↓
11-Hydroxylase deficiency	↓	↓
Cushing's syndrome:		
Adrenal tumor or hyperplasia	N	N
Ectopic ACTH production	N or ↓	N or ↓
"Pseudoaldosteronism"—a familial renal tubular disorder	↓	↓
Factitious—licorice ingestion	↓	↓
NORMOTENSIVE		
Syndrome of juxtaglomerular hyperplasia (Bartter's syndrome)	↑	↑
Renal tubular acidosis	↑	↑
Familial periodic paralysis	↑ with attack	N
Secondary aldosteronism:		
Cirrhosis with ascites	↑	↑
Congestive heart failure	↑	↑

and should be diagnostic, with lateralization of an elevated aldosterone level in patients with a solitary adenoma. An additional helpful finding is a postural rise in levels of plasma aldosterone, which is characteristic of patients with idiopathic hyperplasia, probably as a consequence of a small increment in angiotensin II levels (Ganguly et al., 1973; Biglieri, 1979). In contrast, plasma aldosterone levels usually decline in patients with solitary adenomas who assume the upright posture; plasma renin levels are markedly suppressed, and the neoplasm is predominantly under the control of the circadian decline in secretion of ACTH. Elevated levels of the aldosterone precursor 18-hydroxycorticosterone have also been reported in patients with an adenoma; normal levels are seen in patients with idiopathic hyperplasia (Ferriss et al., 1978b).

Two uncommon types of adrenal hyperplasia resulting from hydroxylation defects in cortisol biosynthesis and associated with hypertension have been described (Table 85–6). Hypokalemia and hypertension are corrected by administration of glucocorticoids. The 17-hydroxylase deficiency described by Biglieri and Mantero (1973) results in impaired cortisol production, increased ACTH secretion, and overproduction of corticosterone and 11-deoxycorticosterone through the unblocked pathway. The latter steroid is a potent mineralocorticoid and leads to hypertension, hypervolemia, and hypokalemia. The expansion of plasma volume suppresses renin secretion, and aldosterone output diminishes. Since the sex steroid pathway is also blocked in the 17-hydroxylase deficiency syndrome, patients also present with sexual immaturity. The 11-hydoxylase deficiency syndrome (New and Seaman, 1970) causes overproduction of 11-deoxycortisol (compound S) and 11-deoxycorticosterone; the latter is thought to be responsible for hypertension. Since the sex pathway is not blocked in this syndrome, increased ACTH secretion leads to increased adrenal androgen production. As a result, virilizing syndromes are seen in female patients and precocious puberty in male subjects. Glucocorticoid administration has also rarely been reported to correct a hypertension-hypokalemia syndrome, although a hydroxylation deficiency has not been identified (so-called glucocorticoid suppressible hyperaldosteronism) (Giebink et al., 1973). The aforementioned hypertension-hypokalemia syndrome that is responsive to glucocorticoid administration should be suspected if the family history is strongly positive, especially for hypertension occurring in young males.

Hypertension and hypokalemic alkalosis may occur in some cases of Cushing's syndrome due to adrenal hyperplasia or tumor; they are most commonly found in patients with excessive ACTH secretion arising in a nonendocrine carcinoma. Although very high levels of cortisol are capable of producing potassium depletion, excessive production of aldosterone and 11-deoxycorticosterone is seen in some cases of adrenal carcinoma (associated with Cushing's syndrome, virilization, or feminization) (Biglieri et al., 1968). Modestly elevated levels of 11-deoxycorticosterone also occur in the adrenal hyperplasia of Cushing's syndrome as a result of excess pituitary ACTH secretion, but hypokalemia and suppressed PRA are not commonly seen.

11-Deoxycorticosterone (DOC)–secreting adenomas have also been reported in hypertensive patients with hypokalemic alkalosis. Plasma renin levels are suppressed while aldosterone levels are not elevated, suggesting the diagnosis of mineralocorticoid excess secondary to a steroid other than aldosterone (Kondo et al., 1976).

Liddle et al. (1964) have described a family with hypertension and hypokalemia simulating primary aldosteronism but with low aldosterone production. The syndrome appears to be a renal tubular disorder marked by an enhanced responsiveness to aldosterone, with a resultant unusual capacity of the kidneys to retain sodium and excrete potassium.

A condition indistinguishable clinically from primary aldosteronism has been found to be produced by the chronic ingestion of large amounts of licorice (Taylor and Bartter, 1977) or chewing tobacco. Glycyrrhizic acid is the culprit ingredient; because of its mineralocorticoid-like effects, production of both renin and aldosterone is suppressed. Similar syndromes have been described following administration of carbenoxolone for gastric ulcer and fluorohydrocortisone for postural hypotension (Chobanian et al., 1979).

Hypersecretion of aldosterone may occur in hypertension of an accelerated form because of stimulation of the zona glomerulosa by high circulating levels of angiotensin II generated by elevated renin levels arising from renal ischemia (so-called *secondary hyperaldosteronism*). The ischemia may result either from extrarenal vascular obstruction or from intrarenal vascular damage (Schambelan and Perloff, 1980). Thus, elevated aldosterone output is found in many patients with malignant hypertension and in some patients with renal artery obstruction or with hypertension complicated by renal impairment. In all these states the finding of high plasma renin levels together with increased aldosterone output provides the main indication that one is dealing with secondary rather than primary aldosteronism (see Fig. 85–24). The fact that hypertension pursues a malignant course and is accompanied by papilledema and, in most cases, by hyponatremia is suggestive, but not conclusive, evidence against the diagnosis of primary aldosteronism. Pathologically, the adrenal glands are hyperplastic or exhibit bilateral nodular hyperplasia. Bilateral total adrenalectomy is not indicated. It has been previously found to ameliorate but not cure the hypertension; hypokalemia, however, is often improved. The use of rapid-sequence pyelography and selective renal angiography is of critical importance in diagnosis. It is to be noted that when the metabolic abnormalities are produced by excessive aldosterone, the administration of spironolactone is capable of blocking the action of aldosterone in the renal tubule and reversing the hypokalemic alkalosis, whether induced by primary or by secondary aldosteronism. On the other hand, correction of the hypertension with spironolactone is usually seen only in primary aldosteronism when the secretion of aldosterone is pathologically related to the hypertension, such as in an aldosterone-producing adenoma.

Hypertension with secondary aldosteronism and biochemical findings characteristic of renal vascular hypertension has been reported in patients with renin-secreting juxtaglomerular cell tumors (Conn, 1977). The diagnosis is usually confirmed by visualization of the tumor by renal arteriography, by a unilateral increase in renal vein renin levels, or by both. Hypertension with elevated renin levels and secondary aldosteronism is also seen as a complication of oral contraceptive therapy.

Treatment. When the cause of hyperaldosteronism is an aldosterone-producing adenoma, the proper treatment is surgical removal of the tumor. In patients with diffuse or nodular bilateral adrenocortical hyperplasia, the source of the stimulus responsible for the hyperplasia is not known; more importantly, response to bilateral adrenalectomy is not predictable. The antihypertensive response to the blockade of aldosterone with spironolactone has also been used to predict the response to surgery. Patients with solitary adenomas generally achieve normalization (50 per cent) or reduction (25 per cent) of blood pressure and correction of hypokalemia (Weinberger et al., 1979). However, hypertension has recurred (without primary aldosteronism) in approximately 40 per cent of patients after the tenth postoperative year (Biglieri el al., 1970a). Patients with bilateral nod-

ular hyperplasia often achieve correction of the hypokalemic syndrome and blood pressure often improves, but patients generally do not become normotensive (Hunt et al., 1975). Preoperative visualization of the adrenal glands and simultaneous adrenal vein sampling may be necessary to definitively localize the source of the hyperaldosteronism whenever an adenoma is not seen on CT scan (Fig. 85–25). When a typical tumor is found, it should be removed by unilateral adrenalectomy or occasionally with partial adrenalectomy (Fig. 85–25). In patients with presumed bilateral adrenocortical hyperplasia, medical management is the treatment of choice.

Preoperative management concentrates on correcting potassium deficits, using supplemental potassium chloride in doses of 40 to 150 mEq per day. A low-sodium diet will aid potassium repletion, and in some cases aldosterone antagonists (spironolactone) or agents that interfere with renal tubular ion transport (triamterene and amiloride) may be helpful.

Patients who have undergone resection of a solitary adenoma have a postoperative diuresis of sodium while retaining potassium. The carbon dioxide content and pH of the blood also return to normal. These shifts are nearly complete by the second or third postoperative week. Polyuria and polydipsia disappear more promptly. In some patients, azotemia, hyponatremia, and hyperkalemia develop during the immediate postoperative period, reflecting transient aldosterone deficiency and suppression of the contralateral adrenal zona glomerulosa. In such cases, replacement therapy with fluorocortisol may be required temporarily, but in most cases management consists of aggressive volume repletion.

In the majority of patients with a solitary aldosterone-producing adenoma, the decline or normalization of blood pressure occurs within 4 months after surgery. In about 15 per cent of patients there is a temporary decline in pressure, but a subsequent gradual rise to preoperative levels occurs even though all abnormalities of electrolyte metabolism have been completely corrected. Thus, it would appear that in some patients the hypertension is fixed, presumably on a renal basis.

TUMORS OF THE ADRENAL CORTEX

NONFUNCTIONING ADRENAL TUMORS

With the widespread use of abdominal CT scanning, many patients with incidental adrenal masses are being diagnosed. This perhaps could be expected, since 10 to 20 per cent of the patients at routine autopsy have benign adrenal cortical adenomas. The differential diagnosis of an incidentally discovered adrenal mass should include a functioning adrenal tumor (such as pheochromocytoma, cortical adenoma, or carcinoma), cyst, nonfunctioning adrenal adenoma or carcinoma, and metastatic carcinoma. No further studies are indicated in patients with known metastatic disease or in whom an adrenal cyst or myelolipoma can be accurately diagnosed by CT scanning. The remaining patients should be evaluated for functioning adrenal tumors by appropriate biochemical testing (urine steroids, catecholamines, and so forth). While functioning adrenal tumors are likely to be associated with an elevated arterial blood pressure, it should be noted that nonfunctioning adenomas discovered at autopsy occur more frequently in patients with essential hypertension. Nonfunctioning tumors present difficult decisions, since 20 per cent of adrenal carcinomas are nonfunctioning; however, the frequency of adrenocortical carcinoma is extremely low compared with the incidence of benign nonfunctioning adenomas. An important finding is the size of the lesion, since most adrenocortical carcinomas are larger than 6 cm when initially discovered, whereas benign large adenomas (i.e., greater than 6 cm in size) are rare in autopsy studies. Thus, nonfunctioning masses greater than 6 cm in size should certainly be removed at the outset (Copeland, 1983). Our own analysis of the experience with adrenal masses (Hussain et al., 1985) suggests that only nonfunctioning masses less than 3.5 cm and nonenhancing after administration of contrast agent should be followed by CT scans (e.g., at 3- to 6-month intervals). A change in the size of the lesion may be an indication for surgery. Of course, the patient's age and overall medical condition should enter into the decision-making. Thus, elderly subjects with severe cardiovascular diseases are likely to be followed with the understanding that the incidence of nonfunctioning adrenal carcinoma is extremely low while the operative risk may be unacceptably high.

The great majority of nonfunctioning tumors of sufficient size to elicit symptoms are malignant. For example, of 35 nonfunctioning tumors reviewed by Rapaport et al. (1956), 33 were considered to be malignant. These tumors occur mainly in adults, particularly from the fourth to seventh decade. Rarely, they may develop in aberrant adrenal tissue. Levels of adrenal cortical steroids are normal. However, detailed study of urinary steroids has sometimes revealed the presence of increased levels of hormonally inactive precursors of the adrenocortical hormones. Symptoms result from progressive enlargement or from metastases; the latter occur mainly to para-aortic lymph nodes, lungs, or liver. Usually a mass is palpable, and on occasion the mass may be mistaken for kidney. Pain in the abdomen or flank is common and may be a helpful localizing sign. Malaise, weight loss, and fever often appear. Adrenal carcinomas tend to be larger than adenomas, and weights up to 1000 gm have been reported. The cut surface is usually lobular and the tissue is soft, friable, and frequently hemorrhagic or necrotic. The stroma usually contains abundant thin-walled blood vessels. Spread may occur by direct growth into adrenal veins and the vena cava. The malignant nature of adrenocortical neoplasms cannot always be determined from the appearance and arrangement of cells alone. Although some show pleomorphism, anaplasia, and abnormal mitotic activity indicative of malignancy, others are indistinguishable from adenomas on cytologic examination, and their true character may be indicated only by the presence of metastases. Other indications of malignancy include capsular invasion, excessive mitoses, giant cells with unusual hyperchromatism, and nuclear-cytoplasmic disproportion.

Primary mesenchymal tumors have been reported as arising in the adrenal cortex. These rare and usually incidental neoplasms have included fibroma, myoma, lipoma, hemangioma, lymphangioma, and fibrosarcoma. *Myelolipoma* is a tumor-like lesion, usually involving the medulla and sometimes the cortex, which is composed of mature fat cells with focal areas of myeloid tissue. The CT scan reveals the low-density factor. The nature of the lesion is in doubt, but it appears to be a type of metaplasia, although it is not associated with extramedullary hematopoiesis elsewhere.

Adrenal cysts at times attain a size sufficiently large to displace the kidney as well as the intestines. CT scanning and ultrasonography are pivotal in the differential diagnosis of these lesions.

FUNCTIONING ADRENAL ADENOMAS

Benign cortisol- and aldosterone-producing adenomas and their management have been discussed previously under Cushing's syndrome and primary aldosteronism.

FUNCTIONING ADRENAL CARCINOMA

Carcinoma of the adrenal cortex is fortunately a rare malignancy, accounting for less than 0.2 per cent of deaths from all cancers. It occurs at any age; perhaps the highest incidence is between the ages of 20 and 50 years, but a significant number of cases occur before the age of 10 years. In all published series, approximately two thirds of the patients have been female, perhaps reflecting the fact that 80 per cent or more of these tumors are functional, and the most common clinical manifestations (virilization or Cushing's syndrome) are more easily observed in female subjects (Richie and Gittes, 1980). On the other hand, in most collected series, the majority of patients with nonfunctioning adrenal carcinoma are males.

Virilizing and Mixed Syndromes. Functioning adrenal carcinomas produce the following syndromes: isosexual precocity in male children, virilization in females, Cushing's syndrome, aldosteronism, and, rarely, hypoglycemia. The combination of Cushing's syndrome and virilization is the most frequent disorder, emphasizing the fact that adrenal carcinomas are less apt to produce a "pure" clinical picture than is seen in adrenal hyperplasia or benign adenomas. When Cushing's syndrome occurs in a child, adrenal carcinoma is the most frequent cause, whereas in the adult female in her reproductive years, adrenal hyperplasia is much more common. Aldosterone-producing tumors are usually benign, but carcinoma is occasionally found. Tumors producing hypoglycemia as the major clinical feature are rare. The hypoglycemia is severe and of the fasting type, resembling that produced by pancreatic islet cell tumors; however, immunoreactive insulin levels are undetectable. In such cases the mechanism of the hypoglycemia is uncertain, but the production of an insulin-like peptide (somatomedin-C) has been reported.

Measurements of plasma and urinary steroids frequently complement the CT scan and provide the key to diagnosis. Although urinary steroid values tend to be high, the output in relation to adrenal mass is usually lower than normal, reflecting inefficient use of steroid precursors. Patients with adrenal cancer commonly excrete large amounts of adrenal androgens, whether the tumor causes Cushing's syndrome, virilization, or feminization (Hutter and Kayhoe, 1966a). Thus, very high levels of plasma DHEA SO_4 and urinary 17-ketosteroids are always suggestive of a malignant tumor; for example, 17-ketosteroids may exceed 1000 mg/24 hr, but values in the range of 50 to 200 mg/24 hr are more frequent. Abnormal excretion of 17-ketosteroids and clinical virilization are not always well correlated, since these steroids are derived from both androgenic and nonandrogenic precursors.

However, virilization in the female in the presence of normal or minimally elevated urinary 17-ketosteroids is very uncommon in adrenal carcinoma and is always suggestive of a testosterone-secreting ovarian lesion. Rarely, a benign adrenal adenoma may secrete testosterone predominantly. It is to be noted that adrenal androgen production may be increased without elevated cortisol production, but the converse is rarely true in carcinoma. In fact, an elevated cortisol level in association with normal or *decreased* adrenal androgen production (because of the feedback suppression of ACTH) favors the diagnosis of a benign cortisol-producing adenoma. Cushing's syndrome is not invariably present when urinary 17-hydroxycorticosteroids are increased in adrenal carcinoma; in fact, compounds that are not derived from cortisol are included in these measurements. For example, tetrahydro-S (tetrahydro-11-deoxycortisol) may be the major 17-hydroxycorticosteroid in the urine of patients with adrenal carcinoma. Lipsett et al. (1963) found elevated values in every one of 13 patients with malignant adrenal tumors. Accordingly, elevated plasma 11-deoxycortisol or urine tetrahydro-11-deoxycortisol levels strongly point toward a diagnosis of adrenal carcinoma, although the diagnosis of congential adrenal hyperplasia (CAH) also needs to be excluded. In contrast to subjects with CAH, stimulation with ACTH or suppression with dexamethasone does not produce a significant change in steroid output in patients with adrenal carcinoma.

Feminizing Syndrome in Males. Most feminizing adrenal tumors occur between 25 and 50 years of age and are malignant (Gabrilove et al., 1965). Gynecomastia is the most frequent finding and is nearly always the presenting complaint (Fig. 85–26*A*). It is usually bilateral but sometimes is more pronounced on one side and may be associated with tenderness and pigmentation of the areolae. Testicular atrophy and a diminished libido or potency occur in approximately half the patients. Arterial hypertension and edema are occasionally found. Some patients with feminizing adrenal carcinoma show clinical features of Cushing's syndrome—moon face, cutaneous striae, osteoporosis, and diabetes. Children with this disorder show, in addition to gynecomastia, acceleration of growth and bone age. These tumors are typically very large and have been palpable in more than 50 per cent of the patients (Fig. 85–26*B*). Most of the tumors are now easily detected by CT imaging techniques.

Feminizing adrenal tumors secrete increased amounts of androstenedione, which is converted peripherally into the estrogens with

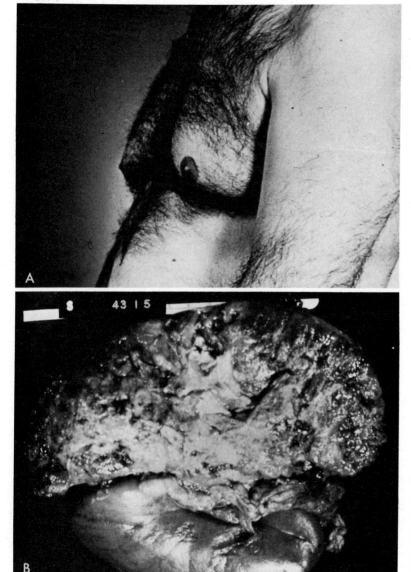

Figure 85–26. *A,* Gynecomastia in male patient with a feminizing cortical carcinoma. *B,* Surgical specimen of the encapsulated adrenal neoplasm surrounding but not grossly invading the kidney. On histologic examination there was microscopic capsular invasion and lymphatic invasion but no lymph node involvement.

the result that blood and urinary estrogens are increased beyond the normal male range. Usually the distribution of estrone, estradiol, and estriol is similar to that of normal males. Estrogen excretion tends to be greater in malignant tumors than in adenomas. Rarely, only urinary estrogen levels are elevated, but adrenal androgen production is also increased in most cases; as previously discussed, very high values of urine 17-ketosteroids and plasma DHEASO$_4$ are characteristic of adrenal carcinoma. The urinary excretion of pregnanetriol and tetrahydro-S (or blood levels of 17α-hydroxyprogesterone and 11-deoxycortisol, respectively) may also be abnormally high, reflecting impairment of hydroxylating enzymes. In approximately half of the patients, cortisol secretion is also increased. Pituitary gonadotropins are usually undetectable, reflecting the suppression of pituitary function by estrogen. Human chorionic gonadotropin production has also been reported in some cases of feminizing adrenal carcinoma; plasma titers of this hormone can serve as a marker for following the response to therapy. The differential diagnosis of feminization in the male should also include testicular and pulmonary neoplasms, which can produce estrogens or chorionic gonadotropins, or both (Gabrilove, 1975).

Metastasis. The most common sites of metastasis of adrenal carcinoma are the lung, liver and lymph nodes (Richie and Gittes, 1980). The para-aortic nodes are most frequently involved, but distant lymphatic spread may occur to the supraclavicular, hilar, or axillary nodes. Adrenal carcinoma frequently extends directly into adjacent structures, especially the kidney. Invasion of the retroperitoneal space is also seen. It is of interest to note that metastases to bone and brain are less common than in renal cell carcinoma.

In rare cases, many years elapse before recurrence or metastatic spread appears. However, the neoplasm is usually highly malignant. At least 50 per cent of the patients are dead within 2 years of the onset of symptoms. The 3-year survival rate is less than 25 per cent. The immediate causes of death are septicemia, hemorrhage from necrotizing tumor, bronchopneumonia, thrombosis of the vena cava (usually associated with marked sodium retention and edema), and inanition.

Treatment. The treatment of adrenal cancer is surgical removal of the lesion. If this can be accomplished, regression of endocrine symptons occurs. The surgical approach may be aided by arteriographic demonstration of the vascular supply (Fig. 85–27). Thoracoabdominal exposure is best for large tumors. Local recurrences of tumor are frequent and tend to develop into large abdominal masses. Palliative excision or radiotherapy of these recurrent lesions can result in considerable decrease in local symptoms. If surgery is elected, adequate preoperative preparation with cortisol is essential, since contralateral adrenal atrophy commonly occurs.

X-ray therapy has not been shown to be effective in inoperable adrenal carcinoma. Chemotherapy, however, has achieved a place in management. The compound mitotane, or o,p'DDD (l,l-dichloro-2-[0-chlorophenyl]-2 [p-chlorophenyl]-ethane), an isomer of the insecticide DDD (Fig. 85–28), has been shown to produce a marked decrease in the secretion of steroids by the adrenal cortex, often associated with focal degenerative lesions of the zona reticularis and zona fasciculata. Hutter and Kay-

Figure 85–27. Selective arteriogram of a large adrenocortical carcinoma. *A,* The selective injection of an inferior artery entering the large left adrenocortical carcinoma, lying in its suprarenal position. A later film (right) shows the adrenographic effect of diffusion of the opaque medium through the lower portion of the tumor. *B,* The selective catheterization and injection of one of the phrenic arteries to this large adrenocortical carcinoma; the illustration on the right shows in detail the upper extension of this large tumor beneath the diaphragm and above the kidney. The normal renal pelvis is seen slightly displaced laterally in its upper calyx.

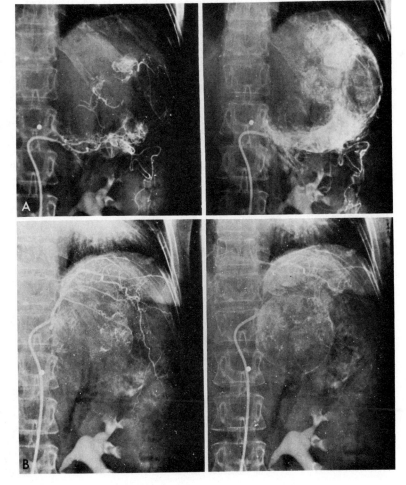

STRUCTURE OF o,p′DDD AND RELATED INSECTICIDES

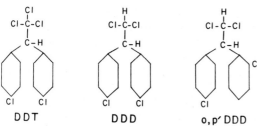

DDT   DDD   o,p′DDD

Figure 85–28. Structure of o,p′DDD and related insecticides.

hoe (1966b) initially summarized the results of o,p′DDD treatment of 138 patients with adrenal carcinoma. An additional large series confirmed their findings (Lubitz et al., 1973). Initial dosage for adults is 2 to 6 gm in divided doses; subsequently, the level is increased until toxicity becomes a limiting factor. The maximal daily dose in most patients is 8 to 10 gm. Toxic side effects are noted in approximately 90 per cent of patients. Drug reactions predominantly involve the gastrointestinal tract, neuromuscular system, and skin. Gastrointestinal disturbances include anorexia, nausea or vomiting, and diarrhea. Central nervous system depression, manifested as lethargy and somnolence, occurs in about one fourth of treated patients but is usually reversible with reduction of dosage. Dizziness, vertigo, muscle tremors, headache, and confusion have also occurred. Cutaneous eruptions appear in about 15 per cent of the patients and are not always dose-related. Other less common changes include visual blurring, diplopia, and lens opacity (which may disappear following withdrawal of the drug). Bone marrow depression and liver damage have not been noted.

O,p′DDD also alters the extra-adrenal metabolism of cortisol so that a smaller fraction is excreted as 17-hydroxycorticosteroids. Therefore, plasma or urinary free cortisol should be monitored to follow the effects of o,p′DDD on the hypercortisolism.

In approximately 70 per cent of patients, urinary steroid values decrease during treatment (Hutter and Kayhoe, 1966b). Urinary 17-ketosteroids, 17-hydroxycorticosteroids, aldosterone, and urinary estrogens may be affected separately or in toto. It is important to note that the fall in steroid excretion may not occur until 3 to 4 weeks of treatment have elapsed. Approximately 35 per cent of treated patients may also be expected to show objective signs of tumor regression, including a reduction in the size of palpable masses, a decrease (or even temporary disappearance) of pulmonary metastatic lesions, diminished pain, and improved strength (Fig. 85–29). It is noteworthy that a good steroid response occurs in all patients who show objective improvement in measurable disease; the converse is not true, since less than half of steroid responders show objective clinical improvement. Furthermore, a demonstrable reduction in tumor growth may be associated with some prolongation of life. Finally, owing to the poor prognosis of patients with adrenal carcinoma, low-dose, long-term o,p′DDD therapy has been recommended as adjuvant therapy

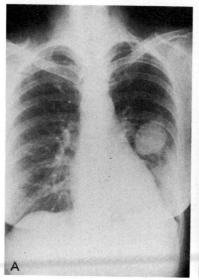
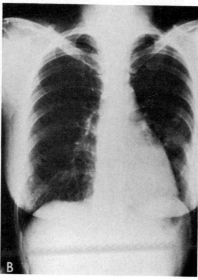

Figure 85–29. A, Roentgenogram of chest showing recurrence of pulmonary metastasis from adrenocortical carcinoma. B, Almost complete disappearance of this following chemotherapy with o,p′DDD. The patient continued to be well 9 years after the original carcinoma of the left adrenal was removed, but recurrence, at 10 years, both pulmonary and abdominal, resulted in death. (From Ney, C., and Friedenberg, R. [Eds.]: Radiographic Atlas of the Genitourinary System. Philadelphia, J. B. Lippincott Company, 1966.)

preoperatively or immediately followintg surgery even in the absence of clinically evident metastases. In one study, mean survival for patients receiving this adjuvant therapy program was longer than for patients treated with surgery or irradiation alone or those treated with o,p'DDD after metastatic disease had become clinically evident.

Other agents have been used for the control of metabolic derangements resulting from steroid-producing lesions. Metyrapone may be used to correct hypercortisolism, but secondary elevations of desoxycorticosterone (DOC) may lead to excessive mineralocorticoid activity. Another compound is aminoglutethimide; *in vitro* and *in vivo* studies indicate that the drug inhibits adrenal steroid synthesis by interfering with the conversion of cholesterol to pregnenolone. As a result, the synthesis of cortisol, aldosterone, and androgens is suppressed. The drug has produced favorable reductions in steroid levels in patients with metastatic adrenocortical carcinoma (Schteingart et al., 1966). Dosage is from 0.75 to 2.0 gm per day. At dose levels of 1.2 gm per day or less, minimal side effects have been encountered. At doses of 1.5 gm per day and over, anorexia, somnolence, fever, vomiting, ataxia, and skin rashes may develop, but these untoward effects disappear following withdrawal of the drug.

THE ADRENAL MEDULLA

"Adrenalin" (or epinephrine) was the first hormone to be isolated and chemically identified, and for many years the physiology of the adrenal medulla was interpreted solely in terms of epinephrine production. The discovery of norepinephrine in adrenergic nerve fibers by von Euler led to a re-evaluation of medullary function, and the existence of two medullary hormones was subsequently established. The classic work of W. B. Cannon emphasized that under conditions of stress "this sympathicoadrenal system is brought prominently and usefully into action in emotional excitement, in vigorous muscular work, asphyxia, low blood pressure, chilling surroundings and hypoglycemia—in brief, it serves effectively in emergencies."

ANATOMY

The adrenal medulla is a functional part of the nervous system and can be regarded as a specialized sympathetic ganglion that is innervated by preganglionic cholinergic neurons.

Embryologically, two cell types, the chromaffinoblast and the neuroblast, differentiate from a common stem cell (the sympathogonia of the primitive neuroectoderm) to form the adrenal medulla. The chromaffinoblast and the neuroblast mature into chromaffin cells and sympathetic ganglion cells, respectively. The chromaffin cell is so named because of its capacity to show brown intracytoplasmic granules on treatment with oxidants (chromates). It has been clearly demonstrated that the granules represent the storage form of catecholamines. Isolated chromaffin granules contain large amounts of adenosine triphosphate (ATP), and there is a molar relationship between total catecholamine and total adenine nucleotide. The molar ratio of catecholamine to ATP is rather constant at about 4:1, suggesting that four positively charged catecholamine molecules bind reversibly with four negatively charged sites on an ATP molecule. When the medullary cell is stimulated to discharge catecholamines by splanchnic nerve stimulation, there is a sharp decrease in the intracellular concentration of both catechol and ATP. Apparently, the hydrolysis of ATP, which releases high-energy bond phosphate, is involved in depolymerization of the granule and the release of catecholamine into the blood.

Histochemical studies indicate the presence of two different chromaffin cell types in the adrenal medulla. One is predominantly epinephrine-secreting, and the other produces norepinephrine. Chromaffin cells are widely distributed in the body at birth, but extra-adrenal chromaffin bodies undergo progressive involution until puberty. Thereafter, chromaffin cells persist in small paraganglionic bodies lying along the retropleural and retroperitoneal sympathetic chains and in the organs of Zuckerkandl, paired structures lying anterior to the abdominal aorta just above the bifurcation.

CATECHOLAMINE BIOSYNTHESIS AND CATABOLISM

By isotopic tracer methods and chromatography the biosynthetic scheme shown in Figure 85–30 has been achieved (Mussachio, 1975). Tyrosine is converted to dihydroxyphenylalanine (dopa), which in turn is converted to dopamine by the enzyme L-dopa decarboxylase. The first step, the meta-hydroxylation to dopa by the mitochondrial enzyme tryosine hydroxylase is rate-limiting for the entire pathway. Dopamine is the first pharmacologically active compound formed in this sequence; it has many of the pharmacologic effects of epinephrine and

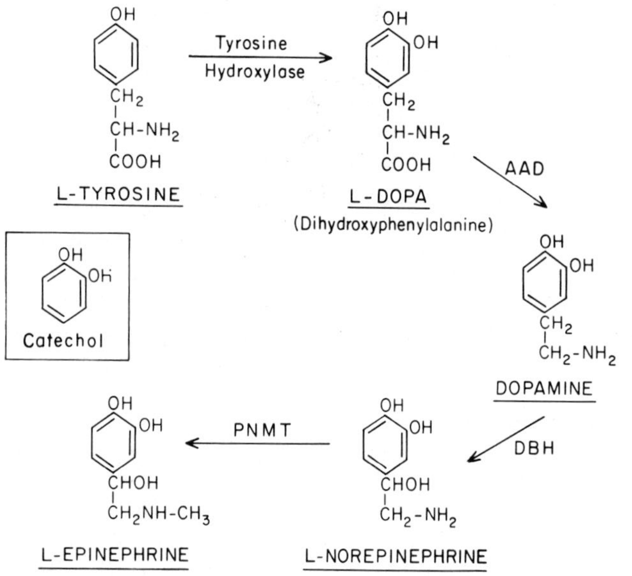

Figure 85–30. Catecholamine biosynthesis (see text for description). Tyrosine hydroxylase is the rate-limiting enzyme for the active pathway. DBH = dopamine-beta-hydroxylase; PNMT = phenyl-ethanolamine-N-methyl transferase; AAD = aromatic L-amino acid decarboxylase.

norepinephrine but is far less potent. The beta-hydroxylation of dopamine to norepinephrine is catalyzed by dopamine-beta-hydroxylase (DBH), an enzyme associated with the granules that store catecholamines. Norepinephrine is converted to epinephrine in those chromaffin cells in the adrenal medulla that can carry out N-methylation. The N-methylation of norepinephrine is controlled by phenylethanolamine-N-methyl transferase (PNMT), an enzyme inducible by high levels of glucocorticoid. Thus, the anatomic localization of the adrenal medulla within the cortex is strategic, in that a supply of steroid-enriched blood is provided for the adrenal medulla and the epinephrine-forming enzyme PNMT. Epinephrine is the major hormone of the adrenal medulla, constituting approximately 80 per cent of its total content of catecholamine. The major source of norepinephrine is the extra-adrenal postganglionic sympathetic neurons. Depolarization of the nerve leads to the discharge of norepinephrine and the soluble portion of DBH from the vesicle into the synaptic cleft by the process of exocytosis (Schober et al., 1977).

The actions of epinephrine and norepinephrine are of brief duration. More than half of intravenously administered catecholamine is metabolized within 2 minutes, and about 10 per cent of administered hormones is excreted in the urine, approximately one half as free hormone and the remainder in conjugated form. Understanding the intermediary metabolism of these hormones is now proving to be of great practical importance in the diagnosis and man-

agement of certain patients with catecholamine-producing tumors. Figure 85–31 summarizes the major routes of epinephrine and norepinephrine catabolism. The most important mechanism in the inactivation of catecholamines is "re-uptake" by storage granules in the postganglionic neuron (Axelrod, 1965). Two degradative mechanisms are enzymatic; one important pathway is via O-methylation through the action of catechol-O-methyl transferase (COMT), which is widely dispersed in body tissues. COMT is present in high concentrations in the liver and kidney; its action is of major importance in the metabolism of circulating catecholamines. Monoamine oxidase (MAO) inactivates catecholamines in most tissues, including sympathetic nerves. About 90 per cent of administered catecholamine is converted into methoxy compounds, of which about 30 per cent is metanephrine plus normetanephrine and about 60 per cent is 3-methoxy-4-hydroxymandelic acid (vanillylmandelic acid, VMA). The latter is formed by the combined action of catechol-O-methyl tranferase and monoamine oxidase. It is to be noted that total bilateral adrenalectomy results in little depression of catecholamine excretion, since approximately 90 per cent of the urinary metabolites are derived from norepinephrine released from extra-adrenal sympathetic nerve endings.

PHYSIOLOGIC EFFECTS

Most of the actions of adrenal medullary hormones can be segregated into five broad areas: a peripheral excitatory action on certain

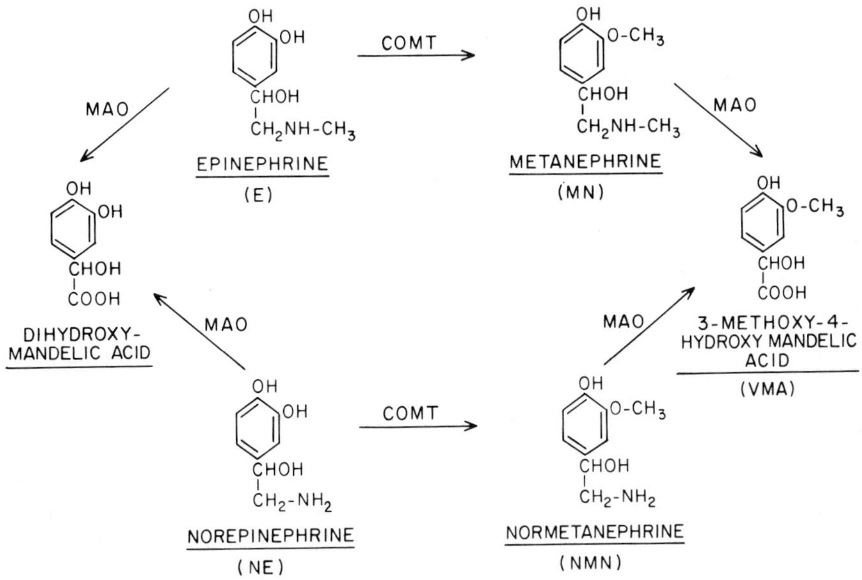

Figure 85–31. Metabolism of epinephrine and norepinephrine (see text for description). COMT = cathechol-O-methyl transferase; MAO = monoamine oxidase.

types of smooth muscles, such as those in blood vessels supplying skin and mucous membranes; a peripheral inhibitory action on certain other types of smooth muscles, such as those in the wall of the gut, in the bronchial tree, and in blood vessels supplying skeletal muscles; a cardiac stimulatory action; metabolic effects; and central nervous system excitation (Landsberg, 1977). The hormones epinephrine and norepinephrine do not show these effects to the same degree. Thus, doses of the two hormones that cause an equal rise in arterial blood pressure have quite different effects on cardiac output, peripheral resistance, heart rate, bronchial musculature, and liver glycogen stores.

Sites of Action. Adrenergic hormones are thought to evoke their characteristic responses through a specialized part of the effector cell termed the receptor. The classification of receptors is descriptive and based on empirically observed responses of different tissues to catecholamine hormones and related compounds. Ahlquist (1948) classified receptor sites as alpha or beta on the basis of their responses to sympathomimetic amines and adrenergic blockers. After the amines were arranged in the order of their potency on a variety of peripheral tissues, two distinct patterns emerged, dividing the tissues into two groups. In one, epinephrine was most potent and isoproterenol least potent; in the other, isoproterenol was most potent and epinephrine least potent. This indicated two types of receptors differing in their affinity for the catecholamines (Lefkowitz, 1977). In gen-

eral, the effect at alpha receptors is excitatory and that at beta receptors is inhibitory, although there are exceptions. Adrenergic blocking agents show high selectivity; for example, phenoxybenzamine (Dibenzyline) acts on alpha receptors, whereas propranolol blocks beta receptors. As a result, the response to blockers is now the main basis for classifying receptor responses. A summary of the two types of adrenergic receptors is given in Table 85–7. Alpha receptors are responsible for vasoconstriction in most areas with increased blood pressure, whereas beta receptors are responsible for an elevated heart rate, increased force of myocardial contraction, and vasodilation in skeletal muscle. Epinephrine and norepinephrine possess both alpha and beta adrenergic effects, although in different degrees; norepinephrine stimulates predominantly alpha receptors, and epinephrine mainly beta receptors.

Beta responses are associated with activation of adenylcyclase; on the other hand, stimulation of alpha receptors is associated with reduction in cyclic AMP concentrations. Moreover, beta-mediated responses may be divided into subgroups: beta-1 receptors, which mediate cardiac stimulation and lipolysis, and beta-2 receptors, which subserve bronchodilatation and vasodilatation. Specific beta-1 and beta-2 agonists and blockers are clinically useful; for example, beta-1 receptor antagonists block the cardiac effects of catecholamines without an associated rise in airway resistance.

Comparative Hormone Effects. The phys-

TABLE 85–7. ADRENERGIC RECEPTORS

Alpha Receptors	Beta Receptors
Vasoconstriction (skin, mucosa, kidney, brain, lung splanchnic)	Intestinal relaxation
Relaxation of gut	Hepatic glycogenolysis
Dilatation of pupil	Increased renin secretion by juxtaglomerular apparatus
Piloerection	Increased insulin secretion
Inhibition of insulin secretion	Lipolysis*
Adrenergic sweating	Cardiac stimulation (increased heart rate, increased myocardial contractility, increased conduction velocity)*
Uterine contraction	Bronchodilatation†
Bladder neck contraction (ejaculation)	Vasodilatation (skeletal muscle and liver)†

*Beta-1 subgroup receptors
†Beta-2 subgroup receptors

iologic effects of the adrenomedullary hormones have been characterized as preparing the organism for emergency responses. The overall effects on the cardiocirculatory system are qualitatively similar to those seen at the beginning of excercise—increase in cardiac output, increase in pulse rate, and rise in blood pressure. Splanchnic vascular constriction (including a reduction in renal blood flow) and dilatation of skeletal muscle vessels produce a redistribution of the enlarged cardiac output. Arteriolar and venoconstriction in most vascular beds are mediated by alpha receptors; skeletal muscle blood flow and cardiac output are regulated by catecholamine beta receptors. Both epinephrine and norepinephrine have a direct inotropic (force of contraction) and chronotropic (rate of contraction) action on the heart. However, the purely vasoconstrictor effect of norepinephrine results in diastolic and systolic hypertension, producing reflex slowing of the heart so that cardiac output is usually unchanged or slightly reduced. The net peripheral vasodilator effect of physiologic doses of epinephrine, due mainly to vasodilatation in skeletal muscle, permits a rise in cardiac output with widening of pulse pressure; systolic pressure rises but diastolic pressure may fall slightly. Cutaneous and renal vasoconstriction occur with both hormones. Both hormones accelerate the rate and increase the depth of respiration. Epinephrine produces a striking excitatory effect on the central nervous system. Much of the smooth muscle of the body, including the nonsphincteric muscle of the gastrointestinal tract, the bronchial tree, and the urinary bladder, is relaxed by epinephrine. Many other types of smooth muscles, including the sphincters of the gastrointestinal tract, the ureters, the erector apparatus of the skin, the dilator of the eyes, and others, are stimulated by epinephrine.

Catecholamines cause increased renin secretion (beta-mediated) by a direct effect on the juxtaglomerular apparatus. Catecholamines also cause bronchodilatation (beta-mediated) and adrenergic sweating (alpha-mediated).

Metabolic effects are mainly mediated by epinephrine, although norepinephrine, in large amounts, elicits the same actions (Landsberg, 1977). One of the major effects is hyperglycemia; blood lactate levels are also increased. Epinephrine promotes formation of cyclic 3′,5′-adenosine monophosphate, which activates phosphorylase, which in turn stimulates glycogenolysis. Catecholamines also stimulate gluconeogenesis, increasing the hepatic production of glucose from amino acid precursors. Epinephrine secretion from the adrenal medulla promptly rises in response to hypoglycemia. Epinephrine via alpha receptors also inhibits insulin release from the beta cells of the pancreatic islets, while glucagon secretion is increased. Epinephrine raises the blood concentration of free fatty acids by increasing the activity of lipase, promoting hydrolysis of triglyceride (beta-mediated). Thus it is seen that catecholamines mobilize both the major energy fuels of the organism. Oxygen consumption may increase as much as 30 per cent in epinephrine-treated subjects; CO_2 production rises even more, resulting in a high respiratory quotient. Much of the calorigenic effect has been ascribed to increased metabolism of lactate; an increase in fat oxidation has also been implicated. Some of the increase in metabolism may also result from increased work of the heart and muscles of respiration.

Epinephrine increases the total leukocyte count and causes eosinopenia. Blood coagulation is accelerated, probably owing to increased activity of factor V. Norepinephrine reduces

TABLE 85–8. MAJOR EFFECTS OF EPINEPHRINE AND NOREPINEPHRINE

	Epinephrine	Norepi-nephrine
Cardiac:		
Heart rate	+	−
Stroke volume	+ +	+ +
Cardiac output	+ + +	0, −
Arrhythmias	+ + + +	+ + + +
Coronary blood flow	+ +	+ + +
Blood pressure:		
Systolic arterial	+ + +	+ + +
Mean arterial	+	+ +
Diastolic arterial	+ ,0, −	+ +
Mean pulmonary	+ +	+ +
Peripheral circulation:		
Total peripheral resistance	−	+ +
Cerebral blood flow	+	0, −
Muscle blood flow	+ +	0, −
Cutaneous blood flow	− −	+ ,0, −
Renal blood flow	−	−
Splanchnic blood flow	+ +	0, +
Metabolic effects:		
Oxygen consumption	+ +	0, +
Blood glucose	+ + +	0, +
Blood lactic acid	+ + +	0, +
Eosinopenic response	+	0
Central nervous system:		
Respiration	+	+
Subjective sensations	+	0, +

+ = increase; 0 = no change; − = decrease.

circulating plasma volume by increasing the transudation of fluid into the tissues as a result of vasoconstriction and a rise of intra-arterial pressure. An infusion of 10 µg/min of norepinephrine in man can cause a 20 per cent reduction of blood volume in approximately 15 minutes (Finnerty et al., 1958). Table 85–8 summarizes the major actions of epinephrine and norepinephrine in man.

Laboratory Evaluation of Adrenergic Function

URINE AND PLASMA CATECHOLAMINE MEASUREMENTS. Adrenergic function is often assessed when there is suspicion of excessive catecholamine biosynthesis, such as in pheo-chromocytoma. In general, measurement of one metabolite (either VMA or metanephrine) plus the total free (unconjugated) urinary catechol-amine excretion diagnoses diseases of adrenergic excess in over 90 per cent of the cases (Sjoerdsma et al., 1966). A summary of recommended methods is given in Table 85–9. In rare instances, fractionating the urine free cate-cholamine level to measure epinephrine and norepinephrine may be helpful if one of these catecholamines is preferentially elevated.

Plasma measurements of norepinephrine and epinephrine have recently become available by the development of highly sensitive radioreceptor assays. Additionally, some studies have suggested that the diagnosis of adrenergic excess can be improved by measuring plasma levels rather than by a timed 24-hour urine collection (Bravo et al., 1979). However, it is emphasized that plasma catecholamines must be collected under rigorously standardized procedures, since stress and postural change can elevate norepinephrine and epinephrine levels well beyond the normal basal recumbent range. Thus, the subject should be recumbent with an indwelling venous catheter and at rest for at least 30 minutes before plasma catecholamines are measured. An additional test that has been suggested is analogous to the dexamethasone-cortisol suppression study, in which clonidine is administered orally and norepinephrine levels are assessed (Bravo et al., 1981) (see Fig. 85–36). In normal individuals, clonidine administration suppresses plasma catecholamines, whereas the levels remain autonomous following α-2-adrenergic stimulation in patients with pheochromocytoma. Plasma dopamine (or urinary homovanillic acid) levels have also been popularly used to diagnose *malignant* medullary tumors, in which the norepinephrine precursor dopamine accumulates (Robinson et al., 1964).

The diagnosis of adrenergic hypofunction is often entertained in patients with severe pos-

TABLE 85–9. CHEMICAL TESTS FOR THE DIAGNOSIS OF PHEOCHROMOCYTOMA

Urine Test	Method	Upper Limit Normal Values (24-hr urine)	Interference
Free catecholamines	Crout (1961)	Total–100 µg NE– 80 µg E – 20 µg	High values with exogenous catecholamines (eye drops, nose drops, bronchodilators, decongestants, alpha-methyldopa, L-dopa); hypoglycemia; acute CNS lesions
Vanillylmandelic acid (VMA)	Pisano et al. (1962)	8 mg	Low values with MAO inhibitors, clofibrate, high values with nalidixic acid
Normetanephrine and metanephrine (NM-M)	Pisano (1960)	1.5 mg	High values with MAO inhibitors, methyldopa, exogenous catecholamines

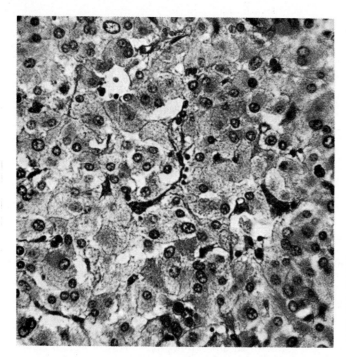

Figure 85–32. Pheochromocytoma of the adrenal in a diabetic patient with persistent hypertension, the neoplastic etiology of which was not recognized before death. Large disorganized adrenal cells surrounding an unusually generous vascular stroma. (Mountainside Hospital, from Campbell, M. F.: Clinical Pediatric Urology. Philadelphia, W. B. Saunders Co., 1956.)

tural hypotensive syndromes. This has been reported in association with central diminution in adrenergic outflow or severe peripheral neuropathy. The proper diagnostic study would include measurement of plasma catecholamines in the recumbent state and immediately following assumption of the upright posture.

PHARMACOLOGIC TESTS. Provocative tests have been largely discarded owing to inherent risks of discharging catecholamines from the tumor. For example, the histamine test has resulted in severe hypertensive crisis, complicated by cerebrovascular accident or myocardial infarction. The phentolamine test has occasionally caused severe hypotensive episodes with secondary vascular shock. On the other hand, the administration of glucagon is relatively free of serious side effects. Provocative testing may be indicated in the rare patient with a truly paroxysmal course (i.e., normal blood pressure and catecholamine levels between paroxysms). A positive test is a pressor response of defined magnitude and the concomitant demonstration of *increased catecholamine excretion during the test*. False positive responses occur in approximately 25 per cent of patients with use of all pharmacologic agents. In patients with a paroxysmal course, an alternative approach is to have the patient collect a fractional urine (6-hour) for catecholamines or, if possible, to measure plasma catecholamines during a paroxysm.

Tumors of the Adrenal Medulla

Clinical considerations are chiefly concerned with medullary tumors. Hypofunction of the adrenal medulla has been implicated in infants with idiopathic spontaneous hypoglycemia. There are also cases of medullary hyperfunction resulting from hyperplasia, primarily in patients with the multiple endocrine neoplasia syndrome (Type II) (DeLellis et al., 1976).

As previously described, chromaffin cells of the adrenal medulla and ganglia of the sympathetic nervous system develop from primitive elements of the neural crest. The sympathogonia may differentiate along the chromaffin line, giving rise to the pheochromoblast and the mature pheochromocyte, or along the neurogenic line to the sympathoblast and finally to the mature ganglion cell. Each of these four types of cells may give rise to tumors: (1) sympathogonioma, an extremely malignant tumor of embryonic life or infancy, characterized by early local invasion and generalized metastases; (2) sympathoblastoma, a common malignant tumor occurring almost exclusively in infancy and childhood; (3) ganglioneuroma, a rare benign tumor composed of sympathetic ganglion cells located within the substance of the adrenal medulla or along the sympathetic chain; and (4) pheochromocytoma, a tumor of pheochromocytes (chromaffin cells), secreting epinephrine and norepinephrine (Fig. 85–32). Ganglioneuromas, neuroblastomas, and pheochromocytomas are all known to produce norepinephrine, epinephrine, or dopamine. In addition to the secretion of catecholamines, tumors arising from neuroectodermal tissues commonly are associated with the ectopic production of polypeptide hormones. Lack of uniformity in the selection of terms designating these different types of lesions has resulted in a number of different names for individual neoplasms in this group (Schwartz et al, 1975). At present, the term "neuroblastoma" is used by most authors to include the histologically similar, highly malignant tumors composed of relatively undifferentiated cells, the sympathogonioma and the sympathoblastoma. When neurofibrils and ganglion cells are also present, the tumor is sometimes designated a ganglioneuroblastoma. A diagnosis of ganglioneuroma (Fig. 85–33) should be restricted to benign tumors with mature ganglion cells.

PHEOCHROMOCYTOMA

Pheochromocytomas are rare, with an estimation that less than 0.1 per cent of hypertensive patients have a chromaffin tumor as the cause of their elevated arterial pressure. However, pheochromocytoma is a curable lesion and is likely to be fatal if the tumor is undiagnosed. Pheochromocytoma may be inherited as a familial autosomal dominant trait (5 per cent); 95 per cent are sporadic. Familial pheochromocytomas are often inherited as part of a pluriglandular neoplastic syndrome (see further on).

Pheochromocytomas may arise wherever chromaffin cells are located. The largest collection of chromaffin tissue is in the adrenal medulla, and approximately 70 per cent of these lesions occur as a discrete, unilateral medullary tumor. Approximately 15 per cent have been found outside the adrenal gland. Fortunately, more than 90 per cent of the ectopic tumors are situated beneath the diaphragm. Almost half of them arise in the superior para-aortic region bounded by the pillars of the diaphragm and the renal pedicles. Many are anterior to the renal pedicle and may be adherent to the renal vein or artery. About one fourth arise in the inferior para-aortic area, near the origin of the inferior mesenteric artery and the aortic bifurcation (organ of Zuckerkandl). Some tumors occur in relationship with the lumbar sympathetic chains. Others have been found in the wall of the urinary bladder. Less than 10 per cent of reported ectopic tumors have occurred in the thorax. Rarely, they have been found at the pulmonary hilum or apex, but the great majority are located posteriorly. One case of intracranial pheochromocytoma has been reported.

Pheochromocytomas are usually round, are often lobulated and highly vascular, and frequently undergo hemorrhagic degeneration with cyst formation. On section they are brown or gray. The histologic appearance is that of adrenal medulla. The cell nuclei are often multiple; cytoplasmic vacuolization is common, and dark staining with chromium salts is characteristic but variable.

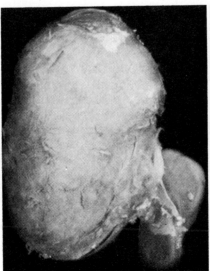 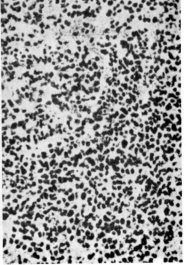

Figure 85–33. Ganglioneuroma in which the tumor is apart from the kidney in a boy of 15 months. *A,* Kidney and tumor showing relationship. *B,* Histology of tumor in *A,* in which large cells like ganglion cells were found in the periphery of the tumor growth. Masses of nerve fibers having a definite neurilemma formed a border like a capsule. In the central portion of the tumor the structure was that of a sympathicoblastoma. In short, the adrenal was part sympatheticoblastoma (embryonal nerve cells) and part ganglioneuroma (adult nerve cells), both tumors being derived from the plenipotential sympathicoblast of the medulla of the adrenal. (Courtesy of Dr. Martha Wollstein, from Campbell, M. F.: Clinical Pediatric Urology. Philadelphia, W. B. Saunders Co., 1956.)

Catecholamine-secreting glomic tissue tumors (chemodectomas) have been described. The embryologic origin of glomic tissue and its relation to chromaffin structures are disputed, but some chemodectomas have given positive chromaffin-staining reactions. Glomic tissue is found at the carotid bifurcation, along the arch of the aorta, at the bulb of the jugular vein, along the femoral vessels, and in the retroperitoneal space. Norepinephrine-secreting tumors of glomic origin have been found in these locations. Clinically, they may be indistinguishable from pheochromocytoma.

In at least 10 per cent of cases, multiple pheochromocytomas are present. The simultaneous occurrence of multiple tumors in different locations follows from the multifocal distribution of chromaffin tissue. Multiple tumors may occur in a single gland, but the common form is bilateral involvement of both adrenal glands. Bilateral adrenal pheochromocytomas are commonly seen in the familial syndromes. The combination of a unilateral medullary tumor plus an extra-adrenal tumor is probably next in frequency; rarely, multiple lesions may all be located outside of the adrenal glands.

The incidence of malignancy has varied in different series. It is to be emphasized that the usual cytologic standards do not hold; capsular and vascular invasion are not adequate criteria for malignancy. Indeed, the only decisive point is usually the development of metastases. In all likelihood, approximately 5 per cent of reported pheochromocytomas have been truly malignant. It is clear that the majority of these lesions secrete catechols and produce hypertension. Malignant tumors tend to be very large. Metastases are found in bones, lungs, liver, and spleen.

Clinical Manifestations

Unlike the normal adrenal medulla, pheochromocytomas characteristically produce large amounts of norepinephrine with lesser and highly variable amounts of epinephrine. Some tumors have been found to produce only norepinephrine, and these are usually extra-adrenal in location. Rarely, epinephrine is the major product, almost invariably in an adrenal pheochromocytoma (Page et al., 1969). Tumors producing dopamine have also been reported. The excessive secretion of pressor amines may be continuous or intermittent. Varying clinical syndromes have been described; paroxysmal hypertension, sustained hypertension, and hypermetabolism (an elevated basal metabolic rate, hyperglycemia, and elevated plasma free fatty acids) (Mellicow, 1977).

Paroxysmal Hypertension. In less than 25 to 30 per cent of cases the hypertension is truly paroxysmal. In these patients the blood pressure will be normal between attacks. Patients with acute paroxysms have an intermittent pattern of hypersecretion and often harbor tumors that are located in the adrenal medulla. The crises may be precipitated by recurring factors (Fig. 85–34), including certain motions of the body, heaving, lifting, coughing or sneezing, defecation, micturition, eating, smoking, alcohol, or anxiety. The appearance of attacks after awakening may be noted. The frequency varies from less than 1 per year to several per day; duration is from seconds to days, but approximately half last 15 minutes or less.

Typical paroxysms are characterized by headache, palpitation (with or without tachycardia), excess sweating, and often severe anxiety. Common also are pallor during the attack, followed by flushing, tremor, nausea and vomiting, weakness, chest pain (sometimes located substernally and constrictive in type), epigastric pain, dizziness, or faintness, paresthesias, pain in the extremities or flank, and sometimes bradycardia. Headaches are usually abrupt in onset, severe, throbbing, and poorly localized. Copius sweating occurs frequently. Dysesthesias may

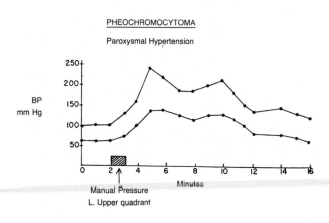

Figure 85–34. Paroxysm of hypertension in a 27-year-old pregnant female. No previous history of hypertension. Paroxysms elicited by changes in position and pressure in left upper quadrant. Episodes accompanied by headache, sweating, palpitations, nausea, epigastric pain, tremor, and anxiety. A 90-gm pheochromocytoma was removed from the area of the splenic plexus.

initiate the episode, followed by pain or cramps in the distal extremities, sometimes reproducing Raynaud's phenomenon. The central feature of these crises is the increase of arterial pressure; on occasion, extreme elevations with diastolic levels up to 180 mm Hg are encountered. Electrocardiographic changes may occur, including disturbances of conduction and of excitability (ventricular tachycardia, nodal rhythm, and multifocal extrasystoles).

In some patients, the disorder retains its typical paroxysmal form throughout its course; in other cases, the paroxysmal disorder changes to sustained hypertension.

Sustained Hypertension. About two thirds of the patients with pheochromocytoma have sustained hypertension (Fig. 85–35). In almost half of this group, the hypertension fluctuates spontaneously or paroxysmal crises are superimposed on the elevated basal level (Gifford et al., 1964). In the remaining patients, the condition is indistinguishable from essential hypertension. In a significant number of these patients the hypertension is severe, with diastolic pressure as high as 140 mm Hg.

Patients with stable hypertension show a tendency toward symptoms of hypermetabolism (tachycardia, increased sweating, recurrent headache, nervousness, and sensitivity to heat.) These patients are especially prone to lose weight. Significant elevations of basal metabolic rate may be encountered, and symptoms and signs may mimic those of hyperthyroidism. Glycosuria and hyperglycemia may occur owing to α-adrenergic suppression of insulin release. Elevated levels of free fatty acids in serum have been demonstrated. Hematocrit values are often elevated, and postural hypotension is common because of the combination of decreased plasma volume and relative insensitivity to postural sympathetic vascular reflexes.

Pheochromocytoma in Children

Pheochromocytomas in children tend to be overlooked. More than 100 cases of pheochromocytomas have been described in children. The youngest patient reported with symptomatic pheochromocytoma was 1 month of age; the average age at diagnosis is 9 years. It is emphasized that a high incidence of bilateral, multiple, and ectopic tumors is characteristic of the disorder in children. Another major feature is the rarity of paroxysmal manifestations; hypertension is nearly always sustained and is often severe. Loss of vision is a frequent early sign. Headaches tend to be severe and may be accompanied by convulsive attacks. The combination of loss of visual acuity, headache, and convulsions often suggests a diagnosis of cerebral tumor; this may be reinforced by finding severe papilledema. Weight loss and excessive sweating are common. Obstruction of the renal artery has occasionally occurred.

Several other diseases encountered in children may involve abnormalities of catecholamine metabolism and may present confusing clinical and laboratory findings.

Neuroblastoma and Ganglioneuroma. These tumors of neural crest origin, long considered to be functionally inactive, are now known to produce increased amounts of norepinephrine, epinephrine, dopamine, and dopa. With neuroblastoma the course is primarily that of a metastatic malignant neoplasm, and hypertension is usually moderate or absent. With ganglioneuroma there is often a distinct syndrome of weight loss, abdominal distention, and chronic diarrhea, frequently associated with hypertension; all of these manifestations are cured with removal of the tumor (see Fig. 85–33). The excretion of catechol metabolites may be high but tends to be variable.

Familial Dysautonomia (Riley-Day Syndrome). This congential disorder of childhood involves defective lacrimation, impaired temperature regulation, loss of pain sensitivity, and hyporeflexia (Riley, 1957). In addition, these children often have hypertension, postural hypotension, and excessive sweating that may be suggestive of pheochromocytoma. It is of note that five of the patients reported by Riley had been mistakenly explored for pheochromocytoma. However, the excretion of catecholamines and their metabolites is usually in the normal range.

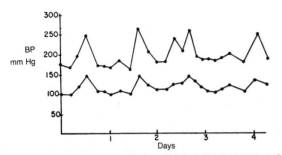

PHEOCHROMOCYTOMA

Sustained Hypertension with Paroxysms

Figure 85–35. A 54-year-old male with a 15-year history of high blood pressure. "Unstable hypertension" and diabetes present for 2 years. On admission the patient showed Grade III retinopathy, congestive heart failure, and jaundice. The only symptoms associated with the paroxysms were increased nervousness and sweating. At surgery, a 40-gm pheochromocytoma was removed from the left adrenal.

Acrodynia. This disease of infancy and childhood is secondary to mercury poisoning. The major features are cutaneous erthyema of the hands and feet with desquamation, painful extremities, photophobia, and listlessness. However, profuse sweating, tachycardia and hypertension also occur, and catecholamine excretion is found to be moderately elevated in some cases.

Familial Pheochromocytoma

The mode of inheritance of familial pheochromocytoma is autosomal dominant with a high degree of penetrance. Certain features set these cases apart from sporadic cases. The incidence of multiple tumors is approximately 50 per cent (usually bilateral pheochromocytomas). Sustained hypertension has been much more common than the paroxysmal type. Certain other disorders have occurred in association with familial pheochromocytoma, including multiple neurofibromatosis; von Hippel–Lindau disease; carcinoma of the thyroid gland; and a triad of familial bilateral pheochromocytomas, medullary thyroid carcinoma, and hyperparathyroidism (so-called Sipple's syndrome or multiple endocrine neoplasia syndromes, Types II and III) (Steiner, 1968; Rashid et al., 1975). Physical findings suggestive of associated diseases include thyroid tumors, neurofibromas, café-au-lait spots, retinal angiomas, and mucosal neuromas. Papillary thyroid carcinoma has occurred in combination with pheochromocytoma, including both familial and nonfamilial instances of the latter. Medullary carcinoma of the thyroid is the most common thyroid tumor seen in association with pheochromocytoma. This tumor is associated with elevated levels of calcitonin, either basally or in response to pentagastrin or combined pentagastrin-calcium infusion. The association of pheochromocytoma, hyperparathyroidism (usually four-gland hyperplasia), and thyroid medullary carcinoma presents as a familial, multiple endocrine neoplasia syndrome of genetic origin (autosomal dominant inheritance). It has recently been found that when patients are screened early, they manifest bilateral adrenal medullary hyperplasia, which is diagnosed earliest by a selective elevation of urinary free epinephrine levels. Some of these patients then progress to develop frank adrenal tumor and pheochromocytoma. Since the syndrome is inherited as an autosomal dominant trait, it is mandatory that all family members be screened for medullary carcinoma of the thyroid, hyperparathyroidism, and pheochromocytoma.

Pheochromocytoma of the Urinary Bladder

Pheochromocytoma of the wall of the urinary bladder produces a distinct clinical syndrome. Typically, paroxysms occur during or shortly after the emptying of an overdistended bladder. Throbbing headaches tend to be a prominent symptom during paroxysms. Painful hematuria occurs in approximately 50 per cent of patients, and other symptoms found in bladder tumors are often present. The tumors are usually small and located in the muscular wall; in some instances, cystoscopy may be normal. The blood pressure response observed during distention of the bladder may be of critical importance in establishing the diagnosis.

Pheochromocytoma and Pregnancy

Establishing the diagnosis of pheochromocytoma ante partum is crucial, since failure to diagnose the tumor is associated with high rates of maternal and fetal mortality (approximately 50 to 60 per cent). Moreover, a substantial reduction in maternal and fetal mortality rates (15 to 20 per cent) is seen when the diagnosis is established ante partum and appropriate therapy is instituted. Fetal wastage is the result of maternal cardiovascular instability and subsequent fetal anoxia. The symptoms and signs of pheochromocytoma during pregnancy are as previously described, but a characteristic finding is hypertension in the supine position, which is probably related to pressure of the uterus on the tumor. The diagnosis should be confirmed by measurements of catecholamine levels in the urine, as previously described. Surgical excision of the tumor is the preferred treatment, but the specific strategy depends on the time of gestation when the diagnosis has been confirmed. It is stressed that all patients should receive preoperative alpha-adrenergic blockage with phenoxybenzamine until blood pressure is controlled. Beta-blockade may also be required to control heart rate or arrhythmias but has the disadvantage of slowing fetal heart rate and increasing myometrial contractility.

If the diagnosis is established early in pregnancy, surgery to remove the tumor is recommended; long-term medical management carries the risk of failure to uniformly control blood pressure, with subsequent maternal or fetal mortality. After the fetus is viable, medical therapy may be necessary to allow the fetus to mature before delivery is undertaken (Griffith et al., 1974). Since spontaneous delivery is associated with high mortality, cesarean section should be performed. Excision of the tumor may be performed at the time of cesarean section or at a later date.

Diagnosis of Pheochromocytoma

In the past, a large proportion of pheochromocytomas were encountered unexpectedly during surgery, or at autopsy. At present time, excellent diagnostic procedures are available. Consequently, the diagnosis depends chiefly on considering the possibility of pheochromocytoma and carrying out appropriate studies.

Chemical Methods Of Diagnosis. The diagnosis of pheochromocytoma depends primarily upon the chemical measurement of catecholamines or their degradation products, or both, in urine or blood. This is best achieved with a carefully timed 24-hour urinary collection, with simultaneous assessment of creatinine to ensure adequacy and accuracy of the 24-hour collection. It is advised that the patient be either symptomatic or hypertensive at the time the urinary collection is performed.

As previously stated, well over 90 per cent of pheochromocytoma patients will be properly identified with a single determination from an accurately collected 24-hour specimen measuring unconjugated catecholamines and one of the metabolites (metanephrine or VMA). It should be noted that commonly used nose drops contain sympathomimetic amines and will interfere with urinary free catecholamine testing. Alpha-methyldopa (Aldomet), used in the treatment of hypertension, also falsely elevates urinary catecholamine measurements; VMA and metanephrine measurements should be used. Reserpine, thiazides, and ganglion-blocking agents (including guanethidine) need not be withdrawn. Monoamine oxidase inhibitors decrease VMA levels, whereas they increase metanephrine levels. Beta-blockade has also been reported to elevate plasma catecholamine levels.

In some patients, the elevation of norepinephrine plus epinephrine output is greater than VMA; in others, the reverse is true. In one series of 64 patients with proved pheochromocytoma, normal values for VMA were found in three cases, for metanephrine in 2 cases, and for catecholamines in 2 cases (Sjoerdsma et al., 1966), but at least one index was abnormal in all the patients. In the majority of those with paroxysmal hypertension, abnormality of one or more of the tests may be detectable between attacks, but in some cases all values are normal in the symptom-free interval. As previously discussed, such patients should keep urine collection bottles at home and begin fractional (4 to 6 hour) collections at the onset of an attack.

Evaluation of Diagnostic Methods. The free or unconjugated catecholamines in urine represent approximately 2 to 4 per cent of the total catecholamines secreted by the adrenal medulla and the sympathetic nervous system. A somewhat larger fraction is present in conjugated form (glucuronides and sulfates). Catechols of dietary origin (bananas and other sources) are present mainly in the conjugated form, so that the measurement of catecholamines in the free state is preferable. An additional advantage of the catecholamine measurement is that it permits separate determination of epinephrine and norepinephrine. This information may be useful, since most tumors that produce mainly epinephrine arise in the adrenal medulla.

False positive reactions in the measurement of VMA ordinarily do not occur, and special diets are not necessary. The O-methylated derivatives of catecholamines (metanephrine and normetanephrine) are not readily separated, and the results are expressed as the total of normetanephrine (NM) plus metanephrine (M). Some laboratories using both methods consider the NM–M procedure simpler and more reliable than the determination of VMA. In some malignant pheochromocytomas, increased plasma dopamine and urinary homovanillic acid levels have been demonstrated, owing to the accumulation of the norepinephrine precursor dopamine (Robinson et al., 1964). Plasma measurements of norepinephrine and epinephrine have recently become available by the development of highly sensitive radioreceptor assays. Additionally, it has been suggested that the diagnosis of adrenergic excess can be improved by measuring plasma levels rather than by a timed 24-hour urine collection (Bravo et al., 1979). However, plasma catecholamines must be collected under rigorously standardized procedures. An additional test in equivocal cases is the clonidine suppression test with measurement of plasma norepinephrine levels (Bravo et al., 1981) (Fig. 85–36). Although uncommon, severe hypotension has been reported following the administration of clonidine in a diagnostic setting. However, it is emphasized that, in the majority of cases, a carefully timed 24-hour urine collection is sufficient to make the diagnosis of an adrenal medullary catecholamine-producing tumor.

Differential Diagnosis of Pheochromocytoma. In patients who complain of paroxysmal symptoms, a variety of syndromes must be considered—most of which are more common than pheochromocytoma but often mimic it.

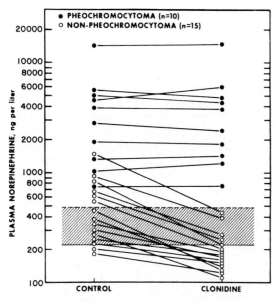

Figure 85–36. Plasma norepinephrine levels in patients with documented (●) or suspected (○) pheochromocytoma before and 3 hours post administration of a single oral dose (0.3 mg) of clonidine. The hatched area represents the levels seen in normal healthy adults. (From Bravo, E. L., et al.: N. Engl. J. Med., *305*:623, 1981.)

Vasodilating headaches (cluster headache, histamine cephalgia) tend to occur episodically in a regular pattern with a sudden onset, almost invariably are unilateral, and are associated with lacrimation, watery nasal discharge, and facial sweating associated with flushing rather than with pallor. Patients receiving monoamine oxidase inhibitors may experience paroxysms following ingestion of indirect-acting sympathomimetic amines (e.g., tyramine found in food by bacterial decarboxylation of tyrosine). *Diencephalic autonomic epileptic seizures* may include all the usual components of pheochromocytoma paroxysms. However, the occurrence of paroxysmal hypertension, headache, diaphoresis, and palpitation during a single epileptic attack must be rare. Confusion with *intracranial tumor* has occurred in pheochromocytoma patients with hypertension. *Acute anxiety* states may be associated with palpitation, tremulousness, weakness, nausea, sweating and labile hypertension, papilledema, and headaches. These findings are usually restricted to those with persistent, severe hypertension, but the hypertension is usually mild and transient and other features of anxiety are usually present. *The menopausal syndrome* with intermittent flushing and sweating may suggest pheochromocytoma when labile hypertension is present. The relief produced by estrogen will settle the

issue. Pressor episodes resembling those of pheochromocytoma, often in association with chest pain, may occur in patients with *coronary artery disease*. The issue is complicated by the fact that angina may occur in patients with pheochromocytoma at the height of an attack.

Certain metabolic disorders require consideration. Some patients with pheochromocytoma and persistent hypertension lose a large amount of weight and complain of heat sensitivity, palpitation, and sweating. Confusion with *thyrotoxicosis* may arise, but specific tests of thyroid function are normal. Since the clinical manifestations of acute *hypoglycemia* are in part those of catecholamine excess, pheochromocytoma may be suspected. The temporal pattern of attacks in both the reactive and the fasting types of hypoglycemia serves to focus attention upon the true cause. In addition, the symptoms are relieved by carbohydrate ingestion, and hypertension is usually not a major problem.

Complications. The principal complications of untreated pheochromocytoma stem from arterial hypertension. Vascular accidents may occur during paroxysms but are unusual. Because the blood pressure is normal between attacks in true paroxysmal disease, vascular changes are not marked. In patients with sustained hypertension, vascular complications are similar to those that occur in essential hypertension of comparable severity and duration. These include retinopathy, cerebrovascular hemorrhage, myocardial infarction, congestive heart failure, and full-blown malignant hypertension. In addition, patients with pheochromocytoma and high circulating levels of catecholamines may develop cardiac arrhythmias, particularly those of ventricular origin.

It has been recognized that cardiomyopathy occurs in some patients with pheochromocytoma (Van Vliet et al., 1966). The myocardial changes are those of fatty degeneration and necrosis of myocardial fibers, usually around small blood vessels, with an associated inflammatory exudate. In another syndrome, idiopathic hypertrophic subaortic stenosis has been reported. Electrocardiographic changes are nonspecific. These syndromes should be suspected in patients with pheochromocytoma who develop congestive heart failure, persistent tachycardia, or acute pulmonary edema. Removal of the catecholamine-producing tumor is often followed by healing of the myocardial lesions.

Hyperglycemia and glycosuria are often present in patients with pheochromocytoma, simulating idiopathic or familial diabetes mellitus (Spergel et al., 1968). Although multiple

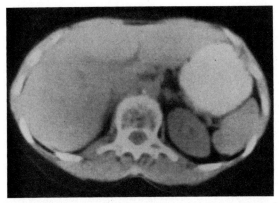

Figure 85–37. Subtle 1-cm left pheochromocytoma imaged by CT scan. The fortuitous separation of the adrenal by fat, especially the left, makes it possible to obtain high resolution for small adrenal masses by this technique.

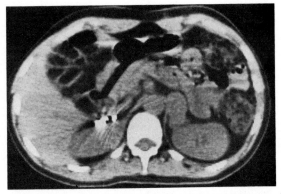

Figure 85–38. Moderate left pheochromocytoma defined by CT. The right side has glares from hemostatic clips used in a prior adrenalectomy for pheochromocytoma 9 years earlier. The patient suffers from von Hippel–Lindau disease, one of a group of neuroectodermal disorders with a higher incidence of pheochromocytoma.

factors may be involved, the major cause is catecholamine-induced inhibition of insulin secretion. Excision of the tumor corrects the abnormality unless underlying genetically determined diabetes is also present.

Treatment of Pheochromocytoma

The definitive treatment of pheochromocytoma is surgical excision of the adrenal medullary tumor(s). This is true for the more than 90 per cent of patients who have benign tumors and in whom the surgical risk is reasonable. For patients with a metastatic malignant pheochromocytoma and for those with presumably benign lesions in whom surgery must be delayed because of severe vascular complications, pharmacologic agents are available that can ameliorate symptoms and reduce arterial blood pressure.

Preoperative Work-up. Once the presence of a pheochromocytoma is biochemically established, certain additional studies should be obtained. Thyroid palpation and parathyroid function should be carefully evaluated because of the occasional association of thyroid carcinoma or hyperparathyroidism. Of great importance is the careful evaluation of the entire cardiovascular system.

Techniques for localization of pheochromocytoma primarily involve CT scanning (Figs. 85–37 to 85–39), since the majority of these tumors are readily demonstrable and are generally greater than 2 cm in size (Stewart et al., 1978). Selective venous sampling for catecholamine levels may also be indicated in certain instances. Arteriography offers a chance of localizing small, highly vascular extraadrenal tumors that cannot be visualized by CT scanning

techniques. It should also be noted that angiography dyes may lead to discharge of catecholamines from a pheochromocytoma; thus, wide fluctuation in blood pressure may be induced and deaths have occurred. Therefore, prior to radiographic contrast study, it is mandatory that pretreatment with the alpha-adrenergic blocker phenoxybenzamine (Dibenzyline) should be instituted in order to guard against a severe hypertensive paroxysm. This drug should be given prophylactically over 5 to 7 days (10 to 40 mg twice daily) until the patient is normotensive.

It is important to emphasize that demonstration of a tumor by radiologic means is no assurance that all tumors have been identified. In the last analysis, the best approach to the problem of locating ectopic and multiple tumors in the abdomen is a careful exploration during

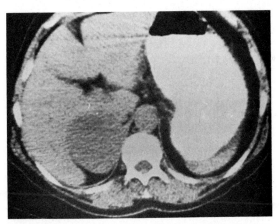

Figure 85–39. Large right adrenal pheochromocytoma obvious on CT scan. A wide thoracoabdominal approach is most useful in such a lesion.

surgery. Except for the rare glomic tumor of the carotid body, extra-abdominal pheochromocytomas will be found only in the thorax, usually in the posterior mediastinum and less commonly on the aortic arch. Most of these are evident on x-rays of the chest; posteroanterior, lateral, and oblique views should be obtained in all cases.

The generalized vasoconstriction produced by elevated norepinephrine levels in patients with pheochromocytoma is associated with a fall in plasma volume; an elevated hematocrit and postural hypotension are associated findings. This hypovolemia also is the major factor producing the hypotension that occurred intra- and postoperatively after removal of the tumor in patients who were not pretreated with alpha-adrenergic blockade. Therefore, plasma volume must be expanded before operation in every case by the use of alpha-blockade. Restriction of sodium intake should also be avoided unless this is medically required (e.g., congestive heart failure).

Preoperative Management. The risk of surgical removal of pheochromocytomas, even in experienced hands, had previously been formidable. The high morbidity and mortality have been mainly attributable to cardiac arrhythmias, hypertensive crises, and vascular shock. However, operative deaths have been virtually eliminated by the development of blocking agents that are capable of modifying the effects of catecholamines (Gitlow et al., 1971).

Once the diagnosis is established, preparation for surgery should begin, even before diagnostic studies are complete.

ALPHA-RECEPTOR BLOCKING AGENTS. Blockade of alpha-adrenergic receptors lowers systolic and diastolic blood pressure, even in the presence of high levels of norepinephrine. The drug of choice is phenoxybenzamine (Dibenzyline). Preoperative use of phentolamine has been discontinued because of its short duration of action and requirement for parenteral administration.

All patients should be treated preoperatively with oral phenoxybenzamine in order to achieve normalization of blood pressure and to guard against severe hypertensive paroxysms. The starting dose is 10 to 20 mg per day in two divided doses; dosage is gradually increased until hypertension is reduced to an acceptable level. Maintenance doses usually range from 40 to 100 mg per day. Side effects include fatigue, nasal congestion, postural hypotension, and compensatory tachycardia. Patients with sustained hypertension are treated until blood pressure returns to near-normal levels for a period of 5 to 7 days; patients with paroxysms are treated until they have been free of severe paroxysmal attacks for a similar period of time. Treatment is continued with full therapeutic doses until the morning of surgery. The result has been better blood pressure control during the operation; fears that bleeding would be excessive have not materialized. Patients have not been refractory to pressor agents, and the hypertensive response to gentle palpation of the tumor has usually not been eliminated. This pressor response to palpation is useful intraoperatively in locating the lesion as well as in searching for multiple tumors at the time of exploration but must not be pursued at the price of increased cardiovascular risk. The pressor response to a discharge of catecholamines also proves that alpha-adrenergic blockade is not complete.

Engelman and Sjoerdsma (1964) have described prolonged treatment with phenoxybenzamine in patients with malignant, metastatic pheochromocytoma for periods of more than 1 year. Spector et al. (1965) have reported on the use of an agent capable of blocking catecholamine synthesis (alpha-methyl-tyrosine) in patients with metastatic pheochromocytoma. This type of therapy remains investigational and can lead to neurologic toxicity (mainly sedation and Parkinsonian-like tremors).

BETA-ADRENERGIC BLOCKERS. Although alpha-adrenergic blockers are of major importance in controlling hypertension, these patients remain susceptible to tachycardias and arrhythmias, especially during surgery (Gitlow et al., 1971). These disturbances result mainly from beta-adrenergic stimulation of the inotropic and chronotropic receptors in the heart. Phenoxybenzamine may reduce the tachycardia of some patients, but its use tends to potentiate the beta-adrenergic actions favoring hypotension and cardiac arrhythmia. The latter are hazardous during operation; ventricular arrhythmias, including bigeminy, multifocal premature beats, and ventricular tachycardia, may occur. As a result, the combined use of alpha- and beta-adrenergic blockers may be indicated under certain circumstances. Preoperatively, a cardiospecific beta-1 receptor antagonist (such as atenolol or metoprolol) is given orally to patients who still have tachycardia or arrhythmias. However, it is stressed that beta-adrenergic blockade should be instituted only after phenoxybenzamine administration has been stabilized. In some cases a moderate rise in blood pressure occurs after beta-blockade has been initiated, requiring a modest increase in the dose of the alpha-blocker phenoxybenzamine. This paradoxical elevation of blood pressure is probably secondary to blockage of beta receptor–mediated vasodilation. Beta-blockers may also be used for arrhythmias that appear *during* surgery. Cardiac rate, blood pressure, and electrocardiogram should be continuously monitored intraoperatively. It should be remembered that when arrhythmias arise during surgery, lidocaine (Xylocaine) is often useful. However, its effects are transient, the action of a single intravenous dose of 50 to 100 mg usually lasting only 15 to 20 minutes. Contraindications to beta-blockade include bronchial asthma or obstruction, heart block, and untreated congestive heart failure. Monoamine oxidase inhibitors, catecholamine-depleting agents (reserpine), and ether anesthesia should be avoided.

Anesthesia. Proper anesthetic management starts preoperatively with sodium pentobarbital to help reduce anxiety. The preferred induction agent is sodium thiopental. Succinylcholine may then be used for intubation. Until recently, halothane had been considered the agent of choice for maintenance of anesthesia because of its ability to suppress sympathoadrenal activity and thereby lower blood pressure. However, its propensity for causing frequent ventricular arrhythmias led to the search for better anesthetic agents. Enflurane (Ethane), an anesthetic agent from the ether group, is nonexplosive, produces excellent muscular relaxation, and does not result in ventricular arrhythmias. Enflurane is now considered the anesthetic agent of choice.

Monitoring. Because of the unpredictable and potentially wide fluctuations in hemodynamic function that may occur during surgery, careful monitoring of the patient is essential. The electrocardiogram should be recorded continuously. Knowledge of arterial blood pressure at all times is also required. This is best accomplished by use of a catheter in the radial artery, providing a visible record of the patient's blood pressure that permits rapid adjustments in medication. The central venous pressure manometer is routinely used, providing an indication of blood volume requirements. Central venous pressure readings are particularly valuable in preventing vascular overloading when large amounts of blood or fluids are being infused.

Surgery. The transabdominal approach is preferred because of the frequent occurrence of extra-adrenal and multiple tumors. We prefer a high transverse abdominal incision (chevron type) or a thoracoabdominal incision on the side

of a large adrenal pheochromocytoma (Gittes, 1983). It is to be emphasized that careful inspection of the entire retroperitoneal area is essential. Both the adrenal glands and all of the para-aortic tissues, including the organ of Zuckerkandl, are explored in sequence. Careful palpation of suspected lesions with continuous monitoring of intra-arterial pressure has aided in locating tumors, particularly when multiple lesions are present.

The right adrenal is exposed by retracting the liver upward, holding the duodenum toward the midline, and retracting the hepatic flexure of the colon downward and mesially. The kidney is displaced gently downward, and the peritoneum is incised just above and lateral to the upper pole of the kidney. The proximity of the right adrenal to the vena cava and its tendency to extend both anteriorly and posteriorly to it should be remembered. The left adrenal is exposed by retracting the splenic flexure of the colon mesially and downward while simultaneously displacing the spleen and fundus of the stomach upward and the tail of the pancreas anteriorly. The peritoneum above and lateral to the kidney is incised, the kidney is moved downward, and the adrenal is brought into view.

Intraoperatively, blood pressure elevations should be titrated into the normal range with a continuous infusion of nitroprusside. This is prepared by adding 50 mg of nitroprusside to 500 ml of 5 per cent dextrose solution. A microdrip regulator should be used to ensure a precise flow rate. The average adult dose is 3 µg per kg per minute (approximately 200 µg per minute); the maximum dose should not exceed 800 µg per minute. Nitroprusside has the advantage of a direct effect on the arterial wall, immediate onset of action, and recovery within 1 to 2 minutes. Moreover, blood pressure control is much smoother with this agent than with the short-acting alpha-blocking agent phentolamine, which cannot be administered as a continuous infusion but rather must be given as intermittent boluses. Another advantage of using nitroprusside is that the infusion can be immediately terminated when the adrenal vein is clamped, thereby preventing exacerbation of a falling blood pressure when the tumor is removed.

Should a reduction of blood pressure fail to occur immediately following resection of the tumor, the presence of an additional undiscovered pheochromocytoma should be suspected and the possibility of antecedent renal ischemia considered. The postadrenalectomy decline in blood pressure should be anticipated; prior to resection of the tumor, generous infusion of crystalloid or transfusion of whole blood should be started, and deliberate overreplacement of estimated blood losses is often desirable. Circulatory overloading is prevented by careful attention to central venous pressure. If arterial pressure falls below 90/60 mm Hg despite fluid replacement, a small amount of norepinephrine can be given intravenously. The intravenous administration of 25 gm of mannitol to obtain improved renal blood flow also merits consideration.

Postoperative Management. Continuous recording of blood pressure should be maintained during the immediate postoperative period in the recovery room. Upon completion of the operation, these patients should be turned and moved with great care, since they are very susceptible to acute hypotension. If the use of peripheral vasoconstrictors has been necessary following the removal of the tumor, efforts to decrease the rate of infusion and to discontinue their use as soon as possible should be made. Once the blood pressure has been stabilized without continuing pressor amine therapy, postoperative management is similar to that of other hypertensive patients undergoing surgical procedures.

In the immediate perioperative period, repeat measurements of urinary catecholamines may be misleading. Catecholamine elevations may persist for a few weeks postoperatively in some patients in whom the lesion was completely resected because of hormonal release from tissue storage sites. However, normal catecholamine levels must ultimately be demonstrated, and periodic measurement is also indicated to rule out metastatic disease or the appearance of another pheochromocytoma. In some cases, particularly with long-standing hypertension, the blood pressure may never return to normal, suggesting that other factors are involved (e.g., essential hypertension, secondary renal hypertension).

References

Ahlquist, R. P.: A study of the adrenotropic receptors. Am. J. Physiol., 153:586, 1948.

Aron, D. C., Tyrrell, J. B., Fitzgerald, P. A. et al.: Cushing's syndrome: Problems in diagnosis. Medicine, 60:25, 1981.

Axelrod, J.: The metabolism, storage and release of catecholamines. Recent Prog. Horm. Res., 21:597, 1965.

Baxter, J. D., and Forsham, P. H.: Tissue effects of glucocorticoids. Am. J. Med., 53:573, 1972.

Baxter, J. D., and Rousseau, G. G.: Glucocorticoid hormone action: An overview. In Baxter, J. D., and Rousseau, G. G. (Eds.). Glucocorticoid Hormone Action. New York, Springer-Verlag, 1979, pp. 1–24.

Beierwaltes, W. H., Lieberman, L. M., Ansari, A. N., et al.: Visualization of human adrenal glands in vivo by scintillation scanning. JAMA, 216:275, 1971.

Beisel, W. R., Cos, J. J., Harton, R., et al.: Physiology of urinary cortisol excretion. J. Clin. Endocrinol. Metab., 24:887, 1964.

Berson, S. A., and Yalow, R. S.: Radioimmunoassay of ACTH in plasma. J. Clin. Invest., 47:2725, 1968.

Besser, G. M., and Edwards, C. R. W.: Cushing's syndrome. Clin. Endocrinol. Metab. 1:451, 1972.

Biglieri, E. G.: Effect of posture on plasma concentrations of aldosterone in hypertension and primary hyperaldosteronism. Nephron, 23:112, 1979.

Biglieri, E. G., and Forsham, P. H.: Studies on the expanded extracellular volume and responses to various stimuli in primary aldosteronism. Am. J. Med., 30:564, 1960.

Biglieri, E. G., and Mantero, F.: The characteristics, course and implications of the 17-hydroxylation deficiency in man. In Finkelstein, M., Jungblut, P., Klopper, A., and Conti, C. (Eds.): Research on Steroids. Vol. 5. Rome, Societa Editrice Universo, 1973, pp. 385–399.

Biglieri, E. G., Schambelan, M., Slaton, P. E., et al.: The intercurrent hypertension of primary aldosteronism. Circ. Res., 27 (Suppl. 1):195, 1970a.

Biglieri, E. G., Slaton, P. E., Schambelan, M., et al.: Hypermineralocorticoidism. Am. J. Med., 45:170, 1968.

Biglieri, E. G., Stockigt, J. R., and Schambelan, M.: A preliminary evlauation for primary aldosteronism. Arch. Intern. Med., 126:1004, 1970b.

Biglieri, E. G., Stockigt, J. R., and Schambelan, M.: Adrenal mineralocorticoids causing hypertension. Am. J. Med., 52:623, 1972.

Bravo, E. L., Tarazi, R. C., Gifford, R. W., et al.: Circulating and urinary catecholamines in pheochromocytoma: Diagnostic and pathophysiologic implications. N. Engl. J. Med., 301:682, 1979.

Bravo, E. L., Tarazi, R. C., Fouad, F. M., et al.: Clonidine-suppression test. N. Engl. J. Med., 305:623, 1981.

Brooks, R. V.: Biosynthesis and metabolism of adrenocortical steroids. In James, V. H. T. (Ed.): The Adrenal Gland. New York, Raven Press, 1979, pp. 149–162.

Byyny, R. L.: Withdrawal from glucocorticoid therapy. N. Engl. J. Med., 295:30, 1976.

Camacho, A. M., and Migeon, C. J.: Testosterone excretion and production rate in normal adults and in patients with congenital adrenal hyperplasia. J. Clin. Endocrinol. Metab., 26:893, 1966.

Campbell, M. F.: Anomalies of the genital tract. In Campbell, M. F., and Harrison, J. H. (Eds.): Urology. 3rd ed. Philadelphia, W. B. Saunders Co., 1970.

Child, D. F., Burke, C. W., Burley, D. M., et al.: Drug control of Cushing's syndrome: Combined aminoglutethimide and metyrapone therapy. Acta Endocrinol., 82:330, 1976.

Chobanian, A. V., Volicer, L., Tifft, C. P., et al.: Mineralocorticoid-induced hypertension in patients with orthostatic hypotension. N. Engl. J. Med., 301:68, 1979.

Chute, R., Soutter, L., and Kerr, W. S., Jr.: Value of thoracoabdominal incision in removal of kidney tumors. N. Engl. J. Med., 241:951, 1949.

Conn, J. W.: Presidential address. Primary aldosteronism, a new clinical entity. J. Lab. Clin. Med., 45:3, 1955.

Conn, J. W.: Primary reninism. In Genest, J., Koiw, E., and Kuchel, O. (Eds): Hypertension. Physiopathology and Treatment. New York, McGraw-Hill, 1977, pp. 840–847.

Conn, J. W., Cohen, E. L., and Rovner, D. R.: Suppression of plasma renin activity in primary aldosteronism. Distinguishing primary from secondary aldosteronism in hypertensive disease. JAMA, *190*:213, 1964a.

Conn, J. W., Knopf, R. F., and Nesbit, R.: Primary aldosteronism: present evaluation of its clinical characteristics and of the results of surgery. *In* Baulieu, E. E., and Robel, P. (Eds.): Aldosterone. Philadelphia, F. A. Davis Co., 1964b, p. 327.

Copeland, P. M.: The incidentally discovered adrenal mass. Ann. Intern Med., *98*:940, 1983.

Crapo, L.: Cushing's syndrome: A review of diagnostic tests. Metabolism, *28*:955, 1979.

Crout, J. R.: Catecholamines in urine. *In* Seligson, D. (Ed.): Standard Methods of Clinical Chemistry. Vol. 3. New York, Academic Press, 1961, pp. 62–80.

Cushing, H.: Pituitary Body, Hypothalamus, and Parasympathetic Nervous System. Springfield, Ill., Charles C Thomas, 1932.

DeLellis, R. A., Wolfe, H. J., Gagel, R. F., et al.: Adrenalmedullary hyperplasia. Am. J. Pathol., *83*:177, 1976.

Dluhy, R. G., Himathongkam, T., and Greenfield, M.: Rapid ACTH test with plasma aldosterone levels: Improved diagnostic discrimination. Ann. Intern. Med., *80*:693, 1974.

Engelman, K., and Sjoerdsma, A.: Chronic medical therapy for pheochromocytoma; a report of four cases. Ann. Intern. Med., *61*:229, 1964.

Exton, J. H.: Regulation of gluconeogenesis by glucocorticoids. *In* Baxter, J. D., and Rousseau, G. E. (Eds.): Glucocorticoid Hormone Action. New York, Springer-Verlag, 1979, pp. 535–546.

Ferriss, J. B., Beevers, D. G., Brown, J. J., et al.: Low-renin ("primary") hyperaldosteronism. Am. Heart J., *95*:64, 1978a.

Ferriss, J. B., Beevers, D. G., Brown, J. J., et al.: Clinical, biochemical and pathological features of low-renin ("primary") hyperaldosteronism. Am. Heart J., *95*:375, 1978b.

Finnerty, F. A., Jr., Bucholz, J. H., and Guildandeu, R.: Blood volumes and plasma protein during levarterenol-induced hypertension. J. Clin. Invest., *37*:425, 1958.

Gabrilove, J. L.: Feminizing interstitial tumor of the testis. Cancer, *35*:1184, 1975.

Gabrilove, J. L., Sharma, D. C., Wotiz, H. H., et al: Feminizing adrenocortical tumors in the male: A review of 52 cases. Medicine, *44*:37, 1965.

Ganguly, A., Melada, G. A., Luetscher, J. A., et al.: Control of plasma aldosterone in primary aldosteronism: Distinction between adenoma and hyperplasia. J. Clin. Endocrinol. Metab., *37*:765, 1973.

Ganong, W. F.: The central nervous system and the synthesis and release of adrenocorticotropic hormone. *In* Nalbandov, A. V. (Ed.): Advances in Neuroendocrinology. Urbana, University of Illinois Press, 1963.

Giebink, G. S., Gotlin, R. W., Biglieri, E. G., et al.: A kindred with familial glucocorticoid-suppressible aldosteronism. J. Clin. Endocrinol. Metab., *36*:715, 1973.

Gifford, R. W., Jr., Kvale, W. F., Maher, F. T., et al.: Clinical features, diagnosis and treatment of pheochromocytoma: A review of 76 cases. Mayo Clin. Proc., *39*:281, 1964.

Gill, G. N.: ACTH regulation of the adenal cortex. *In* Gill, G. N. (Ed.): *In* Pharmacology of Adrenal Cortical Hormones, New York, Pergamon Press, 1979, pp. 35–66.

Gitlow, S. E., Pertsemlidis, D., and Bertani, L. M.: Management of patients with pheochromocytoma. Am. Heart J., *82*:557, 1971.

Gittes, R. F.: Surgery for pheochromocytoma. *In* Glenn, J.

F. (Ed.): Urologic Surgery. Third ed. Philadelphia, J. B. Lippincott, 1983, pp. 47–54.

Gordon, R. D., Kuchel, O., Liddle, G. W., et al: Role of the sympathetic nervous system in regulating renin and aldosterone production in man. J. Clin. Invest., *46*:599, 1967.

Granner, D. K.: The role of glucocorticoids as biological amplifiers. *In* Baxter, J. D., and Rousseau, G. G. (Eds.): Glucocorticoid Hormone Action. New York, Springer-Verlag, 1979, pp. 593-611.

Griffith, M. I., Felts, J. H., James, F. M., et al.: Successful control of pheochromocytoma in pregnancy. JAMA, *229*:437, 1974.

Hoffman, K.: Relations between chemical structure and function of adrenocorticotropin and melanocyte-stimulating hormones. *In* Handbook of Physiology, Section 7: Endocrinology, Vol. 4. American Physiological Society, Baltimore, The Williams & Wilkins Co., 1974, pp. 29–59.

Hogan, T. F., Citrin, D. L., Johnson, B. M., et al.: O,P'-DDD (mitotane) therapy of adrenal cortical carcinoma. Cancer, *42*:2177, 1978.

Hunt, T. K., Schambelan, M., and Biglieri, E. G.: Selection of patients and operative approach in primary aldosteronism. Ann. Surg., *182*:353, 1975.

Hussain, S., Belldegrun, A., Seltzer, S., et al.: Differentiation of malignant from benign adrenal masses: Predictive indices on computed tomography. Am. J. Roentgenol., *144*:61, 1985.

Hutter, A. M., and Kayhoe, D. E.: Adrenal cortical carcinoma. Clinical features of 138 patients. Am. J. Med., *41*:572, 1966a.

Hutter, A. M., and Kayhoe, D. E.: Adrenal cortical carcinoma. Results of treatment with o,p'DDD in 138 patients. Am. J. Med., *41*:581, 1966b.

Ingle, D. J.: Some studies on the role of the adrenal cortex in organic metabolism. Ann. N. Y. Acad. Sci., *50*:576, 1949.

Ito, T., Woo, J., Haning, R., et al.: A radioimmunoassay for aldosterone in human peripheral plasma including a comparison of alternate techniques. J. Clin. Endocrinol., *34*:106, 1972.

Jacobs, H. S., and Nabarro, J. D. N.: Tests of hypothalamic-pituitary-adrenal function in man. Q. J. Med., *38*:475, 1969.

Kem, D. C., Weinberger, M. H., Mays, D. M., et al.: Saline suppression of plasma aldosterone in hypertension. Arch. Intern. Med., *128*:380, 1971.

Kondo, K., Saruta, T., Saito, I., et al.: Benign desoxycorticosterone-producing adrenal tumor. JAMA, *236*:1042, 1976.

Korenman, S. G., and Lipsett, M. B.: Is testosterone glucuronide uniquely derived from plasma testosterone? J. Clin. Invest., *43*:2125, 1964.

Krieger, D. T.: Rhythms in CRF, ACTH, and corticosteroids. *In* Krieger, D. T. (Ed.): Endocrine Rhythms. New York, Raven Press, 1979, pp. 123–142.

Landsberg, L.: Catecholamines. Clin. Endocrinol. Metab., *6*:523, 1977.

Lefkowitz, R. J.: Biochemical properties of alpha- and beta-adrenergic receptors and their relevance to the clinician. Cardiovasc. Med., *2*:573, 1977.

Liddle, G. W.: Test of pituitary-adrenal suppressibility in the diagnosis of Cushing's syndrome. J. Clin. Endocrinol. Metab., *20*:1539, 1960.

Liddle, G. W.: Cushing's syndrome. *In* Eisenstein, A. B. (Ed).: The Adrenal Cortex. Boston, Little Brown & Co., 1967, p. 523.

Liddle, G. W., Bledsoe, T., and Coppage, W. S.: A familial renal disorder simulating primary aldosteronism but with negligible aldosterone secretion. *In* Baulieu, E. E., and Robel, P. (Eds.): Aldosterone. Philadelphia, F. A. Davis Co., 1964, p. 353.

Liddle, G. W., Estep, H., Kendall, J. W., Jr., et al: Clinical application of a new test of pituitary reserve. J. Clin. Endocrinol. Metab., *19*:875, 1959.

Linde, R., Coulam, C., Battino, R., et al.: Localization of aldosterone-producing adenoma by computed tomography. J. Clin. Endocrinol. Metab., *49*:642, 1979.

Linfoot, J. A.: Heavy ion therapy: Alpha particle therapy of pituitary tumors. *In* Linfoot, J. A. (Ed.): Recent Advances in the Diagnosis and Treatment of Pituitary Tumors. New York, Raven Press, 1979, pp. 245–267.

Lipsett, M. B., Hertz, R., and Ross, G. T.: Clinical and pathological aspects of adrenocortical carcinoma. Am. J. Med., *35*:374, 1963.

Lubitz, J. A., Freeman, L., and Okun, R.: Mitotane use in inoperable adrenal cortical carcinoma. JAMA, *223*:1109, 1973.

Ludens, J. H., and Fanestil, D. D.: The mechanism of aldosterone function. *In* Gill, G. N. (Ed.): Pharmacology of Adrenal Cortical Hormones. New York, Pergamon Press, 1979, pp. 143–184.

Luetscher, J. A., Hancock, E. N., Camargo, C. A., et al.: Conjugation of 1,2-³H-aldosterone in human liver and kidneys and renal extraction of aldosterone and labeled conjugates from blood plasma. J. Clin. Endocrinol. Metabol., *25*:628, 1965.

Luton, J. P., Mahoudeau, J. A., Bouchard, P., et al.: Treatment of Cushing's disease by o,p'-DDD: Survey of 62 cases. N. Engl. J. Med., *300*:459, 1979.

McKenna, T. J., Island, D. P., Nicholson, W. E., and Liddle, G. W.: Dopamine inhibits angiotensin-stimulated aldosterone biosynthesis in bovine adrenal cells. J. Clin. Invest., *64*:287, 1979.

Mellicow, M. M.: One hundred cases of pheochromocytoma. Cancer, *40*:1987, 1977.

Migeon, C.: Adrenal androgens in man. Am. J. Med., *53*:606, 1972.

Miller, W. L., Johnson, L. K., Baxter, J. D., and Roberts, J. L.: Processing of the precursor to corticotropin and beta-lipotropin in man. Proc. Natl. Acad. Sci., *77*:5211, 1980.

Moll, G. W., and Rosenfield, R. L.: Testosterone binding and free plasma androgen concentrations under physiological conditions: Characterization by flow dialysis technique. J. Clin. Endocrinol. Metab., *49*:730, 1979.

Moore, F. D.: Bodily changes in surgical convalescence. I. The normal sequence—observations and interpretation. Ann. Surg., *137*:289, 1953.

Moore, T. J., Dluhy, R. G., Williams, G. H., et al: Nelson's syndrome: frequency, prognosis and effect of prior pituitary irradiation. Ann. Intern. Med., *85*:731, 1976.

Murphy, B. E. P.: Clinical evaluation of urinary cortisol determinations by competitive protein-binding radioassay. J. Clin. Endocrinol. Metab., *28*:434, 1968.

Mussachio, J. M.: Enzymes involved in the biosynthesis and degradation of catecholamines. *In* Iversen, L. L., Iversen, S. D., and Snyder, S. H. (Eds.): Handbook of Psychopharmacology, Vol. 3. New York, Plenum Publishing Co., 1975, p. 1.

Netter, F. H.: Ciba Collection of Medical Illustrations. Vol. 4: Endocrine System and Selected Metabolic Diseases. Summit, N. J., Ciba Pharmaceutical, 1965, pp. 77–81.

Neville, A. M., and Mackay, A. M.: The structure of the human adrenal cortex in health and disease. Clin. Endocrinol. Metab., *1*:361, 1972.

New, M. I., and Seaman, M. P.: Secretion rates of cortisol and aldosterone precursors in various forms of congen-

ital adrenal hyperplasia. J. Clin. Endocrinol. Metab., *30*:361, 1970.

Nicolis, G. L., Mitty, H. A., Modlinger, R. S., et al.: Percutaneous adrenal venography: A clinical study of 50 patients. Ann. Intern. Med., *76*:899, 1972.

Orth, D. N., and Liddle, G. W.: Results of treatment in 108 patients with Cushing's syndrome. N. Engl. J. Med., *285*:243, 1971.

Page, L. B., Raker, J. W., and Berberith, F.R.: Pheochromocytoma with predominant epinephrine secretion. Am. J. Med., *47*:648, 1969.

Peterson, R. E.: Metabolism of adrenocorticosteroids in man. Ann. N.Y. Acad. Sci., *82*:846, 1959.

Peterson, R. E.: Metabolism of adrenal cortisol steroids. *In* Christy, N. P. (Ed.): The Human Adrenal Cortex. New York, Harper & Row, 1971, pp. 87–189.

Pisano, J. J.: A simple analysis for normetanephrine and metanephrine in urine. Clin. Chim. Acta, *5*:406, 1960.

Pisano, J. J., Crout, J. R., and Abraham, D.: Determination of 3-methoxy-4-hydroxymandelic acid in urine. Clin. Chim. Acta, 7:285, 1962.

Plotz, C. M., Knowlton, A. I., and Ragan, C.: The natural history of Cushing's syndrome. Am. J. Med., *13*:597, 1952.

Rabinowe, S. L., Jackson, R. A., et al.: Ia-positive T lymphocytes in recently diagnosed idiopathic Addison's disease. Am. J. Med., *77*:587, 1984.

Rapaport, E., Goldberg, M. B., et al.: Mortality in surgically treated adrenocortical tumors. Postgrad. Med., *11*:325, 1956.

Rashid, M., Khairi, A., et al.: Mucosal neuroma, pheochromocytoma and medullary thyroid carcinoma: Multiple endocrine neoplasia, Type 3. Medicine, *54*:89, 1975.

Richie, J. P., and Gittes, R. F.: Carcinoma of the adrenal cortex. Cancer, *45*:1957, 1980.

Riley, C. M.: Familial dysautonomia. *In* Levine, S. Z. (Ed.): Advances in Pediatrics. Chicago, Year Book Medical Publishers, 1957, p. 157.

Robinson, R., Smith, P., and Whittaker, S. R. F.: Secretion of catecholamines in malignant pheochromocytoma. Br. Med. J., *1*:422, 1964.

Ruder, H. J., Guy, R. L., and Lipsett, M. B.: A radioimmunoassay for cortisol in plasma and urine. J. Clin. Endocrinol. Metab., *35*:219, 1972.

Ryan, K. J.: Metabolism of C-16–oxygenated steroids by human placenta: the formation of estriol. J. Biol. Chem., *234*:200, 1959.

Sandberg, A. A., and Slaunwhite, W. R., Jr.: Physical state of adrenal cortical hormones in plasma. *In* Christy, N. P. (Ed.): The Human Adrenal Cortex. New York, Harper & Row, 1971, p. 69.

Schambelan, M., and Perloff, D.: Renovascular hypertension and renal parenchymal hypertension. *In* Brenner, B. M., and Rector, F. C., Jr. (Eds.): The Kidney. Philadelphia, W. B. Saunders Co., 1980, pp. 1719-1741.

Schambelan, M., Stockigt, J. R., and Biglieri, E. G.: Isolated hypoaldosteronism in adults, a renin deficiency syndrome. N. Engl. J. Med., *287*:573, 1972.

Schober, R., Nitsch, C., Rinne, U., et al.: Calcium-induced displacement of membrane-associated particles upon aggregation of chromaffin granules. Science, *195*:495, 1977.

Schteingart, D. E., Cash, R., and Conn, J. W.: Aminoglutethimide and metastatic adrenal cancer: maintained reversal (six months) of Cushing's syndrome. JAMA, *198*:1007, 1966.

Schwartz, E. L., Mao, P., Hermied, O., et al.: Catecholamine-secreting paraganglioma. The problem of classification. Arch. Intern. Med., *135*:978, 1975.

Selye, H.: Textbook of Endocrinology. Montreal, University of Montreal, 1947.

Silber, R. H., and Porter, C. C.: The determination of 17,21-dihydroxy-20-ketosteroids in urine and plasma. J. Biol. Chem., *210*:923, 1954.

Singer, W., Kovacs, K., Ryan, N., et al.: Ectopic ACTH syndrome: Clinicopathological correlations. J. Clin. Pathol., *31*:591, 1978.

Sjoerdsma, A., Engelman, K., et al.: Pheochromocytoma: Current concepts of diagnosis and treatment. Ann. Intern. Med., *65*:1302, 1966.

Soffer, L. J., Dorfman, R. I., and Gabrilove, J. L.: The Human Adrenal Gland. Philadelphia Lea & Febiger, 1961.

Spector, S., Sjoerdsma, A., and Udenfriend, S.: Blockage of endogenous norepinephrine synthesis by alpha-methyl-tyrosine, an inhibitor of tyrosine hydroxylase. J. Pharmacol. Exp. Ther., *147*:86, 1965.

Spergel, G., Bleicher, S. J., and Ertel, N. H.: Carbohydrate and fat metabolism in patients with pheochromocytoma. N. Engl. J. Med., *228*:803, 1968.

Staub, J. J., Noelpp, B., Girard, J.: The short metyrapone test: Comparison of the plasma ACTH response to metyrapone and insulin-induced hypoglycemia. Clin. Endocrinol., *10*:595, 1979.

Steiner, A. L., Goodman, A. D., and Powers, S. R.: Study of a kindred with pheochromocytoma, medullary thyroid carcinoma, hyperparathyroidism and Cushing's disease: Multiple endocrine neoplasia, type 2. Medicine, *47*:371, 1968.

Stewart, B. H., Bravo, E. L., Haaga, J., et al.: Localization of pheochromocytoma by computed tomography. N. Engl. J. Med., *229*:460, 1978.

Stockigt, J. R., Hewett, M. J., Topliss, D. J., et al: Renin and renin substrate in primary adrenal insufficiency: Contrasting effects of glucocorticoid and mineralocorticoid deficiency. Am. J. Med., *6*:915, 1979.

Streeten, D. H. P., Stevenson, C. T., et al: The diagnosis of hypercortisolism. Biochemical criteria differentiating patients from lean and obese normal subjects and from females on oral contraceptives. J. Clin. Endocrinol. Metab. *29*:1191, 1969.

Tait, J. F., and Horton, R.: The in vivo estimation of blood production and interconversion rates of androstenedione and testosterone and the calculation of their secretion rates. *In* Pincus, G., and Nakao, T. (Eds.): Dynamics of Steroid Metabolism. New York, Academic Press, 1965, p. 393.

Tarazi, R. C., Frohlich, E. D., and Dustan, H. P. : Plasma volume in men with essential hypertension. N. Engl. J. Med., *278*:762, 1968.

Taylor, A. A., and Bartter, F. C.: Hypertension in licorice intoxication, acromegaly, and Cushing's syndrome. *In* Genest, J., Koiw, E., and Kuchel, O. (Eds.): Hypertension: Physiopathology and Treatment. New York, McGraw-Hill, 1977, pp. 755–767.

Thorn, G. W., Forsham, P. H., et al.: Advances in the diagnosis and treatment of adrenal cortical insufficiency. Am. J. Med., *10*:595, 1951.

Tobian, L.: Interrelationships of electrolytes, juxtaglomerular cells and hypertension. Physiol. Rev., *40*:280, 1960.

Tyrrell, J. B.: Cushing's disease. Press Conc. Intern. Med., *13*:5, 1980.

Tyrrell, J. B., Brooks, R. M., Fitzgerald, P. A., et al.: Cushing's disease: Selective trans-sphenoidal resection of pituitary adenomas. N. Engl. J. Med., *298*:753, 1978.

Vale, W., Spiess, J., Rivier, C., and Rivier, J.: Characterization of a 41-residue ovine hypothalamic peptide that stimulates secretion of corticotropin and β-endorphin. Science, *213*:1394, 1981.

Van Vliet, P. D., Burchell, H. B., and Titus, J. C.: Focal myocarditis associated with pheochromocytoma. N. Engl. J. Med., *274*:1102, 1966.

Villee, D. B.: The development of steroidogenesis. Am. J. Med., *53*:533, 1972.

Weinberger, M. H., Grim, C. E., Hollifield, J. W., et al.: Primary aldosteronism: Diagnosis, localization and treatment. Ann. Intern. Med., *90*:386, 1979.

Weitzman, E. D., Fukushima, D., Nogeire, C., et al: Twenty-four hour pattern of the episodic secretion of cortisol in normal subjects. J. Clin. Endocrinol. Metab., *33*:14, 1971.

Williams, G. H., and Dluhy, R. G.: Aldosterone biosynthesis: Interrelationship of regulatory factors. Am. J. Med., *53*:595, 1972.

Wilson, J. D.: The pathogenesis of benign prostatic hypertrophy. Am. J. Med., *68*:745, 1980.

INDEX

Note: Page numbers in *italics* refer to illustrations. Page numbers followed by t refer to tables.

i